Medical-Surgical Nursing Review and Resource Manual

2nd Edition

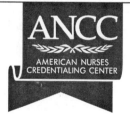

ANCC
AMERICAN NURSES
CREDENTIALING CENTER

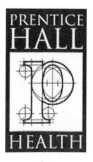

PRENTICE
HALL
HEALTH

Library of Congress Cataloging-in-Publication Data

Medical-surgical nursing review and resource manual. -- 2nd ed.
    p. ; cm.

Includes index.

1. Nursing--Examinations, questions, etc. 2. Surgical nursing--Examinations, questions, etc. I. American Nurses Credentialing Center. Institute for Credentialing Innovation.

[DNLM: 1. Education, Continuing, Nursing. 2. Perioperative Nursing--methods. WY 18.5 M489 2007]

Published by: American Nurses Credentialing Center
                     Institute for Credentialing Innovation

                     8515 Georgia Avenue, Suite 400
                     Silver Spring, MD   20910-3492

                     www.nursecredentialing.org

ISBN-13: 978-0-9793811-0-2   ISBN-10: 0-9793811-0-X

RT55.M47 2007   610.73076--dc22   2007018723

Medical-Surgical Nursing Review and Resource Manual, 2nd Edition

July 2007

Please direct your comments and/or queries to:
revmanuals@ana.org

The health care services delivery system is a volatile marketplace demanding superior knowledge, clinical skills, and competencies from all registered nurses. Autonomy in nursing practice, and nurse career marketability and mobility in the new century hinge on affirming the profession's formative philosophy which places a priority on a lifelong commitment to the principles of education and professional development. The knowledge base of nursing theory and practice is expanding, and, while care has been taken to ensure the accuracy and timeliness of the information presented in the *Medical-Surgical Nursing Review and Resource Manual,* clinicians are advised to always verify the most current national treatment guidelines and recommendations, and to practice in accordance with professional standards of care used with regard to the unique circumstances that apply in each practice situation. In addition, every effort has been made in this text to insure accuracy and, in particular, to confirm that drug selections and dosages are in accordance with current recommendations and practice, including the ongoing research, changes to government regulations, and the developments in product information provided by pharmaceutical manufacturers. However, it is the responsibility of each nurse practitioner (NP) to verify drug product information and to practice in accordance with professional standards of care. In addition, the editors wish to note that provision of information in this text does not imply an endorsement of any particular products, procedures or services. As a review text, this content is provided at a level that describes what a family NP should know upon entry into practice. NPs may object, for religious or other reasons, to the provisions of certain services. That decision, too, must be left to the individual NP.

Therefore, the authors, editors, American Nurses Association (ANA), American Nurses Association's Publishing (ANP), American Nurses Credentialing Center (ANCC), and the Institute for Credentialing Innovation cannot accept responsibility for errors or omissions, or for any consequences or liability, injury, and/or damages to persons or property from application of the information in this manual, and make no warranty, express or implied, with respect to the contents of the Medical-Surgical Nursing Review and Resource Manual.

Published by: The Institute for Credentialing Innovation
8515 Georgia Avenue, Suite 400
Silver Spring, MD 20910-3402
www.nursecredentialing.org

This second edition of the Medical-Surgical Nursing Review and Resource manual is a compilation of materials from two outstanding review resources for the medical/surgical nurse. Page 1–61 are compiled from ANCC's *Cardiac Vascular Nursing Review and Resource Manual, 2nd Edition.*

Pages 65–961 are compiled with permission from Pearson/Prentice Hall's ***Medical-Surgical Nursing: Critical Thinking in Client Care, 3rd Edition*** by Priscilla Lemone and Karen Burke.

Introduction to the Continuing Education (CE) Contact Hour Application Process for *Medical-Surgical Nursing Review and Resource Manual, 2nd Edition*

The Institute for Credentialing Innovation now offers the continuing education contact hours for this manual online at www.NursingWorld.org, the American Nurses Association's Web site. This process involves answering approximately 25 to 30 questions that test knowledge of the information contained within this manual. The continuing education contact hours can be completed at any time, and a certificate can be printed from the Web site immediately upon successful completion of the test.

The *Medical-Surgical Nursing Review and Resource Manual* is designed to meet the following objectives:

1. Describe the key components, including risk assessment, health history, and ethical issues, for care of medical-surgical clients.
2. Analyze the pharmacologic and invasive and noninvasive treatments for selected diseases.
3. Discuss the nurse's role in care of acute and chronically ill patients with selected diseases.

Upon completion of this manual and the online CE test, a nurse can receive a total of 88 continuing education contact hours at a price of $88. The entire process—online test and evaluation form—must be completed by December 31, 2010 in order to receive credit. To begin the process, please e-mail revmanuals@ana.org *or* go to the ANCC Web site at www.nursecredentialing.org for specific instructions. Your patience with this new process is greatly appreciated.

Inquiries or Comments

If you have any questions about the CE contact hours, please e-mail The Institute at revmanuals@ana.org. You may also mail any comments to Editor/Project Manager, at the address listed below.

Duplicate CE Certificates

Once you have successfully passed the CE test on NursingWorld, you may go back and re-print your certificate as often as you wish.

The Institute for Credentialing Innovation
American Nurses Credentialing Center
Attn: Editor/Project Manager
8515 Georgia Avenue, Suite 400
Silver Spring, MD   20910-3492
Fax: (301) 628-5342

The American Nurses Association is accredited as a provider of continuing nursing education by the American Nurses Credentialing Center's Commission on Accreditation and approved by the California Board of Registered Nursing, Provider Number CEP6178.

Contents

Section III – Special Considerations

section one

Considerations for Practice

Ethical and Legal Issues

Ethics

1. Ethics is the systematic study of moral conduct and provides the framework for studying and examining moral dilemmas.
2. Bioethics, also called biomedical ethics or medical ethics, is the study of moral conduct within the context of health care.
3. Morality refers to norms about right and wrong human conduct that form a social consensus.
   a. Moral virtues are socially valued character traits.
   b. Five moral virtues for health professionals
      1) Compassion combines active regard for another's welfare with an emotional response of sympathy, tenderness, and discomfort at another's misfortune or suffering.
      2) Discernment involves the ability to make judgments and decisions without being unduly influenced by extraneous considerations (e.g., fears, personal attachments).
      3) Trustworthiness involves ability and strength of character, dependability, and reliability.
      4) Integrity involves firm adherence to moral and ethical principles.
      5) Conscientiousness involves careful, dependable, and competent practice.

Ethical Principles

1. Beneficence means to do good.
   a. Promote the well-being of the patient.
   b. Prevent harm.
2. Nonmaleficence means to refrain from harm.
   a. Obligates the clinician to avoid inflicting harm directly or intentionally.
   b. Balanced with beneficence – maximize benefits while minimizing harm.
3. Autonomy refers to the human right to make one's own decisions. Clinicians show respect for autonomy when they engage in the following behaviors.

    a.   Tell the truth.

    b.   Respect the privacy of others.

    c.   Protect confidential information.

    d.   Obtain consent for interventions with patients.

    e.   When asked, help others make important decisions.

    4.   Justice is the principle of fairness.

    a.   To treat equals equally.

    b.   To refrain from discrimination.

Code of Ethics for Nurses

Table 1-1 lists the 9 provisions of the Code. The full document includes interpretative statements related to each provision.

Table 1-1. Code of Ethics for Nurses

1. The nurse, in all professional relationships, practices with compassion and respect for the inherent dignity, worth, and uniqueness of every individual, unrestricted by considerations of social or economic status, personal attributes, or the nature of the health problem.

2. The nurse's primary commitment is to the patient, whether an individual, family, group, or community.

3. The nurse promotes, advocates for, and strives to protect the health, safety, and rights of the patient.

4. The nurse is responsible and accountable or individual nursing practice and determines the appropriate delegation of tasks consistent with the nurses obligation to provide optimum patient care.

5. The nurse owes the same duties to self as to others, including the responsibility to preserve integrity and safety, to maintain competence, and to continue personal and professional growth.

6. The nurse participates in establishing, maintaining, and improving health care environments and conditions of employment conducive to the provision of quality health care and consistent with the values of the profession through individual and collective action.

7. The nurse participated is the advancement of the profession through contributions to practice, education, administration, and knowledge development.

8. The nurse collaborates with other health professionals and the public in promoting community, national, and international efforts to meet health needs.

9. The profession of nursing, as represented by associations and their members, is responsible for articulating nursing values, for maintaining the integrity of the profession and its practice, and for shaping social policy.

Selected Issues in Clinical Practice

Informed consent is based on respect for autonomy. There are five elements of informed consent.

1. Decisional capacity includes the ability to understand and make decisions.
   a. Decisional capacity is specific, not global. It depends on the match between the patient's abilities and the specific decision-making task.
   b. Decisional capacity may vary over time and be intermittent.
      1) Physiological (e.g., illness, hypoxia) and situational factors (e.g., medically uninformed person admitted to the Emergency Department) may affect decision-making capacity.
      2) If the patient's decision-making capacity can not be established initially, it is appropriate to assess his or her understanding, deliberative capacity, and coherence over time, and to consult with an expert when necessary.
      3) Surrogate decision-makers are authorized to make decisions for patients when decisional capacity is impaired.
         a) If possible, the surrogate decision-maker is required to make the decision that the incompetent patient would have made if competent. This is the "substituted judgment" standard. Surrogates may have written evidence of a person's wishes (e.g., a living will or letter), verbal evidence (i.e., conversations), or they may make inferences based on the person's history of relevant choices.
         b) If the surrogate has no way of knowing what choice a person would have made, then the 'best interests' standard should be used. That is, the surrogate should choose the option that appears to be in the best interests of the patient. Hence, surrogates are held to a higher standard of decision-making than competent individuals are held. Competent individuals may make health care choices that are eccentric, poorly reasoned, biased, etc., but, unless evidence exists to support such a choice, a surrogate is compelled ethically and legally to act in the patient's best interests.
      4) The order of surrogate authority varies slightly by state but generally specifies the following list in descending order of priority:
         a) Court-appointed guardian
         b) Durable power of attorney
         c) Spouse
         d) Adult children (usually requires unanimous consensus)
         e) Parents (usually requires unanimous consensus)
         f) Adult siblings (usually requires unanimous consensus)
2. Disclosure includes a core set of information about the treatment or research procedure, including the following:
   a. Facts or descriptions that patients usually consider relevant in making a decision to refuse or consent (e.g., risks, benefits).
   b. Information the clinician believes to be relevant (e.g., alternate treatments).
   c. The clinician's recommendation.
   d. The purpose of seeking consent.

e. The nature and limits of consent (e.g., research studies that include the right to withdraw from study without penalty).

f. Patients have the right to refuse to be informed regarding their health care decisions, however, in that situation, the clinician should document the refusal in the medical record.

3. Understanding is difficult to assess. Patients and research subjects should understand, at least, what the clinician or researcher believes the patient needs to understand to authorize the procedure.

4. Voluntariness implies that the patient agrees to the intervention without undue influence.

5. Consent is the acceptance or refusal of the treatment or research study after the patient is adequately informed.

a. Consent can be withdrawn at any time.

b. A written form documenting that consent has occurred is required for some health care decisions such as sterilization, injection of a radioactive substance, surgery, etc. Which procedures and decisions require written evidence of consent is usually mandated by institutional policies and, occasionally, by law.

c. All health care should be delivered using the model of informed consent, including nursing controlled activities such as ambulation following surgery, preoperative teaching, etc. Written evidence of consent for such non-invasive activities is not required.

Advance directives – a person while competent, can complete a directive documenting his or her health care wishes or values, or selecting a surrogate to make decisions during periods of incapacity.

1. Living wills are directives that specify preferred treatment during periods of incapacity. They represent written evidence of a patient's wishes.

2. Durable power of attorney for health care (DPAHC) is a legal document in which one person assigns authority to another to act as his or her surrogate if he or she is unable to make health care decisions.

a. Other types of durable powers of attorney exist, but in general, only the DPAHC includes health care decision-making authority.

3. The Patient Self-Determination Act of 1990 requires health care facilities to develop programs to inform patients and staff about advance directives.

Access to care is a major ethical and political issue confronting the US and is based in the principle of justice.

1. Access is limited, in part, by economic considerations. Different insurance plans provide different reimbursement for, and different access to care.

a. Approximately 18% of the non-elderly US population lack health insurance of any kind.

b. Approximately 25% of the US population has publicly supported care (e.g., Medicare, Medicaid) or insurance unconnected to employment.

c. Approximately 60% of the US population has employer-based insurance.

2. Principle of justice – fair distribution of resources; equals are treated equally – implies a right to health care.

3. The dilemma confronting the US is how to fund and distribute health care fairly.

Nurse/health care team/patient relationships

1. Veracity obligates the nurse to be truthful with patients and members of the health care team. A current example is the increased emphasis on the need to disclose health care errors to one's colleagues, the institution, the patient, and, in some cases, to government agencies.

2. Privacy obligates the clinician to appropriately restrict access to the patient and to the health record. A current privacy issue is the need to restrict clinicians' access to the electronic medical records of any patients with whom they are not directly involved in care. This includes hospitalized colleagues, employees, public figures, and family or friends.

3. Confidentiality requires clinicians to share information about the patient only with the patient and those health professionals who are involved in caring for the patient.

4. Fidelity refers to faithfulness in keeping a promise. The nurse makes an implied promise to care for a patient based on the social contract that the profession of nursing has established with the public. Fidelity requires that the nurse put the patient's interests above other interests, such as financial, personal, or other people involved in the patient's care or life.

5. The five moral virtues described above are essential to effective team function.

Questions about **withholding and withdrawing treatment** derive from the principles of beneficence and nonmaleficence.

1. Medical futility is a controversial concept.
   a. Quantitative medical futility describes a situation where research and practice would suggest that there is less than a 1% chance that the treatment will have the intended effect (e.g., CPR in a cachectic patient with metastasized cancer). Quantitatively futile treatments are not obligatory.
   b. Qualitative futility describes situations where the treatment will have the intended effect but will not achieve a desired benefit (i.e., tube feeding a patient who has suffered a severe stroke will provide nutrition but will not restore neurological function).

2. Ordinary versus extraordinary treatments.
   a. The traditional rule is that extraordinary treatment can be withheld but ordinary treatment cannot.
   b. The distinction between ordinary and extraordinary treatments is not clear and of uncertain moral and ethical meaning.

3. Double-effect – A single act may have two effects, one beneficial and one harmful. For example, a patient, requiring high doses of a narcotic analgesic for pain control (intended beneficial effect), may be at risk for respiratory depression (unintended harmful effect).
   a. Is there an alternate treatment that provides the intended effect (pain control) without the unintended effect (respiratory depression)?
   b. Is the treatment provided for its intended effect (pain control, not respiratory depression)?
   c. Does the intended effect (pain control) outweigh the unintended effect (respiratory depression)?

Ethical Reasoning

Application of a systematic way of thinking about an ethical dilemma will help to reach a conclusion. Steps in the reasoning process include:

1. Review facts and assumptions about the case or situation.
   a. Clinical data and treatment options
   b. Relevant law
   c. Patient preferences and beliefs
   d. Goal of treatment
2. Define the ethical dilemma in specific terms.
   a. An ethical dilemma requires a choice between courses of action that involve fundamental concepts of right and wrong.
   b. Ethical dilemmas usually involve concepts of rights, duties, and responsibilities.
   c. An ethical dilemma is not a difference of opinion about treatment or different appraisals of clinical facts.
3. List possible courses of action.
4. Choose a course of action, considering:
   a. Patient preferences
   b. Professional standards
   c. Relevant law
   d. Personal values and principles
5. Evaluate the choice.
   a. Consistent with ethical principles?
   b. Consistent with decisions made in similar cases?
   c. Consistent with values and principles of those affected, i.e. , culturally sensitive?
   d. Consequences of the decision?

Ethical Decision-Making Resources

1. Ethics committees are multidisciplinary groups that are responsible to review ethical dilemmas and advise clinicians.
2. Ethics consultation services provide "on-call" assistance to patients, families, and clinicians when confronted by ethical dilemmas.
3. Formal educational programs in ethics provide clinicians with an understanding and a framework for decision-making.
4. Policies related to ethical issues (e.g., Do Not Attempt Resuscitation policy) guide institutional practices.

Patient's Rights

1. Patient's rights are derived from the ethical theory of Liberal Individualism
2. In 1990, the American Hospital Association codified the following in the Patient's Bill of Rights.
   a. Right to considerate and respectful care

b. Right to information about diagnosis, treatment, and prognosis

c. Right to make decisions about the plan of care

d. Right to have advance directives

e. Right to privacy

f. Right to confidentiality

g. Right to review clinical records

h. Right to responsible care and services, including the right to transfer

i. Right to information about business relationships among the hospital, educational institutions, and payers that might influence care and treatment

j. Right to reasonable continuity of care

k. Right to be informed of hospital policies and procedures that regulate patient care, treatment, and responsibilities. Includes the right to grievance and dispute resolution.

Regulation of Nursing Practice

Professional Regulation

1. Professional practice standards are authoritative statements by which the nursing profession describes the responsibilities of nurses.

   a. **Standards of care** describe a competent level of nursing care as demonstrated by the nursing process. (Includes assessment, diagnosis, outcome identification, planning, implementation, and evaluation.)

   b. **Standards of professional performance** describe a competent level of behavior in the professional role. (Includes activities related to quality of care, performance appraisal, education, collegiality, ethics, collaboration, research, and resource utilization.)

2. Nursing's social policy statement describes the discipline of nursing, its scope, and the profession's responsibility to society.

   a. The 1980 Social Policy Statement defined nursing as "the diagnosis and treatment of human responses to actual or potential health problems."

   b. Since that time, definitions of nursing have acknowledged four essential features:

      1) Attention to the full range of human experiences and responses to health and illness (i.e., not limited to actual or potential health problems)

      2) Integration of objective data with understanding of the patient's subjective experience.

      3) Use of scientific knowledge in the process of diagnosis and treatment.

      4) Provision of caring relationships that facilitate healing.

   c. Scope of basic nursing practice involves promoting, supporting, and restoring health; preventing illness; and assisting with activities that contribute to a peaceful death.

      1) Nurses in basic practice coordinate care, prepare patients for tests and procedures, and monitor the patient's response to various treatments.

      2) Nurses in basic practice provide care in a variety of settings, including hospitals, homes, schools, places of employment, correctional facilities, nursing homes, and community-based health care facilities.

Professional Certification

1. Private (not governmental) agencies sponsor programs to certify that individuals meet certain criteria and are prepared to practice in that discipline or clinical area.
2. Certification recognizes specialized knowledge and skills beyond that which is required for safe, basic practice.

Legal Regulation of Nursing Practice

1. Protects the public health, safety, and welfare.
   a. All states require licensure for nursing practice (e.g., registered nurse, licensed practical nurse).
   b. Most states have additional requirements for advanced clinical nursing practice (i.e., nurse practitioner, clinical nurse specialist, nurse anesthetist, and nurse midwife).
2. Nurse practice acts are state laws that grant the right to practice nursing to individuals who meet predetermined standards (e.g., education).
   a. Regulatory boards (e.g., Board of Nursing [BON]) are created under the nurse practice acts and govern nursing practice in the state.
   b. The BON is responsible for the following:
      1) Determining eligibility for licensing and relicensing.
      2) Approving and supervising educational programs.
      3) Enforcing the statutes (i.e., the nurse practice acts and the BON regulations).
      4) Writing rules and regulations governing the practice of nursing.
   c. Basic grounds for disciplinary action:
      1) Fraud in obtaining a license.
      2) Unprofessional, illegal, dishonorable, or immoral conduct.
      3) Performance of specific actions prohibited by the acts.
      4) Conviction of a felony or crime of moral turpitude.
      5) Drug or alcohol addiction rendering the individual incapable of performing duties.
   d. Possible sanctions, if found guilty of the above, include:
      1) Revocation of license.
      2) Suspension of license for a specified period of time.
      3) Suspension of license for an unspecified period of time with the opportunity to reapply after a specified program of study or treatment.
      4) Prohibition of work in specified settings.

Legal Aspects

Individual Accountability

1. The individual is personally responsible for his or her own actions.
2. The person who actually causes the harm has the primary responsibility.
3. Duty to communicate may be most important duty of the nurse.
   a. Communicate change in the patient's condition to the physician.
   b. Communicate concern about impaired practice to the nurse manager or supervisor.

   c.   Communicate concerns about short staffing to the appropriate person whenever the situation occurs.

Employer and Supervisor Accountability

1. An employer is liable for the actions of its employees within their scope of employment.
   a. The employer may not be responsible if the employee is acting beyond his or her scope of employment.
   b. Employer and supervisor responsibility does not eliminate individual responsibility.
2. A supervisor may be liable for harm caused by an incompetent nurse, if the supervisor failed to assess the nurse's ability; if the employee has a known problem that can affect performance (e.g., alcoholism); or if the supervisor failed to provide adequate supervision.
3. A health care facility is obligated to carefully monitor the credentials and competence of employees and independent contractors.

Independent Contractor Accountability

1. The independent contractor is responsible for his or her own actions.
2. The health care facility or organization may be liable also if it had reason to know that the independent contractor was incompetent and failed to act.

Torts

1. A tort is a civil action for financial damages for injury to a person, property, or reputation.
2. Negligence, an unintentional tort, is the most common cause of cases involving nurses.
   a. Failure to adhere to the standard of nursing care (negligent practice) results in harm to the patient.
   b. Four elements must be proved to establish a claim of negligence
      1) Duty
         a) It must be proved that the nurse had a duty (responsibility) to care for the patient.
         b) The scope or limits of that duty must be proved. Published standards of care and the actions of a "reasonably prudent nurse" (expert witness) are used to establish scope of duty.
      2) Breach of duty – it must be proved that the nurse deviated in some manner from the standard of care.
      3) Injury or harm to the patient must result. Harm may be physical, emotional, or financial.
      4) Causation – the breach of duty must be proved to be the proximate cause of injury.
   c. In order to protect yourself against negligent practice:
      1) Know your practice area and remain current.
      2) Know your abilities and limitations.
      3) Know and follow the standards of care in your area.
      4) Know and follow your facility's policies and procedures.
      5) Know your patients and their families, and build good relationships with them.

    d. Statute of limitations specifying the time limits within which a suit must be filed can:

       1) Be established under state law.

       2) Vary by nature of the complaint. In most states, a complaint of negligence must be entered within two years of the time the patient (or patient's representative) becomes aware of the injury.

3. Torts result generally in financial settlements. The BON may take action regarding licensure in addition to the financial settlements resulting from a successful civil tort (malpractice) claim. Crimes carry the possibility of jail sentences.

4. In some states, Good Samaritan Laws extend a degree of immunity to persons providing care gratuitously in an emergency situation.

    a. Actions are protected (in most states) if they are offered in good faith and are not reckless.

5. Intentional torts contain purposeful action and the intent to do an act – the intent does not have to be hostile or malicious. There must be an understanding that the harmful outcome is highly likely or that the act was done with reckless disregard for the interest of the patient.

    a. Assault and battery.

       1) An assault is a credible threat that causes another to become apprehensive of being touched in a manner that is offensive, insulting, provoking, or physically injurious.

       2) If the threat (assault) is carried out, the act is battery.

    b. Defamation is the wrongful injury to the reputation of another person.

       1) Oral defamation is libel.

       2) Written defamation is slander.

       3) Statement must be made to a third person; statements made directly to the person are not defamatory.

       4) Best protection against defamation: truth and privilege.

          a) True statements are not basis for legal action.

          b) A privileged statement is one that could be considered defamatory in other situations, but is not because of a legally recognized higher duty that the person making the communication must honor.

    c. Invasion of privacy occurs when an unauthorized person has access to confidential information.

       1) Information about a patient is confidential and should not be released without permission of the patient.

       2) Mandatory reporting of communicable diseases, suspicion of child or elder abuse, and other matters required by law to be reported to the appropriate officials is not invasion of privacy.

          a) Disclosure to the general public, media, or other interested parties is invasion of privacy.

          b) Clinicians who give access to information about patients for whom they do not have direct responsibility are invading the privacy of those patients and may be subject to institutional or civil penalty.

    d. Fraud and misrepresentation are false or misleading statements that the patient relies on to his or her detriment.

    e. False imprisonment is the unlawful restriction of the freedom of a person, including physical restraint.

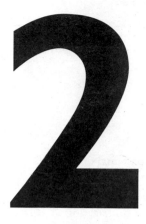

Ethics

Nursing and Health

Nursing Theory

Theory is to nursing practice as a road map is to a cross-country car trip. Theory, like a road map, provides direction to facilitate successful outcomes.

1. Theory is a set of concepts, definitions, and propositions that project a systematic view of phenomena by defining specific interrelationships among the concepts for purposes of describing, explaining, and predicting phenomena.

2. A concept is a word or phrase that describes an abstract idea or mental image of a phenomenon. Concepts are the building blocks of theory. For example, concepts with special relevance to nursing are "health" and "cardiovascular fitness."

3. A proposition is a statement about a concept or the relationship between two or more concepts. For example, a descriptive proposition related to health is "health is more than the absence of disease." A relational proposition is "cardiovascular fitness is a component of health."

4. The purpose of theory is to describe, explain, or predict phenomena. Theory serves the discipline of nursing in several ways:
   a. As an organized reservoir for knowledge and research findings.
   b. To explain observations and predict outcomes.
   c. To stimulate new directions in practice and research.
   d. To develop research questions for testing.

5. Theory improves nursing practice by increasing understanding of phenomena; this understanding influences behavior. Learning to think differently about phenomena enables one to try different approaches.

Health and Illness

Health and illness are key concepts in nursing theory, research, and practice. In 1974, the World Health Organization (WHO) defined health as follows: "Health is a state of complete physical, mental, and social well-being, and not merely the absence of disease and infirmity."

1. This definition changed the conceptualization of health from an illness model to a competence model. Health became a positive condition to be attained.

2. Four general conceptualizations of health are found in the nursing literature.
    a. Clinical: Health is the absence of disease or injury.
    b. Role: Health is the ability to perform role functions.
    c. Adaptive: Health is adaptation or adjustment to life's demands.
    d. Eudaemonistic: Health is the expression of the maximum potential of the individual. The WHO definition is an example of eudaimonistic definition.

3. Holistic theorists define health as a state or process in which the individual experiences a sense of well-being and the integration of body, mind, and spirit interacting harmoniously with the environment.

4. Illness and disease are different concepts. Illness is the subjective experience of the symptoms and suffering to which the individual assigns meaning. Disease is a discrete entity causing specific symptoms.
    a. Some scholars conceptualize health and illness as existing on a single continuum, from optimum health to terminal illness.
    b. Others conceptualize health and illness on two distinct, but interacting, continua. One continuum ranges from no illness to terminal illness; the other from optimum health to poor health.

Human Behavior

Theories of human behavior have been used to describe, explain, or predict health-related behavior. Theories and models that focus on individuals describe, explain, or predict the choices that individuals make about health-related behavior.

Maslow's Hierarchy of Needs

Maslow's hierarchy depicts human need as a pyramid with survival needs at the base and the most sophisticated needs at the apex of the pyramid. As needs are met at each level, the next higher level provides motivation for behavior. Layers of the pyramid, from most basic to most sophisticated are:

1. Physiological survival needs – food, air, sleep, and shelter;
2. Safety needs – freedom from fear of threat to survival;
3. Belonging needs – affiliation and love; and
4. Self-actualization needs – maximizing one's potential and achieving personal fulfillment.

Social Cognitive Theory

Social Cognitive Theory (SCT) examines the mental processes through which thoughts, beliefs, and attitudes are converted into behavior. Perceived self-efficacy is a significant determinant of behavior.

1. Perceived self-efficacy is an individual's assessment of his or her ability to perform the actions necessary to achieve a desired outcome.
2. Perceived self-efficacy is a thought or belief that is unrelated to actual skill-level.

3. Perceived self-efficacy is behavior specific – an individual's perceived self-efficacy for engaging in exercise may differ from his perceived self-efficacy for dietary change.

4. Efficacy information is obtained from four sources.

   a. Mastery experience is the most powerful source and comes from engaging in the behavior and evaluating personal performance.

   b. Vicarious experience comes from watching others perform a task and hearing their self-evaluation and feedback.

   c. Physiological cues provide information to the individual through his level of autonomic arousal. People use physiological cues related to anxiety, fear, and tranquility to judge their competence.

   d. Verbal or social persuasion is information presented by others to convince the individual that he or she possesses the capacity to carry out a specific course of action. Verbal or social persuasion is the least powerful source of efficacy information.

5. SCT and perceived self-efficacy have been used in several studies of the resumption of activity after an acute cardiac event. In general, perceived self-efficacy for a specific behavior is moderately-to-highly correlated with achievement of the behavior.

Health Belief Model

The Health Belief Model (HBM) explains why healthy people use health-protecting and disease-preventing services. The HBM has been refined and extended to explain individual responses to preventive services and illness treatment.

1. In the HBM, three sets of variables interact and determine individual response.

   a. Individual perceptions

      1) Perceived vulnerability of the individual

      2) Perceived seriousness of the disease

      3) Perceived benefits of preventive action

      4) Perceived barriers to preventive action

   b. Modifying factors

      1) Demographics: Age, gender, and ethnicity

      2) Psychosocial characteristics: Personality, social class, and peer group pressure

      3) Structural characteristics: Knowledge about the disease and prior experience with disease

   c. Cues to action

      1) Media campaigns

      2) Advice from others

      3) Postcard reminders

2. The interaction of individual perceptions, modifying factors, and cues to action determines whether or not a person engages in a health-promoting behavior.

3. The HBM has been used to explain health-related behavior and to guide program development to increase the likelihood of success.

4. Across studies, perceived barriers to preventive action have been most consistently associated with health-promoting behaviors. When perceived barriers are high, the likelihood of adopting the preventive behavior is low.

5. The HBM has been criticized for several reasons:

    a. It places responsibility for action exclusively on the individual.

    b. It focuses on avoiding negative behavior, as opposed to embracing positive health behaviors.

    c. The motivation for behavior change comes from perceived threat or fear related to illness.

Health Promotion Model

The Health Promotion Model (HPM) focuses on health-seeking rather than disease-preventing behaviors.

1. In the HPM, two sets of variables interact and determine individual commitment to action:

    a. Individual characteristics and experiences (including expectations).

    b. Behavior-specific thoughts and feelings

        1) Perceived benefits of action

        2) Perceived barriers to action

        3) Perceived self-efficacy

        4) Activity-related affect.

2. The commitment to action may be modified or broken by competing demands and preferences.

3. In general, studies that used the HPM produced evidence that supports the relationships between perceived self-efficacy; benefits of, and barriers to, action; and health-related behavior.

Transtheoretical Model

The Transtheoretical Model (TTM) describes a 6-stage process of behavior change. The motivation to change, and effective interventions to promote change, differ by stage. Progression through the stages is not linear. The average person goes through the stages several times before behavior change is achieved.

1. In the **precontemplation** stage, the client has no intention of changing.

    a. The client may deny that change is needed, blame others for the problem, or feel overwhelmed and demoralized.

    b. Clinicians are most effective if they are empathetic and patient while offering hope for change.

2. In the **contemplation** stage, the client acknowledges the need to change but is ambivalent and anxious about the change.

    a. Clinicians can provide information, acknowledge ambivalence, help clarify goals, and eliminate barriers to change.

3. In the **preparation** stage, the client begins to explore different options or ways to change the behavior. He or she is actively planing to change within the next month.

    a. Clinicians can assist the client to make realistic plans about how to handle relapse while focusing on the future and the benefits of change.

4. In the **action** stage, the client changes the behavior.

    a. Clinicians assist the client to substitute alternate behaviors. Affirmation and support are helpful at this stage.

5. In the **maintenance** stage, the client continues the change. If a lapse occurs, it may result in fear and decreased self-efficacy.

    a. Clinicians assist the client to view a lapse as a learning opportunity without imposing guilt. A lapse is not a defeat.

6. In the **termination** stage, the client revises his self-image and the former behavior is no longer a threat.

    a. Clinicians remain alert to risks for old behavior and continue to promote the client's self-efficacy for the behavior.

7. The TTM developed through studying the process of smoke cessation with adults. Subsequent studies have shown its applicability to exercise and other behavior changes.

Community-level Behavior Change

Social Ecology Theory

Social Ecology Theory (SET) examines the way people influence, and are influenced by, their environment and pays particular attention to the interface between person and environment.

1. Responsibility for health is shared between individuals and community systems.

2. Health promoting strategies are developed through community action and public policy.

Programs based on SET focus on creating healthier communities to produce healthier people.

    a. The role of the clinician is consultant and supporter of the change process.

    b. The Minnesota Heart Health Program is an example of a community-based behavior change program. Strategies employed included community-level health education programs related to smoke cessation, exercise, and nutrition.

Organizational Change

Lewin's Planned Change

Lewin's process of planned change is the classic theory of organizational change.

1. Successful change involves unfreezing existing structures, introducing the change and moving to a new level, and re-freezing the structures to incorporate the change.

2. Successful change requires identifying forces driving the change and those restraining the change. Change is accomplished by strengthening driving forces and reducing restraining forces.

Strategies for Organizational Change

Strategies for organizational change reflect individual change theories.

1. Empirical–rational strategies for organizational change reflect the Theory of Reasoned Action.

    a. The logic is as follows: Organizations are comprised of people. People are rational. To create change, provide education and disseminate knowledge. Once the people see the benefit, they will adopt the change.

2. Normative–reeducative strategies of organizational change reflect social cognitive theory.

3. Power–coercive strategies of organizational change reflect motivational theories. The impetus for change is authority or organizational power. Change occurs because it reduces pain or harm as opposed to increasing pleasure or benefit.

Barriers to Organizational Change

Forces restraining acceptance of organizational change include the following:

1. Threat to self-interest – the change will be harmful in some way.
2. Inaccurate perceptions of the effect the change will have.
3. Disagreement about the value of the change.
4. Low tolerance for change and uncertainty, which may be related to lack of self-confidence.
5. Time – a system that has been stable for a long time is resistant to change.

Drivers for Organizational change

Forces facilitating acceptance of organizational change include the following:

1. People believe that the change is their idea or agrees with their ideas.
2. People are part of the change process.
3. Other people who are important to the individual support the change.
4. The change reduces burden or work.
5. The change is introduced as a pilot with evaluation.
6. The change is implemented using skillful, enthusiastic leadership that emphasizes communication and participation.

Family Dynamics

1. Families are important in nursing practice. Families are conceptualized as the context within which the individual exists and as the client for therapeutic intervention.
2. Family may be defined as a small group of intimates related biologically, legally or emotionally – a family is as it defines itself.
3. Cardiovascular and other health risk factors cluster within families. The Framingham Heart Study found a higher than expected concordance between spouses for blood pressure, cholesterol, triglyceride, blood sugar, smoking, and pulmonary function.

Family Systems Theory

1. Members of the family interact as a functional whole. Change in one element of the family system affects the whole system.
   a. The family as a whole is greater than (and different from) the sum of its parts.
   b. Individuals are best understood within the family context.
2. The family system is in contact with the environment, and with input and output across its boundaries.
   a. Families function to transmit culture.
   b. Family members occupy a variety of roles and functions that may assume varying importance at different familial developmental stages.

  c. Family members, especially the spouse, are the most important source of social support.

   1) Social support has a direct effect on health.

   2) The quality of family relationships has an indirect effect on health by buffering stress.

3. Problems and symptoms occurring within family members reflect the family's adaptation to its total structure and environment at a given point in time.

4. Adaptive efforts of family members effect the biological, interpersonal, and intrapsychic connections with the family (nuclear and extended) and the society.

  a. Concurrent events in different parts of the family are connected in some way.

5. There are normative expectations related to timing of major transitions within the family, such as leaving home, marriage, and childbirth.

  a. "On time" events create less strain within the family than "off time" events.

Family Life Cycle

1. As with individuals, family development follows a predictable course.

  a. Unattached young adult

  b. Newly married couple

  c. Family with young children

  d. Family with adolescent children

  e. Family with adult children who have moved out

  f. Later life family

2. Families oscillate between periods of closeness (centripetal) and periods of distance (centrifugal). These periods reflect the needs of the family within its developmental stage. For example, a family with young children requires high cohesion (centripetal), while a family with adult children requires more distance (centrifugal).

Family Response to Serious Illness

Family response to serious illness depends on when the illness occurs within the family life cycle, which family member falls ill, and the family's usual coping style. For example, a myocardial infarction may have different meaning to a family with young children versus a later life family. Family stress related to role change may differ by whether it is the husband or the wife who becomes ill.

Crisis Theory

Crisis is a response to hazardous events and is experienced as a painful state. A situation becomes a crisis because the individual perceives it as threatening in a highly significant way. Clinicians describe crisis as a clinical syndrome involving emotional upset, increased tension, unpleasant affect, ineffective coping strategies, and impaired functioning.

1. Life events associated with loss and threat can precipitate situational crisis.

  a. Examples include death, divorce, major illness, job loss, rape, and trauma.

  b. Positive events, such as marriage and childbirth, create conflicts that can lead to crisis. For example, differences in values related to family or religion. The arrival of the first child creates major change in the couple's relationship, which can cause conflict and stress related to loss.

2. Developmental crises occur at predictable points in which new behavior must be learned in order for the individual to move to the next level. Erickson identified three developmental tasks with potential for crisis that occur in adulthood:

   a. Intimacy versus isolation in young adults

   b. Generativity versus self-absorption in middle-aged adults

   c. Hope versus despair in older adults

3. Crisis occurs when the usual coping strategies are unable to control effectively or resolve the tension generated by the situation. Each person usually functions within a specific range of effectiveness and personal satisfaction. In a crisis, there is overwhelming emotional distress that interferes with effective problem solving.

   a. A crisis is self-limited and some resolution occurs in four to ten weeks.

   b. All of the person's energy and resources focus on resolution of the crisis and reduction of the pain.

4. The person in crisis is generally more open to accepting help. Minimal help may produce meaningful results.

Crisis Intervention

1. Crisis intervention consists of short-term psychotherapy with specific goals:

   a. To keep the individual safe – prevent harm to self or others.

   b. To return the individual to the pre-crisis level of functioning or higher.

   c. To enhance the coping techniques and self-esteem.

2. Crisis intervention techniques include reassurance, suggestion, support, environmental manipulation, and psychotropic medications.

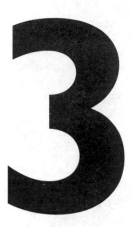

Leadership

Leadership is the personal characteristics or qualities that the leader uses to influence others to achieve an identified goal. Key attributes of a leader that promote the achievement of the identified goal are:

1. The leader works effectively with members of the group or team.
2. The leader facilitates communication among members of the group or team.
3. The leader motivates the members of the group or team.

Leadership Styles

1. Autocratic leadership uses power to influence group members. The leader makes the decision and gives minimal consideration to the ideas or suggestions of members.
2. Participative leadership uses the democratic process for decisionmaking with group members. The leader encourages the participation of members and provides consistent feedback.
3. Laissez-faire leadership uses minimal guidance and provides little feedback to group members. The leader is unwilling to make decisions and consequently does not initiate change.
4. Transactional leadership focuses on daily activities and is comfortable with the status quo. The leader rewards group members for work completed and deals with problems after they have occurred.
5. Transformational leadership articulates a vision and commitment to the organization's goals. The leader empowers members to achieve the goals and vision.

Leadership in Cardiovascular Care

Cardiovascular (CV) nurses assume a leadership role as they coordinate care. The complexity of cardiac and vascular care is increasing and there is a great need for interdisciplinary collaboration to meet patient care needs. Participative and transformational leadership styles facilitate group or team processes to achieve desired outcomes in patient care.

Team Building

Team building involves many factors that promote good working relationships among team members. Teams collaborate to promote the efficiency of the organization and to optimize patient outcomes. Teams develop the highest potential of its members so that they contribute in significant ways, accept more responsibility, and share a commitment to the organizational goals and structure.

Team

1. A team is a group of people committed to an identified, shared purpose, with common goals, complementary or shared skills, and a similar approach to completing the work. Each member is accountable to the team for the completion of assigned tasks.

2. Attributes of a successful team include the ability to self-regulate, awareness of team member roles including strengths and weaknesses, adaptability to changing events, accountability for evaluating actions, and responsibility for revising the plan as necessary.

Team Building Models

1. The Traditional Model of Team Effectiveness views the team as a series of components that include team building, team processes, and team effectiveness. This model examines the symptoms of team effectiveness, but does not look at the actual reasons, such as motivation or cognitive processes, that drive the team towards attainment of its goals.

    a. Assumptions are that the team is passive, stable, and a behavioral entity.

    b. Team building is geared towards redesigning behavioral processes by examining the signs of team effectiveness, rather than the causes.

    c. Team processes include communication, social integration, role clarification, and goal setting.

    d. Process, attitudinal, and perceptual indicators measure team effectiveness.

2. Cognitive Motivational Model of Team Effectiveness (CoMMTE) is based on the premise that each of the variables (i.e., assumptions, team causes, team processes, team effectiveness, and team building) are interdependent and can be used to evaluate and redesign team developed interventions.

    a. CoMMTE assumes that the team is an active, dynamic, fluid, and cognitive-motivational entity.

    b. Team causes or purposes include shared goals and actions, the ability to evaluate its actions, and to redesign its interventions.

    c. Team processes are self-regulated and have diagnostic perogative.

    d. Team effectiveness is measured by the achievement of results.

    e. Team building focuses on redesigning cognitive functioning by analyzing team effectiveness.

Benefits of Team Building in Health Care

1. Nursing, medicine, and other health care professionals must provide integrated care that supports optimal use of health care resources to improve patient outcomes.

2. Collaboration among nurses provides continuity of care by focusing on a plan that promotes teamwork to enhance positive patient outcomes and to coordinate care delivery.

3. Interdisciplinary collaboration involves the joint contributions of professionals from other disciplines, such as nursing and medicine, working towards the common goals of

improving quality of care and outcomes for patients.

4. Teams can streamline health care services for patients while avoiding duplication or gaps in their care.

Team Building and Teamwork

1. Clear expectations about the roles, skills, and goals of the team and its members enhance teamwork, reduce conflict, and promote success.
2. Participative learning experiences foster collaboration among the members of the team.
3. Effective communication among team members promotes team effectiveness.
4. Support, encouragement, respect, and commitment among members facilitate teamwork.
5. Recognition of one member of the team as the leader by other members enhances group processes.

Barriers to Team Building and Team Work

1. Health care professionals have not been taught about teamwork or team building.
2. Sex role stereotyping and gender hierarchy have a negative effect on interdisciplinary groups.
3. Role status of team members has the potential to impede communication within the group.
4. Team members with traditional views of organizational roles may have difficulty with teamwork.
5. Situations that promote lack of communication, support, and respect for team members impair teamwork.

Team Building for CV Care

1. The formation of teams and subsequent team building are beneficial for the management of acute and chronically ill patients with cardiac and vascular health problems.
2. Decreased length of stay for cardiac surgical patients mandates that health care services are coordinated within the hospital among nursing, cardiology, cardiac surgery, anesthesia, physical therapy, dietary, and respiratory therapy. The development of fast track protocols for early extubation and discharge of these patients required interdisciplinary collaboration.
3. The formation of teams to address the needs of hospitalized CV "outliers" has also been effective. Nurses used primary nursing to manage the nursing care needs, while interdisciplinary teams developed clinical pathways. For example, the development of ventilator weaning and extubation protocols has decreased the duration of mechanical ventilation and hospitalization for patients after cardiac surgery.
4. Teamwork has also been effective in coordinating the care of patients with chronic CV diseases, such as heart failure. Intra- and interdisciplinary team efforts provide continuity in the transition from hospital to home.

Case Management

Definitions

Nursing uses case management to coordinate the care of patients. Case management is defined differently by different professional organizations.

1. The Case Management Society of America states that case management is "a collective process which assesses, plans, implements, coordinates, monitors, and evaluates the options and services required to meet an individual's health needs using communications and available resources to promote quality, cost-effective outcomes. " This definition, while broad enough to encompass the different disciplines involved in case management, does not address nursing's unique role.

2. The American Nurses Credentialing Center defines nursing case management as "a dynamic and systematic collaborative approach to providing and coordinating health care services to a defined population. It is a participative process to identify and facilitate options and services for meeting individuals' health needs, while decreasing fragmentation and duplication of care, and enhancing quality, costeffective clinical outcomes."

Case Management Models

1. Nursing case management models evolved from primary nursing and were traditionally used in acute care settings.
   a. Nurse case managers coordinate each patient's care throughout hospitalization as the patient moves to different locations throughout the institution.
   b. Nursing case management plans use diagnostic related grouping (DRG) length of stay, critical pathway reports, and variance analysis, along with interdisciplinary collaborative group practice arrangements, to provide health care services to these patients.

2. Community-based case management models use case managers to coordinate the care of patients from the hospital to the community or long-term care settings, if indicated. These patients have chronic health conditions and need long-term health care services. Community-based models provide care and resources to high-risk patients across the continuum of care.

3. Case management models have been modified to accomodate the needs of patients in a variety of community settings.
   a. Long-term health care models are used for prior authorization screening or direct service.
   b. Rehabilitation case management targets chronic medical or psychosocial health problems that have a longer recovery or treatment time than acute health problems.
   c. Occupational health care models focus on employee health with return to work and wellness as the major goals.
   d. Private case management involves subcontracting with individuals or groups for the coordination of services, advocacy, and counseling.
   e. Insurance case management emphasizes the linkage of resources for patient care but is not involved with direct care.
   f. Managed care and health maintenance organization (HMO) case management models monitor access to services and advocate cost effective alternatives to services. In some cases, permission for costly services is required but not necessarily granted.

Role of Case Managers

1. Establish a professional case management relationship with the patient and family.
2. Assist the patient and family in adapting to the health problem.
3. Advocate for the patient and family.
4. Ensure that patient and family education needs associated with the health problems are met.
5. Manage, coordinate, and facilitate the health care services that the patient and family need.
6. Make sure that health care services are appropriate, delivered within the required time frames, and coordinated across the continuum of care.
7. Evaluate the quality and cost-effectiveness of health care services delivered to patients and their family.

Total Quality Management

1. Total quality management (TQM) is a way to run complex organizations to achieve the aims or mission of the organization.
2. TQM emphasizes empowerment of employees
   a. An underlying principle is that most people are trying quite hard to do their best work, further the mission of the organization, and meet the needs of the customers.
3. TQM recognizes that an organization or department has multiple customers who may have competing needs.
   a. A customer is anyone who depends on a department to provide a service. Customers of nursing service include patients and families (external), but also physicians and other clinicians (internal).
   b. TQM focuses on meeting the needs of both internal and external customers.
4. Quality problems occur when good people get caught in broken processes or systems that don't work.
   a. The people doing the work have the most information about how the work gets done.
   b. Quality is cost effective. Fewer resources are required to do the job right the first time, than are required to do it multiple times until it is right.
5. A key strategy of TQM is to involve the worker in improving the work processes through continuous quality improvement.

Continuous Quality Improvement

1. Continuous quality improvement (CQI) is an approach to improve quality that focuses on how the work gets done (process) rather than on who is doing the work (people).
2. A process is a sequence of actions leading to an outcome that is important to customers (i.e., patients) who depend on the process.
3. It often happens with complex processes that no one individual or department understands the whole process. Therefore, CQI requires an interdepartmental team.

a. Suppose, for example, that it took too long for a patient who was experiencing a stroke to get from the Emergency Department (ED) to the angiography suite where a thrombolytic agent could be administered. A CQI team formed to address this quality problem might require representation from the ED, business office (patient registration), nursing (triage), medicine, transportation, and radiology.

4. CQI empowers health care workers to reduce the cost and improve the quality of their work.

Shewart Cycle

1. Shewart Cycle (also known as the Deming Cycle) is the planning and improvement process most commonly used in US health care organizations today. The cycle has four steps: plan, do, check, act (PDCA).

2. The CQI team plans change by studying the process, deciding what could improve it, and identifying data to be used in monitoring the process.

3. The team tests the proposed change by doing a small-scale trial or data simulation exercise.

The team checks the effects of the trial by studying the results and modifies the planned change, if necessary.

4. The team acts to improve the process by implementing the change.

5. The cycle repeats continuously. Small changes are implemented and evaluated until the process is as efficient as can be achieved.

In the time transferring the client from ED to angiography suite example:

a. **Plan:** The team measured the average time from ED check-in to throbolytic injection. They studied the process and determined that time waiting for transport was a critical factor.

b. **Do:** The team assigned a transporter to the ED for one month and continued to monitor time to thrombolytic injection.

c. **Check:** Pre- and post-intervention data were analyzed and the team found that time to throbolytic injection was reduced by twenty-five minutes. The team consensus was that further reduction was possible.

d. **Act:** The one-month trial of the transporter was extended another month and preprinted physician orders were implemented as well. Time-to-thrombolytic-injection data were gathered continually.

e. **Repeat:** The data showed further reduction in time. The team continued to examine the process to identify further potential improvement.

CQI Relies on Data

1. Quality issues are identified from data.

2. Local and national data are used to establish benchmarks for quality care.

3. Data are collected and analyzed to determine the effect of the change on the process of care.

Barriers to Implementing CQI Programs

1. Organizational barriers include:

a. Resistance to change.

    b.   Culture is so deeply engrained that the behavioral change is in conflict with the organization's philosophy.

    c.   There is limited time for the change to take place.

    d.   Lack of organizational support for CQI.

2.   Management barriers include:

    a.   Management not accepting role change associated with CQI.

    b.   Organization's goals not clearly communicated to management.

    c.   Lack of managerial support.

3.   Process barriers include:

    a.   Data are not available.

    b.   National or local benchmarks have not been defined.

4.   CQI team barriers include:

    a.   Inadequate team building.

    b.   Key departments not represented.

    c.   Lack of understanding by team members of the CQI process.

    d.   Personal agendas.

Outcome Evaluation

Outcome evaluation is important for patients, health care providers, and the health care system. It can be used to evaluate the effect of care on the patient's recovery from cardiac and vascular procedures. This process can also be used to enhance the knowledge of health care providers, establish the criteria for clinical decisionmaking, evaluate the effectiveness of interventions, and to identify areas for improvement.

An outcome is a change in status between two points in time. The change may be positive or negative.

1.   Frequently used patient outcomes include the following examples:

    a.   Morbidity or incidence of complications

    b.   Mortality

    c.   Hemodynamic parameters (e.g., pulmonary artery pressures, central venous pressures)

    d.   Laboratory values (e.g., blood sugar, prothrombin time, international normalized ratio [INR])

    e.   Symptoms (e.g., nausea, vomiting, pain, fatigue, angina, anxiety, depression)

    f.   Functional status (e.g., activities of daily living, sexuality, family function, employment)

2.   Frequently used health care provider outcomes include the following examples

    a.   Change in knowledge or skill-level

    b.   Compliance with practice standards

3.   Frequently used system outcomes include the following examples:

    a.   Service utilization

    b.   Length of hospital stay or duration of services

    c.   Cost of care or services

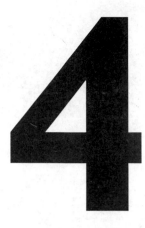

Research

Problem Identification

Sources of Ideas for Research Problems

1. Clinical practice
   a. The idea emerges: For example, how can the nurse relieve patient and family anxiety about early hospital discharge?
   b. Brainstorm with colleagues: Do others perceive anxiety about early discharge to be a problem? Why is it a problem? Does it have bad outcomes?
   c. Review the literature: Has the question been answered? Is the answer definitive? Are observable variables suggested or supported by the literature?
   d. Identify variables: What concepts contained in the questions have the ability to vary?
      1) Possible patient-related variables: Age, gender, procedure, and pre-hospitalization anxiety.
      2) Possible nurse-related variables: Age, gender, education, and experience.
      3) Possible system-related variables: Discharge planning procedure, length of hospital stay, and referral to home care.
2. Continuous quality improvement trends
3. Theory
   a. Some scholars believe that the purpose of nursing research is to generate and test theory, and research that is unrelated to theory is trivial.
4. Literature
5. Priorities set by professional organizations and funding agencies
6. Conferences with, and input from, colleagues

Problem Evaluation

1. Does the problem occur frequently? If not, does it occur infrequently, but have a significant effect on outcome?
2. Can the problem or question be answered by collecting observable data?

3. Will answering the question result in better care?
4. Are the resources necessary to answer the question available? Is it feasible, practical?
5. Is the question ethical? Will some good come to the participant or society? Are the risks outweighed by the benefits of participation?
6. Is the nurse's level of interest in the question sufficient to sustain the effort?

Stating the Question or Problem

1. A research question is a concise statement, worded in the present tense, that includes one or more variables (or concepts) .
2. Kinds of research questions:
   a. Descriptive: For example, "How is anxiety related to early discharge manifested in patients and families?"
   b. Exploratory or relational: For example, "What is the relationship between pre-discharge anxiety and post-discharge behavior?"
   c. Predictive: For example, "Does self-efficacy, pre-discharge anxiety, or family structure best predict post-discharge behavior?"
   d. Experimental or quasi-experimental: If one can predict the outcome, the next step would be to modify the outcome. If one knew, for example, that self-efficacy predicted post-discharge behavior, then one could prescribe a self-efficacy enhancement intervention to influence post-discharge behavior.

Research Method

The research question and the existing knowledge about the phenomena of interest determine the research method used.

1. Qualitative methods are inductive; quantitative methods are deductive.
2. Qualitative methods are used in the following situations.
   a. When the question is broad and little is known about the subject. For example, "How do mid-life women decide to use natural, as opposed to pharmaceutical, estrogen replacement?"
   b. To achieve a deep, rich understanding of the phenomena – discovery, exploration, and description of the phenomena. For example, "What factors contribute to women's delay in seeking emergency care when experiencing symptoms of myocardial infarction?"
   c. In combination with quantitative methods – for triangulation or as a complement.
   d. For instrument development.
   e. To generate hypotheses about relationships for subsequent testing.
3. Quantitative methods are used to:
   a. Explain and predict phenomena.
   b. Generate evidence of cause and effect.
   c. Test theory or instruments.
   d. Evaluate the effectiveness of interventions.

Qualitative Methods

General Characteristics

1. Qualitative methods allow the researcher to gain insight through discovering meaning.
2. Qualitative methods are a way to explore the richness and complexity of phenomenon.
3. Qualitative data are expressed in words rather than numbers.
4. Data collection and analysis occur concurrently.
5. Theoretical or purposive sampling is used. Using insights from the data, the researcher selects informants with particular characteristics to increase theoretical understanding of the phenomenon.
6. Researchers are concerned with the trustworthiness of qualitative studies

Assuring Trustworthiness

1. Credibility is the truth-value of the study. It has been compared to the internal validity of a study using quantitative methods. When assessing the credibility of the study, the reviewer considers the period of engagement with the study, the use of multiple data sources (triangulation), and if the researcher checked with the informants and included their response before publishing the study.
2. Transferability of a study has been compared to the external validity of a study using quantitative methods. In general, the result of a qualitative study is deep, rich description of a phenomenon or process. Results are not directly transferable to other settings or populations. The understanding gained may be used to inform other studies or practices.
3. Dependability of a study has been compared to the reliability of a quantitative study. The researcher maintains scrupulous records about methods and decisions that can be reviewed and verified in a process audit.
4. Confirmability of a study has been compared to the objectivity of a quantitative study. The issue here is the extent to which the meanings assigned to the data are grounded in the events and the culture rather than in the researcher's experience. "Would another analyst find similar meaning in the data?"

Phenomenological Research

Phenomenological research is used to describe experiences as they are lived from the perspective of the study participant.

1. Phenomenology is not just a research method, but also a philosophy that guides the research process.
2. The first step in conducting a phenomenological study is to identify the phenomena of interest.
3. The research question asks "What is the human experience and meaning of this phenomena?"
4. Sampling requires locating and identifying people living with the phenomena who are willing to share their thoughts, feelings, and experiences with the researcher.
5. Data are generated and collected through observation, interview, videotape, and descriptions written by participants.

6. Analysis consists of attaching meaning to statements and the outcome is a theoretical statement responding to the research question.
   a. Excerpts from the data are used to support the theoretical statement.
   b. Many nurses are familiar with Benner's phenomenological study of nursing knowledge acquisition, *From Novice to Expert.*

Grounded Theory

Grounded theory is a research method used to understand basic social processes. It has its roots in sociology.

1. The first step is to identify the social process of interest.
2. Data are generated and collected through participant-observation and intensive interviewing.
3. Data are coded and categorized.
   a. Constant comparative analysis compares each piece of data with every other piece.
   b. The categories are found within the data – not preconceived.
   c. Data are collected until all of the characteristics of the category are revealed.
4. The outcome is a theory explaining the social process of interest that is grounded in the data from which it was derived.

Ethnography

Ethnography is a research method used to understand a culture (or subculture) from its own perspective. Ethnography has its roots in anthropology.

1. The first step with ethnography is to identify the culture to be studied.
2. Literature review provides a background for the study.
   a. The researcher seeks a general understanding of the phenomena to be examined specifically within the culture.
   b. Studies of health-behavior and experiences of homeless people may use ethnographic methods, for example.
3. Data generation and collection require access to the culture and key informants.
   a. Key informants are members of the culture who are willing to share their knowledge of the culture and the phenomena.
   b. The researcher becomes immersed in the culture through active participation.
4. Data are collected through observation and interview.
5. Analysis involves identifying meaning attached to the data and events by the informants. Members of the culture validate meaning before the results are final.
6. The outcome is detailed description of the phenomena as experienced within the culture.

Historiography

Historiography examines past events.

1. The first step is to select the topic and questions to be examined.
2. Next the researcher must identify sources of data and obtain access to these sources.

a. Data may include letters, memos, and mementos.

3. Analysis involves synthesis of the data collected.

4. The outcome is a cogent retelling of historical events and their meaning.

a. Examples of historical studies include *We Band of Angels* and *Critical Care Nursing*.

Content Analysis

Content analysis is a method used to classify words in text by their theoretical importance.

1. Content analysis differs from other qualitative methods as it uses numbers to represent frequency, order, or intensity of words, phrases, or sentences.

2. Content analysis is sometimes used in historical research.

3. Theoretically significant categories are identified. Data are classified into categories and the number of data segments assigned to the category is determined.

4. Descriptive statistics may be used to count and summarize data.

Quantitative Methods

General Concerns and Issues

1. Variables

   a. An independent variable is the stimulus or activity that is manipulated by the researcher to create an effect on the dependent variable.

      1) Control is very important in experimental and quasi-experimental designs.

      2) The greater the amount of control the researcher has, the stronger the evidence from the study.

   b. A dependent variable is the response, behavior, or outcome that the researcher wants to predict or explain.

   c. Extraneous variables are all of the other factors that can vary and may influence the dependent variable.

      1) The researcher uses research design amd statistical methods to reduce the effect of extraneous variables.

   d. Demographic variables are characteristics of the subjects that are collected for descriptive purposes.

2. Causality – support for causal relationships.

   a. Correlation or association alone does not prove causality.

   b. Three conditions must be met to establish causality:

      1) Strong correlation between the proposed cause and effect.

      2) Proposed cause must precede the effect in time.

      3) Proposed cause must be present every time the effect occurs.

   c. Multicausality – multiple factors contribute to the effect or outcome.

   d. Probability addresses relative, rather than absolute, causality. It describes the likelihood that one factor caused another.

3. Validity of a study is a measure of the truth or accuracy of the study. There are multiple aspects of validity that contribute to strength of the evidence provided by a study.

a. Statistical conclusion validity is concerned with whether the conclusions made through statistical analyses accurately reflect the real world.

    1) Type I error occurs when the researcher concludes that there is a difference between two groups when in reality there is no difference.

        a) The risk of Type I error increases when the researcher conducts multiple statistical analyses of relationships or differences.

        b) Some relationships or differences may be found by chance within the sample that do not reflect true population relationships or differences.

    2) Type II error occurs when the researcher concludes that there is no difference between two samples when there is a true difference.

        a) Low statistical power is the most common cause of Type II error.

b. Internal validity is the extent to which the effect detected in a study results from the relationship between the independent and dependent variable, and not from some extraneous factor.

c. Construct validity is the quality of the fit between the definition of a concept of interest and its method of measurement.

d. External validity describes the extent to which study findings can be generalized beyond the sample used in the study.

Quantitative Designs

1. Descriptive designs are used when the purpose is to delineate characteristics of a sample or setting. The purpose is to avoid generalizing to a larger population.

2. Correlational designs study a population by systematically examining a representative sample. Findings may be generalized to the population represented by the sample.

a. Crosssectional designs collect data at one point in time.

b. Longitudinal designs collect data at more than one point in time.

c. Correlational designs may be used also to describe relationships between, or among, factors when the intent is not to make inferences about a larger population.

3. Quasi-experimental and experimental designs are used to test hypotheses about causal relationships.

a. Control is a basic characteristic of experimental and quasi-experimental designs. Control is the ability of the researcher to manipulate the independent variable and to eliminate, hold constant, or measure the effect of extraneous variables.

b. Elements of a true experimental design include the following:

    1) At least two groups – experimental and control.

    2) Random assignment of the sample to the experimental and control groups.

    3) Pre-tests before the manipulation of the independent variable.

    4) Post-tests following manipulation of the independent variable.

c. When all four elements cannot be met, the design is quasi-experimental.

Sampling

Sampling involves selecting a group of people or elements to participate in a study.

1. Population refers to the entire set of people or elements that meet the sampling criteria.

Accessible population refers to the set of people or elements that meet the sampling criteria to which the researcher can gain access.

2. Sampling criteria are the characteristics essential for inclusion in the target population.

   a. Inclusion criteria are characteristics that must be present for a subject to be included in the population.

   b. Exclusion criteria are characteristics that, when present, cause a subject to be excluded from the population.

3. Representativeness is the extent to which the sample is like the population.

4. Adequate sample size for a study is determined by the anticipated effect size, power of the statistical tests, and significance level.

   a. Effect size is the amount of an impact or the strength of the relationship between the independent and dependent variables.

   b. Power is the capacity of the statistical test to detect significant differences or relationships that exist between groups in the sample. The minimal acceptable power for a study is .80, meaning there is an 80% probability of correctly discerning a difference between two groups.

   c. The significance level is set by the researcher and determines the probability of making a Type I error (concluding that there is a difference between two groups when in reality there is no difference). In general, researchers use a probability of .05 or less when analyzing data. When a test of difference is significant at the .05 level, the researcher may conclude that there is a 95% probability that the two groups are different.

Sampling Error

Parameters describe population characteristics or attributes; statistics describe sample characteristics.

1. Sampling error is the difference between a sample statistic and a population parameter.

   a. If the sample does not reflect the population, sampling error will be large.

   b. Random variation is the expected difference that occurs when one measures a variable in different subjects from the same sample.

   c. Systematic variation occurs when subjects vary in some specific way from the population as a whole.

2. Random sampling is a way to assure that every individual in the population has an equal chance to be selected into the sample.

   a. Random sampling assures that the sample represents the population and minimizes systematic variation.

   b. Random samples include simple random samples, stratified random samples, and cluster samples.

3. In non-probability sampling, every individual in the population does not have an equal chance to be selected.

   a. Non-probability sampling reduces the likelihood that the sample represents the population. There is an increased risk of systematic variation.

   b. Non-probability samples include convenience and quota samples.

      1) Random assignment to a group is used in an attempt to control systematic bias within convenience samples.

Measurement

Measurement is the process of assigning numbers to objects, events, or situations according to a rule.

1. Levels of measurement
    a. Nominal scale is the lowest level of measurement. Numbers function as labels or categories and cannot be used for calculation. For example, the numbers on baseball players' shirts are labels only. And, when the variable gender is measured using 1 for female and 2 for male, the numbers represent categories only.
        1) The categories are mutually exclusive.
        2) All of the data fit in one of the categories (exhaustive).
    b. Ordinal scale represents sequence or order – members of a set are placed in order from most to least with respect to some characteristic. For example, a graduating student may be first or tenth in a class. The number is significant in terms of relative position.
        1) Categories are mutually exclusive and exhaustive.
        2) Categories can be placed in order, but intervals are not equal.
    c. Interval scale has order and equal numerical distance between intervals. For example, temperature is measured on an interval scale. The difference between seventy degrees and eighty degrees is the same as the difference between fifty degrees and sixty degrees. A temperature of zero degrees does not indicate the absence of temperature, however.
        1) Categories are mutually exclusive and exhaustive.
        2) Categories can be placed in order.
        3) Intervals are equal, but the scale does not contain absolute zero.
    d. Ratio scale is the highest form of measurement and exists on a continuum. Weight, length, and volume are examples of ratiolevel measurements. Zero represents the absence of weight, length, or volume. Because absolute zero is contained in the scale, one can say that ten pounds is twice as heavy as five pounds.
        1) Categories are mutually exclusive and exhaustive.
        2) Categories can be placed in order.
        3) Intervals are equal.
        4) Scale contains absolute zero.

Measurement Issues

It is not possible to measure a concept perfectly. Measurement error is the difference between the concept in reality and as it is measured by an instrument.

There are three components to a measured score: the true score, the observed score, and the error score. The observed score equals the true score plus the error score.

There are two components to the error score – random error and systematic error.

1. Random error causes the observed score to vary around the true score.
    a. According to measurement theory, the sum of random errors is zero. Some observed scores will be higher than the true scores and some will be lower, but, taken together, the errors will add up to zero.

b. Random error is not correlated with the true score. Random error will not cause the mean score to be higher or lower than the true mean, but will increase the amount of unexplained variance around the true mean. Random error cannot be eliminated.

2. Systematic error causes the observed score to vary from the true score in a consistent (systematic) way. For example, a scale that consistently weighs subjects as two pounds heavier than their true weight adds systematic error. Systematic error effects mean scores.

   a. The goal in measurement is to reduce systematic error as much as possible.

3. Reliability of a measure reflects the consistency or reproducibility of scores obtained with the measure.

   a. Reliability testing provides an indication of the amount of random error inherent in the measurement of the concept within the sample.

   b. Reliability of a measure is expressed as a correlation coefficient with 1.00 representing perfect reliability and 0.00 representing no reliability.

   c. Estimates of reliability are specific to the sample being tested.

      1) Reliability testing is performed on each instrument used in a study before other statistical analyses are done.

      2) A reliability coefficient of 0.80 is the minimal acceptable level for established instruments. For newly developed instruments, a reliability coefficient of 0.70 may be accepted.

4. Validity of a measure reflects the extent to which an instrument represents the concept being measured within the specific situation. Validity of a measure determines the appropriateness, meaningfulness, and usefulness of inferences made from scores on the measure.

   a. Systematic error reduces the validity of measures.

   b. Evidence for the validity of an instrument develops through repeated use over time in a variety of situations. Traditionally, the various means of accumulating evidence have been grouped into categories. The use of category labels does not indicate different kinds of validity, but different types of evidence.

      1) Content-related evidence examines the extent to which the method of measurement includes representative elements from a domain of content.

         a) Content-related evidence often relies on expert judgment to identify appropriate elements for inclusion.

         b) Factor analysis is a statistical method that examines clusters of relationships among items. Once the clusters are identified mathematically, the analyst explains theoretically why the items grouped as they did.

      2) Criterion-related evidence examines the performance of an instrument in comparison with other measures, preferably a "gold standard."

      3) Evidence of validity accrues from differential predictions of future or concurrent events.

         a) The ability to predict future performance.

         b) The ability to differentiate between groups known to be high and low in the concept of interest.

5. Sensitivity is the ability of a measure to detect relevant change in the concept.

Data Collection Strategies

1. Observation
   a. Answers questions about overt human behavior – actions, facial expressions, body language, etc.
   b. Allows phenomena to be studied in their natural environment.
2. Self-report – interviews, questionnaires, and surveys.
   a. Answers questions about facts, beliefs, feelings, and attitudes.
   b. Individuals may be unwilling or unable to answer the questions. Questions may not be answered truthfully.
3. Existing data – public records, medical records, national databases.
   a. Existing data may be used to answer a new question. For example, an investigator might use census data to explore a health-related question.
   b. Personal health (medical) records are often used in case studies. Health records may contain biases of the health care clinician.
4. Physiological measures – blood pressure, heart rate, blood tests, etc.

Protection of Human Rights

1. Informed consent
2. Anonymity and confidentiality
3. Risks and benefits

Data Analysis

1. The research question, methods used to obtain data, and characteristics of the data determine the appropriate statistical tests to be used.
2. Descriptive statistics provide precise, standard ways to summarize and communicate complex information about a sample.
   a. Measures of central tendency
      1) The mode is the numerical value or score that occurs with the highest frequency.
      2) The median is the score at the exact center of the distribution. Exactly 50% of scores is above the median and 50% of the scores is below the median.
      3) The mean is the sum of scores divided by the number of scores included in the sum.
   b. Shape of the distribution
      1) Symmetry – left side of the curve is a mirror image of the right side of the curve. When a curve is symmetrical all three measures of central tendency are equal. When a curve is not symmetrical, it is skewed.
         a) Positive skew – the largest portion of data falls below the mean; the curve has a tail extending to the right.
         b) Negative skew – the largest portion of data falls above the mean; the curve has an initiating tail.
      2) Modality – a curve may be unimodal, bimodal or multimodal. Symmetric curves are usually unimodal.

     3) Kurtosis – describes the peakedness of the curve, which is related to the spread or variability of the scores.

  c. Measures of dispersion

     1) The range is the mathematical difference between the highest and lowest scores.

     2) The standard deviation is the average amount by which scores vary around the mean.

     3) The variance is the average of the squared standard deviations. It is frequently used in statistics, but is difficult to interpret as a measure of dispersion.

  d. Measures of association

     1) Contingency tables or cross tabulations allow visual comparison of summary data related to two variables within the sample.

       a) Contingency tables are used to examine nominal or ordinal level data.

       b) Chi-square is a statistic designed to test for differences between cells in contingency tables.

     2) Correlation coefficients provide information about the direction, strength, and shape of relationships. Values range from −1.00 (a perfect and inverse correlation) to +1.00 (a perfect and positive correlation).

3. Inferential statistics allow the investigator to go beyond description of the sample and make probabilistic inferences about the population.

  a. Parametric statistics require assumptions about the distribution of data – normality and homogeneity of variance, for example.

  b. Non-parametric statistics make no assumptions about the shape of the distribution.

     1) Non-parametric statistics are particularly relevant when the distribution is not normal or the sample size is small.

     2) Non-parametric statistics are commonly used to analyze nominal and ordinal-level data.

  c. Hypothesis testing of differences and association between variables.

     1) Tests of difference

       a) Parametric: t-test, ANOVA

       b) Non-parametric: Mann Whitney U test, sign test

     2) Tests of association

       a) Parametric: Pearson correlation coefficients.

       b) Non-parametric: Spearman and Kendall correlation coefficients.

Evidence-based Practice

Evidence-based practice is the synthesis and use of scientific information (i.e., evidence) to direct practice.

Sources and Kinds of Evidence

1. National guidelines may be research based, represent the consensus of experts, or more commonly, both.

a. The Agency for Healthcare Policy and Research, now the Agency for Healthcare Research and Quality, published practice guidelines that summarized evidence related to specific topics. Some guidelines are now outdated and archived, but can be viewed online from the Web sites (www. ahrq. gov or www. guideline. gov) . Evidence-based guidelines:

   1) Contain comprehensive review and summary of existing research.

   2) Rate the quality of the evidence; place highest value on evidence from randomized clinical trials (RCT) .

      a) Strongest evidence rating A – results of two or more RCTs.

      b) Rating B – results of two or more controlled clinical trials.

      c) Rating C – results of one controlled trial, two case series or descriptive studies, or expert opinion.

   3) Expert panel makes practice recommendations based on evaluation of the evidence.

2. Professional organizations publish research-based protocols. For example, Nurses Improve the Care to the Hospitalized Elders (NICHE), sponsored by the Hartford Foundation at NYU.

3. Research utilization: Before using research in practice, a comprehensive analysis should be performed.

   a. Locate relevant clinical nursing research.

   b. Critique the research to determine transferablity, feasibility, and readiness for use in practice.

      1) Assess quality of the research – the strength of the evidence and applicability to clinical practice.

      2) Studies that have been replicated generate more confidence in outcomes.

4. Local data – Continuous Quality Improvement (CQI)

   a. Revise systems and processes on the basis of data about the process itself.

   b. CQI measures the current status, locates comparative data, and establishes benchmarks.

   c. Change in practice is initiated; data continue to be gathered and analyzed; additional change is implemented as indicated.

   d. The improvement process is continuous and cyclical.

Outcomes Evaluation

The growing expense of health care led to focus on outcomes – how to maximize the benefit associated with the resources used in health care.

An outcome is a change in patient health status between two or more points in time.

1. Health status encompasses physiologic, functional, cognitive, emotional, and behavioral health.

2. Outcomes can be positive, negative, or neutral changes in health status.

Outcome is a function of baseline condition of the individual and treatment factors. Frequently used outcome measures:

1. Patient satisfaction measures.
2. Functional health status.
3. Mortality rates.

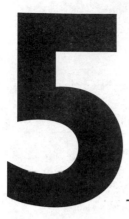

Education and Counseling

Adult Learning

Adult learning is a persistent change in behavior based on experience.

Characteristics of Adult Learners
1. Adult learners have problems to solve and learn best when content is related to the immediate need, problem, or deficit.
   a. Adult learners are self-directed.
   b. Adult learners are motivated and have a need to know.
2. Adult learners have life experiences that can hinder or facilitate learning.
   a. Learning is enhanced when new content builds on past experience and is related to something the learner knows.

Domains of Learning
1. Cognitive learning deals with the intellectual or knowledge area and involves acquiring facts, reaching conclusions, or making decisions.
2. Affective learning consists of changing the attitudes, feelings, and interests the individual has toward an object or idea.
3. Psychomotor learning involves mastering physical skills or motor activities.

Conditions for Learning
1. Learning depends on three conditions: motivation to learn, ability to learn, and the learning environment.
2. Motivation describes the effect of internal and external forces on the individual that initiate, direct, and maintain behavior.
   a. Motivation to learn is based on previous knowledge, attitudes, and sociocultural factors.
   b. Motivation is the willingness of the individual to learn.
   c. Six theories of motivation offer insight about why people may learn or change.
      1) A desired behavior is reinforced or rewarded.

      2) A behavior change satisfies a need for food, shelter, love, or self-esteem.

      3) Changing the behavior relieves cognitive dissonance.

          a) Cognitive dissonance is the tension felt when a deeply held belief is challenged by an inconsistent behavior.

      4) The causal explanations or attributions an individual makes about the situation can affect his or her motivation to change.

          a) For example, patients who attribute their heart attack to a high-fat diet may be more likely to change their diet than those who attribute their heart attack to bad luck or genetics.

          b) Locus of control is a key concept in attribution theory.

3. People with an internal locus of control attribute success or failure to their own efforts.

4. People with an external locus of control attribute success or failure to external factors, such as luck, fate, or difficulty of the task.

    1) Individual differences in personality may influence motivation to learn or change.

      a) Optimism is a personality trait that has been positively associated with information seeking and changing behavior.

      b) Learned helplessness causes a person to believe he or she will fail no matter what is tried, thus making the person less likely to learn or change.

      c) Coping style may be a part of personality structure, although coping style may also be learned.

    2) The individual's perceived ability to achieve the goal affects motivation.

      a) Self-efficacy is correlated positively with activity level after a heart attack.

5. Ability to learn reflects the learner's developmental level, physical wellness, and intellectual thought processes.

  a. Developmental level refers to the stage of life of the individual. Each stage is accompanied by developmental tasks and concerns. For example, a young adult is concerned with establishing intimacy and close personal relationships. An older adult understands his or her purpose in life and seeks to share accumulated wisdom.

    1) Literacy level involves reading, comprehension, problem solving, math calculation, and the application of these abilities.

      a) Illiteracy is found among all ethnic groups and at all socioeconomic levels.

      b) Health literacy is the level of literacy required to function in the health environment. Health literacy cannot be predicted from educational level.

      c) Cues to low health literacy include the following behaviors:

          1) Withdrawing or avoiding learning situations.

          2) Excuses when asked to review printed material – too tired, forgot my glasses, gave it to my partner to take home, for example.

          3) Listening and observing very carefully to memorize how things work.

    2) Language. Does the learner speak and understand English? If not, are the interpreter's skills sufficient to explain?

  b. Physical wellness includes the required level of strength, coordination, and sensory acuity for learning.

1) Physical size and strength must match the task to be performed or the equipment to be used.

2) Coordination is the dexterity required for complex motor skills. Consider, for example, the dexterity required to prepare and administer insulin injections. If dexterity is inadequate, an alternate method of administration must be found.

3) The sensory acuity level needed to receive information and respond appropriately to teaching includes vision, hearing, touch, taste, and smell.

    a) Instructor awareness can compensate for some reduced or impaired sensory acuity.

c. Multiple intellectual processes are necessary for learning to occur. For example, the ability to pay attention, to understand language, to manipulate symbols, to retrieve information from memory, and to transfer learning to novel situations.

1) Intellectual ability can be affected by health status (e.g., person with receptive aphasia due to a stroke), developmental stage (e.g., child versus adult), and genetic factors (e.g., person with Down's syndrome).

6. The environment can have a significant impact on the ability to learn. Many factors may need to be addressed to facilitate learning and minimize barriers to learning.

a. Teacher/learner ratio.

1) Some individuals may learn better in a group, but a group may be too distracting for others.

2) Some may learn better in small, interactive groups, while others learn better in large groups where there is more anonymity.

3) Groups provide the opportunity for adult learners to learn from one another's experiences and understanding of the material presented.

4) Much patient education is presented in a one-to-one (e.g., nurse to patient) session. One-to-one teaching is sometimes called counseling. It tends to be more responsive to individual concerns and approaches.

b. Privacy and the assurance of confidentiality are necessary when addressing sensitive issues (e.g., HIV status, genetic counseling).

c. Comfortable physical environment

1) Moderate temperature

2) Sufficient lighting that minimizes glare

3) Minimal extraneous noise

4) Adequate ventilation

5) Appropriate and comfortable furniture

Patient Education Process

The patient education process parallels the nursing process.

Assessment

Assessment data are used to define learning needs and develop a teaching plan to meet the needs of the individual.

1. Assessment of need to learn.
   a. What does the patient know, feel, and believe about his or her health condition?
   b. What does he or she need to know?
2. Assessment of motivation to learn.
   a. What motivates this person to learn or change?
      1) The learner with an internal locus of control may be eager to change his or her health behavior because the change will enhance feelings of control.
      2) The learner with an external locus of control may be difficult to involve in learning and behavior change. He or she does not believe that individual behavior affects health status.
      3) The learner who believes someone else controls his or her health (e.g., the nurse or a family member) may expect "someone else" to correct the condition.
   b. Are there health-related cultural beliefs that may affect learning? Who should be included in the teaching and decisionmaking processes?
3. Assessment of readiness to learn.
   a. Are there attitudes or beliefs that may hinder the ability to learn?
      1) Some individuals deny or do not believe that health behaviors effect health status, (e.g., individuals who continue to smoke with peripheral vascular disease). Others believe that it does not matter what they do; illness is going to happen anyway.
      2) Perceived benefits of changing behaviors differ among learners. Some individuals may not want to devote the time and energy to change a behavior that they do not believe will improve their quality of life. Others may feel that any effort to change is good.
      3) Teaching strategies and techniques used for affective learning (changing attitudes and beliefs) differ from those used for cognitive learning (attaining facts and information).
   b. Does the learner have the necessary energy and endurance or will fatigue hinder learning?
      1) Patient fatigue often limits the amount of information that can be presented in one session.
   c. Is the learner comfortable?
      1) Is pain controlled and the patient mentally alert?
      2) Does the patient feels safe with the instructor and in the setting?
         a) Privacy and confidentiality assured.
         b) Patient perceives the instructor as knowledgeable.
   d. Are there sensory impairments for which the instructor must compensate?
   e. Does the patient have the physical maturity and coordination needed to learn psychomotor skills?

Diagnostic Statement and Objectives

1. Nursing diagnoses provide broad diagnostic statements. The following North American Nursing Diagnosis Association (NANDA) diagnoses may require educational intervention.

    a.   Deficient knowledge (specify)

    b.   Ineffective coping

    c.   Ineffective health maintenance

    d.   Noncompliance

2.   Learning objectives are developed in the cognitive (facts and information), affective (attitudes and beliefs), and psychomotor (skills) domains.

3.   Learning objectives are developed in behavioral terms that specify performance, conditions, and outcome.

    a.   Performance: Action verbs describe what the learner will do. For example, make a list or solve a problem.

    b.   Conditions: Identify specific circumstances that will be included in the action. For example, place, time of day, or equipment and tools to be used.

    c.   Criteria: Indicate how achievement of the objective will be evaluated or measured. For example, test score, accuracy, or frequency.

4.   Although objectives are developed and written by the instructor, they must be relevant to the learner. Mutual objective setting helps to assure relevance.

Intervention: Teaching-Learning

1.   The role of the instructor is to facilitate learning. The role of the student is to learn.

2.   Structured teaching has been shown to be more effective than unstructured teaching.

3.   The instructor selects teaching strategies that help the learner to achieve his or her objectives.

4.   Teaching strategies may be more or less effective depending upon the learning domain, learner characteristics, the learning environment, and the skill of the instructor.

    a.   Lecture is used commonly when teaching groups.

       1) Lecture is an effective method for presenting facts (cognitive learning), but is less effective for affective or psychomotor learning.

       2) Lecture combined with discussion is more effective than lecture alone.

          a) Discussion allows the learner to express personal feelings and concerns, to ask questions, and to clarify misunderstandings.

    b.   Question and answer (Q & A) sessions focus the discussion on specific learner needs.

       1) Q & A sessions can facilitate both cognitive and affective learning.

       2) Q & A sessions are effective in teaching groups and in one-to-one teaching.

          a) In groups, individuals may learn from others' questions.

       3) Q & A sessions require active learner participation.

       4) Q & A sessions are not effective unless the learner has prior knowledge about the subject. The learner must know enough to recognize and ask questions.

    c.   Demonstration with repeat demonstration is an effective strategy for teaching psychomotor skills.

       1) Explanation while slowly demonstrating the skill evolves into offering cues to the learner while he or she practices the skill.

       2) Repeated practice with praise reinforces the behavior and helps the learner to move toward independent functioning.

   3) Supervised repeat demonstration assists with evaluation of learning.

   4) Demonstration/repeat demonstration is effective with small groups and in one-on-one teaching.

d. Role-playing is an effective strategy for teaching in the affective domain (i.e., attitudes and beliefs).

   1) The learner responds to a stimulus based on his or her experience while the teacher offers guidance and feedback.

   2) The role-playing may need to be repeated several times before the learner is able to internalize the behavior.

   3) In role-modeling, the instructor may take the role of the patient and demonstrate an appropriate response.

e. Oral or written tests may be used for evaluation of cognitive and psychomotor learning.

   1) Tests can be used as a part of assessment (pretests) and as an evaluation method to check progress.

   2) Oral tests may be better than written tests when literacy is a concern.

   3) Some learners are intimidated by written tests.

f. Simulation or case study method can be used to teach and evaluate the application of material to different situations.

   1) Simulation may be computer-based or may use actors to create the scenario.

   2) The scenario is presented and the learner interacts with the computer or actor.

   3) Solutions and recommendations offered by the learner in response to the scenarios allow instructors to evaluate the effectiveness of their teaching.

g. Teaching tools include books, pamphlets, pictures, films, slides, audio and video tapes, models, programmed instruction, and computer-assisted learning modules.

   1) Selection of effective teaching tools depends on the planned instructional method, learning needs assessed, and the learning ability of the student.

   2) The instructor must evaluate tools for content, format, reading level, and appropriateness of illustrations before use.

      a) Content must match the patient's reading level and present the subject material clearly and logically.

         1) Avoid technical language.

         2) Standardized assessment formulas can be used to establish readability, (e.g., SMOG).

      b) Content must be relevant to the situation and contain accurate, current information.

      c) Format of the materials affects learning. In general, materials should:

         1) Be organized with important general points presented first.

         2) Progress to specific information based on general points.

         3) Be logical and "user friendly" (e.g., Q & A format.)

      d) Illustrations enhance learning by emphasizing and reinforcing the written message. They increase motivation by attracting attention, adding variety, and providing breaks in the text.

h. Illustrations should focus on the crucial aspects of the content.

      1) Effective illustrations:

        a) Are simple, uncluttered, and labeled legibly.

        b) Graphic symbols may help if there are language barriers

        c) Colors should be accurate and portray a realistic image.

      2) Learner interpretation of illustrations may be influenced by literacy level, cultural beliefs, and prior experience.

   i. Layout and design of printed material can greatly influence its effectiveness.

      1) Font should be clear and easy to read.

      2) Type size should be 12–14 point, especially for the older learner.

      3) Maintain case contrast, avoid all capitals. Use bold or underline for emphasis.

      4) Ink color should offer sufficient contrast with the paper color.

      5) Glossy paper may produce glare and make reading difficult.

      6) Adequate spacing of text, illustrations, and "white space" makes the materials easier to read.

Evaluation and Reteaching

1. Evaluation is used to measure learning and health-related outcomes, monitor performance, and determine competence. Information gathered during evaluation is used to redirect teaching with the goal of improving responses and outcomes.

2. Direct and indirect measurement are used for evaluation.

   a. Direct measurement involves observing the learner and recording behaviors. The observer may use tools to guide the observations and rate behavior, such as:

      1) Rating scales (e.g., Likert, numerical [1–10, 0–5, 1–100] or visual analog scales).

      2) Checklists of required behaviors.

      3) Anecdotal notes (i.e., written observations of behavior).

   b. Indirect measurement makes the assumption that learning has occurred when learners have achieved a predetermined level. Indirect measurement does not measure behavior directly.

      1) Oral questioning is a flexible form of indirect measurement.

        a) Oral questioning allows immediate feedback to the learner and the correction by the instructor of areas of weakness.

        b) Oral questioning may be difficult for the learner if oral expression or language is a problem.

      2) Written tests are an indirect measure of cognitive learning. The most effective tests are well written, based on identified learning objectives, and involve increasing levels of difficulty.

Documentation

1. In the clinical recored, document the content presented, written materials provided, and the patient's understanding of the information.

Patient Education and Counseling

1. Knowledge is necessary, but not sufficient, to change health behavior.
2. Patient education and counseling often occur in busy practice settings.

Strategies

1. Several patient education/counseling strategies have been described that can be implemented in brief periods of time during routine health visits.

    a. Frame the teaching to match the patient's perceptions.

    b. Fully inform patients of the purposes and expected effects of interventions and when to expect these effects. For example, when a smoker quits smoking, risk for cardiac and vascular mortality drops significantly in the first year, and then more gradually through ensuing years.

    c. Suggest small changes rather than large ones. Loss of three to four pounds in four weeks is better than recommending loss of twenty-five pounds in six months.

    d. Be specific. If a patient is walking a mile a day, three days a week, recommend increasing frequency to five days a week.

    e. It is sometimes easier to add new behaviors than to eliminate established behaviors. It may be easier to add moderate exercise than to reduce caloric intake.

    f. Link new behaviors to established behaviors. For example, linking riding an exercise bicycle for thirty minutes to watching the evening news.

    g. Use the power of the profession. Direct, explicit, simple measures are powerful. For example, the message "You have smoked your last cigarette" may be effective if given by a trusted health professional.

    h. Get explicit commitments from the patient.

    i. Use a combination of strategies. Educational efforts that incorporate individual counseling, group classes, and written materials are more likely to be effective than single strategies.

    j. Involve office staff. Patient education and counseling is a shared responsibility of physicians, nurses, health educators, dietitians, and allied health professionals. The provision of educational materials in the waiting area may stimulate interest and discussion of health-related topics.

    k. Refer – an increasing number of educational programs are available through community agencies, national voluntary organizations, and health facilities.

    l. Monitor progress through follow-up contact. Inquire at each visit about progress and challenges. Telephone calls initiated by the professional to the patient to assess progress may provide external motivation for change.

Health Self-Management

Health self-management issues include health maintenance, disease prevention, and health promotion.

Health Maintenance

Health maintenance activities are behaviors that maintain or improve health over time. Health maintenance depends on three characteristics: perception of health, motivation to change when needed, and adherence to prescribed interventions.

1. Perception of health involves one's understanding of current health status and having the knowledge to manage positive health behaviors.

    a. Health perceptions include the importance of health, the ability to control health, and the benefits of, and barriers to, healthy behavior.

    b. Factors affecting health perception include age and developmental stage, personality characteristics and physical wellness. These factors are discussed in Section 1C of the Conditions For Learning section at the beginning of this chapter.

2. Motivation to change is determined by the responsibility that the learner assumes for health. Factors that may affect motivation to change are discussed in Section 1C(1) of the Conditions For Learning section at the beginning of this chpater.

3. Adherence to (or compliance with) prescribed intervention requires making the decision to change or comply, setting goals, and making the actual therapeutic lifestyle changes.

    a. Making a decision and commitment to change may be difficult to achieve, but it is an essential first step.

    b. Need to set goals that are realistic and achievable. Failure occurs when the goals are unrealistic and too difficult to achieve.

    c. Making and maintaining lifestyle changes over time is often difficult.

        1) Negative life events (e.g., the death of a spouse, family member, or close friend) can weaken the patient's resolve and old behaviors may resurface.

        2) The professional helps the patient to view the reoccurrence of old behavior as a temporary lapse rather than as a failure.

    d. A positive social support system helps the patient focus on the treatment goals.

Disease Prevention

Disease prevention is the organized effort to limit the development and progression of lifestyle-related illness. Three areas of disease prevention are primary, secondary, and tertiary.

1. Primary prevention precedes the occurrence of disease and is used with healthy populations.

    a. Primary prevention aims to decrease the probability of disease.

    b. Primary prevention includes immunizations, health education programs, and fitness activities such as eating a healthy diet, avoiding alcohol and tobacco products, and exercising regularly.

2. Secondary prevention involves screening to detect and treat disease in its earliest stages, (i.e., before symptoms are present).

    a. Early detection and treatment are associated with improved health outcomes and reduced morbidity and mortality.

    b. Secondary prevention includes screening programs, such as cholesterol screening, vision/hearing screening, and blood pressure screening.

3. Tertiary prevention attempts to reduce complications and disability from established disease, thereby improving quality of life.

   a. In rehabilitation, the goal is to minimize residual dysfunction and to maximize functional level.

   b. An example of tertiary prevention is a Cardiac Rehabilitation Program that includes lifestyle changes such as altering dietary and exercise habits, remodeling attitude, and modifying response to stress.

Health Promotion

Health promotion refers to risk reduction strategies applied at the population level (macro level) . Nurses have major roles as educators for the prevention of disease and enhancement of quality of life and as citizens to influence health policy.

1. Passive health promotion requires no action by the individual. For example:

   a. Fluoridation of municipal drinking water.

   b. Fortification of milk with vitamin D.

   c. Addition of iodine to table salt.

2. Active health promotion is the adoption of and participation in health programs by the individual (micro level). For example:

   a. Achieving and maintaining an ideal weight.

   b. Eating a healthy diet.

   c. Not smoking or using tobacco.

   d. Exercising regularly.

   e. Reducing stress.

Discharge Planning

Discharge planning facilitates the patient's transition between settings along the continuum of care. Discharge planning usually begins with admission to an institutional setting (hospital or nursing home) and continues until full recovery occurs, or the patient's condition is stabilized at the highest possible functional level.

Key Elements

Key elements addressed in discharge planning include changes in the patient's condition, coordination and facilitation of care, and negotiation of roles and responsibilities.

1. Transitions involve changes in patient condition. These changes may require adjustment by patients and their families.

   a. Mobility may be altered due to disease, surgery, or trauma. For example, an independent elderly patient may require a walker after surgery for an injured hip.

   b. Self-concept may change and need to be addressed. For example, a person may feel 'damaged' and less confident after myocardial infarction (MI) or heart surgery.

   c. Role-performance may be altered permanently or temporarily after a stroke or aneurysm repair. The person may be unable to return to his or her former occupation, and roles within the family and community may need to be renegotiated.

    d.   Similarly, self-care deficits may be present for the stroke patient either short- or long-term.

2. Coordination of care is the identification, implementation, and direction of treatment prior to discharge.

    a.   In the acute care setting, coordination of care is facilitated by the use of multidisciplinary care paths or critical pathways.

        1)   Care paths or critical pathways sequence interventions to achieve expected outcomes over a projected length of stay for specific case types.

        2)   If care is provided according to these guidelines, and variance from the guidelines is addressed promptly, the patient will be discharged in a timely manner, and in as healthy a condition as possible.

    b.   Home care and long-term care agencies use similar case-specific, clinical guidelines for care coordination.

3. Facilitation of care and discharge requires the anticipation of discharge needs upon admission.

    a.   Initial assessment of potential discharge needs is done when the patient is admitted to the facility or service.

    b.   Initial assessment of family resources and caregiving ability must occur also.

4. Negotiation is the process by which discharge goals and roles and responsibilities are determined or assigned.

    a.   Negotiation may be formal or informal.

    b.   Negotiation may be necessary in the following examples.

        1)   The patient who is unable to manage at home may need supportive care (e.g., a visiting nurse, temporary nursing home placement, or outpatient rehabilitation).

        2)   The patient's health problems may require more family involvement (e.g., 24-hour supervision). The family may select a responsible person, or multiple family members may agree to be present for specified times.

Levels of Discharge Planning

Levels of discharge planning vary based on patient needs, family support, and financial resources. There are three levels of discharge planning currently used in hospitals: basic, simple, and complex.

1. Basic discharge planning may require only patient teaching.

    a.   The clinical nurse may do the teaching (e.g., wound care or medication actions).

    b.   Specialists (e.g., dietitians, enterostomal nurses, lactation nurses, diabetic educators) may be involved with the teaching.

2. Simple discharge planning involves referring the patient to community resources. This usually involves giving the necessary information to the patient or family, such as:

    a.   Sources for durable medical equipment.

    b.   Private-pay, in-home service agencies.

    c.   Sources for outpatient therapies (e.g., speech, physical or occupational therapy).

3. Complex discharge planning involves interdisciplinary collaboration, coordination, and negotiation. The discharge planner, the patient (when possible), and the family work together with community-based, sub-acute, or long-term care services to formulate the most appropriate discharge plan.

    a. Community-based care may be needed when the patient remains in the home environment, but requires supervision or therapy on an intermittent basis. For example:

        1) Day care programs for the cognitively impaired adults

        2) Home care services may include nurses, aides, therapists, and durable medical equipment companies.

    b. Sub-acute care is designed for patients who are too ill to be discharged from the hospital to a traditional extended care facility or home. There are four types of sub-acute care facilities.

        1) Transitional units are an alternative to continued hospital stays for patients with complex nursing or medical care needs (e.g., deep wound management, complicated vascular, or cardiac surgery).

        2) General units are for stable patients who require a moderate level of care (e.g., long-term intravenous therapy).

        3) Chronic units are for patients with little or no hope of recovery (e.g., ventilator-dependent patients).

        4) Long-term transitional units are for patients with medically complex conditions when recovery is expected (e.g., acute ventilator support with difficulty weaning).

    c. Nursing homes offer care to patients experiencing debilitating acute or chronic illnesses (e.g., multiple sclerosis, muscular dystrophy, surgery, or trauma).

        1) Skilled nursing facilities provide care that requires licensed health care professionals, such as nurses or therapists (e.g., tube feedings, care of stage three and four wounds).

        2) Nursing facilities care for patients who cannot independently perform activities of daily living.

        3) Residential facilities such as assisted-living centers and group homes offer supervision of patients who are fairly independent and able to perform most or all self-care activities.

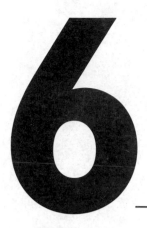

Community
Health Practice

Community health practice provides the organizational structure, health care resources, and interdisciplinary collaboration to promote healthy people and communities.

Community health providers focus on individuals, families, populations, and the community using public health science.

Community health practice involves the identification of needs, and improvement of health, for people in communities.

Community health principles promote the positive connections between populations, their environment, and health of the community.

Community Health Clients

1. Individuals
2. Families
3. Populations are composed of people who occupy or live in a certain area, but can also include those with similar attributes or characteristics. The homeless and frail elders are examples of vulnerable populations.
4. Aggregates are groupings of individuals who are loosely associated with one another by characteristics such as by age, gender, race, risk factors, or health problems. Women with heart disease and people who smoke cigarettes are examples of aggregates.

Types of Communities

1. Geographic communities are defined by the boundaries of towns, cities, or neighborhoods.
2. Common interest communities are collections of people with similar interests or goals that are usually health related, such as smoking cessation or 911 emergency care for acute coronary syndromes.
3. Community of solution is a group of people who come together to solve a problem, such as the lack of health care for indigent populations.

Building a Healthy Community

People work together in a group to identify the needs of the community.
The group identifies and agrees on goals.

The group reaches consensus on the strategies to achieve the goals.
The group collaborates on the actions to attain the desired outcomes.

Levels of Prevention

1. Primary prevention includes actions used to keep an illness from occurring.
   a. Altering the susceptibility of people to illness.
   b. Decreasing exposure to substances that may cause disease.
   c. Examples are public education on risk factors for coronary heart disease (CHD) or strategies for smoking cessation.
2. Secondary prevention includes those actions that are used in the early detection and treatment of health problems. These actions may include hypertension or cholesterol screening, for example.
3. Tertiary prevention includes actions to decrease the severity of health problems that have occurred.
   a. The goals are to minimize disability and to preserve or restore function.
   b. These actions may include treatment and rehabilitation for those people who are recovering from a stroke, for example.

Components of Community Health Practice

Health Promotion

1. Health promotion involves efforts to promote optimal health in individuals, families, populations, and communities to:
   a. Increase the period of healthy living for people of all age groups.
   b. Decrease health disparities in groups of people, especially for those at high risk for health problems, such as cardiovascular diseases.
      1) For example, black women have a higher risk for stroke than white women. A program directed specifically to black women might be used to reduce this disparity.
   c. Increase access to clinical preventive services for all people to decrease the incidence, or increase early detection, of health problems.

Disease Management (DM)

This component of community health practice focuses on disease and illness.
1. Treatment of usually chronic diseases, according to clinical guidelines that have been shown to be effective for a majority of the people with the disease.
2. Goal of DM is to prevent medical crises through education, monitoring, and early intervention.
3. DM has demonstrated benefit in populations with diabetes, hypertension, CHD, and heart failure.
4. DM may be accomplished in several ways.
   a. Nursing and other health care services may be provided to people with the disease such as home visits from a health care agency, clinics at a homeless shelter or mobile van, or screening, education, counseling, and referrals offered at neighborhood health centers.

b. People may be offered assistance to obtain treatment such as nutritional counseling for those affected by elevated cholesterol or appointments with cardiologists for problems such as hypertension.

Rehabilitation

This component focuses on reducing disability and restoring function for individuals, families, populations, and communities.

1. Interventions include cognitive and functional assessment, realistic goal setting, counseling and intensive education, physical occupational and speech therapy, environmental modification, and outcome evaluation.

2. Health care organizations involved in rehabilitation include subacute hospitals, long-term care facilities, and home care agencies.

3. For some people and their families, participation in groups such as "The Mended Hearts" provides needed support and guidance as they recover from cardiovascular procedures.

Program Development

1. Community health providers develop programs for individuals, families, populations, and communities. Programs may also be aimed at the people involved with building healthy communities such as the lay public, interdisciplinary health care providers, and administrators of health care agencies.

2. These programs may focus on screening people for health problems, educating people about risk factors or diseases that may impact their health, and teaching community health providers about changes in care delivery or community issues. For example, a community education program that highlights the symptoms of myocardial infarction and emergency care may be developed to increase the public's awareness of this health problem and to improve survival by prompt treatment.

Practice Evaluation

1. Practice evaluation involves the analysis of community health practice and, if indicated, the identification of need for change.

2. There are several types of evaluation that may be used for this process.

   a. Outcome evaluation involves analysis of the impact of community health practice on patient/family knowledge, incidence of disease, recovery from illness, health care visits, and complications. This process can be used to evaluate the quality of care based on the numbers of positive and negative outcomes.

   b. Structure and process evaluation involves the formation and operation of a treatment plan with established performance standards.

      1) Structures include the resources to meet the identified needs of the community or goals of the plan. Structures include provider qualifications, licensing, certification, and program funding.

      2) Process is the way in which services are delivered.

Community Health Nursing

1. Community health nursing synthesizes theories from public health science, nursing science, and community health practice to address the needs of communities and vulnerable populations.
2. Community health nurses use the nursing process to identify client, family, and group needs, set goals, plan and provide services, and evaluate the impact of their care.
   a. They formulate health promotion strategies for clients, families, and groups.
   b. Community health nurses encourage client and family self-care and independence.
   c. They use aggregate data and analysis to guide and evaluate their work with groups and populations.
3. Community health nurses work collaboratively with health care providers from other disciplines to manage the care of clients.

Roles of Community Health Nurses

1. The clinician role includes the care that is provided to individuals, families, groups, and populations. Health care services are focused on holistic practices that integrate principles of health promotion, disease management, and rehabilitation.
2. The educator role includes the instruction and counseling of individuals, families, groups, and populations. Community health nurses incorporate principles of adult learning into the educator role. They evaluate the effect of their teaching through program evaluation.
3. The collaborator role includes working with health care providers from other disciplines and with different groups of people to meet the needs of individuals, families, groups, and populations.
4. The researcher role involves examining community health problems by collecting and analyzing data. Data collection and analysis may be for continuous quality improvement or to answer a research question.
5. The leadership role focuses on initiating healthful change with different groups within the community. Community health nurses facilitate the achievement of goals by guiding the work of the group. Additionally, community health nurses have a leadership role beyond the community by influencing health policies at the state and federal levels.

Practice Settings

1. Homes.
2. Ambulatory care sites such as outpatient departments of hospitals, clinics, neighborhood health centers, day care centers, senior centers, health departments, migrant camps, and homeless shelters.
3. Public and private schools (e.g., preschool, elementary, middle, secondary vocational, technical, specialized schools, and colleges).
4. Occupational health sites, such as clinics in industry.
5. Residential settings including hospice, halfway houses, camps, assisted living, and long-term care facilities.
6. Parishes.

Emerging Needs of Aggregates

1. Aging of the population will have a major impact on community health nursing.

   a. The number of people age 65 years and older in the US will more than double to 70 million by the year 2030, while the numbers of centenarians will increase from 65,000 to 381,000 people.

   b. Many elderly have at least one chronic health problem that requires monitoring by health care providers.

   c. The increased acuity of illness in the elderly, together with the shortened length of hospital stays, will continue to impact community health practice.

2. Increasing cultural diversity of the population is having a significant influence on community health nursing.

   a. The US is becoming more racially and ethnically diverse. The number of minorities living in the US has been projected to increase to 22% by 2020.

   b. Community health nurses and other clinicians need to be culturally competent to meet the needs of the growing African-American, Hispanic, Asian, and other populations.

3. The community mental health movement will continue to affect the responsibilities of community health nurses.

   a. There will be increasing numbers of people needing mental health and substance abuse services in diverse community health settings such as clinics, halfway houses, and residential facilities.

4. Communicable diseases will have a substantial effect on the practice of community health nurses as treatment changes occur. Additionally, there exists the possibility of the emergence of new diseases and the increased virulence of existing health conditions that will affect community health practice.

5. Bioterrorism is a renewed area of concern for the US.

   a. The exact risks associated with the use of biochemical weapons are not known.

   b. Bioterrorism could result in epidemics with the potential to infect large segments of the population because of the delayed onset of symptoms for certain diseases and the increased mobility of people.

Healthy People 2010

This document identifies goals and objectives that target changes specific to age, gender, and race to improve the health of the US over the next decade. *Healthy People 2010* incorporates previous initiatives such as the 1979 Surgeon General's Report, and *Healthy People and Healthy People 2000: National Health Promotion and Disease Prevention Objectives. Healthy People 2010* is available online at www.health.gov/healthypeople.

Goals

Increase quality and years of healthy life
Eliminate health disparities

Focus Areas

Approximately 467 objectives were formulated within 28 focus areas. The objectives include interventions intended to achieve the goals by the year 2010.

The focus areas of interest for cardiac and vascular nurses include diabetes, heart disease and stroke, physical activity and fitness, and tobacco use.

Leading Health Indicators

1. Reflect the major health concerns in the US at the beginning of the 21st century.
2. Will be used to measure the health of the US over the next decade.
3. The leading health indicators are:
   a. Physical activity
   b. Overweight and obesity
   c. Tobacco use
   d. Substance abuse
   e. Responsible sexual behavior
   f. Mental health
   g. Injury and violence
   h. Environmental quality
   i. Immunization
   j. Access to health care

People, communities, professional organizations, and federal agencies are involved with *Healthy People 2010* and with measuring the improvement in the health of the people of the US.

Community Initiatives

National Organizations

1. The American Heart Association (AHA), a national voluntary organization, has sponsored several national campaigns to reduce the risk of cardiovascular disease (CVD) for individuals and communities.
   a. "My Heart Watch" is a community education program for preventing heart attack and stroke that includes risk assessment tools, cardiovascular health information, and chat rooms.
   b. "Take Wellness to Heart" is an initiative that is focused on increasing the awareness of women about their risk for heart disease and stroke.
   c. "Operation Heartbeat" is a community education program designed to increase community knowledge and support for emergency care related to cardiac arrest.
2. The National Heart, Lung, and Blood Institute sponsors several national initiatives that are focused on the goals of *Healthy People 2010* and community education.
   a. "Act in Time to Heart Attack Signs" is a public education campaign to increase awareness about emergency care of heart attack victims.
   b. "National High Blood Pressure Education Program" is to increase public awareness of hypertension and its treatment.
   c. "Detection, Evaluation, and Treatment of High Blood Cholesterol in Adults (Adult Treatment Panel III)" is a national cholesterol education program to decrease the morbidity and mortality associated with CHD by lowering blood cholesterol.

d. "Obesity Education Initiative" is to decrease the incidence of obesity and physical inactivity, thus reducing the risk for CVD and diabetes.

e. "Developing a Woman's Heart Health Education Action Plan" is a new cardiovascular education program for women, especially those at high risk.

State and Local Initiatives

State and local chapters of voluntary organizations such as the AHA promote cardiovascular initiatives through public and professional involvement in community education programs.

Other organizations, such as schools and health care agencies, are involved with community education programs to reduce the risk of cardiovascular diseases by increasing the public's awareness and by implementing screening initiatives.

Many state governments are using *Healthy People 2010* as a framework for building healthy communities. They are using the leading health indicators and objectives to promote healthy living for the people in their respective states and to reduce disparities in health. Another focus of the *Healthy People 2010* initiative is to make the community a healthier place to live.

section two

Assessment of Body Systems

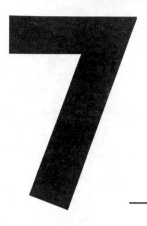

Assessing Clients with Cardiac Disorders

The heart, a muscular pump, beats an average of 70 times per minute, or once every 0.86 seconds, every minute of a person's life. This continuous pumping moves blood through the body, nourishing tissue cells, and removing wastes. Deficits in the structure or function of the heart affect all body tissues. Changes in cardiac rate, rhythm, or output may limit almost all human functions, including self-care, mobility, and the ability to maintain fluid volume status, respirations, tissue perfusion, and comfort. Cardiac changes may also affect self-concept, sexuality, and role performance.

Review of Anatomy and Physiology

The heart is a hollow, cone-shaped organ approximately the size of an adult's fist, weighing less than one pound. It is located in the mediastinum of the thoracic cavity, between the vertebral column and the sternum, and is flanked laterally by the lungs. Two-thirds of the heart mass lies to the left of the sternum; the upper base lies beneath the second rib, and the pointed apex is approximate with the fifth intercostal space, midpoint to the clavicle.

The Pericardium

The heart is covered by a double layer of fibroserous membrane, the pericardium. The pericardium encases the heart and anchors it to surrounding structures, forming the pericardial sac. The snug fit of the pericardium prevents the heart from overfilling with blood. The *parietal pericardium* is the outermost layer. The *visceral pericardium* (or *epicardium*) adheres to the heart surface. The small space between the visceral and parietal layers of the pericardium is called the pericardial cavity. A serous lubricating fluid produced in this space cushions the heart as it beats.

Layers of the Heart Wall

The heart wall consists of three layers of tissue: the epicardium, the myocardium, and the endocardium. The outermost epicardium is the same structure as the visceral pericardium. The middle layer of the heart wall, the myocardium, consists of specialized cardiac muscle cells (myofibrils) that provide the bulk of contractile heart muscle. The innermost layer, the endocardium, is a sheath of endothelium that lines the inside of the heart's chambers and great vessels.

Chambers and Valves of the Heart

The heart has four hollow chambers, two upper atria and two lower ventricles. They are separated longitudinally by the interventricular septum.

The right atrium receives deoxygenated blood from the veins of the body: The superior vena cava returns blood from the body area above the diaphragm, the inferior vena cava returns blood from the body below the diaphragm, and the coronary sinus drains blood from the heart. The left atrium receives freshly oxygenated blood from the lungs through the pulmonary veins.

The right ventricle receives deoxygenated blood from the right atrium and pumps it through the pulmonary artery to the lungs for oxygenation. The left ventricle receives the freshly oxygenated blood from the left atrium and pumps it out the aorta to the arterial circulation.

Each of the heart's chambers is separated by a valve which allows unidirectional blood flow to the next chamber or great vessel. The atria are separated from the ventricles by the two atrioventricular (AV) valves; the tricuspid valve is on the right side, and the bicuspid (or mitral) valve is on the left. The flaps of each of these valves are anchored to the papillary muscles of the ventricles by the *chordae tendineae*. These structures control the movement of the AV valves to prevent backflow of blood.

The ventricles are connected to their great vessels by the semilunar valves. On the right, the pulmonary valve joins the right ventricle with the pulmonary artery. On the left, the aortic valve joins the left ventricle to the aorta.

Closure of the AV valves at the onset of contraction produces the first heart sound, or S_1 (characterized by the syllable "lub"); closure of the semilunar valves at the onset of relaxation produces the second heart sound, or S_2 (characterized by the syllable "dub").

Systemic and Coronary Circulation

Because each side of the heart both receives and ejects blood, the heart is often described as a double pump. Pulmonary circulation begins with the right heart. Deoxygenated blood from the venous system enters the right atrium through two large veins, the superior and inferior venae cavae, and is transported to the lungs via the pulmonary artery and its branches. After oxygen and carbon dioxide are exchanged in the capillaries of the lungs, oxygen-rich blood returns to the left atrium through several pulmonary veins. Blood is then pumped out of the left ventricle through the aorta and its major branches to supply all body tissues. This second circuit of blood flow is called the systemic circulation.

While this continuous circulation of blood through the heart meets the body's oxygen needs, the heart muscle itself is supplied by its own network of vessels through the coronary circulation. The left and right coronary arteries originate at the base of the aorta and branch out to encircle the myocardium. While ventricular contraction delivers blood through the pulmonary and systemic circuits as described above, it is during ventricular relaxation that the coronary arteries fill with oxygen-rich blood. Then, after the blood perfuses the heart muscle, the cardiac veins drain the blood into the coronary sinus, which empties into the right atrium of the heart.

The Cardiac Cycle and Cardiac Output

The contraction and relaxation of the heart constitutes one heartbeat and is called the **cardiac cycle**. Ventricular filling is followed by ventricular **systole,** a phase during which the ventricles contract and eject blood into the pulmonary and systemic circuits. Systole is followed by a relaxation phase known as **diastole,** during which the ventricles refill, the atria contract, and the myocardium is perfused. Normally, the complete cardiac cycle occurs about 70 to 80 times per minute, measured as the heart rate (HR).

Each contraction ejects a certain volume of blood, called the **stroke volume (SV).** Stroke volume ranges from 60 to 100 mL/beat and averages about 70 mL/beat in an adult. The **cardiac output (CO)** is the amount of blood pumped by the ventricles into the pulmonary and systemic circulations in one minute. Multiplying the stroke volume by the heart rate determines the cardiac output: **CO X HR = SV.**

The average adult cardiac output ranges from 4 to 8 L/min. **Ejection fraction (EF)** is the percentage of total blood in the ventricle at the end of the diastole ejected from the heart with each beat. The normal ejection fraction ranges from 50% to 70%. Cardiac output is an indicator of how well the heart is functioning as a pump: If the heart cannot pump effectively, cardiac output and tissue perfusion are decreased. Body tissues that do not receive enough blood and oxygen (carried in the blood on hemoglobin) become **ischemic** (deprived of oxygen). If the tissues do not receive enough blood flow to maintain the functions of the cells, the cells die.

Activity level, metabolic rate, physiologic and psychologic stress responses, age, and body size all influence cardiac output. In addition, cardiac output is determined by the interaction of four major factors: heart rate, preload, afterload, and contractility. Changes in each of these variables influence cardiac output intrinsically, and each also can be manipulated to affect cardiac output. The heart's ability to respond to the body's changing need for cardiac output is called **cardiac reserve.**

Heart Rate

Heart rate is affected by both direct and indirect autonomic nervous system stimulation. Direct stimulation is accomplished through the innervation of the heart muscle by sympathetic and parasympathetic nerves. The sympathetic nervous system increases the heart rate, whereas the parasympathetic vagal tone slows the heart rate. Reflex regulation of heart rate in response to systemic blood pressure also occurs through activation of sensory receptors, known as baroreceptors or pressure receptors, located in the carotid sinus, aortic arch, venae cavae, and pulmonary veins.

If heart rate increases, cardiac output increases (up to a point) even if there is no change in stroke volume. However, rapid heart rates decrease the amount of time available for ventricular filling during diastole. Cardiac output then falls because decreased filling time decreases stroke volume. Coronary artery perfusion also decreases, because the coronary arteries fill primarily during diastole. Cardiac output decreases during bradycardia if stroke volume stays the same, because the number of cardiac cycles is decreased.

Preload

Preload is the amount of cardiac muscle fiber tension, or stretch, that exists at the end of diastole, just before contraction of the ventricles. Preload is influenced by venous return and the compliance of the ventricles. It is related to the total volume of blood in the ventricles: The greater the volume, the greater the stretch of the cardiac muscle fibers, and the greater the force with which the fibers contract to accomplish emptying. This principle is called *Starling's law of the heart.*

This mechanism has a physiologic limit. Just as continuous overstretching of a rubber band causes the band to relax and lose its ability to recoil, overstretching of the cardiac muscle fibers eventually results in ineffective contraction. Disorders, such as renal disease and congestive heart failure, result in sodium and water retention and increased preload. Vasoconstriction also increases venous return and preload.

Too little circulating blood volume results in a decreased venous return and, therefore, a decreased preload. A decreased preload reduces stroke volume and thus cardiac output. Decreased preload may result from hemorrhage or maldistribution of blood volume, as occurs in third spacing.

Afterload

Afterload is the force the ventricles must overcome to eject their blood volume. It is the pressure in the arterial system ahead of the ventricles. The right ventricle must generate enough tension to open the pulmonary valve and eject its volume into the low-pressure pulmonary arteries. Right ventricle afterload is measured as pulmonary vascular resistance (PVR). The left ventricle, in contrast, ejects its load by overcoming the pressure behind the aortic valve. Afterload of the left ventricle is measured as systemic vascular resistance (SVR). Arterial pressures are much higher than pulmonary pressures; thus, the left ventricle has to work much harder than the right ventricle.

Alterations in vascular tone affect afterload and ventricular work. As the pulmonary or arterial blood pressure increases (e.g., through vasoconstriction), PVR and/or SVR increases, and the work of the ventricles increases. As workload increases, consumption of myocardial oxygen also increases. A compromised heart cannot effectively meet this increased oxygen demand, and a vicious cycle ensues. By contrast, a very low afterload decreases the forward flow of blood into the systemic circulation and the coronary arteries.

Contractility

Contractility is the inherent capability of the cardiac muscle fibers to shorten. Poor contractility of the heart muscle reduces the forward flow of blood from the heart, increases the ventricular pressures from accumulation of blood volume, and reduces cardiac output. Increased contractility may overtax the heart.

The Conduction System of the Heart

The cardiac cycle is perpetuated by a complex electrical circuit, commonly known as the intrinsic conduction system of the heart. Cardiac muscle cells possess an inherent characteristic of self-excitation, which enables them to initiate and transmit impulses independent of a stimulus. However, specialized areas of myocardial cells typically exert a controlling influence in this electrical pathway.

One of these specialized areas is the sinoatrial (SA) node, located at the junction of the superior vena cava and right atrium. The SA node acts as the normal "pacemaker" of the heart, usually generating an impulse 60 to 100 times per minute. This impulse travels across the atria via internodal pathways to the atrioventricular (AV) node, in the floor of the interatrial septum. The very small junctional fibers of the AV node slow the impulse, slightly delaying its transmission to the ventricles. It then passes through the bundle of histidine at the atrioventricular junction and continues down the interventricular septum through the right and left bundle branches and out to the Purkinje fibers in the ventricular muscle walls.

This path of electrical transmission produces a series of changes in ion concentration across the membrane of each cardiac muscle cell. The electrical stimulus increases the permeability of the cell membrane, creating an action potential (electrical potential). The result is an exchange of sodium, potassium, and calcium ions across the cell membrane, which changes the intracellular electrical charge to a positive state. This process of depolarization results in myocardial contraction. As the ion exchange reverses and the cell returns to its resting state of electronegativity, the cell is repolarized, and cardiac muscle relaxes. The cellular action potential serves as the basis for electrocardiography (ECG), the recording of the electrical impulses that immediately precede contraction of the heart muscle.

Clinical Indicators of Cardiac Output

For many critically ill clients, invasive hemodynamic monitoring catheters are used to measure cardiac output in quantifiable numbers. However, advanced technology is not the only way to identify and assess compromised blood flow. Because cardiac output perfuses the body's tissues, clinical indicators of low cardiac output may be manifested by changes in organ function that result from compromised blood flow. For example, a decrease in blood flow to the brain presents as a change in level of consciousness. Other clinical manifestations of decreased cardiac output are discussed in Chapters 8 and 39.

Cardiac index (CI) is the cardiac output adjusted for the client's body size, also called the client's body surface area (BSA). Because it takes into account the client's BSA, the cardiac index provides more meaningful data about the heart's ability to perfuse the tissues and therefore is a more accurate indicator of the effectiveness of the circulation.

BSA is stated in square meters (m²), and cardiac index is calculated as CO divided by BSA. Cardiac measurements are considered adequate when they fall within the range of 2.5 to 4.2 L/min/m². For example, two clients are determined to have a cardiac output of 4 L/min. This parameter is within normal limits. However, one client is 5 feet, 2 inches (157 cm) tall and weighs 120 lb (54.5 kg), with a BSA of 1.54 m². This client's cardiac index is 4 ÷ 1.54, or 2.6 L/min/m². The second client is 6 feet, 2 inches (188 cm) tall and weighs 280 lb (81.7 kg), with a BSA of 2.52 m². This client's cardiac index is 4 ÷ 2.52, or 1.6 L/min/m². The cardiac index results show that the same cardiac output of 4 L/min is adequate for the first client but grossly inadequate for the second client.

Assessing Cardiac Function

Conduct both a health assessment interview to collect subjective data and a physical assessment to collect objective data.

The Health Assessment Interview

This section provides guidelines for collecting subjective data through a health assessment interview specific to cardiac function. A health assessment interview to determine problems with cardiac function may be conducted as part of a health screening or a total health assessment, or it may focus on a chief complaint, such as chest pain. If the client has a problem with cardiac function, analyze its onset, characteristics, course, severity, precipitating and relieving factors, and any associated symptoms, noting the timing and circumstances. For example, ask the client:

- What is the location of the chest pain you experienced? Did it move up to your jaw or into your left arm?

- What type of activity brings on your chest pain?
- Have you noticed any changes in your energy level?
- Have you felt lightheaded during the times your heart is racing?

The interview begins by exploring the client's chief complaint (e.g., chest pain, palpitations, or shortness of breath). Describe the client's symptoms in terms of location, quality or character, timing, setting or precipitating factors, severity, aggravating and relieving factors, and associated symptoms.

Explore the client's history for heart disorders such as angina, heart attack, congestive heart failure (CHF), hypertension (HTN), and valvular disease. Ask the client about previous heart surgery or illnesses, such as rheumatic fever, scarlet fever, or recurrent streptococcal throat infections. Also, ask about the presence and treatment of other chronic illnesses such as diabetes mellitus, bleeding disorders, or endocrine disorders. Review the client's family history for coronary artery disease (CAD), HTN, stroke, hyperlipidemia, diabetes, congenital heart disease, or sudden death.

Ask the client about past or present occurrence of various cardiac symptoms, such as chest pain, shortness of breath, difficulty breathing, cough, palpitations, fatigue, lightheadedness or dizziness, fainting, heart murmur, blood clots, or swelling. Because cardiac function affects all other body systems, a full history may need to explore other related systems, such as respiratory function and/or peripheral vascular function.

Review the client's personal habits and nutritional history, including body weight; eating patterns; dietary intake of fats, salt, fluids; dietary restrictions; hypersensitivities or intolerances to food or medication; and the use of caffeine and alcohol. If the client uses tobacco products, ask about type (cigarettes, pipe, cigars, snuff), duration, amount, and efforts to quit. If the client uses street drugs, ask about type, method of intake (e.g., inhaled or injected), duration of use, and efforts to quit. Include questions about the client's activity level and tolerance, recreational activities, and relaxation habits. Assess the client's sleep patterns for interruptions in sleep due to dyspnea, cough, discomfort, urination, or stress. Ask how many pillows the client uses when sleeping. Also consider psychosocial factors that may affect the client's stress level: What is the client's marital status, family composition, and role within the family? Have there been any changes? What is the client's occupation, level of education, and socioeconomic level? Are resources for support available? What is the client's emotional disposition and personality type? How does the client perceive his or her state of health or illness, and how able is the client to comply with treatment?

Physical Assessment

Physical assessment of cardiac function may be performed either as part of a total assessment or alone for clients with suspected or known problems with cardiac function. Assess the heart through inspection, palpation, and auscultation over the precordium (the area of the chest wall overlying the heart).

The equipment needed for an examination of the heart includes a stethoscope with a diaphragm and a bell, a good light source, and a ruler. Before the examination, collect all the equipment, and explain the examination to the client to decrease anxiety. A quiet environment is essential to hear and assess heart sounds accurately.

The client may sit or lie in the supine position. Movements over the precordium may be more easily seen with tangential lighting (in which the light is directed at a right angle to the area being observed, producing shadows). Assess the following types of movements.

- **Apical impulse** is a normal, visible pulsation (thrust) in the area of the midclavicular line in the left fifth intercostal space. It can be seen on inspection in about half of the adult population.
- **Retraction** is a pulling in of the tissue of the precordium; a slight retraction just medial to the midclavicular line at the area of the apical impulse is normal and is more likely to be visible in thin clients.
- **Lift** is a more sustained thrust than normal.
- **Heave** is an excessive thrust.

Apical Impulse Assessment with Abnormal Findings (✓)

- First using palmar surface and then repeating with finger pads, palpate the precordium for symmetry of movement and the apical impulse for location, size, amplitude, and duration. To locate the apical impulse, ask the client to assume a left lateral recumbent position. Simultaneous palpation of the carotid pulse may also be helpful. The apical impulse is not palpable in all clients.
  - ✓ An enlarged or displaced heart is associated with an apical impulse lateral to the midclavicular line (MCL) or below the fifth left intercostal space (ICS).
  - ✓ Increased size, amplitude, and duration of the point of maximal impulse (PMI) are associated with left ventricular volume overload (increased preload) in conditions such as HTN and aortic stenosis, and in pressure overload (increased afterload) in conditions such as aortic or mitral regurgitation.
  - ✓ Increased amplitude alone may occur with hyperkinetic states, such as anxiety, hyperthyroidism, and anemia.
  - ✓ Decreased amplitude is associated with a dilated heart in cardiomyopathy.
  - ✓ Displacement alone may also occur with dextrocardia, diaphragmatic hernia, gastric distention, or chronic lung disease.
  - ✓ A **thrill** (a palpable vibration over the precordium or an artery) may accompany severe valve stenosis.
  - ✓ A marked increase in amplitude of the PMI at the right ventricular area occurs with right ventricular volume overload in atrial septal defect.
  - ✓ An increase in amplitude and duration occurs with right ventricular pressure overload in pulmonic stenosis and pulmonary hypertension. A lift or heave may also be seen in these conditions (and in chronic lung disease).
  - ✓ A palpable thrill in this area occurs with ventricular septal defect.
- Palpate the subxiphoid area with the index and middle finger.
  - ✓ Right ventricular enlargement may produce a downward pulsation against the fingertips.
  - ✓ An accentuated pulsation at the pulmonary area may be present in hyperkinetic states.
  - ✓ A prominent pulsation reflects increased flow or dilation of the pulmonary artery.
  - ✓ A thrill may be associated with aortic or pulmonary stenosis, aortic stenosis, pulmonary HTN, or atrial septal defect.

✓ Increased pulsation at the aortic area may suggest aortic aneurysm.

✓ A palpable second heart sound (S^2) may be noted with systemic HTN.

Cardiac Rate and Rhythm Assessment with Abnormal Findings (✓)

- Auscultate heart rate.
  ✓ A heart rate exceeding 100 beats per minute (BPM) is **tachycardia.** A heart rate less than 60 BPM is **bradycardia.**

- Simultaneously palpate the radial pulse while listening to the apical pulse.
  ✓ If the radial pulse falls behind the apical rate, the client has a **pulse deficit,** indicating weak, ineffective contractions of the left ventricle.

- Auscultate heart rhythm.
  ✓ **Dysrhythmias** (abnormal heart rate or rhythm) may be regular or irregular in rhythm; their rates may be slow or fast. Irregular rhythms may occur in a pattern (e.g., an early beat every second beat, called *bigeminy*), sporadically, or with frequency and disorganization (e.g., atrial fibrillation). A pattern of gradual increase and decrease in heart rate that is within normal heart rate and that correlates with inspiration and expiration is called sinus arrhythmia.

Heart Sounds Assessment with Abnormal Findings (✓)

- Identify S_1 (first heart sound) and note its intensity. At each auscultatory area, listen for several cardiac cycles.
  ✓ An accentuated S_1 occurs with tachycardia, states in which cardiac output is high (fever, anxiety, exercise, anemia, hyperthyroidism), complete heart block, and mitral stenosis.
  ✓ A diminished S_1 occurs with first-degree heart block, mitral regurgitation, CHF, coronary artery disease, and pulmonary or systemic HTN. The intensity is also decreased with obesity, emphysema, and pericardial effusion. Varying intensity of S_1 occurs with complete heart block and grossly irregular rhythms.

- Listen for splitting of S_1.
  ✓ Abnormal splitting of S_1 may be heard with right bundle branch block and premature ventricular contractions.

- Identify S_2 (second heart sound) and note its intensity.
  ✓ An accentuated S_2 may be heard with HTN, exercise, excitement, and conditions of pulmonary HTN such as mitral stenosis, CHF, and cor pulmonale.
  ✓ A diminished S_2 occurs with aortic stenosis, a fall in systolic blood pressure (shock), pulmonary stenosis, and increased anterioposterior chest diameter.

- Listen for splitting of S_2.
  ✓ Wide splitting of S_2 is associated with delayed emptying of the right ventricle resulting in delayed pulmonary valve closure (e.g., mitral regurgitation, pulmonary stenosis, and right bundle branch block).
  ✓ Fixed splitting occurs when right ventricular output is greater than left ventricular output and pulmonary valve closure is delayed (e.g., with atrial septal defect and right ventricular failure).

- ✓ Paradoxical splitting occurs when closure of the aortic valve is delayed (e.g., left bundle branch block).
- Identify extra heart sounds in systole.
  - ✓ Ejection sounds (or clicks) result from the opening of deformed semilunar valves (e.g., aortic and pulmonary stenosis).
  - ✓ A midsystolic click is heard with mitral valve prolapse (MVP).
- Identify the presence of extra heart sounds in diastole.
  - ✓ An opening snap results from the opening sound of a stenotic mitral valve.
  - ✓ A pathologic S_3 (a third heart sound that immediately follows S_2), or *ventricular gallop*, results from myocardial failure and ventricular volume overload (e.g., CHF, mitral or tricuspid regurgitation).
  - ✓ An S_4 (a fourth heart sound that immediately precedes S_1), or *atrial gallop*, results from increased resistance to ventricular filling after atrial contraction (e.g., HTN, CAD, aortic stenosis, and cardiomyopathy).
  - ✓ A less common right-sided S_4 occurs with pulmonary HTN and pulmonary stenosis.
  - ✓ A combined S_3 and S_4 is called a summation gallop and occurs with severe CHF.
- Identify extra heart sounds in both systole and diastole.
  - ✓ A pericardial friction rub results from inflammation of the pericardial sac, as with pericarditis.

Murmur Assessment with Abnormal Findings (✓)

- Identify any **murmurs.** Note location, timing, presence during systole or diastole, and intensity. Use the following scale to grade murmurs:

  I = Barely heard
  II = Quietly heard
  III = Clearly heard
  IV = Loud
  V = Very loud
  VI = Loudest; may be heard with stethoscope off the chest. A thrill may accompany murmurs of grade IV to grade VI.

- Note pitch (low, medium, high), and quality (harsh, blowing, or musical). Note pattern/shape, crescendo, decrescendo, and radiation/transmission (to axilla, neck).
  - ✓ Midsystolic murmurs are heard with semilunar valve disease (e.g., aortic and pulmonary stenosis) and with hypertrophic cardiomyopathy.
  - ✓ Pansystolic (holosystolic) murmurs are heard with AV valve disease (e.g., mitral and tricuspid regurgitation, ventricular septal defect).
  - ✓ A late systolic murmur is heard with MVP.
  - ✓ Early diastolic murmurs occur with regurgitant flow across incompetent semilunar valves (e.g., aortic regurgitation).
  - ✓ Middiastolic and presystolic murmurs, such as with mitral stenosis, occur with turbulent flow across the AV valves.
  - ✓ Continuous murmurs throughout systole and all or part of diastole occur with patent ductus arteriosus.

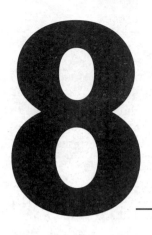

Nursing Care of Clients with Coronary Heart Disease

Changes in the conduction of electrical impulses through the heart, impaired blood flow to the myocardium, and structural changes in the heart itself affect the heart's ability to fulfill its major purpose: to pump enough blood to meet the body's demand for oxygen and nutrients. Disruptions in cardiac function affect other organ systems as well, potentially leading to organ system failure and death.

Cardiovascular disease (CVD) is a generic term for disorders of the heart and blood vessels. CVD is the leading cause of death and disability in the United States. Over 60 million people have some type of cardiovascular disease. The economic costs of CVD, both direct and indirect, to the nation are estimated at $329 billion annually (National Heart, Lung, and Blood Institute [NHLBI], 2002).

On an encouraging note, however, the incidence of new CVD cases per year is decreasing. Public education aimed at reducing fat intake, increasing exercise, and lowering cholesterol levels have made people more aware of risk factors associated with CVD. The mortality rate from heart disease peaked in 1963 and has shown a slow, but steady, decline since that time.

This chapter focuses on disorders of myocardial blood flow (coronary heart disease) and cardiac rhythm. Disorders of cardiac structure and function are discussed in Chapter 9. Review the normal anatomy and physiology and nursing assessment of the heart in Chapter 7 before proceeding with this chapter.

Disorders of Myocardial Perfusion

The Client with Coronary Heart Disease
Coronary heart disease (CHD), or *coronary artery disease (CAD),* affects 12.6 million people in the United States and causes more than 500,000 deaths annually (NHLBI, 2002). CHD is caused by impaired blood flow to the myocardium (Porth, 2002). Accumulation of atherosclerotic plaque in the coronary arteries is the usual cause. Coronary heart disease may be asymptomatic, or may lead to angina pectoris, myocardial infarction (MI or heart attack), dysrhythmias, heart failure, and even sudden death.

Many risk factors for CHD can be controlled through lifestyle modification. In fact, with increased public awareness of risk factors related to CHD, mortality rates are declining by about 3.3% per year. Nevertheless, CHD remains a major public health problem. Heart disease is the leading cause of death for all U.S. ethnic groups, except Asian females (NHBLI, 2002). Nurses are in a prime position to encourage and support positive lifestyle changes by teaching and promoting healthy living practices. Individual choices can, and do, affect health.

The highest incidence of CHD is in the Western world, mainly in white males age 45 and older. Both men and women are affected by coronary heart disease; in women, however, the onset is about ten years later because of the heart-protective effects of estrogen. After menopause, women's risk is equal to that of men.

The causes of atherosclerosis are not known, but certain risk factors have been linked with the development of atherosclerotic plaques. The Framingham Heart Study provided vital research into the relationship between risk factors and the development of heart disease. Research into CHD is ongoing, looking at causative factors, manifestations, and protective measures for many populations.

Risk Factors

Risk factors for CHD are frequently classified as *nonmodifiable*, those factors that cannot be changed, and *modifiable*, those factors that can be changed.

Nonmodifiable

Age is a nonmodifiable risk factor. Over 50% of heart attack victims are 65 or older; 80% of deaths due to myocardial infarction occur in this age group. *Gender, race,* and *genetic factors* also are nonmodifiable risk factors for CHD. Men are affected by CHD at an earlier age than women. African-Americans have a higher incidence of hypertension, which contributes to more rapid development of atherosclerosis.

Modifiable

Modifiable risk factors include lifestyle factors and pathologic conditions that predispose the client to developing CHD. Pathologic conditions often can be controlled. Behavioral or lifestyle factors can be controlled or completely eliminated. Lifestyle changes require significant commitment by the client; ongoing support from the health care team is vital for success.

Pathologic Conditions

Disease conditions that contribute to CHD include hypertension, diabetes mellitus, and hyperlipidemia. Elevated homocystine levels and the metabolic syndrome are emerging risk factors. Although these conditions are not a matter of choice, they are modifiable risk factors that can often be controlled through medication, weight control, diet, and exercise.

Hypertension is consistent blood pressure readings greater than 140 mmHg systolic or 90 mmHg diastolic. Hypertension is common, affecting more than one-third of people over age 50 in the United States. Its prevalence is higher in African-Americans than in Hispanics, and higher in Hispanics than in white Americans (NHLBI, 2002).

Diabetes mellitus contributes to CHD in several ways. Diabetes is associated with higher blood lipid levels, a higher incidence of hypertension, and obesity—all risk factors in their own right. In addition, diabetes affects blood vessels, contributing to the process of atherosclerosis. Hyperglycemia, altered platelet function, and elevated fibrinogen levels also are thought to play a role.

Hyperlipidemia is an abnormally high level of blood lipids and lipoproteins. Lipoproteins carry cholesterol in the blood. Low-density lipoproteins (LDLs) are the primary carriers of cholesterol. High levels of LDL (Memory cue: LDLs = **l**ess **d**esirable **l**ipoproteins) promote atherosclerosis because LDL deposits cholesterol on artery walls. Table 8-1 lists desirable and high-risk levels for total and LDL cholesterol. In contrast, high-density lipoproteins (HDLs = **h**ighly **d**esirable **l**ipoproteins) help clear cholesterol from the arteries, transporting it to the liver for excretion. HDL levels above 35 mg/dL appear to reduce the risk of CHD. Triglycerides, compounds of fatty acids bound to glycerol and used for fat storage by the body, are carried on very low-density lipoprotein (VLDL) molecules. Elevated triglyerides also contribute to the risk for CHD.

Recent research demonstrates a link between elevated serum *homocysteine levels* and CHD. Until menopause, women have lower homocysteine levels than men, which may partially explain their lower risk for CHD. Homocysteine levels are negatively correlated with serum folate and dietary folate intake; that is, increasing folate intake lowers homocysteine levels.

Metabolic syndrome is another emerging risk factor for CHD. Metabolic syndrome is a group of related risk factors occurring in the same individual: abdominal obesity, hyperlipidemia, hypertension, insulin resistance, and an increased tendency toward clotting and inflammation. The metabolic syndrome appears to significantly increase the risk for premature CHD.

Risk factors unique to women include *premature menopause, oral contraceptive use,* and *hormone replacement therapy (HRT).* At menopause, serum HDL levels drop and LDL levels rise, increasing the risk of CHD. Early menopause (natural or surgically induced) increases the risk of CHD and MI. Women who have a bilateral oophorectomy before age 35 without hormone replacement are eight times more likely to have an MI than women experiencing natural menopause. Estrogen replacement therapy reduces the risk of CHD and MI in these women. Oral contraceptives, by contrast, increase the risk for myocardial infarction, particularly in women who also smoke. This increased risk is due to the tendency of oral contraceptives to promote clotting, and their effects on blood pressure, serum lipids, and glucose tolerance (Woods, Froelicher, & Motzer, 2000). The Women's Health Initiative randomized trial of HRT showed an increased risk for CHD in previously healthy women taking a commonly prescribed combination of estrogen and progestin (Writing Group, 2002). This well-controlled research study was terminated early when it showed a small but significant increase risk for CHD, stroke, pulmonary embolism, and invasive breast cancer in women taking HRT.

Table 8-1. Classification of Serum Cholesterol Values*

	Total Cholesterol (mg/dL)	**LDL Cholesterol (mg/dL)**
Optimal		Less than 100
Desirable	Under 200	100–129
Borderline High	200 to 239	130 to 159
High	240 or higher	160 or higher
Very High		190

*As defined by the National Blood, Lung, and Heart Institute's National Cholesterol Education Program.

Lifestyle Factors

Cigarette smoking is an independent risk factor for CHD, responsible for more deaths from CHD than from lung cancer or pulmonary disease (Woods et al., 2000). The male cigarette smoker has two to three times the risk of developing heart disease than the nonsmoker; the female who smokes has up to four times the risk. For both men and women who stop smoking, the risk of mortality from CHD is reduced by half. Second-hand (or environmental) tobacco smoke also increases the risk of death from CHD, by as much as 30% (Woods et al., 2000). Tobacco smoke promotes CHD in several ways. Carbon monoxide damages vascular endothelium, promoting cholesterol deposition. Nicotine stimulates catecholamine release, increasing blood pressure, heart rate, and myocardial oxygen use. Nicotine also constricts arteries, limiting tissue perfusion (blood flow and oxygen delivery). Further, nicotine reduces HDL levels and increases platelet aggregation, increasing the risk of thrombus formation.

Obesity (body weight greater than 30% over ideal body weight), increased body mass index (BMI), and fat distribution affect the risk for CHD. Obese people have higher rates of hypertension, diabetes, and hyperlipidemia. In the Framingham study, obese men over age 50 had twice the incidence of CHD and acute MI of those who were within 10% of their ideal weight. Central obesity, or intra-abdominal fat, is associated with an increased risk for CHD. The best indicator of central obesity is the waist circumference. A waist-to-hip ratio of greater than 0.8 (women) or 0.9 (men) increases the risk for CHD.

Physical inactivity is associated with higher risk of CHD. Research data indicate that people who maintain a regular program of physical activity are less prone to developing CHD than sedentary people. Cardiovascular benefits of exercise include increased availability of oxygen to the heart muscle, decreased oxygen demand and cardiac workload, and increased myocardial function and electrical stability. Other positive effects of regular physical activity include decreased blood pressure, blood lipids, insulin levels, platelet aggregation, and weight.

Diet may be a risk factor for CHD, independent of fat and cholesterol intake. Diets high in fruits, vegetables, whole grains, and unsaturated fatty acids appear to have a protective effect. The underlying factors are not clear, but probably relate to nutrients such as antioxidants, folic acid, other B vitamins, omega-3 fatty acids, and other unidentified micronutrients (National Cholesterol Education Program, 2001).

Physiology Review

The two main coronary arteries, the left and the right, supply blood, oxygen, and nutrients to the myocardium. They originate in the root of the aorta, just outside the aortic valve. The *left main coronary artery* divides to form the anterior descending and circumflex arteries. The *anterior descending* artery supplies the anterior interventricular septum and the left ventricle. The *circumflex* branch supplies the left lateral wall of the left ventricle. The *right coronary artery* supplies the right ventricle and forms the posterior descending artery. The *posterior descending* artery supplies the posterior portion of the heart.

Blood flow through the coronary arteries is regulated by several factors. Aortic pressure is the primary factor. Other factors include the heart rate (most flow occurs during diastole, when the muscle is relaxed), metabolic activity of the heart, blood vessel tone (constriction), and collateral circulation. Although there are no connections between the large coronary arteries, small arteries are joined by **collateral channels.** If large vessels are gradually occluded, these channels enlarge, providing alternative routes for blood flow (Porth, 2002).

Pathophysiology

Atherosclerosis

Coronary atherosclerosis is the most common cause of reduced coronary blood flow. **Atherosclerosis** is a progressive disease characterized by *atheroma* (plaque) formation, which affects the intimal and medial layers of large and midsize arteries.

Atherosclerosis is initiated by unknown precipitating factors that cause lipoproteins and fibrous tissue to accumulate in the arterial wall. Although the precise mechanisms are unknown, the most accepted theory is that atherosclerosis begins with an injury to or inflammation of endothelial cells lining the artery. Endothelial damage promotes platelet adhesion and aggregation, and attracts leukocytes to the area.

At the injury site, *atherogenic* (atherosclerosis-promoting) lipoproteins collect in the intimal lining of the artery. Macrophages migrate to the injured site as part of the inflammatory process. Contact with platelets, cholesterol, and other blood components stimulates smooth muscle cells and connective tissue within the vessel wall to proliferate abnormally. Although blood flow is not affected at this stage, this early lesion appears as a yellowish fatty streak on the inner lining of the artery. Fibrous plaque develops as smooth muscle cells enlarge, collagen fibers proliferate, and blood lipids accumulate. The lesion protrudes into the arterial lumen and is fixed to the inner wall of the intima. It may invade the muscular media layer of the vessel as well. The developing plaque not only gradually occludes the vessel lumen, but also impairs the vessel's ability to dilate in response to increased oxygen demands. Fibrous plaque lesions often develop at arterial bifurcations or curves or in areas of narrowing. As the plaque expands, it can produce severe stenosis or total occlusion of the artery.

The final stage of the process is the development of *atheromas,* complex lesions consisting of lipids, fibrous tissue, collagen, calcium, cellular debris, and capillaries. These calcified lesions can ulcerate or rupture, stimulating thrombosis. The vessel lumen may be rapidly occluded by the thrombus, or it may embolize to occlude a distal vessel.

Plaque formation may be *eccentric,* located in a specific, asymmetric region of the vessel wall, or *concentric,* involving the entire vessel circumference. Manifestations of the process usually do not appear until about 75% of the arterial lumen has been occluded.

Myocardial Ischemia

Myocardial cells become ischemic when the oxygen supply is inadequate to meet metabolic demands. The critical factors in meeting metabolic demands of cardiac cells are coronary perfusion and myocardial workload (Copstead & Banasik, 2000). The oxygen content of the blood is a contributing factor.

Myocardial cells have limited supplies of adenosine triphosphate (ATP) for energy storage. When myocardial workload increases or the supply of blood and oxygen falls, cellular ATP stores are quickly depleted, affecting their contractility. Cellular metabolism switches from an efficient aerobic process to anaerobic metabolism. Lactic acid accumulates, and cells are damaged. If blood flow is restored within 20 minutes, aerobic metabolism and contractility are restored, and cellular repair begins (McCance & Huether, 2002). Continued ischemia results in cell necrosis and death (infarction).

Coronary heart disease is generally divided into two categories, chronic ischemic heart disease and acute coronary syndromes. *Chronic ischemic heart disease* includes stable and vasospastic angina, and silent myocardial ischemia. *Acute coronary syndromes* range from unstable angina to myocardial infarction (Porth, 2002). These disorders are discussed in the following sections of this chapter.

Collaborative Care

Care of clients with coronary heart disease focuses on aggressive risk factor management to slow the atherosclerotic process and maintain myocardial perfusion. Until manifestations of chronic or acute ischemia are experienced, the diagnosis often is presumptive, based on history and the presence of risk factors.

Diagnostic Tests

Laboratory testing is used to assess for risk factors such as an abnormal blood lipid profile (elevated triglyceride and LDL levels and decreased HDL levels).

- *Total serum cholesterol* is elevated in hyperlipidemia. A *lipid profile* includes triglyceride, HDL, and LDL levels as well, and enables calculation of the ratio of HDL to total cholesterol. The ratio should be at least 1:5, with 1:3 being the ideal ratio. Elevated lipid levels are associated with an increased risk of atherosclerosis. For the most accurate results, dietary cholesterol intake should be consistent for three weeks prior to testing, and the client should fast for ten to twelve hours before the sample is drawn. Alcohol intake and many medications can affect results.

Diagnostic tests to identify subclinical (asymptomatic) CHD may be indicated when multiple risk factors are present.

- *C-reactive protein* is a serum protein associated with inflammatory processes. Recent evidence suggests that elevated blood levels of this protein may be predictive of CHD.
- The *ankle-brachial blood pressure index (ABI)* is an inexpensive, noninvasive test for peripheral vascular disease that may be predictive of CHD.
- *Exercise ECG testing* may be performed. ECGs are used to assess the response to increased cardiac workload induced by exercise. The test is considered "positive" for CHD if myocardial ischemia is detected on the ECG (depression of the ST segment by greater than 3 mm), the client develops chest pain, or the test is stopped due to excess fatigue, dysrhythmias, or other symptoms before the predicted maximal heart rate is achieved.
- *Electron beam computed tomography (EBCT)* creates a three-dimensional image of the heart and coronary arteries that can reveal plaque and other abnormalities. This noninvasive test requires no special preparation, and can identify clients at risk for developing myocardial ischemia.
- *Myocardial perfusion imaging* (see the section on angina that follows) may be used to evaluate myocardial blood flow and perfusion, both at rest and during stress testing (exercise or mental stress). These diagnostic tests are further explained in the section on angina. Perfusion imaging studies are costly, and, therefore, not recommended for routine CHD risk assessment.

Risk Factor Management

Conservative management of CHD focuses on risk factor modification, including smoking, diet, exercise, and management of contributing conditions.

Smoking

Smoking cessation rapidly reduces the risk for CHD and improves cardiovascular status. People who quit reduce their risk by 50%, regardless of how long they smoked before quitting. For women, the risk becomes equivalent to a nonsmoker within three to five years of smoking cessation (Woods et al., 2000). In addition, stopping smoking improves HDL levels, lowers LDL levels, and reduces blood viscosity. All smokers are advised to quit. Health promotion activities focus on preventing children, teenagers, and adults from starting to smoke.

Diet

Dietary recommendations by the National Cholesterol Education Program (2001) include reduced saturated fat and cholesterol intake, and strategies to lower LDL levels. Most fats are a mixture of saturated and unsaturated fatty acids. The highest proportions of saturated fat are found in whole-milk products, red meats, and coconut oil. Nonfat dairy products, fish, and poultry as primary protein sources are recommended. Solidified vegetable fats (e.g., margarine, shortening) contain *trans* fatty acids, which behave more like saturated fats. Soft margarines and vegetable oil spreads contain low levels of trans fatty acids, and should be used instead of butter, stick margarine, and shortening. Monounsaturated fats, found in olive, canola, and peanut oils, actually lower LDL and cholesterol levels. Certain cold-water fish, such as tuna, salmon, and mackerel, contain high levels of omega-3 (or n-3) fatty acids, which help raise HDL levels, and decrease serum triglycerides, total serum cholesterol, and blood pressure.

In addition, increased intake of soluble fiber (found in oats, psyllium, pectin-rich fruit, and beans) and insoluble fiber (found in whole grains, vegetables, and fruit) is recommended. Folic acid and vitamins B_6 and B_{12} affect homocystine metabolism, reducing serum levels. Leafy green vegetables (e.g., spinach and broccoli) and legumes (e.g., black-eyed peas, dried beans, and lentils) are rich sources of folate. Meat, fish, and poultry are rich in vitamins B_6 and B_{12}. Vitamin B_6 is also found in soy products; B_{12} is in fortified cereals. Increased intake of antioxidant nutrients (vitamin E, in particular) and foods rich in antioxidants (fruits and vegetables) appears to increase HDL levels and have a protective effect on CHD.

In middle-aged and older adults, moderate alcohol intake may reduce the risk for CHD (National Cholesterol Education Program, 2001). Consumption of no more than two drinks per day for men or one drink per day for women is recommended. A drink is 5 ounces of wine, 12 ounces of beer, or 1 1/2 ounces of whiskey. People who do not drink alcohol, however, should not be encouraged to start consuming it as a heart-protective measure.

People who are overweight or obese are encouraged to lose weight through a combination of reduced calorie intake (maintaining a nutritionally sound diet) and increased exercise. High-protein, high-fat weight loss programs are not recommended for weight reduction.

Exercise

Regular physical exercise reduces the risk for CHD in several ways. It lowers VLDL, LDL, and triglyceride levels, and raises HDL levels. Regular exercise reduces the blood pressure and insulin resistance. Unless contraindicated, all clients are encouraged to participate in at least 30 minutes of moderately intense physical activity 5 to 6 days each week.

Hypertension

Although hypertension often cannot be prevented or cured, it can be controlled. Hypertension control (maintaining a blood pressure lower than 140/90 mmHg) is vital to reduce its atherosclerosis-promoting effects and to reduce the workload of the heart. Management strategies include reducing sodium intake, increasing calcium intake, regular exercise, stress management, and medications.

Diabetes

Diabetes increases the risk of CHD by accelerating the atherosclerotic process. Weight loss (if appropriate), reduced fat intake, and exercise are particularly important for the diabetic client. Because hyperglycemia apparently also contributes to atherosclerosis, consistent blood glucose management is vital.

Medications

Drug therapy to lower total serum cholesterol and LDL levels and to raise HDL levels now is an integral part of CHD management. It is used in conjunction with diet and other lifestyle changes, and is based on the client's overall risk for CHD.

Drugs used to treat hyperlipidemia act specifically by lowering LDL levels. The goal of treatment is to achieve an LDL level of < 130 mg/dL. Medications to treat hyperlipidemia are not inexpensive; the cost–benefit ratio needs to be considered, as long-term treatment may be required. The four major classes of cholesterol-lowering drugs are statins, bile acid sequestrants, nicotinic acid, and fibrates. The nursing implications and client teaching for these drug classes are outlined in the Medication Administration table on the next page.

The statins, including lovastatin (Mevacor), pravastatin (Pravachol), simvastatin (Zocor), and others, are first-line drugs for treating hyperlipidemia. They effectively lower LDL levels and may also increase HDL levels. The statins can cause myopathy; all clients are instructed to report muscle pain and weakness or brown urine. Liver function tests are monitored during therapy, as these drugs may increase liver enzyme levels.

The other cholesterol-lowering drugs, such as the bile acid sequestrants, nicotinic acid, and fibrates, are primarily used when combination therapy is required to effectively lower serum cholesterol levels. They also may be used for selected clients, such as younger adults, women who wish to become pregnant, or to specifically lower triglyceride levels.

Clients at high risk for MI are often started on prophylactic low-dose aspirin therapy. The dose ranges from 80 to 325 mg/day (Tierney et al., 2001). Aspirin is contraindicated, however, for clients who have a history of aspirin sensitivity, bleeding disorders, or active peptic ulcer disease. Angiotensin-converting enzyme (ACE) inhibitors also may be prescribed for high-risk clients, including diabetics with other CHD risk factors.

Complementary Therapies

Diet and exercise programs that emphasize physical conditioning and a low-fat diet rich in antioxidants have been shown to be effective in managing CHD. Supplements of vitamins C, E, B_6, and B_{12}, and folic acid may be beneficial. Other potentially helpful complementary therapies include herbals, such as ginkgo biloba, garlic, curcumin, and green tea; and consumption of red wine, foods containing bioflavonoids, and nuts. Behavioral therapies of benefit for clients with CHD include relaxation and stress management, guided imagery, treatment of depression, anger/hostility management, and meditation, tai chi, and yoga.

Nursing Care

Health Promotion

Present information about healthy lifestyle habits to community and religious groups, school children (kindergarten through twelfth grade), and through the print media. In promoting healthy lifestyle habits, nurses can positively affect the incidence, morbidity, and mortality from CHD.

Strongly encourage all clients to avoid smoking in the first place, and to stop all forms of tobacco use. Discuss the adverse effects of smoking and the benefits of quitting. Provide information about dietary recommendations to maintain a healthy weight and optimal cholesterol levels. Discuss the benefits and importance of regular exercise. Finally, encourage clients with cardiovascular risk factors to undergo regular screening for hypertension, diabetes, and hyperlipidemia.

Assessment

Nursing assessment for CHD focuses on identifying risk factors.

* *Health history:* current manifestations such as chest pain or heaviness, shortness of breath, weakness; current diet, exercise patterns, and medications; smoking history and pattern of alcohol intake; history of heart disease, hypertension, or diabetes; family history of CHD or other cardiac problems.
* *Physical examination:* current weight and its appropriateness for height; body mass index; waist-to-hip ratio; blood pressure; strength and equality of peripheral pulses.

Table 8-2. Medication Administration—Cholesterol-Lowering Drugs

Statins

Lovastatin (Mevacor)
Pravastatin (Pravachol)
Simvastatin (Zocor)
Fluvastatin (Lescol)
Atorvastatin (Lipitor)

Statins inhibit the enzyme HMG-CoA reductase in the liver, lowering LDL synthesis and serum levels. The statins are first-line treatment for elevated LDL, used in conjunction with diet and lifestyle changes. Although their side effects are minimal, they may cause increased serum liver enzyme levels and myopathy.

Nursing Responsibilities
* Monitor serum cholesterol and liver enzyme levels before and during therapy. Report elevated liver enzyme levels.
* Assess for muscle pain and tenderness. Monitor CPK level if present.
* If taking digoxin concurrently, monitor for and report digoxin toxicity.

Client and Family Teaching
* Promptly report muscle pain, tenderness, or weakness; skin rash or hives, or changes in skin color; abdominal pain, nausea, or vomiting.
* Do not use these drugs if you are pregnant or plan to become pregnant.
* Inform your doctor if you are taking any other medications concurrently.

Continued on the next page

Table 8-2. Continued

Nicotinic Acid

Niacin (Nicobid, Nicolar, Niaspan, others)

Nicotinic acid in both prescription and nonprescription forms lowers total and LDL cholesterol and triglyceride levels. The crystalline form and Niaspan, a prescription extended release tablet, also raise HDL levels. Because the doses required to achieve significant cholesterol-lowering effects are associated with multiple side effects, nicotinic acid generally is used in combination therapy, particularly with the statin drugs.

Nursing Responsibilities
• Give oral preparations with meals and accompanied by a cold beverage to minimize GI effects.
• Administer with caution to clients with active liver disease, peptic ulcer disease, gout, or type 2 diabetes.
• Monitor blood glucose, uric acid levels, and liver function tests during treatment.

Client and Family Teaching
• Flushing of face, neck, and ears may occur within two hours following dose; these effects generally subside as treatment continues. Alcohol use during nicotinic acid therapy may worsen this effect.
• Report weakness or dizziness with changes in posture (lying to sitting; sitting to standing) to your doctor. Change positions slowly to reduce the risk of injury.

Bile Acid Sequestrants

Cholestyramine (Questran)
Colestipol (Colestid)
Colesevelam (Welchol)

Bile acid sequestrants lower LDL levels by binding bile acids in the intestine, reducing its reabsorption and cholesterol production in the liver. They are used in combination therapy regimens and for women who are considering pregnancy. Their primary disadvantages are inconvenience of administration due to bulk and gastrointestinal side effects such as constipation.

Nursing Responsibilities
• Mix cholestyramine and colestipol powders with four to six ounces of water or juice; administer once or twice a day as ordered with meals.
• Store in a tightly closed container.

Client and Family Teaching
• Promptly report constipation, severe gastric distress with nausea and vomiting, unexplained weight loss, black or bloody stools, or sudden back pain to your doctor.
• Drinking ample amounts of fluid while taking these drugs reduces problems of constipation and bloating.
• Do not omit doses as this may affect the absorption of other drugs you are taking.

Table 8-2. Continued

Fibric Acid Derivatives

Gemfibrozil (Lopid)
Fenofibrate (Tricor)
Clofibrate (Atromid-S)

The fibrates are used to lower serum triglyceride levels; they have only a slight to modest effect on LDL. They affect lipid regulation by blocking triglyceride synthesis. They are used to treat very high triglyceride levels, and may be used in combination with statins.

Nursing Responsibilities
• Monitor serum LDL and VLDL levels, electrolytes, glucose, liver enzymes, renal function tests, and CBC during therapy. Report abnormal values.
• Up to two months of treatment may be required to achieve a therapeutic effect; rebound, with decreasing benefit, may occur in the second or third month of treatment.

Client and Family Teaching
• Take with meals if the drug causes gastric distress.
• Promptly report flulike symptoms (fatigue, muscle aching, soreness, or weakness) to your doctor.
• Do not use this drug if you are pregnant or plan to become pregnant. Use reliable birth control measures while taking this drug.
• Contact your doctor before stopping this drug and before taking any over-the-counter preparations.

Nursing Diagnoses and Interventions

Imbalanced Nutrition: More than Body Requirements

This nursing diagnosis may be appropriate for clients who are obese, have a waist-to-hip ratio greater than 0.8 (female) or 0.9 (male), or whose diet history or serum cholesterol levels indicate a need to reduce fat and cholesterol intake.

• Encourage assessment of food intake and eating patterns to help identify areas that can be improved. *Clients often are unaware of their fat and cholesterol intake, particularly when many meals are eaten away from home. Careful assessment increases awareness and allows the client to make conscious changes.*

• Discuss American Heart Association and therapeutic lifestyle change (TLC) dietary recommendations, emphasizing the role of diet in heart disease. Provide guidance regarding specific food choices with healthy alternatives. *Specific diet information and suggestions help the client make better food choices.*

• Refer to clinical dietitian for diet planning and further teaching. Suggest cookbooks that offer low-fat recipes to encourage healthier eating, and provide American Heart Association and American Cancer Society recipe pamphlets and information on low-fat eating. *These resources provide tools for the client to use as eating patterns change.*

• Encourage gradual but progressive dietary changes. *Drastic changes in eating patterns may cause frustration and discourage the client from maintaining a healthy diet over the long term.*

- Discourage use of high-fat, low-carbohydrate, or other fad diets for weight loss. *These diets may adversely affect serum cholesterol and triglyceride levels, and often are too drastic to maintain over the long term.*

- Encourage reasonable goals for weight loss (e.g., 1.0 to 1.5 lb per week and a 10% weight loss over six months). Provide information about weight loss programs and support groups such as Weight Watchers and Take Off Pounds Sensibly (TOPS). *Gradual but steady weight loss is more likely to be sustained. Recognized programs that emphasize healthy eating provide support and incentive for making lifetime dietary changes.*

Ineffective Health Maintenance

Clients with risk factors for CHD may be unable to identify or independently manage their risk factors.

- Discuss risk factors for CHD, stressing that changing or managing those factors that can be modified reduces the client's overall risk for the disease. *Clients with significant nonmodifiable risk factors may be discouraged, reducing their ability to eliminate or control modifiable risk factors.*

- Discuss the immediate benefits of smoking cessation. Provide resource materials from the American Heart Association, the American Lung Association, and the American Cancer Society. Refer to a structured smoking cessation program to increase the likelihood of success in quitting. *Long-time smokers may assume that the damage from smoking has already been done, and quitting would not be "worth the price."*

- Help the client identify specific sources of psychosocial and physical support for smoking cessation, dietary, and lifestyle changes. *Support persons, groups, and aids, such as nicotine patches, help the client achieve success and provide encouragement during difficult times, such as withdrawal symptoms.*

- Discuss the benefits of regular exercise for cardiovascular health and weight loss. Help identify favorite forms of exercise or physical activity. Encourage planning for thirty minutes of continuous aerobic activity (i.e., walking, running, bicycling, swimming) four to five times a week. Encourage identification of an "exercise buddy" to help maintain motivation. *Engaging in preferred activities with a partner maintains motivation and increases the likelihood of maintaining an exercise program. Encourage continuation of the plan, even when days are missed. Exercise is cumulative, so increasing the duration of exercise on subsequent days can "make up" for a lost day.*

- Provide information and teaching about prescribed medications such as cholesterol-lowering drugs. Discuss the relationship between hypertension, diabetes, and CHD. *Teaching is important to promote understanding of and compliance with the prescribed drug regimen.*

Home Care

Encourage participation in some form of cardiac rehabilitation program. Formal programs provide comprehensive assessment of, interventions for, and teaching of clients with cardiac disease. Monitored exercise and information about risk factors help clients identify ways to lower their risk for CHD.

Because clients themselves are primarily responsible for maintaining the lifestyle changes necessary to reduce the risk of CHD, provide teaching and support as outlined in the previous section. Assist the client to make healthy choices and reinforce positive changes. Emphasize the importance of regular follow-up appointments to monitor progress.

The Client with Angina Pectoris

Angina pectoris, or *angina,* is chest pain resulting from reduced coronary blood flow, which causes a temporary imbalance between myocardial blood supply and demand. The imbalance may be due to coronary heart disease, atherosclerosis, or vessel constriction that impairs myocardial blood supply. Hypermetabolic conditions such as exercise, thyrotoxicosis, stimulant abuse (e.g., cocaine), hyperthyroidism, and emotional stress can increase myocardial oxygen demand, precipitating angina. Anemia, heart failure, or pulmonary diseases may affect blood and oxygen supplies as well, causing angina.

Pathophysiology

The imbalance between myocardial blood supply and demand causes temporary and reversible myocardial ischemia. **Ischemia,** deficient blood flow to tissue, may be caused by partial obstruction of a coronary artery, coronary artery spasm, or a thrombus. Obstruction of a coronary artery deprives cells in the region of the heart normally supplied by that vessel of oxygen and nutrients needed for metabolic processes. Cellular processes are compromised. Reduced oxygen causes cells to switch from aerobic metabolism to anaerobic metabolism. Anaerobic metabolism causes lactic acid to build up in the cells. It also affects cell membrane permeability, releasing substances such as histamine, kinins, and specific enzymes that stimulate terminal nerve fibers in the cardiac muscle and send pain impulses to the central nervous system. The pain radiates to the upper body because the heart shares the same dermatome as this region. Return of adequate circulation provides the nutrients needed by cells, and clears the waste products. More than 30 minutes of ischemia irreversibly damages myocardial cells (necrosis).

Three types of angina have been identified:

- *Stable angina* is the most common and predictable form of angina. It occurs with a predictable amount of activity or stress, and is a common manifestation of CHD. Stable angina usually occurs when the work of the heart is increased by physical exertion, exposure to cold, or by stress. Stable angina is relieved by rest and nitrates.

- *Prinzmetal's (variant) angina* is atypical angina that occurs unpredictably (unrelated to activity), and often at night. It is caused by coronary artery spasm with or without an atherosclerotic lesion. The exact mechanism of coronary artery spasm is unknown. It may result from hyperactive sympathetic nervous system responses, altered calcium flow in smooth muscle, or reduced prostaglandins to promote vasodilation.

- *Unstable angina* occurs with increasing frequency, severity, and duration. Pain is unpredictable and occurs with decreasing levels of activity or stress and may occur at rest. Clients with unstable angina are at risk for myocardial infarction.

- *Silent myocardial ischemia,* or asymptomatic ischemia, is thought to be common in people with CHD. Silent ischemia may occur with either activity or with mental stress. Mental stress increases the heart rate and blood pressure, increasing myocardial oxygen demand (McCance & Huether, 2002).

Manifestations

The cardinal manifestation of angina is chest pain. The pain typically is precipitated by an identifiable event, such as physical activity, strong emotion, stress, eating a heavy meal, or exposure to cold. The classic sequence of angina is activity–pain, rest–relief. The client may describe the pain as a tight, squeezing, heavy pressure, or constricting sensation. It characteristically begins beneath the sternum and may radiate to the jaw, neck, or arm. Less characteristically, the pain may be felt in the jaw, epigastric region, or back. Anginal pain usually lasts less than 15 minutes and is relieved by rest. Additional manifestations of angina include dyspnea, pallor, tachycardia, and great anxiety and fear. The manifestations of angina are summarized in Table 8-3.

Table 8-3. Manifestations of Angina

Chest pain:	Substernal or precordial (across the chest wall); may radiate to neck, arms, shoulders, or jaw
Quality:	Tight, squeezing, constricting, or heavy sensation; may also be described as burning, aching, choking, dull, or constant
Associated manifestations:	Dyspnea, pallor, tachycardia, anxiety, and fear
Precipitating factors:	Exercise or activity, strong emotion, stress, cold, or heavy meal
Relieving factors:	Rest, position change; nitroglycerine

Collaborative Care

Acute angina care focuses on relieving pain and restoring coronary blood flow. Long-term management is directed at the causes of impaired myocardial blood supply. As for CHD, risk factor management is a vital component of care for the client with angina (see the preceding section of this chapter).

Diagnostic Tests

The diagnosis of angina is based on past medical history and family history, a comprehensive description of the chest pain, and physical assessment findings. Laboratory tests may confirm the presence of risk factors, such as an abnormal blood lipid profile and elevated blood glucose. Diagnostic tests provide information about overall cardiac function.

Common diagnostic tests to assess for coronary heart disease and angina include electrocardiography, stress testing, nuclear medicine studies, echocardiography (ultrasound), and coronary angiography.

Electrocardiography   A resting ECG may be normal, may show nonspecific changes in the ST segment and T wave, or may show evidence of previous myocardial infarction. Characteristic ECG changes are seen during anginal episodes. During periods of ischemia, the ST segment is depressed or downsloping, and the T wave may flatten or invert. These changes reverse when ischemia is relieved. For more details about the ECG, its waveforms, and its uses, see the section of this chapter about dysrhythmias.

Stress Electrocardiography   Stress electrocardiography (exercise stress test) uses ECGs to monitor the cardiac response to an increased workload during progressive exercise.

Radionuclide Testing   Radionuclide testing is a safe, noninvasive technique to evaluate myocardial perfusion and left ventricular function. The amount of radioisotope injected is very small; no special radiation precautions are required during or after the scan. Thallium-201 or a technetium-based radiocompound is injected intravenously, and the heart is scanned with a radiation detector. Ischemic or infarcted cells of the myocardium do not take up the substance normally, appearing as a "cold spot" on the scan. If the ischemia is transient, these spots gradually fill in, indicating the reversibility of the process. With severe ischemia or a myocardial infarction, these areas may remain devoid of radioactivity.

Left ventricular function can also be evaluated. Whereas the ejection fraction, or portion of blood ejected from the left ventricle during systole, normally increases during exercise, it may actually decrease in coronary heart disease and stress-induced ischemia.

Radionuclide testing may be combined with pharmacologic stress testing for clients who are physically unable to exercise or to detect subclinical myocardial ischemia. A vasodilator is injected to induce the same ischemic changes that occur with exercise in the diseased heart. Coronary arteries unaffected by atherosclerosis dilate in response to the drugs, increasing blood flow to already well-perfused tissue. This reduces flow to ischemic muscle, called *myocardial steal syndrome.*

Echocardiography   *Echocardiography* is a noninvasive test that uses ultrasound to evaluate cardiac structure and function. High-frequency sound waves emitted from a transducer are reflected off of heart structures back to the transducer as echoes. These echoes are displayed on a screen. Echocardiography is usually performed with the transducer held to the chest wall. It may be done at rest, during supine exercise, or immediately following upright exercise to evaluate movement of the myocardial wall and assess for possible ischemia or infarction.

Transesophageal echocardiography (TEE) uses ultrasound to identify abnormal blood flow patterns as well as cardiac structures. In TEE, the probe is on the tip of an endoscope inserted into the esophagus, positioning it close to the posterior heart (especially the left atrium and the aorta). It avoids interference by breasts, ribs, or lungs.

Coronary Angiography   *Coronary angiography* is the gold standard for evaluating the coronary arteries. Guided by fluoroscopy, a catheter introduced into the femoral or brachial artery is threaded into the coronary artery. Dye is injected into each coronary opening, allowing visualization of the main coronary branches and any abnormalities, such as stenosis or obstruction. Narrowing of the vessel lumen by more than 50% is considered significant; most lesions that cause symptoms involve more than 70% narrowing. Vessel obstructions are noted on a coronary artery "map" that provides a guide for tracking disease progression and for elective treatment with angioplasty or cardiac surgery. During angiogram, the drug ergonovine maleate may be injected to induce coronary artery spasm and diagnose Prinzmetal's angina.

Medications

Drugs may be used for both acute and long-term relief of angina. (See Table 8-4.) The goal of drug treatment is to reduce oxygen demand and increase oxygen supply to the myocardium. Three main classes of drugs are used to treat angina: nitrates, beta blockers, and calcium channel blockers.

Nitrates
Nitrates, including nitroglycerin and longer-acting nitrate preparations, are used to treat acute anginal attacks and prevent angina.

Sublingual nitroglycerin is the drug of choice to treat acute angina. It acts within one to two minutes, decreasing myocardial work and oxygen demand through venous and arterial dilation, which in turn reduce preload and afterload. It may also improve myocardial oxygen supply by dilating collateral blood vessels and reducing stenosis. Rapid-acting nitroglycerin is also available as a buccal spray in a metered system. For some clients, this may be easier to handle than small nitroglycerin tablets.

Longer-acting nitroglycerin preparations (oral tablets, ointment, or transdermal patches) are used to prevent attacks of angina, not to treat an acute attack. The primary problem with long-term nitrate use is the development of *tolerance,* a decreasing effect from the same dose of medication. Tolerance can be limited by a dosing schedule that allows a nitrate-free period of at least eight to ten hours daily. This is usually scheduled at night, when angina is less likely to occur.

Headache is a common side effect of nitrates, and may limit their usefulness. Nausea, dizziness, and hypotension are also common effects of therapy.

Beta Blockers

Beta blockers, including propranolol, metoprolol, nadolol, and atenolol, are considered first-line drugs to treat stable angina. They block the cardiac-stimulating effects of norepinephrine and epinephrine, preventing anginal attacks by reducing heart rate, myocardial contractility, and blood pressure, thus reducing myocardial oxygen demand. Beta blockers may be used alone or with other medications to prevent angina.

Beta blockers are contraindicated for clients with asthma or severe COPD (see Chapter 15) because they may cause severe bronchospasm. They are not used in clients with significant bradycardia, or AV conduction blocks, and are used cautiously in heart failure, Beta blockers are not used to treat Prinzmetal's angina because they may make it worse.

Calcium Channel Blockers

Calcium channel blockers reduce myocardial oxygen demand and increase myocardial blood and oxygen supply. These drugs, which include verapamil, diltiazem, and nifedipine, lower blood pressure, reduce myocardial contractility, and, in some cases, lower the heart rate, decreasing myocardial oxygen demand. They are also potent coronary vasodilators, effectively increasing oxygen supply. Like beta blockers, calcium channel blockers act too slowly to effectively treat an acute attack of angina; they are used for long-term prophylaxis. Because they may actually increase ischemia and mortality in clients with heart failure or left ventricular dysfunction, these drugs are not usually prescribed in the initial treatment of angina. They are used cautiously in clients with dysrhythmias, heart failure, or hypotension.

Aspirin

The client with angina, particularly unstable angina, is at risk for myocardial infarction because of significant narrowing of the coronary arteries. Low-dose aspirin (80 to 325 mg/day) is often prescribed to reduce the risk of platelet aggregation and thrombus formation.

Revascularization Procedures

Several procedures may be used to restore blood flow and oxygen to ischemic tissue. Nonsurgical techniques include transluminal coronary angioplasty, laser angioplasty, coronary atherectomy, and intracoronary stents. Coronary artery bypass grafting (CABG) is a surgical procedure that may be used.

Table 8-4. Medication Administration—Antianginal Medications

Organic Nitrates

Nitroglycerin (Nitropaste, Nitro-Dur, Nitro-Bid, Nitrol, Transderm-Nitro, Nitrogard, Nitrodisc, Tridil)
Isosorbide dinitrate (Isordil)
Isosorbide mononitrate (ISMO)
Amyl nitrite

Nitrates dilate both arterial and venous vessels, depending on the dose. Coronary artery vasodilation increases blood flow and myocardial oxygen supply. Venous dilation allows peripheral blood pooling, reducing venous return, preload, and cardiac work. Arterial dilation reduces vascular resistance and afterload, also reducing cardiac work. Sublingual nitroglycerin (NTG) tablets are used to treat and prevent acute anginal attacks (when taken prophylactically before activity). Nitrates are administered sublingually, by buccal spray, or intravenously for immediate effect; or orally or topically for sustained effect.

Nursing Responsibilities

- Dilute intravenous nitroglycerin before infusing; use only glass bottles for the mixture. Nitroglycerin adheres to PVC bags and tubing, affecting the amount of drug that is delivered. Use non-PVC infusion tubing.
- Wear gloves when applying nitroglycerin paste or ointment to prevent absorbing the drug through the skin. Measure dose carefully and spread evenly in a two-by-three inch area.
- Remove nitroglycerin patches or ointment at night to help prevent tolerance.

Client and Family Teaching

- Use only the sublingual, buccal, and spray forms of nitrates to treat acute angina.
- If the first nitrate dose does not relieve angina within five minutes, take a second dose. After five more minutes, you may take a third dose if needed. If the pain is unrelieved or lasts for twenty minutes or longer, seek medical assistance immediately.
- Carry a supply of nitroglycerin tablets with you. Dissolve sublingual nitroglycerin tablets under the tongue or between the upper lip and gum. Do not eat, drink, or smoke until the tablet is completely dissolved.
- Keep sublingual tablets in their original amber glass bottle to protect them from heat, light, and moisture. Replace your supply every six months.
- You may experience a burning or tingling sensation under the tongue and develop a transient headache when you take the drug. These are expected; the headache will diminish over time.
- Use caution when standing from a sitting position; nitroglycerine may make you lightheaded.
- Rotate ointment or transdermal patch application sites. Apply to a hairless area; spread ointment evenly without rubbing or massaging. Remove the patch or residual ointment at bedtime daily. Apply a fresh dose in the morning.
- If you are using a long-acting nitrate, keep a supply of immediate-acting nitrates to treat acute angina.

Continued on the next page

Table 8-4. Continued

Beta Blockers

Atenolol (Tenormin)
Metoprolol (Lopressor)
Propranolol (Inderal)
Nadolol (Corgard)

Beta blockers decrease cardiac workload by blocking beta receptors on the heart muscle, decreasing heart rate, contractility, myocardial oxygen consumption, and blood pressure. Beta blockers also reduce *reflex tachycardia,* which may develop with other antianginal drugs. Beta blockers are frequently prescribed as antianginal and antihypertensive agents.

Nursing Responsibilities
- Document heart rate and blood pressure before administering the medication. Withhold drug if the heart rate is below 50 BPM or the blood pressure is below prescribed limits. Notify the physician.
- Assess for and report possible contraindications to therapy, including heart failure, bradycardia, AV block, asthma, or COPD.
- Do not abruptly discontinue these drugs after long-term therapy, as this can increase heart rate, contractility, and blood pressure, and cause fatal dysrhythmia, myocardial infarction, or stroke.

Client and Family Teaching
- Beta blockers help prevent angina, but will not relieve an acute attack. Keep a supply of fast-acting nitrates on hand for acute anginal attacks.
- Do not suddenly stop taking this medication. Discuss discontinuing this medication with your doctor.
- Take your pulse daily. Do not take the drug, and contact your doctor, if your heart rate is below 50 BPM. Check your blood pressure frequently.
- Report a slow or irregular pulse, swelling or weight gain, or having difficulty breathing to your doctor.

Calcium Channel Blockers

Nifedipine (Adalat, Procardia)
Diltiazem (Cardizem)
Verapamil (Isoptin, Calan)
Bepridil (Vascor)
Felodipine (Plendil)
Isradipine (DynaCirc)
Nicardipine (Cardene)
Nimodipine (Nimotop)

Calcium channel blockers are used to control angina, hypertension, and dysrhythmias. By blocking the entry of calcium into cells, these drugs reduce contractility, slow the heart rate and conduction, and cause vasodilation. Calcium channel blockers increase myocardial oxygen supply by dilating the coronary arteries; they decrease the workload of the heart by lowering vascular resistance and oxygen demand. Calcium channel blockers are often prescribed for clients with coronary artery spasm (Prinzmetal's angina).

Table 8-4. Continued

Nursing Responsibilities

- Do not mix verapamil in any solution containing sodium bicarbonate. Administer IV push verapamil over two to three minutes.
- Document blood pressure and heart rate before administering the drug. Withhold the drug if the heart rate is below 50 BPM. Notify the physician.
- The nifedipine capsule may be punctured and administered by extracting the liquid with a syringe and squirting the dose under the client's tongue. (Discard the needle first!)
- Use caution when giving a calcium channel blocker with other cardiac depressants, such as beta blockers. Concomitant administration with nitrates may cause excessive vasodilation.
- Manifestations of toxicity include nausea, generalized weakness, signs of decreased cardiac output, hypotension, bradycardia, and AV block. Report these findings immediately. Maintain intravenous access, and slowly administer intravenous calcium chloride. Do not infuse large volumes of fluid to treat hypotension as heart failure may result.

Client and Family Teaching

- Take your pulse before taking the drug. Do not take the drug, and notify physician, if your heart rate drops below 50 BPM.
- Keep a fresh supply of immediate-acting nitrate available to treat acute anginal attacks. Calcium channel blockers will not work fast enough to relieve an acute attack.

Percutaneous Coronary Revascularization

Percutaneous coronary revascularization (PCR) are procedures used to restore blood flow to the ischemic myocardium in clients with CHD. Approximately 600,000 PCR procedures are done annually in the United States. PCR is used to treat clients with:

- Moderately severe, chronic stable angina unrelieved by medical therapy.
- Mild angina but objective evidence of coronary ischemia.
- Unstable angina.
- Acute myocardial infarction (Braunwald et al., 2001).

PCR procedures are similar to the procedure used for coronary angiography. A catheter introduced into the arterial circulation is guided into the opening of the narrowed coronary artery. A flexible guidewire is inserted through the catheter lumen into the affected vessel. The guidewire is then used to thread an angioplasty balloon, arterial stent, or other therapeutic device into the narrowed segment of the artery. The procedure is performed in the cardiac catheterization laboratory using local anesthesia. The hospital stay is short (one to two days), minimizing costs.

For *balloon angioplasty* (also called percutaneous transluminal coronary angioplasty or PTCA), a balloon-tipped catheter is threaded over the guidewire, with the balloon positioned across the area of narrowing. The balloon is inflated in a step-by-step fashion for about 30 seconds to 2 minutes to compress the plaque against the arterial wall, with a goal of reducing the vessel obstruction to less than 50% of the arterial lumen. When used alone, balloon angioplasty is associated with a relatively high risk of abrupt vessel closure and restenosis. Its primary current use is in combination with stent placement or atherectomy.

Intracoronary stents are metallic scaffolds used to maintain an open arterial lumen. Stents reduce the rate of restenosis following angioplasty by about one-third, and are now used in 70% to 80% of all PCR procedures (Braunwald et al., 2001). The stent is placed over a balloon catheter, guided into position, and expanded as the balloon is inflated. It then remains in the artery as a prop after the balloon is removed. Endothelial cells will completely line the inner wall of the stent to produce a smooth inner lining. Antiplatelet medications (aspirin and ticlopidine) are given following stent insertion to reduce the risk of thrombus formation at the site.

In contrast to balloon and stent procedures which enlarge the artery by displacing plaque, *atherectomy* procedures remove plaque from the identified lesion. The directional atherectomy catheter shaves the plaque off vessel walls using a rotary cutting head, retaining the fragments in its housing and removing them from the vessel. Rotational atherectomy catheters pulverize plaque into particles small enough to pass through the coronary microcirculation. Laser atherectomy devices use laser energy to remove plaque.

Complications following PCR procedures include hematoma at the catheter insertion site, pseudoaneurysm, embolism, hypersensitivity to contrast dye, dysrhythmias, bleeding, vessel perforation, and restenosis, or reocclusion of the treated vessel.

Coronary Artery Bypass Grafting

Surgery for coronary heart disease involves using a section of a vein or an artery to create a connection (or bypass) between the aorta and the coronary artery beyond the obstruction. This, then, allows blood to perfuse the ischemic portion of the heart. The internal mammary artery in the chest and the saphenous vein from the leg are the vessels most commonly used for coronary artery bypass grafting (CABG).

Bypass grafts are safe and effective. Angina is totally relieved or significantly reduced in 90% of clients who undergo complete revascularization. While anginal pain may recur within three years, it rarely is as severe as before surgery. Coronary artery bypass graft has a positive effect on mortality in many cases. It is recommended for clients who have multiple vessel disease and impaired left ventricular function or diabetes, and for clients who have significant obstruction of the left main coronary artery (Braunwald et al., 2001).

A median sternotomy is used to access the heart. The heart is usually stopped during surgery. The *cardiopulmonary bypass (CPB) pump* is used to maintain perfusion to the rest of the organs during open-heart surgery. Venous blood is removed from the body through a cannula placed in the right atrium or the superior and inferior venae cavae. Blood then circulates through the CPB pump, where it is oxygenated, its temperature regulated, and is filtered. Oxygenated blood is returned to the body through a cannula in the ascending aorta. Cardiopulmonary bypass enables surgeons to operate on a quiet heart and a relatively bloodless field. Hypothermia can be maintained to reduce the metabolic rate and decrease oxygen demand during surgery.

When the saphenous vein is used, it is excised from its normal attachments in the leg, flushed with a cold heparinized saline solution, and then reversed so that its valves do not interfere with blood flow. It is *anastomosed* (grafted) to the aorta and the coronary artery, distal to the occlusion. This provides a bridge or conduit for blood flow past the obstruction. If the internal mammary artery (IMA) is used, its distal end is excised and anatomosed to the coronary artery distal to the obstruction. The IMA often is used to revascularize the left coronary artery, because of the greater oxygen demand of the left ventricle.

Once grafting is completed, cardiopulmonary bypass is discontinued and the client is rewarmed. Rewarming stimulates the heart to resume beating. Temporary pacing wires are sutured in place and passed through the chest wall in case temporary pacing is necessary. Chest tubes are placed in the pleural space and mediastinum to drain blood and reestablish negative pressure in the thoracic cavity. The sternum is closed using heavy wires and bone wax, the skin is closed with sutures or staples, and sterile dressings are applied over sternal and leg incisions.

Minimally Invasive Coronary Artery Surgery

Minimally invasive coronary artery surgery is a potential future alternative to CABG. Two approaches may be used: *port-access coronary artery bypass* uses several small holes, or "ports" in the chest wall to access vessels for connection to the CPB pump and the surgical site; CPB is avoided altogether using the *minimally invasive coronary artery bypass (MIDCAB)* approach. With MIDCAB, a small surgical incision and several chest wall ports are used to graft a chest wall artery to the affected coronary vessel while the heart continues to beat.

Transmyocardial Laser Revascularization

A new development in myocardial revascularization techniques is called *transmyocardial laser revascularization (TMLR)*. In this procedure, a laser is used to drill tiny holes into the myocardial muscle itself to provide collateral blood flow to ischemic muscle. Clients whose coronary artery obstructions are too diffuse to bypass are candidates for this new surgical treatment.

Nursing Care

Health Promotion

In addition to health promotion measures identified for CHD, emphasize the importance of active CHD risk factor management to slow progression of the disease. Encourage clients to stop smoking. Discuss the use of cholesterol-lowering drug therapy with clients who have hypercholesterolemia. Encourage regular aerobic exercise and a diet based on American Heart Association or National Cholesterol Education Program guidelines.

Assessment

Focused assessment data for the client with angina includes the following:

- *Health history:* chest pain, including type, intensity, duration, frequency, aggravating factors and relief measures; associated symptoms; history of other cardiovascular disorders, peripheral vascular disease, or stroke; current medications and treatment; usual diet, exercise, and alcohol intake patterns; smoking history; use of other recreational drugs.
- *Physical assessment:* vital signs and heart sounds; strength and equality of peripheral pulses; skin color and temperature (central and peripheral); physical appearance during pain episode (e.g., shortness of breath, apparent anxiety, color, diaphoresis).

Nursing Diagnoses and Interventions

The focus of nursing care for clients with angina is similar to the collaborative care focus: to reduce myocardial oxygen demand and improve the oxygen supply. Angina usually is treated in community settings; the primary nursing focus is education. High-priority nursing problems for clients with angina include ineffective cardiac tissue perfusion and management of the prescribed therapeutic regimen.

Ineffective Tissue Perfusion: Cardiac

The pain of angina results from impaired blood flow and oxygen supply to the myocardium. Nursing interventions can both prevent ischemia and shorten the duration of pain.

- Keep prescribed nitroglycerin tablets at the client's side so one can be taken at the onset of pain. *Anginal pain indicates myocardial ischemia. Nitroglycerin reduces cardiac work and may improve myocardial blood flow, relieving ischemia and pain.*

- Start oxygen at 4 to 6 L/min per nasal cannula or as prescribed. *Supplemental oxygen reduces myocardial hypoxia.*

- Space activities to allow rest between them. *Activity increases cardiac work and may precipitate angina. Spacing of activities allows the heart to recover.*

- Teach about prescribed medications to maintain myocardial perfusion and reduce cardiac work. Emphasize that long-acting nitrates, beta blockers, and calcium channel blockers are used to *prevent* anginal attacks, not to *treat* an acute attack. *It is important for the client to understand the purpose and use of prescribed drugs to maintain optimal myocardial perfusion.*

- Instruct to take sublingual nitroglycerin before engaging in activities that precipitate angina (e.g., climbing stairs, sexual intercourse). *This prophylactic dose of nitroglycerin helps maintain cardiac perfusion when increased work is anticipated, preventing ischemia and chest pain.*

- Encourage to implement and maintain a progressive exercise program under the supervision of the primary care provider or a cardiac rehabilitation professional. *Exercise slows the atherosclerotic process and helps develop collateral circulation to the heart muscle.*

- Refer to a smoking cessation program as indicated. *Nicotine causes vasoconstriction and increases the heart rate, decreasing myocardial perfusion and increasing cardiac workload.*

Risk for Ineffective Therapeutic Regimen Management

Denial may be strong in the client with angina pectoris. Because many people think of the heart as the locus of life itself, problems such as angina remind people of their mortality, an uncomfortable fact. Denial may lead to "forgetting" to take prescribed medications or to attempting activities that will precipitate angina. Some clients, by contrast, may become "cardiac cripples," afraid to engage in activities because of anticipated chest pain. Their inactivity may actually hasten the atherosclerotic process and inhibit collateral circulation development, worsening angina.

- Assess knowledge and understanding of angina. *Assessment allows tailoring of teaching and interventions to the needs of the client.*

- Teach about angina and atherosclerosis as needed, building on current knowledge base. *This can help the client understand that angina is a manageable disease and that pain can usually be controlled and the disease progress slowed.*

- Provide written and verbal instructions about prescribed medications and their use. *Written instructions reinforce teaching and are available to the client for future reference.*

- Stress the importance of taking chest pains seriously while maintaining a positive attitude. *Although it is vital to recognize the significance of chest pain and deal with it appropriately, it is also important to maintain a positive outlook.*

- Refer to a cardiac rehabilitation program or other organized activities and support groups for clients with coronary artery disease. *Programs such as these help the client develop risk factor management strategies, maintain a program of supervised activity, and gain coping skills.*

Home Care

Many clients with stable angina manage their pain effectively, continuing to live active and productive lives. To promote effective management of this disorder, include the following topics in teaching for home care.

- Coronary heart disease and the processes that cause chest pain, including the relationship between the pain and reduced blood flow to the heart muscle.
- Use and effects (desired and adverse) of prescribed medications; importance of not discontinuing medications abruptly.
- Nitroglycerine use for acute angina: Always carry several tablets (not the entire supply); prophylactic use before activities that often cause chest pain; take tablet at first indication of pain, rather than waiting to see if the pain develops; seek immediate medical assistance if three nitroglycerin tablets over 15 to 20 minutes do not relieve the pain.
- The importance of calling 911 or going to the emergency department immediately for unrelieved chest pain.
- Appropriate storage of nitroglycerin: This unstable compound needs to be stored in a cool, dry, dark place; no more than a 6-month supply should be kept on hand.

For the client who has undergone cardiac surgery, also include the following:
- Respiratory care, activity, and pain management.
- The importance of actively participating in rehabilitation.
- Manifestations of infection or other potential complications and their management.

The Client with Acute Myocardial Infarction

An **acute myocardial infarction (AMI),** necrosis (death) of myocardial cells, is a life-threatening event. If circulation to the affected myocardium is not promptly restored, loss of functional myocardium affects the heart's ability to maintain an effective cardiac output. This may ultimately lead to cardiogenic shock and death.

Heart disease remains the leading cause of death in the United States. Of the major heart diseases, myocardial infarction (MI) or *heart attack,* and other forms of ischemic heart disease cause the majority of deaths. Annually, approximately 650,000 people in the United States experience their first MI; another 450,000 suffer an MI subsequent to the initial one. Nearly 530,000 people died of coronary heart disease in 2000, with most of these deaths related to MI (NHLBI, 2002).

The majority of deaths from MI occur during the initial period after symptoms begin: approximately 60% within the first hour, and 40% prior to hospitalization. Heightening public awareness of the manifestations of MI, the importance of seeking immediate medical assistance, and training in cardiopulmonary resuscitation (CPR) techniques are vital to decrease deaths due to MI.

Myocardial infarction rarely occurs in clients without preexisting coronary heart disease. While no specific cause has been identified, the risk factors for MI are those for coronary heart disease: age, gender, heredity, race; smoking, obesity, hyperlipidemia, hypertension, diabetes, sedentary lifestyle, diet, and others.

Pathophysiology

Atherosclerotic plaque may form stable or unstable lesions. *Stable* lesions progress by gradually occluding the vessel lumen, whereas *unstable* (or *complicated*) lesions are prone to rupture and thrombus formation. Stable lesions often cause angina (discussed in the previous section); unstable lesions often lead to **acute coronary syndromes,** or acute ischemic heart diseases. Acute coronary syndromes include unstable angina, myocardial infarction, and sudden cardiac death (McCance & Huether, 2002).

Myocardial infarction occurs when blood flow to a portion of cardiac muscle is blocked, resulting in prolonged tissue ischemia and irreversible cell damage. Coronary occlusion is usually caused by ulceration or rupture of a complicated atherosclerotic lesion. When an atherosclerotic lesion ruptures or ulcerates, substances are released that stimulate platelet aggregation, thrombin generation, and local vasomotor tone. As a result, a thrombus (clot) forms, occluding the vessel and interrupting blood flow to the myocardium distal to the obstruction.

Cellular injury occurs when the cells are denied adequate oxygen and nutrients. When ischemia is prolonged, lasting more than 20 to 45 minutes, irreversible hypoxemic damage causes cellular death and tissue necrosis. Oxygen, glycogen, and ATP stores of ischemic cells are rapidly depleted. Cellular metabolism shifts to an anaerobic process, producing hydrogen ions and lactic acid. Cellular acidosis increases cells' vulnerability to further damage. Intracellular enzymes are released through damaged cell membranes into interstitial spaces.

Cellular acidosis, electrolyte imbalances, and hormones released in response to cellular ischemia affect impulse conduction and myocardial contractility. The risk of dysrhythmias increases, and myocardial contractility decreases, reducing stroke volume, cardiac output, blood pressure, and tissue perfusion.

The subendocardium suffers the initial damage, within 20 minutes of injury, because this area is the most susceptible to changes in coronary blood flow. If blood flow is restored at this point, the infarction is limited to subendocardial tissue (a *subendocardial* or *non Q wave infarction*). The damage progresses to the epicardium within one to six hours. When all layers of the myocardium are affected, it is known as a *transmural infarction.* A significant Q wave develops with a transmural infarction, so this also may be called a *Q wave MI.* Complications, such as heart failure, are more frequently associated with Q wave MIs; however, clients with non Q wave MIs frequently experience recurrent ischemia or subsequent MI within weeks or months of the event (Woods et al., 2000).

The necrotic, infarcted tissue is surrounded by regions of injured and ischemic tissues. Tissue in this ischemic area is potentially viable; restoration of blood flow minimizes the amount of tissue lost. This surrounding tissue also undergoes metabolic changes. It may be *stunned,* its contractility impaired for hours to days following reperfusion, or *hibernating,* a process that protects myocytes until perfusion is restored. *Myocardial remodeling* also may occur, with cellular hypertrophy and loss of contractility in regions distant from the infarction. Rapid restoration of blood flow limits these changes (McCance & Huether, 2002).

When a larger artery is compromised, *collateral vessels* connecting smaller arteries in the coronary system dilate to maintain blood flow to the cardiac muscle. The degree of collateral circulation helps determine the extent of myocardial damage from ischemia. Acute occlusion of a coronary artery without any collateral flow results in massive tissue damage and possible death. Progressive narrowing of the larger coronary arteries allows collateral vessels to develop and enlarge, meeting the demand for blood flow. Good collateral circulation can limit the size of an MI.

Myocardial infarction usually affects the left ventricle because it is the major "workhorse" of the heart; its muscle mass is greater, as are its oxygen demands.

Myocardial infarctions are described by the damaged area of the heart. The coronary artery that is occluded determines the area of damage. Occlusion of the left anterior descending (LAD) artery affects blood flow to the anterior wall of the left ventricle (an *anterior MI*) and part of the interventricular septum. Occlusion of the left circumflex artery (LCA) causes a *lateral MI*. *Right ventricular, inferior,* and *posterior infarcts* involve occlusions of the right coronary artery (RCA) and posterior descending artery (PDA). Occlusion of the left main coronary artery is the most devastating, causing ischemia of the entire left ventricle, and a grave prognosis. Identifying the infarct site helps predict possible complications and determine appropriate therapy.

Cocaine-Induced MI

Acute myocardial infarction may develop due to cocaine intoxication. Cocaine increases sympathetic nervous system activity by both increasing the release of catecholamines from central and peripheral stores and interfering with the reuptake of catecholamines. This increased catecholamine concentration stimulates the heart rate and increases its contractility, increases the automaticity of cardiac tissues and the risk of dysrhythmias, and causes vasoconstriction and hypertension. The client with cocaine-induced MI may present with an altered level of consciousness, confusion and restlessness, seizure activity, tachycardia, hypotension, increased respiratory rate, and respiratory crackles.

Manifestations

Pain is a classic manifestation of myocardial infarction. Chest pain due to MI is more severe than anginal pain. However, it is not the intensity of the chest pain that distinguishes MI from angina, but its duration and its continuous nature. The onset of pain is sudden and, usually, is not associated with activity. In fact, most MIs occur in the early morning. Clients with a history of angina may have more frequent anginal attacks in the days or weeks prior to an MI. Chest pain may be described as crushing and severe; as a pressure, heavy, or squeezing sensation; or as chest tightness or burning. The pain often begins in the center of the chest (*substernal*), and may radiate to the shoulders, neck, jaw, or arms. It lasts more than 15 to 20 minutes and is not relieved by rest or nitroglycerin.

Women and older adults often experience atypical chest pain, presenting with complaints of indigestion, heartburn, nausea, and vomiting. Up to 25% of clients with acute MI deny chest discomfort (Woods et al., 2000).

Compensatory mechanisms cause many of the other symptoms of MI. Sympathetic nervous system stimulation causes anxiety, tachycardia, and vasoconstriction. This results in cool, clammy, mottled skin. Pain and blood chemistry changes stimulate the respiratory center, causing tachypnea. The client often has a sense of impending doom and death. Tissue necrosis causes an inflammatory reaction that increases the white blood cell count and elevates the temperature. Serum cardiac enzyme levels rise as enzymes are released from necrotic cardiac cells.

Other manifestations may vary, depending on the location and amount of infarcted tissue. Hypertension, hypotension, or signs of heart failure may develop. Vagal stimulation may cause nausea and vomiting, bradycardia, and hypotension. Hiccuping may develop due to diaphagmatic irritation. If a large vessel is occluded, the first sign of MI may be sudden death. Typical manifestations of MI are listed in Table 8-3.

The risk of complications associated with myocardial infarction is related to the size and location of the MI.

Dysrhythmias

Dysrhythmias, disturbances or irregularities of heart rhythm, are the most frequent complication of MI. Dysrhythmias are discussed in detail in the next section of this chapter.

Infarcted tissue is *arrhythmogenic;* that is, it affects the generation and conduction of electrical impulses in the heart, increasing the risk of dysrhythmias. Premature ventricular contractions (PVCs) are common following an MI, developing in more than 90% of clients with an acute MI. While not dangerous in themselves, they may be predictive of more dangerous dysrhythmias, such as ventricular tachycardia or ventricular fibrillation (Woods et al., 2000). The risk of ventricular fibrillation is greatest the first hour after MI; it is a frequent cause of sudden cardiac death associated with acute MI. Its incidence declines with time. If the infarct affects a conduction pathway, electrical conduction may be affected. Any degree of atrioventricular (AV) block may occur following MI, especially when the anterior wall is infarcted. First-degree and Mobitz I (Wenckebach) blocks are most common, although complete heart block may develop. Bradydysrhythmias (abnormal slow rhythms) also may develop, particularly when the inferior wall of the ventricle is affected.

Pump Failure

Myocardial infarction reduces myocardial contractility, ventricular wall motion, and compliance. Impaired contractility and filling may produce heart failure. The risk of heart failure is greatest when large portions of the left ventricle are infarcted. Heart failure may be more severe with an anterior infarction. Loss of 20% to 30% of the left ventricular muscle mass may cause manifestations of left-sided heart failure, including dyspnea, fatigue, weakness, and respiratory crackles on auscultation. Inferior or right ventricular MI may lead to right-sided heart failure with manifestations, such as neck vein distention and peripheral edema. Hemodynamic monitoring is often initiated for clients with evidence of heart failure. Heart failure and its manifestations are discussed in greater depth in Chapter 9.

CARDIOGENIC SHOCK. *Cardiogenic shock,* impaired tissue perfusion due to pump failure, results when functioning myocardial muscle mass decreases by more than 40%. The heart is unable to pump enough blood to meet the needs of the body and maintain organ function. Low cardiac output, due to cardiogenic shock, also impairs perfusion of the coronary arteries and myocardium, further increasing tissue damage. Mortality from cardiogenic shock is greater than 70%, although this can be reduced by prompt intervention with revascularization procedures. See Chapter 40 for a more extensive discussion of cardiogenic shock.

Infarct Extension

Approximately 10% of clients experience extension or reinfarction in the area of the original infarction during the first 10 to 14 days after an MI. *Extension* of the MI is characterized by increased myocardial necrosis from continued blood flow impairment and ongoing injury. *Expansion* of the MI is described as a permanent expansion of the infarcted area from thinning and dilation of the muscle. Infarct extension and expansion may cause manifestations, such as continuing chest pain, hemodynamic compromise, and worsening heart failure.

Structural Defects

Necrotic muscle is replaced by scar tissue that is thinner than the ventricular muscle mass. This can lead to such complications as ventricular aneurysm, rupture of the interventricular septum or papillary muscle, and myocardial rupture. A *ventricular aneurysm* is an outpouching of the ventricular wall. It may develop when a large section of the ventricle is replaced by scar tissue. Because it does not contract during systole, stroke volume decreases. Blood may pool within the aneurysm, causing clots to form. Ischemia of the papillary muscle or chordae tendineae may cause structural damage leading to papillary muscle dysfunction or rupture. This affects AV valve function (usually the mitral valve), causing *regurgitation,* backflow of blood into the atria during systole. The interventricular septum may perforate or rupture due to ischemia and infarction. Myocardial rupture is a risk between four and seven days after MI, when the injured tissue is soft and weak. This potential complication of MI is often fatal.

Pericarditis

Tissue necrosis prompts an inflammatory response. *Pericarditis,* inflammation of the pericardial tissue surrounding the heart, may complicate AMI, usually within two to three days. Pericarditis causes chest pain that may be aching or sharp and stabbing, aggravated by movement or deep breathing. A *pericardial friction rub* may be heard on auscultation of heart sounds.

Dressler's syndrome, thought to be a hypersensitivity response to necrotic tissue or an autoimmune disorder, may develop days to weeks after AMI. It is a symptom complex characterized by fever, chest pain, and dyspnea. Dressler's syndrome may spontaneously resolve or recur over several months, causing significant discomfort and distress.

Collaborative Care

Immediate treatment goals for the MI client are to:
- Relieve chest pain.
- Reduce the extent of myocardial damage.
- Maintain cardiovascular stability.
- Decrease cardiac workload.
- Prevent complications.

Slowing the process of coronary heart disease and reducing the risk of future MI is a major long-term management goal for the client.

Rapid assessment and early diagnosis is important in treating AMI. "Time is muscle" is a medical truism for the client with AMI. The evolution of an AMI is dynamic: The quicker the artery is reopened (medically, surgically, or spontaneously), the more myocardium can be salvaged. Survival and long-term outcomes following AMI are improved by rapidly restoring blood flow to the "stunned" myocardium surrounding the infracted tissue, reducing myocardial oxygen demand and limiting the accumulation of toxic by-products of necrosis and reperfusion (Braunwald et al., 2001). The American Heart Association (AHA) recommends initiation of definitive treatment within one hour of entry into the health care system.

The major problem interfering with timely reperfusion is delay in seeking medical care following the onset of symptoms. Up to 44% of clients with symptoms of chest discomfort or pain wait more than four hours before seeking treatment. Many factors are cited as reasons for treatment delay, including advanced age, the perception of the seriousness of symptoms, denial, access to medical care, the availability of an emergency response system, and in-hospital delays (see the Nursing Research section below). Immediate evaluation of the client presenting with manifestations of myocardial infarction is essential to early diagnosis and treatment.

Diagnostic Tests

Diagnostic testing is used to establish the diagnosis of AMI.

Serum Cardiac Markers

Serum cardiac markers are proteins released from necrotic heart muscle. The proteins most specific for diagnosis of MI are the creatine phosphokinase (CK or CPK) and cardiacspecific troponins (see Table 8-5).

- *Creatine phosphokinase* is an important enzyme for cellular function found principally in cardiac and skeletal muscle and the brain. CK levels rise rapidly with damage to these tissues, appearing in the serum 4 to 6 hours after AMI, peaking within 12 to 24 hours, and then declining over the next 48 to 72 hours. The CK level correlates with the size of the infarction; the greater the amount of infarcted tissue, the higher the serum CK level.

- CK-MB (also called MB-bands) is a subset of CK specific to cardiac muscle. This isoenzyme of CK is considered the most sensitive indicator of MI. Elevated CK alone is not specific for MI; elevated CK-MB greater than 5% is considered a positive indicator of MI. CK-MB levels do not normally rise with chest pain from angina or causes other than MI.

- Cardiac muscle troponins, *cardiac-specific troponin T (cT_nT)* and *cardiac-specific troponin I (cT_nI)*, are proteins released during myocardial infarction that are sensitive indicators of myocardial damage. These proteins are part of the actin-myocin unit in cardiac muscle and, normally, are not detectable in the blood. With necrosis of cardiac muscle, troponins are released and blood levels rise. The specificity of cT_nT and cT_nI to cardiac muscle necrosis makes these markers particularly useful when skeletal muscle trauma contributes to elevated CK levels (e.g., when CPR has been performed or traumatic injury occurred at the time of the MI). They are sensitive enough to detect very small infarctions that do not cause significant CK elevation. Both cT_nT and cT_nI remain in the blood for 10 to 14 days after an MI, making them useful to diagnose MI when medical treatment is delayed.

Serum levels of cardiac markers are ordered on admission and for three succeeding days. Serial blood levels help establish the diagnosis and determine the extent of myocardial damage.

Other laboratory tests may include the following:

- *Myoglobin* is one of the first cardiac markers to be detectable in the blood after an MI. It is released within a few hours of symptom onset. Its lack of specificity to cardiac muscle and rapid excretion (blood levels return to normal within 24 hours) limit its use, however (Braunwald et al., 2001).

- *Complete blood count (CBC)* shows an elevated white blood cell (WBC) count due to inflammation of the injured myocardium. The *erythrocyte sedimentation rate (ESR)* also rises because of inflammation.

- *Arterial blood gases* (ABGs) may be ordered to assess blood oxygen levels and acid-base balance.

Electrocardiography, echocardiography, and myocardial nuclear scans are the most common diagnostic tests performed when AMI is suspected. With the exception of the ECG, the timing of these tests depends on the client's immediate condition. Hemodynamic monitoring may be initiated in the unstable client following MI.

- The *electrocardiogram* reflects changes in conduction due to myocardial ischemia and necrosis. Characteristic ECG changes seen in AMI include T wave inversion, elevation of the ST segment, and formation of a Q wave. Ischemic changes in the heart are seen as depression of the ST segment or inversion of the T wave. With myocardial injury, elevation of the ST segment occurs. Significant Q wave development indicates a transmural, or full-thickness infarction. Myocardial damage can be localized using the 12-lead ECG. See the next section of this chapter for more information about ECGs.

• *Echocardiography* is a noninvasive test to evaluate cardiac wall motion and left ventricular function. Images are produced as ultrasound waves strike cardiac structures and are reflected back through a transducer. Echocardiography can be done at the bedside.

• *Radionuclide imaging* may be done to evaluate myocardial perfusion. These studies cannot differentiate between an acute MI and old scar tissue, but do help identify the specific area of myocardial ischemia and damage. Several isotopes may be used. Thallium-201 collects in normally perfused myocardium; ischemic areas appear blue or as "cold" spots when the heart is scanned for radioactivity. In contrast, technetium-99m pyrophosphate, another commonly used radioisotope, accumulates in ischemic tissue and appears red, or "hot."

• *Hemodynamic monitoring* may be initiated when AMI significantly affects cardiac output and hemodynamic status.

Table 8-5. Cardiac Markers

Marker	Normal Level	Primary Tissue Location	Significance of Elevation	Changes Occuring with MI		
				Appears	Peaks	Duration
CK (CPK)	Male: 12 to 80 U/L Female: 10 to 70 U/L	Cardiac muscle, skeletal muscle, brain	Injury to muscle cells	3 to 6 hours	12 to 24 hours	24 to 48 hours
CK-MB	0% to 3% of total CK	Cardiac muscle	MI, cardiac ischemia, myocarditis, cardiac contusion, defibrillation	4 to 8 hours	18 to 24 hours	72 hours
cT_nT	<0.2 mcg/L	Cardiac muscle	Acute MI, unstable angina	2 to 4 hours	24 to 36 hours	10 to 14 days
cT_nI	<3.1 mcg/L	Cardiac muscle	Acute MI, unstable angina	2 to 4 hours	24 to 36 hours	7 to 10 days

Medications

Aspirin, a platelet inhibitor, is now considered an essential part of treating AMI. A 160 to 325 mg aspirin tablet is given by emergency personnel, with the instructions that it is to be chewed (for buccal absorption). This initial dose is followed by a daily oral dose of 160 to 325 mg of aspirin.

Other medications are used to help reduce oxygen demand and increase oxygen supply. Thrombolytic agents, analgesics, and antidysrhythmic agents are among the principal classes of drugs used.

Thrombolytic Therapy

Thrombolytic agents, drugs that dissolve or break up blood clots, are first-line drugs used to treat acute MI. These drugs activate the fibrinolytic system to lyse or destroy the clot, restoring blood flow to the obstructed artery. Early thrombolytic administration (within the first six hours of MI onset) limits infarct size, reduces heart damage, and improves outcomes. Activation of the fibrinolytic system can cause multiple complications; approximately 0.5% to 5% of clients receiving thrombolytic drugs experience serious bleeding complications. Not every client is a candidate for thrombolytic therapy; for example, it is contraindicated in clients with known bleeding disorders, history of cerebrovascular disease, uncontrolled hypertension, pregnancy, or recent trauma or surgery of the head or spine (Tierney et al., 2001).

Four thrombolytic agents are commonly used today. Among the four, little difference in effectiveness has been demonstrated; there are, however, big differences in cost. Streptokinase, a biologic agent derived from group C *Streptococcus* organisms, is the least expensive of the drugs. Its primary drawback is the risk of a severe hypersensitivity reaction, including anaphylaxis. Streptokinase is administered by intravenous infusion. Anisoylated plasminogen streptokinase activator complex (APSAC) is a related drug that can be administered by bolus over two to five minutes. It has many of the same effects as streptokinase, but is considerably more expensive. Tissue plasminogen activator (t-PA) and reteplase are more effective in reestablishing myocardial perfusion, especially when the pain developed more than three hours previously. These drugs, however, are the most expensive. Nursing care of the client receiving a thrombolytic agent is outlined on the next page.

Analgesia

Pain relief is vital in treating the client with AMI. Pain stimulates the sympathetic nervous system, increasing the heart rate and blood pressure and, in turn, myocardial workload. Sublingual nitroglycerin may be given (up to three 0.4-mg doses at 5-minute intervals). In addition to pain relief, nitroglycerin may decrease myocardial oxygen demand and increase the supply of oxygen to the myocardium by dilating collateral vessels. Morphine sulfate is the drug of choice for pain and sedation. Following an initial intravenous dose of 4 to 8 mg, small doses (2 to 4 mg) may be repeated intravenously every five minutes until pain is relieved. It is important to assess frequently for pain relief and possible adverse effects of analgesia, such as excessive sedation. Antianxiety agents such as diazepam (Valium) may also be administered to promote rest.

Antidysrhythmics

Dysrhythmias are a common complication of AMI, particularly in the first 12 to 24 hours. Antidysrhythmic medications are used as needed to treat dysrhythmias. They also may be given prophylactically to prevent dysrhythmias. Ventricular dysrhythmias are treated with a class I or class III antidysrhythmic drug (see the Medication Administration Table on page 852). Symptomatic bradycardia (bradycardia with associated hypotension and other signs of low cardiac output) is treated with intravenous atropine, 0.5 to 1 mg. Intravenous verapamil or the short-acting beta blocker esmolol (Brevibloc) may be ordered to treat atrial fibrillation or other supraventricular tachydysrhythmias.

Other Medications

Beta blockers such as propranolol (Inderal), atenolol (Tenormin), and metoprolol (Lopressor) reduce pain, limit infarct size, and decrease the incidence of serious ventricular dysrhythmias in AMI. These drugs decrease the heart rate, reducing cardiac work and myocardial oxygen demand. Initial doses are given intravenously. Oral beta blocker therapy is continued to reduce the risk of reinfarction and death related to cardiovascular causes (Braunwald et al., 2001).

Angiotensin-converting enzyme (ACE) inhibitors also reduce mortality associated with AMI. These drugs reduce ventricular remodeling following an MI, reducing the risk for subsequent heart failure. They also may reduce the risk of reinfarction (Braunwald et al., 2001).

Intravenous nitroglycerin may be administered for the first 24 to 48 hours to reduce myocardial work. Nitroglycerin is a peripheral and arterial vasodilator that reduces afterload. It dilates coronary arteries and collateral channels in the heart, increasing coronary blood flow to save myocardial tissue at risk. Nitrates may, however, cause reflex tachycardia or excessive hypotension, so close monitoring is necessary during administration. See Table 8-4 for the nursing implications of these drugs.

Anticoagulants and other antiplatelet medications often are prescribed to maintain coronary artery patency following thrombolysis or a revascularization procedure. Abciximab (ReoPro) suppresses platelet aggregation and reduces the risk of reocclusion following angioplasty. It also improves vessel opening with thrombolytic therapy, permitting lower doses of thrombolytic drugs (Lehne, 2001). Standard or low-molecular-weight heparin preparations often are given to clients with AMI. Heparin helps establish and maintain patency of the affected coronary artery. It also is used, along with long-term warfarin, to prevent systemic or pulmonary embolism in clients with significant left ventricular impairment or atrial fibrillation following AMI.

Clients with pump failure and hypotension may receive intravenous dopamine, a vasopressor. At low doses (less than 5 mg/kg/min), it improves blood flow to the kidneys, preventing renal ischemia and possible acute renal failure. With increasing doses, dopamine increases myocardial contractility and causes vasoconstriction, improving blood pressure and cardiac output.

Antilipemic agents are used for the client with hyperlipidemia. A stool softener, such as docusate sodium, is prescribed to maintain normal bowel function and reduce straining.

Medical Management

The client with a suspected or confirmed MI is monitored continuously. Care is provided in the intensive coronary care unit for the first 24 to 48 hours, after which time less intensive monitoring (e.g., telemetry) may be required. An intravenous line is established to allow rapid administration of emergency medications.

Bed rest is prescribed for the first 12 hours to reduce the cardiac workload. The bedside commode generally is allowed; studies have shown this to be less stressful than using a bedpan. If the client's condition is stable, sitting in a chair at the bedside is permitted after 12 hours. Activities are gradually increased as tolerated. A quiet, calm environment with limited outside stimuli is preferred. Visitors are limited to promote rest. Oxygen is administered by nasal cannula at 2 to 5 L/min to improve oxygenation of the myocardium and other tissues.

A liquid diet is often prescribed for the first 4 to 12 hours to reduce gastric distention and myocardial work. Following that, a low-fat, low-cholesterol, reduced-sodium diet is allowed.

Sodium restrictions may be lifted after two to three days if no evidence of heart failure is present. Small, frequent feedings are often recommended. Drinks containing caffeine, and very hot and cold foods may also be limited.

Revascularization Procedures

Many clients with AMI are treated with immediate or early percutaneous coronary revascularization (PCR), such as angioplasty and stent placement. PCR may follow thrombolytic therapy or be used in place of thrombolytic therapy to restore blood flow to ischemic myocardium. When compared with thrombolytic therapy, prompt PCR reduces hospital mortality (Braunwald et al., 2001). In some cases, CABG surgery may be performed. The choice of procedure depends on the client's age and immediate condition, the time elapsed from the onset of manifestations, and the extent of myocardial disease and damage. These procedures and related nursing care are covered in more depth in the preceding section on angina.

Other Invasive Procedures

For clients with large MIs and evidence of pump failure, invasive devices may be used to temporarily take over the function of the heart, allowing the injured myocardium to heal. The intra-aortic balloon pump is widely used to augment cardiac output. Ventricular assist devices are indicated for clients requiring more or longer term artificial support than the intra-aortic balloon pump provides.

Intra-Aortic Balloon Pump

The *intra-aortic balloon pump (IABP),* also called intra-aortic balloon counterpulsation, is a mechanical circulatory support device that may be used after cardiac surgery or to treat cardiogenic shock following AMI. The IABP temporarily supports cardiac function, allowing the heart gradually to recover by decreasing myocardial workload and oxygen demand and increasing perfusion of the coronary arteries.

A catheter with a 30 to 40 mL balloon is introduced into the aorta, usually via the femoral artery. The balloon catheter is connected to a console that regulates the inflation and deflation of the balloon. The IABP catheter inflates during diastole, increasing perfusion of the coronary and renal arteries, and deflates during systole, decreasing afterload and cardiac workload. The inflation–deflation sequence is triggered by the ECG pattern. During the most acute period, the balloon inflates and deflates with each heart beat (1:1 ratio), providing maximal assistance to the heart. As the client's condition improves, the IABP is weaned to inflate–deflate at varying intervals (e.g., 1:2, 1:4, 1:8). This provides a continually decreasing amount of support as the heart muscle recovers. When mechanical assistance is no longer required, the IABP catheter is removed.

Ventricular Assist Devices

Use of *ventricular assist devices (VADs)* to aid the failing heart is becoming more common with advances in technology. Whereas the IABP can supplement cardiac output by approximately 10% to 15%, the VAD temporarily takes partial or complete control of cardiac function, depending on the type of device used. VADs may be used as temporary or complete assist in AMI and cardiogenic shock when there is a chance for recovery of normal heart function after a period of cardiac rest. The device also may be used as a bridge to heart transplant. Nursing care for the client with a VAD is supportive and includes assessing hemodynamic status and for complications associated with the device. Clients with VAD are at considerable risk for infection; strict aseptic technique is used with all invasive catheters and dressing changes. Pneumonia also is a risk due to immobility and ventilatory support. Mechanical failure of the VAD is a life-threatening event that requires immediate intervention (Urden, Stacy, & Lough 2002).

Cardiac Rehabilitation

Cardiac rehabilitation is a long-term program of medical evaluation, exercise, risk factor modification, education, and counseling designed to limit the physical and psychological effects of cardiac illness and improve the client's quality of life (Woods et al., 2000). Cardiac rehabilitation begins with admission for a cardiac event, such as AMI or a revascularization procedure. Phase one of the program is the inpatient phase. A thorough assessment of the client's history, current status, risk factors, and motivation is obtained. During this phase, activity progresses from bed rest to independent performance of activities of daily living (ADLs) and ambulation within the facility. Both subjective and objective responses to increasing activity levels are evaluated. Excess fatigue, shortness of breath, chest pain, tachypnea, tachycardia, or cool, clammy skin indicate activity intolerance. Phase two, immediate outpatient cardiac rehabilitation, begins within three weeks of the cardiac event. The goals for the outpatient program are to increase activity level, participation, and capacity; improve psychosocial status and treat anxiety or depression; and provide education and support for risk factor reduction. Continuation programs, phase three of cardiac rehabilitation, are directed at providing a transition to independent exercise and exercise maintenance. During this final phase, the client may "check in" every three months to evaluate risk factors, quality of life, and exercise habits (Woods et al., 2000).

Nursing Care

Health Promotion

Health promotion activities to prevent acute myocardial infarction are those outlined for coronary heart disease and angina in previous sections of this chapter. In addition, discuss risk factor management, use of prescribed medications, and cardiac rehabilitation to reduce the risk of complications or future infarctions.

Assessment

Nursing assessment for the client with AMI must be both timely and ongoing. Assessment data related to AMI includes the following:

- *Health history:* complaints of chest pain, including its location, intensity, character, radiation, and timing; associated symptoms such as nausea, heartburn, shortness of breath, and anxiety; treatment measures taken since onset of pain; past medical history, especially cardiac related; chronic diseases; current medications and any known allergies to medications; smoking history and use of recreational drugs and alcohol.

- *Physical examination:* general appearance including obvious signs of distress; vital signs; peripheral pulses; skin color, temperature, moisture; level of consciousness; heart and breath sounds; cardiac rhythm (on beside monitor); bowel sounds, abdominal tenderness.

Nursing Diagnoses and Interventions

Priorities of nursing care include relieving chest pain, reducing cardiac work, and promoting oxygenation. Psychosocial support is especially important, because an acute myocardial infarction can be devastating, bringing the client face-to-face with his or her own mortality for the first time.

Acute Pain

Chest pain occurs when the oxygen supply to the heart muscle does not meet the demand. Myocardial ischemia and infarction cause pain, as does reperfusion of an ischemic area following thrombolytic therapy or emergent PTCA. Pain stimulates the sympathetic nervous system, increasing cardiac work. Pain relief is a priority of care for the client with AMI.

- Assess for verbal and nonverbal signs of pain. Document characteristics and the intensity of the pain, using a standard pain scale. Verify nonverbal indicators of pain with the client. *Frequent, careful pain assessment allows early intervention to reduce the risk of further damage. Pain is a subjective experience; its expression may vary with location and intensity, previous experiences, and cultural and social background. Pain scales provide an objective tool for measuring pain and a way to assess pain relief or reduction.*

- Administer oxygen at 2 to 5 L/min per nasal cannula. *Supplemental oxygen increases oxygen supply to the myocardium, decreasing ischemia and pain.*

- Promote physical and psychologic rest. Provide information and emotional support. *Rest decreases cardiac workload and sympathetic nervous system stimulation, promoting comfort. Information and emotional support help decrease anxiety and provide psychologic rest.*

- Titrate intravenous nitroglycerin as ordered to relieve chest pain, maintaining a systolic blood pressure greater than 100 mmHg. *Nitroglycerin decreases chest pain by dilating peripheral vessels, reducing cardiac work, and dilating coronary vessels, including collateral channels, improving blood flow to ischemic tissue.*

- Administer 2 to 4 mg morphine by intravenous push for chest pain as needed. *Morphine is an effective narcotic analgesic for chest pain. It decreases pain and anxiety, acts as a venodilator, and decreases the respiratory rate. The resulting reduction in preload and sympathetic nervous system stimulation reduces cardiac work and oxygen consumption.*

Ineffective Tissue Perfusion

Cardiac muscle damage affects its compliance, contractility, and the cardiac output. The extent of the effect on tissue perfusion depends on the location and amount of damage. Anterior wall infarcts have a greater effect on cardiac output than do right ventricular infarcts. Infarcted muscle also increases the risk for cardiac dysrhythmias, which can also affect the delivery of blood and oxygen to the tissues.

- Assess and document vital signs. Report increases in heart rate and changes in rhythm, blood pressure, and respiratory rate. *Decreased cardiac output activates compensatory mechanisms that may cause tachycardia and vasoconstriction, increasing cardiac work.*

- Assess for changes in level of consciousness (LOC); decreased urine output; moist, cool, pale, mottled or cyanotic skin; dusky or cyanotic mucous membranes and nail beds; diminished to absent peripheral pulses; delayed capillary refill. *These are manifestations of impaired tissue perfusion. A change in LOC is often the first manifestation of altered perfusion because brain tissue and cerebral function depends on a continuous supply of oxygen.*

- Auscultate heart and breath sounds. Note abnormal heart sounds (e.g., an S_3 or S_4 gallop or a murmur) or adventitious lung sounds. *Abnormal heart sounds or adventitious lung sounds may indicate impaired cardiac filling or output, increasing the risk for decreased tissue perfusion.*

- Monitor ECG rhythm continuously. *Dysrhythmias can further impair cardiac output and tissue perfusion.*

- Monitor oxygen saturation levels. Administer oxygen as ordered. Obtain and assess ABGs as indicated. *Oxygen saturation is an indicator of gas exchange, tissue perfusion, and* the effectiveness of oxygen administration. ABGs provide a more precise measurement of blood oxygen levels and allow assessment of acid-base balance.

- Administer antidysrhythmic medications as needed. *Dysrhy-thmias affect tissue perfusion by altering cardiac output.*

- Obtain serial CK, isoenzyme, and troponin levels as ordered. *Levels of cardiac markers, CK isoenzymes in particular, correlate with the extent of myocardial damage.*

- Plan for invasive hemodynamic monitoring. *Hemodynamic monitoring facilitates AMI management and treatment evaluation by providing a means of assessing pressures in the systemic and pulmonary arteries, the relationship between oxygen supply and demand, cardiac output, and cardiac index.*

Ineffective Coping

Coping mechanisms help a person deal with a life-threatening event or with acute changes in health. However, certain coping mechanisms may be detrimental to restoring health, particularly if the client relies on them for a prolonged period. Denial, for example, is a common coping mechanism among post–MI clients. In the initial stages, denial can reduce anxiety. Continued denial, however, can interfere with learning and compliance with treatment.

- Establish an environment of caring and trust. Encourage the client to express feelings. *Establishing a trusting nurse–client relationship provides a safe environment for the client to discuss feelings of helplessness, powerlessness, anxiety, and hopelessness. The nurse may then be able to provide additional resources to meet the client's needs.*

- Accept denial as a coping mechanism, but do not reinforce it. *Denial may initially help by diminishing the psychological threat to health, decreasing anxiety. However, its prolonged use can interfere with acceptance of reality and cooperation, possibly delaying treatment and hindering recovery.*

- Note aggressive behaviors, hostility, or anger. Document any failure to comply with treatments. *These signs can indicate anxiety and denial.*

- Help the client identify positive coping skills used in the past (e.g., problem-solving skills, verbalization of feelings, asking for help, prayer). Reinforce use of positive coping behaviors. *Coping behaviors that have been successful in the past can help the client deal with the current situation. These familiar methods can decrease feelings of powerlessness.*

- Provide opportunities for the client to make decisions about the plan of care, as possible. *This promotes self-confidence and independence. Participating in care planning gives the client a sense of control and the opportunity to use positive coping skills.*

- Provide privacy for the client and significant other to share their questions and concerns. *Privacy provides an opportunity for the client and partner to share their feelings and fears, offer support and encouragement to one another, relieve anxiety, and establish effective coping methods.*

Fear

The fear of death and disability can be a paralyzing emotion that adversely affects the client's recovery from acute myocardial infarction.

- Identify the client's level of fear, noting verbal and nonverbal signs. *This information enables the nurse to plan appropriate interventions. Clients may not voice concerns; attention to nonverbal indicators is important. Controlling fear helps decrease sympathetic nervous system responses and catecholamine release that may increase feelings of fear and anxiety.*

- Acknowledge the client's perception of the situation. Allow to verbalize concerns. *A sudden change in health status causes anxiety and fear of the unknown. Verbalizing these fears may help the client cope with change and allow the health care team to provide information and correct misconceptions.*
- Encourage questions and provide consistent, factual answers. Repeat information as needed. *Accurate and consistent information can reduce fear. Honest explanations help strengthen the client-nurse relationship and help the client develop realistic expectations. Anxiety and fear decrease the ability to concentrate and retain information; therefore, information may need to be repeated.*
- Encourage self-care. Allow the client to make decisions regarding the plan of care. *This promotes personal responsibility for health and allows some control over the situation. Clients' confidence increases as their dependence decreases.*
- Administer antianxiety medications as ordered. *These medications promote rest and relaxation and decrease feelings of anxiety, which may act as barriers to health restoration.*
- Teach nonpharmacologic methods of stress reduction (e.g., relaxation techniques, mental imagery, music therapy, breathing exercises, meditation, massage). *Stress management techniques can help reduce tension and anxiety, provide a sense of control, and enhance coping skills.*

Home Care

Cardiac rehabilitation begins with admission to the health care facility and continues through the inpatient stay and after discharge into the rehabilitative period. The emphasis is on realistic application of information to maintain lifestyle changes.

Assessing readiness to learn is an important first step in preparing for home care. The client in strong denial may not identify any relevance to the information being taught. Evaluate ability to learn, assessing physiologic and psychologic health, beliefs regarding personal responsibility for health, and expectations of the health care system. Also assess developmental level, ability to perform psychomotor skills, cognitive function, learning disabilities, existing knowledge base, and the influence of previous learning experiences. Provide written material to supplement teaching and encourage questions.

Include the following topics in teaching for home care.

- The normal anatomy and physiology of the heart, and the specific area of heart damage
- The process of CHD and implications of MI
- Purposes and side effects of prescribed medications
- The importance of complying with the medical regimen and cardiac rehabilitation program and of keeping follow-up appointments
- Information about community resources, such as the local chapter of the American Heart Association

After discharge, follow up by telephone within one week and periodically thereafter during the recovery period. Provide telephone numbers of resource personnel who are available to respond to questions and concerns after discharge. Because the client who has had an MI is at high risk for sudden cardiac death, encourage family members to learn CPR and provide information about community resources for CPR training.

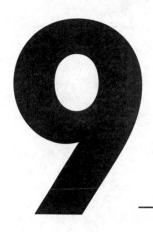

Nursing Care of Clients with Cardiac Disorders

Cardiac disorders affect the structure and/or function of the heart. These disorders interfere with the heart's primary purpose: to pump enough blood to meet the body's demand for oxygen and nutrients. Disruptions in cardiac function affect the functioning of other organs and tissues, potentially leading to organ system failure and death.

Heart failure is the most common cardiac disorder. Other cardiac disorders discussed in this chapter include structural cardiac disorders, such as valve disorders and cardiomyopathy, and inflammatory cardiac disorders, such as endocarditis and pericarditis. Before continuing with this chapter, please review the heart's anatomy and physiology and nursing assessment in Chapter 7.

Heart Failure

Heart failure, the inability of the heart to pump enough blood to meet the metabolic demands of the body, is the end result of many conditions. Frequently, it is a long-term effect of coronary heart disease and myocardial infarction when left ventricular damage is extensive enough to impair cardiac output (see Chapter 8). Other diseases of the heart may also cause heart failure, including structural and inflammatory disorders. In normal hearts, failure can result from excessive demands placed on the heart. Heart failure may be acute or chronic.

The Client with Heart Failure

As mentioned, heart failure is the inability of the heart to function as a pump to meet the needs of the body. As a result, cardiac output falls, leading to decreased tissue perfusion. The body initially adjusts to reduced cardiac output by activating inherent compensatory mechanisms to restore tissue perfusion. These normal mechanisms may result in vascular congestion—and hence, the commonly used term *congestive heart failure (CHF)*. As these mechanisms are exhausted, heart failure ensues, with increased morbidity and mortality.

Heart failure is a disorder of cardiac function. It frequently is due to *impaired myocardial contraction,* which may result from coronary heart disease and myocardial ischemia or infarct or from a primary cardiac muscle disorder, such as cardiomyopathy or myocarditis. Structural cardiac disorders, such as valve disorders or congenital heart defects, and hypertension can also lead to heart failure when the heart muscle is damaged by the long-standing *excessive workload* associated with these conditions. Other clients without a primary abnormality of myocardial function may present with manifestations of heart failure due to *acute excess demands* placed on the myocardium, such as volume overload, hyperthyroidism, and massive pulmonary embolus. Hypertension and coronary heart disease are the leading causes of heart failure in the United States. The high prevalence of hypertension in African-Americans contributes significantly to their risk for and incidence of heart failure.

Nearly 5 million people in the United States are currently living with heart failure; approximately 550,000 new cases of heart failure are diagnosed annually (American Heart Association [AHA], 2001). Its incidence and prevalence increase with age: Less than 5% of people between ages 55 and 64 have heart failure, whereas 6% to 10% of people older than 65 are affected (Hunt et al., 2001). The prognosis for a client with heart failure depends on its underlying cause and how effectively precipitating factors can be treated. Most clients with heart failure die within eight years of the diagnosis. The risk for sudden cardiac death is dramatically increased, occurring at a rate six to nine times that of the general population (AHA, 2001).

Physiology Review

The mechanical pumping action of cardiac muscle propels the blood it receives to the pulmonary and systemic vascular systems for reoxygenation and delivery to the tissues. *Cardiac output (CO)* is the amount of blood pumped from the ventricles in one minute. Cardiac output is used to assess cardiac performance, especially left ventricular function. Effective cardiac output depends on adequate functional muscle mass and the ability of the ventricles to work together. Cardiac output normally is regulated by the oxygen needs of the body: As oxygen use increases, cardiac output increases to maintain cellular function. *Cardiac reserve* is the ability of the heart to increase CO to meet metabolic demand. Ventricular damage reduces the cardiac reserve.

Cardiac output is a product of heart rate and stroke volume. *Heart rate* affects cardiac output by controlling the number of ventricular contractions per minute. It is influenced by the autonomic nervous system, catecholamines, and thyroid hormones. Activation of a stress response (e.g., hypovolemia or fear) stimulates the sympathetic nervous system, increasing the heart rate and its contractility. Elevated heart rates increase cardiac output. Very rapid heart rates, however, shorten ventricular filling time (diastole), reducing stroke volume and cardiac output. On the other hand, a slow heart rate reduces cardiac output simply because of fewer cardiac cycles.

Stroke volume is the volume of blood ejected with each heartbeat; it is determined by preload, afterload, and myocardial contractility. *Preload* is the volume of blood in the ventricles at end-diastole (just prior to contraction). The blood in the ventricles exerts pressure on the ventricle walls, stretching muscle fibers. The greater the blood volume, the greater force with which the ventricle contracts to expel the blood. Enddiastolic volume (EDV) depends on the amount of blood returning to the ventricles (*venous return*), and the distensibility or stiffness of the ventricles (*compliance*).

Afterload is the force needed to eject blood into the circulation. This force must be great enough to overcome arterial pressures within the pulmonary and systemic vascular systems. The right ventricle must generate enough force to open the pulmonary valve and eject its blood into the pulmonary artery. The left ventricle ejects its blood into the systemic circulation by overcoming the arterial resistance behind the aortic valve. Increased systemic vascular resistance increases afterload, impairing stroke volume and increasing myocardial work.

Contractility is the natural ability of cardiac muscle fibers to shorten during systole. Contractility is necessary to overcome arterial pressures and eject blood during systole. Impaired contractility affects cardiac output, by reducing stroke volume. The *ejection fraction (EF)* is the percentage of blood in the ventricle that is ejected during systole. A normal ejection fraction is approximately 60%.

Pathophysiology

When the heart begins to fail, mechanisms are activated to compensate for the impaired function and maintain the cardiac output. The primary compensatory mechanisms are (1) the Frank Starling mechanism; (2) neuroendocrine responses including activation of the sympathetic nervous system and the renin-angiotensin system; and (3) myocardial hypertrophy.

Decreased cardiac output initially stimulates aortic baroreceptors, which in turn stimulate the sympathetic nervous system (SNS). SNS stimulation produces both cardiac and vascular responses through the release of norepinephrine. Norepinephrine increases heart rate and contractility by stimulating cardiac beta receptors. Cardiac output improves as both heart rate and stroke volume increase. Norepinephrine also causes arterial and venous vasoconstriction, increasing venous return to the heart. Increased venous return increases ventricular filling and myocardial stretch, increasing the force of contraction (the Frank-Starling mechanism). Overstretching the muscle fibers past their physiologic limit results in an ineffective contraction.

Blood flow is redistributed to the brain and the heart to maintain perfusion of these vital organs. Decreased renal perfusion causes renin to be released from the kidneys. Activation of the renin-angiotensin system produces additional vasoconstriction and stimulates the adrenal cortex to produce aldosterone and the posterior pituitary to release antidiuretic hormone (ADH). Aldosterone stimulates sodium reabsorption in renal tubules, promoting water retention. ADH acts on the distal tubule to inhibit water excretion and causes vasoconstriction. The effect of these hormones is significant vasoconstriction and salt and water retention, with a resulting increase in vascular volume. Increased ventricular filling increases the force of contraction, improving cardiac output. The increased vascular volume and venous return also increase atrial pressures, stimulating the release of an additional hormone, *atrial natriuretic factor (ANF)* or *atriopeptin*. Atrial natriuetic factor balances the effects of the other hormones to a certain extent, promoting sodium and water excretion and inhibiting the release of norepinephrine, renin, and ADH. This hormone is thought to be a natural preventive that delays severe cardiac decompensation.

Ventricular remodeling occurs as the heart chambers and myocardium adapt to fluid volume and pressure increases. The chambers dilate to accommodate excess fluid resulting from increased vascular volume and incomplete emptying. Initially, this additional stretch causes more effective contractions. *Ventricular hypertrophy* occurs as existing cardiac muscle cells enlarge, increasing their contractile elements (actin and myosin) and force of contraction.

Although these responses may help in the short-term regulation of cardiac output, it is now recognized that they hasten the deterioration of cardiac function. The onset of heart failure is heralded by *decompensation,* the loss of effective compensation. Heart failure progresses due to the very mechanisms that initially maintained circulatory stability.

The rapid heart rate shortens diastolic filling time, compromises coronary artery perfusion, and increases myocardial oxygen demand. Resulting ischemia further impairs cardiac output. Beta-receptors in the heart become less sensitive to continued SNS stimulation, decreasing heart rate and contractility. As the beta-receptors become less sensitive, norepinephrine stores in the cardiac muscle become depleted. In contrast, alpha-receptors on peripheral blood vessels become increasingly sensitive to persistent stimulation, promoting vasoconstriction and increasing afterload and cardiac work.

Initially, ventricular hypertrophy and dilation increase cardiac output, but chronic distention causes the ventricular wall eventually to thin and degenerate. The purpose of hypertrophy is thus defeated. In addition, chronic overloading of the dilated ventricle eventually stretches the fibers beyond the optimal point for effective contraction. The ventricles continue to dilate to accommodate the excess fluid, but the heart loses the ability to contract forcefully. The heart muscle may eventually become so large that the coronary blood supply is inadequate, causing ischemia.

Chronic distention exhausts atrial stores of ANF. The effects of norepinephrine, renin, and ADH prevail, and the renin-angiotensin pathway is continually stimulated. This mechanism ultimately raises the hemodynamic stress on the heart by increasing both preload and afterload. As heart function deteriorates, less blood is delivered to the tissues and to the heart itself. Ischemia and necrosis of the myocardium further weaken the already failing heart, and the cycle repeats.

In normal hearts, the cardiac reserve allows the heart to adjust its output to meet metabolic needs of the body, increasing the cardiac output by up to five times the basal level during exercise. Clients with heart failure have minimal to no cardiac reserve. At rest, they may be unaffected; however, any stressor (e.g., exercise, illness) taxes their ability to meet the demand for oxygen and nutrients. Manifestations of activity intolerance when the person is at rest indicate a critical level of cardiac decompensation.

Classifications

Heart failure is commonly classified in several different ways, depending on the underlying pathology. Classifications include systolic versus diastolic failure, left-sided versus right-sided failure, high-output versus low-output failure, and acute versus chronic failure.

Systolic Versus Diastolic Failure

Systolic failure occurs when the ventricle fails to contract adequately to eject a sufficient blood volume into the arterial system. Systolic function is affected by loss of myocardial cells due to ischemia and infarction, cardiomyopathy, or inflammation. The manifestations of systolic failure are those of decreased cardiac output: weakness, fatigue, and decreased exercise tolerance.

Diastolic failure results when the heart cannot completely relax in diastole, disrupting normal filling. Passive diastolic filling decreases, increasing the importance of atrial contraction to preload. Diastolic dysfunction results from decreased ventricular compliance due to hypertrophic and cellular changes and impaired relaxation of the heart muscle. Its manifestations result from increased pressure and congestion behind the ventricle: shortness of breath, tachypnea, and respiratory crackles if the left ventricle is affected; distended neck veins, liver enlargement, anorexia, and nausea if the right ventricle is affected. Many clients have components of both systolic and diastolic failure.

Left-Sided Versus Right-Sided Failure

Depending on the pathophysiology involved, either the left or the right ventricle may be primarily affected. In chronic heart failure, however, both ventricles typically are impaired to some degree. Coronary heart disease and hypertension are common causes of *left-sided heart failure*, whereas *right-sided heart failure* often is caused by conditions that restrict blood flow to the lungs, such as acute or chronic pulmonary disease. Left-sided heart failure also can lead to right-sided failure as pressures in the pulmonary vascular system increase with congestion behind the failing left ventricle.

As left ventricular function fails, cardiac output falls. Pressures in the left ventricle and atrium increase as the amount of blood remaining in the ventricle after systole increases. These increased pressures impair filling, causing congestion and increased pressures in the pulmonary vascular system. Increased pressures in this normally low-pressure system increase fluid movement from the blood vessels into interstitial tissues and the alveoli.

The manifestations of left-sided heart failure result from pulmonary congestion and decreased cardiac output. Fatigue and activity intolerance are common early manifestations. Dizziness and syncope may also result from decreased cardiac output. Pulmonary congestion causes dyspnea, shortness of breath, and cough. The client may develop **orthopnea** (difficulty breathing while lying down), prompting use of two or three pillows or a recliner for sleeping. Cyanosis from impaired gas exchange may be noted. On auscultation of the lungs, inspiratory crackles (rales) and wheezes may be heard in lung bases. An S_3 gallop may be present, reflecting the heart's attempts to fill an already distended ventricle.

In right-sided heart failure, increased pressures in the pulmonary vasculature or right ventricular muscle damage impair the right ventricle's ability to pump blood into the pulmonary circulation. The right ventricle and atrium become distended, and blood accumulates in the systemic venous system. Increased venous pressures cause abdominal organs to become congested and peripheral tissue edema to develop.

Dependent tissues tend to be affected because of the effects of gravity; edema develops in the feet and legs, or if the client is bedridden, in the sacrum. Congestion of gastrointestinal tract vessels causes anorexia and nausea. Right upper quadrant pain may result from liver engorgement. Neck veins distend and become visible even when the client is upright due to increased venous pressure.

High-Output Failure

Clients in hypermetabolic states (e.g., hyperthyroidism, infection, anemia, or pregnancy) require increased cardiac output to maintain blood flow and oxygen to the tissues. If the increased blood flow cannot meet the oxygen demands of the tissues, compensatory mechanisms are activated to further increase cardiac output, which in turn further increases oxygen demand. Thus, even though cardiac output is high, the heart is unable to meet increased oxygen demands. This condition is known as *high-output failure*.

Acute Versus Chronic Failure

Acute failure is the abrupt onset of a myocardial injury, such as a massive MI, resulting in suddenly decreased cardiac function and signs of decreased cardiac output. *Chronic failure* is a progressive deterioration of the heart muscle due to cardiomyopathies, valvular disease, or CHD.

Manifestations and Complications

In addition to the previous manifestations for the various classifications of heart failure, other signs and symptoms commonly are seen.

A fall in cardiac output activates mechanisms that cause increased salt and water retention. This causes weight gain and further increases pressures in the capillaries, resulting in edema. *Nocturia,* voiding more than one time at night, develops as edema fluid from dependent tissues is reabsorbed when the client is supine. **Paroxysmal nocturnal dyspnea (PND),** a frightening condition in which the client awakens at night acutely short of breath, also may develop. Paroxysmal nocturnal dyspnea occurs when edema fluid that has accumulated during the day is reabsorbed into the circulation at night, causing fluid overload and pulmonary congestion. Severe heart failure may cause dyspnea at rest as well as with activity, signifying little or no cardiac reserve. Both an S_3 and an S_4 gallop may be heard on auscultation.

The compensatory mechanisms initiated in heart failure can lead to complications in other body systems. Congestive hepatomegaly and splenomegaly caused by engorgement of the portal venous system results in increased abdominal pressure, ascites, and gastrointestinal problems. With prolonged right-sided heart failure, liver function may be impaired. Myocardial distention can precipitate dysrhythmias, futher impairing cardiac output. Pleural effusions and other pulmonary problems may develop. Major complications of severe heart failure are cardiogenic shock and acute pulmonary edema, a medical emergency described in the next section of this chapter.

Collaborative Care

The main goals for care of heart failure are to slow its progression, reduce cardiac workload, improve cardiac function, and control fluid retention. Treatment strategies are based on the evolution and progression of heart failure.

Diagnostic Tests

Diagnosis of heart failure is based on the history, physical examination, and diagnostic findings.

- *Atrial natriuretic factor (ANF),* also called atrial natriuretic hormone (ANH), and *B-type natriuretic peptide (BNP)* are hormones released by the heart muscle in response to changes in blood volume. Blood levels of these hormones increase in heart failure.
- *Serum electrolytes* are measured to evaluate fluid and electrolyte status. Serum osmolarity may be low due to fluid retention. Sodium, potassium, and chloride levels provide a baseline for evaluating the effects of treatment.
- *Urinalysis, blood urea nitrogen (BUN),* and serum *creatinine* are obtained to evaluate renal function.
- *Liver function tests* including ALT, AST, LDH, serum bilirubin, and total protein and albumin levels, are obtained to evaluate possible effects of heart failure on liver function.
- In acute heart failure, *arterial blood gases (ABGs)* are drawn to evaluate gas exchange in the lungs and tissues.
- *Chest X-ray* may show pulmonary vascular congestion and cardiomegaly in heart failure.
- *Electrocardiography* is used to identify ECG changes associated with ventricular enlargement and to detect dysrhythmias, myocardial ischemia, or infarction.

- *Echocardiography with Doppler flow studies* are performed to evaluate left ventricular function. Echocardiography uses ultrasound waves reflected off cardiac structures to produce images of the heart. The transducer which generates and receives the reflected waves may be placed on the chest wall *(transthoracic echocardiography)*. For more accurate evaluation of the posterior surface of the heart, the transducer may be on the distal end of an endoscope inserted into the esophagus *(transesophageal echocardiography)*. Doppler flow studies use ultrasound waves reflecting off red blood cells to measure the velocity of blood flow across valves, within cardiac chambers, and through the great vessels.
- *Radionuclide imaging* is used to evaluate ventricular function and size (see Chapter 8).

Table 9-1. Medication Administration Heart Failure

Angiotensin-Converting Enzyme (ACE) Inhibitors

Enalapril (Vasotec)	Lisinopril (Prinivil, Zestril)
Captopril (Capoten)	Fosinopril (Monopril)
Moexipril (Univasc)	Quinapril (Accupril)
Ramipril (Altace)	Trandolapril (Mavik)

ACE inhibitors prevent acute coronary events and reduce mortality in heart failure. ACE inhibitors interfere with production of angiotensin II, resulting in vasodilation, reduced blood volume, and prevention of its effects in the heart and blood vessels. In heart failure, ACE inhibitors reduce afterload and improve cardiac output and renal blood flow. They also reduce pulmonary congestion and peripheral edema. ACE inhibitors suppress myocyte growth and reduce ventricular remodeling in heart failure.

Nursing Responsibilities
- Do not give these drugs to women in the second and third trimesters of pregnancy.
- Carefully monitor clients who are volume depleted or who have impaired renal function.
- Use an infusion pump when administering ACE inhibitors intravenously.
- Monitor blood pressure closely for two hours following first dose and as indicated thereafter.
- Monitor serum potassium levels; ACE inhibitors can cause hyperkalemia.
- Monitor white blood cell (WBC) count for potential neutropenia. Report to the physician.

Client and Family Teaching
- Take the drug at the same time every day to ensure a stable blood level.
- Monitor your blood pressure and weight weekly. Report significant changes to your doctor.
- Avoid making sudden position changes; for example, rise from bed slowly. Lie down if you become dizzy or lightheaded, particularly after the first dose.
- Report any signs of easy bruising and bleeding, sore throat or fever, edema, or skin rash. Immediately report swelling of the face, lips, or eyelids, and itching or breathing problems.
- A persistent, dry cough may develop. Contact your doctor if this becomes a problem.
- Take captopril or moexipril one hour before meals.

Continued on the next page

Table 9-1. Continued

Diuretics

Chlorothiazide (Diuril)	Spironolactone (Aldactone)
Furosemide (Lasix)	Triamterene (Dyrenium)
Ethacrynic acid (Edecrin)	Amiloride (Midamor)
Bumetanide (Bumex)	Acetazolamide (Diamox)
Hydrochlorothiazide (HydroDIURIL)	

Diuretics act on different portions of the kidney tubule to inhibit the reabsorption of sodium and water and promote their excretion. With the exception of the potassium-sparing diuretics—spironolactone, triamterene, and amiloride—diuretics also promote potassium excretion, increasing the risk of hypokalemia. Spironolactone, an aldosterone receptor blocker, reduces symptoms and slows progression of heart failure. Aldosterone receptors in the heart and blood vessels promote myocardial remodeling and fibrosis, activate the sympathetic nervous system, and promote vascular fibrosis (which decreases compliance) and baroreceptor dysfunction (Lehne, 2001).

Nursing Responsibilities

- Obtain baseline weight and vital signs.

- Monitor blood pressure, intake and output, weight, skin turgor, and edema as indicators of fluid volume status.

- Assess for volume depletion, particularly with loop diuretics (furosemide, ethacrynic acid, and bumetanide): dizziness, orthostatic hypotension, tachycardia, muscle cramping.

- Report abnormal serum electrolyte levels to the physician. Replace electrolytes as indicated.

- Do not administer potassium replacements to clients receiving a potassium-sparing diuretic.

- Evaluate renal function by assessing urine output, BUN, and serum creatinine.

- Administer intravenous furosemide slowly, no faster than 20 mg/minute. Evaluate for signs of ototoxicity. Do not administer this drug or ethacrynic acid concurrently with aminoglycoside antibiotics (e.g., gentamycin) which are also ototoxic.

Client and Family Teaching

- Drink at least six to eight glasses of water per day.

- Take your diuretic at times that will be the least disruptive to your lifestyle, usually in the morning and early afternoon if a second dose is ordered. Take with meals to decrease gastric upset.

- Monitor your blood pressure, pulse, and weight weekly. Report significant weight changes to your doctor.

- Report any of the following to your doctor: severe abdominal pain, jaundice, dark urine, abnormal bleeding or bruising, flulike symptoms, signs of hypokalemia, hyponatremia, and dehydration (thirst, salt craving, dizziness, weakness, rapid pulse). See Chapter 39 for manifestations of electrolyte imbalances.

- Avoid sudden position changes. You may experience dizziness, lightheadedness, or feelings of faintness.

- Unless you are taking a potassium-sparing diuretic, integrate foods rich in potassium into your diet (see Chapter 39). Limit sodium use.

Table 9-1. Continued

Positive Inotropic Agents

Digitalis Glycosides

Digoxin (Lanoxin)

Digitalis improves myocardial contractility by interfering with ATPase in the myocardial cell membrane and increasing the amount of calcium available for contraction. The increased force of contraction causes the heart to empty more completely, increasing stroke volume and cardiac output. Improved cardiac output improves renal perfusion, decreasing renin secretion. This decreases preload and afterload, reducing cardiac work. Digitalis also has electrophysiologic effects, slowing conduction through the AV node. This decreases the heart rate and reduces oxygen consumption.

Nursing Responsibilities
- Assess apical pulse before administering. Withhold digitalis and notify the physician if heart rate is below 60 BPM and/or manifestations of decreased cardiac output are noted. Record apical rate on medication record.
- Evaluate ECG for scooped (spoon-shaped) ST segment, AV block, bradycardia, and other dysrhythmias (especially PVCs and atrial tachycardias).
- Report manifestations of digitalis toxicity: anorexia, nausea, vomiting, abdominal pain, weakness, vision changes (diplopia, blurred vision, yellow-green or white halos seen around objects), and new-onset dysrhythmias.
- Assess potassium, magnesium, calcium, and serum digoxin levels before giving digitalis. Hypokalemia can precipitate toxicity even when the serum digitalis level is in the "normal" range.
- Monitor clients with renal insufficiency or renal failure and older adults carefully for digitalis toxicity.
- Prepare to administer digoxin immune fab (Digibind) for digoxin toxicity.

Client and Family Teaching
- Take your pulse daily before taking your digoxin. Do not take the digoxin if your pulse is below 60 or if you are weak, fatigued, lightheadeded, dizzy, short of breath, or having chest pain. Notify your physician immediately.
- Contact your doctor if you develop manifestations of digitalis toxicity: palpitations, weakness, loss of appetite, nausea, vomiting, abdominal pain, blurred or colored vision, double vision.
- Avoid using antacids and laxatives; they decrease digoxin absorption.
- Notify your physician immediately if you develop manifestations of potassium deficiency: weakness, lethargy, thirst, depression, muscle cramps, or vomiting.
- Incorporate foods high in potassium into your diet: fresh orange or tomato juice, bananas, raisins, dates, figs, prunes, apricots, spinach, cauliflower, and potatoes.

Continued on the next page

Table 9-1. Continued

Sympathomimetic Agents

Dopamine (Inotropin)   Dobutamine (Dobutrex)

Sympathomimetic agents stimulate the heart, improving the force of contraction. Dobutamine is preferred in managing heart failure because it does not increase the heart rate as much as dopamine, and it has a mild vasodilatory effect. These drugs are given by intravenous infusion and may be titrated to obtain their optimal effects.

Phosphodiesterase Inhibitors

Amrinone (Inocor)   Milrinone (Primacor)

Phosphodiesterase inhibitors are used in treating acute heart failure to increase myocardial contractility and cause vasodilation. The net effects are an increase in cardiac output and a decrease in afterload.

Nursing Responsibilities

- Use an infusion pump to administer these agents. Monitor hemodynamic parameters carefully.
- Avoid discontinuing these drugs abruptly.
- Change solutions and tubing every 24 hours.
- Amrinone is given as an intravenous bolus over two to three minutes, followed by an infusion of 5 to 10 mg/kg/min.
- Amrinone may be infused full strength or diluted in normal saline or half-strength saline. Do not mix this drug with dextrose solutions. After dilution, amrinone can be piggybacked into a line containing a dextrose solution.
- Monitor liver function and platelet counts; amrinone may cause hepatotoxicity and thrombocytopenia.

Client and Family Teaching

- Notify the nursing staff if you experience abdominal pain or notice a skin rash or bruising.

The Client with Pulmonary Edema

Pulmonary edema is an abnormal accumulation of fluid in the interstitial tissue and alveoli of the lung. Both cardiac and noncardiac disorders can cause pulmonary edema. Cardiac causes include acute myocardial infarction, acute heart failure, and valvular disease. *Cardiogenic pulmonary edema,* the focus of this section, is a sign of severe cardiac decompensation. Noncardiac causes of pulmonary edema include primary pulmonary disorders, such as acute respiratory distress syndrome (ARDS), trauma, sepsis, drug overdose, or neurologic sequelae.

Pulmonary edema is a medical emergency: The patient is literally drowning in the fluid in the alveolar and interstitial pulmonary spaces. Its onset may be acute or gradual, progressing to severe respiratory distress. Immediate treatment is necessary.

Pathophysiology

In cardiogenic pulmonary edema, the contractility of the left ventricle is severely impaired. The ejection fraction falls as the ventricle is unable to eject the blood that enters it, causing a sharp rise in end-diastolic volume and pressure. Pulmonary hydrostatic pressures rise, ultimately exceeding the osmotic pressure of the blood. As a result, fluid leaking from the pulmonary capillaries congests interstitial tissues, decreasing lung compliance, and interfering with gas exchange. As capillary and interstitial pressures increase further, the tight junctions of the alveolar walls are disrupted, and the fluid enters the alveoli, along with large red blood cells and protein molecules. Ventilation and gas exchange are severely disrupted, and hypoxia worsens.

Manifestations

The client with acute pulmonary edema presents with classic manifestations (see section below). Dyspnea, shortness of breath, and labored respirations are acute and severe, accompanied by orthopnea, inability to breathe when lying down. Cyanosis is present, and the skin is cool, clammy, and diaphoretic. A productive cough with pink, frothy sputum develops due to fluid, RBCs, and plasma proteins in the alveoli and airways. Crackles are heard throughout the lung fields on auscultation. As the condition worsens, lung sounds become harsher. The client often is restless and highly anxious, although severe hypoxia may cause confusion or lethargy.

As noted earlier, pulmonary edema is a medical emergency. Without rapid and effective intervention, severe tissue hypoxia and acidosis will lead to organ system failure and death.

Collaborative Care

Immediate treatment for acute pulmonary edema focuses on restoring effective gas exchange and reducing fluid and pressure in the pulmonary vascular system. The client is placed in an upright sitting position with the legs dangling to reduce venous return by trapping some excess fluid in the lower extremities. This position also facilitates breathing.

Diagnostic testing is limited to assessment of the acute situation. *Arterial blood gases (ABGs)* are drawn to assess gas exchange and acid-base balance. Oxygen tension (PaO_2) is usually low. Initially, carbon dioxide levels ($PaCO_2$) may also be reduced because of rapid respirations. As the condition progresses, the $PaCO_2$ rises and respiratory acidosis develops. *Oxygen saturation* levels also are continuously monitored. The *chest X-ray* shows pulmonary vascular congestion and alveolar edema. Provided the client's condition allows, *hemodynamic monitoring* is instituted. In cardiogenic pulmonary edema, the pulmonary artery wedge pressure (PAWP) is elevated, usually over 25 mmHg. Cardiac output may be decreased.

Morphine is administered intravenously to relieve anxiety and improve the efficacy of breathing. It also is a vasodilator that reduces venous return and lowers left atrial pressure. Although morphine is very effective for clients with cardiogenic pulmonary edema, its antidote, naloxone, is kept readily available in case respiratory depression occurs.

Oxygen is administered using a positive pressure system that can achieve a 100% oxygen concentration. A continuous positive airway pressure (CPAP) mask system may be used, or the client may be intubated and mechanical ventilation employed. Positive pressure increases alveolar pressures and gas exchange while decreasing fluid diffusion into the alveoli.

Potent loop diuretics such as furosemide, ethacrynic acid, or bumetanide are administered intravenously to promote rapid diuresis. Furosemide is also a venous dilator, reducing venous return to the heart. Vasodilators such as intravenous nitroprusside are given to improve cardiac output by reducing afterload. Dopamine or dobutamine and, possibly, digoxin are administered to improve the myocardial contractility and cardiac output. Intravenous aminophylline may be used cautiously to reduce bronchospasm and decrease wheezing.

When the client's condition has stabilized, further diagnostic tests may be done to determine the underlying cause of pulmonary edema, and specific treatment measures directed at the cause instituted.

Nursing Care

Nursing care of the client with acute pulmonary edema focuses on relieving the pulmonary effects of the disorder. Interventions are directed toward improving oxygenation, reducing fluid volume, and providing emotional support.

The nurse often is instrumental in recognizing early manifestations of pulmonary edema and initiating treatment. As with many critical conditions, emergent care is directed toward the ABCs: airway, breathing, and circulation.

Nursing Diagnoses and Interventions

Impaired Gas Exchange
Accumulated fluid in the alveoli and airways interfere with ventilation of and gas exchange within the alveoli.

- Ensure airway patency.
- Assess respiratory status frequently, including rate, effort, use of accessory muscles, sputum characteristics, lung sounds, and skin color. *The status of a client in acute pulmonary edema can change rapidly for the better or worse.*
- Place in high-Fowler's position with the legs dangling. *The upright position facilitates breathing and decreases venous return.*
- Administer oxygen as ordered by mask, CPAP mask, or ventilator. *Supplemental oxygen promotes gas exchange; positive pressure increases the pressure within the alveoli, airways, and thoracic cavity, decreasing venous return, pulmonary capillary pressure, and fluid leak into the alveoli.*
- Encourage to cough up secretions; if necessary, provide nasotracheal suctioning. *Coughing moves secretions from smaller airways into larger airways where they can be suctioned out if necessary.*

Decreased Cardiac Output
Cardiogenic pulmonary edema usually is caused by either an acute decrease in myocardial contractility or increased workload that exceeds the ability of the left ventricle.

- Monitor vital signs, hemodynamic status, and rhythm continuously. *Acute pulmonary edema is a critical condition, and cardiovascular status can change rapidly.*

- Assess heart sounds for possible S₃, S₄, or murmurs. *These abnormal heart sounds may be due to excess work or may indicate the cause of the acute pulmonary edema.*

- Initiate an intravenous line for medication administration. Administer morphine, diuretics, vasodilators, bronchodilators, and positive inotropic medications (e.g., digoxin) as ordered. *These drugs reduce cardiac work and improve contractility.*

- Keep accurate intake and output records. Restrict fluids as ordered. *Fluids may be restricted to reduce vascular volume and cardiac work.*

Fear

Acute pulmonary edema is a very frightening experience for everyone (including the nurse).

- Provide emotional support for the client and family members. *Fear and anxiety stimulate the sympathetic nervous system, which can lead to ineffective respiratory patterns and interfere with cooperation necessary for care measures.*

- Explain all procedures and the reasons to the client and family members. Keep information brief and to the point. Use short sentences and a reassuring tone. *Anxiety and fear interfere with the ability to assimilate information; brief, factual information and reassurance reduce anxiety and fear.*

- Maintain close contact with the client and family, providing reassurance that recovery from acute pulmonary edema is often as dramatic as its onset.

- Answer questions, and provide accurate information in a caring manner. *Knowledge reduces anxiety and psychologic stress associated with this critical condition.*

Home Care

During the acute period, teaching is limited to immediate care measures. Once the acute episode of pulmonary edema has resolved, teach the client and family about its underlying cause and prevention of future episodes. If pulmonary edema follows an acute MI, include information related to CHD and the AMI, as well as information related to heart failure. Review the teaching and home care for clients with these disorders for further information.

Disorders of Cardiac Structure

The Client with Valvular Heart Disease

Proper heart valve function ensures one-way blood flow through the heart and vascular system. **Valvular heart disease** interferes with blood flow to and from the heart. Acquired valvular disorders can result from acute conditions, such as infective endocarditis, or from chronic conditions, such as rheumatic heart disease. Rheumatic heart disease is the most common cause of valvular disease (McCance & Huether, 2002). Acute myocardial infarction can also damage heart valves, causing tearing, ischemia, or damage to the papillary muscles that affects valve leaflet function. Congenital heart defects may affect the heart valves, often with no manifestations until adulthood. Aging affects heart structure and function, and also increases the risk for valvular disease.

Physiology Review

The heart valves direct blood flow within and out of the heart. The valves are fibroelastic tissue supported by a ring of fibrous tissue (the annulus) which provides support.

The atrioventricular (AV) valves, the **mitral** (or *bicuspid*) **valve** on the left and the **tricuspid valve** on the right, separate the atria from the ventricles. These valves normally are fully open during diastole, allowing blood to flow freely from the atria into the ventricles. Rising pressure within the ventricles at the onset of systole (contraction) closes the AV valves, creating the S_1 heart sound ("lub"). The leaflets of the AV valves are connected to ventricular papillary muscles by fibrous *chordae tendineae*. The chordae tendineae prevent the valve leaflets from bulging back into the atria during systole.

The semilunar valves, the **aortic** and **pulmonic valves,** separate the ventricles from the great vessels. They open during systole, allowing blood to flow out of the heart with ventricular contraction. As the ventricle relaxes and intraventricular pressure falls at the beginning of diastole, the higher pressure within the great vessels (the aorta and pulmonary artery) closes these valves, creating the S_2 heart sound ("dup").

Pathophysiology and Manifestations

Valvular heart disease occurs as two major types of disorders: stenosis and regurgitation. **Stenosis** occurs when valve leaflets fuse together and cannot fully open or close. The valve opening narrows and becomes rigid. Scarring of the valves from endocarditis or infarction, and calcium deposits can lead to stenosis. Stenotic valves impede the forward flow of blood, decreasing cardiac output because of impaired ventricular filling or ejection and stroke volume. Because stenotic valves also do not close completely, some backflow of blood occurs when the valve should be fully closed.

Regurgitant valves (also called *insufficient* or *incompetent* valves) do not close completely. This allows **regurgitation,** or backflow of blood, through the valve into the area it just left. Regurgitation can result from deformity or erosion of valve cusps caused by the vegetative lesions of bacterial endocarditis, by scarring or tearing from myocardial infarction, or by cardiac dilation. As the heart enlarges, the valve *annulus* (supporting ring of the valve) is stretched, and the valve edges no longer meet to allow complete closure.

Valvular disease causes hemodynamic changes both in front of and behind the affected valve. Blood volume and pressures are reduced in front of the valve, because flow is obstructed through a stenotic valve and backflow occurs through a regurgitant valve. By contrast, volumes and pressures characteristically increase behind the diseased valve. These hemodynamic changes may lead to pulmonary complications or heart failure. Higher pressures and compensatory changes to maintain cardiac output lead to remodeling and hypertrophy of the heart muscle.

Stenosis increases the work of the chamber behind the affected valve as the heart attempts to move blood through the narrowed opening. Excess blood volume behind regurgitant valves causes dilation of the chamber. In mitral stenosis, for example, the left atrium hypertrophies to generate enough pressure to open and deliver its blood through the narrowed mitral valve. Not all of the blood is delivered before the valve closes, leaving blood to accumulate in the left atrium. This chamber dilates to accommodate the excess volume.

Eventually, cardiac output falls as compensatory mechanisms become less effective. The normal balance of oxygen supply and demand is upset, and the heart begins to fail. Increased muscle mass and size increase myocardial oxygen consumption. The size and workload of the heart exceed its blood supply, causing ischemia and chest pain. Eventually, necrosis occurs and functional muscle is lost. Contractile force, stroke volume, and cardiac output decrease. High pressures on the left side of the heart are reflected backward into the pulmonary system, causing pulmonary edema, pulmonary hypertension, and, eventually, right ventricular failure.

Valvular disorders interfere with the smooth flow of blood through the heart. The flow becomes turbulent, causing a **murmur,** a characteristic manifestation of valvular disease.

Blood forced through the narrowed opening of a stenotic valve, or regurgitated from a higher pressure chamber through an incompetent valve, creates a jet stream effect (much like water spurting out of a partially occluded hose opening). The physical force of this jet stream damages the endocardium of the receiving chamber, increasing the risk for infective endocarditis.

The higher pressures on the left side of the heart subject its valves (the mitral and aortic valves) to more stress and damage than those on the right side of the heart (the tricuspid and pulmonic). Pulmonic valve disease is the least common of the valvular disorders.

Mitral Stenosis

Mitral stenosis narrows the mitral valve, obstructing blood flow from the left atrium into the left ventricle during diastole. It is usually caused by rheumatic heart disease or bacterial endocarditis; it rarely results from congenital defects. It affects females more frequently (66%) than males (Braunwald et al., 2001). Mitral stenosis is chronic and progressive.

In mitral valve stenosis, fibrous tissue replaces normal valve tissue, causing valve leaflets to stiffen and fuse. Resulting changes in blood flow through the valve lead to calcification of the valve leaflets. As calcium is deposited in and on the valve, the leaflets become more rigid and narrow the opening further. As the valve leaflets become less mobile, the chordae tendineae fuse, thicken, and shorten. Thromboemboli may form on the calcified leaflets.

The narrowed mitral opening impairs blood flow into the left ventricle, reducing end-diastolic volume and pressure, and decreasing stroke volume. The narrowed opening also forces the left atrium to generate higher pressure to deliver blood to the left ventricle. This leads to left atrial hypertrophy. The left atrium also dilates as obstructed blood flow increases its volume. As the resistance to blood flow increases, high atrial pressures are reflected back into the pulmonary vessels, increasing pulmonary pressures. Pulmonary hypertension increases the workload of the right ventricle, causing it to dilate and hypertrophy. Eventually, heart failure occurs.

Mitral stenosis may be asymptomatic or cause severe impairment. Its manifestations depend on cardiac output and pulmonary vascular pressures. Dyspnea on exertion (DOE) is typically the earliest manifestation. Others include cough, hemoptysis, frequent pulmonary infections such as bronchitis and pneumonia, paroxysmal nocturnal dyspnea, orthopnea, weakness, fatigue, and palpitations. As the stenosis worsens, manifestations of right heart failure, including jugular venous distension, hepatomegaly, ascites, and peripheral edema develop. Crackles may be heard in the lung bases. In severe mitral stenosis, cyanosis of the face and extremities may be noted. Chest pain is rare but may occur.

On auscultation, a loud S_1, a split S_2, and a mitral opening snap may be heard. The opening snap reflects high left atrial pressure. The murmur of mitral stenosis occurs during diastole, and is typically low-pitched, rumbling, crescendo-decrescendo. It is heard best with the bell of the stethoscope in the apical region. It may be accompanied by a palpable thrill (vibration).

Atrial dysrhythmias, particularly atrial fibrillation, are common due to chronic atrial distention. Thrombi may form and subsequently embolize to the brain, coronary arteries, kidneys, spleen, and extremities—potentially devastating complications.

Women with mitral stenosis may be asymptomatic until pregnancy. As the heart tries to compensate for increased circulating volume (30% more in pregnancy) by increasing cardiac output, left atrial pressures rise, tachycardia reduces ventricular filling and stroke volume, and pulmonary pressures increase. Sudden pulmonary edema and heart failure may threaten the lives of the mother and fetus.

Mitral Regurgitation

Mitral regurgitation or *insufficiency* allows blood to flow back into the left atrium during systole because the valve does not close fully. Rheumatic heart disease is a common cause of mitral regurgitation. Men develop mitral regurgitation more frequently than women. Degenerative calcification of the mitral annulus may cause mitral regurgitation in older women. Processes that dilate the mitral annulus or affect the supporting structures, papillary muscles, or the chordae tendineae may cause mitral regurgitation (e.g., left ventricular hypertrophy and MI). Congenital defects also may cause mitral regurgitation.

In mitral regurgitation, blood flows into both the systemic circulation and back into the left atrium through the deformed valve during systole. This increases left atrial volume. The left atrium dilates to accommodate its extra volume, pulling the posterior valve leaflet further away from the valve opening and worsening the defect. The left ventricle dilates to accommodate its increased preload and low cardiac output, further aggravating the problem.

Mitral regurgitation may be asymptomatic or cause symptoms such as fatigue, weakness, exertional dyspnea, and orthopnea. In severe or acute regurgitation, manifestations of left-sided heart failure develop, including pulmonary congestion and edema. High pulmonary pressures may lead to manifestations of right-sided heart failure.

The murmur of mitral regurgitation is usually loud, high pitched, rumbling, and holosystolic (occurring throughout systole). It is often accompanied by a palpable thrill and is heard most clearly at the cardiac apex. It may be characterized as a cooing or gull-like sound or have a musical quality (Braunwald et al., 2001).

Mitral Valve Prolapse

Mitral valve prolapse (MVP) is a type of mitral insufficiency that occurs when one or both mitral valve cusps billow into the atrium during ventricular systole. MVP is more common in young women between ages 14 and 30; its incidence declines with age. Its cause often is unclear. It also can result from acute or chronic rheumatic damage, ischemic heart disease, or other cardiac disorders. It commonly affects people with inherited connective tissue disorders such as Marfan syndrome. Mitral valve prolapse usually is benign, but about 0.01% to 0.02% of people with MVP have thickened mitral leaflets and a significant risk of morbidity and sudden death.

Excess collagen tissue in the valve leaflets and elongated cordae tendineae impair closure of the mitral valve, allowing the leaflets to billow into the left atrium during systole. Some ventricular blood volume regurgitates into the left atrium.

Mitral valve prolapse usually is asymptomatic. A midsystolic ejection click or murmur may be audible. A high-pitched late systolic murmur, sometimes described as a "whoop" or "honk," due to the regurgitation of blood through the valve, may develop in MVP. Atypical chest pain is the most common symptom of MVP. It may be left sided or substernal, and is frequently related to fatigue, not exertion. Tachydysrhythmias may develop with MVP, causing palpitations, lightheadedness, and syncope. Increased sympathetic nervous system tone may cause a sense of anxiety (Woods et al., 2000).

Mitral valve prolapse increases the risk for bacterial endocarditis. Progressive worsening of regurgitation can lead to heart failure. Thrombi may form on prolapsed valve leaflets; embolization may cause transient ischemic attacks (TIAs).

Aortic Stenosis

Aortic stenosis obstructs blood flow from the left ventricle into the aorta during systole. Aortic stenosis is more common in males (80%) than females (Braunwald et al., 2001). Aortic stenosis may be idiopathic, or due to a congenital defect, rheumatic damage, or degenerative changes. When rheumatic heart disease is the cause, mitral valve deformity is also often present. Rheumatic heart disease destroys aortic valve leaflets, with fibrosis and calcification causing rigidity and scarring. In the older adult, calcific aortic stenosis may result from degenerative changes associated with aging. Constant "wear and tear" on this valve can lead to fibrosis and calcification. Idiopathic calcific stenosis generally is mild and does not impair cardiac output.

As aortic stenosis progresses, the valve annulus decreases in size, increasing the work of the left ventricle to eject its volume through the narrowed opening into the aorta. To compensate, the ventricle hypertrophies to maintain an adequate stroke volume and cardiac output. Left ventricular compliance also decreases. The additional workload increases myocardial oxygen consumption, which can precipitate myocardial ischemia. Coronary blood flow may also decrease in aortic stenosis. As left ventricular end-diastolic pressure increases because of reduced stroke volume, left atrial pressures increase. These pressures also affect the pulmonary vascular system; pulmonary vascular congestion and pulmonary edema may result.

Aortic stenosis may be asymptomatic for many years. As the disease progresses and compensation fails, usually between age 50 and 70 years, obstructed cardiac output causes manifestations of left ventricular failure. Dyspnea on exertion, angina pectoris, and exertional syncope are classic manifestations of aortic stenosis. Pulse pressure, an indicator of stroke volume, narrows to 30 mmHg or less. Hemodynamic monitors show increased left atrial pressure and pulmonary artery wedge pressure, as well as decreased stroke volume and cardiac output.

Aortic stenosis produces a harsh systolic murmur best heard in the second intercostal space to the right of the sternum. This crescendo-decrescendo murmur is produced by turbulence of blood entering the aorta through the stenotic valve. A palpable thrill is often felt. The murmur may radiate to the carotid arteries. Ventricular hypertrophy displaces the cardiac impulse to the left of the midclavicular line. As aortic stenosis progresses, S_3 and S_4 heart sounds may be heard, indicating heart failure and reduced left ventricular compliance.

As cardiac output falls, tissue perfusion decreases. Late in the disease, pulmonary hypertension and right ventricular failure develop. Untreated, symptomatic aortic stenosis has a poor prognosis; 10% to 20% of these clients experience sudden cardiac death (Braunwald, et al., 2001).

Aortic Regurgitation

Aortic regurgitation, also called *aortic insufficiency,* allows blood to flow back into the left ventricle from the aorta during diastole. It is more common in males (75%) in its "pure" form; in females, it is commonly associated with coexisting mitral valve disease. Most aortic regurgitation (67%) results from rheumatic heart disease (Braunwald et al., 2001). Other causes include congenital disorders, infective endocarditis, blunt chest trauma, aortic aneurysm, syphilis, Marfan syndrome, and chronic hypertension.

In aortic regurgitation, thickened and contracted valve cusps, scarring, fibrosis, and calcification impede complete valve closure. Chronic hypertension and aortic aneurysm may dilate and stretch the aortic valve opening, increasing the degree of regurgitation.

In aortic regurgitation, volume overload affects the left ventricle as blood from the aorta adds to blood received from the atrium during diastole. This increases diastolic left ventricular pressure. Increased preload causes more forceful contractions and a high stroke volume. With time, muscle cells hypertrophy to compensate for increased cardiac work and afterload; eventually this hypertrophy compromises cardiac output and increases regurgitation.

High left-ventricular pressures increase left atrial workload and pressure. This pressure is transmitted to the pulmonary vessels causing pulmonary congestion. The workload of the right ventricle increases as a result, and right-sided heart failure may develop. Acute aortic regurgitation from traumatic injury or infective endocarditis causes a rapid decline in hemodynamic status from acute heart failure and pulmonary edema, because compensatory mechanisms do not have time to develop.

Aortic regurgitation may be asymptomatic for many years, even when severe. The increased stroke volume may cause complaints of persistent palpitations, especially when recumbent. A throbbing pulse may be visible in arteries of the neck; the force of contraction may cause a characteristic head bob (Musset's sign) and shake the whole body. Other symptoms include dizziness, and exercise intolerance.

Fatigue, exertional dyspnea, orthopnea, and paroxysmal nocturnal dyspnea are common in aortic regurgitation. Anginal pain may result from excessive cardiac work and decreased coronary perfusion. Unlike CAD, angina often occurs at night and may not respond to conventional therapy.

The murmur of aortic regurgitation is heard during diastole as blood flows back into the left ventricle from the aorta. It is a "blowing," high-pitched sound heard most clearly at the third left intercostal space. A palpable thrill and ventricular heave may be noted. An S_3 and S_4 may be heard as the heart fails and ventricular compliance diminishes. The apical impulse is displaced to the left.

High systolic and low diastolic pressures cause a widened pulse pressure. The arterial pressure waveform has a rapid upstroke and quickly collapsing downstroke, known as a *water-hammer pulse.* It is caused by the force of rapid and early delivery of the stroke volume into the aorta.

Tricuspid Valve Disorders

Tricuspid stenosis obstructs blood flow from the right atrium to the right ventricle. It usually results from rheumatic heart disease; mitral stenosis often occurs concurrently with tricuspid stenosis.

Fibrosed, retracted tricuspid valve cusps and fused leaflets narrow the valve orifice and prevent complete closure. Right ventricular filling is impaired during diastole, and during systole, some blood regurgitates back into the right atrium. Pressure in the right atrium increases, and it enlarges in response to the increased pressure and workload. This increased right atrial pressure is reflected backward into the systemic circulation. Right ventricular stroke volume decreases, reducing the volume delivered to the pulmonary system and left heart. Stroke volume, cardiac output, and tissue perfusion fall.

Manifestations of tricuspid stenosis relate to systemic congestion and right-sided heart failure. They include increased central venous pressure, jugular venous distention, ascites, hepatomegaly, and peripheral edema. Low cardiac output causes fatigue and weakness. The low-pitched, rumbling diastolic murmur of tricuspid stenosis is most clearly heard in the fourth intercostal space at the left sternal border or over the xiphoid process.

Tricuspid regurgitation usually occurs secondarily to right ventricular dilation. Stretching distorts the valve and its supporting structures, preventing complete valve closure. Left ventricular failure is the usual cause of right ventricular overload; pulmonary hypertension is another cause. The valve may also be damaged by rheumatic heart disease, infective endocarditis, inferior MI, trauma, or other conditions.

Tricuspid regurgitation allows blood to flow back into the right atrium during systole, increasing right atrial pressures. Increased right atrial pressure causes manifestations of right-sided heart failure, including systemic venous congestion and low cardiac output. Atrial fibrillation due to atrial distention is common. The retrograde flow of blood over the deformed tricuspid valve causes a high-pitched, blowing systolic murmur heard over the tricuspid or xiphoid area.

Pulmonic Valve Disorders

Pulmonic stenosis obstructs blood flow from the right ventricle into the pulmonary system. It usually is a congenital disorder, although rheumatic heart disease or cancer also may cause pulmonic stenosis. The right ventricle hypertrophies to generate the pressure needed to pump blood into the pulmonary system. The right atrium also hypertrophies to overcome the high pressures generated in the right ventricle. Right-sided heart failure occurs when the ventricle can no longer generate adequate pressure to force blood past the narrowed valve opening.

Pulmonic stenosis typically is asymptomatic unless severe. Dyspnea on exertion and fatigue are early signs. As the condition progresses, right-sided heart failure develops, with peripheral edema, ascites, hepatomegaly, and increased venous pressures. Turbulent blood flow caused by the narrowed valve generates a harsh, systolic crescendo-decrescendo murmur heard in the pulmonic area, the second left intercostal space.

Pulmonic regurgitation is more common than pulmonary stenosis. It is a complication of pulmonary hypertension, which stretches and dilates the pulmonary orifice, causing incomplete valve closure. Infective endocarditis, pulmonary artery aneurysm, and syphilis may also cause pulmonic regurgitation.

Incomplete valve closure allows blood to flow back into the right ventricle during diastole, decreasing blood flow to the pulmonary circuit. The extra blood increases right ventricular end-diastolic volume. When the ventricle can no longer compensate for the increased volume, right-sided heart failure develops. The murmur of pulmonic regurgitation is a high-pitched, decrescendo, blowing sound heard along the left sternal border during diastole.

Collaborative Care

A heart murmur identified during routine physical examination often is the initial indication of valvular disease. If no symptoms are present, close observation for disease progression and prophylactic therapy to prevent infection of the diseased heart may be the only treatment. Manifestations of heart failure are treated with diet and medications. When medical management is no longer effective, surgery is considered.

Diagnostic Tests

The following diagnostic tests help to identify and diagnose valvular disease.

*   *Echocardiography* is used routinely to diagnose valvular disease. Thickened valve leaflets, vegetations or growths on valve leaflets, myocardial function, and chamber size can be determined, and pressure gradients across valves and pulmonary artery pressures can be estimated. Either transthoracic or transesophageal echocardiography may be used.

*   *Chest X-ray* can identify cardiac hypertrophy, chamber and great vessel enlargement, and dilation of the pulmonary vasculature. Calcification of the valve leaflets and annular openings may also be visible.

*   *Electrocardiography* can demonstrate atrial and ventricular hypertrophy, conduction defects, and dysrhythmias associated with valvular disease.

*   *Cardiac catheterization* may be used to assess contractility and to determine the pressure gradients across the heart valves, in the heart chambers, and in the pulmonary system.

Medications

Heart failure resulting from valvular disease is treated with diuretics, ACE inhibitors, vasodilators, and possibly digitalis glycosides. Digitalis increases the force of myocardial contraction to maintain cardiac output. Diuretics, ACE inhibitors, and vasodilators reduce preload and afterload.

In clients with valvular disorders, atrial distention often causes atrial fibrillation. Digitalis or small doses of beta blockers are given to slow the ventricular response. Anticoagulant therapy is added to prevent clot and embolus formation, a common complication of atrial fibrillation as blood pools in the noncontracting atria. Anticoagulant therapy is also required following insertion of a mechanical heart valve.

Valvular damage increases the risk for infective endocarditis as altered blood flow allows bacterial colonization. Antibiotics are prescribed prophylactically prior to any dental work, invasive procedures, or surgery to minimize the risk of bacteremia (bacteria in the blood) and subsequent endocarditis.

Percutaneous Balloon Valvuloplasty

Percutaneous balloon valvuloplasty is an invasive procedure performed in the cardiac catheterization laboratory. A balloon catheter similar to that used in coronary angioplasty procedures is inserted into the femoral vein or artery. Guided by fluoroscopy, the catheter is advanced into the heart and positioned with the balloon straddling the stenotic valve. The balloon is then inflated for approximately 90 seconds to divide the fused leaflets and enlarge the valve orifice. Balloon valvuloplasty is the treatment of choice for symptomatic mitral valve stenosis. It is used to treat children and young adults with aortic stenosis, and may be indicated for older adults who are poor surgical risks, and as a "bridge to surgery" when heart function is severely compromised (Braunwald, et al., 2001). Nursing care of the client with a balloon valvuloplasty is similar to that of the client following coronary revascularization.

Surgery

Surgery to repair or replace the diseased valve may be done to restore valve function, alleviate symptoms, and prevent complications and death. Ideally, diseased valves are repaired or replaced before cardiopulmonary function is severely compromised. The diseased valve is repaired when possible, because the risk for surgical mortality and complications is lower than with valve replacement.

Reconstructive Surgery

Valvuloplasty is a general term for reconstruction or repair of a heart valve. Methods include "patching" the perforated portion of the leaflet, resecting excess tissue, debriding vegetations or calcification, and other techniques. Valvuloplasty may be used for stenotic or regurgitant mitral and tricuspid valves, mitral valve prolapse, and aortic stenosis. Common valvuloplasty procedures include the following:

* *Open commissurotomy,* surgical division of fused valve leaflets, is done to open stenotic valves. Fused commissures (junctions between valve leaflets or cusps) are incised, and calcium deposits are debrided as needed.

* *Annuloplasty* repairs a narrowed or an enlarged or dilated valve annulus, the supporting ring of the valve. A prosthetic ring may be used to resize the opening, or stitches and purse-string sutures may be used to reduce and gather excess tissue. Annuloplasty may be used for either stenotic or regurgitant valves.

Valve Replacement

Valve replacement is indicated when manifestations of valve dysfunction develop, preferably before left heart function is seriously impaired. In general, three factors determine the outcome of valve replacement surgery: (1) heart function at the time of surgery: (2) intraoperative and postoperative care, and (3) characteristics and durability of the replacement valve.

Many different prosthetic heart valves are available, including mechanical and biologic tissue valves. Selection depends on the valve hemodynamics, resistance to clot formation, ease of insertion, anatomic suitability, and client acceptance (Meeker & Rothrock, 1999). The client's age, underlying condition, and contraindications to anticoagulation, such as a desire to become pregnant, are also considered in selecting the appropriate prosthesis.

Biologic tissue valves may be *heterografts,* excised from a pig or made of calf pericardium, or *homografts* from a human (obtained from a cadaver or during heart transplant). Biologic valves allow more normal blood flow and have a low risk of thrombus formation. As a result, long-term anticoagulation rarely is necessary. They are less durable, however, than mechanical valves. Up to 50% of biologic valves must be replaced by fifteen years.

Mechanical prosthetic valves have the major advantage of long-term durability. These valves are frequently used when life expectancy exceeds ten years. Their major disadvantage is the need for lifetime anticoagulation to prevent the development of clots on the valve.

Most mechanical valves are either a tilting disk or a ball and cage design. The tilting-disc valve designs are frequently used because they have a lower profile than the caged-ball types, allowing blood to flow through the valve with less obstruction. The St. Jude bileaflet design has good hemodynamics and low risk for clot formation. Both biologic and mechanical valves increase the risk of endocarditis, although its incidence is fairly low.

Nursing Care

Health Promotion

Preventing rheumatic heart disease is a key element in preventing heart valve disorders. Rheumatic heart disease is a consequence of rheumatic fever (see previous section of this chapter), an immune process that may be a sequela to hemolytic streptococcal infection of the pharynx (strep throat). Early treatment of strep throat prevents rheumatic fever. Teach individual clients, families, and communities about the importance of timely and effective treatment of strep throat. Emphasize the importance of completing the full prescription of antibiotics to prevent development of resistant bacteria. Prophylactic antibiotic therapy before invasive procedures to prevent infectious endocarditis is an important health promotion measure for clients with preexisting heart disease.

Assessment

Assessment data related to valvular heart disease includes the following:

- *Health history:* complaints of decreasing exercise tolerance, dyspnea on exertion, palpitations; history of frequent respiratory infections; previous history of rheumatic heart disease, endocarditis, or a heart murmur.

- *Physical examination:* vital signs; skin color and temperature, evidence of clubbing or peripheral edema; neck vein distention; breath sounds; heart sounds and presence of S_3, S_4, or murmur; timing, grade, and characteristics of any murmur; palpate for cardiac heave and thrills; abdominal contour, liver and spleen size.

Nursing Diagnoses and Interventions

Nursing priorities include maintaining cardiac output, managing manifestations of the disorder, teaching about the disease process and its management, and preventing complications. Nursing care of the client undergoing valve surgery is similar to that of the client having other types of open-heart surgery, with increased attention to anticoagulation and preventing endocarditis.

Decreased Cardiac Output

Nearly all valve disorders affect ventricular filling and/or emptying, reducing cardiac output. Stenosis of the AV valves impairs ventricular filling and increases atrial pressures. Regurgitation of these valves reduces cardiac output as a portion of the blood in the ventricle regurgitates into the atria during systole. Stenosis of the semilunar valves obstructs ventricular outflow to the great vessels; regurgitation allows blood to flow back into the ventricles, creating higher filling pressures. When compensatory measures fail, heart failure develops.

- Monitor vital signs and hemodynamic parameters, reporting changes from the baseline. *A fall in systolic blood pressure and tachycardia may indicate decreased cardiac output.*

Increasing pulmonary artery and pulmonary wedge pressures may also indicate decreased cardiac output, causing increased congestion and pressure in the pulmonary vascular system.

- Monitor intake and output; weigh daily. Report weight gain of three to five pounds within 24 hours. *Fluid retention is a compensatory mechanism that occurs when cardiac output decreases; 2.2 lb. (1 kg.) of weight equals 1 L of fluid.*

- Restrict fluids as ordered. *Fluid intake may be restricted to reduce cardiac workload and pressures within the heart and pulmonary circuit.*

- Monitor oxygen saturation continuously and arterial blood gases as ordered. Report oxygen saturation less than 95% (or as specified) and abnormal ABG results. *Oxygen saturation levels and ABGs allow assessment of oxygenation.*

- Elevate the head of the bed. Administer supplemental oxygen as ordered. *These measures improve alveolar ventilation and oxygenation.*

- Provide for physical, emotional, and mental rest. *Physical and psychologic rest decreases the cardiac workload.*

- Administer prescribed medications as ordered to reduce cardiac workload. *Diuretics, ACE inhibitors, and direct vasodilators may be prescribed to reduce fluid volume and afterload, reducing cardiac work.*

Activity Intolerance

Altered blood flow through the heart impairs delivery of oxygen and nutrients to the tissues. As the heart muscle fails, and is unable to compensate for altered blood flow, tissue perfusion is further compromised. Dyspnea on exertion is often an early symptom of valvular disease.

- Monitor vital signs before and during activities. *A change in heart rate of more than 20 BPM, a change of 20 mmHg or more in systolic BP, and complaints of dyspnea, shortness of breath, excessive fatigue, chest pain, diaphoresis, dizziness, or syncope may indicate activity intolerance.*

- Encourage self-care and gradually increasing activities as allowed and tolerated. Provide for rest periods, uninterrupted sleep, and adequate nutritional intake. *Gradual progression of activities avoids excessive cardiac stress. Encouraging self-care increases the client's self-esteem and sense of power. Adequate rest and nutrition facilitate healing, decrease fatigue, and increase energy reserves.*

- Provide assistance as needed. Suggest use of a shower chair, sitting while brushing hair or teeth, and other energy-saving measures. *Reducing energy expenditure helps maintain a balance of oxygen supply and demand.*

- Consult with cardiac rehabilitation specialist or physical therapist for in-bed exercises and an activity plan. *In-bed exercises may help improve strength.*

- Discuss ways to conserve physical energy at home. *Information provides practical ways to deal with activity limitations and empowers the client to manage these limitations.*

Risk for Infection

Damaged and deformed valve leaflets, and turbulent blood flow through the heart, significantly increase the risk of infective endocarditis. Invasive diagnostic and monitoring lines (e.g., cardiac catheterization, hemodynamic monitoring) and disrupted skin with surgery also increase the risk of infection.

- Use aseptic technique for all invasive procedures. *Invasive procedures breach the body's protective mechanisms, potentially allowing bacteria to enter. Aseptic technique reduces this risk.*

- Assess wounds and catheter sites for redness, swelling, warmth, pain, or evidence of drainage. *These signs of inflammation may signal infection.*

- Administer antibiotics as ordered. Ensure completion of the full course. *Antibiotics are used to prevent and treat infection. Completion of the full course of therapy prevents drug-resistant organisms from multiplying.*

- Monitor WBC and differential. Notify physician of leukocytosis or leukopenia. *A high WBC and increased percentage of immature WBCs (bands) may indicate bacterial infection; a low WBC count may indicate an impaired immune response and increased susceptibility to infection.*

Ineffective Protection

Anticoagulant therapy commonly is prescribed for clients with chronic atrial fibrillation, a history of emboli, and following valve replacement surgery. Although chronic anticoagulant therapy decreases the risk of clots and emboli, it increases the risk for bleeding and hemorrhage.

- Test stools and vomitus for occult blood. *Bleeding due to excessive anticoagulation may not be apparent.*

- Instruct client to avoid using aspirin or other nonsteroidal anti-inflammatory drugs (NSAIDs). Encourage reading ingredient labels on over-the-counter drugs; many contain aspirin. *Aspirin and other NSAIDs interfere with clotting and may potentiate the effects of the anticoagulant therapy.*

  - Advise using a soft-bristled toothbrush, electric razor, and gentle touch when cleaning fragile skin. *These measures decrease the risk of skin or gum trauma and bleeding.*

Home Care

For most clients, valvular disease is a chronic condition. The client has primary responsibility for managing effects of the disorder. To prepare the client and family for home care, discuss the following topics.

- Management of symptoms, including any necessary activity restrictions or lifestyle changes.

- The importance of adequate rest to prevent fatigue.

- Diet restrictions to reduce fluid retention and symptoms of heart failure.

- Information about prescribed medications, including purpose, desired and possible adverse effects, scheduling, and possible interactions with other drugs.

- The importance of keeping follow-up appointments to monitor the disease and its treatment.

- Notifying all health care providers about valve disease or surgery to facilitate prescription of prophylactic antibiotics before invasive procedures or dental work.

- Manifestations to immediately report to the health care provider: increasing severity of symptoms, especially of worsening heart failure or pulmonary edema; signs of transient ischemic attacks or other embolic events; evidence of bleeding, such as joint pain, easy bruising, black and tarry stools, bleeding gums, or blood in the urine or sputum.

Provide referrals to community resources such as home maintenance services, home health services, and structured cardiac rehabilitation programs. Refer the client and family (especially the primary food preparer) to a dietitian or nutritionist for teaching and assistance with menu planning.

The Client with Cardiomyopathy

The **cardiomyopathies** are disorders that affect the heart muscle itself. They are a diverse group of disorders that affect both systolic and diastolic functions. Cardiomyopathies may be either primary or secondary in origin. Primary cardiomyopathies are idiopathic; their cause is unknown. Secondary cardiomyopathies occur as a result of other processes, such as ischemia, infectious disease, exposure to toxins, connective tissue disorders, metabolic disorders, or nutritional deficiencies. In many cases, the cause of cardiomyopathy is unknown. In 1999, more than 27,000 deaths were directly attributed to cardiomyopathy. Mortality associated with cardiomyopathy is higher in older adults, men, and African-Americans (AHA, 2001).

Pathophysiology and Manifestations

The cardiomyopathies are categorized by their pathophysiology and presentation into three groups: dilated, hypertrophic, and restrictive.

Dilated Cardiomyopathy

Dilated cardiomyopathy is the most common type of cardiomyopathy, accounting for 87% of cases (AHA, 2001). The cause of dilated cardiomyopathy is unknown, although alcohol and cocaine abuse, chemotherapeutic drugs, pregnancy, and systemic hypertension may contribute to its development. Some cases of dilated cardiomyopathy are genetic; it can be transmitted in an autosomal dominant, autosomal recessive, or X-linked pattern (Porth, 2002).

In dilated cardiomyopathy, heart chambers dilate and ventricular contraction is impaired. Both end-diastolic and end-systolic volumes increase, and the left ventricular ejection fraction is substantially reduced, decreasing cardiac output. Left ventricular dilation is prominent; left ventricular hypertrophy is usually minimal. The right ventricle also may be enlarged. Extensive interstitial fibrosis (scarring) is evident; necrotic myocardial cells also may be seen (Braunwald, et al., 2001).

Manifestations of dilated cardiomyopathy develop gradually. Heart failure often develops years after the onset of dilation and pump failure. Both right- and left-sided failure occur, with dyspnea on exertion, orthopnea, paroxysmal nocturnal dyspnea, weakness, fatigue, peripheral edema, and ascites. Both S_3 and S_4 heart sounds are commonly heard, as well as an AV regurgitation murmur. Dysrhythmias are common, including supraventricular tachycardias, atrial fibrillation, and complex ventricular tachycardias. Untreated dysrhythmias can lead to sudden death (Porth, 2002). Mural thrombi (blood clots in the heart wall) may form in the left ventricular apex and embolize to other parts of the body.

The prognosis of dilated cardiomyopathy is grim; most clients get progressively worse and 50% die within five years after the diagnosis; 75% die within ten years (AHA, 2001).

Hypertrophic Cardiomyopathy

Hypertrophic cardiomyopathy is characterized by decreased compliance of the left ventricle and hypertrophy of the ventricular muscle mass. This impairs ventricular filling, leading to small end-diastolic volumes, and low cardiac output. About half of all clients with hypertrophic cardiomyopathy have a family history of the disease. It is genetically transmitted in an autosomal dominant pattern (Braunwald, et al., 2001).

The pattern of left ventricular hypertrophy is unique in that the muscle may not hypertrophy "equally." In a majority of clients, the interventricular septal mass, especially the upper portion, increases to a greater extent than the free wall of the ventricle. The enlarged upper septum narrows the passageway of blood into the aorta, impairing ventricular outflow. For this reason, this disorder is also known as *idiopathic hypertrophic subaortic stenosis (IHSS)* or *hypertrophic obstructive cardiomyopathy (HOCM)*.

Hypertrophic cardiomyopathy may be asymptomatic for many years. Symptoms typically occur when increased oxygen demand causes increased ventricular contractility. They may develop suddenly during or after physical activity; in children and young adults, sudden cardiac death may be the first sign of the disorder. Hypertrophic cardiomyopathy is the probable or definite cause of death in 36% of young athletes who die suddenly (AHA, 2001). It is hypothesized that sudden cardiac death is due to ventricular dysrhythmias or hemodynamic factors. Predictors of sudden cardiac death in this population include age of less than thirty years, a family history of sudden death, syncopal episodes, severe ventricular hypertrophy, and ventricular tachycardia seen on ambulatory ECG monitoring (Braunwald, et al., 2001). For a brief synopsis of a nursing research study regarding family presence during CPR and invasive procedures, see the section at the end of this chapter.

The usual manifestations of hypertrophic cardiomyopathy are dyspnea, angina, and syncope. Angina may result from ischemia due to overgrowth of the ventricular muscle, coronary artery abnormalities, or decreased coronary artery perfusion. Syncope may occur when the outflow tract obstruction severely decreases cardiac output and blood flow to the brain. Ventricular dysrhythmias are common; atrial fibrillation may also develop. Other manifestations of hypertrophic cardiomyopathy include fatigue, dizziness, and palpitations. A harsh, crescendo-decrescendo systolic murmur of variable intensity heard best at the lower left sternal border and apex is characteristic in hypertrophic cardiomyopathy. An S_4 may also be noted on auscultation.

Restrictive Cardiomyopathy

The least common form of cardiomyopathy, *restrictive cardiomyopathy* is characterized by rigid ventricular walls that impair diastolic filling. Causes of restrictive cardiomyopathy include myocardial fibrosis and infiltrative processes, such as amyloidosis. Fibrosis of the myocardium and endocardium causes excessive stiffness and rigidity of the ventricles. Decreased ventricular compliance impairs filling, with decreased ventricular size, elevated end-diastolic pressures, and decreased cardiac output. Contractility is unaffected, and the ejection fraction is normal. The manifestations of restrictive cardiomyopathy are those of heart failure and decreased tissue perfusion. Dyspnea on exertion and exercise intolerance are common. Jugular venous pressure is elevated, and S_3 and S_4 are common. The prognosis for restrictive cardiomyopathy is poor. Most clients die within three years, and the systemic nature of the underlying disease process precludes effective treatment.

Collaborative Care

With the exception of treating an underlying cause, little can be done to treat either dilated or restrictive cardiomyopathies. For these disorders, treatment focuses on managing heart failure and treating dysrhythmias. Refer to the section of this chapter on heart failure and Chapter 29 for specific treatment strategies. Treatment of hypertrophic cardiomyopathy focuses on reducing contractility and preventing sudden cardiac death. Strenuous physical exertion is restricted, as it may precipitate dysrhythmias or sudden cardiac death. Dietary and sodium restrictions may help diminish the manifestations.

Diagnostic Tests

Diagnosis begins with a history and physical assessment to rule out known causes of heart failure. Other tests may include the following:

- *Echocardiography* is done to assess chamber size and thickness, ventricular wall motion, valvular function, and systolic and diastolic function of the heart.
- *Electrocardiography and ambulatory ECG monitoring* demonstrate cardiac enlargement and detect dysrhythmias.
- *Chest X-ray* shows cardiomegaly, enlargement of the heart, and any pulmonary congestion or edema.
- *Hemodynamic studies* are used to assess cardiac output and pressures in the cardiac chambers and pulmonary vascular system.
- *Radionuclear scans* help identify changes in ventricular volume and mass, as well as perfusion deficits.
- *Cardiac catheterization* and *coronary angiography* may be done to evaluate coronary perfusion, the cardiac chambers, valves, and great vessels for function and structure, pressure relationships, and cardiac output.
- *Myocardial biopsy* uses the tranvenous route to obtain myocardial tissue for biopsy. The cells are examined for infiltration, fibrosis, or inflammation.

Medications

The drug regimen used to treat heart failure also is used for dilated or restrictive cardiomyopathy. This includes ACE inhibitors, vasodilators, and digitalis (see previous section of this chapter). Beta blockers also may be used with caution in clients with dilated cardiomyopathy. Anticoagulants are given to reduce the risk of thrombus formation and embolization. Antidysrhythmic drugs are avoided if possible due to their tendency to precipitate further dysrhythmias (Braunwald, et al., 2001).

Beta blockers are the drugs of choice to reduce anginal symptoms and syncopal episodes associated with hypertrophic cardiomyopathy. The negative inotropic effects of beta blockers and calcium channel blockers decrease the myocardial contractility, decreasing obstruction of the outflow tract. Beta blockers also decrease heart rate and increase ventricular compliance, increasing diastolic filling time and cardiac output. Vasodilators, digitalis, nitrates, and diuretics are contraindicated. Amiodarone may be used to treat ventricular dysrhythmias (Braunwald, et al., 2001).

Surgery

Without definitive treatment, clients with cardiomyopathy develop end-stage heart failure. Cardiac transplant is the definitive treatment for dilated cardiomyopathy. Ventricular assist devices may be used to support cardiac output until a donor heart is available. Transplantation is not a viable option for restrictive cardiomyopathy, because transplantation does not eliminate the underlying process causing infiltration or fibrosis, and, eventually, the transplanted organ is affected as well. See the section on heart failure for more information about cardiac transplantation.

In severely symptomatic clients with obstructive hypertrophic cardiomyopathy, excess muscle may be surgically resected from the aortic valve outflow tract. The septum is incised, and tissue is removed. This procedure provides lasting improvement in about 75% of clients (Braunwald, et al., 2001).

An implantable cardioverter-defibrillator (ICD) often is inserted to treat potentially lethal dysrhythmias, reducing the need for antidyrhythmic medications. A dual-chamber pacemaker may also be used for to treat hypertrophic cardiomyopathy.

Nursing Care

Nursing assessment and care for clients with dilated and restrictive cardiomyopathy is similar to that for clients with heart failure. Teaching about the disease process and its management is vital. Some degree of activity restriction often is necessary; assist to conserve energy while encouraging self-care. Support coping skills and adaptation to required lifestyle changes. Provide information and support for decision making about cardiac transplantation, if that is an option. Discuss the toxic and vasodilator effects of alcohol, and encourage abstinence. See the nursing care section for heart failure for nursing diagnoses and suggested interventions.

The client with hypertrophic cardiomyopathy requires care similar to that provided for myocardial ischemia; nitrates and other vasodilators, however, are avoided. If surgery is performed, nursing care is similar to that for any client undergoing open-heart surgery or cardiac transplant. Discuss the genetic transmission of hypertrophic cardiomyopathy, and suggest screening of close relatives (parents and siblings).

Provide pre- and postoperative care and teaching as appropriate for clients undergoing invasive procedures or surgery for cardiomyopathy.

Nursing diagnoses that may be appropriate for clients with cardiomyoapathy include:
- *Decreased cardiac output* related to impaired left ventricular filling, contractility, or outflow obstruction.
- *Fatigue* related to decreased cardiac output.
- *Ineffective breathing pattern* related to heart failure.
- *Fear* related to risk for sudden cardiac death.
- *Ineffective role performance* related to decreasing cardiac function and activity restrictions.
- *Anticipatory grieving* related to poor prognosis.

Home Care

Cardiomyopathies are chronic, progressive disorders generally managed in home and community care settings, unless surgery or transplant are planned, or end-stage heart failure develops. When teaching the client and family about home care, include the following topics:

- Activity restrictions and dietary changes to reduce manifestations and prevent complications.
- Prescribed drug regimen, its rationale, intended and possible adverse effects.
- The disease process, its expected ultimate outcome, and treatment options.
- Cardiac transplantation, including the procedure, the need for lifetime immunosuppression to prevent transplant rejection, and the risks of postoperative infection and long-term immunosuppression.
- Symptoms to report to the physician or for which immediate care is needed.
- Cardiopulmonary rescusitation procedures and available training sites.
- Refer the client and family for home and social services and counseling as indicated. Provide community resources such as support groups or the AHA.

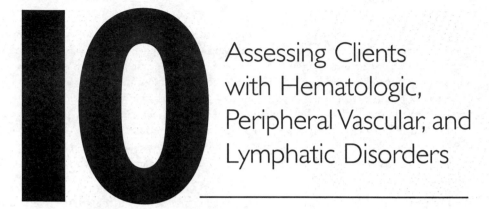

Assessing Clients with Hematologic, Peripheral Vascular, and Lymphatic Disorders

As the heart ejects blood with each beat, a closed system of blood vessels transports oxygenated blood to all body organs and tissues and then returns it to the heart for reoxygenation in the lungs. This branching network of vessels is called the peripheral vascular system. Systemic circulation is made possible by the vessels of the peripheral vascular system: the arteries, veins, and capillaries. The lymphatic system is a special vascular system that helps maintain sufficient blood volume in the cardiovascular system by picking up excess tissue fluid and returning it to the bloodstream.

Review of Anatomy and Physiology

Arterial and Venous Networks

The two main components of the peripheral vascular system are the arterial network and the venous network. The arterial network begins with the major arteries that branch from the aorta. These major arteries branch into successively smaller arteries, which in turn subdivide into the smallest of the arterial vessels, called arterioles. The smallest arterioles feed into beds of hairlike capillaries in the body's organs and tissues.

In the capillary beds, oxygen and nutrients are exchanged for metabolic wastes, and deoxygenated blood begins its journey back to the heart through venules, the smallest vessels of the venous network. Venules join the smallest of veins, which in turn join larger and larger veins. The blood transported by the veins empties into the superior and inferior venae cavae entering the right side of the heart.

Structure of Blood Vessels

The structure of blood vessels reflects their different functions within the circulatory system. Except for the tiniest vessels, blood vessel walls have three layers: the tunica intima, the tunica media, and the tunica adventitia. The tunica intima, the innermost layer, is made of simple squamous epithelium (the endothelium); this provides a slick surface to facilitate the flow of blood. In arteries, the middle layer, or tunica media, is made of smooth muscle and is thicker than the tunica media of veins. This makes arteries more elastic than veins and allows the arteries to alternately expand and recoil as the heart contracts and relaxes with each beat, producing a pressure wave, which can be felt as a **pulse** over an artery. The smaller arterioles are less elastic than arteries but contain more smooth muscle, which promotes their constriction (narrowing) and dilation (widening). In fact, arterioles, rather than arteries, exert the major control over arterial blood pressure. The tunica adventitia, or outermost layer, is made of connective tissue and serves to protect and anchor the vessel. Veins have a thicker tunica adventitia than do arteries.

Blood in the veins travels at a much lower pressure than blood in the arteries. Veins have thinner walls, a larger lumen, and greater capacity, and many are supplied with valves that help blood flow against gravity back to the heart. The "milking" action of skeletal muscle contraction (called the *muscular pump*) also supports venous return. When skeletal muscles contract against veins, the valves proximal to the contraction open, and blood is propelled toward the heart. The abdominal and thoracic pressure changes that occur with breathing (called the *respiratory pump*) also propel blood toward the heart.

The tiny capillaries, which connect the arterioles and venules, contain only one thin layer of tunica intima that is permeable to the gases and molecules exchanged between blood and tissue cells. Capillaries typically are found in interwoven networks. They filter and shunt blood from terminal arterioles to postcapillary venules.

Physiology of Arterial Circulation

The factors that affect arterial circulation are blood flow, peripheral vascular resistance, and blood pressure. **Blood flow** refers to the volume of blood transported in a vessel, in an organ, or throughout the entire circulation over a given period of time. It is commonly expressed as liters or milliliters per minute or cubic centimeters per second.

Peripheral vascular resistance (PVR) refers to the opposing forces or impedance to blood flow as the arterial channels become more and more distant from the heart. Peripheral vascular resistance is determined by three factors:

- *Blood viscosity:* The greater the viscosity, or thickness, of the blood, the greater its resistance to moving and flowing.
- *Length of the vessel:* The longer the vessel, the greater the resistance to blood flow.
- *Diameter of the vessel:* The smaller the diameter of a vessel, the greater the friction against the walls of the vessel and, thus, the greater the impedance to blood flow.

Blood pressure is the force exerted against the walls of the arteries by the blood as it is pumped from the heart. It is most accurately referred to as mean arterial pressure (MAP). The highest pressure exerted against the arterial walls at the peak of ventricular contraction (systole) is called the systolic blood pressure. The lowest pressure exerted during ventricular relaxation (diastole) is the diastolic blood pressure.

Mean arterial blood pressure is regulated mainly by cardiac output (CO) and peripheral vascular resistance (PVR), as represented in this formula: MAP = CO ¥ PVR. For clinical use, the MAP may be estimated by calculating the diastolic blood pressure plus one-third of the pulse pressure (the difference between the systolic and diastolic blood pressure).

Factors Influencing Arterial Blood Pressure

Blood flow, peripheral vascular resistance, and blood pressure, which influence arterial circulation, are in turn influenced by various factors. The sympathetic and parasympathetic nervous systems are the primary mechanisms that regulate blood pressure. Stimulation of the sympathetic nervous system exerts a major effect on peripheral resistance by causing vasoconstriction of the arterioles, thereby increasing blood pressure. Parasympathetic stimulation causes vasodilation of the arterioles, lowering blood pressure. Baroreceptors and chemoreceptors in the aortic arch, carotid sinus, and other large vessels are sensitive to pressure and chemical changes and cause reflex sympathetic stimulation, resulting in vasoconstriction, increased heart rate, and increased blood pressure.

The kidneys help maintain blood pressure by excreting or conserving sodium and water. When blood pressure decreases, the kidneys initiate the renin-angiotensin mechanism. This stimulates vasoconstriction, resulting in the release of the hormone aldosterone from the adrenal cortex, increasing sodium ion reabsorption and water retention. In addition, pituitary release of antidiuretic hormone (ADH) promotes renal reabsorption of water. The net result is an increase in blood volume and a consequent increase in cardiac output and blood pressure.

Temperatures may also affect peripheral resistance: Cold causes vasoconstriction, whereas warmth produces vasodilation. Many chemicals, hormones, and drugs influence blood pressure by affecting cardiac output and/or peripheral vascular resistance. For example, epinephrine causes vasoconstriction and increased heart rate; prostaglandins dilate blood vessel diameter (by relaxing vascular smooth muscle); endothelin, a chemical released by the inner lining of vessels, is a potent vasoconstrictor; nicotine causes vasoconstriction; and alcohol and histamine cause vasodilation.

Dietary factors, such as intake of salt, saturated fats, and cholesterol, elevate blood pressure by affecting blood volume and vessel diameter. Race, gender, age, weight, time of day, position, exercise, and emotional state may also affect blood pressure. These factors influence the arterial pressure; systemic venous pressure, though it is much lower, is also influenced by such factors as blood volume, venous tone, and right atrial pressure.

The Lymphatic System

The structures of the lymphatic system include the lymphatic vessels and several lymphoid organs. The lymphatic vessels, or lymphatics, form a network around the arterial and venous channels and interweave at the capillary beds. They collect and drain excess tissue fluid, called lymph, that "leaks" from the cardiovascular system and accumulates at the venous end of the capillary bed. The lymphatics return this fluid to the heart through a one-way system of lymphatic venules and veins that eventually drain into the right lymphatic duct and left thoracic duct, both of which empty into their respective subclavian veins. Lymphatics are a low-pressure system without a pump; their fluid transport depends on the rhythmic contraction of their smooth muscle and the muscular and respiratory pumps that assist venous circulation.

The organs of the lymphatic system are the lymph nodes, the spleen, the thymus, the tonsils, and the Peyer patches of the small intestine. Lymph nodes are small aggregates of specialized cells that assist the body's immune system by removing foreign material, infectious organisms, and tumor cells from lymph. Lymph nodes are distributed along the lymphatic vessels, forming clusters in certain body regions, such as the neck, axilla, and groin. The spleen, the largest lymphoid organ, is in the upper left quadrant of the abdomen under the thorax. The main function of the spleen is to filter the blood by breaking down old red blood cells and storing or releasing to the liver their by-products, such as iron. The spleen also synthesizes lymphocytes, stores platelets for blood clotting, and serves as a reservoir of blood. The thymus gland is in the lower throat and is most active in childhood, producing hormones, such as thymosin, that facilitate the immune action of lymphocytes. The tonsils of the pharynx and Peyer patches of the small intestine are lymphoid organs that protect the upper respiratory and digestive tracts from foreign pathogens.

Assessing Peripheral Vascular and Lymphatic Function

The nurse conducts both a health assessment interview to collect subjective data and a physical assessment to collect objective data.

The Health Assessment Interview

This section provides guidelines for collecting subjective data through a health assessment interview specific to the functions of the peripheral vascular system and the lymphatic system.

The Peripheral Vascular System The health assessment of the peripheral vascular system may focus on the client's chief complaint, such as swelling or pain in the legs, or it may be part of a full cardiovascular assessment. If the client has a chief complaint, analyze its onset, characteristics and course, severity, precipitating and relieving factors, and any associated symptoms, noting the timing and circumstances. For example, ask the client the following:

- Does the leg pain occur only with activities such as walking, or also during rest?
- Do your ankles swell at the end of the day, after sitting for prolonged periods, or after sleeping all night?
- Does temperature or the position of your body affect the symptoms?

Next, explore the client's medical and family history for any cardiovascular disorders, such as heart disease, arteriosclerosis, peripheral vascular disease (PVD), stroke, hypertension (HTN), hyperlipidemia (elevated fat in blood) and blood clots, or other chronic illnesses (e.g., diabetes). Ask about past surgery of the heart or blood vessels, or tests to evaluate their function, and about any medications that affect circulation or blood pressure.

Continue the assessment interview with a review of symptoms. Ask the client about past or present pain, burning, numbness, or tingling in the limbs or digits; leg fatigue or cramps; changes in skin color or temperature, texture of hair, ulcers or skin irritation, varicose veins, phlebitis (inflamed veins) or edema (swelling). Explore the client's nutritional history for intake of protein, vitamins and minerals, salt, fats, and fluid. Quantify any consumption of caffeine and alcohol, and history of smoking (in pack years) or other tobacco use. Assess the client's activity level for exercise habits and tolerance.

It is important to consider socioeconomic factors that may precipitate or aggravate circulatory problems (e.g., inadequate clothing, shoes, or shelter) and occupational factors, such as prolonged standing or sitting, or exposure to temperature extremes. Also assess psychosocial factors that may affect the client's stress level and emotional state.

The Lymphatic System

The health assessment of the lymphatic system includes a review of specific lymphatic findings, such as lymph node enlargement or swollen glands, as well as other more general complaints about infection or impaired immunity, such as fever, fatigue, or weight loss. If a health problem exists, analyze its onset, characteristics, severity, and precipitating and relieving factors, noting the timing and circumstances. For example, ask the client the following:

- Did you notice that the glands in your neck became swollen after an infection?
- Have you noticed increased fatigue or weakness?
- Have you ever been exposed to radiation?

Explore the client's history for chronic illnesses (e.g., cardiovascular disease, renal disease, cancer, tuberculosis, HIV infection), predisposing factors (e.g., surgery, trauma, infection, blood transfusions, intravenous drug use), and environmental exposure (e.g., radiation, toxic chemicals, travelrelated infectious disease). Review the family history for any incidence of cancer, anemia, or blood dyscrasias. Ask the client about past or present bleeding (e.g., from the nose, gums, or mouth; from vomiting; from the rectum; bruising) and associated symptoms (e.g., pallor, dizziness, fatigue, difficulty breathing); lymph node changes (e.g., enlargement, pain or tenderness, itching, warmth); swelling of extremities; and recurrent irritations or infections. Lastly, an assessment of the client's socioeconomic status, lifestyle, intravenous drug use, and sexual practices may be significant in determining risk for diseases associated with impaired lymphatic function.

Physical Assessment: The Peripheral Vascular System

Physical assessment of the peripheral vascular system can be performed as part of the full cardiovascular assessment, or alone for clients who have known or suspected peripheral vascular disease or who are at risk for circulatory complications (e.g., clients who have undergone surgery or are immobile). The techniques used to assess the peripheral vascular system include auscultation of blood pressure, palpation of the major pulse points of the body, and inspection of the skin for such changes as edema, ulcerations, or alterations in color and temperature. Recommended equipment for this assessment includes a stethoscope, a tape measure, and a metric ruler. The client may be assessed in the supine, sitting, or standing positions. Table 10-1 reviews guidelines for blood pressure measurement.

Blood Pressure and Pulse Pressure Assessment with Abnormal Findings (✓)
- Auscultate blood pressure in each arm with the client seated.
    - ✓ Consistent BP readings over 140/90 in adults under age 40 is considered hypertension.
    - ✓ BP under 90/60 is considered hypotension.
    - ✓ An **auscultatory gap**—a temporary disappearance of sound between the systolic and diastolic BP—may be a normal variation, or it may be associated with systolic HTN or a drop in diastolic BP due to aortic stenosis.
    - ✓ **Korotkoff sounds** (see Table 10-1) may be heard down to zero with cardiac valve replacements, hyperkinetic states, thyrotoxicosis, and severe anemia, as well as after vigorous exercise.
    - ✓ The sounds of aortic regurgitation may obscure the diastolic BP.
    - ✓ A difference of over 10 mmHg between arms suggests arterial compression on the side of the lower reading, aortic dissection, or coarctation of the aorta.

- Auscultate blood pressure in each arm with the client standing. If orthostatic changes occur, measure the BP with the client supine, legs dangling, and again with the client standing, one to three minutes apart.
  - ✓ A decrease in systolic BP of over 10 to 15 mmHg and a drop in diastolic BP on standing is called **orthostatic hypotension.** Causes include antihypertensive medications, volume depletion, peripheral neurovascular disease, prolonged bed rest, and aging.
- Observe the pulse pressure. The **pulse pressure** is the difference between the systolic and diastolic BP. For example, if the BP is 140/80, the pulse pressure is 60. A normal pulse pressure is one-third the systolic measurement.
  - ✓ A widened pulse pressure with an elevated systolic BP occurs with exercise, arteriosclerosis, severe anemia, thyrotoxicosis, and increased intracranial pressure.
  - ✓ A narrowed pulse pressure with a decreased systolic BP occurs with shock, cardiac failure, and pulmonary embolus.

Table 10-1. Guidelines for Blood Pressure Monitoring

Review of Korotkoff Sounds

The first sound heard is the systolic pressure; at least two consecutive sounds should be clear. If the sound disappears, and then is heard again 10 to 15 mm later, an auscultatory gap is present; this may be a normal variant, or it may be associated with hypertension. The first diastolic sound is heard as a muffling of the Korotkoff sound and is considered the best approximation of the true diastolic pressure. The second diastolic sound is the level at which sounds are no longer heard.

The American Heart Association recommends documenting all three readings when measuring blood pressure, for example, 120/72/64. If only two readings are documented, the systolic and the second diastolic pressure are taken, for example, 120/64.

Technique Reminders

- < Choose a cuff of an appropriate size: The cuff should snugly cover two-thirds of the upper arm, and the bladder should completely encircle the arm. The bladder should be centered over the brachial artery, with the lower edge 2 to 3 cm above the antecubital space.
- < The client's arm should be slightly flexed and supported (on a table or by the examiner) at heart level.
- < To determine how high to inflate the cuff, palpate the brachial pulse, and inflate the cuff to the point on the manometer at which the pulse is no longer felt; then, add 30 mmHg to this reading, and use the sum as the target for inflation. Wait 15 seconds before reinflating the cuff to auscultate the BP.
- < To recheck a BP, wait at least 30 seconds before attempting another inflation.
- < Always inflate the cuff completely, then deflate it. Once deflation begins, allow it to continue; do not try to reinflate the cuff if the first systolic sound is not heard or if the cuff inadvertently deflates.
- < The bell of the stethoscope more effectively transmits the low-pitched sounds of BP.

Table 10-1. Continued

Sources of Error

< Falsely high readings can occur if the cuff is too small, too loose, or if the client supports his or her own arm.

< Falsely low readings can occur if a standard cuff is used on a client with thin arms.

< Inadequate inflation may result in underestimation of the systolic pressure or overestimation of the diastolic pressure if an auscultatory gap is present.

< Rapid deflation and repeated or slow inflations (causing venous congestion) can lead to underestimation of the systolic BP and overestimation of the diastolic BP.

Factors Altering Blood Pressure

< A change from the horizontal to upright position causes a slight decrease (5 to 10 mm) in systolic BP; the diastolic BP remains unchanged or rises slightly.

< BP taken in the arm is lower when the client is standing.

< If the BP is taken with the client in the lateral recumbent position, a lower BP reading may be obtained in both arms; this is especially apparent in the right arm with the client in the left lateral position.

< Factors that increase BP include exercise, caffeine, cold environment, eating a large meal, painful stimuli, and emotions.

< Factors that lower BP include sleep (by 20 mmHg) and very fast, slow, or irregular heart rates.

< BP tends to be higher in taller or heavier clients.

Alternative Methods of Blood Pressure Measurement

< The palpatory method may be necessary if severe hypotension is present and the BP is inaudible. Palpate the brachial pulse, and inflate the cuff 30 mm above the point where the pulse disappears; deflate the cuff, and note the point on the manometer where the pulse becomes palpable again. Record this as the palpatory systolic BP.

< Leg BP measurement may be needed when there is injury of the arms or to rule out coarctation of the aorta or aortic insufficiency when arm diastolic BP is over 90 mmHg. Place the client in the prone or supine position with the leg slightly flexed. Place a large leg cuff on the thigh with the bladder centered over the popliteal artery. Place the bell of the stethoscope over the popliteal space. Normal leg systolic BP is higher than arm BP; diastolic BP should be equal to or lower than arm BP. Abnormally low leg BP occurs with aortic insufficiency and coarctation of the aorta.

Skin Assessment with Abnormal Findings (✓)

• Inspect the color of the skin.

   ✓ Pallor reflects constriction of peripheral blood flow (e.g., due to syncope or shock) or decreased circulating oxyhemoglobin (e.g., due to anemia).

   ✓ Central cyanosis of the lips, earlobes, oral mucosa, and tongue suggests chronic cardiopulmonary disease.

Artery and Vein Assessment with Abnormal Findings (✓)

- Palpate the temporal arteries.
    - ✓ Redness, swelling, nodularity, and variations in pulse amplitude may occur with temporal arteritis.
- Inspect and palpate the carotid arteries. Note symmetry, the pulse rate, rhythm, volume, and amplitude. Note any variation with respiration. Describe all pulses as increased, normal, diminished, or absent. Scales ranging from 0 to 4+ are sometimes used as follows:

    0 = Absent
    1+ = Diminished
    2+ = Normal
    3+ = Increased
    4+ = Bounding

    - ✓ A unilateral pulsating bulge is seen with a tortuous or kinked carotid artery.
    - ✓ Alterations in pulse rate or rhythm are due to cardiac dysrhythmias.
    - ✓ An absent pulse indicates arterial occlusion.
    - ✓ A hypokinetic (weak) pulse is associated with decreased stroke volume. This may be due to congestive heart failure (CHF), aortic stenosis, or hypovolemia; to increased peripheral resistance, which may result from cold temperatures; or to arterial narrowing, commonly found with atherosclerosis.
    - ✓ A hyperkinetic (bounding) pulse occurs with increased stroke volume and/or decreased peripheral resistance. This may result from states in which cardiac output is high or from aortic regurgitation. It also may occur with anemia, hyperthyroidism, bradycardia, or reduced compliance, as with atherosclerosis.
    - ✓ A bigeminal pulse is marked by decreased amplitude of every second beat. This may be due to premature contractions (usually ventricular).
    - ✓ Pulsus alternans is a regular pulse with alternating strong and weak beats. This may be due to left ventricular failure and severe HTN.
    - ✓ The waterhammer pulse (collapsing pulse) has a greater than normal amplitude with a sharp rise and fall. It occurs with aortic insufficiency.
    - ✓ Pulsus bisferiens has two main peaks in amplitude ("double beat") and occurs with combined aortic stenosis and regurgitation, pericardial effusion, and constructive pericarditis.
    - ✓ Pulsus paradoxus is a pulse in which the amplitude is diminished or absent during inspiration and exaggerated during expiration. Pulsus paradoxus occurs with cardiac tamponade, constrictive pericarditis, and severe chronic lung disease.
    - ✓ A palpable thrill over the carotid artery suggests arterial narrowing, as with atherosclerosis.
- Auscultate the carotid arteries, using the bell of the stethoscope.
    - ✓ A murmuring or blowing sound heard over stenosed peripheral vessels is known as a bruit. A bruit heard over the middle to upper carotid artery suggests atherosclerosis.
- Inspect and palpate the internal and external jugular veins for venous pressure.

✓ An increase in jugular venous pressure over 3 cm and located above the sternal angle reflects increased right atrial pressure. This occurs with right ventricular failure or, less commonly, with constrictive pericarditis, tricuspid stenosis, and superior venae cavae obstruction.

- If venous pressure is elevated, assess the hepatojugular reflex. (Compress the liver in the right upper abdominal quadrant with the palm of the hand for 30 to 60 seconds while observing the jugular veins.)

  ✓ A decrease in venous pressure reflects reduced left ventricular output or blood volume.

  ✓ Unilateral neck vein distention suggests local compression or anatomic anomaly.

  ✓ A rise in the column of neck vein distention over 1 cm with liver compression indicates right heart failure.

Upper Extremity Assessment with Abnormal Findings (✓)

- Inspect and palpate the arms, noting size and symmetry, skin color, and temperature.

  ✓ Unilateral swelling with venous prominence occurs with venous obstruction.

  ✓ Extreme localized pallor of the fingers is seen with Raynaud disease.

  ✓ Cyanosis of the nailbeds reflects chronic cardiopulmonary disease.

  ✓ Cold temperature of the hands and fingers occurs with vasoconstriction.

- Palpate the nail beds for capillary refill. (Apply pressure to the client's fingertips. Watch for blanching of the nail beds. Release the pressure. Note the time it takes for capillary refill, indicated by the return of pink color on release of the pressure.)

  ✓ Capillary refill that takes more than two seconds reflects circulatory compromise, such as hypovolemia or anemia.

- Assess venous pattern and pressure. (Elevate one of the client's arms over the head for a few seconds. Slowly lower the arm. Observe the filling of the client's hand veins.)

  ✓ Distention of hand veins at elevations over 9 cm above heart level reflects an increase in systemic venous pressure.

- Palpate the radial and brachial pulses. Note rate, rhythm, volume amplitude, symmetry, variations with respiration.

  ✓ Alterations in pulse rate or rhythm are due to cardiac dysrhythmias, such as atrial fibrillation, atrial flutter, and premature ventricular contractions. A pulse rate over 100 beats per minute is tachycardia; a pulse rate below 60 BPM is bradycardia.

  ✓ A pulse deficit (slower radial rate than apical rate) occurs with dysrhythmias and CHF.

  ✓ Irregularities of rhythm produce early beats and pauses (skipped beats) in the pulse, which may be regular in pattern, sporadic, or grossly irregular.

  ✓ Diminished or absent radial pulses may be due to thromboangitis obliterans (Buerger disease) or acute arterial occlusion.

  ✓ A weak and thready pulse, often with tachycardia, reflects decreased cardiac output.

  ✓ A bounding pulse occurs with hyperkinetic states and atherosclerosis.

  ✓ Unequal pulses between extremities suggest arterial narrowing or obstruction on one side.

✓ In sinus dysrhythmia (a normal variant, especially in young adults), the pulse rate increases with inspiration and decreases with expiration.

- If arterial insufficiency is suspected, palpate the ulnar pulse and perform the Allen test:
    - Have the client make a tight fist.
    - Compress both the radial and ulnar arteries.
    - Have the client open the hand to a slightly flexed position.
    - Observe for pallor and manifestations of pain.
    - Release the ulnar artery and observe for the return of pink color within three to five seconds.
    - Repeat the procedure on the radial artery.
    - ✓ The normal ulnar artery may or may not have a palpable pulse.
    - ✓ Persistent pallor with the Allen test suggests ulnar artery occlusion.

- Inspect and palpate each leg, noting size, shape, and symmetry; arterial pattern; skin color, temperature, and texture; hair pattern; pigmentation; rashes; ulcers, sensation; and capillary refill.
    - ✓ Chronic arterial insufficiency may be due to arteriosclerosis or autonomic dysfunction, or to acute occlusion resulting from thrombosis, embolus, or aneurysm.
    - ✓ Signs of arterial disruption include pallor, dependent rubor (dusky redness); cool to cold temperature; and atrophic changes, such as hair loss with shiny and smooth texture, thickened nails, sensory loss, slow capillary refill, and muscle atrophy.
    - ✓ Ulcers with symmetric margins, a deep base, black or necrotic tissue, and absence of bleeding may occur at pressure points on or between the toes, on the heel, on the lateral malleolar or tibial area, over the metatarsal heads, or along the side or sole of the foot.
    - ✓ Gangrene due to complete arterial occlusion presents as black, dry, hard skin; pregangrenous color changes include deep cyanosis and purple-black discoloration.

Lower Extremity Assessment with Abnormal Findings (✓)

- With the client supine, assess the venous pattern of the legs. Repeat with the client standing.
    - ✓ Signs of venous insufficiency include swelling, thickened skin, cyanosis, stasis dermatitis (brown pigmentation, erythema, and scaling), and superficial ankle ulcers located predominantly at the medial malleolus with uneven margins, ruddy granulation tissue, and bleeding. Varicose veins appear as dilated, tortuous, and thickened veins, which are more prominent in a dependent position.

- Palpate the femoral, popliteal, posterior tibial, and dorsalis pedis pulses for volume, amplitude, and symmetry.
    - ✓ Diminished or absent leg pulses suggest partial or complete arterial occlusion of the proximal vessel and are often due to arteriosclerosis obliterans.
    - ✓ Increased and widened femoral and popliteal pulsations suggest aneurysm.
    - ✓ Absence of a posterior tibial pulse with signs and symptoms of arterial insufficiency is usually due to acute occlusion by thrombosis or embolus.
    - ✓ Diminished or absent pedal pulses are often due to popliteal occlusion associated with diabetes mellitus.

- If pulses are diminished, observe for postural color changes. Elevate both legs 60 degrees, and observe the color of the soles of the feet. Have the client sit and dangle the legs; note the return of color to the feet.

  ✓ Extensive pallor on elevation is suggestive of arterial insufficiency.

  ✓ Rubor (dusky redness) of the toes and feet along with delayed venous return (over 45 seconds) suggests arterial insufficiency.

- If arterial insufficiency is suspected, auscultate the femoral arteries.

  ✓ Femoral bruits suggest arterial narrowing due to arteriosclerosis.

- Inspect and gently palpate the calves.

  ✓ Redness, warmth, swelling, tenderness, and cords along a superficial vein suggest thrombophlebitis or deep vein thrombosis (DVT).

- Inspect and palpate for edema. Use your thumb to compress the dorsum of the client's foot, around the ankles, and along the tibia. A depression in the skin that does not immediately refill is called pitting edema. Edema can be graded on a scale of from 1+ to 4+:

1+ (–2mm depression)	No visible change in the leg; slight pitting
2+ (–4mm depression)	No marked change in the shape of the leg; pitting slightly deeper
3+ (–6mm depression)	Leg visibly swollen; pitting deep
4+ (–8mm depression)	Leg very swollen; pitting very deep

  ✓ Edema may be caused by disease of the cardiovascular system such as CHF; by renal, hepatic, or lymphatic problems; or by infection.

  ✓ Venous distention suggests venous insufficiency or incompetence.

Abdominal Assessment with Abnormal Findings (✓)

- Inspect and palpate the abdominal aorta. Note size, width, and any visible pulsations or bulging.

  ✓ A pulsating mass in the upper abdomen suggests an aortic aneurysm, particularly in the older adult.

  ✓ An aorta greater than 2.5 to 3 cm in width reflects pathologic dilation, most likely due to arteriosclerosis.

- Auscultate the epigastrium and each abdominal quadrant, using the bell of the stethoscope.

  ✓ Abdominal bruits reflect turbulent blood flow associated with partial arterial occlusion.

  ✓ A bruit heard over the aorta suggests an aneurysm.

  ✓ A bruit heard over the epigastrium and radiating laterally, especially with HTN, suggests renal artery stenosis.

  ✓ Bruits heard in the lower abdominal quadrants suggest partial occlusion of the iliac arteries.

Physical Assessment: The Lymphatic System

Physical assessment of the lymphatic system is usually integrated into the assessment of other body systems. For example, the tonsils are observed with the pharynx during the head and neck assessment; the regional lymph nodes are evaluated with corresponding body regions (e.g., occipital, auricular, and cervical nodes are evaluated with assessment of the head and neck, axillary nodes with assessment of the breast or thorax, epitrochlear node with assessment of the peripheral vascular exam of the arms, and inguinal nodes with assessment of the abdomen); the spleen can be palpated during the abdominal assessment. The techniques of inspection and palpation are used for the lymphatic examination; a tape measure and metric ruler may be helpful.

Skin Assessment with Abnormal Findings (✓)

- Inspect the skin of the extremities and over the regional lymph nodes, noting any edema, erythema, red streaks, or skin lesions.

    ✓ **Lymphangitis** (inflammation of a lymphatic vessel) may produce a red streak with induration (hardness) following the course of the lymphatic collecting duct; infected skin lesions may be present, particularly between the digits.

    ✓ **Lymphedema** (swelling due to lymphatic obstruction) occurs with congenital lymphatic anomaly (Milroy disease) or with trauma to the regional lymphatic ducts from surgery or metastasis (e.g., arm lymphedema after radical mastectomy with axillary node removal).

    ✓ Edema of lymphatic origin is usually not pitting, and the skin may be thickened; one example is the taut swelling of the face and body that occurs with myxedema, associated with hypothyroidism.

Lymph Node Assessment with Abnormal Findings (✓)

- Palpate the regional lymph nodes of the head and neck, axillae, arms, and groin.

    Use firm, circular movements of the finger pads and note size, shape, symmetry, consistency, delineation, mobility, tenderness, sensation, and condition of overlying skin.

    ✓ **Lymphadenopathy** refers to the enlargement of lymph nodes (over 1 cm) with or without tenderness. It may be caused by inflammation, infection, or malignancy of the nodes or the regions drained by the nodes.

    ✓ Lymph node enlargement with tenderness suggests inflammation (lymphadenitis). With bacterial infection, the nodes may be warm and matted with localized swelling.

    ✓ Malignant or metastatic nodes may be hard, indicating lymphoma; rubbery, indicating Hodgkin disease; or fixed to adjacent structures. Usually, they are not tender.

    ✓ Ear infections and scalp and facial lesions, such as acne, may cause enlargement of the preauricular and cervical nodes.

    ✓ Anterior cervical nodes are enlarged and infected with streptococcal pharyngitis and mononucleosis.

    ✓ Lymphadenitis of the cervical and submandibular nodes occurs with herpes simplex lesions.

    ✓ Brain tumors may metastasize to the occipital nodes.

    ✓ Enlargement of supraclavicular nodes, especially the left, is highly suggestive of metastatic disease from abdominal and thoracic cancer.

    ✓ Axillary lymphadenopathy is associated with breast cancer.

✓ Lesions of the genitals may produce enlargement of the inguinal nodes.

✓ Persistent generalized lymphadenopathy is associated with acquired immune deficiency syndrome (AIDS) and AIDS-related complex (ARC).

Spleen Assessment with Abnormal Findings (✓)

• Palpate for the spleen, in the upper left quadrant of the abdomen.

✓ A palpable spleen in the left upper abdominal quadrant of an adult may indicate abnormal enlargement (splenomegaly) and may be associated with cancer, blood dyscrasias, and viral infection, such as mononucleosis.

• Percuss for splenic dullness in the lowest left intercostal space (ICS) at the anterior axillary line or in the ninth to tenth ICS at the midaxillary line.

✓ A dull percussion note in the lowest left ICS at the anterior axillary line or below the tenth rib at the midaxillary line suggests splenic enlargement.

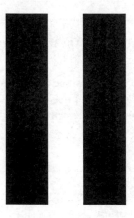

Nursing Care of Clients with Hematologic Disorders

Disorders affecting the blood and blood-forming organs have effects that range from minor disruptions in daily activities to major life-threatening crises. Clients with hematologic disorders need holistic nursing care, including emotional support and care for problems involving major body systems.

Blood is an exchange medium between the external environment and the body's cells. Blood consists of plasma, solutes (e.g., proteins, electrolytes, and organic constituents), red blood cells, white blood cells, and platelets, which are fragments of cells.

The *hematopoietic* (blood-forming) system includes the bone marrow (myeloid) tissues, where blood cells form, and the lymphoid tissues of the lymph nodes, where white blood cells mature and circulate. All blood cells originate from cells in the bone marrow called **stem cells,** or *hemocytoblasts.* Regulatory mechanisms cause stem cells to differentiate into families of parent cells, each of which gives rise to one of the formed elements of the blood (red blood cells, platelets, and white cells).

Red Blood Cell Disorders

Red blood cells (RBCs), and the hemoglobin molecules they contain, are required for oxygen transport to body tissues. Hemoglobin also binds with some carbon dioxide, carrying it to the lungs for excretion. Abnormal numbers of RBCs, changes in their size and shape, or altered hemoglobin content or structure can adversely affect health. Anemia, the most common RBC disorder, is an abnormally low RBC count or reduced hemoglobin content. Polycythemia is an abnormally high RBC count.

Physiology Review of Red Blood Cells

The red blood cell (**erythrocyte**) is shaped like a biconcave disk. This unique shape increases the surface area of the cell and allows the cell to pass through very small capillaries without disrupting the cell membrane. RBCs are the most common type of blood cell.

Hemoglobin is the oxygen-carrying protein within RBCs. It consists of the heme molecule and globin, a protein molecule. Globin is made of four polypeptide chains—two alpha chains and two beta chains. Each of the four polypeptide chains contains a heme unit containing an iron atom. The iron atom binds reversibly with oxygen, allowing it to transport oxygen as *oxyhemoglobin* to the cells. Hemoglobin is synthesized within the RBC. The rate of synthesis depends on the availability of iron (Porth, 2002).

Normal adult laboratory values for red blood cells are defined and identified in Table 11-1. The size, color, and shape of stained RBCs also may be analyzed. RBCs may be *normocytic* (normal size), smaller than normal (*microcytic*), or larger than normal (*macrocytic*). Their color may be normal (*normochromic*) or diminished (*hypochromic*).

Table 11-1. **Normal Laboratory Values for Red Blood Cells**

Laboratory Test	Normal Range	Definition
Red blood cell (RBC) count		
• Men	4.2–5.4 million/mm³	Number of circulating RBCs
• Women	3.6–5.0 million/mm³	per mm³ of blood
Reticulocytes	1.0%–1.5% of total RBC	Number of immature RBCs per mm³ of blood
Hemoglobin (Hgb)		
• Men	14–16.5 g/dL	Amount of Hgb per dL (100 mL)
• Women	12–15 g/dL	of blood
Hematocrit (Hct)		
• Men	40%–50%	Packed volume of RBCs in 100 mL
• Women	37%–47%	of blood expressed as a percentage
Mean corpuscular volume (MCV)	85–100 fL/cell	Average volume of individual RBCs
Mean corpuscular Hgb concentration (MCHC)	31–35 g/dL	Average concentration or percentage of hemoglobin per RBC
Mean corpuscular Hgb (MCH)	27–34 pg/cell	Calculated average weight of hemoglobin per RBC

Red Blood Cell Production and Regulation

In adults, RBC production (**erythropoiesis**) begins in red bone marrow of the vertebrae, sternum, ribs, and pelvis, and is completed in the blood or spleen. *Erythroblasts* begin forming hemoglobin while they are in the bone marrow, a process that continues throughout RBC lifespan. Erythroblasts differentiate into *normoblasts*. As these slightly smaller cells mature, their nucleus and most organelles are ejected, eventually causing normoblasts to collapse inward and assume the characteristic biconcave shape of RBCs. The cells enter the circulation as *reticulocytes,* which fully mature in about 48 hours. The complete sequence from stem cell to RBC takes three to five days.

Tissue hypoxia is the stimulus for RBC production. The hormone *erythropoietin* is released by the kidneys in response to hypoxia. It stimulates the bone marrow to produce RBCs. However, the process of RBC production takes about five days to maximize. During periods of increased RBC production, the percentage of reticulocytes in the blood exceeds that of mature cells.

Red Blood Cell Destruction

RBCs have a life span of about 120 days. Old or damaged RBCs are *lysed* (destroyed) by phagocytes in the spleen, liver, bone marrow, and lymph nodes. The process of RBC destruction is called **hemolysis.** Phagocytes save and reuse amino acids and iron from heme units in the lysed RBCs. Most of the heme unit is converted to bilirubin, an orange-yellow pigment that is removed from the blood by the liver and excreted in the bile.

During disease processes causing increased hemolysis or impaired liver function, bilirubin accumulates in the serum, causing a yellowish appearance of the skin and sclera (*jaundice*).

The Client with Anemia

Anemia is an abnormally low number of circulating RBCs, low hemoglobin concentration, or both. Decreased numbers of circulating RBCs is the usual cause of anemia. This may result from blood loss, inadequate RBC production, or increased RBC destruction. Insufficient or defective hemoglobin within RBCs contributes to anemia. Depending on its severity, anemia may affect all major organ systems.

Pathophysiology and Manifestations

A number of different pathologic mechanisms can lead to anemia. Regardless of the cause, every type of anemia reduces the oxygen-carrying capacity of the blood, leading to tissue hypoxia. The resulting manifestations depend on the severity of the anemia, how quickly it develops, and other factors such as age and health status.

When anemia develops gradually and the RBC reduction is moderate, successful compensatory mechanisms may result in few symptoms except when the oxygen needs of the body increase due to exercise or infection. Symptoms develop as RBCs are further reduced. Pallor of the skin, mucous membranes, conjunctiva, and nail beds develops as a result of blood redistribution to vital organs and lack of hemoglobin. As tissue oxygenation decreases, the heart and respiratory rates rise. Tissue hypoxia may cause angina, fatigue, dyspnea on exertion, and night cramps. It also stimulates erythropoietin release; increased erythropoietin activity may cause bone pain. Cerebral hypoxia can lead to headache, dizziness, and dim vision. Heart failure may develop in severe anemia.

With rapid blood loss, blood volume is decreased as well as the oxygen-carrying capacity of the blood. Signs of circulatory shock may occur. With chronic bleeding, fluid shifts from the interstitial spaces into the vessels, maintaining blood volume. Blood viscosity is reduced, which may result in a systolic heart murmur.

Anemia is categorized by cause: blood loss, nutritional, hemolytic, and bone marrow suppression. The pathophysiology of these types of anemias follows.

Blood Loss Anemia

When anemia results from acute or chronic bleeding, RBCs and other blood components are lost from the body. With acute blood loss, circulating volume decreases, increasing the risk for shock and circulatory failure (see Chapter 6). Fluid shifts from the interstitial spaces into the vascular compartment to maintain blood volume, diluting the cellular components of the blood and reducing its viscosity. In acute blood loss, circulating RBCs are of normal size and shape, but the hemoglobin and hematocrit are reduced. If sufficient iron is available, the number of circulating RBCs returns to normal within 3 to 4 weeks after the bleeding episode. Chronic blood loss, on the other hand, depletes iron stores as RBC production attempts to maintain the RBC supply. The resulting RBCs are microcytic (small) and hypochromic (pale).

Nutritional Anemias

Nutritional anemias result from nutrient deficits that affect RBC formation (erythropoiesis) or hemoglobin synthesis. The nutrient deficit may be caused by inadequate diet, malabsorption, or an increased need for the nutrient. The most common types of nutritional anemias are iron deficiency anemia, vitamin B_{12} anemia, and folic acid deficiency anemia. Vitamin B_{12} and folic acid anemias are sometimes called megaloblastic anemias, as enlarged nucleated RBCs called megaloblasts are seen in these anemias.

Iron Deficiency Anemia

Iron deficiency anemia is the most common type of anemia. It develops when the supply of iron is inadequate for optimal RBC formation. The body cannot synthesize hemoglobin without iron. Iron deficiency anemia results in fewer numbers of RBCs, microcytic and hypochromic RBCs, as well as malformed RBCs (poikilocytosis).

Excessive iron loss due to chronic bleeding is the usual cause of iron deficiency anemia in adults. Menstrual blood loss is the most common cause in adult females. Iron deficiency anemia also may result from inadequate dietary iron intake (less than 1 mg/day), malabsorption, or the increased iron requirements associated with pregnancy and lactation. Table 11-1 summarizes common causes of iron deficiency anemia.

Iron deficiency anemia is particularly common in older adults. Chronic, occult (hidden) blood loss may occur from slowly bleeding ulcers, gastrointestinal inflammation, hemorrhoids, and cancer. Inadequate dietary iron intake also contributes to anemia in the older adult. Access to transportation may limit fresh food consumption, a factor contributing to poor iron intake among all adults, especially people with limited or fixed incomes.

Table 11-2. Causes of Iron Deficiency Anemia

< Dietary deficiencies
< Decreased absorption
   a. Partial or total gastrectomy
   b. Chronic diarrhea
   c. Malabsorption syndromes
< Increased metabolic requirements
   a. Pregnancy
   b. Lactation
< Blood loss
   a. Gastrointestinal bleeding (especially due to ulcers or chronic aspirin use)
   b. Menstrual losses
< Chronic hemoglobinuria

In addition to the general manifestations of anemia described earlier, chronic iron deficiency may lead to brittle, spoon-shaped nails; cheilosis (cracks at the corners of the mouth); a smooth, sore tongue; and pica (a craving for unusual substances, such as clay or starch).

The primary treatment for iron deficiency anemia is increased dietary intake of iron-rich foods and oral or parenteral iron supplements.

Vitamin B$_{12}$ Deficiency Anemia

Vitamin B$_{12}$ is necessary for DNA synthesis and is almost exclusively found in foods derived from animals. **Vitamin B$_{12}$ deficiency** occurs when inadequate vitamin B$_{12}$ is consumed, or, more commonly, when it is poorly absorbed from the gastrointestinal tract. Deficiency of this vitamin impairs cell division and maturation, especially in rapidly proliferating red blood cells. As a result, macrocytic, misshapen (oval rather than concave) RBCs with thin membranes are produced. Great numbers of these large, immature RBCs enter the circulation. These cells are fragile, incapable of carrying adequate amounts of oxygen, and have a shortened life span.

Failure to absorb dietary vitamin B$_{12}$ is called **pernicious anemia.** It develops due to lack of *intrinsic factor,* a substance secreted by the gastric mucosa. Intrinsic factor binds with vitamin B$_{12}$ and travels with it to the ileum, where the vitamin is absorbed. In the absence of intrinsic factor, vitamin B$_{12}$ cannot be absorbed into the body.

Vitamin B$_{12}$ deficiency may also result from other malabsorption disorders and dietary factors. Resection of the stomach or ileum, loss of pancreatic secretions, and chronic gastritis can affect vitamin B$_{12}$ absorption. Dietary deficiencies of vitamin B$_{12}$ are rare, usually occurring only among strict vegetarians.

Manifestations of vitamin B$_{12}$ deficiency anemia develop gradually as bodily stores of the vitamin are depleted. Pallor or slight jaundice and weakness develop. In pernicious anemia, a smooth, sore, beefy red tongue and diarrhea may occur. Because vitamin B$_{12}$ is important for neurologic function, *paresthesias* (altered sensations, such as numbness or tingling) in the extremities and problems with *proprioception* (the sense of one's position in space) develop. These manifestations may progress to difficulty maintaining balance due to spinal cord damage. Central nervous system manifestations of relatively short duration (six months or less) are reversible with treatment, but may be permanent if treatment is delayed (Tierney, et al, 2001).

When the anemia results from insufficient dietary intake of vitamin B$_{12}$, clients are instructed to increase their intake of foods containing the vitamin, such as meats, eggs, and dairy products. Vitamin B$_{12}$ supplements may be ordered for severe anemia or for clients who are strict vegetarians. Parenteral vitamin B$_{12}$ replacement is required when malabsorption disorders or lack of intrinsic factor is the cause. Parenteral replacement therapy must be continued for life.

Folic Acid Deficiency Anemia

Like vitamin B$_{12}$, folic acid is required for DNA synthesis and normal maturation of red blood cells. **Folic acid deficiency anemia** is characterized by fragile, megaloblastic cells. Folic acid is found in green leafy vegetables, fruits, cereals, and meats, and is absorbed from the intestines.

Folic acid deficiency anemia due to inadequate intake is more common among people who are chronically undernourished. This includes older adults, alcoholics, and drug addicts.

Alcoholics are especially at risk because alcohol suppresses folate metabolism, which forms folic acid. Increased folic acid requirements may also lead to anemia. Pregnant women are at the greatest risk. Infants and teenagers can develop temporary folic acid deficiencies during periods of rapid growth. Impaired folic acid absorption and metabolism can cause folic acid deficiency anemia. Malabsorption disorders such as celiac sprue (a hereditary gastrointestinal disorder characterized by inability to metabolize amino acids found in gluten), and certain medications, such as methotrexate and some chemotherapeutic agents, may be implicated. Causes of folic acid deficiency anemia are summarized in Table 11-3.

Table 11-3. Causes of Folic Acid Deficiency Anemia

Inadequate dietary intake

At risk:

a. Older adults

b. Alcoholics

c. Clients receiving total parenteral nutrition

Increased metabolic requirements

At risk:

a. Pregnant women

b. Infants and teenagers

c. Clients undergoing hemodialysis

d. Clients with forms of hemolytic anemia

Folic acid malabsorption and impaired metabolism

a. Celiac sprue

b. Chemotherapeutic agents, folate antagonists (methotrexate, pentamidine), or anticonvulsants

c. Alcoholism

The manifestations develop gradually as folic acid stores are depleted. Signs and symptoms may include pallor, progressive weakness and fatigue, shortness of breath, and heart palpitations. Manifestations similar to those associated with vitamin B_{12} anemia, such as glossitis, cheilosis, and diarrhea, are common. No neurologic symptoms occur with folic acid deficiency anemia, helping differentiate it from vitamin B_{12} deficiency anemia. These two nutritional anemias do, however, sometimes coexist.

Among the undernourished, adding foods containing folic acid to the diet usually corrects the anemia. Other clients often require oral folic acid supplements. Depending on the cause of the deficiency, folate replacement may continue for a short or an expended period of time. Folate supplements are recommended for all women who can become pregnant and during pregnancy. Folate deficiency is strongly associated with neural tube defects such as meningomyelocele. The neural tube develops early in the process of fetal development, often before pregnancy is recognized.

Hemolytic Anemias

Hemolytic anemias are characterized by premature destruction (*lysis*) of RBCs. When RBCs break down, iron and other by-products of their destruction remain in the plasma. RBC lysis may occur within the circulatory system or due to phagocytosis by cells of the reticuloendothelial system. In response to hemolysis, the hematopoietic activity of bone marrow increases, leading to increased reticulocytes in circulating blood. Most types of hemolytic anemia are characterized by normocytic and normochromic RBCs.

There are many different causes of hemolytic anemias. The cause may be *intrinsic,* arising from disorders within the RBC itself, or *extrinsic,* originating outside the RBC. Intrinsic disorders include cell membrane defects, defects in hemoglobin structure and function, and inherited enzyme deficiencies. Extrinsic causes of hemolytic anemia include drugs, bacterial and other toxins, and trauma. This section discusses sickle cell anemia, thalassemia, acquired hemolytic anemia, and glucose-6-phosphate dehydrogenase anemia.

Sickle Cell Anemia

Sickle cell anemia is a hereditary, chronic hemolytic anemia. It is characterized by episodes of *sickling,* during which RBCs become abnormally crescent shaped. The disorder is transmitted as an autosomal recessive genetic defect. This defect causes synthesis of an abnormal form of hemoglobin (HbS) within red blood cells. Sickle cell anemia can significantly shorten life span, with most deaths occurring due to infection (McCance & Huether, 2002).

The disease is most common among people of African descent. In the United States, 7% to 13% of blacks carry the defective gene, having inherited it from one parent (McCance & Huether, 2002). These people have *sickle cell trait.* About 40% of their hemoglobin is HbS (Porth, 2002). They are likely to remain asymptomatic unless stressed by severe hypoxia. Less than 1% of African-Americans are homozygous for the disorder; that is, they have inherited a defective gene from both parents. These people have *sickle cell disease;* nearly all their hemoglobin is HbS (Porth, 2002). They are at risk for **sickle cell crisis,** severe episodes of fever and intense pain that are the hallmark of this disorder.

The HbS gene changes the structure of the beta chain of the hemoglobin molecule. When hypoxemia develops and HbS is deoxygenated, it crystallizes into rodlike structures. Clusters of these rods form long chains that deform the erythrocyte into a crescent or sickle shape. The sickled cells tend to clump together and obstruct capillary blood flow, causing ischemia and possible infarction of surrounding tissue.

When normal oxygen tension is restored, the sickled RBCs resume their normal shape; that is, they "unsickle." Repeated episodes of sickling and unsickling weaken RBC cell membranes. The weakened RBCs are hemolyzed and removed. Consequently, the normal life span of RBCs is greatly reduced in sickle cell anemia, increasing the demand for RBC production. Conditions likely to trigger sickling include hypoxia, low environmental or body temperature, excessive exercise, anesthesia, dehydration, infections, or acidosis.

The acute and chronic manifestations of sickle cell anemia arise from episodes of RBC sickling. Sickling causes general manifestations of hemolytic anemia, including pallor, fatigue, jaundice, and irritability. Extensive sickling can precipitate a crisis due to occluded circulation, impaired erythropoiesis, or sequestration of large amounts of blood in the liver or spleen.

A vasoocclusive or thrombotic crisis occurs when sickling develops in the microcirculation. Obstruction of blood flow triggers vasospasm that halts all blood flow in the vessel. Lack of blood flow leads to tissue ischemia and infarction. Vasoocclusive crises are painful and last an average of four to six days. Infarction of small vessels in the extremities causes painful swelling of the hands and feet; large joints also may be affected. Priapism (persistent, painful erection of the penis) may develop. Abdominal pain may signal infarction of abdominal organs and structures. Stroke may result from cerebral vessel occlusion (McCance & Huether, 2002). Repeated infarcts associated with sickling can affect the structure and function of nearly every organ system.

Compromised erythropoiesis can lead to profound *aplastic anemia* in sickle cell disease due to the shortened RBC life span. *Sequestration crises* are marked by pooling of large amounts of blood in the liver and spleen. This sickle cell crisis only occurs in children.

There is no cure for this disease; treatment is primarily supportive. Treatment for sickle cell crisis includes rest, oxygen, and analgesics for pain. Adequate hydration is essential to improve blood flow, reduce pain, and prevent renal damage. Precipitating factors are treated, and folic acid supplements may be given to meet the increased demands for RBC production. Blood transfusions may be necessary during surgery or pregnancy. Genetic counseling is recommended for people at risk for sickle cell anemia.

Thalassemia

Thalassemia is an inherited disorder of hemoglobin synthesis in which either the alpha or beta chains of the hemoglobin molecule are missing or defective. This leads to deficient hemoglobin production and fragile hypochromic, microcytic RBCs called *target cells* because of their distinctive bull's-eye appearance.

Thalassemia usually affects certain populations. People of Mediterranean descent (southern Italy and Greece) are more likely to have beta-defect thalassemias (often called *Cooley anemia* or Mediterranean anemia). People of Asian ancestry, especially from Thailand, the Philippines, and China, more often have alpha-defect thalassemia. Africans and African-Americans may have both alpha- and beta-defect thalassemia. As with sickle cell anemia, only one defective beta chain-forming gene may be present (*beta-thalassemia minor*), causing mild symptoms, or both may be defective (*beta-thalassemia major*), leading to more severe symptoms. Children with thalassemia major rarely reach adulthood, although repeated blood transfusions may extend their lifespan (McCance & Huether, 2002). Four genes are responsible for alpha chain formation; one, two, three, or all four, may be defective. In the latter case (*alpha-thalassemia major*), death is inevitable and usually occurs in utero. Genetic studies and counseling are recommended for people at risk for this illness.

People with thalassemia minor often are asymptomatic. When manifestations do occur, they include mild to moderate anemia, mild splenomegaly, bronze skin coloring, and bone marrow hyperplasia. The major form of the disease causes severe anemia, heart failure, and liver and spleen enlargement from increased red cell destruction. Fractures of the long bones, ribs, and vertebrae may result from bone marrow expansion and thinning due to increased hematopoiesis. Accumulation of iron in the heart, liver, and pancreas following repeated transfusions for treatment may eventually cause failure of these organs.

Acquired Hemolytic Anemia *Acquired hemolytic anemia* results from hemolysis due to factors outside of the RBC. Causes of acquired hemolytic anemias include:

- Mechanical trauma to RBCs produced by prosthetic heart valves, severe burns, hemodialysis, or radiation.
- Autoimmune disorders.
- Bacterial or protozoal infection.
- Immune-system-mediated responses, such as transfusion reactions.
- Drugs, toxins, chemical agents, or venoms.

The manifestations of acquired hemolytic anemia depend on the extent of hemolysis and the body's ability to replace destroyed RBCs. The anemia itself often is mild to moderate as erythropoiesis increases to replace the destroyed RBCs. The spleen enlarges as it removes damaged or destroyed RBCs. If the breakdown of heme units exceeds the liver's ability to conjugate and excrete bilirubin, jaundice develops. When the condition is severe, bone marrow expands, and bones may be deformed or may develop pathologic fractures. The severity of generalized manifestations of anemia (tachycardia, pallor, etc.) depends on the degree of anemia and deficiency of tissue oxygenation.

Glucose-6-Phosphate Dehydrogenase (G6PD) Anemia

Glucose-6-phosphate dehydrogenase (G6PD) anemia is caused by a hereditary defect in RBC metabolism. It is relatively common in people of African and Mediterranean descent. The defective gene is located on the X chromosome and therefore affects more males than females. There are many variations of this genetic defect.

G6PD is an enzyme that catalyzes glycolysis, the process in which an RBC derives cellular energy. A defect in G6PD action causes direct oxidation of hemoglobin, damaging the RBC. Hemolysis usually occurs only when the affected person is exposed to stressors (e.g., drugs such as aspirin, sulfonamides, or vitamin K derivatives) that increase the metabolic demands on RBCs. The G6PD deficiency impairs the necessary compensatory increase in glucose metabolism and causes cellular damage. Damaged RBCs are destroyed over a period of seven to twelve days.

When exposed to a stressor triggering G6PD anemia, symptoms develop within several days. These may include pallor, jaundice, hemoglobinuria (hemoglobin in the urine), and an elevated reticulocyte count. As new RBCs develop, counts return to normal.

Aplastic Anemia

In **aplastic anemia,** the bone marrow fails to produce all three types of blood cells, leading to *pancytopenia.* Normal bone marrow is replaced by fat. Fortunately, aplastic anemia is rare. *Fanconi anemia* is a rare aplastic anemia caused by defects of DNA repair. The underlying cause of about 50% of acquired aplastic anemia is unknown (*idiopathic aplastic anemia*). Other cases follow stem cell damage caused by exposure to radiation or certain chemical substances such as benzene, arsenic, nitrogen mustard, certain antibiotics (especially chloramphenicol), and chemotherapeutic drugs (McCance & Huether, 2002). Aplastic anemia also may occur with viral infections, such as mononucleosis, hepatitis C, and HIV disease (Porth, 2002). Anemia develops as the bone marrow fails to replace RBCs that have reached the end of their life span. Remaining RBCs are normochromic and normocytic.

Manifestations of aplastic anemia vary with the severity of the pancytopenia. Its onset usually is insidious, but may be sudden. Manifestations include fatigue, pallor, progressive weakness, exertional dyspnea, headache, and, ultimately, tachycardia and heart failure. Platelet deficiency leads to bleeding problems. A deficiency of white blood cells increases the risk of infection, causing manifestations such as fever.

Treatment focuses on removing the causative agent, if known, and using blood transfusions. Transfusions may be discontinued as soon as the bone marrow resumes blood cell production. Complete recovery may take months. Bone marrow transplant may be the treatment of choice in some instances.

Collaborative Care

Ensuring adequate tissue oxygenation is the priority of care in treating anemia. Specific therapy is determined by the underlying cause of the disorder. Usual treatments include medications, dietary modifications, blood replacement, or supportive interventions.

Diagnostic Tests

When anemia is suspected, the following laboratory and diagnostic tests may be ordered.

* *Complete blood count (CBC)* is done to determine blood cell counts, hemoglobin, hematocrit, and red blood cell indices (see Table 11–1).

* *Iron levels* and *total iron-binding* capacity are performed to detect iron deficiency anemia. A low serum iron concentration and elevated total iron-binding capacity are indicative of iron deficiency anemia.

* *Serum ferritin* is low due to depletion of the total iron reserves available for hemoglobin synthesis. Ferritin is an iron-storage protein produced by the liver, spleen, and bone marrow. Ferritin mobilizes stored iron when metabolic needs are higher than dietary intake.

* *Sickle cell test* is a screening test to evaluate hemolytic anemia and detect HbS.

* *Hemoglobin electrophoresis* separates normal hemoglobin from abnormal forms. It is used to evaluate hemolytic anemia, diagnose thalassemia, and differentiate sickle cell trait from sickle cell disease (Malarkey & McMorrow, 2000).

* *Schilling test* measures vitamin B_{12} absorption before and after intrinsic factor administration to differentiate between pernicious anemia and intestinal malabsorption of the vitamin. A 24-hour urine sample is collected following administration of radioactive vitamin B_{12}. Lower than normal levels of the tagged B_{12} when intrinsic factor is given concurrently indicate malabsorption rather than pernicious anemia.

* *Bone marrow examination* is done to diagnose aplastic anemia. In aplastic anemia, normal marrow elements are significantly decreased as they are replaced by fat cells.

* *Quantitative assay of G6PD* may be performed to confirm a diagnosis of glucose-6-phosphate dehydrogenase deficiency.

Medications

Medications used to treat anemia depend on its cause. Iron replacement therapy is ordered for iron deficiency anemia. Supplemental iron may be given by mouth or intramuscularly. Parenteral vitamin B_{12} is given when malabsorption or lack of intrinsic factor leads to vitamin B_{12} deficiency anemia. Folic acid is ordered for women of childbearing age, pregnant women, and clients with folic acid deficiency or sickle cell anemia to meet the increased demands of the bone marrow. Hydroxyurea, a drug that promotes fetal hemoglobin production, may be prescribed for clients with sickle cell disease. Resulting increased levels of fetal hemoglobin interfere with the sickling process and reduce the incidence of painful crises (Braunwald et al., 2001). Nursing implications for clients receiving iron, vitamin B_{12}, and folic acid are found in Table 11-4.

Immunosuppressive therapy with antithymocyte globulin (ATG), corticosteroids, and cyclosporine may be used to treat aplastic anemia. Androgens may stimulate blood cell production in some clients with aplastic anemia. See Chapter 9 for more information about immunosuppression.

Dietary Therapy

Dietary modifications are recommended for nutritional deficiency anemias, such as iron deficiency anemia, vitamin B_{12} deficiency anemia, or folic acid deficiency anemia.

Blood Transfusion

Blood transfusions may be indicated to treat anemias resulting from major blood loss, such as from trauma or major surgery, and severe anemia regardless of cause. Blood transfusions are fully discussed in Chapter 40.

Table 11-4. Medication Administration—Drugs to Treat Anemia

Iron Sources

> Ferrous sulfate (Feosol, Fer-in-sol)
> Ferrous gluconate (Fergon, Ferralet, Fertinic)
> Iron dextran injection (Imferon)
> Iron polysaccharide

Iron preparations are normally taken by mouth and are absorbed from the gastrointestinal tract. They are given to treat anemias resulting from iron deficiency or blood loss. When absorbed, iron combines with transferrin. This complex then is transported to the bone marrow and incorporated into hemoglobin.

Nursing Responsibilities
- Prior to giving the drug, assess for use of drugs that might interact with iron (e.g., antacids, allopurinol, chloramphenicol, tetracyclines, vitamin E), gastrointestinal bleeding, and manifestations of anemia.
- Administer iron preparations with orange juice to enhance absorption.
- If using an elixir, give it through a straw to prevent staining the teeth.
- Monitor for manifestations of iron toxicity: nausea, diarrhea, or constipation; symptoms of anaphylactic shock (extreme cases).
- Monitor hemoglobin and reticulocyte counts.
- If the client is also taking tetracyclines, schedule the dose of iron 2 hours before tetracycline (iron reduces the absorption of tetracycline).

Client and Family Teaching
- Gastrointestinal side effects may be reduced by taking iron with food (but not milk, which decreases absorption).
- Stools may be dark green or black; this is harmless.
- Increase fluids and fiber in diet to decrease constipation.

Continued on the next page

Table 11-4. Continued

Vitamin B$_{12}$ Sources

Cyanocobalamin (Kaybovite [oral], Anacobin [parenteral], Bedoz)

Cyanocobalamin is used to treat vitamin B$_{12}$ deficiencies or malabsorption and pernicious anemia. It is rapidly absorbed when administered orally or by injection, and it is stored in the liver. Intrinsic factor is necessary for absorption from the gastrointestinal tract.

Nursing Responsibilities
- Do not expose crystalline injection to light.
- Assess for other drugs that might interfere with the therapeutic response: chloramphenicol, cimetidine, colchicine, and timed-release potassium decrease its effectiveness.
- Do not mix cyanocobalamin in a syringe with other medications.
- Administer parenteral doses intramuscularly or deep subcutaneously to decrease local irritation.
- Monitor hemoglobin, RBC counts, reticulocyte counts, and potassium levels.

Client and Family Teaching
- A burning sensation with injection is temporary.
- Avoid alcohol, which interferes with absorption.
- If used to treat pernicious anemia, the medication must be taken for life.

Folic Acid Sources

Folic acid (Folvite, novofolacid)

Synthetic folic acid is used to treat folic acid deficiency and megaloblastic or macrocytic anemia. It is absorbed from the gastrointestinal tract and stored in the liver.

Nursing Responsibilities
- Prior to giving the medication, assess for use of drugs that alter its effect: corticosteroids, methotrexate, oral contraceptives, phenytoin, sulfonamides.
- Do not mix folic acid with other medications in the same syringe.
- Monitor for possible hypersensitivity response of skin rash.

Client and Family Teaching
- Large doses of folic acid may cause the urine to become darker yellow.
- Excess alcohol intake increases folic acid requirements.

Complementary Therapies

Complementary health care practitioners may recommend specific plant enzymes to treat nutritional anemias. Plant enzymes are believed to aid digestion of proteins, fats, and carbohydrates, facilitating absorption of their nutrients. Therapy is determined by the specific type of anemia. Plant enzymes should not be used alone to treat anemia, and it is important to check for possible interactions with prescribed medications before starting therapy.

Nursing Care

Health Promotion

Nursing measures to prevent anemia focus on teaching good dietary habits to all clients, regardless of age. Stress the importance of consuming adequate amounts of iron, folate, and the B vitamins. Provide a list of dietary sources of these nutrients. Discuss alternate iron sources with vegetarian clients, and teach them that foods high in vitamin C enhance the absorption of iron from grains, legumes, and other sources. Emphasize the importance of adequate iron intake in women of childbearing age and older adults. Stress the increased need for these nutrients during pregnancy, and discuss strategies to ensure an adequate intake.

Assessment

Assessment data to collect for clients with suspected anemia includes:

- *Health history:* complaints of shortness of breath with activity, fatigue, weakness, dizziness or fainting, palpitations; history of previous anemia, bleeding episodes; menstrual history (if appropriate); medications; chronic diseases; usual diet and patterns of alcohol intake or cigarette smoking.
- *Physical examination:* general appearance, skin color; vital signs including temperature; heart and lung sounds; peripheral pulses, capillary refill; abdominal tenderness; obvious bleeding or bruising.

Nursing Diagnoses and Interventions

Anemia affects circulating oxygen levels and tissue oxygenation. Priority nursing diagnoses include activity intolerance, altered oral mucous membranes, and self-care deficits. With acute blood-loss anemia, risk for insufficient cardiac output also is a priority. Clients with sickle cell disease have specific needs related to the effects of the disease on tissue perfusion; see the section on disseminated intravascular coagulation (DIC) later in this chapter for nursing interventions appropriate to ineffective tissue perfusion, associated pain, and maintaining oxygenation.

Activity Intolerance

Anemia causes weakness and shortness of breath on exertion. These symptoms are due to decreased circulating oxygen levels secondary to low hemoglobin levels. Weakness, fatigue, and/or vertigo may occur even during activities of daily living, including those associated with self-care, home life, job performance, and social roles.

- Help identify ways to conserve energy when performing necessary or desired activities. *Modifying the approach to a particular activity may reduce cardiorespiratory symptoms and activity-related fatigue. Alternative ways of performing tasks (e.g., sitting when performing hygiene care and kitchen tasks) may reduce oxygen demands. In some cases, assistance from others is necessary to conserve energy and reduce symptoms.*
- Help the client and family establish priorities for tasks and activities. *Because family members may need to assume responsibility for additional tasks, the plan's success depends on mutually established goals.*

- Assist to develop a schedule of alternating activity and rest periods throughout the day. *Rest periods decrease oxygen needs, reducing strain on the heart and lungs, and allowing restoration of homeostasis before further activities.*
- Encourage eight to ten hours of sleep at night. *Rest decreases oxygen demands and increases available energy for morning activities.*
- Monitor vital signs before and after activity. *Vital signs provide a measure of activity tolerance. Increased heart and respiratory rates or a change in blood pressure may indicate intolerance of the activity.*
- Discontinue activity if any of the following occurs.
  a. Complaints of chest pain, breathlessness, or vertigo
  b. Palpitations or tachycardia that does not return to normal within four minutes of resting
  c. Bradycardia
  d. Tachypnea or dyspnea
  e. Decreased systolic blood pressure

These changes may signify cardiac decompensation due to insufficient oxygenation. The intensity, duration, or frequency of the activity needs to be reduced.

- Instruct the client not to smoke. *Smoking causes vasoconstriction and increases carbon monoxide levels in the blood, interfering with tissue oxygenation.*

Impaired Oral Mucous Membrane

Glossitis and cheilosis may occur with nutritional deficiencies of iron, folate, and vitamin B_{12}. The tongue and lips become very red, and fissures or cracks may form at the corners of the mouth.

- Monitor condition of lips and tongue daily. *Glossitis and cheilosis increase the risk for bleeding and infection and may require medical treatment. Pain and discomfort may interfere with oral intake, further worsening the nutritional deficiency.*
- Use a mouthwash of saline, saltwater, or half-strength peroxide and water to rinse the mouth every two to four hours. Avoid alcohol-based mouthwashes. *This cleanses and soothes oral mucous membranes. Alcohol-based mouthwashes further irritate and dry oral tissues.*
- Provide frequent oral hygiene (after each meal and at bedtime) with a soft bristle toothbrush or sponge. *Removing food debris from painful fissures promotes comfort. A soft toothbrush reduces irritation or bleeding of oral mucosa. Keeping the oral cavity clean also reduces the risk of infection.*
- Apply a petroleum-based lubricating jelly or ointment to the lips after oral care. *Lubricating ointment helps to retain moisture, facilitate healing, and protect the lips from other drying agents.*
- Instruct to avoid hot, spicy, or acidic foods. *Such foods may further irritate and dry mucous membranes.*
- Encourage soft, cool, bland foods. *Foods that are soothing to the mucous membranes promote comfort and help maintain adequate food and fluid intake. Minimizing oral pain may also promote compliance with oral care routines.*
- Encourage eating four to six small meals daily with high protein and vitamin content. *Small, frequent meals may be better tolerated, increasing intake. Nutrient-rich meals promote healing of the mucous membranes.*

Risk for Decreased Cardiac Output

Cardiac output may be affected by acute bleeding and volume loss or by heart failure resulting from severe anemia. In addition, impaired tissue oxygenation leads to an increased respiratory rate and dyspnea.

- Monitor vital signs, breath sounds, and apical pulse. *Increased cardiac workload can affect the blood pressure, heart, and respiratory rates. Increased blood flow can lead to heart murmur or abnormal heart sounds such as S_3 or S_4. Tachypnea and dyspnea may affect the depth of respirations, alveolar ventilation, and blood and tissue oxygenation.*

- Assess for pallor, cyanosis, and dependent edema. *Blood is shunted to the vital organs, causing vasoconstriction of skin vessels. This, in addition to lower levels of hemoglobin, cause pallor. Cyanosis, especially of the lips and nail beds, indicates inadequate oxygenation of blood. Dependent edema occurs in response to right ventricular failure.*

Self-Care Deficit

Energy expenditures for activities of daily living (ADLs) may cause oxygen demands to exceed supply in the client with severe anemia.

- Assist with ADLs, such as bathing, grooming, and eating, as needed. *Assistance decreases energy expenditures and tissue requirements for oxygen, reducing cardiac workload.*

- Discuss the importance of rest periods prior to such activities as dressing. *Rest reduces oxygen demand and cardiac workload. The person who is able to perform self-care in activities of daily living maintains independence, self-esteem, and morale.*

Home Care

With the exception of anemia resulting from acute hemorrhage, most clients with anemia are treated in the home and community setting. Include the following topics when preparing the client and family for home care.

- Nutritional strategies to address deficiencies
- Prescribed medications, vitamins, or mineral supplements and their appropriate use, intended effect, possible adverse effects, and interactions with food or other medications
- Energy conservation strategies
- Other recommended treatment measures and follow-up
- If the anemia is genetically transmitted, such as sickle cell anemia, include inheritance patterns of the disorder, symptoms of crisis, and manifestations to report to the physician.

Provide referrals for counseling to facilitate decisions about pregnancy as indicated. Also refer for nutritional assistance and teaching, home health care, or assistance with self-care and home maintenance activities as indicated. Older adults with nutritional anemias may benefit from community services such as senior meals or Meals-on-Wheels.

Platelet and Coagulation Disorders

Platelet and coagulation disorders affect **hemostasis,** control of bleeding. Hemostasis is a series of complex interactions between platelets and clotting mechanisms that maintains a relatively steady state of blood volume, blood pressure, and blood flow through injured vessels.

Physiology Review

Platelets

Platelets, or **thrombocytes,** are cell fragments that have no nucleus and cannot replicate. They are metabolically active, however, producing ATP and releasing mediators required for clotting. Platelets are formed in the bone marrow as pinched-off portions of large megakaryocytes. Platelet production is controlled by *thrombopoietin,* a protein produced by the liver, kidney, smooth muscle, and bone marrow. The number of circulating platelets controls thrombopoietin release. Once released from the bone marrow, platelets remain in the spleen for about eight hours before entering the circulation. Platelets live up to ten days in circulation. There are about 250,000 to 400,000 platelets in each milliliter of blood. An excess of platelets is *thrombocytosis.* A deficit of platelets is *thrombocytopenia.*

Hemostasis

Hemostasis, or blood clotting, is a complex process that controls bleeding and clotting. The five stages to hemostasis are: (1) vessel spasm, (2) formation of the platelet plug, (3) development of an insoluble fibrin clot, (4) clot retraction, and (5) clot dissolution.

Vessel Spasm   When a blood vessel is damaged, thromboxane A_2 (TXA_2) is released from platelets and cells, causing *vessel spasm.* This spasm constricts the damaged vessel for about one minute.

Formation of the Platelet Plug   Platelets attracted to the damaged vessel wall change from smooth disks to spiny spheres. Receptors on the activated platelets bind with *von Willebrand factor,* a protein molecule, and exposed collagen fibers at the site of injury to form the *platelet plug.* The platelets release adenosine diphosphate (ADP) and TXA_2 to activate nearby platelets, adhering them to the developing plug. Activation of the clotting pathway on the platelet surface converts fibrinogen to fibrin. Fibrin, in turn, forms a meshwork that binds the platelets and other blood cells to form a stable plug.

Blood Coagulation   The process of **coagulation** creates a meshwork of fibrin strands that cements the blood components to form an insoluble clot. Coagulation requires many interactive reactions and two clotting pathways. The slower intrinsic pathway is activated when blood contacts collagen in the injured vessel wall; the faster extrinsic pathway is activated when blood is exposed to tissues. The final outcome of both pathways is fibrin clot formation. Each procoagulation substance is activated in sequence; the activation of one coagulation factor activates another in turn.

Clot Retraction   After the clot is stabilized (within about 30 minutes), trapped platelets contract, much like muscle cells. Platelet contraction squeezes the fibrin strands, pulling the broken portions of the ruptured blood vessel closer together. Growth factors released by the platelets stimulate cell division and tissue repair of the damaged vessel.

Clot Dissolution   *Fibrinolysis,* the process of clot dissolution, begins shortly after the clot has formed, restoring blood flow and promoting tissue repair. Like coagulation, fibrinolysis requires a sequence of interactions between activator and inhibitor substances. Plasminogen, an enzyme that promotes fibrinolysis, is converted into plasmin, its active form, by chemical mediators released from vessel walls and the liver. Plasmin dissolves the clot's fibrin strands and certain coagulation factors. Stimuli such as exercise, fever, and vasoactive drugs promote plasminogen activator release. The liver and endothelium also produce fibrinolytic inhibitors.

The Client with Thrombocytopenia

Thrombocytopenia is a platelet count of less than 100,000 per milliliter of blood. It can lead to abnormal bleeding. A continuing decline in circulating platelets to less than 20,000/mL can lead to spontaneous bleeding and hemorrhage from minor trauma. Bleeding due to platelet deficiency usually occurs in small vessels, causing manifestations such as *petechiae* (small red or purple spots that do not blanch with pressure) and *purpura* (purple bruising). The mucous membranes of the nose, mouth, GI tract, and vagina often bleed. Serious and potentially fatal bleeding occurs when the platelet count is less than 10,000/mL.

Thrombocytopenia results from one of three mechanisms: decreased production, increased sequestration in the spleen, or accelerated destruction. Primary thrombocytopenia that leads to increased platelet destruction is discussed below. Secondary thrombocytopenia may be caused by aplastic anemia, bone marrow malignancy, infection, radiation therapy, or drug therapy. Platelet sequestration usually is due to an enlarged spleen. Up to 80% of platelets may be removed from circulation with significant splenomegaly (Porth, 2002). Finally, thrombocytopenia may result from premature platelet destruction associated with disseminated intravascular coagulation (DIC).

Pathophysiology and Manifestations

The two types of primary thrombocytopenia are immune thrombocytopenic purpura and thrombotic thrombocytopenic purpura.

Immune Thrombocytopenic Purpura

Immune thrombocytopenic purpura (ITP), also known as *idiopathic thrombocytopenic purpura*, is an autoimmune disorder in which platelet destruction is accelerated. In its chronic form, ITP typically affects young adults between age 20 and 40; women are affected more often than men. Acute ITP is more common in children, and often follows a viral illness. Acute ITP typically lasts only one to two months (McCance & Huether, 2002).

In ITP, proteins on the platelet cell membrane stimulate autoantibody production, usually IgG antibodies. These autoantibodies adhere to the platelet membrane. Although the platelets function normally, the spleen reacts to them as being foreign and destroys the altered platelets after only one to three days of circulation.

The manifestations of ITP are due to bleeding from small vessels and mucous membranes. Petechiae and purpura develop, often on the anterior chest, arms, neck, and oral mucous membranes. Bruising also may be apparent. As bleeding progresses, epistaxis (nosebleed), hematuria, excess menstrual bleeding, and bleeding gums occur. Spontaneous intracranial bleeding is rare, but does occur. Associated symptoms include weight loss, fever, and headache.

Thrombotic Thrombocytopenic Purpura

Thrombotic thrombocytopenic purpura (TTP) is a rare disorder in which thrombi occlude arterioles and capillaries of the microcirculation. Many organs are affected, including the heart, kidneys, and brain. The incidence of TTP is increasing (McCance & Huether, 2002). Its cause is unknown. Platelet aggregation is a key feature of the disorder. As RBCs circulate through partially occluded vessels, they fragment, leading to hemolytic anemia (Porth, 2002).

TTP may be acute, the more common and severe form, or chronic. Acute idiopathic TTP may be fatal within months, if untreated. The manifestations of TTP include purpura and petechiae, and neurologic symptoms such as headache, seizures, and altered consciousness.

Collaborative Care

The diagnosis of thrombocytopenia is based on history, manifestations, and diagnostic test results. Management focuses on treating or removing any causative factors and treating the platelet deficiency.

Diagnostic Tests

The following diagnostic tests are used to identify thrombocytopenia.

- *CBC* evaluates all cellular components of the blood, as well as the hemoglobin and hematocrit.
- *Platelet count* is decreased.
- *Antinuclear antibodies (ANA)* are measured to assess for autoantibodies.
- *Serologic studies* for hepatitis viruses, cytomegalovirus (CMV), Epstein-Barr virus, toxoplasma, and HIV may be done.
- *Bone marrow examination* evaluates for aplastic anemia and megakaryocyte production.

Medications

Oral glucocorticoids, such as prednisone, are prescribed to suppress the autoimmune response. Many clients who respond to glucocorticoid treatment relapse when the drug is withdrawn, however. Immunosuppressive drugs such as azathioprine, cyclophosphamide, and cyclosporine may be used.

Treatments

Platelet transfusions may be required to treat acute bleeding due to thrombocytopenia. Platelets are prepared from fresh whole blood; one unit contains 30 to 60 mL of platelet concentrate. The expected increase in platelets after one unit is infused is 10,000/mL. *Plasmapheresis*, or *plasma exchange therapy*, is the primary treatment for acute thrombotic thrombocytopenic purpura. The client's plasma is removed and replaced with fresh frozen plasma to remove autoantibodies, immune complexes, and toxins.

Surgery

A *splenectomy* (surgical removal of the spleen) is the treatment of choice if the client with ITP relapses when glucocorticoids are discontinued. The spleen is the site of platelet destruction and antibody production. This surgery often cures the disorder, although relapse may occur years after splenectomy.

Nursing Care

Assessment

- Health history: complaints of bruising with minor or no trauma, bleeding gums, nosebleed, heavy or prolonged menstrual periods, black, tarry, or bloody stools, hematemesis, headache, fever, or neurologic symptoms; recent weight loss; recent viral or other illness; current and recent medications; exposure to toxins

- Physical examination: skin and mucous membranes for color, temperature, petechiae, purpura, or bruises; vital signs; weight; mental status and level of consciousness; heart and breath sounds; abdominal exam; body fluids for occult blood

Nursing Diagnoses and Interventions

Inadequate platelets impair hemostasis, placing the client at risk for bleeding. Bleeding gums, an early sign of the disorder, affects oral mucous membrane integrity as well.

Ineffective Protection

Bleeding is a serious complication associated with thrombocytopenia. As platelet counts (measured in cubic millimeters) decrease, the risk of bleeding increases: The risk is minimal with counts greater than 50,000 mm³; moderate when the count is between 20,000 and 50,000 mm³; and significant when the count falls below 20,000 mm³.

- Monitor vital signs, heart and breath sounds every four hours. Frequently assess for other manifestations of bleeding:
  a. Skin and mucous membranes for petechiae, ecchymoses, and hematoma formation
  b. Gums, nasal membranes, and conjunctiva for bleeding
  c. Overt or occult blood in emesis, urine, or stool
  d. Vaginal bleeding
  e. Prolonged bleeding from puncture sites
  f. Neurologic changes: headache, visual changes, altered mental status, decreasing level of consciousness, seizures
  g. Abdominal: epigastric pain, absence of bowel sounds, increasing abdominal girth, abdominal guarding or rigidity

Early identification of bleeding is important to prevent serious blood loss and shock.

- Apply pressure to puncture sites for 3 to 5 minutes; apply pressure to arterial blood gas sites for 15 to 20 minutes. *Pressure promotes hemostasis and clot formation.*
- Instruct to avoid forcefully blowing the nose or picking crusts from the nose, straining to have a bowel movement, and forceful coughing or sneezing. *These activities increase the risk of external and internal bleeding.*

Impaired Oral Mucous Membranes

Thrombocytopenia frequently leads to bleeding of the gums and oral mucosa. As a result, risk for infection and impaired nutrition increases.

- Frequently assess the mouth for bleeding. Inquire about oral pain or tenderness. *Breakdown of oral mucous membranes increases the risk of infection and bleeding, and causes discomfort with eating.*
- Encourage use of a soft-bristle toothbrush or sponge to clean teeth and gums. *Hard bristles may abrade oral mucosa, causing bleeding and increasing the risk of infection.*
- Instruct to rinse the mouth with saline every two to four hours. Apply petroleum jelly to lips as needed to prevent dryness and cracking. *Saline mouth rinses and petroleum jelly help maintain oral tissue integrity and promote cleansing and healing.*

- Instruct to avoid alcohol-based mouthwashes, very hot foods, alcohol, and crusty foods. Teach to drink cool liquids at least every two hours. *Avoiding foods and liquids that traumatize oral mucosa increases comfort; fluid intake prevents dehydration and helps maintain mucous membrane integrity.*

Home Care

In the adult, ITP often is a chronic disorder that the client and family must learn to manage. Secondary thrombocytopenia may be either acute or chronic. Discuss the following topics when preparing the client and family for home care:

- Nature of the disorder, its usual course, and the treatment plan
- Use, desired and potential adverse effects of prescribed medications
- Risks and benefits of surgery or treatments, such as plasma replacement therapy
- The importance of follow-up tests and visits for care
- Measures to reduce the risk of bleeding: safety measures such as a soft-bristle toothbrush, electric razor, avoidance of contact sports and hazardous activities, and avoiding medications that further interfere with platelet function.

Refer for home health or other community services (e.g., housekeeping, shopping) as indicated.

The Client with Disseminated Intravascular Coagulation

Disseminated intravascular coagulation (DIC) is a disruption of hemostasis characterized by widespread intravascular clotting and bleeding. It may be acute and life threatening or relatively mild. DIC is a clinical syndrome that develops as a complication of a wide variety of other disorders. Sepsis is the most common cause of DIC. Gram-negative and gram-positive bacteria as well as viruses, fungi, and protozoal infections may lead to DIC (McCance & Huether, 2002).

Pathophysiology

DIC is triggered by endothelial damage, release of tissue factors into the circulation, or inappropriate activation of the clotting cascade by an endotoxin. Both the intrinsic and the extrinsic clotting cascade may be activated, although the extrinsic cascade usually is the one activated. Extensive thrombin entering the systemic circulation overwhelms natural anticoagulants, leading to unrestricted clot formation (McCance & Huether, 2002). Clotting may be localized to an individual organ, or widespread with deposition of small thrombi and emboli throughout the microvasculature (Braunwald, et al., 2001). The widespread clotting consumes clotting factors and activates fibrinolytic processes with anticoagulant production. As a result, hemorrhage occurs.

The sequence of DIC follows:

1. Endothelial damage, tissue factors, or toxins stimulate the clotting cascade.
2. Excess thrombin within the circulation overwhelms naturally occurring anticoagulants.
3. Widespread clotting occurs within the microvasculature.

4. Thrombi and emboli impair tissue perfusion, leading to ischemia, infarction, and necrosis.
5. Clotting factors (including platelets) are consumed faster than they can be replaced.
6. Clotting activates fibrinolytic processes which begin to break down clots.
7. Fibrin degradation products (*FDPs*, potent anticoagulants) are released, contributing to bleeding.
8. Clotting factors are depleted, the ability to form clots is lost, and hemorrhage occurs.

Manifestations

The manifestations of DIC result from both clotting and bleeding, although bleeding is more obvious, especially in acute DIC. Bleeding ranges from oozing blood following an injection to frank hemorrhage from every body orifice. Chronic DIC may be asymptomatic, or may present with peripheral cyanosis, thrombosis, and pregangrenous changes in the fingers and toes, nose, and genitalia (Braunwald et al., 2001).

Collaborative Care

Treatment of DIC is directed toward treating the underlying disorder and preventing further bleeding or massive thrombosis. Treatment stabilizes the client, reduces complications, and allows recovery to occur; it does not cure DIC (Braunwald, et al., 2001).

Diagnostic Tests

Diagnostic tests are used to confirm the diagnosis of DIC and evaluate the risk for hemorrhage.

- *CBC and platelet count* are used to evaluate the hemoglobin, hematocrit, and number of circulating platelets. *Schistocytes*, fragmented RBCs, may be noted due to cell trapping and damage within fibrin thrombi. The platelet count is decreased.
- *Coagulation studies* show prolonged *prothrombin time (PT), partial thromboplastin time (PTT)*, and *thrombin time*, and a low *fibrinogen level* due to depletion of clotting factors. The fibrinogen level helps predict bleeding in DIC: As it falls, the risk of bleeding increases (Braunwald, et al., 2001).
- *Fibrin degradation products (FDPs)* or *fibrin split products (FSPs)* are increased due to the fibinolysis that occurs with DIC.

Treatments

When bleeding is the major manifestation of DIC, fresh frozen plasma and platelet concentrates are given to restore clotting factors and platelets. Heparin, although controversial, may be administered. Heparin interferes with the clotting cascade and may prevent further clotting factor consumption due to uncontrolled thrombosis. It is used when bleeding is not controlled by plasma and platelets, as well as when the client has manifestations of thrombotic problems, such as acrocyanosis and possible gangrene. Long-term heparin therapy (administered by injection or continuous infusion using a portable pump) may be necessary for clients with chronic DIC.

Nursing Care

Assessment

Nurses can be instrumental in identifying early manifestations of DIC, facilitating timely intervention. Focused nursing assessment for DIC includes:

- *Health history:* recent abortion (spontaneous or therapeutic) or current pregnancy; presence of a known malignant tumor; history of abnormal bleeding episodes or a hematologic disorder.

- *Physical examination:* bleeding from puncture wounds (e.g., injections), IV sites, incisions; hematuria, obvious or occult blood in emesis or stool, epistaxis, other abnormal bleeding; vital signs; heart and breath sounds; abdominal assessment including girth, contour, bowel sounds, tenderness or guarding to palpation; color, temperature, skin condition of hands, feet, and digits; petechiae or purpura of skin, mucous membranes.

Nursing Diagnoses and Interventions

Clients with acute DIC often are critically ill, with multiple nursing care needs. Priority nursing diagnoses discussed in this section focus on impaired tissue perfusion and gas exchange, pain, and fear. Septic shock may precipitate DIC; hemorrhagic shock may occur as a complication of DIC. See Chapter 40 for nursing diagnoses and interventions related to these problems.

Ineffective Tissue Perfusion

Thrombi and emboli forming throughout the microcirculation affect the perfusion of multiple organs and tissues. Additionally, bleeding due to clotting factor consumption affects cardiac output and blood flow to these tissues.

- Assess extremity pulses, warmth, and capillary refill. Monitor level of consciousness (LOC) and mental status. *Monitoring central and peripheral tissue perfusion facilitates early treatment of impaired perfusion.*

- Carefully reposition at least every two hours. *Position changes facilitate circulation and tissue perfusion, as well as provide an opportunity to assess for purpura, pallor, and bleeding.*

- Discourage crossing the legs, and do not elevate the knees on the bed or with a pillow. *These positions may impair arterial and venous flow to the lower legs and feet, increasing vascular stasis and the risk for thrombosis.*

- Minimize use of tape on the skin, using binders, nonadhesive dressings, and other devices as needed. *Preventing skin trauma reduces the risk for bleeding and potential infection.*

Impaired Gas Exchange

Microclots in the pulmonary vasculature are likely to interfere with gas exchange in the client with DIC.

- Monitor oxygen saturation continuously. Administer oxygen as ordered. *Oxygen saturation levels are a noninvasive means of assessing gas exchange. Supplemental oxygen promotes gas exchange and reduces cardiac work, relieving dyspnea.*

- Place in Fowler or high-Fowler position as tolerated. *Elevating the head of the bed improves diaphragmatic excursion and alveolar ventilation.*

- Maintain bed rest. *Bed rest reduces oxygen demands and cardiac work.*
- Encourage deep breathing and effective coughing. *Increased respiratory depth and clearance of secretions from airways improves alveolar ventilation and oxygenation.*
- Cautious nasotracheal suctioning may be instituted if cough is ineffective or an endotracheal tube is in place. *Removal of secretions facilitates ventilation and oxygenation. However, care must be used to minimize suction-induced hypoxia and airway trauma.*
- Administer analgesics and antianxiety drugs as needed to control pain and anxiety. Provide reassurance and comfort measures. *Pain and anxiety increase the respiratory rate and decrease the depth of respirations, reducing effective ventilation and gas exchange.*

Pain

Both the underlying cause of DIC and tissue ischemia from microvascular clots can cause pain. Identifying the etiology of pain is important to identify potential complications or harmful effects of DIC and to institute effective treatment.

- Use a standard pain scale chart to evaluate and monitor pain and analgesic effectiveness. *Monitoring pain and response to medication facilitates development of an appropriate and effective treatment plan.*
- Handle extremities gently. *Gentle handling reduces the risk of further injury to and pain in ischemic tissues.*
- Apply cool compresses to painful joints. *Application of cold decreases pain through the gate-control mechanism, inhibiting the dorsal horn of the spinal cord and reducing the sensation of pain.*

Fear

The underlying serious illness and a complication such as DIC results in an uncertain prognosis, often accompanied by fear.

- Encourage the client and family to verbalize concerns. *This helps the client and family identify their concerns and frame questions.*
- Answer questions truthfully. *Providing honest answers is vital to developing a therapeutic nurse-client relationship. Accurate responses allow the client and family to set priorities as they plan for an uncertain future.*
- Help the client and family identify coping strategies to manage this significant situational stressor. *Implementing past effective coping methods may provide the skills to manage the current crisis.*
- Provide emotional support. *The presence of a caring nurse helps reduce the fear and anxiety associated with a crisis.*
- Maintain a calm environment. *A calm environment provides reassurance that the situation is in control, reduces anxiety, and promotes rest.*
- Respond promptly when the client calls for help. *Prompt responses to expressed needs helps develop a trusting relationship and a sense of confidence that assistance is readily available.*
- Teach relaxation techniques. *Relaxation techniques can reduce muscle tension and other signs of anxiety. Gaining control over physical responses can help the client gain a sense of control over the situation.*

Home Care

Although the immediate crisis of acute DIC is resolved prior to discharge, the client may have some continuing effects of the disorder, such as impaired tissue integrity of distal extremities. Teach the client and family about specific care needs, such as foot care or dressing changes. Provide instruction about any continuing medications and follow-up care.

Clients with chronic DIC may require continuing heparin therapy, using either intermittent subcutaneous injections or a portable infusion pump. Teach the client and family members how to administer the injection or manage the infusion pump. Provide a referral to home health care or a home intravenous management service for assistance. Discuss the manifestations of excessive bleeding or recurrent clotting that need to be reported to the physician.

The Client with Hemophilia

Hemophilia is a group of hereditary clotting factor disorders that lead to persistent and sometimes severe bleeding. Although often considered a disease of children, hemophilia may be diagnosed in adults. Deficiencies of three clotting factors, VIII, IX, and XI, account for 90% to 95% of the bleeding disorders collectively called hemophilia (McCance & Huether, 2002).

Pathophysiology

Hemophilia A (or *classic hemophilia*) is the most common type of hemophilia, caused by deficiency or dysfunction of clotting factor VIII. The estimated incidence of hemophilia A is 1 in 10,000 male births. It is transmitted as an X-linked recessive disorder from mothers to sons. The genetic defect of hemophilia A on the X chromosome may cause deficient factor VIII production or a defective form of the protein. When the concentration of the clotting factor is 5% to 35% of normal, the disease is *mild*. Bleeding is infrequent, and usually associated with trauma. Concentrations of 1% to 5% of normal result in *moderate* disease. Again, bleeding usually occurs secondarily to trauma. *Severe* hemophilia occurs when concentrations are less than 1% of normal. Bleeding is frequent, often occurring without trauma (Braunwald, et al., 2001; McCance & Huether, 2002).

Hemophilia B (also called *Christmas disease*), accounts for about 15% of cases, and is caused by a deficiency in factor IX. Despite the difference in clotting factor deficits, hemophilia A and B are clinically identical. Hemophilia B also is transmitted from mother to son as an X-linked recessive disorder.

Von Willebrand disease, often considered as a type of hemophilia, is the most common hereditary bleeding disorder (Porth, 2002). It is caused by a deficit of or defective von Willebrand (vW) factor, a protein that mediates platelet adhesion (Tierney, et al., 2001). Reduced levels of factor VIII often also are present, because vW factor carries factor VIII. This clotting disorder is transmitted in an autosomal dominant pattern, and affects men and women equally. Bleeding associated with von Willebrand disease is rarely severe. It often is diagnosed when prolonged bleeding follows surgery or a dental extraction.

Factor XI deficiency (or *hemophilia C*) is inherited in an autosomal recessive pattern, and most often affects Ashkenazi Jews (Braunwald, et al., 2001). It is usually a mild disorder, identified when postoperative bleeding is prolonged. A comparison of the types of hemophilia is found in Table 11-5.

People with hemophilia form a platelet plug at the site of bleeding, but the clotting factor deficit impairs formation of a stable fibrin clot. The effect of vW factor deficiency is somewhat different, in that platelet aggregation at the site of injury is impaired. In either case, prolonged or extensive bleeding may result. Often bleeding occurs in response to injury or as a result of surgery. However, a severe clotting factor deficit can lead to spontaneous bleeding into the joints (*hemarthrosis*), deep tissues, and central nervous system. Hemarthrosis often causes joint deformity and disability, usually of the elbows, hips, knees, and ankles.

Manifestations

The following are manifestations of hemophilia:

- Hemarthrosis
- Easy bruising and cutaneous hematoma formation with minor trauma (e.g., an injection)
- Bleeding from the gums and prolonged bleeding following minor injuries or cuts
- Gastrointestinal bleeding, with hematemesis (vomiting blood), occult blood in the stools, gastric pain, or abdominal pain
- Spontaneous hematuria or epistaxis (nosebleed)
- Pain or paralysis due to the pressure of hematomas on nerves.

Intracranial hemorrhage is a potentially life-threatening manifestation of hemophilia.

Table 11-5. Types of Hemophilia

Type/Name	Deficiency	Characteristics	Treatment
Hemophilia (Classic hemophilia)	Factor VIII	Transmitted by females; occurs primarily in males; bleeding time normal; coagulation time prolonged	Factor VIII concentrate or cryoprecipitate
Hemophilia B	Factor IX	Transmitted by females; occurs primarily in males; bleeding time normal; coagulation time prolonged	Factor IX (Christmas disease concentrate)
von Willebrand disease	vW factor Factor VIII	Occurs in both females and males; bleeding time and coagulation time are both prolonged	Cryoprecipitate and DDAVP
Factor XI deficiency	Factor XI	Occurs in both males and females; the activated partial thromboplastin time is prolonged	Fresh frozen plasma

Collaborative Care

Treatment of hemophilia focuses on preventing and/or treating bleeding, primarily by replacing deficient clotting factors. Specific treatment depends on the severity of the disorder and the specific factor deficiency. Care may be complicated by hepatitis or HIV disease in people with hemophilia treated with clotting factor concentrates prepared from multiple units of donated blood. Today, routine testing of all blood, improved blood donor screening, and current methods of treating hemophilia have significantly reduced the risk for these bloodborne diseases.

Diagnostic Tests

The following laboratory tests may be ordered.

- *Serum platelet levels* are measured and are usually normal.
- **Coagulation studies** such as APTT, bleeding time, and prothrombin time are used to screen for hemophilia when abnormal bleeding occurs. APTT is increased in all types of hemophilia. Prothrombin time is unaffected in these disorders but may be measured to rule out other disorders. Bleeding time is prolonged in von Willebrand disease, but normal in hemophilia A and B.
- *Factor assays* are performed; factor VIII is decreased in hemophilia A and often in von Willebrand disease, factor IX is decreased in hemophilia B, and factor XI in hemophilia C.
- *Amniocentesis* or *chorionic villus sampling* are used to identify the genetic defect of hemophilia when there is a known family history of the disease.

Medications

Deficient clotting factors are replaced regularly, as a prophylactic measure before surgery and dental procedures, and to control bleeding. Clotting factors may be given as fresh-frozen plasma, cryoprecipitates, or concentrates. Factor levels are measured on a regular basis to determine whether the treatment is adequate. Clotting factors are often self-administered and may be taken either on a regular or intermittent schedule.

Fresh-frozen plasma replaces all clotting factors (including both factor VIII and factor IX) except platelets. When the cause of bleeding is not yet determined, fresh-frozen plasma may be administered intravenously until a definitive diagnosis is made.

Hemophilia A is usually treated with either heat-treated factor VIII concentrate (heat treating reduces the risk of transmitting disease) or recombinant factor VIII. Although recombinant factor VIII, produced using recombinant DNA technology, eliminates the risk of viral disease transmission, its use is limited by cost. The dose of factor VIII is determined by the severity of the deficit and the presence or prospect of active bleeding (e.g., planned surgery).

Desmopressin acetate (DDAVP, Stimate) may be given to people with mild hemophilia A or von Willebrand disease prior to minor surgeries. This drug causes release of factor VIII and will raise blood levels by two- or threefold for several hours, reducing the risk of bleeding and the need for clotting factor concentrate (Tierney, et al., 2001).

Factor IX concentrate (administered intravenously) is used to treat hemophilia B. Because factor IX concentrates also contain a number of other proteins, there is risk of thrombosis with recurrent use. They are used judiciously, only when needed. Products produced by recombinant technology, or that are monoclonally purified, carry a lower risk of stimulating thrombus formation (Braunwald, et al., 2001). Fresh-frozen plasma replaces factor XI and is used when necessary. It may be given daily until the risk for bleeding decreases.

Factor VIII concentrates contain functional vW factor, and may be used to treat von Willebrand disease. Aspirin is avoided in all types of hemophilia.

Nursing Care

Health Promotion
Encourage clients with a family history of hemophilia or bleeding disorders to seek genetic counseling during their family planning process. Although tests are available for the hemophilia gene, the technology to correct the disorder in utero does not yet exist.

Assessment
While severe hemophilia usually is diagnosed in childhood, milder cases may not be identified until surgery, invasive dental work, or a traumatic injury causes extensive or prolonged bleeding. Focused assessment related to hemophilia includes the following:

- *Health history:* previous bleeding episodes with or without trauma; history of easy bruising, hematomas, epistaxis, bleeding gums, hematuria, vomiting blood, or joint pain; aspirin use; family history of hemophilia or bleeding disorders.
- *Physical examination:* vital signs; bruising or bleeding of skin or mucous membranes; mental status; abdominal assessment; presence of joint deformity, decreased range of motion.

Nursing Diagnoses and Interventions
Impaired blood clotting, the need for continuing care and disease management, and the risk for genetic transmission of hemophilia are priority problems for the client with hemophilia.

Ineffective Protection
The inability to form stable clots and stem bleeding from injured blood vessels creates a significant risk for the client with hemophilia. Nursing care measures focus on preventing injury and protecting the skin from damage.

- Monitor for signs of bleeding, including hematomas, ecchymoses, and purpura, as well as surface oozing or bleeding. Check emesis and stool for occult blood. *Bleeding may occur in cutaneous tissues as well as internal organs. Bleeding in the upper gastrointestinal tract may not be readily apparent in the stool.*
- Notify the physician of any apparent bleeding. *Prompt intervention with administration of clotting factor concentrate decreases the risk of hemorrhage and subsequent hypovolemia.*
- Avoid intramuscular injections, rectal temperatures, and enemas. *These can pose a risk of tissue and vascular trauma, which can precipitate bleeding.*
- Use safety measures in personal care. For example, use an electric razor rather than a razor blade to shave. *Use of an electric razor minimizes the opportunity to develop superficial cuts that may result in bleeding.*
- If bleeding occurs, control blood loss using gentle pressure, ice, or a topical hemostatic agent, such as absorbable gelatin sponge, microfibrillar collagen hemostat, or topical thrombin. *Direct pressure occludes bleeding vessels. Ice, a vasoconstrictor, may facilitate bleeding control, as do topical hemostatic agents.*

- Instruct the client to avoid activities that increase the risk of trauma, including contact sports, physical exertion associated with job performance, and to eliminate safety hazards in the home. *Depending on the severity of the clotting factor deficit, even minor trauma can lead to serious bleeding episodes. Safer activities, such as noncontact sports (e.g., swimming, golf), and occupations that do not require physical labor may be substituted.*

Risk for Ineffective Health Maintenance

Hemophilia is a chronic disorder, requiring active management to prevent and control bleeding and complications. Frequent visits to the physician or clinic may be necessary. In addition, the client may need to learn to self-administer clotting factors and measures to prevent complications. The lifelong nature of the disorder may interfere with compliance, especially during early adulthood.

- Assess knowledge of disorder and the related treatments. *Assessment allows identification of knowledge gaps and provides a basis on which to provide additional information. Impaired disease management may be due to lack of knowledge or a conscious decision not to follow the recommendations of the health care provider.*
- Provide information about the bleeding disorder and prescribed medications and treatments. *Individualized instruction is more effective than general, possibly irrelevant information.*
- Provide emotional support, expressing confidence in the client's self-care abilities. *Emotional support helps the client incorporate the care regimen into his or her lifestyle.*
- Provide supervised learning and practice opportunities for administering clotting factors and topical hemostatic agents. *Successful practice sessions instill confidence in the ability to manage care and provide an opportunity for questions and exploring alternatives.*

Home Care

Discuss the following topics when preparing the client with a bleeding disorder and the family for home care.

- Recognizing the manifestations of internal bleeding: pallor, weakness, restlessness, headache, disorientation, pain, swelling. These manifestations require emergency medical care and should be reported immediately.
- Applying cold packs and immobilizing the joint for 24 to 48 hours if hemarthrosis occurs
- Using analgesics for pain; avoiding prescription and over-the-counter drugs containing aspirin
- Ensuring a safe home environment (e.g., padding sharp edges of furniture, using transition lighting or a night light; avoiding scatter rugs, and wearing protective gloves when working in the house or yard)
- Using safe grooming practices such as electric razors
- Wearing a MedicAlert bracelet in case of accident
- Practicing good dental hygiene to decrease potential tooth decay and extractions. If dental procedures are necessary, discuss the need for prophylactic factor administration with the dentist and physician.
- Following safer-sex practices
- Preparing and administering intravenous medications

Refer the client and family to a local hemophilia or bleeding disorders support group. Provide contact information for national organizations and information clearinghouses, such as:

National Hemophilia Foundation
112 West 32nd Street, New York, NY 10001
1-800-42-HANDI • www.hemophilia.org

White Blood Cell and Lymphoid Tissue Disorders

Disorders of the white blood cells and lymphoid tissue include infectious mononucleosis, the leukemias, multiple myeloma, and malignant lymphomas (Hodgkin disease and non-Hodgkin lymphoma). A review of the physiology of white blood cells and lymphoid tissues precedes discussion of the diseases.

Physiology Review

White Blood Cells

White blood cells (WBCs), also called leukocytes, are a part of the body's defense against microorganisms. On average, there are 5,000 to 10,000 WBCs per cubic millimeter of blood, accounting for about 1% of total blood volume. **Leukocytosis** is a higher than normal WBC count; **leukopenia** is a WBC count that is lower than normal.

WBCs originate from hemopoietic stem cells in the bone marrow. These stem cells differentiate into the various types of white blood cells.

The two basic types of WBCs are granular leukocytes (or *granulocytes*) and nongranular leukocytes. Granulocytes have horseshoe-shaped nuclei and contain large granules in the cytoplasm. Stimulated by granulocyte-macrophage colony-stimulating factor (GM-CSF) and granulocyte colony-stimulating factor (G-CSF), granulocytes mature fully in the bone marrow before being released into the bloodstream. Following are the three types of granulocytes.

- Neutrophils (also called polymorphonuclear [*PMNs*] or segmented [*segs*] leukocytes) comprise 60% to 70% of the total circulating WBCs. Their nuclei are divided into three to five lobes. Neutrophils are active phagocytes, the first cells to arrive at a site of injury. Their numbers increase during inflammation. Immature forms of neutrophils (*bands*) are released during inflammation or infections. Neutrophils have a life span of only about 10 hours and are constantly being replaced.
- *Eosinophils* comprise 1% to 3% of circulating WBCs, but are found in large numbers in the mucosa of the intestines and lungs. Their numbers increase during allergic reactions and parasitic infestations.
- *Basophils,* which comprise less than 1% of the WBC count, contain histamine, heparin, and other inflammatory mediators. Basophils increase in numbers during allergic and inflammatory reactions.

Nongranular WBCs (agranulocytes) include the monocytes and lymphocytes. They enter the bloodstream before final maturation.

- *Monocytes* are the largest of the WBCs. They comprise approximately 3% to 8% of the total WBC count. Monocytes contain powerful bactericidal substances and proteolytic enzymes. They are phagocytic cells that mature into macrophages. Macrophages dispose of foreign and waste material, especially in inflammation. They are an active part of the immune response.

- *Lymphocytes* comprise 20% to 30% of the WBC count. Lymphocytes mature in lymphoid tissue into B cells and T cells. B cells are involved in the humoral immune response and antibody formation, whereas T cells take part in the cell-mediated immunity process (see Chapter 9). Plasma cells (which arise from B cells) are lymphoid cells found in bone marrow and connective tissue; they also are involved in immune reactions.

Lymphoid Tissues and Organs

Lymphoid tissues are connective tissues that contain billions of lymphocytes. *Lymphoid organs* include the bone marrow, thymus, lymph nodes, associated lymphoid tissues, and the spleen. New lymphocytes are created and differentiated in the *central* or *primary* lymphoid organs, the bone marrow and thymus. Lymphocytes and other WBCs are formed in the bone marrow. While still immature, some lymphocytes migrate to the thymus. In the thymus, they further differentiate to become active immune cells (T cells or T lymphocytes).

The *peripheral* or *secondary* lymphoid organs (the lymph nodes, associated lymphoid tissues, and spleen) have an active role in immune function (see Chapter 9). The lymph circulation returns interstitial fluids to the circulatory system. Lymph nodes filter and process lymph drainage. They contain multiple lymphocytes and macrophages, so all lymph is exposed to many immunocompetent cells. Lymphoid tissue is also found in many organs, such as the gastrointestinal tract, tonsils, adenoids, and airways. This tissue, called mucosa-associated lymphoid tissue (MALT), helps prevent microorganisms from entering the body.

The spleen is the largest lymphatic organ. It stores and processes blood, removing aged RBCs and processing their hemoglobin. The spleen contains phagocytic cells that help clear bloodborne pathogens.

The Client with Neutropenia

Leukopenia is a decrease in the total circulating white blood cell count. Although any type of WBC may be affected, neutrophils, which make up the majority of WBCs, are affected most often. *Neutropenia* is a decrease in circulating neutrophils, usually less than 1500 cells/µm. Neutropenia may be either congenital or acquired, developing secondarily to prolonged infection, hematologic disorders, starvation, or autoimmune disorders, such as rheumatoid arthritis. *Agranulocytosis* is severe neutropenia, with less than 200 cells/µm. Numbers of other granulocytes also are reduced. It is usually due to impaired leukocyte formation in the bone marrow or increased cell destruction in circulating blood. Chemotherapy and other drugs can suppress the bone marrow. Agranulocytosis significantly increases the risk for infection. *Aplastic anemia* affects production of all blood cells, resulting in anemia, thrombocytopenia, and agranulocytosis.

Neutrophils are an integral component of the immune response. The manifestations of neutropenia reflect the resulting impaired immunity and inflammatory response. Opportunistic bacterial, fungal, and protozoal infections develop, commonly affecting the respiratory tract and mucosa of the mouth, GI tract, and vagina. Malaise, chills, and fever with extreme weakness and fatigue are common manifestations.

Hematopoietic growth factors such as GM-CSF are administered to stimulate granulocyte maturation and differentiation. Infections are treated with antibiotic therapy.

The primary nursing care focus is protecting the client from infection.

The Client with Infectious Mononucleosis

Infectious mononucleosis is characterized by invasion of B cells in the oropharyngeal lymphoid tissues by the Epstein-Barr virus (EBV). This disease is usually benign and self-limiting. It often affects young adults between the ages of 15 and 30. The virus is present in saliva, which appears to be the primary mode of transmission. As a result, infectious mononucleosis is often called the "kissing disease."

When the virus enters the body, unaffected B cells produce antibodies against the virus, and T cells directly attack the virus. Infected B cells are destroyed as the virus replicates. The proliferation of B and T cells, as well as the removal of dead and damaged leukocytes, is responsible for the swelling of lymphoid tissues.

The incubation period for infectious mononucleosis is four to eight weeks. Its onset is insidious, with headache, malaise, and fatigue. Fever, sore throat, and cervical lymphadenopathy (lymph node enlargement and pain) lasting one to three weeks is common. Symptom severity varies from person to person. Lymph node involvement may be generalized; about 50% of people with infectious mononucleosis develop an enlarged spleen (splenomegaly).

Laboratory findings include increased lymphocytes and monocytes, with about 20% of the cells atypical in form. Early in the infection, the WBC count usually is normal or low, but by the second week it increases and remains elevated for four to eight weeks. Platelet counts are often low during the illness.

Recovery occurs in two to three weeks; however, debility and lethargy may last for up to three months. The treatment includes bed rest and analgesic agents to alleviate the symptoms. Nursing care is primarily educational to prevent further spread of the disease.

The Client with Leukemia

Leukemia (literally, "white blood") is a group of chronic malignant disorders of white blood cells and white blood cell precursors. In leukemia, the usual ratio of red to white blood cells is reversed. Leukemias are characterized by replacement of bone marrow by malignant immature white blood cells, abnormal immature circulating WBCs, and infiltration of these cells into the liver, spleen, and lymph nodes throughout the body.

Although leukemia is often thought of as a childhood disease, it is diagnosed ten times more often in adults than children. An estimated 30,800 new cases of leukemia occur yearly; approximately half are chronic leukemia and half are acute leukemia. In 2002, approximately 21,700 people died of leukemia (American Cancer Society [ACS], 2002). The highest incidence of leukemia is found in the United States, Canada, Sweden, and New Zealand (McCance & Huether, 2002).

Although the cause of most leukemias is unknown, certain risk factors have been identified. The incidence of leukemia is higher in people with Down syndrome and certain other genetic disorders. Exposure to ionizing radiation and certain chemicals such as benzene (present in gasoline and cigarette smoke) increases the risk for leukemia, as does treatment for other cancers. Some leukemias are known to be caused by a retrovirus, human T-cell leukemia/lymphoma virus-1 (HTLV-1) (ACS, 2002).

Leukemias are classified by their acuity and by the predominant cell type involved. The *acute* leukemias are characterized by an acute onset, rapid disease progression, and immature or undifferentiated blast cells. *Chronic* leukemias, on the other hand, have a gradual onset, prolonged course, and abnormal mature-appearing cells. *Lymphocytic* (or *lymphoblastic*) leukemias involve immature lymphocytes and their precursor cells in the bone marrow. Lymphocytic leukemias infiltrate the spleen, lymph nodes, CNS, and other tissues. *Myelocytic* (or *myeloblastic*) leukemias involve myeloid stem cells in the bone marrow, interfering with the maturation of all types of blood cells, including granulocytes, RBCs, and thrombocytes (Porth, 2002). Acute lymphoblastic leukemia is the most common type of leukemia in children. In adults, acute myeloblastic leukemia and chronic lymphocytic leukemia are the most common types (McCance & Huether, 2002). In summary, the general types of leukemia are as follows:

- Acute lymphocytic (lymphoblastic) leukemia (ALL)
- Chronic lymphocytic leukemia (CLL)
- Acute myelocytic (myeloblastic) leukemia (AML)
- Chronic myelocytic (myelogenous) leukemia (CML)

This general system of classifying leukemias does not differentiate subtypes of acute leukemias. The French-American-British (FAB) system for classifying acute leukemias further differentiates acute leukemias by the predominant cell involved and the degree of cell differentiation (Table 11-3).

Without treatment, leukemia is invariably fatal, usually due to complications of leukemic cell infiltration of bone marrow or vital organs. With treatment, prognosis varies. The 5-year survival rate is 46% (ACS, 2002). The types, pathology, manifestations, and treatment for the major leukemias are outlined in Table 11-7.

Pathophysiology and Manifestations

Leukemia begins with malignant transformation of a single stem cell. Leukemic cells proliferate slowly, but do not differentiate normally. They have a prolonged life span and accumulate in the bone marrow. As they accumulate, they compete with the proliferation of normal cells. Leukemic cells do not function as mature WBCs, and are ineffective in the inflammatory and immune processes. Leukemic cells replace normal hematopoietic elements in the marrow. Because erythrocyte- and platelet-producing cells are crowded out, severe anemia, splenomegaly, and bleeding difficulties result.

Leukemic cells leave the bone marrow and travel through the circulatory system, infiltrating other body tissues such as the central nervous system, testes, skin, gastrointestinal tract, and the lymph nodes, liver, and spleen. Death usually is due to internal hemorrhage and infections.

Table 11-6. FAB Classification of Acute Leukemia

Type	Class	Predominant Cells	Prognosis
Acute Lymphocytic	L_1	Immature lymphoblasts	>90% remission rate in children
Leukemia (ALL)	L_2	Mature lymphoblasts	Relapse common after 2 or more years of remission
	M_0	Undifferentiated cells	Poor
Acute Myelocytic	M_1	Immature myeloblasts	Good; complete response in $\geq$65%
Leukemia	M_2	Mature myeloblasts	Good for 2 or more years of remission
	M_3	Promyelocytes	Good in adults
	M_4	Myelocytes and monocytes	Poorest in adults
	M_5	Poorly or well-differentiated monocytes	Poor
	M_6	Predominant eythroblasts	Variable
	M_7	Megakaryocytes	

The general manifestations of leukemia (regardless of type) result from anemia, infection, and bleeding. These include pallor, fatigue, tachycardia, malaise, lethargy, and dyspnea on exertion. Infection may cause fever, night sweats, oral ulcerations, and frequent or recurrent respiratory, urinary, integumentary, or other infections. Increased bleeding due to thrombocytopenia leads to bruising; petechiae; bleeding gums; and bleeding within specific organs and tissues.

Other manifestations result from leukemic cell infiltration, increased metabolism, and increased leukocyte destruction. Infiltration of the liver, spleen, lymph nodes, and bone marrow causes pain and tissue swelling in the involved areas. Meningeal infiltration may cause manifestations of increased intracranial pressure, such as headache, altered level of consciousness, cranial nerve impairment, nausea, and vomiting. Infiltration of the kidneys may affect renal function, with decreased urine output and increased blood urea nitrogen and creatinine. Increased metabolism causes heat intolerance, weight loss, dyspnea on exertion, and tachycardia. Destruction of large numbers of WBCs releases substantial amounts of uric acid into the circulation; uric acid crystals may obstruct renal tubules, causing renal insufficiency.

Acute Myelocytic Leukemia

Acute myelocytic leukemia (AML) is characterized by uncontrolled proliferation of myeloblasts (the precursors of granulocytes) and hyperplasia of the bone marrow and spleen. AML accounts for most acute leukemia in adults. Treatment induces complete remission in 70% of clients, although only about 25% achieve cure or long-term remission (Porth, 2002).

The manifestations of AML result from neutropenia and thrombocytopenia. Decreased neutrophils lead to recurrent severe infections, such as pneumonia, septicemia, abscesses, and mucous membrane ulceration. The manifestations of thrombocytopenia include petechiae, purpura, and ecchymoses (bruising), epistaxis (nosebleeds), hematomas, hematuria, and gastrointestinal bleeding. Bone infarctions or subperiosteal infiltrates of leukemic cells may cause bone pain. Anemia is a late manifestation, causing fatigue, headaches, pallor, and dyspnea on exertion. Death usually results from infection or hemorrhage.

Bone marrow aspiration shows a proliferation of immature WBCs. The CBC shows thrombocytopenia and normocytic, normochromic anemia.

Table 11-7. Major Types of Leukemia

Classification	Characteristics	Manifestations	Treatment
Acute lymphoblastic leukemia (ALL)	Primarily affects children and young adults; leukemic cells may infiltrate CNS	Recurrent infections; bleeding; pallor, bone pain, weight loss, sore throat, fatigue, night sweats, weakness	Chemotherapy; bone marrow transplant (BMT), or stem cell transplant (SCT)
Chronic lymphocytic leukemia (CLL)	Primarily affects older adults; insidious onset and slow, chronic course	Fatigue; exercise intolerance; lymphadenopathy and splenomegaly; recurrent infections, pallor, edema, thrombophlebitis	Often requires no treatment; chemotherapy; BMT
Acute myelocytic leukemia (AML)	Common in older adults, may affect children and young adults. Strongly associated with toxins, genetic disorders, and treatment of other cancers	Fatigue, weakness, fever; anemia; headache, bone and joint pain; abnormal bleeding and bruising; recurrent infection; lymphadenopathy, splenomegaly, and hepatomegaly	Chemotherapy; SCT
Chronic myelocytic leukemia (CML)	Primarily affects adults; early course slow and stable, progressing to aggressive phase in 3–4 years	Early: Weakness, fatigue, dyspnea on exertion; possible splenomegaly Later: fever, weight loss, night sweats	Interferon-α; chemotherapy, SCT

Chronic Myelocytic Leukemia

Chronic myelocytic leukemia (CML) is characterized by abnormal proliferation of all bone marrow elements. CML is usually associated with a chromosome abnormality called the Philadelphia chromosome, a translocation of chromosome 22 to chromosome 9. This type of leukemia constitutes approximately 20% of adult leukemias. It usually affects clients over age 50; its incidence is higher in men than in women. Ionizing radiation and exposure to chemicals are implicated as causes of CML.

People with CML are often asymptomatic in the early stages and, in fact, are often diagnosed when a routine blood test reveals abnormal cell counts. Anemia causes weakness, fatigue, and dyspnea on exertion. The spleen often is enlarged, causing abdominal discomfort. Within three to four years, disease progresses to a more aggressive phase. Rapid cell proliferation and hypermetabolism cause fatigue, weight loss, sweating, and heat intolerance. Finally, the disease evolves to acute leukemia, with blast cell proliferation and constitutional symptoms. Survival following the onset of this final stage averages only two to four months (Porth, 2002).

Acute Lymphocytic Leukemia

Acute lymphocytic leukemia (ALL) is the most common type of leukemia in children and young adults. ALL causes abnormal proliferation of lymphoblasts in the bone marrow, lymph nodes, and spleen.

The onset of ALL is usually rapid. Lymphoblasts proliferating in bone marrow and peripheral tissues crowd the growth of normal cells. Normal hematopoiesis is suppressed, leading to thrombocytopenia, leukopenia, and anemia. Manifestations of infections, bleeding, and anemia develop. Bone pain resulting from rapid generation of marrow elements, lymphadenopathy, and liver enlargement are also common. Infiltration of the central nervous system causes headaches, visual disturbances, vomiting, and seizures.

The CBC shows an elevated WBC count with increased lymphocytes on the differential. RBC and platelet counts are decreased. Bone marrow studies reveal a hypercellular marrow with growth of lymphoblasts. Combination chemotherapy produces complete remission in 80% to 90% of adults with ALL.

Chronic Lymphocytic Leukemia

Chronic lymphocytic leukemia (CLL) is characterized by proliferation and accumulation of small, abnormal, mature lymphocytes in the bone marrow, peripheral blood, and body tissues. The abnormal cells are usually B-lymphocytes that are unable to produce adequate antibodies to maintain normal immune function. CLL occurs more commonly in adults, especially in older adults (median age 65). CLL is the least common type of the major leukemias.

CLL has a slow onset and is often diagnosed during a routine physical examination. If symptoms are present, they usually include vague complaints of weakness or malaise. Possible clinical findings include anemia, infection, and enlarged lymph nodes, spleen, and liver. As in other leukemias, bone marrow hyperplasia is present. Erythrocyte and platelet counts are reduced. Leukocyte counts may either be elevated or reduced, but abnormal cells are always present. In CLL, years may elapse before treatment is required. Survival of this disease averages approximately seven years.

Collaborative Care

Treatment for leukemia focuses on achieving remission or cure and relieving symptoms. The methods of treatment may include chemotherapy, radiation therapy, and bone marrow or stem cell transplantation. Cure is more often achieved in children with acute leukemia than in adults, although long-term remissions (disease-free periods with no signs or symptoms) can often be achieved.

Diagnostic Tests

The following diagnostic tests are ordered when leukemia is suspected.

- *CBC* with differential is done to evaluate cell counts, hemoglobin and hematocrit levels, and the number, distribution, and morphology (size and shape) of WBCs.

- *Platelets* are measured to identify possible thrombocytopenia secondary to the leukemia and the risk of bleeding.
- *Bone marrow examination* provides information about cells within the marrow, the type of erythropoiesis, and the maturity of erythropoietic and leukopoietic cells.

Chemotherapy

Single agent or combination chemotherapy is used to treat most types of leukemia, with the goal of eradicating leukemic cells and producing remission. Combination chemotherapy reduces drug resistance and toxicity, and interrupts cell growth at various stages of the cell cycle, producing complimentary effect of the drugs used.

Chemotherapy for leukemia generally is divided into the induction phase and postremission therapy. During *induction,* drug doses are high to eradicate leukemic cells from the bone marrow. Also, these high doses often damage stem cells and interfere with production of normal blood cells. Circulating mature blood cells are not affected because they are no longer dividing. The degree of bone marrow suppression is influenced by a number of factors, including age, nutritional status, concurrent chronic diseases such as impaired liver or renal function, the drug and drug dose, and prior treatment.

Colony-stimulating factors (CSFs), also called hematopoietic growth factors, often are administered to "rescue" the bone marrow following induction chemotherapy. CSFs are cytokines that regulate the growth and differentiation of blood cells. Factors that support neutrophil maturation, *granulocyte-macrophage CSF (GM-CSF)* and *granulocyte CSF (G-CSF)* are commonly used. Bone pain is a common side effect of therapy with these agents. Clients also may experience fevers, chills, anorexia, muscle aches, and lethargy (Braunwald, et al., 2001).

Once remission has been achieved, postremission chemotherapy is continued to eradicate any additional leukemic cells, prevent relapse, and prolong survival. A single chemotherapeutic agent, combination therapy, or bone marrow transplant may be used for postremission treatment.

Radiation Therapy

Radiation therapy damages cellular DNA. While the cell continues to function, it cannot divide and multiply. Cells that divide rapidly, such as bone marrow and cancer cells (radiosensitive cells), respond quickly to radiation therapy. Although normal cells are affected, they are better able to recover from the damage caused by the radiation than are cancer cells.

Bone Marrow Transplant

Bone marrow transplant (BMT) is the treatment of choice for some types of leukemia (see Table 11-4). BMT often is used in conjunction with or following chemotherapy or radiation. There are two major categories of BMT: In allogeneic BMT, the bone marrow of a healthy donor is infused into the client with the illness; in autologous BMT, the client is infused with his or her own bone marrow.

Allogeneic BMT

Allogeneic BMT uses bone marrow cells from a donor (often from a sibling with closely matched tissue antigens; closely matched unrelated donors may also be used). Prior to allogeneic BMT, high doses of chemotherapy and/or total body irradiation are used to destroy leukemic cells in the bone marrow. Then donor marrow is infused through a central venous line. Prior to BMT and reestablishment of bone marrow function, the client is critically ill and at significant risk for infection and bleeding due to depletion of WBCs and platelets.

Allogeneic BMT may precipitate *graft-versus-host disease (GVHD)*, which develops in 25% to 60% of all clients receiving an allogeneic BMT. In GVHD, immune cells of the donated bone marrow identify the recipient's body tissue as foreign. Consequently, T lymphocytes in the donated marrow attack the liver, skin, and gastrointestinal tract, causing skin rashes, and progressing to desquamation (loss of skin), diarrhea, gastrointestinal bleeding, and liver damage. GVHD is treated with antibiotics and steroids; immunosuppressant drugs, such as thalidomide and immunotoxin (Xomazyme), may be used, if necessary.

Autologous BMT

Autologous BMT uses the client's own bone marrow to restore bone marrow function after chemotherapy or radiation. This procedure is often called *bone marrow rescue*. In autologous BMT, about 1 L of bone marrow is aspirated (usually from the iliac crests) during a period of disease remission. The bone marrow is then frozen and stored for use after treatment. If relapse occurs, lethal doses of chemotherapy or radiation are given to destroy the immune system and malignant cells, and to prepare space in the bone marrow for new cells. The filtered bone marrow is then thawed and infused intravenously through a central line. The infused marrow cells slowly become a part of the client's bone marrow, the neutrophil count increases, and normal hematopoiesis takes place.

As in allogeneic BMT, the client is critically ill during the period of bone marrow destruction and immunosuppression. The client is hospitalized in a private room for six to eight weeks or more. Potential complications include malnutrition, infection, and bleeding.

Stem Cell Transplant

Allogeneic **stem cell transplant (SCT)** is an alternative to bone marrow transplant. SCT results in complete and sustained replacement of the recipient's blood cell lines (WBCs, RBCs, and platelets) with cells derived from the donor stem cells.

Donors must have tissue that is closely matched with that of the recipient. Prior to harvesting, hematopoietic growth factors, including G-CSF and GM-CSF, are administered to the donor for four to five days. This increases the concentration of stem cells in peripheral blood, allowing it to be used for the transplant instead of bone marrow. Peripheral blood is removed and white cells are separated from the plasma, then administered via a large central venous catheter. Large concentrations of stem cells are also present in umbilical cord blood. This may be stored and used in some cases (Braunwald, et al., 2001).

The recipient undergoes similar treatment prior to SCT as for BMT. The risks for infection and other complications, as well as GVHD, are similar.

Biologic Therapy

Cytokines, such as interferons and interleukins, are biologic agents that may be used to treat some leukemias. These agents modify the body's response to cancer cells; in some cases, they are cytotoxic as well. Interferons are a complex group of messenger proteins normally produced in response to antigens, such as viruses (see Chapter 42). They have multiple effects, including moderating immune function and inhibiting abnormal cell proliferation and growth. Interferon-α may be used to treat some leukemias, particularly CML. Side effects commonly associated with interferon therapy include flulike symptoms, persistent fatigue and lethargy, weight loss, and muscle and joint pain.

Complementary Therapies

Although many complementary and alternative medicine therapies have been purported to treat cancer in general, at this time, none have been shown to have sustained benefit in treating leukemia.

Nursing Care

Health Promotion

Health promotion activities related to leukemia include teaching about leukemia risk factors, particularly those that can be controlled. Discuss the potential dangers of exposure to ionizing radiation and certain chemicals, such as benzene. Encourage all clients to avoid smoking cigarettes. Discuss genetic counseling with clients at high risk for having a child with Down syndrome (over age 35).

Assessment

Focused assessment data related to leukemia includes:

* *Health history:* complaints of fatigue, weakness, dyspnea on exertion, frequent infections, sore throat, night sweats, bleeding gums, or nose bleeds; recent weight loss; exposure to ionizing radiation (multiple X-rays, residence near a site of radiation or atomic testing) or chemicals (occupational); prior treatment for cancer; history of an immune disorder.
* *Physical examination:* skin and mucous membranes for bruising, purpura, petechiae, ulcers or lesions; pallor; vital signs, including orthostatic vitals; heart and lung sounds; abdominal examination; stool for occult blood.

Nursing Diagnoses and Interventions

When caring for the client with leukemia, the nurse considers the chronic and life-threatening nature of the disease as well as the effects of treatment. Priority nursing problems may include: risk for infection, imbalanced nutrition, impaired oral mucous membranes, impaired protection (bleeding), and grieving.

Risk for Infection

Changes in white blood cell function impair the immune and inflammatory responses in leukemia, increasing the risk for infection. WBCs may be immature and ineffective, or, in some cases, deficient. Chemotherapy or radiation therapy further depresses bone marrow function, and increases the risk for infection.

* Promptly report manifestations of infection: fever, chills, throat pain, cough, chest pain, burning on urination, purulent drainage, and itching and burning in vaginal or rectal areas.*Prompt reporting allows timely intervention to prevent overwhelming infection and sepsis.*
* Institute infection protection measures.
  a. Maintain protective isolation as indicated.
  b. Ensure meticulous handwashing among all people in contact with the client.

c. Assist as needed with appropriate hygiene measures.

d. Restrict visitors with colds, flu, or infections.

e. Provide oral hygiene after every meal.

f. Avoid invasive procedures when possible, including injections, intravenous catheters, catheterizations, and rectal and vaginal procedures. When necessary, use strict aseptic technique for all invasive procedures and monitor carefully for infection.

These precautions minimize exposure to bacterial, viral, and fungal pathogens. Infection is the major cause of death in clients with leukemia. Mucous membranes are especially susceptible to breakdown and infection as a result of tissue damage from chemotherapy or radiation.

• Monitor vital signs including temperature and oxygen saturation every four hours. Report temperature spikes with chilling, tachypnea, tachycardia, restlessness, change in Pao_2, and hypotension. The inflammatory response may be impaired in leukemia, masking signs of infection until sepsis develops, indicated by manifestations like those above.

• Monitor neutrophil levels (measured in cubic millimeters) for relative risk for infection:

2000 to 2500: no risk

1000 to 2000: minimal risk

500 to 1000: moderate risk

Below 500: severe risk

Neutrophils are the first line of defense against infection. As levels decrease, the risk for infection increases.

• Explain infection precautions and restrictions and their rationale; explain that these measures are usually temporary. *Client and family understanding increases compliance and lowers the risk of infection.*

Imbalanced Nutrition: Less Than Body Requirements

The client with leukemia may have difficulty meeting nutritional needs due to increased metabolism, fatigue, loss of appetite from radiation, nausea and vomiting from chemotherapy, or painful oral mucous membranes that make chewing and swallowing difficult and/or painful.

• Weigh regularly and evaluate weight loss over time to determine degree of malnutrition. A weight loss of 10% to 20% may indicate malnutrition. *A minimum intake of nutrients is necessary for health and tissue repair; cancer increases metabolic needs over this basal requirement. Weight loss occurs when metabolic requirements are not met. Both the disease process and its treatment can interfere with nutrient intake.*

• Address causative or contributing factors to inadequate food and fluid intake.

a. Provide mouth care before and after meals; use a soft toothbrush or sponges as necessary.

b. Provide liquids with different textures and tastes.

c. Increase liquid intake with meals.

d. Reduce intake of milk and milk products, which makes mucus more tenacious.

e. Assist to a sitting position for eating.

f. Ensure that the environment is clean and odor-free.

g. Provide medications for pain or nausea 30 minutes before meals, if prescribed.

h. Provide rest periods before meals.

i. Offer small, frequent meals including low-fat, high kilocalorie (kcal) foods throughout the day.

j. Provide commercial supplements, such as Ensure.

k. Avoid painful or unpleasant procedures immediately before or after meals.

l. Suggest measures to improve food tolerance, such as eating dry foods when arising, consuming salty foods if allowed, and avoiding very sweet, rich, or greasy foods.

Anorexia, nausea and vomiting, diarrhea, stomatitis, taste changes, and dysphagia often make eating difficult during cancer treatment when good nutrition is most important. Maintaining nutritional status decreases morbidity and mortality by preventing weight loss, improving the response to treatment, minimizing adverse effects, and improving quality of life. Small, frequent meals are often better tolerated, especially high-protein, high-kcal foods.

Impaired Oral Mucous Membrane

Stomatitis, inflammation and ulceration of the oral mucous membrane, is common in leukemia. Chemotherapy can further impair the integrity of constantly dividing oral tissues.

- Inspect the buccal region, gums, sublingual area, and the throat daily for swelling or lesions. Ask about oral pain or burning. *Breakdown of the oral mucous membrane increases the risk of infection and bleeding, causes pain and discomfort with eating and swallowing, and may cause swelling that interferes with the airway.*

- Culture any oral lesions. *Herpes simplex virus and Candida (yeast) are more common in clients with neutropenia. Herpes lesions are usually red, raised, fluid-filled blisters; Candida causes a white coating and patches of white plaque.*

- Assist with mouth care and oral rinses with saline or a solution of hydrogen peroxide and water (1:1 or 1:3 hydrogen peroxide and water) every two to four hours. Apply petroleum jelly to the lips to prevent dryness and cracking. *These measures help prevent infection and increase comfort.*

- Encourage use of soft-bristle toothbrush or sponge to clean teeth and gums. *Toothbrushes with hard bristles may abrade inflamed mucosa, causing bleeding and increasing the risk of infection.*

- Administer medications as ordered to treat infection or relieve pain. *Topical antifungal agents, such as nystatin, may be prescribed to treat Candida infections. Topical anesthetics, such as lidocaine, may be prescribed to relieve comfort and facilitate good oral care.*

- Instruct client to avoid alcohol-based mouthwashes, citrus fruit juices, spicy foods, very hot or very cold foods, alcohol, and crusty foods. Suggest bland, cool foods and cool liquids at least every two hours. *Avoiding mucosa-traumatizing foods and liquids increases comfort; bland, cool foods and liquids cause the least pain. Intake of adequate fluids is necessary to prevent dehydration.*

Ineffective Protection

Bleeding is the second most common cause of leukemia deaths. As platelet counts decrease, the risk of bleeding increases (see preceding section on thrombocytopenia).

- Assess vital signs every four hours and body systems every shift for bleeding.

    a. Skin and mucous membranes for petechiae, ecchymoses, and purpura

    b. Gums, nasal membranes, and conjunctiva for bleeding

    c. Vomitus, stool, and urine for visible or occult blood

    d. Vaginal bleeding

    e. Prolonged bleeding from puncture sites

    f.   Neurologic changes, such as headache, visual changes, altered mentation, decreased level of consciousness, seizures

    g.   Abdomen for complaints of epigastric pain, diminished bowel sounds, increasing abdominal girth, rigidity or guarding

Early identification of bleeding helps prevent significant blood loss and potential shock. Internal hemorrhage may lead to tachycardia, hypotension, pallor, and diaphoresis. Bleeding into the lungs may cause dyspnea; bleeding into the abdomen causes increased girth, pain, and guarding. Intracranial bleeding affects mental status and level of consciousness.

- Avoid invasive procedures, such as using rectal thermometers and suppositories, vaginal douches, suppositories, or tampons, urinary catheterization, and parenteral injections, if possible. Diagnostic procedures, such as biopsy or lumbar puncture, should not be done if the platelet count is less than 50,000. *Invasive procedures can cause tissue trauma and bleeding. Procedures that use large-bore needles should be delayed until the platelet count is increased.*

- Apply pressure to injection sites for 3 to 5 minutes, and to arterial punctures for 15 to 20 minutes. *Pressure prevents prolonged bleeding by prompting hemostasis and clot formation.*

- Instruct to avoid forcefully blowing or picking the nose, forceful coughing or sneezing, and straining to have a bowel movement. *These activities can damage mucous membranes, increasing the risk for bleeding.*

Anticipatory Grieving

The diagnosis of cancer and a potentially life-threatening illness causes actual or perceived losses, such as loss of function, independence, normal appearance, friends, self-esteem, and self. Grieving is the emotional response to those losses. The adaptive process of mourning a loss and resolving grief is called grief work; grief work cannot begin until a loss is acknowledged. See Chapter 43 for a detailed discussion of grief and loss.

- Discuss roles of the client and family and ways in which they managed stressful situations in the past. Assess coping strategies and their effectiveness. Help identify sources of strength and support. Discuss changing roles resulting from leukemia diagnosis, and its effect on spiritual, social, and economic status, and usual lifestyle. Evaluate cultural or ethnic factors that affect grief reactions. *Grieving is a normal response to a real or potential loss that begins at the time of diagnosis. The timing, duration, and intensity of grief and responses to grief may differ among family members. Share information on diagnosis, role change, and physical loss among all family members to build the foundation for mutual understanding and trust.*

- Use therapeutic communication skills to facilitate open discussion of losses and provide permission to grieve. *Encouraging discussion about the meaning of the loss helps decrease some of the anxiety associated with loss. This, in turn, allows the client and family to examine the current situation and compare it with past situations that they have coped with successfully.*

- Provide information about agencies that offer support in dealing with grief, and make referrals as indicated. Consider self-help groups, cancer support groups, and bereavement groups. *Participating in support groups with others who are anticipating or experiencing a similar loss can decrease feelings of isolation.*

Home Care

Client and family teaching for home care after treatment for leukemia focuses on encouraging self-care, providing information about the disease and the treatment, preventing infection and injury, and promoting nutrition. Teaching techniques for each of these areas are as follows:

Encouraging Self-Care

- Hygiene measures and energy conservation during self-care activities
- Oral hygiene including using a soft-bristle toothbrush several times daily; avoid flossing
- Reporting lesions, bleeding, or signs of infection promptly
- Maintaining a balance of rest and activity

Information about Leukemia and Treatment

- Bone marrow function, the pathophysiology of leukemia, and potential complications of leukemia
- Prognosis for the specific type of leukemia
- Treatment measures, such as chemotherapy, radiation, bone marrow or stem cell transplant, their purpose and effects, where treatment is available, and potential adverse effects or risks
- Community, regional, and national resources for people with leukemia

Preventing Infection and Injury

- Handwashing and other measures to reduce exposure to pathogens, such as avoiding people who are ill and avoiding crowds
- Avoiding foodborne illnesses by washing fruits and vegetables, proper food storage
- Dental hygiene measures
- Avoiding immunizations
- Manifestations to report: fever, chills, burning on urination, foul-smelling urine, vaginal or rectal discharge, skin lesions
- Avoiding contact sports or strenuous exercise if platelet count is low
- Using an electric razor for shaving, avoiding rectal or vaginal suppositories, vaginal tampons, or enemas
- Increasing dietary fiber and using a bulk-forming laxative as needed to prevent straining
- Avoiding over-the-counter or prescription drugs that interfere with platelet function
- The importance of reporting any bleeding (nosebleeds, rectal bleeding, vomiting blood, excessive menstrual periods, blood in the urine, bleeding gums, bruises, or collections of blood under the skin) or changes in behavior to the health care provider

Promoting Nutrition

- Eating several small, low-fat, high-calorie meals and drinking five to eight glasses of water daily
- Reporting continued weight loss, loss of appetite, or inability to eat for 24 hours
- Discussing dietary needs with the dietitian

Assistance with physical care, finances, and transportation may be required following discharge. Refer the client and family to social services, support groups, home care services as needed, and other agencies that can provide needed services, such as local chapters of the American Cancer Society, which can provide hospital beds and transportation for outpatient cancer treatment.

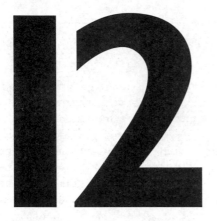

Nursing Care of Clients with Peripheral Vascular Disorders

The major processes that interfere with peripheral blood and lymphatic flow fluid include constriction, obstruction, inflammation, and vasospasm. These conditions lead to disorders of blood pressure regulation, peripheral artery function, aortic structure, venous circulation, and lymphatic circulation.

A holistic approach is important when caring for clients with disorders of the peripheral vascular and lymphatic systems. The focus of care is on teaching long-term care measures, pain relief, improving peripheral blood and lymphatic circulation, preventing tissue damage, and promoting healing. The prescribed treatment may have emotional, social, and economic effects on the client and family.

Disorders of Blood Pressure Regulation

Blood flows through the circulatory system from areas of higher pressure to areas of lower pressure. The amount of pressure in any portion of the vascular system is affected by a number of factors, including blood volume, vascular resistance, and cardiac output. The **blood pressure** is the tension or pressure exerted by blood against arterial walls. A certain amount of pressure within the system is necessary to maintain open vessels, capillary perfusion, and oxygenation of all body tissues. Excess pressure, however, has harmful effects, increasing the workload of the heart, altering the structure of the vessels, and affecting sensitive body tissues such as the kidneys, eyes, and central nervous system.

This section focuses on **hypertension,** or excess pressure in the arterial portion of systemic circulation. Excessively low blood pressure, *hypotension,* is discussed in the shock section of Chapter 40. Altered pulmonary vascular pressures are discussed in Chapter 15.

Physiology Review

Blood flow through the circulatory system requires *sufficient blood volume* to fill the blood vessels and *pressure differences* within the system that allow blood to move forward. The arterial, or supply side, of the circulation has relatively high pressures created by the thick elastic walls of the arteries and arterioles. On the other hand, the venous, or return side of the system, is a low pressure system of thin-walled, distensible veins. Blood flows through the capillaries linking these two systems from the higher pressure arterial side to the lower pressure venous side.

The arterial blood pressure is created by the ejection of blood from the heart during systole (*cardiac output* or *CO*) and the tension, or resistance to blood flow, created by the elastic arterial walls (*systemic vascular resistance or SVR*). The blood pressure rises as the heart contracts during systole, ejecting its blood. This pressure wave, or the **systolic blood pressure,** is felt as the peripheral pulse and heard as the Korotkoff sounds during blood pressure measurement. In healthy adults the average systolic pressure is 120 mmHg. During diastole, or cardiac relaxation and filling, elastic arterial walls maintain a minimum pressure, the **diastolic blood pressure,** to maintain blood flow through the capillary beds. The average diastolic pressure in a healthy adult is 80 mmHg. The difference between the systolic and diastolic pressure, normally about 40 mmHg, is known as the **pulse pressure.** The **mean arterial pressure (MAP)** is the average pressure in the arterial circulation throughout the cardiac cycle. The formula MAP = CO X SVR is often used to show the relationships between factors determining the blood pressure.

Cardiac output is determined by the blood volume and the ability of the ventricles to fill and effectively pump that blood. A number of factors contribute to systemic vascular resistance, including vessel length, blood viscosity, and vessel diameter and distensibility (compliance). While vessel length and blood viscosity remain relatively constant, vessel diameter and compliance are subject to normal regulatory activities and disease.

The arterioles normally determine the SVR as their diameter changes in response to a variety of stimuli:

- *Sympathetic nervous system (SNS)* stimulation. Baroreceptors in the aortic arch and carotid sinus signal the SNS via the cardiovascular control center in the medulla when the MAP changes. A drop in MAP stimulates the SNS, increasing the heart rate, cardiac output, and constricting arterioles (except in skeletal muscle). As a result, BP rises. A rise in MAP has the opposite effect, decreasing the heart rate and cardiac output, and causing arteriolar vasodilation.

- *Circulating epinephrine and norepinephrine* from the adrenal cortex (e.g., the fight-or-flight response) have the same effect as SNS stimulation.

- *Renin-angiotensin-aldosterone system* responds to renal perfusion. A drop in renal perfusion stimulates renin release. Renin converts angiotensinogen to angiotensin I, which is subsequently converted to angiotensin II in the lungs by angiotensin-converting enzyme (ACE). Angiotensin II is a potent vasoconstrictor. It also promotes sodium and water retention both directly and by stimulating the adrenal medulla to release aldosterone. Both SVR and CO increase, raising BP.

- *Atrial natriuretic peptide* is released from atrial cells in response to stretching by excess blood volume. It promotes vasodilation and sodium and water excretion, lowering BP.

- *Adrenomedullin* is a peptide synthesized and released by endothelial and smooth muscle cells in blood vessels. It is a potent vasodilator.

- *Vasopressin or antidiuretic hormone* (from the posterior pituitary gland) promotes water retention and vasoconstriction, raising BP.

- *Local factors,* such as inflammatory mediators and various metabolites, can promote vasodilation, affecting BP.

In addition to the above, the primary factor affecting vessel compliance is the extent of arteriosclerosis (hardening of the arteries) and atherosclerosis (plaque accumulation).

The Client with Primary Hypertension

Primary hypertension, also known as *essential hypertension,* is a persistently elevated systemic blood pressure. About 50 million people in the United States have hypertension. More than 90% of these have primary hypertension, which has no identified cause.

Hypertension primarily affects middle-aged and older adults: 38% of people age 50 to 59 and 71% of people age 80 and older are hypertensive (National Heart, Lung, and Blood Institute [NHLBI], 2002). Hypertension is often called a "silent killer," because affected people often have no symptoms of the disease. Awareness and effective treatment of hypertension have significantly improved. Thirty years ago, only 51% of people with hypertension were aware of their condition and only 16% were effectively treated and controlled. In 1994, 88% of people with hypertension were aware of the disease, and 65% were effectively treated and controlled (NHLBI, 2002).

The prevalence of hypertension is significantly higher in African-Americans than in Caucasians and Hispanics. More than 35% of African-American adults are hypertensive, whereas less than 25% of adult Caucasians and Hispanic people are affected. In Caucasians and Hispanics, more males than females are hypertensive; in African-Americans the prevalence in men and women is nearly equal (NHLBI, 2002). Essential hypertension affects people of all income groups, causing significant financial repercussins, because of its effects on other body systems: cerebrovascular accident (stroke), coronary artery disease, and chronic renal failure.

Hypertension is defined as systolic blood pressure of 140 mmHg or higher, or diastolic pressure of 90 mmHg or higher, based on the average of three or more readings taken on separate occasions (NHLBI, 2002). Exceptions include clients being treated for hypertension and an initial reading of a systolic pressure of 210 mmHg or higher and/or a diastolic blood pressure of 120 mmHg or higher. Table 12–1 identifies classifications of blood pressure for adults age 18 and older as defined by the Joint National Committee.

A number of risk factors have been identified for primary hypertension. Genetics play a role, as do environmental factors.

- *Family history.* Studies show a genetic link in 30% to 40% of primary hypertension (Porth, 2002). Genes involved in the renin-angiotensin-aldosterone system and others that affect vascular tone, salt and water transportation in the kidney, obesity, and insulin resistance are likely involved in the development of hypertension.
- *Age.* The incidence of hypertension rises with increasing age. Aging affects baroreceptors involved in blood pressure regulation as well as arterial compliance. As the arteries become less compliant, pressure within the vessels increases. This is often most apparent as a gradual increase in the systolic pressure with aging. Systolic hypertension increases the risk for cerebrovascular accident (stroke).
- *Race.* Essential hypertension is more common and severe in blacks than in people of other ethnic backgrounds. This may relate to the genes controlling the reninangiotensin-aldosterone system, although the exact mechanism for this increased risk is not yet understood.
- *Mineral intake.* High sodium intake often is associated with fluid retention. Although salt and water retention increase blood volume and cardiac output, it is not clear how

salt intake contributes to the onset of hypertension or why some people are affected, but others are not. Increased sodium intake does not cause hypertension, nor does the blood pressure fall with salt restriction in all hypertensive clients. Low potassium, calcium, and magnesium intakes also contribute to hypertension by unknown mechanisms. The ratio of sodium to potassium intake appears to play a role; possibly through the effects of increased potassium intake on sodium excretion. Potassium also may reduce vasoconstriction related to norepinephrine and other vasoactive substances (Porth, 2002). The link between low calcium and magnesium intakes and hypertension is unclear.

- *Obesity.* Central obesity (fat cell deposits in the abdomen), determined by an increased waist-to-hip ratio, has a stronger correlation with hypertension than body mass index or skinfold thickness. Although a clear correlation exists between obesity and hypertension, the relationship may be one of common cause: Genetic factors appear to play a role in the common triad of obesity, hypertension, and insulin resistance.

- *Insulin resistance.* Insulin resistance, with resulting hyperinsulinemia, is linked with hypertension by an unknown mechanism. Activation of the sympathetic nervous system, vascular smooth muscle growth due to excess insulin, the effect of insulin on renal regulation of sodium and water, and changes in cell membrane transport of sodium and calcium have been proposed as mechanisms in this relationship.

- *Excess alcohol consumption.* Regular consumption of three or more drinks a day increases the risk of hypertension. Decreasing or discontinuing alcohol consumption reduces the blood pressure, particularly systolic readings. Lifestyle factors associated with excessive alcohol intake (obesity and lack of exercise) may contribute to hypertension as well.

- *Smoking.* In recent years, a relationship between serum norepinephrine levels (elevated by smoking) and hypertension has been documented. The goal of ongoing research is to clarify the long-term effects of smoking on blood pressure.

- *Stress.* Physical and emotional stress cause transient elevations of blood pressure, but the role of stress in primary hypertension is less clear. Blood pressure normally fluctuates throughout the day, increasing with activity, discomfort, or emotional responses, such as anger. Frequent or continued stress may cause vascular smooth muscle hypertrophy or affect central integrative pathways of the brain (Porth, 2002).

Table 12-1. Classification of Blood Pressure for Adults Age 18 and Older*

Category	Systolic (mmHg)		Diastolic (mmHg)
Optimal	<120	and	<80
Normal	<130	and	<85
High-normal	130–139	or	85–89
Hypertension[‡]			
Stage 1	140–159	or	90–99
Stage 2	160–179	or	100–109
Stage 3	≥180	or	≥110

*When systolic and diastolic blood pressures fall into different categories, the higher category is used to classify blood pressure status.

‡*Based on the average of two or more readings taken at each of two or more visits after an initial screening.*

Note. Adapted from *The Sixth Report of the Joint National Committee on Prevention, Detection, Education, and Treatment of High Blood Pressure,* NIH Publication No. 98-4080 by NHLBI, 1997, Bethesda, MD: National Institutes of Health. Available: http://www.nhlbi.nih.gov/guidelines/hypertension

Pathophysiology

Primary hypertension is thought to develop from a complex interaction of factors that regulate cardiac output and systemic vascular resistance. These interactions may include:

- Sympathetic nervous system overactivity with overstimulation of α- and β-adrenergic receptors, resulting in vasoconstriction and increased cardiac output.
- Renin-angiotensin-aldosterone system overactivity affects vasomotor tone and salt and water excretion. In addition, angiotensin II mediates arteriolar remodeling, which permanently increases SVR.
- Other chemical mediators of vasomotor tone and blood volume, such as atrial natriuretic peptide (factor), also play a role by affecting vasomotor tone and sodium and water excretion.
- The interaction between insulin resistance and endothelial function may be a primary cause of hypertension. Insulin resistance decreases the release of nitric oxide and other endogenous vasodilators, affects renal function, and increases sympathetic nervous system activity (McCance & Huether, 2002).

The result is sustained increases in blood volume and peripheral resistance. The cardiovascular system adapts to increased blood volume by increasing cardiac output. Autoregulatory mechanisms in the systemic arteries react to the increased volume, causing vasoconstriction. The increased systemic vascular resistance causes hypertension. Sustained hypertension, in turn, affects the cardiovascular system. The rate of atherosclerosis accelerates, increasing the risk for coronary heart disease and stroke. The workload of the left ventricle increases, leading to ventricular hypertrophy, which then increases the risk for coronary heart disease, dysrhythmias, and heart failure. Hypertension can also lead to nephrosclerosis and renal insufficiency (Porth, 2002).

Manifestations

The early stages of primary hypertension typically are asymptomatic, marked only by elevated blood pressure. Blood pressure elevations are initially transient, but eventually become permanent. When symptoms do appear, they are usually vague. Headaches, usually in the back of the head and neck, may be present on awakening, and subside during the day. Other symptoms result from target organ damage, and may include nocturia, confusion, nausea and vomiting, and visual disturbances. Examination of the retina of the eye may reveal narrowed arterioles, hemorrhages, exudates, and papilledema (swelling of the optic nerve).

Collaborative Care

Hypertension management focuses on reducing the blood pressure to less than 140 mmHg systolic and 90 mmHg diastolic. *The Sixth Report of the Joint National Committee on Prevention, Detection, Evaluation, and Treatment of High Blood Pressure* (NHLBI, 1997) recommends a treatment plan based on cardiovascular disease risk factors, the presence or absence of target organ damage, and blood pressure levels (Table 12–2). Emphasis is placed on adherence to the treatment plan to prevent long-term consequences of hypertension (e.g., stroke, heart failure, renal failure). Both pharmacologic and nonpharmacologic approaches are used. There is no cure for hypertension, but it can be controlled.

Table 12-2. Recommended Hypertension Treatment

Stage	Risk Group A*	Risk Group B**	Risk Group C***
High-normal (130–139/85–89)	Lifestyle modification	Lifestyle modification	Drug therapy plus lifestyle modification
Stage 1 (140–159/90–99)	Lifestyle modification for up to 12 months, then drug therapy	Lifestyle modification for up to 6 months, then drug therapy	Drug therapy plus lifestyle modification
Stages 2 and 3 (>160/>100)	Drug therapy plus lifestyle modification	Drug therapy plus lifestyle modification	Drug therapy plus lifestyle modification

*Risk Group A: High normal blood pressure or stage 1, 2, or 3 hypertension; no clinical cardiovascular disease, target organ damage, or other risk factors

**Risk Group B: Hypertension; no clinical cardiovascular disease or target organ damage, one or more major risk factors such as smoking, hyperlipidemia, older age (>60 years), male gender or postmenopausal female, family history of cardiovascular disease

***Risk Group C: Hypertension; clinical cardiovascular disease or target organ damage; presence of diabetes with or without other risk factors

Note: Adapted from *The Sixth Report of the Joint National Committee on Prevention, Detection, Evaluation, and Treatment of High Blood Pressure*, NIH Publication No. 98-4080 by the NHLBI, 1997, Bethesda, MD: National Institutes of Health. Available: http://www.nhlbi.nih.gov/guidelines/hypertension

Diagnostic Tests

There are no specific diagnostic tests for essential hypertension. Diagnostic testing focuses on identifying possible causes of secondary hypertension and determining target organ damage and other cardiovascular risk factors. Routine laboratory tests such as urinalysis, complete blood count, and blood chemistries (including electrolytes, glucose, and cholesterol levels) are done before treatment is started.

Lifestyle Modifications

Lifestyle modifications generally are recommended for all clients with high normal blood pressure or intermittent or sustained hypertension. These modifications include weight loss, dietary changes, restricted alcohol use and cigarette smoking, increased physical activity, and stress reduction.

Diet

Dietary approaches to managing hypertension focus on reducing sodium intake, maintaining adequate potassium and calcium intakes, and reducing total and saturated fat intake. A mild to moderate sodium restriction (no added salt) lowers blood pressure and potentiates the effect of antihypertensive drugs for most hypertensive clients. The DASH (Dietary Approaches to Stop Hypertension) diet has proven beneficial effects in lowering blood pressure. This diet focuses on whole foods rather than individual nutrients. It is rich in fruits and vegetables (up to ten servings per day), and low in total and saturated fats.

Weight loss is recommended for clients who are obese. A balanced diet such as the DASH diet is recommended for weight loss. See Table 12-3.

Table 12-3. DASH Diet

- Grains – 7 to 8 servings per day

- Vegetables – 4 to 5 servings per day

- Fruits – 4 to 5 servings per day

- Nonfat/lowfat milk – 2 to 3 servings per day

- Lean meat (including fish and poultry) – 2 or fewer servings per day

- Nuts, seeds, and dry beans – 4 to 5 servings per week

- Calories – 2000 per day

Alcohol and Cigarette Use

The recommended alcohol intake for clients with hypertension is no more than 15 mL of ethanol per day. This translates to 12 oz. of beer, 5 oz. of wine, or 1 oz. of whiskey. Women and lighter-weight people should reduce this limit by half. Although alcohol withdrawal may increase blood pressure, this is usually temporary and diminishes as abstinence or restricted intake continues.

Although nicotine is a vasoconstrictor, substantial data linking smoking to hypertension are lacking. A definitive link exists between smoking and heart disease, however. Clients who smoke are strongly urged to quit. Smoking also reduces the effect of some antihypertensive medications, such as propranolol (Inderal). Smoking cessation aids, such as nicotine patches and gum contain, lower amounts of nicotine and usually do not raise blood pressure.

Physical Activity

Regular exercise, such as walking, cycling, jogging, or swimming, reduces blood pressure and contributes to weight loss, stress reduction, and feelings of overall well-being. Previously sedentary clients are encouraged to engage in aerobic exercise for 30 to 45 minutes per day, most days of the week. Isometric exercise, such as weight training, may not be appropriate, as it can raise the systolic blood pressure.

Stress Reduction

Stress stimulates the sympathetic nervous system, increasing vasoconstriction, systemic vascular resistance, cardiac output, and the blood pressure. Regular, moderate exercise is the treatment of choice for reducing stress in hypertensive clients. Relaxation techniques, such as biofeedback, therapeutic touch, yoga, and meditation, to relax both mind and body, may also lower blood pressure, although their effect has not been proven in hypertension management.

Medications

Current pharmacologic treatment of hypertension involves using one or more of the following drug classes: diuretics, beta-adrenergic blockers, centrally acting sympatholytics, vasodilators, angiotensin-converting enzyme (ACE) inhibitors, and calcium channel blockers. These drug classes have different sites of action.

Treatment usually is initiated using a single antihypertensive drug at a low dose. The dose is slowly increased until optimal blood pressure control is achieved. If the drug does not effectively lower the blood pressure, or has troubling side effects, a different drug from another class of antihypertensive medications is substituted. If, on the other hand, the drug is tolerated well, but has not lowered blood pressure to the desired level, a second drug from another class may be added to the treatment regimen.

A diuretic or a beta blocker often is prescribed initially for uncomplicated hypertension. These drugs lower blood pressure and reduce the risk of complications, such as heart failure and stroke. Diuretics are the preferred treatment for isolated systolic hypertension in older adults. ACE inhibitors also are commonly used in initial treatment of hypertension, particularly for clients who are diabetic or who have heart failure or a history of MI.

Other factors considered in selecting drugs for treating hypertension include demographic characteristics of the client, concurrent conditions, quality of life, cost, and possible interactions among prescribed drugs. In general, diuretics and calcium channel blockers are more effective for treating hypertension in blacks than beta blockers or ACE inhibitors. Beta blockers are preferred to treat hypertension with concurrent coronary heart disease and angina, but are contraindicated for clients who have asthma or depression. Beta blockers also reduce exercise tolerance and may adversely affect lifestyles of some clients.

Thiazide diuretics, such as hydrochlorothiazide (HydroDIURIL), are widely used to control hypertension. In major clinical studies, single therapy with diuretics controlled blood pressure in about 50% of the clients and reduced hypertension-linked morbidity and mortality related to coronary heart disease. Diuretics control hypertension primarily by preventing tubular reabsorption of sodium, thus promoting sodium and water excretion and reducing blood volume. Thiazide diuretics also reduce systemic vascular resistance through an unknown mechanism. Diuretics are particularly effective for blacks and for clients who are obese, older, or who have increased plasma volume or low renin activity. The adverse effects of diuretics are generally dose related. In addition to hypokalemia, diuretics may affect serum levels of glucose, triglycerides, uric acid, low-density lipoproteins, and insulin. More information about diuretics can be found in Chapters 24 and 39.

Treatment of clients in risk group C is generally more aggressive to minimize the risk of MI, heart failure, or stroke. When the average blood pressure is greater than 200/120, immediate therapy, and possible hospitalization, is vital.

After a year of effective hypertension control, an effort may be made to reduce the dosage and number of drugs. This is known as step-down therapy. It is more successful in clients who have made lifestyle modifications. Careful blood pressure monitoring is necessary during and after step-down therapy, as the blood pressure often rises again to hypertensive levels.

Nursing Care

Health Promotion

Health promotion teaching and activities focus on the modifiable risk factors for hypertension. Advise all clients (as well as children and adolescents) to stop or never start smoking. Discuss the risks of obesity, excess alcohol intake, and a sedentary lifestyle with clients. Encourage all clients to eat a diet rich in fruits and vegetables and low in total and saturated fat. Discuss the potential benefits of maintaining an adequate calcium and potassium intake, and provide lists of foods containing these nutrients. Advise all clients to remain active and engage in aerobic exercise for four or more days a week. Discuss the stress reducing benefits of exercise.

Table 12-4. Medication Administration – Antihypertensive Drugs

Alpha-Adrenergic Blockers

> Doxazosin (Cardura)
> Prazosin (Minipress)
> Terazosin (Hytrin)

Alpha-adrenergic blocking agents block alpha receptors in vascular smooth muscle, decreasing vasomotor tone and vasoconstriction. They also reduce serum levels of low-density (LDL) and very low-density lipoproteins (VLDL). However, vasodilation may cause orthostatic hypotension and reflex stimulation of the heart, resulting in tachycardia and palpitations. A beta blocker may be ordered to minimize this effect.

Nursing Responsibilities
- Give the first dose at bedtime to minimize risk of fainting (called "first-dose syncope"). If the first dose is given in the daytime (or if the dose is increased), instruct patient to remain in bed for three to four hours.
- Assess blood pressure and apical pulse before each dose and as indicated thereafter.

Client and Family Teaching
- There is a risk of fainting after taking the first dose of this drug. Take the drug at bedtime to reduce this risk, and do not drive or engage in other hazardous activities for 12 to 24 hours after the first dose.

Continued on the next page

Table 12-4. Continued

- This drug may cause dizziness or lightheadedness. Change positions slowly, and sit down if you become dizzy or lightheaded.
- Notify your primary care provider if you develop nasal congestion or impotence while taking this drug.
- Notify your primary care provider before discontinuing this medication.

Angiotensin-Converting Enzyme (ACE) Inhibitors

Benazepril (Lotensin)
Moexipril (Univasc)

Captopril (Capoten)
Perindopril (Aceon)

Enalapril (Vasotec)
Quinapril (Accupril)

Fosinopril (Monopril)
Ramipril (Altace)

Lisinopril (Zestril)
Trandolapril (Mavik)

Angiotensin II Receptor Blockers

Eprosartan (Teveten)
Losartan (Cozaar)

Irbersartan (Avapro)
Valsartan (Diovan)

Candesartan (Atacand)

The ACE inhibitors lower blood pressure by preventing conversion of angiotensin I to angiotensin II. This in turn prevents vasoconstriction and sodium and water retention. Angiotensin II receptor blockers (ARBs) have the same effect, but they act by blocking the effect of angiotensin II on receptors. Both ACE inhibitors and ARBs are less effective for African-American patients and are contraindicated for pregnant women (Lehne, 2001). Their primary adverse effects are persistent cough, first-dose hypotension, and hyperkalemia.

Nursing Responsibilities
- Assess blood pressure and WBC before giving the first dose. Monitor blood pressure for two hours after the first dose and on a regular basis thereafter.
- Administer by mouth one hour before meals; tablets may be crushed.
- Report changes in WBC or differential, hyperkalemia, or changes in BUN or serum creatinine to the primary care provider.
- Do not administer to clients with renal artery stenosis or who are pregnant.
- Immediately report and treat manifestations of angioedema (giant wheals and edema of the tongue, glottis, and pharynx). Initiate resuscitation measures as needed. Discontinue drug immediately and do not use in the future.

Table 12-4. Continued

Client and Family Teaching

- Report peripheral edema, signs of infection, or difficulty breathing to your primary care provider.
- Change position (lying to sitting and sitting to standing) slowly to prevent dizziness; sit down if dizziness or lightheadedness develops.
- Do not take a potassium supplement or use a potassium-based salt substitute while taking this drug unless prescribed by your physician.
- Notify your physician if you become pregnant while taking this drug. Although it is safe early in pregnancy, taking the drug during the second and third trimesters may harm the fetus.

Beta-Adrenergic Blocking Agents

Acebutolol (Sectral)
Nadolol (Corgard)

Atenolol (Tenormin)
Penbutolol (Levatol)

Betaxolol (Kerlone)
Pindolol (Visken)

Bisoprolol (Zebeta)
Propranolol (Inderal)

Carteolol (Cartrol)
Timolol (Blocadren)

Metoprolol tartrate (Lopressor)

Beta-adrenergic blockers are commonly used to control hypertension. Beta blockers reduce blood pressure by preventing beta-receptor stimulation in the heart, thereby decreasing heart rate and cardiac output. Beta blockers also interfere with renin release by the kidneys, decreasing the effects of angiotensin and aldosterone. Potential adverse effects of beta blockers include bronchospasm, fatigue, sleep disturbances, nightmares, bradycardia, heart block, worsening of heart failure, gastrointestinal disturbances, impotence, and increased triglyceride levels.

Nursing Responsibilities
- Before giving initial dose, assess for contraindications to beta blockers such as asthma, chronic lung disease, bradycardia, or heart block.
- Assess blood pressure and apical pulse before giving; notify primary care provider if vital signs are outside established parameters.
- Report adverse effects, such as bradycardia, decreased cardiac output (fatigue, dyspnea with exertion, hypotension, decreased level of consciousness), heart failure, heart block, bronchoconstriction (wheezing, dyspnea), or altered blood glucose levels (in diabetic clients).
- Carefully monitor responses of the older client.

Continued on the next page

Table 12-4. Continued

Client and Family Teaching

- Monitor blood pressure and pulse daily as instructed.
- Change position (lying to sitting and sitting to standing) slowly to prevent dizziness and possible falls.
- Report effects such as fatigue, lethargy, and impotence to your primary care provider.
- Notify your physician if you become short of breath, develop a cough, or experience swelling of your extremities.
- If you have diabetes, check blood glucose levels more frequently as hypoglycemia may develop with few symptoms.
- Talk to your primary care provider before taking any over-the-counter medications.
- Carry an adequate supply of the drug when traveling. Do not stop taking this drug without notifying your primary care provider.

Calcium Channel Blockers

Amlodipine (Norvasc)
Nifedipine (Procardia)

Diltiazem (Cardizem)
Nimodipine (Nimotop)

Felodipine (Plendil)
Nisoldipine (Sular)

Isradipine (DynaCirc)
Verapamil (Isoptin)

Nicardipine (Cardene)

Calcium channel blockers inhibit the flow of calcium ions across the cell membrane of vascular tissue and cardiac cells. In doing so, they relax arterial smooth muscle, lowering peripheral resistance through vasodilation. Calcium channel blockers can cause reflex tachycardia, and some (e.g., verapamil and diltiazem) may impair cardiac function, worsening heart failure.

Nursing Responsibilities

- Assess blood pressure, apical pulse, and liver and renal function tests prior to giving these drugs.
- Calcium channel blockers may be given orally or intravenously.
- Do not administer verapamil or diltiazem to clients with severe hypotension, sinus, or atrioventricular blocks. Administer with caution to clients also taking digoxin or a beta blocker.
- Periodically monitor blood pressure and apical pulse during therapy. Promptly report signs of bradycardia, AV block, or heart failure to the physician.

Client and Family Teaching

- Take blood pressure and pulse daily as taught. Notify your physician if your pulse is less than 60 BPM or your blood pressure is not within the specified range.

Table 12-4. Continued

- This drug may cause constipation. Drink six to eight glasses of water each day, and increase fiber in diet.
- Report shortness of breath, weight gain, or swelling in feet or ankles to your primary care provider.

Centrally Acting Sympatholytics

Clonidine (Catapres)
Guanfacine (Tenex)

Guanabenz (Wytensin
Methyldopa (Aldomet)

The centrally acting sympatholytics stimulate the a_2 receptors in the CNS to suppress sympathetic outflow to the heart and blood vessels. A fall in cardiac output and vasodilation result, reducing blood pressure. Dry mouth and sedation are common adverse effects. Severe reflex hypertension may occur if abruptly discontinued. Clonidine is contraindicated during pregnancy; methyldopa is contraindicated for clients with active liver disease.

Nursing Responsibilities
- Assess for contraindications to therapy. Obtain baseline blood pressure, CBC, Coomb test, and liver function studies.
- Administer oral doses at bedtime to minimize effects of sedation.
- Methyldopa may be given intravenously for hypertensive emergencies.
- Apply transdermal clonidine patch to dry, hairless area of intact skin on the chest or upper arm. Assess for rash, which indicates allergy, at area of application.
- Promptly report changes in laboratory values to the physician. Discontinue methyldopa if manifestations of liver dysfunction develop.

Client and Family Teaching
- Relieve dry mouth by sipping water or chewing sugarless gum.
- Take with meals if gastric upset or nausea develop.
- Change position (lying to sitting and sitting to standing) slowly to prevent dizziness and possible falls.
- Do not suddenly discontinue medication or skip doses; this could cause serious hypertension.
- Report mental depression or decreased mental acuity to your health care provider.
- Side effects, such as dry mouth, nausea, and dizziness, tend to diminish over time.
- Do not drive a car if the medications cause drowsiness.

Vasodilators

Hydralazine (Apresoline)
Minoxidil (Loniten)

Vasodilators reduce blood pressure by relaxing vascular smooth muscle (especially in the arterioles), and decreasing peripheral vascular resistance. These drugs are often prescribed in

Continued on the next page

Table 12-4. Continued

combination with a diuretic or beta blocker, because they can cause reflex tachycardia and fluid retention. Because these drugs can have significant toxic effects, they are not routinely used to manage chronic hypertension.

Nursing Responsibilities
- Hydralazine may be given orally or intravenously; minoxidil is given orally.
- Assess blood pressure and pulse before giving the drug, and monitor during therapy as indicated. Report tachycardia or hypotension to the physician.
- Report peripheral edema and manifestations of volume overload and heart failure.
- Immediately report muffled heart sounds or paradoxical pulse as pericardial effusion and possible cardiac tamponade may develop during minoxidil therapy.
- Discontinue hydralazine and report manifestations of a SLE-like syndrome: muscle or joint pain, fever, or symptoms of nephritis or pericarditis.

Client and Family Teaching
- Change position (lying to sitting and sitting to standing) slowly to prevent dizziness and possible falls.
- Report muscle, joint aches, and fever to your health care provider.
- Headache, palpitations, and rapid pulse may develop, but should abate in about ten days.
- Do not discontinue the medication without talking to your health care provider.
- Minoxidil may cause excessive hair growth. Contact your physician if this becomes troublesome.

Assessment
Focused assessment of the client with hypertension includes:

- *Health history:* complaints of morning headache, cervical pain; cardiovascular or central nervous system manifestations; history of hypertension, renal disease, diabetes; family history of high blood pressure, heart failure, or kidney disease; current medications.
- *Physical examination:* vital signs including blood pressure in both arms, apical and peripheral pulses; ophthalmologic exam of retinal fundus.

Nursing Diagnoses and Interventions
All clients with primary hypertension and their families need significant teaching to manage this chronic condition. Health maintenance is a high-priority problem. Depending on the stage of hypertension and concurrent illnesses, other appropriate nursing diagnoses may include imbalanced nutrition, fluid volume excess, and risk for noncompliance.

Ineffective Health Maintenance
Unhealthy lifestyle and behaviors can lead to health problems such as hypertension. When hypertension has been identified, knowledge of the disease and its management is vital for the client. Willingness to take responsibility for hypertension management is central to effective blood pressure control. Adopting healthy lifestyle changes enhances drug therapy;

in some cases, the need for medications may be eliminated or reduced. Because hypertension is often an asymptomatic disease and many antihypertensive drugs have unpleasant side effects, it is vital that the client understand the chronic progressive nature of the disease and its long-term consequences.

- Assist with identifying current behaviors that contribute to hypertension. *The client must first identify contributory behaviors before he or she can change them. Using knowledge of hypertension risk factors, the nurse can help identify behaviors and factors contributing to hypertension that can be changed. Including the family in this process is important to reduce potential sabotage of the client's efforts to adopt healthier behaviors.*

- Assist in developing a realistic health maintenance plan. *Preparing a health maintenance plan for the client does little to encourage personal responsibility for health. However, nurses can guide clients in developing realistic goals and expectations for the treatment plan and modifying risk factors, such as smoking, exercise, diet, and stress.*

- Help the client and family identify strengths and weaknesses in maintaining health. *Discussing areas of the health maintenance plan that are working well, and those that present difficulties, can help to identify necessary changes in the plan and additional strategies for implementing it.*

Risk for Noncompliance

Noncompliance, or failure to follow the identified treatment plan, is a continuing risk for any client with a chronic disease. Recommended lifestyle changes such as diet, exercise, restricted alcohol intake, stress reduction, and smoking cessation often are difficult to maintain on a continuing basis. In addition, prescribed medications may have undesirable effects, whereas hypertension itself often has no symptoms or noticeable effects.

- Inquire about reasons for noncompliance with recommended treatment plan. Listen openly and without judging. *Nonthreatening discussion of factors contributing to noncompliance validates the client's self-esteem and partnership in the treatment plan.*

- Evaluate knowledge of hypertension, its long-term effects, and treatment. Provide additional information and reinforce teaching as needed. *Knowledge increases the sense of control, which also increases the likelihood of compliance with treatment.*

- Assist to develop realistic short-term goals for lifestyle changes. *Attempting to lose weight, exercise daily, stop smoking, and dramatically change the diet all at the same time may be overwhelming, leading to a sense of failure. Smaller, gradual changes are more easily incorporated into lifestyle and daily activities, improving compliance.*

- Help the client identify cues and develop reminders (e.g., written notes, a medication box filled weekly) to assist with maintaining a schedule for exercise and medications. *Cues and other devices provide helpful reminders of activities and schedules until they are incorporated into habits.*

- Reassure the client that relapse into old habits and behaviors is common. Encourage avoiding feelings of guilt associated with relapse, and use the circumstance to renew efforts to comply with treatment. *Guilt and feelings of failure can lead to further noncompliance unless the event is used to identify reasons for noncompliance and ways to prevent it from recurring in the future.*

Imbalanced Nutrition: More Than Body Requirements

The relationship between obesity, excess alcohol intake, and hypertension is well documented. Hypertension is particularly associated with central obesity, identified by waist circumference greater than hip circumference. While weight loss is difficult and takes commitment to changing eating and exercise habits, it is possible for most clients to achieve.

- Assess usual daily food intake, and discuss possible contributing factors to excess weight, such as sedentary lifestyle, or using food as a reward or stress reliever. Inquire about diversional activities, exercise patterns, and previous weight reduction efforts (e.g., participation in weight reduction programs or using fad or crash diets). *Assessment data provides clues about contributing factors to obesity, the client's knowledge base about the relationship between eating and exercise habits and weight, and safe weight loss strategies. This provides direction for further teaching and for developing a realistic weight reduction plan.*

- Mutually determine with the client a realistic target weight (e.g., loss of 10% of current body weight over a 6-month period). Regularly monitor weight. Encourage a system of nonfood rewards for achieving small, incremental goals. *Setting weight loss goals helps formalize the process and provides motivation for continued progress. Developing realistic goals may be difficult; unrealistic goals, however, set the client up for failure. Continuous incremental weight loss provides reassurance that it can be achieved and promotes permanent weight reduction.*

- Refer to a dietitian for information about low-fat, low-calorie foods and eating plans. Focus on changing eating habits as opposed to "following a diet." *Focusing on changing eating habits promotes the sense that low-fat, low-calorie eating patterns should become a part of lifestyle, rather than a short-term measure to be endured until the weight loss goal is achieved.*

- Recommend participating in an approved weight loss program such as Weight Watchers, Overeaters Anonymous, or Take off Pounds Sensibly (TOPS). *Organized weight loss programs provide structure for a balanced weight reduction program, as well as mutual support from others trying to lose weight.*

Excess Fluid Volume

Excess fluid volume often contributes to hypertension by increasing the cardiac output. A number of factors associated with hypertension can cause excess fluid volume, including sodium retention and disruption of the renin-angiotensin-aldosterone system. In addition, some antihypertensive drugs, such as calcium channel blockers and vasodilators, can contribute to excess fluid in the interstitial spaces and peripheral edema.

- Monitor intake and output, and weigh daily (if in an acute or long-term care facility) or weekly (in the community). *Rapid weight changes (over days) reflect fluid balance than more accurately intake and output records. One liter of fluid weighs 1 kg (2.2 lb). Weight changes and intake and output records help monitor the effects of therapy.*

- Monitor for peripheral edema (sacral edema in the bedridden client). *Drugs, such as vasodilators, can cause fluid accumulation in interstitial tissues, leading to peripheral or dependent edema. Adding a diuretic to the treatment plan may be necessary.*

- Refer to a dietitian for teaching about a restricted sodium diet. Discuss the relationship between sodium intake and fluid retention. Provide opportunities to choose low-sodium foods from simulated menus. Support efforts, and reassure that lifestyle changes, such as consuming less sodium, take time. *Knowledge provides the power to take control of sodium intake. Patience and perseverance are needed to succeed; positive reinforcement of efforts to change long-standing dietary patterns is important.*

- Discuss the importance of adhering to treatment plans, such as dietary restrictions and medication schedules. *Understanding the rationale for treatment measures promotes the client's sense of control and encourages compliance with the treatment regimen.*

The Client with Secondary Hypertension

Secondary hypertension is elevated blood pressure resulting from an identifiable underlying process. It accounts for only 5% to 10% of identified cases of hypertension. Kidney disease and coarctation of the aorta are common causes of secondary hypertension. In older adults, renovascular disease is the most common cause of sudden hypertension. The pathophysiology of selected causes of secondary hypertension are summarized below.

- *Kidney disease.* Any disease that affects renal blood flow (e.g., renal artery stenosis) or renal function (e.g., glomerulonephritis, renal failure) can lead to hypertension. Disruption of the blood supply stimulates the renin-angiotensinaldosterone system, with resulting vasoconstriction and sodium and water retention. Altered kidney function affects the elimination of water and electrolytes, leading to hypertension.

- *Coarctation of the aorta.* Coarctation of the aorta is narrowing of the aorta, usually just distal to the subclavian arteries. Reduced renal and peripheral blood flow stimulates the renin-angiotensin-aldosterone system and local vasocontrictive responses, raising the blood pressure. A marked difference between pressures in the upper and lower extremities is common, with weak pulses and poor capillary refill in the lower extremities.

- *Endocrine disorders.* Adrenal gland disorders such as Cushing syndrome and primary aldosteronism can cause hypertension. A rare tumor of the adrenal medulla, pheochromocytoma, causes persistent or intermittent hypertension. Other endocrine disorders, such as hyperthyroidism and pituitary disorders, can also lead to hypertension.

- *Neurologic disorders.* Increased intracranial pressure causes an elevated blood pressure as the body attempts to maintain cerebral blood flow. Disorders that interfere with autonomic nervous system regulation, such as high spinal cord injury, may allow the sympathetic nervous system to predominate, increasing systemic vascular resistance and blood pressure.

- *Drug use.* Estrogen and oral contraceptive use may lead to hypertension, possibly by prompting sodium and water retention and affecting the renin-angiotensin-aldosterone system. Stimulant drugs, such as cocaine and methamphetamines, increase systemic vascular resistance and cardiac output, resulting in hypertension.

- *Pregnancy.* About 10% of all pregnant women are hypertensive. Hypertension may predate pregnancy or occur as a direct response to the pregnancy. The mechanism of pregnancy-induced hypertension (PIH) is unclear. It is a significant cause of maternal and fetal morbidity and mortality and requires careful perinatal management.

The pattern of secondary hypertension varies, depending on its cause. Pheochromocytoma may cause attacks of hypertension that last for minutes to hours, accompanied by anxiety, palpitations, diaphoresis, pallor, and nausea and vomiting. Primary aldosteronism may cause hypertension, weakness, paresthesias, polyuria, and nocturia (see Chapter 26). Symptoms of kidney disease accompany hypertension when a renal disorder is the cause.

The following diagnostic tests may be ordered to differentiate primary from secondary hypertension.

- *Renal function studies* and *urinalysis* to identify renal causes of hypertension. Elevated serum creatinine and BUN, reduced creatinine clearance, and hematuria, proteinuria, and casts often indicate kidney disease.
- *Serum potassium* is decreased in hyperaldosteronism.
- *Blood chemistries,* including serum electrolytes, glucose, and lipid studies are done to detect abnormalities indicative of endocrine or cardiovascular disease.
- *Intravenous pyelography (IVP), renal ultrasonography, renal arteriography,* and *CT* or *MRI* may be done when secondary hypertension is suspected.

Collaborative and nursing care for the client with secondary hypertension is the same as that for primary hypertension, discussed in the previous section. In addition, the underlying process is treated. See chapters covering specific disorders for more information about treatment measures.

The Client with Hypertensive Crisis

Some clients with hypertension may, for reasons not clearly understood, develop rapid, significant elevations in systolic and/or diastolic pressures. In a *hypertensive emergency,* the systolic pressure may be greater than 240 mmHg and the diastolic pressure higher than 130 mmHg. Immediate treatment (within 1 hour) is vital to prevent cardiac, renal, and vascular damage, and reduce morbidity and mortality. Most hypertensive emergencies occur when clients suddenly stop taking their medications or their hypertension is poorly controlled.

Malignant hypertension is a hypertensive emergency, marked by a diastolic pressure greater than 120 mmHg. It most commonly affects younger clients (30 to 50 years old), black men, pregnant women with toxemia, and people with collagen and/or renal disease (Porth, 2002). Malignant hypertension must be rapidly diagnosed and aggressively (yet carefully) treated to prevent encephalopathy and irreversible renal and cardiac failure (Tierney, et al., 2001). Intense cerebral artery spasms help protect the brain from excess pressure; however, cerebral edema often develops. It may cause manifestations such as headache, confusion, swelling of the optic nerve (papilledema), blurred vision, restlessness, and motor and sensory deficits (Porth, 2002). Prolonged malignant hypertension damages walls of the arterioles and renal blood vessels, and may lead to intravascular coagulation and acute renal failure.

The goal of care in hypertensive emergencies is to reduce the blood pressure by no more than 25% within minutes to 2 hours, then toward 160/100 within 2 to 6 hours. It is important to avoid rapid or excessive blood pressure decreases that may lead to renal, cerebral, or cardiac ischemia (NHLBI, 1997). Blood pressure is monitored frequently (every 5 to 30 minutes) during a hypertensive emergency. The BUN, serum creatinine, calcium, and total protein levels are carefully monitored to help determine the prognosis for recovery. Drug treatment for malignant hypertension includes parenteral administration of a rapidly acting antihypertensive, such as the potent vasodilator sodium nitroprusside (Nipride). Management also focuses on treating any underlying or coexisting heart, kidney, and CNS disorders.

Nursing care for the client with a hypertensive emergency focuses on continuous monitoring of the blood pressure and titrating drugs (administered by intravenous bolus or infusion) as ordered to achieve desired blood pressure. Avoiding excessive or very rapid blood pressure reductions is as important as achieving the desired blood pressure readings. Reassure the client and family of the rapid effect of prescribed drugs. Provide psychologic and emotional support as needed. Maintain an attitude of confidence that the treatment will achieve the desired effect. Following resolution of the hypertensive crisis, review causes of the crisis. Teach the client and family measures to effectively manage hypertension and prevent future hypertensive emergencies.

Disorders of the Aorta and Its Branches

The aorta and its branches may be affected by occlusions, aneurysms, and inflammations. These disorders may be chronic or acute and life threatening (e.g., a thoracic dissection). This section focuses on aneurysms of the aorta and its branches.

The Client with an Aneurysm

An **aneurysm** is an abnormal dilation of a blood vessel, commonly at a site of a weakness or a tear in the vessel wall. Aneurysms commonly affect the aorta and peripheral arteries, because of the high pressure in these vessels. An aneurysm also may develop in the ventricular wall, usually affecting the left ventricle. Most arterial aneurysms are caused by arteriosclerosis or atherosclerosis; trauma may also lead to aneurysm formation.

Arterial aneurysms are most common in men over age 50, most of whom are asymptomatic at the time of diagnosis. Hypertension is a major contributing factor in the development of some types of aortic aneurysms.

Pathophysiology and Manifestations

Aneurysms form due to weakness of the arterial wall. *True aneurysms* are caused by slow weakening of the arterial wall due to the long-term, eroding effects of atherosclerosis and hypertension. True aneurysms affect all three layers of the vessel wall, and most are fusiform and circumferential. *Fusiform aneurysms* are spindle shaped and taper at both ends. *Circumferential* aneurysms involve the entire diameter of the vessel. They generally grow slowly but progressively. Their length and diameter vary considerably among clients. A large fusiform aneurysm may affect most of the ascending aorta as well as a large portion of the abdominal aorta.

False aneurysms, also known as traumatic aneurysms, are caused by a traumatic break in the vessel wall rather than weakening of the vessel. They often are *saccular,* shaped like small outpouchings (sacs) on a portion of the vessel wall. A *berry aneurysm* is a type of saccular aneurysm. They are often small (less than 2 cm in diameter), caused by congenital weakness in the tunica media of the artery. Berry aneurysms are commonly found in the circle of Willis.

Dissecting aneurysms are unique, developing when a break or tear in the tunica intima and media allows blood to invade or *dissect* the layers of the vessel wall. The blood usually is contained by the adventitia, forming a saccular or longitudinal aneurysm.

Aneurysms affect different segments of the aorta and its branches. Their manifestations generally are due to pressure of the aneurysm on adjacent structures.

Thoracic Aortic Aneurysms

Thoracic aortic aneurysms account for about 10% of aortic aneurysms. They usually result from weakening of the aortic wall by arteriosclerosis and hypertension (Tierney, et al., 2001). Other causes include trauma, coarctation of the aorta, tertiary syphilis, fungal infections, and Marfan syndrome. The syphilis spirochete can invade and weaken aortic smooth muscle, causing an aneurysm to develop as long as 20 years after the primary infection. Marfan syndrome fragments elastic fibers of the aortic media, weakening the vessel wall.

Thoracic aneurysms frequently are asymptomatic. When present, symptoms vary by the location, size, and growth rate of the aneurysm. Substernal, neck, or back pain may occur. Pressure on the trachea, esophagus, laryngeal nerve, or superior vena cava may cause dyspnea, stridor, cough, difficult or painful swallowing, hoarseness, edema of the face and neck, and distended neck veins.

Aneurysms of the ascending aortic arch typically cause angina. Aneurysms of the aortic arch often cause dysphagia, dyspnea, hoarseness, confusion, and dizziness. Aneurysms of the thoracic aorta tend to enlarge progressively and may rupture, causing death.

Abdominal Aortic Aneurysms

Abdominal aortic aneurysms are associated with arteriosclerosis and hypertension. Increasing age and smoking are believed to contribute as well. Most abdominal aortic aneurysms are found in adults over age 70. The vast majority (over 90%) develop below the renal arteries, usually where the abdominal aorta branches to form the iliac arteries.

Most abdominal aneurysms are asymptomatic, but a pulsating mass in the mid and upper abdomen and a bruit over the mass are found on exam. When pain is present, it may be constant or intermittent, usually felt in the midabdominal region or lower back. Its intensity may range from mild discomfort to severe pain. Pain intensity often correlates with the size and severity of the aneurysm. Severe pain may indicate impending rupture.

Sluggish blood flow within the aneurysm may cause thrombi (blood clots) to form. These can become emboli (circulating clots), traveling to the lower extremities and occluding peripheral arteries. The aneurysm may also rupture, with hemorrhage and hypovolemic shock. Rupture causes death before hospitalization in up to 50% of all clients; others die before surgery. Only about 10% to 20% of clients survive rupture of an abdominal aortic aneurysm.

Popliteal and Femoral Aneurysms

Most popliteal and femoral aneurysms are due to arteriosclerosis. They are often bilateral and usually affect men.

Popliteal aneurysms may be asymptomatic. Manifestations, if any, are due to decreased blood flow to the lower extremity and include **intermittent claudication** (cramping or pain in the leg muscles brought on by exercise and relieved by rest), rest pain, and numbness. A pulsating mass may be palpable in the popliteal fossa (behind the knee). Thrombosis and embolism are complications; gangrene may result, often necessitating amputation.

A *femoral aneurysm* usually is detected as a pulsating mass in the femoral area. The manifestations are similar to those of popliteal aneurysms, resulting from impaired blood flow. Femoral aneurysms may rupture.

Aortic Dissections

Dissection is a life-threatening emergency caused by a tear in the intima of the aorta with hemorrhage into the media. The hemorrhage dissects or splits the vessel wall, forming a blood-filled channel between its layers. Dissection can occur anywhere along the aorta. *Type A dissection* (also called *proximal dissection*) affects the ascending aorta; *type B dissection* (*distal dissection*) is limited to the descending aorta.

Hypertension is a major predisposing factor for aortic dissection. Other risk factors include male gender, advancing age, Marfan syndrome, pregnancy, congenital defects of the aortic valve, coarctation of the aorta, and inflammatory aortitis (Braunwald, et al., 2001).

Dissection of the thoracic aortic walls progresses along the length of the vessel, moving both proximally and distally. As the aneurysm expands, pressure may prevent the aortic valve from closing or may occlude the branches of the aorta. Descending aortic dissection may extend into the renal, iliac, or femoral arteries.

The primary symptom of an aortic dissection is sudden, excruciating pain. The pain, often described as a ripping or tearing sensation, is usually over the area of dissection. Thoracic dissections cause chest or back pain. Other symptoms may include syncope, dyspnea, and weakness. The blood pressure may initially be increased, but rapidly falls and is often inaudible as the dissection occludes blood flow. Peripheral pulses are absent for the same reason.

Complications develop if major arteries are affected. Obstruction of the carotid artery causes neurologic symptoms, such as weakness or paralysis. The myocardium, kidneys, or bowel may become ischemic or infarct. Acute aortic regurgitation may develop with dissection of the ascending aorta. With treatment, the long-term prognosis is generally good, although the in-hospital mortality rate following surgery is 15% to 20% (Braunwald, et al., 2001).

Collaborative Care

Most aneurysms are asymptomatic, detected through a routine physical examination. Treatment depends on the size of the aneurysm. Small, asymptomatic aneurysms are often not treated; large aneurysms at risk for rupture require surgery.

Diagnostic Tests

Diagnostic studies done to establish the diagnosis and determine the size and location of the aneurysm may include:

- *Chest X-ray* to visualize thoracic aortic aneurysms.
- *Abdominal ultrasonography* to diagnose abdominal aortic aneurysms.
- *Transesophageal echocardiography* to identify the specific location and extent of a thoracic aneurysm and to visualize a dissecting aneurysm.
- *Contrast-enhanced CT* or *MRI* allows precise measurements of aneurysm size.
- *Angiography* uses contrast solution injected into the aorta or involved vessel to visualize the precise size and location of the aneurysm.

Medications

Thoracic aortic aneurysms are treated with long-term beta-blocker therapy, and additional antihypertensive drugs as needed, to control heart rate and blood pressure.

Clients with aortic dissection are initially treated with intravenous beta blockers, such as propranolol (Inderal), metoprolol (Lopressor), labetalol (Normodyne), or esmolol (Brevibloc) to reduce the heart rate to about 60 BPM. Sodium nitroprusside (Nipride) infusion is started concurrently to reduce the systolic pressure to 120 mmHg or less. Calcium channel blockers may also be used. Direct vasodilators such as diazoxide (Hyperstat) and hydralazine (Apresoline) are avoided, as they may actually worsen the dissection (Braunwald, et al., 2001). Constant monitoring of vital signs, hemodynamic pressures (via Swan-Ganz catheter; see Chapter 9 for more information about hemodynamic hydrostatic pressure monitoring), and urine output are vital to ensure adequate perfusion of vital organs.

Following surgical correction of an aneurysm, anticoagulant therapy may be initiated. Heparin therapy is used initially, with conversion to oral anticoagulation prior to discharge. Many clients are maintained indefinitely on anticoagulant therapy; others may use lifelong, low-dose aspirin therapy to reduce the risk of clot formation.

Surgery

Operative repair of aortic aneurysms is indicated when the aneurysm is symptomatic or expanding rapidly. Thoracic aneurysms more than 6 cm in diameter are surgically repaired; asymptomatic abdominal aneurysms greater than 5 cm in diameter may be repaired, depending on the client's operative risk factors. Type A dissections are repaired as soon as feasible; type B dissections may be surgically repaired, depending on the extent of involvement and risk for rupture (Braunwald, et al., 2001).

An open surgical procedure, in which the aneurysm is excised and replaced with a synthetic fabric graft, is the standard treatment for expanding abdominal aortic aneurysms. Although the aneurysm walls may be excised, they usually are left intact and used to cover the graft. Surgical repair of thoracic aneurysms is similar, but more complex, due to major vessels exiting at the aortic arch. Cardiopulmonary bypass is required if the ascending aorta is involved. The aortic valve may also be replaced during surgery.

Endovascular stent grafts are increasingly being used to treat abdominal aortic aneurysms. The stent, which consists of a metal sheath covered with polyester fabric, is placed percutaneously using fluoroscopy to guide its placement. Both straight and bifurcated grafts are available. This option may be preferred in clients who have a high surgical risk (Meeker & Rothrock, 1999).

Nursing Care

Assessment

Focused assessment for the client with a suspected aortic aneurysm includes:

- *Health history:* complaints of chest, back, or abdominal pain; extremity weakness; shortness of breath, cough, difficult or painful swallowing, hoarseness; history of hypertension, coronary heart disease, heart failure, or peripheral vascular disease.
- *Physical examination:* vital signs, including blood pressure in upper and lower extremities; peripheral pulses; skin color and temperature; neck veins; abdominal exam, including gentle palpation for masses and auscultation for bruits; neurologic exam, including level of consciousness, sensation, and movement of extremities.

Nursing Diagnoses and Interventions

Nursing care for clients with an aneurysm of the aorta, or its branches, focuses on monitoring and maintaining tissue perfusion, relieving pain, and reducing anxiety. Nursing care usually is acute, precipitated by a complication or surgical repair of the aneurysm.

Risk for Ineffective Tissue Perfusion

Clients with aortic aneurysms are at risk for impaired tissue perfusion due to aneurysm rupture with resulting hemorrhage and lack of blood flow to tissues distal to the rupture. In addition, thrombi often form within the aneurysm and may become emboli, obstructing distal arterial blood flow.

• Implement interventions to reduce the risk of aneurysm rupture:

    a. Maintain bed rest with legs flat.

    b. Maintain a calm environment, implementing measures to reduce psychologic stress.

    c. Prevent straining during defecation and instruct to avoid holding the breath while moving.

    d. Administer beta blockers and antihypertensives as prescribed.

Activity, stress, and the Valsalva maneuver increase blood pressure, increasing the risk of rupture. Elevating or crossing the legs restricts peripheral blood flow and increases pressure in the aorta or iliac arteries. Beta blockers and antihypertensives are often ordered to reduce pressure in the dilated vessel.

• Continuously monitor cardiac rhythm. Report complaints of chest pain or changes in ECG tracing. Administer oxygen as indicated. *Aortic dissection and repair place the client at significant risk for myocardial infarction (MI), a major cause of postoperative mortality and morbidity (Braunwald, et al., 2001). Rapid identification and treatment of this complication can reduce the risk of death or long-term adverse effects of MI.*

Risk for Injury Potent antihypertensive drugs are often given intravenously to reduce the pressure on an expanding or dissecting aneurysm. Continuous monitoring of infusions and hemodynamic parameters, such as arterial pressure, pulmonary pressures, and cardiac output, is vital to ensure that adequate tissue perfusion is maintained during infusions of these potent drugs.

• Continuously monitor arterial pressure and hemodynamic parameters as indicated. Promptly report results outside the specified parameters to the physician. *Many of the drugs used are effective within minutes. Responses vary among individuals, particularly in the older adult, necessitating continuous monitoring.*

• Monitor urine output hourly. Report output less than 30 mL/hr. *The kidneys are very sensitive to reduced perfusion pressure; inadequate renal blood flow can lead to acute renal failure.*

Anxiety

Clients with aortic aneurysms often are highly anxious because of the urgent nature of the disorder. The nurse must manage the anxiety levels of both the client and family members to effectively address physiologic care needs. Stress reduction is also necessary to help maintain the blood pressure within desired limits.

• Explain all procedures and treatments, using simple and understandable terms. *Simplified explanations are necessary when anxiety levels interfere with learning and understanding.*

• Respond to all questions honestly, using a calm, empathetic, but matter-of-fact manner. *Honesty with the client and family promotes trust and provides reassurance that the true nature of the situation is not being "hidden" from them.*

- Provide care in a calm, efficient manner. *Using a calm manner, even during preparations for emergency surgery, reassures the client and family that although the situation is critical, the staff is prepared to handle things effectively.*
- Spend as much time as possible with the client. Allow supportive family members to remain with the client when possible. *The presence of a health professional and supportive family member reassures the client that he or she is not alone in facing this crisis.*

Home Care

Topics to discuss when preparing clients and their families for home care depend on the treatment plan. Discuss the following topics when surgical repair is not immediately planned and the aneurysm will be monitored:

- Measures to control hypertension, including lifestyle and prescribed drugs
- The benefits of smoking cessation
- Manifestations of increasing aneurysm size or complications to report to the physician

Following surgery, discuss the following topics in preparing the client and family for home care.

- Wound care and preventing infection; manifestations of impaired healing or infection to be reported
- Prescribed antihypertensive and anticoagulant medications and their expected and unintended effects
- The importance of adequate rest and nutrition for healing
- Measures to prevent constipation and straining at stool, such as increasing fluid and fiber in the diet
- The importance of avoiding prolonged sitting, lifting heavy objects, engaging in strenuous exercise, and having sexual intercourse until approved by the physician (usually 6 to 12 weeks)
- Signs and symptoms of complications to report to the physician

Provide referrals to a home health agency or community health service as necessary. Referrals are especially important for older adults and their caregivers, who may require additional assistance with the complex care needs.

Disorders of Venous Circulation

The two primary categories of venous system disorders are occlusive disorders and those related to ineffective venous blood flow. Impaired venous blood flow can lead to stasis and clotting, as well as tissue changes associated with venous congestion.

Physiology Review

The venous system is a low-pressure system in comparison with the arterial circulation. Veins and venules are thin-walled, distensible vessels. While they contain smooth muscle that allows them to contract or expand, the media (muscle layer) of veins is significantly thinner than that of arteries. The low pressures in the venous system allow it to serve as a reservoir for blood. Stimulation by the sympathetic nervous system causes veins to contract, helping maintain vascular volume. The low pressure venous system relies on skeletal muscle contractions and pressure changes in the abdomen and thorax to facilitate blood return to the heart. Unlike arteries, veins of the extremities contain valves to prevent retrograde blood flow.

The Client with Venous Thrombosis

Venous thrombosis (also known as *thrombophlebitis*) is a condition in which a blood clot (thrombus) forms on the wall of a vein, accompanied by inflammation of the vein wall and some degree of obstructed venous blood flow.

Venous thrombi are more common than arterial thrombi, because of lower pressures and flow within the venous system (McCance & Huether, 2002). Thrombi can form in either superficial or deep veins. **Deep venous thrombosis (DVT)** is a common complication of hospitalization, surgery, and immobilization. Obstetric and orthopedic procedures carry a higher risk for venous thrombosis; it may develop in more than 50% of clients having orthopedic surgery, particularly surgeries involving hip or knee (Braunwald, et al., 2001). Other significant risk factors for venous thrombosis include abdominal or thoracic surgery, certain cancers, trauma, pregnancy, and use of oral contraceptives or hormone replacement therapy.

Pathophysiology and Manifestations

Three pathologic factors, called *Virchow triad*, are associated with thrombophlebitis: stasis of blood, vessel damage, and increased blood coagulability. Vessel trauma stimulates the clotting cascade. Platelets aggregate at the site, particularly when venous stasis is present. Platelets and fibrin form the initial clot. Red blood cells are trapped in the fibrin meshwork, and the thrombus propagates (grows) in the direction of blood flow. The inflammatory response is triggered, causing tenderness, swelling, and erythema in the area of the thrombus. Initially the thrombus floats within the vein. Pieces of the thrombus may break loose and travel through the circulation as emboli. Fibroblasts eventually invade the thrombus, scarring the vein wall and destroying venous valves. Although patency of the vein may be restored, valve damage is permanent, affecting directional flow (Tierney, et al., 2001).

Deep Vein Thrombosis

The deep veins of the legs, primarily in the calf, and the pelvis provide the most hospitable environment for venous thrombosis. Approximately 80% of deep vein thromboses begin in the deep veins of the calf, often propagating into the popliteal and femoral veins (Tierney, et al., 2001). DVT usually is asymptomatic; in some clients, a pulmonary embolism may be the first indication.

When present, the manifestations of DVT are primarily due to the inflammatory process accompanying the thrombus. Calf pain, which may be described as tightness or a dull, aching pain in the affected extremity, particularly upon walking, is the most common symptom. Tenderness, swelling, warmth, and erythema may be noted along the course of involved veins. The affected extremity may be cyanotic and often is edematous. Rarely, a cord may be palpated over the affected vein. A positive Homans sign (pain in the calf when the foot is dorsiflexed) is an unreliable indicator of DVT.

Complications The major complications of deep vein thrombosis are chronic venous insufficiency (see the next section of this chapter) and pulmonary embolism. Pulmonary embolism occurs when the clot fragments or breaks loose from the vein wall. As the clot travels, it moves through progressively larger veins and into the right side of the heart. From there it enters the pulmonary circulation, where it eventually occludes arterial flow to a portion of the lungs. The result is a mismatch between ventilation (air flow) and perfusion (blood flow) in a portion of the lungs. The effect on gas exchange depends on the size of the embolism and the vessel it occludes. See Chapter 15 for more information about pulmonary emboli.

Superficial Vein Thrombosis

Venous catheters and infusions are the primary risk factors for superficial venous thrombosis. Superficial vein thrombosis may also develop in conjunction with thromboangitis obliterans, varicose veins, or deep vein thrombosis. It may develop spontaneously in pregnant women or following delivery. In some cases, superficial venous thrombosis of the long saphenous vein is the earliest sign of an abdominal cancer such as pancreatic cancer (Tierney, et al., 2001).

Superficial vein thrombosis is marked by pain and tenderness at the site of the thrombus. A reddened, warm, tender cord extending along the affected vein can be palpated. The area surrounding the vein may be swollen and red.

Table 12-5. Manifestations of Venous Thrombosis

Deep Vein Thrombosis

- Usually asymptomatic
- Dull, aching pain in affected extremity, especially when walking
- Possible tenderness, warmth, erythema along affected vein
- Cyanosis of affected extremity
- Edema of affected extremity

Superficial Vein Thrombosis

- Localized pain and tenderness over the affected vein
- Redness and warmth along the course of the vein
- Palpable cordlike structure along the affected vein
- Swelling and redness of surrounding tissue

Collaborative Care

It is important to differentiate venous thrombosis from other causes of extremity pain, such as cellulitis, muscle strain, contusion, and lymphedema. The history, physical examination, and diagnostic tests are used to establish the diagnosis. Treatment focuses on preventing further clotting or extension of the clot and addressing underlying causes.

Diagnostic Tests

- *Duplex venous ultrasonography* is a noninvasive test used to visualize the vein and measure the velocity of blood flow in the veins. Although the clot often cannot be visualized directly, its presence can be inferred by an inability to compress the vein during the examination.

- *Plethysmography* is a noninvasive test that measures changes in blood flow through the veins. It is often used in conjunction with Doppler ultrasonography. Plethysmography is most valuable in diagnosing thromboses of larger or more superficial veins.
- *Magnetic resonance imaging (MRI)* is another noninvasive means of detecting deep vein thrombosis. It is particularly useful when thrombosis of the vena cavae or pelvic veins is suspected.
- *Ascending contrast venography* uses an injected contrast medium to assess the location and extent of venous thrombosis. Although invasive, expensive, and uncomfortable, contrast venography is the most accurate diagnostic tool for venous thrombosis. It is used when the results of less invasive tests leave the diagnosis unclear (Tierney, et al., 2001).

Prophylaxis

Medications and other measures are used to prevent venous thrombosis when the risk is high. Low-molecular-weight heparins prevent deep vein thrombosis in clients who are undergoing general or orthopedic surgery, experiencing acute medical illness, or on prolonged bed rest. Oral anticoagulation may also be used as a prophylactic measure in clients with fractures or who are undergoing orthopedic surgery.

Elevating the foot of the bed with the knees slightly flexed promotes venous return. Early mobilization and leg exercises, such as ankle flexion and extension, assist venous flow by muscle compression. Intermittent pneumatic compression devices applied to the legs are effective to prevent DVT. They are also used when anticoagulation is contraindicated, due to the increased risk for bleeding (Braunwald, et al., 2001). Elastic stockings are also used to prevent venous thrombosis in clients at risk.

Medications

Anticoagulants to prevent clot propagation and enable the body's own lytic system to dissolve the clot are the mainstay of treatment for venous thrombosis. Thrombolytic drugs, such as streptokinase or tissue plasminogen activator (t-PA), may accelerate the process of clot lysis and prevent damage to venous valves. There is, however, no evidence that thrombolytic therapy is more effective in preventing pulmonary embolism than anticoagulants (Braunwald, et al., 2001). It also significantly increases the risk for bleeding and hemorrhage.

Nonsteroidal anti-inflammatory agents, such as indomethacin (Indocin) or naproxen (Naprosyn), may be ordered to reduce inflammation in the veins and provide symptomatic relief, particularly for clients with superficial vein thrombosis.

Anticoagulants Anticoagulants are given to prevent clot extension and reduce the risk of subsequent pulmonary embolism. Anticoagulation is initiated with unfractionated heparin or low-molecular-weight (LMW) heparin. Following an initial intravenous bolus of 7,500 to 10,000 units of unfractionated heparin, a continuous heparin infusion of 1000 to 1500 IU per hour is started. The dosage is calculated to maintain the activated partial thromboplastin time (aPTT) at approximately twice the control or normal value. An infusion pump is used to deliver the prescribed dosage. Frequent monitoring of the infusion is an important nursing responsibility. Subcutaneous heparin injections may be used as an alternate to intravenous infusion in some instances.

LMW heparins are increasingly used to prevent and treat venous thrombosis. They do not require the close laboratory monitoring of unfractionated heparins. LMW heparin is administered subcutaneously in fixed doses once or twice daily, allowing the option of outpatient treatment. LMW heparins have additional advantages, in that they are more effective and carry lower risks for bleeding and thrombocytopenia than conventional, unfractionated heparins.

Oral anticoagulation with warfarin may be initiated concurrently with heparin therapy. Overlapping heparin and warfarin therapy for four to five days is important because the full anticoagulant effect of warfarin is delayed, and it may actually promote clotting during the first few days of therapy (Tierney, et al., 2001). Warfarin doses are adjusted to maintain the international normalized ratio (INR) at 2.0 to 3.0 (Braunwald, et al., 2001).

Once this level is achieved, the heparin is discontinued and a maintenance dose of warfarin is prescribed to prevent recurrent thrombosis. Anticoagulation generally is continued for at least three months. When DVT is recurrent or risk factors, such as altered coagulability or cancer, are present, anticoagulant therapy may be prolonged. Regular follow-up is necessary to be sure prothrombin times (INR) remain within the desirable range for anticoagulation. See the Medication Administration Table below for the nursing implications for anticoagulant therapy.

Table 12-6. Medication Administration — Anticoagulant Therapy

Heparin

Heparin interferes with the clotting cascade by inhibiting the effects of thrombin and preventing the conversion of fibrinogen to fibrin. This prevents the formation of a stable fibrin clot. At therapeutic levels, heparin prolongs the thrombin time, clotting time, and activated partial thromboplastin time. When given intravenously, its effect is immediate. Given subcutaneously, its onset of action is within one hour. When heparin is discontinued, clotting times return to normal within two to six hours (Spratto & Woods, 2003).

Nursing Responsibilities
- Assess for history of unexplained or active bleeding. Assess laboratory results for abnormal clotting profile or evidence of active bleeding.
- Give a test dose as indicated to clients with a history of multiple allergies or a history of asthma.
- Administer by deep subcutaneous injection; abdominal sites are preferred. Avoid injecting within two inches of the umbilicus. Rotate sites. Do not aspirate prior to injecting or massage after the injection.
- Intravenous solutions may be diluted with dextrose, normal saline, or Ringer's solution. Use an infusion pump.
- Keep protamine sulfate, a heparin antagonist, available to treat excessive bleeding.
- Monitor and report abnormal laboratory results and aPTT values outside the desired range.
- Promptly report evidence of bleeding, such as hematemesis, hematuria, bleeding gums, or unexplained abdominal or back pain.

Client and Family Teaching
- Report unusual bleeding or excessive menstrual flow.

Table 12-6. Continued

- Use an electric razor and a soft-bristle toothbrush; prevent injury by clearing pathways, using a night light, and other measures. Do not consume alcohol.
- Avoid contact sports while on anticoagulant therapy.
- Do not consume large amounts of food rich in vitamin K (yellow and dark green vegetables).
- Do not use aspirin or NSAIDs while on heparin therapy, unless advised to do so by your physician.
- Wear a MedicAlert tag and advise all health care providers (including dentists and podiatrists) of therapy.

Low-Molecular-Weight Heparins

Ardeparin (Normiflo)
Enoxaparin (Lovenox)

Dalteparin (Fragmin)
Tinzaparin (Innohep)

LMW heparins are the most bioavailable fraction of heparin. They provide a more precise and predictable anticoagulant effect than unfractionated heparins. Like unfractionated heparin, LMW heparin prevents conversion of prothrombin to thrombin, liberation of thromboplastin from platelets, and formation of a stable clot. LMW heparins cannot be used interchangeably with each other, or with unfractionated heparin.

Nursing Responsibilities
- Assess for evidence of active bleeding, a history of bleeding disorders or thrombocytopenia, or sensitivity to heparin, sulfites, or pork products.
- Monitor for unusual or masked bleeding. PT and aPTT levels may be within normal levels even in the presence of hemorrhage.
- Administer by deep subcutaneous injection into abdominal wall, thigh, or buttocks. Rotate sites. Do not aspirate or massage.

Client and Family Teaching
- Subcutaneous self-administration technique, timing of doses, and site rotation. Do not rub site after administering to minimize bruising.
- Do not take aspirin, NSAIDs, or other over-the-counter drugs, unless recommended by your physician.
- Promptly report excessive bruising or bleeding, chest pain, difficulty breathing, itching, rash, or swelling to your health care provider.
- Keep follow-up appointments as scheduled.

Oral Anticoagulant

Warfarin (Coumadin)

Warfarin interferes with synthesis of vitamin K–dependent clotting factors by the liver, leading to depletion of these factors. It has no effect on already circulating clotting factors or on existing clots. Warfarin inhibits extension of existing thrombi and the formation of new clots. Its action is cumulative and more prolonged than that of heparin.

Continued on the next page

Table 12-6. Continued

Nursing Responsibilities
- Assess laboratory results and history for evidence of abnormal bleeding.
- Multiple drugs affect the metabolism and protein binding of warfarin; note all medications and assess for interactions with warfarin.
- Do not give during pregnancy as warfarin may cause congenital malformations.
- Oral tablets may be crushed and given without regard to meals.
- Dilute intravenous warfarin with supplied diluent; administer within four hours by direct intravenous injection at a rate of 25 mg/min.
- Keep vitamin K available to reverse effects of warfarin in the event of excessive bleeding or hemorrhage.
- Monitor PT or INR; report values outside the desired range.

Client and Family Teaching
- Do not take your prescribed dose and notify your physician immediately if bleeding occurs (hematemesis, bright red or black tarry feces, hematuria, bleeding gums, excessive bruising, etc.). Report rash or manifestations of hepatitis (dark urine, malaise, yellow skin or sclera).
- Take your warfarin at the same time every day; do not change brands as their effects may differ.
- Menstrual bleeding may be slightly increased; contact your health care provider if it increases significantly. Use reliable birth control to prevent pregnancy while taking warfarin. Immediately contact your health care provider if you think you may be pregnant.
- Take precautions to prevent injury and bleeding: use a soft toothbrush and electric razor, wear shoes, and use a night light. Avoid participating in contact sports.
- Do not smoke, use alcohol, or take any over-the-counter drugs, unless specifically recommended by your health care provider. Notify all health care providers, including dentists and podiatrists, of therapy. Wear a MedicAlert tag.
- Obtain lab tests as scheduled and keep all scheduled follow-up appointments.

Treatments

Treatment of venous thrombosis also includes measures to relieve symptoms and reduce inflammation. With superficial vein thrombosis, applying warm, moist compresses over the affected vein, extremity rest, and anti-inflammatory agents usually provide relief of symptoms.

Bed rest may be ordered for deep vein thrombosis. The duration of bed rest typically is determined by the extent of leg edema. The legs are elevated 15 to 20 degrees, with the knees slightly flexed, above the level of the heart to promote venous return and discourage venous pooling. Elastic antiembolism stockings (TEDS) or pneumatic compression devices are also frequently ordered to stimulate the muscle-pumping mechanism that promotes the return of blood to the heart. When permitted, walking is encouraged while avoiding prolonged standing or sitting. Crossing the legs also is avoided, as are tight-fitting garments or stockings that bind.

Surgery

Venous thrombosis usually is effectively treated with conservative measures and anticoagulation. In some cases, however, surgery is required to remove the thrombus, prevent its extension into deep veins, or prevent the effects of embolization.

Venous thrombectomy is done when thrombi lodge in the femoral vein and their removal is necessary to prevent pulmonary embolism or gangrene. Successful thrombus removal rapidly improves venous circulation. The duration of this effect varies.

When venous thrombosis is recurrent and anticoagulant therapy is contraindicated, a filter may be inserted into the vena cava to capture emboli from the pelvis and lower extremities, preventing pulmonary embolism. Several different filters are available. The Greenfield filter is widely used for its ability to trap emboli within its apex while maintaining patency of the vena cava. The filter can be inserted under fluoroscopy with local anesthesia. Mortality and morbidity associated with the filter are very low (Meeker & Rothrock, 1999).

Extensive thrombosis of the saphenous vein may necessitate ligation and division of the saphenous vein where it joins the femoral vein to prevent clot extension into the deep venous system. A vein affected by septic venous thrombosis is excised to control the infection. Antibiotic therapy also is initiated.

Nursing Care

Health Promotion

Prevention of venous thrombosis is an important component of nursing care for all at-risk clients. Position clients to promote venous blood flow from the lower extremities, with the feet elevated and the knees slightly bent. Avoid placing pillows under the knees and positions in which the hips and knees are sharply flexed. Use a recliner chair or foot stool when sitting. Ambulate clients as soon as possible, and maintain a regular schedule of ambulation throughout the day. Teach ankle flexion and extension exercises, and frequently remind clients to perform them. Apply elastic hose and pneumatic compression devices when appropriate. Instruct clients to avoid crossing legs when in bed or sitting. Inquire about possible prophylactic heparin or warfarin therapy for clients undergoing orthopedic surgery or other high-risk procedures. Frequently assess intravenous sites. Change the site and catheter as dictated by agency protocol, and if evidence of local inflammation is noted.

Assessment

Assess clients at risk for venous thrombosis for manifestations and risk factors.

*   *Health history:* complaints of leg or calf pain, its duration and characteristics, and the effect of walking on the pain; history of venous thrombosis or other clotting disorders; current medications.
*   *Physical examination:* inspect affected extremity for redness, edema; palpate for tenderness, warmth, cordlike structures; body temperature.

Nursing Diagnoses and Interventions

In addition to the preventive measures identified earlier, priority nursing diagnoses for the client with venous thrombosis relate to pain, maintenance of tissue perfusion and integrity, and the potential adverse effects of prescribed treatments.

Pain

The pain associated with venous thrombosis results from inflammation of the involved vein. It may be aggravated by use of the involved extremity. Associated edema and swelling may contribute to discomfort. Measures to reduce the inflammation often help relieve the pain.

- Regularly assess pain location, characteristics, and level using a standardized pain scale. Report increasing pain or changes in its location or characteristics. *Tissue substances released during the inflammatory process can stimulate pain receptors. In addition, localized swelling presses on pain-sensitive structures in the area of the inflammation, contributing to discomfort. As inflammation and swelling are reduced, pain should abate. Continued or increasing pain may indicate extension of the thrombosis. Sudden chest pain may indicate a pulmonary embolism, necessitating immediate intervention.*

- Measure calf and thigh diameter of the affected extremity on admission, and daily thereafter. Report increases promptly. *The inflammatory process causes vasodilation and increases vessel permeability, causing edema of the affected extremity. Baseline and subsequent measurements provide a measure of treatment effectiveness.*

- Apply warm, moist heat to affected extremity at least four times daily, using warm, moist compresses or an aqua-K pad. *Moist heat penetrates tissues to a greater depth. Warmth promotes vasodilation, allowing reabsorption of excess fluid into the circulation. Vasodilation also reduces resistance within the affected vessel, reducing pain. As edema subsides, pressure on surrounding tissues is relieved, thereby reducing pain.*

- Maintain bed rest as ordered. *Using leg muscles during walking exacerbates the inflammatory process and increases edema. This, in turn, increases venous compression and pain.*

Ineffective Tissue Perfusion: Peripheral

As thrombi develop, they occlude the lumen of the vein and obstruct blood flow. In addition, the accompanying inflammatory response may precipitate vessel spasms, further impairing arterial and venous blood flow and tissue perfusion. Impaired tissue perfusion, in turn, deprives tissues of nutrients and oxygen. As a result, distal tissues of the affected extremity are at risk for ulceration and infection.

- Assess skin of the affected lower leg and foot at least every eight hours; more often as indicated. *Frequent assessment is important to rapidly detect early signs of tissue breakdown and implementation of measures to protect vulnerable tissues. Early intervention allows healing and restoration of tissue integrity; allowed to continue, the process can lead to necrosis and potential gangrene.*

- Elevate extremities at all times, keeping knees slightly flexed and legs above the level of the heart. *Elevation of the extremities promotes venous return and reduces peripheral edema. Knee flexion promotes muscle relaxation.*

- Use mild soaps, solutions, and lotions to clean the affected leg and foot daily. Pat dry after washing, and apply a nonalcohol-based lotion or moisturizing cream. *Daily hygiene with nondrying soaps and solutions removes potential pathogens from the skin surface, and maintains skin integrity and the first line of defense against infection. Caustic or harsh soaps or solutions can dry and crack the skin. Dry, cracked skin permits bacteria and other microorganisms to enter and infect the tissue, potentially leading to ulceration and venous gangrene.*

- Use egg crate mattress or sheepskin on the bed as needed. *Egg crate mattresses and sheepskins distribute weight more evenly, preventing excess pressure on affected tissues.*
- Encourage frequent position changes, at least every two hours while awake. *Frequent position changes reduce pressure on bony prominences and edematous tissue, reducing the risk of tissue breakdown.*

Ineffective Protection

Anticoagulant therapy interferes with the body's normal clotting mechanisms, increasing the risk for bleeding and hemorrhage.

- Monitor laboratory results, including the INR (prothrombin time), aPTT, hemoglobin, and hematocrit as indicated. Report values outside the normal or desired range. *Coagulation studies are used to monitor the effect of anticoagulant medications. Values within the desired range prevent further clot development while carrying a low risk for bleeding and hemorrhage. A fall in the hemoglobin and hematocrit may indicate undetected bleeding.*

Impaired Physical Mobility

Although prolonged bed rest rarely is required, it is associated with many problems, including constipation, joint contractures, muscle atrophy, and boredom. Nursing care goals include maintaining joint range of motion, minimizing muscle atrophy, and reducing boredom.

- Encourage active range-of-motion exercises at least every eight hours. Provide passive range of motion as needed. *Range-of-motion exercises maintain joint mobility and prevent contractures. Active range of motion (performed by the client) also helps prevent muscle atrophy and preserve function. While passive range-of-motion exercises do not prevent muscle atrophy, they do maintain joint mobility.*
- Encourage frequent position changes, deep breathing, and coughing. *Prolonged immobility can lead to impaired airway clearance and respiratory complications, such as atelectasis or pneumonia. Turning, coughing, and deep breathing facilitate expulsion of secretions from the respiratory tract, airway clearance, and alveolar ventilation.*
- Encourage increased fluid and dietary fiber intake. *Constipation is a frequent complication of immobility due to decreased gastrointestinal motility and loss of abdominal muscle strength. Increasing fluid and fiber intake helps maintain soft, easily expelled stools.*
- Assist with and encourage ambulation as allowed. *Ambulation promotes venous blood flow, helps maintain muscle tone and joint mobility, and increases the sense of well-being.*
- Encourage diversional activities, such as reading, handiwork or other hobbies, television or video games, and socializing. *Boredom may lead to dozing and inertia, with little physical movement or mental stimulation, increasing the risk for complications of immobility.*

Risk for Ineffective Tissue Perfusion: Cardiopulmonary

A thrombus that forms in the deep veins of the legs or pelvis may break loose or fragment, becoming an embolism. Emboli that originate in the venous system usually become trapped in the pulmonary circulation (pulmonary embolism). Gas exchange in the affected area is impaired as blood flow ceases, or is reduced to an area of the lungs that is well ventilated.

- Frequently assess respiratory status, including rate, depth, ease, and oxygen saturation levels. *A mismatch of ventilation and perfusion can significantly affect gas exchange, leading to rapid, shallow respirations, dyspnea and air hunger, and a fall in oxygen saturation levels.*
- Initiate oxygen therapy, elevate the head of the bed, and reassure the client who is experiencing manifestations of pulmonary embolism. *Oxygen therapy and elevating the head of the bed promote ventilation and gas exchange in those alveoli that are well perfused, helping maintain tissue oxygenation. Reassurance helps reduce anxiety and slow the respiratory rate, promoting greater respiratory depth and alveolar ventilation.*

Home Care

Treatment measures for venous thrombosis may be initiated and carried out on an outpatient basis or continued for an extended period of time following hospital discharge. Include the following topics when teaching for home care:

- Explanation of the disease process
- Treatment measures, including laboratory tests and their purposes, medications and adverse effects that should be reported
- Appropriate methods of heat application
- Prescribed activity restrictions
- Measures to prevent future episodes of venous thrombosis
- The importance of follow-up visits and laboratory tests as scheduled

Refer clients for community nursing services for continued assessment and reinforcement of teaching. Provide referrals for assistance with ADLs and home maintenance services as indicated. Consider referral for physical therapy if needed.

The Client with Chronic Venous Insufficiency

Chronic venous insufficiency is a disorder of inadequate venous return over a prolonged period. Deep vein thrombosis is the most frequent cause of chronic venous insufficiency. Other conditions, such as varicose veins or leg trauma, may contribute; in some instances, it develops without an identified precipitating cause (Braunwald, et al., 2001; Tierney, et al., 2001).

Pathophysiology

Following DVT, large veins may remain occluded, increasing the pressure in other veins of the extremity. This increased pressure distends the veins, separating valve leaflets and impairing their ability to close. DVT also damages valve leaflets, causing them to thicken and contract. The result is impaired unidirectional blood flow and deep vein emptying (Porth, 2002).

When venous valves are incompetent, the muscle-pumping action produced during activity cannot propel blood back to the heart. Venous blood collects and stagnates in the lower leg (*venous stasis*). Venous pressures in the calf and lower leg increase, particularly during ambulation. This increased pressure impairs arterial circulation to the lower extremities as well. The body's ability to provide sufficient oxygen and nutrients to the cells and remove metabolic waste products diminishes. Eventually, there is so little oxygen and nutrients that cells begin to die. The skin atrophies, and subcutaneous fat deposits necrose. Breakdown of red blood cells in the congested tissues causes brown skin pigmentation (Porth, 2002). Venous stasis ulcers develop. Congested tissues impair the body's ability to increase the supply of oxygen, nutrients, and metabolic energy to heal the ulcer. As a result, the condition worsens and, over time, the ulcers enlarge. The congested venous circulation also prevents the blood from mounting effective inflammatory and immune responses, significantly increasing the risk for infection in the ulcerated tissue (McCance & Huether, 2002).

Manifestations

Manifestations of chronic venous insufficiency include lower leg edema, itching, and discomfort of the affected extremity that increase with prolonged standing. The extremity is cyanotic. Recurrent stasis ulcers develop, usually forming just above the ankle, on the medial or anterior aspect of the leg. They heal poorly, forming scar tissue that breaks down easily. Tissue surrounding the ulcer is shiny, atrophic, and cyanotic, and there is a brownish pigmentation to the skin. Other skin changes may develop as well, such as eczema or stasis dermatitis. Necrosis and fibrosis of subcutaneous tissue causes the affected area of the leg to feel hard and somewhat leathery to the touch, but even the slightest trauma to the area can produce serious tissue breakdown.

Table 12-7. Comparison of Arterial and Venous Leg Ulcers

Factor	Arterial Ulcers	Venous Ulcers
Location	Toes, feet, shin	Over medial or anterior ankle
Ulcer appearance	Deep, pale	Superficial, pink
Skin appearance	Normal to atrophic Pallor on elevation Rubor on dependency	Brown discoloration Stasis dermatitis Cyanosis on dependency
Skin temperature	Cool	Normal
Edema	Absent or mild	May be significant
Pain	Usually severe Intermittent claudication Rest pain	Usually mild Aching pain
Gangrene	May occur	Does not occur
Pulses	Decreased or absent	Normal

Table 12-8. Manifestations of Chronic Venous Insufficiency

- Lower extremity edema that worsens with standing
- Itching, dull leg discomfort or pain that increases with standing
- Thin, shiny, atrophic skin
- Cyanosis and brown skin pigmentation of lower leg and foot
- Possible weeping dermatitis
- Thick, fibrous (hard) subcutaneous tissue
- Recurrent ulcerations of medial or anterior ankle

Collaborative Care

Collaborative care for the client with venous insufficiency focuses on relieving symptoms, promoting adequate circulation, and healing and preventing tissue damage.

The history and physical examination often establish the diagnosis of chronic venous insufficiency. Because a history of deep vein thrombosis is a major risk factor, careful evaluation of the past medical history and questioning of the client is important. There are no specific diagnostic tests to confirm the diagnosis of chronic venous insufficiency.

Conservative management of venous insufficiency focuses on reducing edema and treating ulcerations. Prolonged standing or sitting is discouraged. Graduated compression hosiery is ordered for daytime use, and frequent elevation of the legs and feet during the day is recommended. At night, the legs and feet should be elevated above the level of the heart by raising the foot of the mattress.

Treatment of associated stasis dermatitis varies, based on the duration of the condition. Wet compresses of boric acid, buffered aluminum actetate (Burrow solution), or isotonic saline solution are applied to acute weeping dermatitis four times a day for one-hour periods. Following the compress, a topical corticosteroid, such as 0.5% hydrocortisone cream, is applied. Bed rest is prescribed during the acute period. Stasis dermatitis that is subsiding or chronic may be treated with a topical corticosteroid, zinc oxide ointment, or a topical broad-spectrum antifungal cream such as clotrimazole (Lotrimin) cream or miconazole (Monistat) cream (Tierney, et al., 2001).

Isotonic saline compresses or wet-to-dry dressings are applied to stasis ulcers to promote healing. A dilute topical antibiotic solution may also be used (Braunwald et al., 2001). The ulcer may be treated by using a semirigid boot applied to the foot and lower leg. This device may be made of Unna paste or Gauzetex bandage. Bony prominences must be well padded. The boot must be changed every one to two weeks, depending on the amount of drainage from the ulcer. This device often allows ambulatory treatment.

A very large, chronic ulcer may require surgery. In this case, the incompetent veins are ligated, the ulcer is excised, and the area is covered with a skin graft (see Chapter 36).

Nursing Care

Nursing care for the client with chronic venous insufficiency is primarily educative and supportive. Client teaching includes the following recommendations:

- Elevate the legs while resting and during sleep.
- Walk as much as possible, but avoid sitting or standing for long periods of time.
- When sitting, do not cross your legs or allow pressure on the back of the knees, such as sitting on the side of the bed.
- Do not wear anything that pinches your legs, such as knee-high hose, garters, or girdles.
- Wear elastic hose as prescribed. The elastic hose should be tighter over the feet than at the top of the leg. Be sure the tops of the elastic hose do not cut into your legs. Put on the hose after you have had your legs elevated.
- Keep the skin on your feet and legs clean, soft, and dry.

The following nursing diagnoses may apply to the client with chronic venous insufficiency.

*   *Disturbed body image* related to edema and stasis ulcers on lower leg
*   *Ineffective health maintenance* related to lack of knowledge about disorder and prescribed treatments
*   *Risk for infection* related to ulcerations
*   *Impaired physical mobility* related to pain and edema in lower legs
*   *Impaired skin integrity* related to presence of stasis ulcers
*   *Ineffective tissue perfusion: Peripheral* related to incompetent venous valves

See other sections of this chapter for specific nursing interventions related to many of these diagnoses.

The Client with Varicose Veins

Varicose veins are irregular, tortuous veins with incompetent valves. Varicosities may develop in any veins, and may be called by other names, such as hemorrhoids in the rectum and varices in the esophagus. Varicosities usually affect the veins of the lower extremities; the long saphenous vein is often affected, and they also may develop in the short saphenous vein.

Varicose veins affect about 2% of people in industrialized nations. They are more common in women over age 35. Studies also suggest that the increased risk for varicose veins in women may relate to venous stasis during pregnancy. Aging is a risk factor, possibly related to decreased exercise and other factors that contribute to venous stasis. People in occupations that involve prolonged standing, such as beauticians, salespeople, and nurses, also have an increased incidence of varicose veins. Race is a risk factor: Whites are more frequently affected than blacks.

Most varicosities occur in the deep veins of the legs. Contributing causes include obesity, venous thrombosis, congenital arteriovenous malformations, or sustained pressure on abdominal veins (as in pregnancy and/or the presence of abdominal tumors). The effects of gravity, produced by long periods of standing, are a major causative factor.

Pathophysiology and Manifestations

Varicose veins are classified as primary (with no involvement of deep veins) or secondary (caused by the obstruction of deep veins). In both cases, long-standing increased venous pressure stretches the vessel wall. This sustained stretching impairs the ability of the venous valves to close, causing them to become incompetent.

The erect position produces a twofold negative effect on the veins. When standing, the leg veins resemble vertical columns and must withstand the full force of venous blood pressure. Prolonged standing, the force of gravity, lack of leg exercise, and incompetent venous valves all weaken the muscle-pumping mechanism, reducing venous blood return to the heart. As standing continues, the amount of blood pooled in the veins increases, further stretching the vessel wall. The venous valves become increasingly incompetent.

Table 12-9. Manifestations of Varicose Veins

- Severe, aching pain in the leg
- Leg fatigue, heaviness
- Itching of the affected leg (stasis dermatitis)
- Feelings of warmth in the leg
- Visibly dilated veins
- Thin, discolored skin above the ankles
- Stasis ulcers

Although varicose veins may be asymptomatic; most cause manifestations, such as severe aching leg pain, leg fatigue, leg heaviness, itching, or feelings of heat in the legs. The degree of valvular incompetence does not seem to correlate well with the extent of symptoms. The menstrual cycle tends to worsen symptoms, suggesting a possible correlation with hormonal factors in women. Assessment reveals obvious dilated, tortuous veins beneath the skin of the upper and lower leg. If varicose veins are long-standing, the skin above the ankles may be thin and discolored, with a brown pigmentation.

Complications of varicose veins include venous insufficiency and stasis ulcers. Chronic stasis dermatitis may also develop. Superficial venous thrombosis may develop in varicose veins, especially during and after pregnancy, following surgery, and in clients on estrogen therapy (oral contraceptives or hormone replacement therapy).

Collaborative Care

Varicose veins usually can be managed using conservative measures, although surgery may be required if symptoms are severe, when complications develop, or for cosmetic reasons.

Diagnostic Tests

While varicose veins often are diagnosed by the history and physical examination, diagnostic tests may be ordered.

- *Doppler ultrasonography* or *duplex Doppler ultrasound* may be performed to identify specific locations of incompetent valves. This test is particularly useful before surgery to identify valves that allow reflux of blood from the femoral, popliteal, or peripheral deep veins into the superficial veins (Tierney, et al., 2001).
- *Trendelenburg test* may be performed to determine the underlying cause of superficial venous insufficiency. The leg is elevated, then an elastic tourniquet is placed around the distal thigh. The varicosities are then observed as the client stands. When valves of the deep veins are incompetent, the veins remain flat on standing; they rapidly distend when the superficial venous valves are the underlying cause.

Treatments

Although there is no real cure for varicose veins, conservative measures are the core of treatment for most clients with uncomplicated varicose veins. These measures often relieve symptoms and prevent complications by improving venous circulation and relieving pressure on venous tissues. Properly fitted graduated compression stockings are commonly prescribed. They compress the veins, propelling blood back to the heart. Compression stockings augment the muscle pumping action of the legs. When worn during times of prolonged standing, and in combination with frequent leg elevation, compression stockings often prevent progression of the condition and development of complications.

Regular, daily walking also is important. Prolonged sitting and standing are discouraged, although elevating the legs for specified periods during the day is beneficial. Leg elevation promotes venous return, prevents venous stasis, and decreases leg heaviness and fatigue.

Compression Sclerotherapy

In compression sclerotherapy, a sclerosing solution is injected into the varicose vein and a compression bandage is applied for a period of time. This obliterates the vein. Venous blood is rerouted through healthy vessels whose valves are not compromised. Compression sclerotherapy may be used to treat small, symptomatic varicosities. It may be the primary treatment, or it may be used in conjunction with varicose vein surgery. While compression sclerotherapy may be done for cosmetic reasons, complications such as phlebitis, tissue necrosis, or infection may occur, and need to be considered prior to the procedures.

Surgery

Surgical treatment of varicose veins generally is reserved for clients who are very symptomatic, experience recurrent superficial venous thrombosis, and/or develop stasis ulcers. The objective of surgery is to remove the diseased veins. It may be considered for cosmetic reasons.

Surgery usually involves extensive ligation and stripping of the greater and lesser saphenous veins (Braunwald et al., 2001). The evening before surgery, the surgeon marks all incompetent superficial and perforating varicose veins with a permanent ink marker. Under either regional or general anesthesia, the greater saphenous vein is removed and the connected smaller tributaries that have not naturally clotted off are tied off. Multiple small incisions may be made over the varicosities, allowing removal of the affected segments of the vein. Incompetent tributaries that communicate with larger vessels are also ligated. For clients with less extensive disease or clients seeking cosmetic improvement, surgery may involve only the removal of the lesser saphenous vein through an incision in the popliteal fossa.

Postoperative care includes applying pressure bandages for a minimum of six weeks, elevating the extremities to minimize postoperative edema, and gradually increasing amounts of ambulation. Sitting and standing are prohibited during the initial recovery period, and are gradually reintroduced as deemed appropriate by the surgeon.

Nursing Care

Health Promotion

Health promotion activities to reduce the incidence of varicose veins include teaching all clients, particularly young women, the benefits of regular exercise continued over the lifetime. Discuss the effect of prolonged sitting or standing on the legs, and encourage the client, whose occupation involves these activities, to periodically get up and move, or to sit with the legs elevated. Encourage all clients to maintain normal weight for their height.

Assessment

Focused assessment of the client with varicose veins includes the following:

- *Health history:* complaints of leg pain, aching, heaviness, or fatigue; ankle swelling; history of venous thrombosis.
- *Physical examination:* visible, dilated, tortuous superficial veins in lower extremities.

Nursing Diagnoses and Interventions

In planning and providing nursing care for clients with varicose veins, emphasis is placed on the importance of health teaching to manage the symptoms of varicose veins, particularly because there is no cure for the disease. Nursing care for clients who have undergone surgical treatment for varicose veins focuses on assessing and promoting wound healing and preventing infection. Nursing diagnoses may include those related to pain, impaired tissue perfusion and skin integrity, and a risk for impaired neurovascular function.

Chronic Pain

Varicose veins can lead to pooling of venous blood in the lower extremities. Venous congestion can cause a dull ache or feeling of pressure in the legs, particularly after prolonged standing. As venous pressure rises, arterial circulation and delivery of oxygen and nutrients to tissues is impaired. Tissue ischemia contributes to the pain. The pain associated with varicose veins tends to be chronic, developing and progressing gradually over a long period of time.

- Assess pain, including its intensity, duration, and aggravating and relieving factors. *Pain assessment allows collaborative planning with the client to identify appropriate interventions.*
- Inquire about current measures being used by the client to manage pain and its effects. Ask about the effectiveness of current management strategies and the desire to change. *Chronic pain management ultimately falls to the client. Strategies to address the pain must meet the client's needs.*
- Teach and reinforce nonpharmacologic pain management strategies, such as progressive relaxation, imagery, deep breathing, distraction, and meditation. *The effectiveness of such strategies is well documented. Nonpharmacologic measures provide a variety of options for controlling pain while maintaining independence. These measures can also reduce reliance on analgesics.*
- Collaborate with the client to establish a pain control plan. *Collaborative planning for pain management increases the client's sense of control and reduces powerlessness. This, in turn, enhances the ability to cope with pain and its effects.*
- Regularly evaluate the effectiveness of planned interventions and pain management strategies. *Regular evaluation allows modification of the care plan as needed, as well as providing a measure of disease progression. Increasing or poorly controlled pain may necessitate additional collaborative interventions to manage the disorder.*

Ineffective Tissue Perfusion: Peripheral

Varicose veins and venous stasis impair delivery of nutrients and oxygen to peripheral tissues as elevated venous pressures interfere with blood flow through the capillary beds. Improving venous blood flow reduces venous pressures and promotes arterial flow to peripheral tissues.

- Assess peripheral pulses, capillary refill, skin color and temperature, and extent of edema. *Assessment of arterial flow and tissue perfusion provide baseline and continuing data for evaluating the effectiveness of interventions.*

- Teach application and use of properly fitted elastic graduated compression stockings. *Elastic compression stockings compress the veins, promoting venous return from the lower extremities. During ambulation, the stockings enhance the blood-pumping action of the muscles. Because elastic stockings inhibit blood flow through small superficial vessels, they should be removed at least once each day for at least 30 minutes.*
- Advise to elevate the legs for 15 to 20 minutes several times a day and to sleep with the legs elevated above the level of the heart. *Elevating the legs promotes venous return, reducing tissue congestion and improving arterial circulation. Improved venous return also increases the cardiac output and renal perfusion, promoting elimination of excess fluid and decreasing peripheral edema.*

Risk for Impaired Skin Integrity

Ineffective venous valve function impairs venous return and increases venous pressures. These increased pressures oppose arterial blood flow and the delivery of oxygen and nutrients to the cells. As a result, tissues are vulnerable to any additional insult, and may break down.

- Assess lower extremity color, temperature, moisture, and for evidence of pressure or breakdown on admission and at each visit. *Initial and continuing assessment allows timely detection of early signs of skin and tissue breakdown. This, in turn, allows early institution of measures to prevent further tissue damage and promote healing.*
- Teach foot and skin care measures, such as daily cleansing with nondrying soap, gentle drying, and lotions to prevent skin dryness and cracking. *Cleansing removes potentially harmful microorganisms and stimulates circulation. Care is taken to keep the skin moist and supple, promoting its function as the first line of defense against infection.*
- Discuss the importance of adequate nutrition and fluid intake. *Adequate nutrients are necessary to maintain tissue integrity and promote healing. A diet high in protein, carbohydrates, and vitamins and minerals promotes growth and maintenance of skin cells, provides energy, and helps prevent skin breakdown. Adequate hydration helps maintain the moisture and turgor of skin, reducing the risk of drying and breakdown.*

Risk for Peripheral Neurovascular Dysfunction

Severe varicose veins can lead to chronic venous insufficiency, impaired arterial circulation, and ultimately, disrupted sensation in the affected extremity. Impaired neurologic function increases the client's risk for injury and infection of the extremity, as minor trauma may go unnoticed.

- Assess circulation, sensation, and movement of the lower extremities. *Disrupted circulation and venous congestion may interfere with sensory and motor function of the affected extremity. The potential for nerve and muscle involvement is especially high in clients with venous stasis ulcers.*
- Teach measures to protect the extremities from injury, such as always wearing shoes or firm slippers, cotton socks to absorb moisture, and testing the temperature of bath water with a thermometer or the upper extremities before stepping in. *Sensation in the lower extremities may be affected by poor circulation, necessitating additional measures to protect the legs and feet from injury.*

Home Care

Most clients with varicose veins provide self-care at home. Include the following topics when preparing the client and family for home care:

- Leg elevation and exercise program
- Application and use of graduated elastic compression stockings
- Foot and leg care (see Table 12-10)
- Measures to avoid injury and skin breakdown
- Symptoms or potential complications to report to the physician

Provide information about suppliers for elastic stockings and any other required supplies. If venous stasis ulcers have developed, consider referral to home health services for regular assessment of healing and additional teaching.

Table 12-10. Foot Care for the Client with Peripheral Vascular Disease

---

1. Keep legs and feet clean, dry, and comfortable.
    - < Wash legs and feet daily in warm water, using mild soap.
    - < Pat dry using a soft towel; be sure to dry between the toes.
    - < Apply moisturizing cream to prevent drying.
    - < Use powder on the feet and between the toes.
    - < Buy shoes in the afternoon (when feet are largest); never buy shoes that are uncomfortable. Be sure toes have adequate room.
    - < Wear a clean pair of cotton socks each day.

2. Prevent accidents and injuries to the feet.
    - < Always wear shoes or slippers when getting out of bed.
    - < Walk on level ground and avoid crowds, if possible.
    - < Do not go barefoot.
    - < Inspect legs and feet daily; use a mirror to examine backs of legs and bottoms of feet.
    - < Have a professional foot care provider trim toenails and care for corns, calluses, ingrown toenails, or athlete's foot.
    - < Always check the temperature of the water before stepping into the tub.
    - < Do not get the legs or tops of the feet sunburned.
    - < Report leg or foot problems (increased pain, cuts, bruises, blistering, redness, or open areas) to your health care provider.

3. Improve blood supply to the legs and feet.
    - < Do not cross legs.
    - < Do not wear garters or knee stockings.
    - < Do not swim or wade in cold water.

13

Assessing Clients with Respiratory Disorders

The respiratory system provides the cells of the body with oxygen and eliminates carbon dioxide, formed as a waste product of cellular metabolism. The events in this process, called respiration, are:

- *Pulmonary ventilation:*   Air is moved into and out of the lungs.
- *External respiration:*   Exchange of oxygen and carbon dioxide occurs between the alveoli and the blood.
- *Gas transport:*   Oxygen and carbon dioxide are transported to and from the lungs and the cells of the body via the blood.
- *Internal respiration:*   Exchange of oxygen and carbon dioxide is made between the blood and the cells.

Review of Anatomy and Physiology

Although the system functions as a whole, this unit contains separate chapters dealing with the upper respiratory system (the nose, pharynx, larynx, and trachea) and the lower respiratory system (the lungs).

The Upper Respiratory System

The upper respiratory system serves as a passageway for air moving into the lungs and carbon dioxide moving out to the external environment. As air moves through these structures, it is cleaned, humidified, and warmed.

The Nose

The nose is the external opening of the respiratory system. The external nose is given structure by the nasal, frontal, and maxillary bones, as well as plates of hyaline cartilage. The nostrils (also called the external nares) are two cavities within the nose, separated by the nasal septum. These cavities open into the nasal portion of the pharynx through the internal nares. The nasal cavities just behind the nasal openings are lined with skin that contains hair follicles, sweat glands, and sebaceous glands. The nasal hairs filter the air as it enters the nares. The rest of the cavity is lined with mucous membranes that contain olfactory neurons and goblet cells that secrete thick mucus. The mucus not only traps dust and bacteria but also contains lysozyme, an enzyme that destroys bacteria as they enter the nose. As mucus and debris accumulate, mucosal ciliated cells move it toward the pharynx, where it is swallowed. The mucosa is highly vascular, warming air that moves across its surface.

Three structures project outward from the lateral wall of each nasal cavity: the superior, middle, and inferior turbinates. The turbinates cause air entering the nose to become turbulent, and also increase the surface area of mucosa exposed to the air. As air moves through this area, heavier particles of debris drop out and are trapped in the mucosa of the turbinates.

The Sinuses

The nasal cavity is surrounded by paranasal sinuses. These openings are located in the frontal, sphenoid, ethmoid, and maxillary bones. Sinuses lighten the skull, assist in speech, and produce mucus that drains into the nasal cavities to help trap debris.

The Pharynx

The pharynx, a funnel-shaped passageway about five inches (13 cm.) long, extends from the base of the skull to the level of the C6 vertebra. The pharynx serves as a passageway for both air and food. It is divided into three regions: the nasopharynx, the oropharynx, and the laryngopharynx.

The nasopharynx serves only as a passageway for air. Located beneath the sphenoid bone and above the level of the soft palate, the nasopharynx is continuous with the nasal cavities. This segment is lined with ciliated epithelium, which continues to move debris from the nasal cavities to the pharynx. Masses of lymphoid tissue (the tonsils and adenoids) are located in the mucosa high in the posterior wall; these tissues trap and destroy infectious agents entering with the air. The auditory (eustachian) tubes also open into the nasopharynx, connecting it with the middle ear.

The oropharynx lies behind the oral cavity and extends from the soft palate to the level of the hyoid bone. It serves as a passageway for both air and food. An upward rise of the soft palate prevents food from entering the nasopharynx during swallowing. The oropharynx is lined with stratified squamous epithelium that protects it from the friction of food and damage from the chemicals found in food and fluids.

The laryngopharynx extends from the hyoid bone to the larynx. It is also lined with stratified squamous epithelium, and serves as a passageway for both food and air. Air does not move into the lungs while food is being swallowed and moved into the esophagus.

The Larynx

The larynx is about two inches (5 cm.) long. It opens superiorly at the laryngopharynx and is continuous inferiorly with the trachea. The larynx provides an airway and routes air and food into the proper passageway. As long as air is moving through the larynx, its inlet is open; however, the inlet closes during swallowing. The larynx also contains the vocal cords, necessary for voice production.

The larynx is framed by cartilages, connected by ligaments and membranes. The thyroid cartilage is formed by the fusion of two cartilages; the fusion point is visible as the Adam's apple. The cricoid cartilage lies below the thyroid cartilage; other pairs of cartilages form the walls of the larynx. The epiglottis, also a cartilage, is covered with mucosa that contains taste buds. This structure normally projects upward to the base of the tongue; however, during swallowing, the larynx moves upward and the epiglottis tips to cover the opening to the larynx. If anything other than air enters the larynx, a cough reflex expels the foreign substance before it can enter the lungs. This protective reflex does not work if the person is unconscious.

The Trachea

The trachea begins at the inferior larynx and descends anteriorly to the esophagus to enter the mediastinum, where it divides to become the right and left primary bronchi of the lungs. The trachea is about four to five inches (12 to 15 cm.) long and one inch (2.5 cm.) in diameter. It contains 16 to 20 C-shaped rings of cartilage joined by connective tissue. The mucosa lining the trachea consists of pseudostratified ciliated columnar epithelium containing seromucous glands that produce thick mucus. Dust and debris in the inspired air are trapped in this mucus, moved toward the throat by the cilia, and then either swallowed or coughed out through the mouth.

The Lower Respiratory System

The lower respiratory system includes the lungs and the bronchi.

The Lungs

The center of the thoracic cavity is filled by the *mediastinum,* which contains the heart, great blood vessels, bronchi, trachea, and esophagus. The mediastinum is flanked on either side by the lungs. Each lung is suspended in its own pleural cavity, with the anterior, lateral, and posterior lung surfaces lying close to the ribs. The hilus, on the mediastinal surface of each lung, is where blood vessels of the pulmonary and circulatory systems enter and exit the lungs. The primary bronchus also enters in this area. The apex of each lung lies just below the clavicle, whereas the base of each lung rests on the diaphragm. The lungs are elastic connective tissue, called stroma, and are soft and spongy.

The two lungs differ in size and shape. The left lung is smaller and has two lobes, whereas the right lung has three lobes. Each of the lung lobes contains a different number of bronchopulmonary segments. These segments are separated by connective tissue. There are eight segments in the two lobes of the left lung and ten segments in the three lobes of the right lung.

The vascular system of the lungs consists of the pulmonary arteries, which deliver blood to the lungs for oxygenation, and the pulmonary veins, which deliver oxygenated blood to the heart. Within the lungs, the pulmonary arteries branch into a pulmonary capillary network that surrounds the avleoli. Lung tissue receives its blood supply from the bronchial arteries and drains by the bronchial and pulmonary veins.

The Pleura

The pleura is a double-layered membrane that covers the lungs and the inside of the thoracic cavities. The *parietal pleura* lines the thoracic wall and mediastinum. It is continuous with the *visceral pleura,* which covers the external lung surfaces. The pleura produces pleural fluid, a lubricating, serous fluid that allows the lungs to move easily over the thoracic wall during breathing. The pleura's two layers also cling tightly together and hold the lungs to the thoracic wall. The structure of the pleura creates a slightly negative pressure in the pleural space (which is actually a potential rather than an actual space), necessary for lung function.

The Bronchi and Alveoli

The trachea divides into right and left primary bronchi. These main bronchi subdivide into the secondary (lobar) bronchi, then branch into the tertiary (segmental) bronchi, and then into smaller and smaller bronchioles, ending in the terminal bronchioles, which are extremely small. These branching passageways collectively are called the bronchial or respiratory tree. From the terminal bronchioles, air moves into air sacs (called respiratory bronchioles), which further branch into alveolar ducts that lead to alveolar sacs and then to the tiny alveoli. During inspiration, air enters the lungs through the primary bronchus and then moves through the increasingly smaller passageways of the lungs to the alveoli, where oxygen and carbon dioxide exchange occurs in the process of external respiration. During expiration, the carbon dioxide is expelled.

Alveoli cluster around the alveolar sacs, which open into a common chamber called the atrium. There are millions of alveoli in each lung, providing an enormous surface for gas exchange. Alveoli have extremely thin walls of a single layer of squamous epithelial cells over a very thin basement membrane. The external surface of the alveoli are covered with pulmonary capillaries. The alveolar and capillary walls form the respiratory membrane. Gas exchange across the respiratory membrane occurs by simple diffusion. The alveolar walls also contain cells that secrete a surfactant-containing fluid, necessary for maintaining a moist surface and reducing the surface tension of the alveolar fluid to help prevent collapse of the lungs.

The Rib Cage and Intercostal Muscles

The lungs are protected by the bones of the rib cage and the intercostal muscles. There are twelve pairs of ribs, which all articulate with the thoracic vertebrae. Anteriorly, the first seven ribs articulate with the body of the sternum. The eighth, ninth, and tenth ribs articulate with the cartilage immediately above the ribs. The eleventh and twelfth ribs are called floating ribs, because they are unattached.

The sternum has three parts: the manubrium, the body, and the xiphoid process. The junction between the manubrium and the body of the sternum is called the manubriosternal junction or the angle of Louis. The depression above the manubrium is called the suprasternal notch.

The spaces between the ribs are called the intercostal spaces. Each intercostal space is named for the rib immediately above it (e.g., the space between the third and fourth ribs is designated as the third intercostal space). The intercostal muscles between the ribs, along with the diaphragm, are called the inspiratory muscles.

Mechanics of Ventilation

Pulmonary ventilation depends on volume changes within the thoracic cavity. A change in the volume of air in the thoracic cavity leads to a change in the air pressure within the cavity. Because gases always flow along their pressure gradients, a change in pressure results in gases flowing into or out of the lungs to equalize the pressure.

The pressures normally present in the thoracic cavity are the intrapulmonary pressure and the intrapleural pressure. The intrapulmonary pressure, within the alveoli of the lungs, rises and falls constantly as a result of the acts of ventilation (inhalation and exhalation). The intrapleural pressure, within the pleural space, also rises and falls with the acts of ventilation, but it is always less than (or negative to) the intrapulmonary pressure. Intrapulmonary and intrapleural pressures are necessary not only to expand and contract the lungs, but also to prevent their collapse.

Pulmonary ventilation has two phases: inspiration, during which air flows into the lungs; and expiration, during which gases flow out of the lungs. The two phases make up a single breath, and normally occur from 12 to 20 times each minute. A single inspiration lasts for about 1 to 1.5 seconds, whereas an expiration lasts for about 2 to 3 seconds.

During inspiration, the diaphragm contracts and flattens out to increase the vertical diameter of the thoracic cavity. The external intercostal muscles contract, elevating the rib cage and moving the sternum forward to expand the lateral and anteroposterior diameter of the thoracic cavity, decreasing intrapleural pressure. The lungs stretch and the intrapulmonary volume increases, decreasing intrapulmonary pressure slightly below atmospheric pressure. Air rushes into the lungs, as a result of this pressure gradient, until the intrapulmonary and atmospheric pressures equalize.

Expiration is primarily a passive process that occurs as a result of the elasticity of the lungs. The inspiratory muscles relax, the diaphragm rises, the ribs descend, and the lungs recoil. Both the thoracic and intrapulmonary pressures increase, compressing the alveoli. The intrapulmonary pressure rises to a level greater than atmospheric pressure, and gases flow out of the lungs.

Factors Affecting Respiration

The rate and depth of respirations are controlled by respiratory centers in the medulla oblongata and pons of the brain and by chemoreceptors located in the medulla and in the carotid and aortic bodies. The centers and chemoreceptors respond to changes in the concentration of oxygen, carbon dioxide, and hydrogen ions in arterial blood. For example, when carbon dioxide concentration increases or the pH decreases, the respiratory rate increases.

In addition, respiratory passageway resistance, lung compliance, lung elasticity, and alveolar surface tension forces affect respiration.

- Respiratory passageway resistance is created by the friction encountered as gases move along the respiratory passageways, by constriction of the passageways (especially the larger bronchioles), by accumulations of mucus or infectious material, and by tumors. As resistance increases, gas flow decreases.

- Lung compliance is the distensibility of the lungs. It depends on the elasticity of the lung tissue and the flexibility of the rib cage. Compliance is decreased by factors that decrease the elasticity of the lungs, block the respiratory passageways, or interfere with movement of the rib cage.

- Lung elasticity is essential for lung distention during inspiration and lung recoil during expiration. Decreased elasticity from disease, such as emphysema, impairs respiration.

- A liquid film of mostly water covers the alveolar walls. At any gas-liquid boundary, the molecules of liquid are more strongly attracted to each other than to gas molecules. This produces a state of tension, called surface tension, that draws the liquid molecules even more closely together. The water content of the alveolar film compacts the alveoli and aids in the lungs' recoil during expiration. In fact, if the alveolar film were pure water, the alveoli would collapse between breaths. Surfactant, a lipoprotein produced by the alveolar cells, interferes with this adhesiveness of the water molecules, reducing surface tension, and helping expand the lungs. With insufficient surfactant, the surface tension forces can become great enough to collapse the alveoli between breaths, requiring tremendous energy to reinflate the lungs for inspiration.

Respiratory Volume and Capacity

Respiratory volume and capacity are affected by gender, age, weight, and health status.

- Tidal volume (TV) is the amount of air (approximately 500 mL) moved in and out of the lungs with each normal, quiet breath.

- Inspiratory reserve volume (IRV) is the amount of air (approximately 2100 to 3100 mL) that can be inhaled forcibly over the tidal volume.

- Expiratory reserve volume (ERV) is the approximately 1000 mL of air that can be forced out over the tidal volume.

- The residual volume is the volume of air (approximately 1100 mL) that remains in the lungs after a forced expiration.

- Vital capacity refers to the sum of TV + IRV + ERV and is approximately 4500 mL in the healthy client.

- About 150 mL of air never reaches the alveoli (the amount remaining in the passageways) and is called anatomical dead space volume.

Oxygen Transport and Unloading

Oxygen is carried in the blood either bound to hemoglobin or dissolved in the plasma. Oxygen is not very soluble in water, so almost all oxygen that enters the blood from the respiratory system is carried to the cells of the body by hemoglobin. This combination of hemoglobin and oxygen is called *oxyhemoglobin.*

Each hemoglobin molecule is made of four polypeptide chains, with each chain bound to an iron-containing heme group. The iron groups are the binding sites for oxygen; each hemoglobin molecule can bind with four molecules of oxygen.

Oxygen binding is rapid and reversible. It is affected by temperature, blood pH, partial pressure of oxygen (PO_2), partial pressure of carbon dioxide (PCO_2), and serum concentration of an organic chemical called 2,3-DPG. These factors interact to ensure adequate delivery of oxygen to the cells.

The relative saturation of hemoglobin depends on the PO_2 of the blood, as illustrated in the oxygen-hemoglobin dissociation curve.

- Under normal conditions, the hemoglobin in arterial blood is 97.4% saturated with oxygen. Hemoglobin is almost fully saturated at a PO_2 of 70 mmHg. As arterial blood flows through the capillaries, oxygen is unloaded, so that the oxygen saturation of hemoglobin in venous blood is 75%.

- The affinity of oxygen and hemoglobin decreases as the temperature of body tissues increases above normal. As a result, less oxygen binds with hemoglobin, and oxygen unloading is enhanced. Conversely, as the body is chilled, oxygen unloading is inhibited.

- The oxygen-hemoglobin bond is weakened by increased hydrogen ion concentrations. As blood becomes more acidotic, oxygen unloading to the tissues is enhanced. The same process occurs when the partial pressure of carbon dioxide increases because this decreases the pH.

- The organic chemical 2,3-DPG is formed in red blood cells and enhances the release of oxygen from hemoglobin by binding to it during times of increased metabolism (as when body temperature increases). This binding alters the structure of hemoglobin to facilitate oxygen unloading.

Carbon Dioxide Transport

Active cells produce about 200 mL of carbon dioxide each minute; this amount is exactly the same as that excreted by the lungs each minute. Excretion of carbon dioxide from the body requires transport by the blood from the cells to the lungs. Carbon dioxide is transported in three forms: dissolved in plasma, bound to hemoglobin, and as bicarbonate ions in the plasma (the largest amount is in this form).

The amount of carbon dioxide transported in the blood is strongly influenced by the oxygenation of the blood. When the Po_2 decreases, with a corresponding decrease in oxygen saturation, increased amounts of carbon dioxide can be carried in the blood. Carbon dioxide entering the systemic circulation from the cells causes more oxygen to dissociate from hemoglobin, in turn allowing more carbon dioxide to combine with hemoglobin and more bicarbonate ions to be generated. This situation is reversed in the pulmonary circulation, where the uptake of oxygen facilitates the release of carbon dioxide.

Assessing Respiratory Function

The nurse assesses the respiratory system both during a health assessment interview to collect subjective data and a physical assessment to collect objective data.

The Health Assessment Interview

This section provides guidelines for collecting subjective data through a health assessment interview specific to the function of the respiratory system. A health assessment interview to determine problems of the respiratory system may be done as part of a health screening or as part of a total health assessment. Alternatively, the interview may focus on a chief complaint, such as difficulty breathing. If the client has a problem of any part of the respiratory system, analyze its onset, characteristics and course, severity, precipitating and relieving factors, and any associated symptoms, noting the timing and circumstances. For example, you may ask the client the following:

- What problems are you having with your breathing? Is your breathing more difficult if you lie flat? Is it painful to breathe in or out?
- When did you first notice that your cough was becoming a problem? Do you cough up mucus? What color is the mucus?
- Have you had nosebleeds in the past?

During the interview, carefully observe the client for difficulty in breathing, pausing to breathe in the middle of a sentence, hoarseness, changes in voice quality, and cough. Ask about present health status, medical history, family health history, and risk factors for illness. These areas of the client's health status include information about the nose, throat, and lungs.

To determine present health status, ask about pain in the nose, throat, or chest. Information about cough includes what type of cough, when it occurs, and how it is relieved. The client should describe any sputum associated with the cough. Is the client experiencing any dyspnea (difficult or labored breathing)? How is the dyspnea associated with activity levels and time of day? Is the client having chest pain? How is this related to activity and time of day? Note the severity, type, and location of the pain. Explore problems with swallowing, smelling, or taste. Also ask about nosebleeds and nasal or sinus stuffiness or pain, and about current medication use, aerosols or inhalants, and oxygen use.

Document past medical history by asking questions about a history of allergies, asthma, bronchitis, emphysema, pneumonia, tuberculosis, or congestive heart failure. Other questions include a history of surgery or trauma to the respiratory structures and a history of other chronic illnesses, such as cancer, kidney disease, and heart disease. If the client has a health problem involving the respiratory system, ask about medications used to relieve nasal congestion, cough, dyspnea, or chest pain. Document a family history of allergies, tuberculosis, emphysema, and cancer.

The client's personal lifestyle, environment, and occupation may provide clues to risk factors for actual or potential health problems. Question the client about a history of smoking and/or exposure to environmental chemicals (including smog), dust, vapors, animals, coal dust, asbestos, fumes, or pollens. Other risk factors include a sedentary lifestyle and obesity. Also ask the client about use of alcohol and substances that are injected, such as heroin, or inhaled, such as cocaine or marijuana.

Physical Assessment

Physical assessment of the respiratory system may be performed as part of a total assessment, or alone for a client with known or suspected problems. Assess the respiratory system through inspection, palpation, percussion, and auscultation of the nose, throat, thorax, and lungs. In addition, note the client's level of consciousness and assess the color of the lips, nail beds, nose, ears, and tongue for signs of respiratory distress.

The equipment needed to assess the respiratory system includes a tongue blade, penlight, nasal speculum, metric ruler, marking pen, and stethoscope with diaphragm. The room should be warm and well lighted. Ask the client to remove all clothing above the waist; give female clients a gown to wear during the examination. Conduct the examination with the client in the sitting position. Prior to the examination, collect all necessary equipment and explain the techniques to the client to decrease anxiety.

The three different types of normal breath sounds are vesicular, bronchovesicular, and bronchial. Assessment of these sounds is discussed in Table 13-1.

Nasal Assessment with Abnormal Findings (✓)

- Inspect the nose for changes in size, shape, or color.
    - ✓ The nose may be asymmetrical as a result of previous surgery or trauma.
    - ✓ The skin around the nostrils may be red and swollen in allergies.
- Inspect the nasal cavity. Use an otoscope with a broad, short speculum. Gently insert the speculum into each of the nares and assess the condition of the mucous membranes and the turbinates.
    - ✓ The septum may be deviated.
    - ✓ Perforation of the septum may occur with chronic cocaine abuse.

✓ Red mucosa indicates infection.

✓ Purulent drainage indicates nasal or sinus infection.

✓ Allergies may be indicated by watery nasal drainage, pale turbinates, and polyps on the turbinates.

• Assess ability to smell. Ask the client to breathe through one nostril while pressing the other one closed. Ask the client to close his or her eyes. Place a substance with an aromatic odor under the client's nose (use ground coffee or alcohol) and ask the client to identify the odor. Test each nostril separately. This test is usually done only if the client has problems with the sense of smell.

Table 13-1. Normal Breath Sounds

Type of Breath Sound	Characteristics
Vesicular	• Soft, low-pitched, gentle sounds • Heard over all areas of the lungs except the major bronchi • Have a 3:1 ratio for inspiration and expiration, with inspiration lasting longer than expiration
Bronchovesicular	• Medium pitch and intensity of sounds • Have a 1:1 ratio, with inspiration and expiration being equal in duration • Heard anteriorly over the primary bronchus on each side of the sternum, and posteriorly between the scapulae
Bronchial	• Loud, high-pitched sounds • Gap between inspiration and expiration • Have a 2:3 ratio for inspiration and expiration, with expiration longer than inspiration • Heard over the manubrium

---

✓ Changes in the ability to smell may be the result of damage to the olfactory nerve or to chronic inflammation of the nose.

✓ Zinc deficiency may also cause a loss of the sense of smell.

Thoracic Assessment with Abnormal Findings (✓)

• Assess respiratory rate.

✓ **Tachypnea** (rapid respiratory rate) is seen in **atelectasis** (collapse of lung tissue following obstruction of the bronchus or bronchioles), pneumonia, asthma, pleural effusion, pneumothorax, and congestive heart failure.

✓ Damage to the brainstem from a stroke or head injury may result in either tachypnea or **bradypnea** (low respiratory rate).

✓ Bradypnea is seen with some circulatory disorders, lung disorders, as a side effect of some medications, and as a response to pain.

✓ **Apnea,** cessation of breathing lasting from a few seconds to a few minutes, may occur following a stroke or head trauma, as a side effect of some medications, or following airway obstruction.

- Inspect the anteroposterior diameter of the chest. The anteroposterior diameter of the chest should be less than the transverse diameter. Normal ratios vary from 1:2 to 5:7.

  ✓ The anteroposterior diameter is equal to the transverse diameter in barrel chest, which typically occurs with emphysema.

- Inspect for intercostal retraction.

  ✓ Retraction of intercostal spaces may be seen in asthma.

  ✓ Bulging of intercostal spaces may be seen in pneumothorax.

- Inspect and palpate for chest expansion. Place your hands with the fingers spread apart palm down on the client's posterolateral chest. Gently press the skin between your thumbs. Ask the client to breathe deeply. As the client inhales, watch your hands for symmetry of movement.

  ✓ Thoracic expansion is decreased on the affected side in atelectasis, pneumonia, pneumothorax, and pleural effusion.

  ✓ Bilateral chest expansion is decreased in emphysema.

- Gently palpate the location and position of the trachea.

  ✓ The trachea shifts to the unaffected side in pleural effusion and pneumothorax and shifts to the affected side in atelectasis.

- Palpate for tactile fremitus. Ask the client to say "ninety-nine" as you palpate at three different levels for a vibratory sensation called tactile fremitus, which occurs as sound waves from the larynx travel through patent bronchi and lungs to the chest wall.

  ✓ Tactile fremitus is decreased in atelectasis, emphysema, asthma, pleural effusion, and pneumothorax. It is increased in pneumonia if the bronchus is patent.

- Percuss the lungs for dullness over shoulder apices and over anterior, posterior, and lateral intercostal spaces.

  ✓ Dullness is heard in clients with atelectasis, lobar pneumonia, and pleural effusion.

  ✓ Hyperresonance is heard in those with chronic asthma and pneumothorax.

- Percuss the posterior chest for diaphragmatic excursion.

Systematic percussion of the posterior chest from a level of lung resonance to the level of diaphragmatic dullness reveals diaphragmatic excursion, a measurement of the level of the diaphragm. First percuss downward over the posterior thorax while the client exhales fully and holds the breath. Mark the spot at which the sound changes from resonant to dull. Then ask the client to inhale and hold the breath while you percuss downward again to note the descent of the diaphragm. Again mark the spot where the sound changes. Measure the difference, which normally varies from about 3 to 5 cm.

  ✓ Diaphragmatic excursion is decreased in emphysema, on the affected side in pleural effusion, and in pneumothorax.

  ✓ A high level of dullness or a lack of excursion may indicate atelectasis or pleural effusion.

Breath Sound Assessment with Abnormal Findings (✓)

* Auscultate the lungs for breath sounds with the diaphragm of the stethoscope by having the client take slow deep breaths through the mouth. Listen over anterior, posterior, and lateral intercostal spaces.

  ✓ Bronchial breath sounds (expiration > inspiration) and bronchovesicular breath sounds (inspiration = expiration) are heard over lungs filled with fluid or solid tissue.

  ✓ Breath sounds are decreased over atelectasis, emphysema, asthma, pleural effusion, and pneumothorax.

  ✓ Breath sounds are increased over lobar pneumonia.

  ✓ Breath sounds are absent over collapsed lung, pleural effusion, and primary bronchus obstruction.

* Auscultate for crackles, wheezes, and friction rubs. If crackles or wheezes are heard, ask the client to cough and note if adventitious sound is cleared.

  ✓ Crackles (short, discrete, crackling or bubbling sounds) may be noted in pneumonia, bronchitis, and congestive heart failure.

  ✓ Wheezes (continuous, musical sounds) may be heard in clients with bronchitis, emphysema, and asthma.

  ✓ A friction rub is a loud, dry, creaking sound that indicates pleural inflammation.

* Auscultate voice sounds where any abnormal breath sound is noted by having client say "ninety-nine" (bronchophony); whisper "one, two, three" (whispered pectoriloquy); and say "ee" (egophony). Normally, these sounds are heard by the examiner, but are muffled.

  ✓ Voice sounds are decreased or absent over areas of atelectasis, asthma, pleural effusion, and pneumothorax.

  ✓ Voice sounds are increased and clearer over lobar pneumonia.

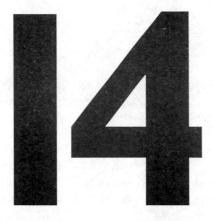

Nursing Care of Clients with Upper Respiratory Disorders

Upper respiratory disorders may affect the nose, paranasal sinuses, tonsils, adenoids, larynx, and pharynx. See Chapter 13 to review the anatomy and physiology of these structures, as well as their assessment. Upper respiratory disorders may be very minor, such as the common cold. However, a patent upper airway is necessary for effective breathing. Acute and even life-threatening problems develop when upper airway patency is affected (e.g., by laryngeal edema). Upper respiratory disorders can affect breathing, communication, and body image. When breathing is compromised because of swelling, bleeding, or accumulation of secretions, fear and anxiety develop.

Nursing care focuses on maintaining the airway, managing pain and symptoms, promoting effective communication, and providing psychologic support for the client and family.

Infectious or Inflammatory Disorders

Constant exposure of the upper respiratory tract to the environment makes it vulnerable to a variety of infectious and inflammatory conditions. Although most upper respiratory infections and inflammations are minor, complications may result. In the frail older adult, the risk of serious problems following an upper respiratory infection can be significant.

Rhinitis, inflammation of the nasal cavities, is the most common upper respiratory disorder. Rhinitis may be either acute or chronic. *Acute viral rhinitis,* or the common cold, is discussed below. Chronic rhinitis includes allergic, vasomotor, and atrophic rhinitis. *Allergic rhinitis,* or hay fever, results from a sensitivity reaction to allergens such as plant pollens. It tends to occur seasonally. The etiology of *vasomotor rhinitis* is unknown. Although its manifestations are similar to those of allergic rhinitis, it is not linked to allergens. *Atrophic rhinitis* is characterized by changes in the mucous membrane of the nasal cavities.

The Client with Viral Upper Respiratory Infection

Viral upper respiratory infections (URIs or the common cold) are the most common respiratory tract infections and are among the most common human diseases. URIs are highly contagious and are prevalent in schools and work environments. The incidence of acute URI peaks during September and late January, coinciding with the opening of schools, as well as toward the end of April. Most adults experience two to four colds each year (Porth, 2002).

Pathophysiology

More than 200 strains of virus cause URI, including rhinoviruses, adenoviruses, parainfluenza viruses, coronaviruses, and respiratory syncytial virus. Occasionally, more than one virus may be present. Viruses causing acute URI spread by aerosolized droplet nuclei during sneezing or coughing or by direct contact. The virus usually spreads when the hands and fingers pick it up from contaminated surfaces and carry it to the eyes and mucous membranes of the susceptible host. Infected clients are highly contagious, shedding virus for a few days prior to and after the appearance of symptoms. Although immunity is produced to the individual virus strain, the number of viruses causing URI ensures that most people continue to experience colds throughout their lifetime.

Viscous mucus secretions in the upper respiratory tract trap invading organisms, preventing contamination of more vulnerable areas. Cells of the upper respiratory tract are infected when the virus attaches to receptors on the cell. Local immunologic defenses, such as secretory IgA antibodies in respiratory secretions, then attempt to inactivate the antigen, producing a local inflammatory response. The mucous membranes of the nasal passages swell and become hyperemic and engorged. Mucus- secreting glands become hyperactive. These responses to the virus produce the typical manifestations of viral URI.

Manifestations

Acute viral upper respiratory infection often presents as the common cold. Nasal mucous membranes appear red (*erythematous*) and *boggy* (swollen). Swollen mucous membranes, local vasodilation, and secretions cause nasal congestion. Clear, watery secretions lead to **coryza** or *rhinorrhea,* profuse nasal discharge. Sneezing and coughing are common. Sore throat is common, and may be the initial symptom. Systemic manifestations of acute viral URI may include low-grade fever, headache, malaise, and muscle aches. Symptoms generally last for a few days up to two weeks. Although acute viral URI is typically mild and self-limited, its effects on the immune defenses of the upper respiratory tract can increase the risk for more serious bacterial infections, such as sinusitis or otitis media.

Collaborative Care

Because most acute viral upper respiratory infections are self-limiting, self-care is appropriate and encouraged. Medical treatment is usually required only when complications, such as sinusitis or otitis media develop.

Diagnosis of acute viral URI is usually based on the history and physical examination. Diagnostic testing may be indicated if a complication, such as bacterial infection, is suspected. A white blood count (WBC) may be ordered to assess for leukocytosis (an elevated WBC). Cultures of purulent discharge may also be obtained.

Treatment is symptomatic. Adequate rest, maintaining fluid intake, and avoiding chills help relieve systemic symptoms, such as fever, malaise, and muscle ache. Instruct clients to cover the mouth and nose with tissue when coughing or sneezing, and to dispose of soiled tissues properly. Additionally, avoiding crowds helps prevent spread of the infection to others.

Medications

Medications may be recommended to shorten the duration of the illness and relieve symptoms. Mild decongestants or over-the-counter antihistamines may help relieve coryza and nasal congestion. Warm saltwater gargles, throat lozenges, or mild analgesics may be used for sore throat. Although no specific antiviral therapy has been shown to be effective, experimental vaccines to prevent acute viral URI are in developmental stages.

Complementary Therapies

Complementary therapies are appropriate for treating most acute viral URI. Herbal remedies, such as Echinacea and garlic, have antiviral and antibiotic effects. Taken at the first sign of infection, Echinacea may reduce the duration and symptoms. The recommended dose of Echinacea varies, depending on the part of the plant used in the preparation. It should not be used for longer than two weeks. It is contraindicated for use during pregnancy and lactation, and in people who have an autoimmune disease such as rheumatoid arthritis.

Aromatherapy with essential oils, such as basil, cedarwood, eucalyptus, frankincense, lavender, marjoram, peppermint, or rosemary, can reduce congestion, and promote comfort and recovery. Teach clients that these essential oils are to be used only for inhalation, not for internal consumption.

Nursing Care

Health Promotion

Clients can limit their incidence of acute viral URI by frequent handwashing and avoiding exposure to crowds. Maintaining good general health and stress-reducing activities support the immune system and help prevent acute viral URI. Teach the client that going out in the rain or cold weather does not cause colds, and that URI are more likely to occur during periods of physical or psychologic stress.

Home Care

The primary nursing role in caring for clients with acute viral URI is educational. Self-care is appropriate for most clients, unless the problem is recurrent or a complication occurs. Acute viral URI may interfere with work and recreational activities. Unless limited by symptoms, normal daily activities and roles usually can be maintained. Additional rest during the acute phase of illness is recommended. Additional fluid intake and a well-balanced diet help support the immune response, hastening recovery.

Include the following topics in teaching clients about home care:

- Using disposable tissues to cover the mouth and nose while coughing or sneezing to reduce airborne spread of the virus.
- Blowing the nose with both nostrils open to prevent infected matter from being forced into the eustachian tubes.
- Washing hands frequently, especially after coughing or sneezing, to limit viral transmission.
- Using over-the-counter preparations for symptomatic relief; precautions related to the sedating effects of antihistamines.
- Limiting use of nasal decongestants to every four hours for only a few days at a time to prevent rebound effect.

The Client with Influenza

Influenza, or *flu,* is a highly contagious viral respiratory disease characterized by coryza, fever, cough, and systemic symptoms, such as headache and malaise. Influenza usually occurs in epidemics or pandemics, although sporadic cases do occur. Localized outbreaks of influenza usually occur about every one to three years. Global epidemics (pandemics) are less frequent, developing every 10 to 15 years until the past two decades. Although influenza tends to be mild and self-limited in healthy adults, older adults and people with chronic heart or pulmonary disease have a high incidence of complications, such as pneumonia, and a higher risk for mortality related to the disease and its complications (Braunwald, et al., 2001).

Pathophysiology

Influenza virus is transmitted by airborne droplet and direct contact. Three major strains of the virus have been identified as influenza A virus, influenza B virus, and influenza C virus. Influenza A is responsible for most infections and the most severe outbreaks of influenza. This is primarily due to its ability to alter its surface antigens, bypassing previously developed immune defenses to the virus. New strains of influenza virus are named according to the strain, geographic origin, and year (e.g., A/Taiwan/89). Outbreaks of influenza B virus are generally less extensive and less severe than those caused by influenza A virus. Illness associated with influenza C virus is mild and often goes unrecognized.

The incubation period for influenza is short, only 18 to 72 hours. The virus infects the respiratory epithelium. It rapidly replicates in infected cells, and is released to infect neighboring cells. Inflammation leads to necrosis and shedding of serous and ciliated cells of the respiratory tract. This allows extracellular fluid to escape, producing rhinorrhea. With recovery, serous cells are replaced more rapidly than ciliated cells, leading to continued cough and coryza. Systemic manifestations of influenza are likely caused by release of inflammatory mediators such as tumor necrosis factor α and interleukin 6 (Braunwald, et al., 2001).

The respiratory epithelial necrosis caused by influenza increases the risk for secondary bacterial infections. Sinusitis and otitis media are frequent complications of influenza. Tracheobronchitis, inflammation of the trachea and bronchi, may develop. While tracheobronchitis is not a serious health risk, its manifestations may persist for up to three weeks.

Influenza is clearly linked to an increased risk for pneumonia, particularly in older adults. Changes in respiratory function associated with aging, including decreased effectiveness of cough and increased residual lung volume, pose little risk in the healthy older adult, but greatly increase the risk for pneumonia associated with influenza. Viral pneumonia is a serious complication that may be fatal. It typically develops within 48 hours of the onset of influenza, often in clients with preexisting heart valve or pulmonary disease. Influenza pneumonia progresses rapidly and can cause hypoxemia and death within a few days. Bacterial pneumonia is more likely to occur in older at-risk adults, but also may affect otherwise healthy adults. It usually presents as a relapse of influenza, with a productive cough and evidence of pneumonia on the chest X-ray. See Chapter 15 for more information about pneumonia.

Reye's syndrome is a rare, but potentially fatal, complication of influenza. Although it is more likely to affect children, it has also been identified in older adults. It is most often associated with influenza B virus. Reye's syndrome develops within two to three weeks after the onset of influenza. It has a 30% mortality rate. Hepatic failure and encephalopathy develop rapidly in clients with Reye's syndrome.

Manifestations

Infection with influenza virus produces one of three syndromes: uncomplicated nasopharyngeal inflammation, viral upper respiratory infection followed by bacterial infection, or viral pneumonia. The onset is rapid; profound malaise may develop in a matter of minutes.

Manifestations of influenza include abrupt onset of chills and fever, malaise, muscle aches, and headache. Respiratory manifestations include dry, nonproductive cough, sore throat, substernal burning, and coryza. Acute symptoms subside within two to three days, although fever may last as long as a week. The cough may be severe and productive. Along with fatigue and weakness, the cough can persist for days or several weeks.

Collaborative Care

Preventing influenza by immunizing at-risk populations is an important aspect of care. Immunization with polyvalent (containing antigens of several viral strains) influenza virus vaccine is about 85% effective in preventing influenza infection for several months to a year (Tierney, et al., 2001). Annual immunization is recommended for at-risk clients, including people over the age of 65; residents of nursing homes; adults and children with chronic cardiopulmonary disorders (e.g., asthma) or chronic metabolic diseases, such as diabetes; and health care workers who have frequent contact with high-risk clients. Additionally, family members of at-risk clients should be vaccinated to reduce the client's risk of exposure. The vaccine is given in the fall, prior to the annual winter outbreak. Medical treatment of influenza focuses on establishing the diagnosis, providing symptomatic relief, and preventing complications.

Diagnostic Tests

The diagnosis of influenza is based on history, clinical findings, and knowledge of an influenza outbreak in the community. A chest X-ray and white blood cell (WBC) count may be done to rule out complications, such as pneumonia. The WBC is commonly decreased in influenza; bacterial infections usually cause increased WBCs.

Medications

Yearly immunization with influenza vaccine is the single most important measure to prevent or minimize symptoms of influenza. Although the vaccine is readily available and inexpensive, only about 30% of at-risk clients are vaccinated each year. Many may fear a reaction from the vaccine, although the vaccines are highly purified and reactions are rare. About 5% of people experience mild symptoms of low-grade fever, malaise, or myalgia for up to 24 hours after vaccination. Because the vaccine is produced in eggs, it should not be given to people who are allergic to egg protein. Serious adverse reactions to influenza vaccine are rare. *Guillain-Barré syndrome,* an acute neurologic disorder characterized by muscle weakness and distal sensory loss, has been associated with certain batches of vaccine.

Amantadine (Symmetrel) or rimantadine (Flumadine) may be used for prophylaxis in unvaccinated people who are exposed to the virus. If the drug is given before, or within 48 hours, of exposure, it inhibits viral shedding and prevents or decreases the symptoms of influenza. If possible, unvaccinated people should receive the vaccine along with the antiviral drug. The drug is continued for several weeks, or for the duration of the influenza outbreak.

Amantadine, rimantadine, and the antiviral drugs zanamivir (Relenza), oseltamivir (Tamiflu), and ribavirin (Virazole) also may be used to reduce the duration and severity of flu symptoms. Both zanamivir and ribavirin are administered by inhalation; the other drugs are given orally. See Chapter 8 for nursing implications for antiviral drugs.

Over-the-counter analgesics, such as aspirin, acetaminophen, or NSAIDs provide symptomatic relief of fever and muscle ache. Antitussives may decrease cough, promoting rest. Antibiotics are not indicated unless secondary bacterial infection occurs.

Nursing Care

Health Promotion
Stress the importance of yearly influenza vaccination for clients in high-risk groups and their families. Teach about spread of the disease, including measures to reduce the risk of contracting influenza, such as avoiding crowds and people who are ill.

Assessment
Unless there is a known outbreak of influenza in the community, it can be difficult to differentiate the manifestations of influenza from those of other URI.

*   *Health history:* known exposure to virus; current symptoms, their onset and duration; presence of dyspnea, chest pain, productive cough, facial pain or pressure in sinus areas; current medications, history of influenza vaccine; chronic diseases such as heart disease, chronic obstructive pulmonary disease (COPD), or diabetes; known medication allergies.
*   *Physical examination:* general appearance; vital signs including temperature; skin color; lung sounds; abdominal exam.

Nursing Diagnoses and Interventions
Although the symptoms of influenza are distressing, most people with the illness provide self-care and do not contact a health care provider. Recommendations to rest in bed during the acute phase of the illness, and limit activities until recovery, are appropriate for influenza.

Severe disease or complications of influenza may necessitate hospitalization for respiratory support and management. For these clients, nursing care focuses on maintaining airway clearance, breathing patterns, and adequate rest.

Ineffective Breathing Pattern
Muscle aches, malaise, and elevated temperature may increase the respiratory rate and alter the depth of respirations, decreasing effective alveolar ventilation. Shallow respirations also increase the risk of *atelectasis,* lack of ventilation in an area of lung.

*   Pace activities to provide for periods of rest. *Tachypnea increases the work of breathing, causing fatigue; fatigue, in turn, can further impair ventilation and reduce the effectiveness of coughing.*

- Elevate the head of the bed. *The upright position improves lung excursion and reduces the work of breathing by lowering the diaphragm, moving abdominal contents downward, creating less resistance to diaphragmatic excursion, and slightly decreasing venous return.*

Ineffective Airway Clearance

Swelling and congestion of mucous membranes, extracellular fluid exudate, and impaired ciliary action due to cell damage increase the risk of impaired airway clearance in influenza. The older adult is at particular risk because of normally reduced ciliary activity and increased lung compliance.

- Maintain adequate hydration. Assess mucous membranes and skin turgor for evidence of dehydration. *Fever and decreased oral fluid intake may lead to dehydration and increased viscosity of secretions. Thick, viscous secretions are more difficult to expectorate.*
- Increase the humidity of inspired air with a bedside humidifier. *Increasing the water content of inhaled air helps loosen thick secretions and soothe mucous membranes.*
- Teach effective cough techniques. Administer analgesics as ordered. *The Huff Cough is effective to maintain open airways and spares energy (see Chapter 36 for client teaching of this technique). Relieving muscle ache increases the ability to cough effectively.*

Disturbed Sleep Pattern

Airway congestion, malaise, muscle aches, and persistent cough may interfere with the ability to rest, increasing fatigue and prolonging recovery.

- Assess sleep patterns using subjective and objective information. *The client may appear to be sleeping but not achieving normal sleep patterns because of influenza symptoms. Both subjective and objective data are important to accurately assess sleep.*
- Provide antipyretic and analgesic medications at, or shortly before, bedtime. *These drugs promote comfort by reducing fever and relieving muscle aches.*

Home Care

Encourage appropriate self-care for clients with influenza. Discuss the following topics related to home care:

- Increase rest during the acute, febrile phase of the illness.
- Maintain a liberal fluid intake, even if anorexic.
- Appropriately use over-the-counter medications for symptom relief.
- Employ hygiene measures, such as using disposable tissues and frequent handwashing, to reduce spread of the disease.
- Know manifestations of potential complications of influenza to report to the primary care provider.

The Client with Laryngeal Obstruction or Trauma

The larynx is the narrowest portion of the upper airway. As such, it is at risk for obstruction. Laryngeal obstruction is a life-threatening emergency. Blows to the neck or other traumatic injuries may damage the larynx, interfering with its patency and function.

Pathophysiology and Manifestations

Laryngeal Obstruction

The larynx may be partially or fully obstructed by aspirated food or foreign objects, or by laryngospasm or edema due to inflammation, injury, or anaphylaxis. Anything that occludes the larynx can obstruct the airway. The most common cause of obstruction in adults is ingested meat that lodges in the airway (the so-called *café coronary*). Risk factors for food aspiration include ingesting large boluses of food and chewing them insufficiently, consuming excess alcohol, and wearing dentures. A foreign body in the larynx causes pain, laryngospasm, dyspnea, and inspiratory stridor. Aspirated foreign bodies may pass through the larynx into the trachea and lungs, causing pneumonitis.

Laryngospasm occurs due to repeated or traumatic intubation attempts, chemical irritation, or hypocalcemia. An acute type I hypersensitivity response may cause anaphylaxis with release of inflammatory mediators leading to angioedema of upper airways and severe laryngeal edema.

The most common manifestations of laryngeal obstruction are coughing, choking, gagging, obvious difficulty breathing with use of accessory muscles, and inspiratory stridor. As the airway is obstructed, signs of asphyxia become apparent. Respirations are labored and noisy with wheezing and stridor. Cyanosis may develop. Respiratory arrest and death may result without prompt treatment.

Laryngeal Trauma

Trauma to the larynx can occur in motor vehicle crashes or assaults (e.g., blows to the neck or attempted strangulation). The larynx may also be traumatized during endotracheal intubation or tracheotomy. Trauma may fracture thyroid and/or cricoid cartilage, resulting in loss of airway patency. Soft-tissue injuries can cause swelling that further impairs the airway. Manifestations of laryngeal trauma may include subcutaneous emphysema or crepitus, voice change, dysphagia and pain with swallowing, inspiratory stridor, hemoptysis, and cough.

Collaborative Care

The treatment goal is to maintain an open airway. If airway obstruction is partial, and the client is able to cough and move air in and out of the lungs, radiologic and laryngoscopic examination may be done to locate the foreign body. An endotracheal tube may be inserted to maintain airflow through the larynx in spasm or an edematous larynx. For anaphylaxis, epinephrine may be administered to reduce laryngeal edema and relieve obstruction.

When airway obstruction is complete, the Heimlich maneuver is performed immediately to clear the obstruction. For the conscious person, the rescuer wraps his or her arms around the victim from behind, places one fist between the umbilicus and xiphoid process, covers the fist with the other hand and forcefully thrusts the hands upward. For the unconscious victim, the rescuer straddles the victim's thighs and delivers thrusts upward and inward on the upper abdomen. These moves are continued until the obstruction is relieved or more definitive care can be given. Endotracheal intubation may be attempted. If intubation is unsuccessful, an immediate cricothyrotomy or tracheotomy must be performed to open the airway.

CT scan is used to identify laryngeal fractures; however, emergency treatment may be required prior to diagnosis to ensure airway patency and preserve life. Soft-tissue injuries may be managed conservatively with bedside humidifier, intravenous fluids, antibiotics, and corticosteroids to reduce edema. More severe injuries require endotracheal intubation or immediate tracheostomy.

Nursing Care

Closely monitor clients at risk for laryngeal obstruction (e.g., following neck trauma, newly extubated clients, and people receiving medications with a high risk of anaphylaxis, such as intravenous antibiotics or radiologic dyes) for manifestations of obstruction, including dyspnea, nasal flaring, tachypnea, anxiety, wheezing, and stridor. Suction the airway as needed; small aspirated foreign bodies might possibly be removed by suctioning. If obstruction is complete, initiate a cardiopulmonary arrest procedure and perform the Heimlich maneuver until the obstruction is relieved or the emergency response team arrives. Prepare to assist with emergency intubation or tracheotomy as needed. Provide emotional support, reassurance, and teaching for the client and family to reduce anxiety.

Health promotion and teaching for home care focus on preventing laryngeal obstruction and early intervention techniques. Everyone should be aware of the risk factors for adult aspiration. Caution clients who wear dentures to take small bites, chewing each bite carefully before swallowing. Discuss the relationship between excessive alcohol intake and food aspiration. Participate in promoting training of the general public in CPR and the Heimlich maneuver. The more people who are adequately trained in emergency procedures, the more likely it is that emergency procedures will be initiated in a timely manner. Clients with a known risk for anaphylaxis, such as people with a previous anaphylactic response and those allergic to bee venom, should wear a MedicAlert tag and carry a bee-sting kit to allow early intervention to prevent severe laryngeal edema and spasm.

The Client with Obstructive Sleep Apnea

Sleep apnea, intermittent absence of airflow through the mouth and nose during sleep, is a serious and potentially life-threatening disorder. It affects at least 2% of middle-aged women and 4% of middle-aged men. Sleep apnea is a leading cause of excessive daytime sleepiness, and may contribute to other problems, such as poor work performance and motor vehicle crashes (Braunwald, et al., 2001; McCance & Huether, 2002).

Types of sleep apnea include obstructive and central. In *obstructive sleep apnea,* the more common type, the respiratory drive remains intact, but airflow ceases due to occlusion of the oropharyngeal airway. *Central sleep apnea* is a neurologic disorder that involves transient impairment of the neurologic drive to respiratory muscles.

In addition to male gender, risk factors for obstructive sleep apnea include increasing age and obesity. Large neck circumference (>17 inches in men and >16 inches in women) is also a known risk factor for obstructive sleep apnea (Porth, 2002). Use of alcohol and other central nervous system depressants may contribute to sleep apnea.

Pathophysiology

During sleep, skeletal muscle tone decreases (except the diaphragm). The most significant decrease occurs during rapid eye movement (REM) sleep (Porth, 2002). Loss of normal pharyngeal muscle tone permits the pharynx to collapse during inspiration as pressure within the airways becomes negative in relation to atmospheric pressure. The tongue is also pulled against the posterior pharyngeal wall by gravity during sleep, causing further obstruction. Obesity or skeletal or soft-tissue changes that decrease inspiratory tone, such as a relatively large tongue in a relatively small oropharynx, contribute to the problem. Airflow obstruction causes the oxygen saturation, PO_2, and pH to fall, and the PCO_2 to rise. This progressive asphyxia causes brief arousal from sleep, which restores airway patency and airflow. Sleep can be severely fragmented as these episodes may occur hundreds of times each night.

Recurrent episodes of apnea and arousal during sleep have secondary physiologic effects. Sleep fragmentation and loss of slow-wave sleep are thought to contribute to neurologic and behavior problems, such as excessive daytime sleepiness, impaired intellect, memory loss, and personality changes. Recurrent nocturnal asphyxia and negative intrathoracic pressure due to airway obstruction increase the workload of the heart. People with coronary heart disease may develop myocardial ischemia and angina. Dysrhythmias, such as significant bradycardia and dangerous tachydysrhythmias, may develop. Left ventricular function may be impaired and heart failure may occur. Systemic blood pressure remains high during sleep and may contribute to systemic hypertension that affects more than 50% of people with obstructive sleep apnea (Braunwald, et al., 2001). Pulmonary hypertension may also develop. Sudden cardiac death is believed to be a potential fatal complication of obstructive sleep apnea.

Manifestations

Narrowed upper airways produce loud snoring during sleep, often years before obstructive sleep apnea occurs. Excessive daytime sleepiness, headache, irritability, and restless sleep also are common manifestations.

Collaborative Care

The goal of care for obstructive sleep apnea is to restore airflow and prevent the adverse effects of the disorder. Sustained weight loss may cure obstructive sleep apnea.

Diagnostic Tests

The diagnosis of obstructive sleep apnea is based on *polysomnography,* an overnight sleep study. Several variables are recorded during the study, including:

- Electroencephalogram and measurements of ocular activity and muscle tone
- Recordings of ventilatory activity and airflow
- Continuous arterial oxygen saturation readings
- Heart rate.

Transcutaneous arterial PCO_2 readings may also be monitored during the study. Because sleep studies are time consuming and expensive, overnight monitoring of oxygen saturation by pulse oximetry may be used to confirm the diagnosis of sleep apnea when symptoms indicate a high probability of the disorder (Braunwald, et al., 2001).

Treatments

Mild to moderate obstructive sleep apnea may be treated by weight reduction, alcohol abstinence, improving nasal patency, and avoiding the supine position for sleep. Although weight reduction often cures the disorder, maintaining optimal weight is difficult. Oral appliances designed to keep the mandible and tongue forward may also be prescribed.

Nasal continuous positive airway pressure (CPAP) is the treatment of choice for obstructive sleep apnea. Positive pressure generated by an air compressor and administered through a tight-fitting nasal mask splints the pharyngeal airway, preventing collapse and obstruction. With proper training, this device is well tolerated by the client. Nasal airways can become dry and irritated with CPAP, so an in-line humidifier or a room humidifier is recommended. A newer device, the BiPaP ventilator, delivers higher pressures during inhalation and lower pressures during expiration, providing less resistance to exhaling.

Surgery

Tonsillectomy and adenoidectomy may relieve upper airway obstruction in some clients. Excision of obstructive tissue from the soft palate, uvula, and posterior lateral pharyngeal wall may be accomplished by *uvulopalatopharyngoplasty (UPPP)*. Although only about 50% of these surgeries are successful in treating sleep apnea, UPPP is useful in selected cases. In severe cases, tracheostomy may also be performed to bypass the area of obstruction.

Nursing Care

Obstructive sleep apnea usually is treated in the home. Nursing care focuses on teaching the client and family about equipment use and strategies to decrease contributing factors such as obesity and alcohol intake. The following nursing diagnoses are appropriate for clients with sleep apnea:

- *Disturbed sleep pattern* related to repeated apneic episodes
- *Fatigue* related to interrupted sleep patterns
- *Ineffective breathing pattern* related to obstruction of upper airway during sleep
- *Impaired gas exchange* related to altered lung ventilation during obstructive episodes
- *Risk for injury* related to daytime somnolence and altered judgment
- *Risk for sexual dysfunction* related to impotence resulting from sleep apnea.

Home Care

Effective sleep apnea management depends on the client's willingness to participate in care. Provide teaching about the following topics:

- Relationship between obesity and sleep apnea
- Plans, resources, and referrals as needed for weight loss (e.g., programs such as Weight Watchers to provide additional support)
- Relationship of alcohol and sedatives to sleep apnea; referral to an alcohol treatment program or Alcoholics Anonymous as indicated

- How to use CPAP if ordered
- The importance of using CPAP continuously at night
- Measures to reduce airway dryness, including supplemental humidity and an adequate fluid intake to maintain moist mucous membranes.

If a support group for people with sleep apnea syndrome is available in the local area, refer the client and family to the group.

15

Nursing Care of Clients with Lower Respiratory Disorders

Many clients in acute care, long-term care, and the community experience acute or chronic disorders affecting the lower respiratory system. These disorders often lead to lost work time and account for a significant portion of health care costs.

Normal function of the lower respiratory system depends on several organ systems: the central nervous system, which stimulates and controls breathing; chemoreceptors in the brain, aortic arch, and carotid bodies, which monitor the pH and oxygen content of blood; the heart and circulatory system, which provide for blood supply and gas exchange; the musculoskeletal system, which provides an intact thoracic cavity capable of expanding and contracting; and the lungs and bronchial tree, which allow air movement and gas exchange. Impaired function of any of these systems affects ventilation and respiration. As a result, tissues may become *hypoxic*, with inadequate oxygen to support metabolic activity.

Disorders of the lower respiratory tract have both local and systemic effects. Local effects include cough, excess mucus production, shortness of breath or **dyspnea** (difficult or labored breathing), **hemoptysis** (bloody sputum), and chest pain. Systemic effects may include fever, anorexia and malaise, **cyanosis** (gray to blue or purple skin color caused by deoxygenated hemoglobin), **clubbing** of fingers and toes (enlargement and blunting of terminal digits), and other manifestations of impaired gas exchange.

Disorders of the lower respiratory system discussed in this chapter include infectious or inflammatory conditions, obstructive and restrictive lung diseases, pulmonary vascular disorders, lung cancer, chest and respiratory trauma, and respiratory failure. Before continuing, review the anatomy, physiology, and assessment of the lower respiratory system in Chapter 34.

Infections and Inflammatory Disorders

Infections and inflammation of the lower respiratory system are common. The respiratory tree is constantly exposed to the environment as air moves into and out of the lower respiratory tract. In addition, the oropharynx is colonized by huge numbers of microorganisms that may be aspirated into the bronchial tree. Both anatomic and physiologic defenses help maintain the sterility of the lower respiratory tract. When these defenses are impaired, the risk for infection increases. For example, drugs, alcohol, or neuromuscular disease may suppress the cough reflex, and the influenza virus can leave the respiratory epithelium vulnerable to bacterial infection. Even in healthy people, microorganisms and other foreign material occasionally enter the bronchial tree and lung parenchyma.

The Client with Acute Bronchitis

Bronchitis, inflammation of the bronchi, may be either an acute or a chronic condition. Acute bronchitis is relatively common in adults. Impaired immune defenses and cigarette smoking increase the risk for acute bronchitis. In otherwise healthy adults, it typically follows a viral upper respiratory infection. Chronic bronchitis is a component of chronic obstructive pulmonary disease (COPD) and is discussed later in this chapter.

Pathophysiology and Manifestations

Infectious bronchitis can be caused by either viruses or bacteria that damage the respiratory mucosa. Inhalation of toxic gases or chemicals can lead to inflammatory bronchitis. In either case, the inflammatory response causes vasodilation and edema of the mucosal lining of the bronchi. Mucosal irritation increases mucus production and initiates the cough reflex.

Acute bronchitis is typically heralded by a nonproductive cough that later becomes productive. The cough often occurs in paroxysms, and may be aggravated by cold, dry, or dusty air. Chest pain, often substernal, is common. Other manifestations include moderate fever and general malaise.

Collaborative Care

The diagnosis of acute bronchitis typically is based on the history and clinical presentation. A chest X-ray may be ordered to rule out pneumonia, because the presenting manifestations can be similar. Other diagnostic testing is rarely indicated. Treatment is symptomatic and includes rest, increased fluid intake, and the use of aspirin or acetaminophen to relieve fever and malaise. Many physicians prescribe a broad-spectrum antibiotic, such as erythromycin or penicillin, because approximately 50% of acute bronchitis is bacterial in origin. An expectorant cough medication is recommended for use during the day and a cough suppressant for night to facilitate rest.

Nursing Care

Nursing interventions for clients with acute bronchitis are primarily educational. Include the following teaching topics:

- Increase fluid intake to keep mucus thin and meet increased needs related to fever.
- Use over-the-counter analgesics and cough preparations containing dextromethorphan for symptom relief.
- Use and effects of any prescribed medications.
- The importance of smoking cessation (as appropriate).

The Client with Pneumonia

Inflammation of the lung parenchyma (the respiratory bronchioles and alveoli) is known as **pneumonia**. Despite significant advances in antibiotic therapy, pneumonia remains the sixth leading cause of death in the United States, and the leading cause of death from infectious disease (Porth, 2002). In 1999, nearly 64,000 deaths in the United States were attributed to pneumonia (NHLBI, 2002). Its incidence and mortality are highest in older adults and people with debilitating diseases. Pneumonia currently accounts for about 10% of adult hospital admissions in the United States.

Pneumonia may be either infectious or noninfectious. Bacteria, viruses, fungi, protozoa, and other microbes can lead to infectious pneumonia. Noninfectious causes include aspiration of gastric contents and inhalation of toxic or irritating gases. Pneumonias often are classified as community acquired, nosocomial (hospital acquired), or opportunistic. Different organisms are implicated in each of these classifications. The most common causative organism for community-acquired pneumonia is *Streptococcus pneumoniae* (also called pneumococcus), a gram-positive bacterium. This organism causes 70% to 75% of all diagnosed cases of pneumonia. *Mycoplasma pneumoniae, Haemophilus influenzae,* and the influenza virus are also leading causes of community-acquired pneumonia. *Staphylococcus aureus* and gram-negative bacteria, such as *Klebsiella pneumoniae, Pseudomonas aeruginosa,* and enteric bacilli, including *Escherichia coli,* are often implicated as nosocomial causes of pneumonia. Organisms, such as *Pneumonocystis carinii,* generally cause infections only in immunocompromised people (opportunistic infections).

Physiology Review

Normally, the lower respiratory tract is sterile. A number of defense mechanisms help maintain this sterile environment. Infectious particles trapped by the mucous membranes of the nose are removed by sneezing, while those deposited in the nasopharynx are usually swallowed or expectorated. Reflex closure of the epiglottis and the branching bronchial tree present anatomic barriers to entry of microorganisms and other possible contaminants. The cilia and mucus that line the respiratory tract, and the cough reflex, serve to trap and eliminate foreign matter that enters the lower respiratory tract. Organisms that make it past these barriers are usually rapidly phagocytized in the alveolus by resident macrophages, then attacked by the inflammatory and immune defenses of the body. Aging impairs these immune responses, increasing the risk for pneumonia.

Pathophysiology

The most common means of entry of pathogens into the lung is aspiration of oropharyngeal secretions containing microbes. Microorganisms may also be inhaled after having been released when an infected person coughs, sneezes, or talks. Contaminated aerosolized water may also be inhaled, an important means of spreading viral and some other types of pneumonia. Finally, bacteria may spread to the lungs through the bloodstream from infection elsewhere in the body.

When the invading microorganisms colonize the alveoli, an inflammatory and immune response is initiated. The antigen-antibody response and endotoxins released by some organisms damage bronchial and alveolar mucous membranes, causing inflammation and edema. Infectious debris and exudate can fill alveoli, interfering with ventilation and gas exchange.

The pathologic process, anatomic location, and manifestations of pneumonias vary according to the infective organism.

Acute Bacterial Pneumonia

Of the bacterial pneumonias, the pathogenesis of pneumococcal (*Streptococcus pneumoniae*) pneumonia is best understood. These bacteria reside in the upper respiratory tract of up to 70% of adults. They may be spread by direct person-to-person contact via droplets. In many cases, infection results from aspiration of resident bacteria. In the lower respiratory tract, the inflammatory response initiated by these organisms causes alveolar edema and the formation of exudate. As alveoli and respiratory bronchioles fill with serous exudate, blood cells, fibrin, and bacteria, *consolidation* (solidification) of lung tissue occurs. The lower lobes of the lungs are usually affected because of gravity. Consolidation of a large portion of an entire lung lobe is known as *lobar pneumonia*. This is the typical pattern for pneumococcal pneumonia. *Bronchopneumonia* is patchy consolidation involving several lobules. Other bacterial pneumonias often present with the patchy involvement of bronchopneumonia; pneumococcal pneumonia may also follow this pattern. The process resolves when macrophages predominate, digesting and removing inflammatory exudate from the infected lung.

Manifestations and Complications

The presentation of bacterial pneumonia is usually acute, with rapid onset of shaking chills, fever, and cough productive of rust-colored or purulent sputum. Chest aching or *pleuritic pain* (sharp localized chest pain that increases with breathing and coughing) is common. Limited breath sounds and fine crackles or rales are heard over the affected area of lung. A pleural friction rub may be audible. If the involved area is large and gas exchange is impaired, dyspnea and cyanosis may be noted.

A more insidious onset, with low-grade fever, cough, and scattered crackles, is more typical of bronchopneumonia. Dyspnea is less commonly seen. The older adult or debilitated client may have atypical manifestations of pneumonia, with little cough, scant sputum, and minimal evidence of respiratory distress. Fever, tachypnea, and altered mentation or agitation may be the primary presenting symptoms.

Pneumococcal pneumonia typically resolves uneventfully; normal lung structure is restored on completion of the process. Local extension of the infection to involve the pleura (*pleuritis*) is the most common complication. Bacteremia can spread the infection to other tissues, leading to meningitis, endocarditis, or peritonitis, and increasing the risk of mortality.

Pneumonias caused by *Staphylococcus aureus* and gram-negative bacteria often cause extensive parenchymal damage with necrosis, lung abscess, and empyema. **Empyema** is accumulation of purulent exudate in the pleural cavity. Progressive destruction of lung tissue and functional impairment is a possible consequence of *Klebsiella* pneumonia.

Legionnaires' Disease

Legionnaires' disease is a form of bronchopneumonia caused by *Legionella pneumophila,* a gram-negative bacterium widely found in water, particularly warm standing water. Legionnaires' disease occurs sporadically and in outbreaks, such as that which occurred at an American Legion convention in 1976, when the disease was first recognized. Contaminated water-cooled air-conditioning systems and other water sources have been implicated in its spread.

Smokers, older adults, and people with chronic diseases or impaired immune defenses are most susceptible to Legionnaires' disease. Symptoms develop gradually, beginning two to ten days after exposure. Dry cough, dyspnea, general malaise, chills and fever, headache, confusion, anorexia and diarrhea, myalgias and arthralgias are common manifestations. Consolidation of lung tissue is patchy or lobar. The mortality rate in Legionnaires' disease is up to 31% without treatment in otherwise healthy people and up to 80% in people who are immunocompromised (Braunwald, et al., 2001).

Primary Atypical Pneumonia

Pneumonia caused by *Mycoplasma pneumoniae* is generally classified as *primary atypical pneumonia,* because its presentation and course significantly differ from other bacterial pneumonias. Mycoplasma infection often causes pharyngitis or bronchitis. When pneumonia develops, patchy inflammatory changes in the alveolar septum and interstitial tissue of the lung occur. Alveolar exudate and consolidation of lung tissue are not features of atypical pneumonia.

Young adults—college students and military recruits in particular—are the primary affected population. Primary atypical pneumonia is highly contagious. Its manifestations resemble those of viral pneumonia; systemic manifestations of fever, headache, myalgias, and arthralgias often predominate. The cough associated with atypical pneumonia is dry, hacking, and nonproductive. Because of the typically mild nature and predominant systemic manifestations, mycoplasmal and viral pneumonia are often referred to as "walking pneumonias."

Viral Pneumonia

Approximately 10% of pneumonias in adults are viral. Influenza and adenovirus are the most common organisms; however, the incidence of cytomegalovirus (CMV) pneumonia is increasing in immunocompromised people. Other viruses such as herpesviruses and measles virus also may cause viral pneumonia. As in primary atypical pneumonia, lung involvement in viral pneumonia is limited to the alveolar septum and interstitial spaces.

Viral pneumonia is typically a mild disease that often affects older adults and people with chronic conditions. It usually occurs in community epidemics. Flulike symptoms of headache, fever, fatigue, malaise, and muscle aching are common, along with a dry cough.

Pneumocystis carinii Pneumonia

As many as 75% to 80% of people with acquired immune deficiency syndrome (AIDS) develop an opportunistic pneumonia caused by *Pneumocystis carinii,* a common parasite found worldwide. Immunity to *P. carinii* is nearly universal, except in immunocompromised people. Opportunistic infection may develop in people treated with immunosuppressive or cytotoxic drugs for cancer or organ transplant, and in people with genetic or acquired immunodeficiency.

Infection with *P. carinii* produces patchy involvement throughout the lungs, causing affected alveoli to thicken, become edematous, and fill with foamy, protein-rich fluid. Gas exchange is severely impaired as the disease progresses.

P. carinii pneumonia (PCP) has an abrupt onset with fever, tachypnea and shortness of breath, and a dry, nonproductive cough. Respiratory distress can be significant, with intercostal retractions and cyanosis.

Aspiration Pneumonia

Aspiration of gastric contents into the lungs results in a chemical and bacterial pneumonia known as *aspiration pneumonia*. Major risk factors for aspiration pneumonia include emergency surgery or obstetric procedures, depressed cough and gag reflexes, and impaired swallowing. Older surgical clients are at significant risk. Enteral nutrition by either nasogastric or gastric tube also increases the risk for aspiration pneumonia. Vomiting is not always apparent; silent regurgitation of gastric contents may occur when the level of consciousness is decreased. Measures to reduce the risk for aspiration pneumonia include minimizing the use of preoperative medications, promoting anesthetic elimination from the body, and preventing nausea and gastric distention.

The low pH of gastric contents causes a severe inflammatory response when aspirated into the respiratory tract. Pulmonary edema and respiratory failure may result. Common complications of aspiration pneumonia include abscesses, bronchiectasis (chronic dilation of the bronchi and bronchioles), and gangrene of pulmonary tissue.

Collaborative Care

Prevention is a key component in managing pneumonia. Identifying vulnerable populations and instituting preventive strategies are measures to reduce the mortality and morbidity associated with pneumonia. With early identification of the infecting organism, appropriate treatment, and support of respiratory function, most clients recover uneventfully. However, pneumonia remains a serious disease with significant mortality, especially in aged and debilitated populations.

Diagnostic Tests

Diagnostic testing for pneumonia focuses on establishing a diagnosis, determining the extent of lung involvement, and identifying the causative organism.

- *Sputum gram stain* rapidly identifies the infecting organisms as gram-positive or gram-negative bacteria. Antibiotic therapy can then be directed at the predominant type of organism until culture and sensitivity results are obtained.
- *Sputum culture and sensitivity* is ordered to identify the infecting organism and determine the most effective antibiotic therapy. When obtaining sputum for culture, it is important to obtain secretions from the lower respiratory tract, not the mouth and nasal passages.
- *Complete blood count (CBC) with white blood cell (WBC) differential* shows an elevated WBC (11,000/mm3 or higher) with increased circulating immature leukocytes (a left shift) in response to the infectious process. White blood cell changes are minimal in viral and other pneumonias.
- *Arterial blood gases (ABGs)* may be ordered to evaluate gas exchange. Alveolar inflammation can interfere with gas exchange across the alveolar-capillary membrane, especially if exudate or consolidation is present. Respiratory secretions or pleuritic pain also can interfere with alveolar ventilation. An arterial oxygen tension (Po_2) of less than 75 to 80 mmHg indicates impaired gas exchange or alveolar ventilation.

- *Pulse oximetry,* a noninvasive method of measuring arterial oxygen saturation, is ordered to continuously monitor gas exchange. The Sao_2 is the percentage of arterial hemoglobin that is saturated or combined with oxygen; it normally is 95% or higher. An Sao_2 of less than 95% may indicate impaired alveolar gas exchange.
- Chest X-ray is obtained to determine the extent and pattern of lung involvement. Fluid, infiltrates, consolidated lung tissue, and atelectasis (areas of alveolar collapse) appear as densities on the film.
- Fiberoptic bronchoscopy may be done to obtain a sputum specimen or remove secretions from the bronchial tree. In this procedure, a flexible bronchoscope is inserted through the mouth and larynx into the tracheobronchial tree, allowing direct visualization of tissues and collection of specimens for analysis. Nursing responsibilities related to bronchoscopy are summarized in the section below.

Immunization

Vaccines offer some degree of protection against the most common bacterial and viral pneumonias.

Pneumococcal vaccine, made of antigens from 23 types of pneumococcus, usually imparts lifetime immunity with a single dose. The vaccine is recommended for people who have a high risk of adverse outcome from bacterial pneumonias: people over age 65; those with chronic cardiac or respiratory conditions, diabetes mellitus, alcoholism, or other chronic diseases; and immunocompromised people.

Influenza vaccine is also recommended for high-risk populations. The predominant strain of influenza virus varies from year to year. A new vaccine formulation is prepared yearly, incorporating antigens of the influenza strains predicted to be the most prevalent for the upcoming flu season (typically the winter months). Vulnerable populations for whom yearly vaccine is recommended include those listed above, as well as health care workers and residents of long-term care facilities. The vaccine contains egg protein, and is not recommended for people who have a severe allergy to eggs or who have previously experienced a severe hypersensitivity response to the vaccine.

Medications

Medications used to treat pneumonia may include antibiotics to eradicate the infection and bronchodilators to reduce bronchospasm and improve ventilation.

Initial antibiotic therapy is based on the results of sputum Gram stain and the pattern of lung involvement shown on the chest X-ray. Typically, a broad-spectrum antibiotic, such as a penicillin, cephalosporin, erythromycin, or aminoglycoside, is ordered until the results of sputum culture and sensitivity tests are available.

When an inflammatory response to the infection causes bronchospasm and constriction, bronchodilators may be ordered to improve ventilation and reduce hypoxia. Bronchodilators generally belong to one of two major groups: the sympathomimetic drugs, such as albuterol sulfate (Proventil) and metaproterenol (Alupent); or the methylxanthines, such as theophylline and aminophylline. Use of these drugs and related nursing implications are discussed in detail in the section on asthma.

An agent to "break up" mucus or reduce its viscosity may be prescribed. Acetylcysteine (Mucomyst), potassium iodide, and guaifenesin (a common ingredient in expectorant cough syrups), help to liquefy mucus, making it easier to expectorate. For many clients, however, increasing fluid intake is an effective means of liquefying mucus.

Table 15-1. Antibiotic Therapy for Selected Pneumonias

Causative Organism	Antibiotic of Choice	Alternative Antibiotics
Streptococcus pneumoniae	Penicillin G or V; doxycycline; amoxicillin	Erythromycin, cephalosporins, fluoroquinolone, vancomycin
Staphylococcus aureus	Penicillinase-resistant penicillin (e.g., nafcillin); vancomycin for methicillin-resistant organisms	Cephalosporins, vancomycin, clindamycin; ciprofloxacin, fluoroquinlones, TMP-SMZ*
Mycoplasma pneumoniae	Erythromycin	Doxycycline, clarithromycin, azithromycin, fluoroquinolone
Klebsiella pneumoniae	Third-generation cephalosporin (with aminoglycoside if severe); methronidazole	Aztreonam, imipenem-cilastatin, fluoroquinolone
Legionella pneumophila	Erythromycin + rifampin; fluoroquinolone	TMP-SMZ*, azithromycin, clarithromycin, ciprofloxacin
Pneumocystis carinii	TMP-SMZ*, pentamidine	Dapsone + trimethoprim, clindamycin + primaquine, trimetrexate + folinic acid

* Trimethoprim-sulfamethoxazole

Treatments

When mucous secretions are thick and viscous, increasing fluid intake to 2500 to 3000 mL per day helps liquefy secretions, making them easier to cough up and expectorate. If the client is unable to maintain an adequate oral intake, intravenous fluids and nutrition may be required.

Incentive spirometry may be used to promote deep breathing, coughing, and clearance of respiratory secretions. Endotracheal suctioning may be required if the cough is ineffective. This invasive technique is discussed in the section describing nursing care for the client with acute respiratory failure. On occasion, bronchoscopy is used to perform pulmonary toilet and remove secretions.

Oxygen Therapy

Oxygen therapy may be indicated for the client who is tachypneic or hypoxemic.

Inflammation of the alveolar-capillary membrane interferes with diffusion of gases across the membrane. Diffusion is affected by several other factors, including the partial pressure of gases on each side of the membrane. Increasing the percentage of inspired oxygen above that of room air (21%) increases the partial pressure of oxygen in the alveoli and enhances its diffusion into the capillaries. Supplemental oxygen therefore improves oxygenation of the blood and tissues in clients with pneumonia.

Depending on the degree of hypoxia, oxygen may be administered by either a low-flow or high-flow system. Low-flow systems include the nasal cannula, simple face mask, partial rebreathing mask, and nonrebreathing mask. A nasal cannula can deliver 24% to 45% oxygen concentrations with flow rates of 2 to 6 L/min. The nasal cannula is comfortable and does not interfere with eating or talking. A simple face mask delivers 40% to 60% oxygen concentrations with flow rates of 5 to 8 L/min. Up to 100% oxygen can be delivered by the nonrebreather mask, the highest concentration possible without mechanical ventilation. When the amount of oxygen delivered must be precisely regulated, a high-flow system such as a Venturi mask is used. The Venturi mask regulates the ratio of oxygen to room air, allowing precise regulation of the oxygen percentage delivered, from 24% to 50%. Severe hypoxia may necessitate intubation and mechanical ventilation. Endotracheal intubation and methods of mechanical ventilation are discussed in the section on respiratory failure.

Chest Physiotherapy

Chest physiotherapy, including percussion, vibration, and postural drainage, may be prescribed to reduce lung consolidation and prevent atelectasis. *Percussion* is performed by rhythmically striking or clapping the chest wall with cupped hands, using rapid wrist flexion and extension. Cupping traps air between the palm and the client's skin, setting up vibrations through the chest wall that loosen respiratory secretions. The trapped air also provides a cushion, preventing injury. When performed correctly, percussion produces a hollow, popping sound. Percussion may also be done using a mechanical percussion cup. The breasts, sternum, spinal column, and kidney regions are avoided during percussion.

Vibration facilitates secretion movement into larger airways. It usually is combined with percussion, although it may be used when percussion is contraindicated or poorly tolerated. Vibration is performed by repeatedly tensing the arm and hand muscles while maintaining firm but gentle pressure over the affected area with the flat of the hand.

Percussion and vibration are done in conjunction with *postural drainage,* which uses gravity to facilitate removal of secretions from a particular lung segment. The client is positioned with the segment to be drained superior to or above the trachea or mainstem bronchus. Drainage of all lung segments requires a variety of positions; rarely do all segments require drainage. Bronchodilators or nebulizer treatments are administered as ordered prior to postural drainage. It is best to perform postural drainage before meals to avoid nausea and vomiting.

Complementary Therapies

Although complementary therapies do not replace conventional treatment for pneumonia, they often promote comfort and speed recovery. The herb Echinacea is widely used to stimulate immune function and treat upper respiratory infections (URIs). Because viral URIs often precede pneumonia, it may be helpful in preventing pneumonia. Goldenseal, which often is sold in combination with Echinaciea, is used to treat bacterial, fungal, and protozoal infections of the mucous membranes of the respiratory tract (Lehne, 2001). Ma huang contains the active ingredient ephedra, which may help relieve bronchospasm and ease breathing. Because the pharmacology of ephedra is identical to ephedrine, this herb should not be used by clients with heart disease, hypertension, diabetes, or prostatic hypertrophy (Lehne, 2001).

Nursing Care

Health Promotion

Health promotion activities focus on pneumonia prevention. Make clients in high-risk groups aware of the benefits of immunizations against influenza and pneumococcal pneumonia. A single dose of pneumococcus vaccine usually produces immunity to most strains of pneumococcal pneumonia, although repeat doses may be needed for older adults and people who are immunosuppressed. (Pneumococcus vaccine is contraindicated for people receiving immunosuppressive therapy.) Annual influenza vaccine helps prevent pneumonia, because pneumonia often occurs as a sequella to influenza.

Additional measures to screen for and detect pneumonia in older adults are appropriate. Frequent pulmonary assessment and aggressive interventions help prevent problems. Restoring and maintaining mobility improves ventilation and helps mobilize secretions. Promoting adequate fluid intake liquefies secretions, making them easier to expectorate.

Assessment

Focused assessment of the client with pneumonia includes the following:

- *Health history:* current symptoms and their duration; presence of shortness of breath or difficulty breathing, chest pain and its relationship to breathing; cough, productive or nonproductive, color, consistency of sputum; other symptoms; recent upper respiratory or other acute illness; chronic diseases such as diabetes, chronic lung disease, or heart disease; current medications; medication allergies.
- *Physical examination:* presentation, apparent distress, level of consciousness; vital signs including temperature; skin color, temperature; respiratory excursion, use of accessory muscles of respiration; lung sounds.

Nursing Diagnoses and Interventions

Clients with lower respiratory disorders such as pneumonia may have multiple nursing care needs, depending on the severity of the illness. Alveolar ventilation and the process of alveolar respiration can be affected by inflammation and secretions. **Hypoxemia**, low levels of oxygen in the blood, and tissue hypoxia may result. Nursing care focuses on supporting optimal respiratory function and promoting rest to reduce metabolic and oxygen needs. Priority nursing diagnoses include: *ineffective airway clearance, ineffective breathing pattern,* and *activity intolerance.*

Ineffective Airway Clearance

The inflammatory response to infection causes tissue edema and exudate formation. In the lungs, the inflammatory response can narrow and potentially obstruct bronchial passages and alveoli. Assessment findings supporting this nursing diagnosis include adventitious breath sounds, such as crackles (rales), rhonchi, and wheezes; dyspnea and tachypnea; coughing; and indicators of hypoxia such as cyanosis, reduced SaO_2 levels, anxiety, and apprehension.

- Assess respiratory status, including vital signs, breath sounds, Sao_2, and skin color at least every 4 hours. *Early identification of respiratory compromise allows intervention before tissue hypoxia is significant.*
- Assess cough and sputum (amount, color, consistency, and possible odor). *Assessment of the cough and nature of sputum produced allow evaluation of the effectiveness of respiratory clearance and the response to therapy.*

- Monitor arterial blood gas results; report increasing hypoxemia and other abnormal results to the physician. *Blood gas changes may be an early indicator of impaired gas exchange due to airway narrowing or obstruction.*
- Place in Fowler's or high-Fowler's position. Encourage frequent position changes and ambulation as allowed. *The upright position promotes lung expansion; position changes and ambulation facilitate the movement of secretions.*
- Assist to cough, deep breathe, and use assistive devices. Provide endotracheal suctioning using aseptic technique as ordered. *Coughing, deep breathing, and suctioning help clear airways.*
- Provide a fluid intake of at least 2500 to 3000 mL per day. *A liberal fluid intake helps liquefy secretions, facilitating their clearance.*
- Work with the physician and respiratory therapist to provide pulmonary hygiene measures, such as postural drainage, percussion, and vibration. *These techniques help mobilize and clear secretions.*
- Administer prescribed medications as ordered, and monitor their effects. *If the infecting organism is resistant to the prescribed antibiotic, little improvement may be seen with treatment. Bronchodilators help maintain open airways but may have adverse effects such as anxiety and restlessness.*

Ineffective Breathing Pattern

Pleural inflammation often accompanies pneumonia, causing sharp localized pain that increases with deep breathing, coughing, and movement, which can lead to rapid and shallow breathing. Distal airways and alveoli may not expand optimally with each breath, increasing the risk for atelectasis and decreasing gas exchange. Fatigue from the increased work of breathing is an additional problem in pneumonia. This, too, can lead to decreased lung inflation and an ineffective breathing pattern.

- Provide for rest periods. *Rest reduces metabolic demands, fatigue, and the work of breathing, promoting a more effective breathing pattern.*
- Assess for pleuritic discomfort. Provide analgesics as ordered. *Adequate pain relief minimizes splinting and promotes adequate ventilation.*
- Provide reassurance during periods of respiratory distress. *Hypoxia and respiratory distress produce high levels of anxiety, which tends to further increase tachypnea and fatigue and decrease ventilation.*
- Administer oxygen as ordered. *Oxygen therapy increases the alveolar oxygen concentration and facilitates its diffusion across the alveolar-capillary membrane, reducing hypoxia and anxiety.*
- Teach slow abdominal breathing. *This breathing pattern promotes lung expansion.*
- Teach use of relaxation techniques, such as visualization and meditation. *These techniques help reduce anxiety and slow the breathing pattern.*

Activity Intolerance

Impaired airway clearance and gas exchange interfere with oxygen delivery to body cells and tissues. At the same time, the infectious process and the body's response to it increase metabolic demands on the cells. The net result of this imbalance between oxygen delivery and oxygen demand is a lack of physiologic energy to maintain normal daily activities.

- Assess activity tolerance, noting any increase in pulse, respirations, dyspnea, diaphoresis, or cyanosis. *These assessment findings may indicate limited or impaired activity tolerance.*
- Assist with self-care activities, such as bathing. *Assistance with activities of daily living reduces energy demands.*
- Schedule activities, planning for rest periods. *Rest periods minimize fatigue and improve activity tolerance.*
- Provide assistive devices, such as an overhead trapeze. *These assistive devices facilitate movement and reduce energy demands.*
- Enlist the family's help to minimize stress and anxiety levels. *Stress and anxiety increase metabolic demands and can decrease activity tolerance.*
- Perform active or passive range of motion (ROM) exercises. *Exercises help maintain muscle tone and joint mobility, and prevent contractures if bed rest is prolonged.*
- Provide emotional support and reassurance that strength and energy will return to normal when the infectious process has resolved and the balance of oxygen supply and demand is restored. *The client may be concerned that activity intolerance will continue to be a problem after the acute infection is resolved.*

Home Care

Clients with pneumonia usually are treated in the community, unless their respiratory status is significantly compromised. Discuss the following topics when preparing the client and family for home care.

- The importance of completing the prescribed medication regimen as ordered; potential drug side effects and their management, including manifestations that necessitate stopping the drug and notifying the physician
- Recommendations for limiting activities and increasing rest
- Maintaining adequate fluid intake to keep mucus thin for easier expectoration
- Ways to maintain adequate nutritional intake, such as small, frequent, well-balanced meals
- The importance of avoiding smoking or exposure to secondhand smoke to prevent further irritation of the lungs
- Manifestations to report to the physician, such as increasing shortness of breath, difficulty breathing, increased fever, fatigue, headache, sleepiness, or confusion
- The importance of keeping all follow-up appointments to ensure disease cure.

Clients with severe respiratory compromise or who are elderly or debilitated may require home care assistance to remain at home. Provide referrals to home intravenous services, home health nursing services, and home maintenance services as indicated. Community services, such as Meals-on-Wheels can provide support to reduce the energy demands of meal preparation.

The Client with Severe Acute Respiratory Syndrome

Severe acute respiratory syndrome (SARS) is a lower respiratory illness of unknown etiology first described in clients in Asia in the fall of 2002. Since then, this emerging disease has been described in clients in North America, Australia, and Europe, although the majority of identified cases are in China (including Hong Kong and Singapore; World Health Organization [WHO], 2003).

The primary population affected by SARS is previously healthy adults age 25 to 70 years. Recent travel (within 10 days of the onset of symptoms) to an area with documented or suspected community transmission of SARS or close contact with a person known or suspected to have SARS are the primary risk factors for this disease.

Pathophysiology and Manifestations

Although not yet proven, the infective agent responsible for SARS is thought to be a newly identified coronavirus. This virus appears to spread by close person-to-person contact. Other potential sources of the infection are through direct contact with an infected person or contaminated object, and exposure of the eyes or mucous membranes to respiratory secretions (Centers for Disease Control and Prevention [CDC], 2003).

The incubation period for SARS is generally 2 to 7 days, although it may be as long as 10 days in some people. Fever higher than 100.4° F (38°C) is typically the initial manifestation of the disease. The high fever may be accompanied by chills, headache, malaise, and muscle aches. After 3 to 7 days, respiratory manifestations of SARS develop, including nonproductive cough, shortness of breath, dyspnea, and possible hypoxemia.

While the majority of people with SARS recover, up to 20% of affected clients require intubation and mechanical ventilation (see the section on respiratory failure). About 3 in 100 clients with SARS die.

Collaborative Care

Prompt identification of SARS, infection control measures, and reporting of the disease are vital to control this potentially deadly disease. Health care providers and public health personnel should report cases of SARS to state and local health departments.

Diagnostic Tests

At this time, no laboratory test is available to diagnose SARS. Initial diagnostic testing for a client with suspected SARS may include the following:

- *Serology tests* for antibodies to the new coronavirus may be available in some research centers.
- *Chest X-ray* may be normal or show interstitial infiltrates in a focal or generalized patchy pattern. In late stages of SARS, consolidation may be evident.
- *Pulse oximetry (oxygen saturation)* often shows hypoxemia in the respiratory phase of the illness.
- *Complete blood count (CBC)* often demonstrates a low lymphocyte count early in the disease. Leukopenia and thrombocytopenia may develop at the peak of the respiratory illness.
- *Creatinine phosphokinase (CPK or CK), ALT,* and *AST* levels may be markedly increased in SARS.
- *Sputum specimen* is obtained. Gram stain and culture are performed on the specimen to rule out other causes of pneumonia.
- *Blood culture* may be done to identify possible bacteremia.

Medications

At this time, no medications have been shown to be consistently effective in treating SARS. Antibiotic and/or antiviral therapy targeted at community-acquired forms of pneumonia may be administered.

Infection Control

Because health care workers are at risk for developing SARS after caring for infected clients, infection control precautions should be immediately instituted when SARS is suspected. Standard precautions are implemented along with contact and airborne precautions. The Centers for Disease Control and Prevention (2003) recommends hand hygiene, gown, gloves, eye protection, and an N95 respirator to prevent transmission of SARS in healthcare settings.

When clients with SARS are managed in the community, they are advised to remain home for ten days after the fever has resolved and until respiratory symptoms are absent or minimal. Members of the household are advised to wash hands frequently or use alcohol-based hand rubs. The client is advised to cover the mouth and nose with tissue when coughing or sneezing and to wear a surgical mask during close contact with uninfected people. Sharing of utensils, towels, and bedding should be avoided. Routine cleaning (e.g., washing with soap and hot water) is adequate to disinfect objects and no special precautions are necessary for disposing of waste.

Treatments

Care of the client with SARS is supportive. Oxygen may be administered to treat hypoxemia. Intubation and mechanical ventilation may be required if respiratory failure or acute respiratory distress syndrome (ARDS) develops.

Nursing Care

Nursing care of the client with SARS focuses on preventing spread of the disease to others and providing respiratory support.

Health Promotion

Advise clients planning elective or nonessential travel to mainland China and Hong Kong, Singapore, and Hanoi, Vietnam, that they may wish to postpone their trips. Use respiratory and contact infection control precautions in addition to standard precautions when caring for all clients with suspected SARS to prevent spread of the disease to health care workers or other clients.

Assessment

Focused assessment data for the client with suspected SARS include the following. For more complete respiratory assessment, see Chapter 13.

* *Health history:* current symptoms, including fever, malaise, shortness of breath, and cough; onset of symptoms; recent international travel or exposure to a person known to have SARS.
* *Physical assessment:* vital signs including temperature; respiratory status, including respiratory rate, depth, and effort; presence of cough; adventitious lung sounds.

Nursing Diagnoses and Interventions

The client with SARS poses a risk for spread of the infection to health care workers and others. In addition, while many people with this disease experience only mild symptoms and recover fully and uneventfully, others develop severe respiratory distress and may require significant respiratory support. Gas exchange may be impaired, leading to significant hypoxemia. In addition to the nursing diagnoses discussed in the previous section on pneumonia, *impaired gas exchange* and *risk for infection* are priority nursing diagnoses.

Impaired Gas Exchange

Although the pathophysiology of SARS is not fully understood, this disorder is known to cause hypoxemia of varying degrees in some clients. Significant hypoxemia may necessitate intubation and mechanical ventilation to support cellular function until recovery occurs.

- Monitor vital signs, color, oxygen saturation, and arterial blood gases. Assess for manifestations, such as anxiety or apprehension, restlessness, confusion or lethargy, or complaints of headache. *These assessment data alert the nurse and care providers to potential hypoxemia or hypercapnia due to impaired gas exchange.*
- Promptly report worsening arterial blood gases and oxygen saturation levels. *Close assessment of these values allows timely intervention as needed.*
- Maintain oxygen therapy and mechanical ventilation as ordered. Hyperoxygenate prior to suctioning. *Oxygen and mechanical ventilation support alveolar gas exchange. Hyperoxygenation prior to suctioning reduces the degree of hypoxemia that occurs during suctioning.*
- Place in Fowler's or high Fowler's position. *Sitting positions decrease pressure on the diaphragm and chest, improving lung ventilation and decreasing the work of breathing.*
- Minimize activities and energy expenditures by assisting with ADLs, spacing procedures and activities, and allowing uninterrupted rest periods. *Rest is vital to reduce oxygen and energy demands.*
- If intubation and mechanical ventilation is necessary, explain the procedure and its purpose to the client and family, providing reassurance that this temporary measure improves oxygenation and reduces the work of breathing. Alert client that talking is not possible while the endotracheal tube is in place, and establish a means of communication. *Thorough explanation is important to relieve anxiety.*

Risk for Infection

The spread of SARS is a risk both in the health care facility and the community in which the client resides. Respiratory and contract precautions are recommended to prevent the spread of SARS via respiratory secretions or contact with the virus.

- Place the client in a private room with airflow control that prevents air within the room from circulating into the hallway or other rooms. A negative flow room in which air is diluted by at least six fresh-air exchanges per hour is recommended. *A negative flow room and multiple fresh-air exchanges dilute the concentration of virus within the room and prevent its spread to adjacent areas.*
- Use standard precautions and respiratory and contact isolation techniques as recommended by the CDC, including wearing respirators, gowns, and eye protection when caring for clients with SARS. *These measures are important to prevent the spread of SARS to others.*

- Discuss the reasons for and importance of respiratory and contact isolation procedures during treatment. *Maintenance of infection control precautions during and immediately following the febrile and respiratory phases of SARS is vital to prevent its spread to health care workers and the community.*
- Place a mask on the client when transporting to other parts of the facility for diagnostic or treatment procedures. *Covering the client's nose and mouth during transport minimizes air contamination and the risk to visitors and personnel.*
- Inform all personnel having contact with the client of the diagnosis. *This allows personnel to take appropriate precautions.*
- Assist visitors to mask prior to entering the room. *Providing visitors with appropriate masks or respirators reduces their risk of infection.*
- Teach the client how to limit transmitting the disease to others:
    a. Always cough and expectorate into tissues.
    b. Dispose of tissues properly, placing them in a closed bag.
    c. Wear a mask if sneezing or unable to control respiratory secretions.
    d. Do not share eating utensils, towels, bedding, or other objects with others, as this disease may also be spread by contact with contaminated objects.

Teaching appropriate precautions helps prevent the spread of SARS to others while allowing as much freedom from restraints as possible.

Home Care

Many clients with SARS experience only mild symptoms and are appropriately cared for in the community. Teaching about home care and infection control precautions is vital to prevent spread of this disease to the community. Include the following topics when teaching for home care:

- The disease, its origin, and how it is spread
- Manifestations of impaired respiratory status to report to the physician
- Preventing spread of the disease to others:
    1. Cover the mouth and nose with tissues when coughing or sneezing. Personally dispose of tissues in a paper bag or the garbage. Wear a surgical mask during close contact with other members of the household.
    2. Limit interactions outside the home; do not go to work, school, or other public areas until you have been free of fever for ten days and your respiratory symptoms are resolving.
    3. Remind all members of the household to wash hands (or use an alcohol-based hand sanitizer) frequently, particularly after direct contact with body fluids.
    4. Do not share eating utensils, towels, or bedding with others. These items can be cleaned with soap and hot water between uses. Clean contaminated surfaces with a household disinfectant.
- Monitoring uninfected members of the household for signs of the illness (instruct client to report fever or respiratory symptoms to the physician).

The Client with Lung Abscess

A **lung abscess** is a localized area of lung destruction or necrosis and pus formation. The most common cause of lung abscess is aspiration and resulting pneumonia. Risk factors, therefore, are those for aspiration: decreased level of consciousness due to anesthesia, injury or disease of the central nervous system, seizure, excessive sedation, or alcohol abuse; swallowing disorders; dental caries; and debilitation secondary to cancer or chronic disease. Lung abscess may also occur as a complication of some types of pneumonia, including those due to *Staphylococcus aureus*, *Klebsiella*, and *Legionella*.

Pathophysiology and Manifestations

A lung abscess forms after lung tissue becomes consolidated (i.e., after alveoli become filled with fluid, pus, and microorganisms). Consolidated tissue becomes necrotic. This necrotic process can spread to involve the entire bronchopulmonary segment and progress proximally until it ruptures into a bronchus. With rupture, the contents of the abscess empty into the bronchus, leaving a cavity filled with air and fluid, a process known as *cavitation*. If purulent material from the abscess is not expectorated, the infection may spread, leading to diffuse pneumonia or a syndrome similar to acute respiratory distress syndrome (ARDS, discussed later in this chapter).

Manifestations of lung abscess typically develop about two weeks after the precipitating event (aspiration, pneumonia, and so on). Their onset may be either acute or insidious. Early symptoms are those of pneumonia: productive cough, chills and fever, pleuritic chest pain, malaise, and anorexia. The temperature may be significantly elevated, 103∞F (39.4∞C) or higher. When the abscess ruptures, the client may expectorate large amounts of foul-smelling, purulent, and possibly blood-streaked sputum. Breath sounds are diminished, and crackles may be noted in the region of the abscess. A dull percussion tone is also present.

Collaborative Care

The diagnosis of lung abscess usually is based on the history and presentation. The CBC may indicate leukocytosis. Sputum culture may not show the organism involved unless rupture occurs. Chest X-ray shows a thick-walled, solitary cavity with surrounding consolidation, although differentiating lung abscess from consolidation can be difficult until cavitation occurs.

Lung abscess is treated with antibiotic therapy, usually intravenous clindamycin (Cleocin), amoxicillin-clavulanate (Augmentin), or penicillin (Tierney, et al., 2001). Postural drainage may be ordered to relieve obstruction and promote drainage. In some cases, bronchoscopy is used to drain the abscess. If the pleural space becomes involved, a chest tube (tube thoracostomy) may be used to drain the abscess. See the section on pneumothorax for further discussion of chest tubes.

Nursing Care

Although most clients with lung abscess recover fully with appropriate antibiotic treatment, rupture and drainage of the abscess into a bronchus is a frightening experience. Nursing care needs of the client relate primarily to maintaining a patent airway and adequate gas exchange. The following nursing diagnoses may be appropriate for the client with lung abscess.

- *Risk for ineffective airway clearance* related to large amounts of purulent drainage in bronchi
- *Impaired gas exchange* related to necrotic and consolidated lung tissue
- *Hyperthermia* related to infectious process
- *Anxiety,* related to copious amounts of purulent sputum.

Client and family teaching focuses on the importance of completing the prescribed antibiotic therapy. Most lung abscesses are successfully treated with antibiotics; however, treatment may last up to one month or more. Emphasize the importance of completing the entire course of therapy to eliminate the infecting organisms. Teach about the medication, including its name, dose, desired and adverse effects. Stress the need to contact the physician if symptoms do not improve or if they become worse. Infection from lung abscess can spread not only to lung and pleural tissue but systemically, causing sepsis. If postural drainage is ordered, teach the client and family how to perform this procedure. When procedures such as bronchoscopy or thoracostomy are performed to drain the abscess, provide preoperative teaching and instruction on postoperative care.

The Client with Tuberculosis

Tuberculosis (TB) is a chronic, recurrent infectious disease that usually affects the lungs, although any organ can be affected. This disease, caused by *Mycobacterium tuberculosis,* is uncommon in the United States, especially among young adults of European descent. Its incidence fell steadily until the mid-1980s, thanks to improved sanitation, surveillance, and treatment of people with active disease. The late 1980s and early 1990s saw a resurgence of the disease, attributed primarily to the HIV/AIDS epidemic, the emergence of multiple-drug-resistant (MDR) strains of TB, and social factors, such as immigration, poverty, homelessness, and drug abuse. Today, the number of people affected by TB in the United States continues to decline, with a total of 15,989 cases reported in 2001 (National Center for HIV, STD, and TB Prevention, 2002). This decline can be attributed to TB-control programs that emphasize promptly identifying new cases and initiating and completing appropriate therapy.

Worldwide, TB continues to be an important health problem. An estimated 8 million cases of TB develop annually, with the vast majority (90%) occurring in developing countries of Asia, Africa, the Middle East, and Latin America. TB accounts for an estimated 2 million deaths each year (Braunwald, et al., 2001).

Today, TB in the United States is a disease primarily affecting immigrants, those infected with HIV, and disadvantaged populations. The TB case rate for foreign-born U.S. residents is more than 8 times higher than that for people born in the United States (NCHSTP 2002). Minority populations are affected to a greater extent than whites—the case rates for blacks, Hispanics, and Native Americans are 7 to 8 times that for whites; for Asians and Pacific Islanders living in the United States, it is more than 20 times higher. Poor urban areas are hit the hardest—areas that are also affected by the epidemics of injection drug use, homelessness, malnutrition, and poor living conditions. Overcrowded institutions also contribute to the spread of TB; transmission in hospitals, homeless shelters, drug treatment centers, prisons, and residential facilities has been documented. People with altered immune function, including older adults and people with AIDS are at particular risk for tuberculosis. Some strains of *M. tb* have become resistant to drugs used to treat the disease.

M. tuberculosis is a relatively slow-growing, slender, rod-shaped, acid-fast organism with a waxy outer capsule, which increases its resistance to destruction. Although the lungs are usually infected, tuberculosis can involve other organs as well. It is transmitted by *droplet nuclei*, airborne droplets produced when an infected person coughs, sneezes, speaks, or sings. The tiny droplets can remain suspended in air for several hours. Infection may develop when a susceptible host breathes in air containing droplet nuclei and the contaminated particle eludes the normal defenses of the upper respiratory tract to reach the alveoli.

The risk for infection is affected by characteristics of the infectious person, the extent of air contamination, duration of exposure, and susceptibility of the host. The number of microbes in the sputum, frequency and force of coughing, and behaviors, such as covering the mouth when coughing, affect the production of droplet nuclei. In a small, closed, or poorly ventilated space, droplet nuclei become more concentrated, increasing the risk of exposure. Prolonged contact, such as living in the same household, increases the risk. Less-than-optimal immune function, a problem for people in lower socioeconomic groups, injection drug users, the homeless, alcoholics, and people with HIV infection, increases the susceptibility of the host.

Pathophysiology

Pulmonary Tuberculosis

Minute droplet nuclei containing one to three bacilli that elude upper airway defense systems to enter the lungs implant in an alveolus or respiratory bronchiole, usually in an upper lobe. As the bacteria multiply, they cause a local inflammatory response. The inflammatory response brings neutrophils and macrophages to the site. These phagocytic cells surround and engulf the bacilli, isolating them and preventing their spread. *M. tb* continues to slowly multiply; some enter the lymphatic system to stimulate a cellular-mediated immune response (see Chapter 42 to review immune responses). Neutrophils and macrophages isolate the bacteria, but cannot destroy them. A granulomatous lesion called a *tubercle*, a sealed-off colony of bacilli, is formed. Within the tubercle, infected tissue dies, forming a cheeselike center, a process called *caseation necrosis*.

If the immune response is adequate, scar tissue develops around the tubercle, and the bacilli remain encapsulated. These lesions eventually calcify and are visible on X-ray. The client, while infected by *M. tb*, does not develop tuberculosis disease. If the immune response is inadequate to contain the bacilli, the disease of tuberculosis can develop. Occasionally, the infection can progress, leading to extensive destruction of lung tissue. In *primary tuberculosis*, granulomatous tissue may erode into a bronchus or into a blood vessel, allowing the disease to spread throughout the lung or other organs. This severe form of tuberculosis is uncommon in adults (Braunwald, et al., 2001).

A previously healed tuberculosis lesion may be reactivated. *Reactivation tuberculosis* occurs when the immune system is suppressed due to age, disease, or use of immunosuppressive drugs. The extent of lung disease can vary from small lesions to extensive cavitation of lung tissue. Tubercles rupture, spreading bacilli into the airways to form satellite lesions and produce tuberculosis pneumonia. Without treatment, massive lung involvement can lead to death, or a more chronic process of tubercle formation and cavitation may result. People with chronic disease continue to spread *M. tb* into the environment, potentially infecting others.

Clients with HIV disease are at high risk for developing active tuberculosis, due to primary infection or reactivation. HIV infection suppresses cellular immunity, which is vital to limiting the replication and spread of *M. tb*.

Manifestations and Complications

The initial infection causes few symptoms and typically goes unnoticed until the tuberculin test becomes positive or calcified lesions are seen on chest X-ray. Manifestations of primary progressive or reactivation tuberculosis often develop insidiously and are initially nonspecific. Fatigue, weight loss, anorexia, low-grade afternoon fever, and night sweats are common. A dry cough develops, which later becomes productive of purulent and/or blood-tinged sputum. It is often at this stage that the client seeks medical attention.

Tuberculosis empyema and bronchopleural fistula are the most serious complications of pulmonary tuberculosis. When a tuberculosis lesion ruptures, bacilli may contaminate the pleural space. Rupture also may allow air to enter the pleural space from the lung, causing pneumothorax.

Extrapulmonary Tuberculosis

When primary disease or reactivation allows live bacilli to enter the bronchi, the disease may spread through the blood and lymph system to other organs. These distant disease metastases may produce an active lesion, or they may become dormant and reactivate at a later time. Extrapulmonary tuberculosis is especially prevalent in people with HIV disease.

Miliary Tuberculosis

Miliary tuberculosis results from hematogenous spread (through the blood) of the bacilli throughout the body. Miliary tuberculosis causes chills and fever, weakness, malaise, and progressive dyspnea. Multiple lesions evenly distributed throughout the lungs are noted on X-ray. The sputum rarely contains organisms. The bone marrow is usually involved, causing anemia, thrombocytopenia, and leukocytosis. Without appropriate treatment, the prognosis is poor.

Genitourinary Tuberculosis

The kidney and genitourinary tract are common extrapulmonary sites for tuberculosis. The organism spreads to the kidney through the blood, initiating an inflammatory process similar to that which occurs in the lungs. Reactivation can occur years after the original infection. As the lesion then enlarges and caseates, a large portion of the renal parenchyma is destroyed. The infection then can spread to rest of the urinary tract, including the ureters and bladder. Scarring and strictures commonly result. In men, the prostate, seminal vesicles, and epididymis may be involved. In women, tuberculosis may affect the fallopian tubes and ovaries.

Manifestations of genitourinary tuberculosis develop insidiously. Symptoms of a urinary tract infection, including malaise, dysuria, hematuria, and pyuria, develop. Flank pain may be present. Men may develop manifestations of epididymitis or prostatitis: perineal, sacral, or scrotal pain and tenderness; difficulty voiding; and fever. Women may have manifestations of pelvic inflammatory disease, impaired fertility, or ectopic pregnancy.

Tuberculosis Meningitis

Tuberculosis meningitis results when tuberculosis spreads to the subarachnoid space. In the United States, this complication most often affects older adults, usually from reactivation of latent disease. Manifestations develop gradually, with listlessness, irritability, anorexia, and fever. Headache and behavior changes are common early symptoms in the older adult. As the disease progresses, the headache increases in intensity, vomiting develops, and the level of consciousness decreases. Convulsions and coma may follow. Without appropriate treatment, neurologic effects may become permanent.

Skeletal Tuberculosis

Tuberculosis of the bones and joints is most likely to occur during childhood, when bone epiphyses are open and their blood supply is rich. The organisms spread via the blood to vertebrae, the ends of long bones, and joints. Immune and inflammatory processes isolate the bacilli, and the disease often becomes evident years or decades later.

Tuberculous spondylitis usually involves the thoracic vertebrae, eroding vertebral bodies and causing them to collapse. Significant kyphosis develops, and the spinal cord may be compressed. The large, weight-bearing joints (hips and knees) are most often affected by tuberculous arthritis, although other joints may be affected, particularly if they have been previously damaged. The involved joint is painful, warm, and tender.

Collaborative Care

Tuberculosis was a major public health concern earlier in this century, before the development of effective sanitation measures and drug treatment. Developing drug-resistant strains, susceptibility of people with HIV disease, and inadequate access to health care for high-risk populations contribute to the continuing significance of tuberculosis as a significant public health threat. Collaborative care, therefore, focuses on the following:

- Early detection
- Accurate diagnosis
- Effective disease treatment
- Preventing tuberculosis spread to others.

Hospitalization is rarely required to treat tuberculosis. With appropriate treatment, clients become noninfective to others fairly rapidly. However, a client with active tuberculosis may be admitted for a concurrent problem or a complication of the disease. Nurses and other health care workers are at risk for exposure if the disease has not yet been diagnosed. When a client with tuberculosis is institutionalized, maintain respiratory isolation to minimize the risk of infection to other clients and to the health care workers.

Noncompliance with prescribed treatment is a major problem in treating active tuberculosis. The client can continue transmitting the disease to others, and drug-resistant strains of bacteria can develop when treatment is incomplete. Tuberculosis must be reported to local and state public health departments, so contacts can be identified and examined. People who share living or work environments with the client can be tested and receive prophylactic treatment. Continuing contact with clients who have active TB is vital to ensure effective cure.

Screening

The tuberculin test is used to screen for tuberculosis infection. A cellular, or delayed hypersensitivity, response to *M. tuberculosis* develops within 3 to 10 weeks after the infection. Injecting a small amount of *purified protein derivative (PPD)* of tuberculin any time thereafter activates this response, attracting macrophages to the area and causing a pronounced local inflammatory response. The amount of induration surrounding the injection site is used to determine infection (see Table 15-2). It is important to remember that a positive response indicates that infection and a cellular (T-cell) response have developed; however, it does not mean that active disease is present or that the client is infectious to others.

Several methods are currently available for tuberculin testing:

- *Intradermal PPD (Mantoux) test:* 0.1 mL of PPD (5 tuberculin units, or TU) is injected intradermally into the dorsal aspect of the forearm. This test is read within 48 to 72 hours, the peak reaction period, and recorded as the diameter of induration (raised area, not erythema) in millimeters.

- *Multiple-puncture (tine) test:* A multiple-puncture device is used to introduce tuberculin into the skin. This test is less accurate than other testing methods. A vesicular reaction is considered positive; any other reaction must be confirmed using a Mantoux test.

Although it is impractical and unnecessary to screen the entire population, the Centers for Disease Control and Prevention (CDC) recommends screening people in the following risk groups:

- People with, or at high risk, for HIV infection.
- Close contacts of people who have or are suspected of having infectious TB.
- People with medical risk factors, such as silicosis, chronic malabsorption, end-stage renal failure, diabetes mellitus, immunosuppression, and hematologic and other malignancies.
- People born in countries with a high prevalence of TB.
- Medically underserved low-income populations, including racial and ethnic minorities.
- Alcoholics and injection drug users.
- Residents and staff of long-term residential facilities, such as long-term care facilities, correctional institutions, and mental health facilities.

False-negative responses are common in people who are immunosuppressed. A two-step procedure may be necessary to elicit a positive response. If the first test elicits a negative response, a second PPD test is given one week later. If the second test also is negative, the client either is free of infection or is *anergic* (unable to react to common antigens). This two-step procedure is recommended for long-term care residents and workers.

Table 15-2. Interpreting Tuberculin Test Results

Area of Induration	Significance
Less than 5 mm	Negative response; does not rule out infection.
5 to 9 mm	Positive for people who: • Are in close contact with a client with infective TB • Have an abnormal chest X-ray • Have HIV infection Negative for all others.

Table 15-2. Continued

10 to 15 mm	Positive for people who have other risk factors: • Birth in a high-incidence country • Low socioeconomic status • African American, Hispanic, Asian American in poverty areas • Injection drug use • Residence in a long-term care facility • Identified local risk factors.
Greater than 15 mm	Positive for all people.

Diagnostic Tests

A positive tuberculin test alone does not indicate active disease. Sputum tests for the bacillus and chest X-rays are routinely used to diagnose and evaluate active disease. A series of three consecutive early-morning sputum specimens is typically examined for bacilli. Use special procedures or personal protective devices when obtaining sputum specimens. If possible, collect specimens in a room equipped with airflow control devices, ultraviolet light, or both. Alternatively, have the client step outside to collect the specimen. Wear a mask capable of filtering droplet nuclei when collecting sputum specimens. Aerosol therapy, percussion, and postural drainage may help the client produce sputum. Occasionally, endotracheal suctioning, bronchoscopy, or gastric lavage may be necessary to obtain a specimen.

* *Sputum smear* is microscopically examined for *acid-fast bacilli. M. tuberculosis* resists decolorizing chemicals after staining. This property is called "acid-fast." The acid-fast smear provides a rapid indicator of the tubercle bacillus.
* *Sputum culture* positive for *M. tuberculosis* provides the definitive diagnosis. However, M. tuberculosis is slow growing, requiring four to eight weeks before it can be detected using traditional culture techniques. Automated radiometric culture systems, such as Bactec, allow detection of *M. tuberculosis* in several days.
* Once the organism is detected, *sensitivity testing* is performed to identify appropriate drug therapy.
* *Polymerase chain reaction (PCR)* permits rapid detection of DNA from *M. tuberculosis.*
* *Chest X-ray* is ordered to diagnose and evaluate TB. Typical findings in pulmonary TB include dense lesions in the apical and posterior segments of the upper lobe and possible cavity formation.

Prior to initiating antituberculosis drug therapy, several additional diagnostic tests may be done to establish baseline data for monitoring potential adverse effects of the drugs.

* *Liver function* tests are obtained prior to treatment with isoniazid (INH) as this drug is hepatotoxic.
* A thorough *vision examination* is done prior to treatment with ethambutol, a commonly used antituberculosis medication. Optic neuritis is a potential adverse effect of this drug. Periodic eye examinations are scheduled during the course of therapy.
* *Audiometric testing* is performed before streptomycin therapy is initiated. Ototoxicity is a significant adverse effect of streptomycin and other aminoglycoside antibiotics. Hearing is also evaluated periodically during the course of therapy to detect any hearing loss.

Medications

Chemotherapeutic medications are used to both prevent and treat tuberculosis infection. Goals of the pharmacologic treatment of TB are to:

- Make the disease noncommunicable to others.
- Reduce symptoms of the disease.
- Effect a cure in the shortest possible time.

Prophylactic treatment is used to prevent active tuberculosis. Clients with a recent skin test conversion from negative to positive are often started on prophylactic therapy, especially when other risk factors are present. Prophylactic therapy is also used for people in close household contact with a person whose sputum is positive for bacilli. Single-drug therapy is effective for prophylactic treatment, whereas treatment of active disease always involves two or more chemotherapeutic medications. For adults, isoniazid (INH), 300 mg per day for a period of 6 to 12 months, is commonly used to prevent active TB.

When isoniazid prophylaxis is contraindicted, bacilli Calmette-Guérin (BCG) vaccine may be prescribed. This vaccine is widely used in developing countries. BCG is made from an attenuated strain of *M. bovis,* a closely related bacillus that causes tuberculosis in cattle. In the United States, BCG vaccine is recommended only for infants, children, and health care workers with a negative tuberculin test who are repeatedly exposed to untreated or ineffectively treated people with active disease. After vaccination with BCG, a positive reaction to tuberculin testing is common. Periodic chest X-rays may be required for screening purposes.

The tuberculosis bacillus mutates readily to drug-resistant forms when only one anti-infective agent is used. Active disease is always treated with concurrent use of at least two antibacterial medications to which the organism is sensitive. The primary antituberculosis drugs can prevent development of resistance because all act by different mechanisms. However, the organism is protected within the tubercule, and six or more months of treatment is necessary to eradicate it.

Newly diagnosed tuberculosis is typically treated with an initial regimen of three oral antitubercular drugs, isoniazid (INH), rifampin, and pyrazinamide, daily for the first two months of treatment. This initial regimen is followed by at least four additional months of therapy with isoniazid and rifampin, given daily or two or three times weekly. In the presence of HIV infection, treatment is continued for at least nine months.

If a drug-resistant strain is suspected, therapy is tailored to the resistance. In some cases, four or more anti-infective drugs may be used.

Antitubercular medications have many adverse and toxic effects. Close monitoring during therapy is necessary. Most have some degree of, or risk for, hepatotoxicity. For this reason, clients should avoid using alcohol and other drugs, such as acetaminophen, or chemicals that can damage the liver. Baseline liver and renal function studies are done prior to initiating therapy. Audiometric testing may also be done before treatment is started, because several commonly used medications can affect hearing. Regular visits to a health care provider are necessary to evaluate regularly for adverse effects. Although none of these drugs have been proved to be teratogenic, potential adverse effects on the fetus are weighed against the benefit to the mother before they are prescribed during pregnancy.

Compliance with the prescribed regimen is also evaluated during follow-up visits. The urine can be examined for color changes characteristic of rifampin and tested for metabolites of

INH. When compliance is a problem, medications are administered under direct supervision. Twice-weekly therapy is more cost-effective in this instance, with a public health nurse watching the client take and swallow the prescribed medication.

Repeat sputum specimens and chest X-rays are used to evaluate the effectiveness of therapy. In most cases, sputum cultures for *M. tuberculosis* are negative within two months of therapy; virtually all clients have negative sputum cultures within three months. If cultures remain positive at three months and beyond, treatment failure and drug resistance are suspected. In this case, cultures of the organism are tested for susceptibility to antitubercular agents, and two or three previously unused drugs are added to the treatment regimen (Braunwald et al., 2001).

With adherence to prescribed treatment, virtually all clients should have negative sputum cultures for *M. tuberculosis* within 3 months. The relapse rate for current treatment regimens is less than 5%. The principal cause of treatment failure is noncompliance (Tierney, et al., 2001).

Table 15-3. Medication Administration — Antituberculosis Drugs

Isoniazid (INH, Laniazid, Nydrazid)

Isoniazid is the drug of choice for tuberculosis prophylaxis and a first-line drug for treating active disease. It is effective against both intracellular and extracellular organisms. Isoniazid is used alone as a prophylactic medication, and in combination with rifampin, ethambutol, or both. A fixed-dose combination form with 150 mg of INH and 300 mg of rifampin (Rifamate) is available as well.

Nursing Responsibilities
- Administer on an empty stomach one hour before or two hours after meals for maximal effect if tolerated; May be given with meals to reduce gastrointestinal effects.
- Monitor for adverse effects.
  a. Numbness and tingling of the extremities (most likely to occur in malnourished, alcoholic, or diabetic clients).
  b. Hepatotoxicity, as evidenced by abnormal liver function studies and scleral jaundice.
  c. Hypersensitivity reactions, such as rash, drug fever, or evidence of anemia, bruising, bleeding, or infection related to agranulocytosis.
- Isoniazid interferes with the metabolism of diazepam (Valium), phenytoin (Dilantin), and carbamazepine. Doses of these drugs may need to be reduced to prevent toxicity.

Client and Family Teaching
- Take the medication as prescribed for the entire treatment period to prevent incomplete eradication of the bacteria and development of resistant strains.
- Take the medication on an empty stomach. If nausea and vomiting occur, take with meals.
- If anorexia, nausea, vomiting, and jaundice (yellowing of the skin and the whites of the eyes) develop, notify your doctor immediately.
- Take pyridoxine as prescribed to prevent peripheral neuropathy.
- Avoid alcohol and other agents that may be harmful to the liver.

Continued on the next page

Table 15-3. Continued

- Notify your doctor if you develop signs of an allergic reaction, such as rash, fever, easy bruising, bleeding gums, or fatigue.
- Use measures to prevent pregnancy while taking INH; this drug may be harmful to the developing fetus.

Rifampin (Rifadin, Rimactane)

Rifampin is commonly used in combination with INH and other antitubercular drugs. It is relatively low in toxicity, although it can cause hepatitis, a flulike immune response, and, rarely, renal failure. Rifampin stimulates the microsomal enzymes of the liver, increasing the rate of metabolism of many drugs and decreasing their effectiveness.

Nursing Responsibilities
- Administer on an empty stomach.
- Monitor CBC, liver function studies, and renal function studies for evidence of toxicity.
- Rifampin reduces the effect of oral contraceptives, quinidine, corticosteroids, warfarin, methadone, digoxin, and hypoglycemics. Monitor for the effectiveness of these drugs.

Client and Family Teaching
- Rifampin causes body fluids, including sweat, urine, saliva, and tears, to turn red-orange. This is not harmful. Avoid wearing soft contact lenses because they may be permanently stained.
- Aspirin may interfere with rifampin absorption and should not be taken concurrently.
- Fever, flulike symptoms, excessive fatigue, sore throat, or unusual bleeding may indicate an adverse reaction to the drug and should be reported to your doctor.

Pyrazinamide (Tebrazid)

Pyrazinamide typically is given with INH and rifampin for the first two months of tuberculosis treatment. Concurrent use of pyrazinamide allows a shorter course of therapy. As with many of the antitubercular agents, pyrazinamide is toxic to the liver. Its other principal adverse effect is hyperuricemia. Gout, however, rarely develops.

Nursing Responsibilities
- Administer with meals to reduce gastrointestinal side effects.
- Monitor liver function studies and serum uric acid levels. Notify the physician if changes are noted.

Client and Family Teaching
- Notify your doctor if you develop loss of appetite, nausea, vomiting, jaundice, or symptoms of gout (a painful, red, hot, swollen joint, often the great toe or elbow).
- While taking this drug, avoid using alcohol or other substances that may be harmful to the liver.

Ethambutol (Myambutol)

Ethambutol is added to the initial treatment regimen or substituted for INH, when an INH-resistant strain of TB is suspected. Ethambutol is a bacteriostatic drug that reduces the development of resistance to the bactericidal first-line agents. Its principal toxic effect

Table 15-3. Continued

is optic neuritis; fortunately, this is reversible. Early signs of optic neuritis include decreased visual acuity and loss of red-green discrimination. This drug may be safe for use in pregnancy.

Nursing Responsibilities
- Record a baseline visual examination prior to therapy. Schedule periodic eye exams during the course of treatment.
- Administer with meals to reduce gastrointestinal side effects.
- Monitor liver and renal function studies and neurologic status while taking this drug. Notify the physician of abnormal findings or significant changes.

Client and Family Teaching
- Monitor vision daily by reading newspapers and looking at the same blue object (using usual corrective lenses, if appropriate). Notify your doctor if changes in vision or color perception occur.

Streptomycin

An aminoglycoside antibiotic, streptomycin is highly effective in treating most mycobacterial infection. Resistance may develop if it is used alone. There are two primary drawbacks to streptomycin: (1) It must be administered parenterally because it is not absorbed in the gastrointestinal tract, and (2) it has toxic effects on the kidneys and ears.

Nursing Responsibilities
- Administer by deep intramuscular injection into a large muscle mass, rotating sites to minimize tissue trauma.
- Monitor urine output, weight, and renal function studies (including BUN and serum creatinine) to detect early signs of nephrotoxicity. Report significant changes to the physician.
- Maintain fluid intake at 2000 to 3000 mL per day to minimize the concentration of drug in the kidney tubules.
- Assess hearing and balance frequently. Have audiometric testing performed as indicated.

Client and Family Teaching
- Maintain a daily fluid intake of at least two to three quarts.
- Weigh yourself on the same scale at least twice a week; report any significant weight gain to your doctor.
- Notify your doctor if hearing acuity decreases, ringing or buzzing sensations in the ear develop, or dizziness occurs.

Nursing Care

Health Promotion

Tuberculosis today presents a greater threat to public health than it does to individuals. Nurses play a key role in maintaining public health. Education and tuberculosis screening are major nursing strategies to prevent TB. Public health teaching includes increasing awareness of tuberculosis as a reemerging threat. Teach clients in all settings how to reduce the spread of

TB by covering their mouths when coughing or sneezing and disposing of sputum appropriately. The benefit of screening programs to identify infected (though not necessarily infective) people also needs to be included in public health education.

The best tuberculosis prevention is early diagnosis of infections and appropriate treatment to achieve cure. BCG vaccine is recommended for infants born in countries where tuberculosis is prevalent, but is not widely used in the United States. It may be administered to health care workers in settings where the risk of infection with MDR strains of *M. tb* is high despite rigorous infection control measures (Braunwald, et al., 2001).

The primary preventive strategy used in the United States is treating people with latent tuberculosis infection demonstrated by a positive tuberculin test. A 9- to 10-month course of treatment with isoniazid reduces the risk of active TB by 90% or more (Braunwald, et al., 2001). Isoniazid is also prescribed prophylactically for people with HIV infection who have been exposed to TB.

Assessment

Focused assessment for the client with suspected TB includes the following:

- *Health history:* complaints of fatigue, weight loss, night sweats, difficulty breathing, cough (productive or nonproductive), bloody sputum, or chest pain; known exposure to TB; most recent tuberculin test and results; living circumstances; alcohol and other recreational drug use.

- *Physical examination:* vital signs including temperature; general appearance; respiratory rate and lung sounds.

Nursing Diagnoses and Interventions

Nursing care related to tuberculosis focuses primarily on infection control and compliance with prescribed treatment.

Deficient Knowledge

Adequate knowledge and information are necessary to manage the disease and prevent its transmission to others. The client needs to understand reasons for prolonged drug therapy and the importance of complying with treatment and follow-up. Antituberculosis drugs are relatively toxic. The client needs to know how to minimize toxicity.

- Assess knowledge about the disease process; identify misperceptions and emotional reactions. *Teaching based on previous learning enhances understanding and retention of information.*

- Assess ability and interest in learning, developmental level, and obstacles to learning. *Assessment allows presentation of information in a manner tailored to the learning needs and style of the client, promoting understanding.*

- Identify support systems, and include partners and other family members in teaching. *A knowledgeable partner provides reinforcement of learning, confirmation of understanding, and encouragement for the client. Including partners also reduces the risk of inadvertent sabotage of the treatment plan.*

- Establish a relationship of mutual trust with the client and partners. *An atmosphere of trust increases receptiveness to teaching and learning.*

- Develop mutually acceptable learning goals with the client and partner. *Working together to identify learning needs and establish goals increases the client's "ownership" and interest in the process.*
- Select appropriate teaching strategies, using learning aids, such as literature and visual materials, that are appropriate for age, level of education, and intellect. *Teaching tailored to the client is more effective and results in better learning.*
- Teach about tuberculosis and the prescribed treatment, including:
  a. Nature of the disease and its spread.
  b. Purpose of treatment and follow-up procedures.
  c. Measures to prevent spreading the disease to others.
  d. Importance of maintaining good general health by eating a well-balanced, high-protein, high-carbohydrate diet; balancing exercise with rest; and avoiding crowds and people with upper respiratory infections.
  e. Names, doses, purposes, and adverse effects of prescribed medications.
  f. Importance of avoiding alcohol and other substances that may damage the liver while taking chemotherapeutic drugs.
  g. Fluid intake needs of 2.5 to 3.0 quarts of fluid per day.
  h. Manifestations to report to the physician: chest pain, hemoptysis, difficulty breathing; anorexia, nausea, or vomiting; yellow tint to skin or sclera; sudden weight gain, swollen feet, ankles, legs, or hands; hearing loss, tinnitus, or vertigo; change in vision or difficulty discriminating colors.

Tuberculosis is a chronic disease requiring lengthy treatment with antitubercular medications. A good understanding of the disease, its treatment, and potential adverse effects of therapy prepares the client to manage care.

- Document teaching and level of understanding. Reinforce teaching and learning as needed. *Teaching is not complete until the client can demonstrate learning of the information.*

Ineffective Therapeutic Regimen Management

The populations at highest risk for developing active tuberculosis—the homeless and members of lower socioeconomic groups—are also at high risk for being unable to manage its complex treatment regimen. Three or more costly medications that may have unpleasant, or even dangerous, side effects are prescribed. Frequent medical follow-up is required. Infectious diseases, such as TB, carry a stigma that may lead to denial of the disease or its seriousness. Alcoholics and IV drug users need to withdraw from their addiction to be successful in treating the disease. The client with HIV infection faces a potentially fatal disease and costly treatment that may well override concerns about tuberculosis management.

- Assess self-care abilities and support systems. *Assessment is used to help determine the client's ability to follow the prescribed regimen.*
- Assess knowledge and understanding of the disease, its complications, treatment, and risks to others. Provide additional teaching and reinforcement as indicated. *Lack of understanding is a barrier to compliance with, and management of, the treatment regimen.*
- Work collaboratively to identify barriers or obstacles to managing the prescribed treatment. *Working collaboratively with the client and other members of the health care team provides insight for overcoming identified barriers to effective treatment.*

- Assist the client, partners (if available), and health care team members to develop a plan for managing the prescribed regimen. *Including the client in developing a plan to manage care increases the sense of control and ownership and helps ensure that personal, cultural, and lifestyle factors are considered. This increases the likelihood of compliance.*

- Provide verbal and written instructions that are clear and appropriate for level of literacy, knowledge, and understanding. *Clearly written directions provide support and reinforcement for the client.*

- Provide active intervention for homeless people, including shelter placement or other housing, and ongoing follow-up by easily accessed health care providers (clinics and public health workers in the neighborhood that do not present transportation or access problems, either real or perceived). *Simple referral will not ensure compliance, especially among disenfranchised populations. Active intervention is needed to help ensure treatment compliance.*

- Refer clients who are unlikely to comply with the treatment regimen to the public health department for management and follow-up. *Because tuberculosis presents a significant public health risk, public health follow-up is essential. In some cases, it is necessary for nurses to administer medications, observing the client swallow all pills.*

Risk for Infection

The spread of tuberculosis is a risk in any facility housing many people. It is especially high in residential care facilities for older clients and for people with AIDS. The increasing incidence of TB among homeless people and members of lower socioeconomic groups increases the risk in hospitals, emergency departments, and public and urgent care clinics. Respiratory precautions are necessary to prevent the spread of TB via microscopic airborne droplets to other clients and to health care workers.

- Place the client in a private room with airflow control that prevents air within the room from circulating into the hallway or other rooms. A negative flow room in which air is diluted by at least six fresh-air exchanges per hour is recommended. *A negative flow room and multiple fresh-air exchanges dilute the concentration of droplet nuclei within the room and prevent their spread to adjacent areas.*

- Use standard precautions and tuberculosis isolation techniques as recommended by the CDC, including wearing masks and gowns when caring for clients who do not reliably cover the mouth when coughing. *These measures are important to prevent the spread of tuberculosis to others.*

- Discuss the reasons for and importance of respiratory isolation procedures during initial hospitalization. When treatment is provided as an outpatient, instruct to avoid crowds and close physical contact and maintain ventilation in living facilities, particularly during the first three weeks of treatment. *These measures help protect others during initial treatment, when sputum is still likely to contain significant numbers of bacilli.*

- Place a mask on the client when transporting to other parts of the facility for diagnostic or treatment procedures. *Covering the client's nose and mouth during transport minimizes air contamination and the risk to visitors and personnel.*

- Inform all personnel having contact with the client of the diagnosis. *This allows personnel to take appropriate precautions.*

- Assist visitors to mask prior to entering the room. *Providing visitors with appropriate masks or respirators reduces their risk of infection.*

- Teach the client how to limit transmitting the disease to others:
  a. Always cough and expectorate into tissues.
  b. Dispose of tissues properly, placing them in a closed bag.
  c. Wear a mask if you are sneezing or unable to control respiratory secretions.
  d. The disease is not spread by touching inanimate objects, so no special precautions are required for eating utensils, clothing, books, or other objects used.

Teaching appropriate precautions helps prevent the spread of tuberculosis to others while allowing as much freedom from restraints as possible.

- Teach how to collect sputum specimens. If necessary, have the client step outside to collect a sputum specimen. *This minimizes the risk of exposure to health care personnel and provides for rapid dilution of any droplet nuclei produced and their exposure to ultraviolet light (which kills the bacteria).*
- Teach the importance of complying with prescribed treatment for the entire course of therapy. *Completion of the entire treatment regimen is important to reduce the risk of relapse and creation of drug-resistant organisms.*

Home Care

Most clients with TB are managed in community settings; few require institutionalization. In addition to the teaching topics and strategies identified above, discuss the following topics when preparing the client and significant others for home care:

- Importance of screening close contacts for infection and possibly prophylactic treatment
- Effect, dose, and timing for all medications, and potential side effects and their management
- Importance of long-term therapy in eradicating the disease
- Principles of good nutrition, dietary guidelines for a client with TB, and other measures to help maintain good health, such as balancing rest with exercise
- Signs and symptoms of complications to report to the physician or health care provider.

Provide referrals as appropriate:

- Smoking cessation clinics or support groups
- Alcohol treatment facilities, Alcoholics Anonymous, other treatment programs or support groups
- Drug treatment facilities, Narcotics Anonymous, other outpatient or inpatient treatment programs or support groups
- Low-cost community clinics and incentive programs for people with TB
- Counseling, support groups, and other community resources that provide additional assistance and support.

The Client with Inhalation Anthrax

Inhalation anthrax is a relatively new potential threat in the United States. This disease rarely affects humans in nature, even though both wild and domestic animals can be infected. However, *Bacillus anthracis,* the spore-forming rod responsible for causing anthrax, has been identified as an agent likely to be used as a biologic weapon. Anthrax spores can be aerosolized so they remain suspended in the air, allowing them to be inhaled into the lungs. Person-to-person transmission does not occur.

Inhalation anthrax causes initial flulike symptoms, including malaise, dry cough, and fever. This is followed by an abrupt onset of severe dyspnea, stridor, and cyanosis. Lymph nodes in the mediastinum and thorax become inflamed and enlarged. Septic shock and/or meningitis may develop. Untreated, death results from hemorrhagic thoracic lymphadenitis and hemorrhagic mediastinitis (Persell, et al., 2002).

Blood cultures and chest X-ray are used to diagnose inhalation anthrax. However, because death can quickly result from the disease, people who are known or suspected to have been exposed to anthrax spores often are treated prophylactically. Ciprofloxacin (Cipro) is used to both prevent and treat inhalation anthrax. Doxycycline (Vibramycin) is an alternative to ciprofloxacin. Although an anthrax vaccine exists, its use at this time is considered experimental (Persell, et al., 2002). See the section on bioterrorism in Chapter 41 for more information about anthrax and the section of this chapter on respiratory failure for nursing care measures for the client with inhalation anthrax.

The Client with a Fungal Infection

Fungal spores are endemic, present in the air everyone breathes. Normal respiratory defense mechanisms allow few of these spores to reach the lungs. If they reach the lungs, pulmonary macrophages and neutrophils efficiently remove them in most people. When they do cause infection, it is typically mild and self-limiting. Most fungi are opportunistic, able to cause infection only in people who are immunocompromised. For this reason, clients with AIDS, renal failure, leukemia, burns, or chronic diseases, as well as people receiving corticosteroids or immunosuppressants, are particularly susceptible to fungal diseases.

Many fungal lung diseases have a geographic distribution pattern. Histoplasmosis and blastomycosis are more common in the southeastern, mid-Atlantic, and central states. California, Arizona, and western Texas are the primary sites for coccidioidomycosis, also known as San Joaquin valley fever (Braunwald, et al., 2001).

The course and manifestations of fungal lung diseases resemble those of tuberculosis. Lung lesions are slow to develop, and symptoms are mild. The fungus can disseminate from the lung to other organs.

Pathophysiology

Histoplasmosis

Histoplasmosis, an infectious disease caused by *Histoplasma capsulatum,* is the most common fungal lung infection in the United States. The organism is found in the soil and is linked to exposure to bird droppings and bats. Infection occurs when the spores are inhaled and reach the alveoli. Most infections develop into *latent asymptomatic disease,* much like tuberculosis, or *primary acute histoplasmosis,* a mild, self-limiting influenzalike illness. Initial chest X-rays are nonspecific; later ones show areas of calcification. *Chronic progressive disease,* usually seen in older adults, typically is limited to the lung but may involve any organ. Progressive lung changes and cavitation occur, with increasing dyspnea and eventual disabling pulmonary disease.

Regional lymph vessels spread the organism from the lungs to other parts of the body, much like the process that occurs in tuberculosis. In the healthy host, normal immune responses inactivate and remove the organism. In the immunocompromised host, however, macrophages remove the fungi, but are unable to destroy them, resulting in *disseminated histoplasmosis*. This type of histoplasmosis is often fatal. Manifestations of fever, dyspnea, cough, weight loss, and muscle wasting are usual. Ulcerations of the mouth and oropharynx may be present, and the liver and spleen are enlarged.

Coccidioidomycosis

Coccidioidomycosis is an infectious disease caused by the fungus *Coccidioides immitis*. This mold grows in the soil of the arid Southwest, Mexico, and Central and South America. When inhaled, the fungus typically causes an acute, self-limiting pulmonary infection that often is asymptomatic and goes unrecognized. If manifestations do occur, they resemble those of influenza, with malaise, fever, body aches, and cough. Pleuritic pain, skin rash, and arthritis of the knees and ankles may also develop. Disseminated disease, which may affect the lymph nodes, meninges, spleen, liver, kidney, skin, and adrenal glands, is rare in immunocompetent people. When it does occur, the mortality rate is high. Meningitis is the usual cause of death.

Blastomycosis

The fungus *Blastomyces dermatitidis* causes the infectious disease blastomycosis. It occurs primarily in the south central and midwestern regions of the United States and in Canada. Men are affected more frequently than women. The lungs are the primary site for the disease, although it may spread to involve the skin, bones, genitourinary system, and, rarely, the central nervous system. Pulmonary symptoms include fever, dyspnea, pleuritic chest pain, and cough, which may become productive of bloody or purulent sputum. If untreated, the disseminated disease is slowly progressive and ultimately fatal.

Aspergillosis

Aspergillus spores are common in the environment, but rarely cause disease except in the immunocompromised. When they do cause infection, *Aspergillus* species invade blood vessels and produce hyphae that branch at acute angles, frequently causing venous or arterial thrombosis. In the lungs, aspergillosis can cause an acute, diffuse, self-limited pneumonitis. The manifestations of pulmonary aspergillosis include dyspnea, nonproductive cough, pleuritic chest pain, chills, and fever. If the organism invades a pulmonary blood vessel, hemoptysis or massive pulmonary hemorrhage can occur. In clients with underlying lung disease, balls of *Aspergillus* hyphae may form within cysts or cavities, usually in the upper lobes of the lung. Symptoms often are milder and more insidious in onset, with fever, weight loss, night sweats, and cough (Braunwald, et al., 2001; Morrison & Lew, 2001).

Collaborative Care

Most fungal lung infections can be diagnosed by microscopic examination of a sputum specimen for the fungus. Blood cultures also may be done, as well as cultures of cerebrospinal fluid if indicated. Chest X-ray may show typical changes in lung tissue or widening of the mediastinum, depending on the infecting organism.

Acute pulmonary histoplasmosis and acute pulmonary coccidioidomycosis usually resolve without treatment, although antifungal drugs may be given to shorten the disease course. Oral itraconazole (Sporanox), a broad-spectrum antifungal agent, is commonly prescribed to treat histoplasmosis. Other fungal lung diseases and clients who are immunocompromised are often treated with intravenous amphotericin B. Surgery (lobectomy) may be indicated for clients with severe hemoptysis associated with aspergillosis.

Nursing Care

Clients with fungal lung infections have different nursing care needs, depending on the disease and their immune status. For most clients, nursing care focuses on education. People living in high-prevalence areas or who have specific risk factors, such as exposure to bird droppings (e.g., cleaning chicken coops, pigeon lofts, or barns where birds roost), decomposed vegetation, rotting wood, or stored grain, need to be aware of the risk, common symptoms, and measures to reduce the risk. Clients with latent histoplasmosis may need education to maintain good general health to prevent reactivation. Teach clients receiving antifungal drugs about the specific drug, its intended and adverse effects, the duration of therapy, and symptoms to report to the physician. Include teaching about any specific precautions such as drug or food interactions. Itraconazole interacts with many medications; verify the safety of concurrent usage with all other prescribed drugs. Its use is contraindicated during pregnancy and lactation; emphasize the importance of effective birth control and of notifying the physician immediately if pregnancy occurs. Amphotericin B is a toxic drug. Administer the intial intravenous dose slowly after premedicating with an antihistamine and antiemetic as ordered to manage its adverse effects. Monitor carefully during infusion and therapy for changes in vital signs, hydration, nutrition, weight, or urine output.

Obstructive Disorders of the Airways

Many pulmonary disorders and diseases can affect the airways. Although their pathophysiology differs, these diseases are characterized by limited airflow. Airflow is limited when:

- Elastic recoil of the lungs is reduced, decreasing the force to push air out.
- Airway lumen are obstructed by secretions, increasing resistance.
- Airway walls are thickened.
- Smooth muscle of the airways is activated, causing bronchoconstriction.
- Interstitial support necessary to maintain airway distention and patency is lost.

Aging contributes to airflow limitation. The number of alveoli decrease, and emphysematous changes (senile emphysema) reduce the surface area for gas exchange. Alveoli become less elastic, causing increased air trapping and dead space.

Limited airflow increases the work of breathing and the residual volume of the lungs as air is trapped behind narrowed or collapsed airways. Inspired air mixes with an abnormally large volume of residual air, effectively reducing the amount of oxygen available in the alveoli. Decreased alveolar ventilation further reduces oxygen available for exchange.

The Client with Asthma

Asthma is a chronic inflammatory disorder of the airways characterized by recurrent episodes of wheezing, breathlessness, chest tightness, and coughing. Inflammation causes increased responsiveness of the airways to multiple stimuli. The widespread airflow obstruction that occurs during acute episodes usually reverses either spontaneously or with treatment.

In the United States, approximately 11 million people experienced at least one asthma attack in the year 2000. Although it is more common in children than adults, about 4% of the adult population is affected. After several years of increase, the prevalence of asthma currently is relatively stable. Asthma is a serious disease, causing more than 4000 deaths in the United States in 1999. Mortality due to asthma is higher in African-Americans than in Caucasians, and higher in females than in males (NHLBI, 2002).

A number of risk factors can be identified for asthma, although many clients develop the disease in the absence of known risk factors. Allergies play a strong role in childhood asthma, although less so in adults. There is a strong genetic component to the disease, although a specific pattern of inheritance has not been identified. Environmental factors, including air pollution and occupational exposure to industrial compounds, may contribute. Respiratory viruses, such as rhinovirus and influenza, can precipitate asthma attacks. Other contributory factors include exercise (particularly in cold air) and emotional stress.

Physiology Review

Airways within the lungs contain crisscrossing strips of smooth muscle that control their diameter. This muscle is innervated by the autonomic nervous system. Parasympathetic (cholinergic) stimulation leads to bronchoconstriction, or narrowing of the airways. Sympathetic stimulation through b_2-adrenergic receptors causes bronchodilation, or expansion of the airways. Slight bronchoconstriction normally predominates. However, when increased airflow is necessary (e.g., during exercise), the parasympathetic system is inhibited, and stimulation of the sympathetic system causes bronchodilation. Inflammatory mediators, such as histamine, released during an antigen-antibody response act directly on bronchial smooth muscle to produce bronchoconstriction.

Pathophysiology

During symptom-free periods, airway inflammation in asthma is subacute or quiet. An acute inflammatory response may be triggered by a variety of factors. Common triggers for an acute asthma attack include exposure to allergens, respiratory tract infection, exercise, inhaled irritants, and emotional upsets.

Childhood asthma (which may continue into adulthood) is most often linked to inhalation of allergens, such as pollen, animal dander, or household dust. Clients with allergic asthma often have a history of other allergies. Environmental pollutants, such as tobacco smoke and irritant gases (e.g., sulfur dioxide, nitrogen dioxide, and ozone), can provoke asthma. Exposure to secondhand smoke as a child is associated with a higher risk for and increased severity of asthma. Agents found in the workplace, such as noxious fumes and gases, chemicals, and dusts, may cause occupational asthma.

Respiratory infections, viral in particular, are a common internal stimulus for an asthmatic attack. Exercise-induced asthma attacks are also common, affecting 40% to 90% of people with bronchial asthma (Porth, 2002). Loss of heat or water from the bronchial surface may contribute to exercise-induced asthma. Exercising in cold, dry air increases the risk of an asthma attack in susceptible people.

Emotional stress is a significant etiologic factor for attacks in as many as half of clients with asthma. Common pharmacologic triggers include aspirin and other NSAIDs, sulfites (which are used as preservatives in wine, beer, fresh fruits, and salad), and beta blockers.

When a trigger such as inhalation of an allergen or irritant, occurs, an *acute* or *early response* develops in the hyperreactive airways predisposed to bronchospasm. Sensitized mast cells in the bronchial mucosa release inflammatory mediators, such as histamine, prostaglandins, and leukotrienes. These mediators stimulate parasympathetic receptors and bronchial smooth muscle to produce bronchoconstriction. They also increase capillary permeability, leading to mucosal edema, and stimulate mucus production.

The attack is prolonged by the *late phase response,* which develops 4 to 12 hours after exposure to the trigger. Inflammatory cells, such as basophils and eosinophils, are activated, which damage airway epithelium, produce mucosal edema, impair mucociliary clearance, and produce or prolong bronchoconstriction. The degree of hyperreactivity depends on the extent of inflammation. Together, bronchoconstriction, edema and inflammation, and mucous secretion narrow the airway. Airway resistance increases, limiting airflow, and increasing the work of breathing.

Limited expiratory airflow traps air distal to the spastic airways. Trapped air mixes with inspired air in the alveoli, reducing its oxygen tension and gas exchange across the alveolar-capillary membrane. Blood flow is reduced to distended alveoli, further affecting gas exchange. As a result, hypoxemia develops. Hypoxemia and increased lung volume due to trapping stimulate the respiratory rate. As a result, the $PaCO_2$ falls, leading to respiratory alkalosis. (See Chapter 5 for more information about acid-base imbalances.)

Manifestations and Complications

An asthma attack is characterized by a subjective sensation of chest tightness, dyspnea, wheezing, and cough (see previous section). The onset of symptoms may be either abrupt or insidious, and an attack may subside rapidly or persist for hours or days. During an attack, tachycardia, tachypnea, and prolonged expiration are common. Diffuse wheezing is heard on auscultation. With more severe attacks, use of accessory muscles of respiration, intercostal retractions, loud wheezing, and distant breath sounds may be noted. Fatigue, anxiety, apprehension, and severe dyspnea that allows speaking only one or two words between breaths, may occur with persistent severe episodes. The onset of respiratory failure is marked by inaudible breath sounds with reduced wheezing and an ineffective cough. Without careful assessment, this apparent relief of symptoms can be misinterpreted as an improvement.

The frequency of attacks and severity of symptoms vary greatly from person to person. Although some people have infrequent, mild episodes, others have nearly continuous manifestations of cough and wheezing with periodic severe exacerbations.

Status asthmaticus is severe, prolonged asthma that does not respond to routine treatment. Without aggressive therapy, status asthmaticus can lead to respiratory failure with hypoxemia, hypercapnia, and acidosis. Endotracheal intubation, mechanical ventilation, and aggressive drug treatment may be necessary to sustain life.

In addition to acute respiratory failure, other complications associated with acute asthma include dehydration, respiratory infection, atelectasis, pneumothorax, and cor pulmonale.

Collaborative Care

The diagnosis of asthma is based primarily on the history and manifestations. Treatment goals are twofold. Daily management focuses on controlling symptoms and preventing acute attacks. During an acute attack, therapy is directed toward restoring airway patency and alveolar ventilation.

Diagnostic Tests

Diagnostic tests are used to determine the degree of airway involvement during and between acute episodes and identify causative factors, such as allergens.

- *Pulmonary function tests (PFTs)* are used to evaluate the degree of airway obstruction. Pulmonary function testing done before and after use of an aerosolized bronchodilator helps determine the reversibility of airway obstruction. The residual volume (RV) of the lungs may be increased, and vital capacity decreased or normal, even during periods of remission. The forced expiratory volume (FEV_1) and peak expiratory flow rate (PEFR) are the most valuable pulmonary function studies to evaluate the severity of an asthma attack and the effectiveness of treatment measures. See Table 15-4.

- *Challenge or bronchial provocation testing* uses an inhaled substance, such as methacholine or histamine, with PFTs to confirm the diagnosis of asthma by detecting airway hyperresponsiveness.

- *ABGs* are drawn during an acute attack to evaluate oxygenation, carbon dioxide elimination, and acid-base status. ABGs initially show hypoxemia with a low Po_2, and mild respiratory alkalosis with an elevated pH and low Pco_2 due to tachypnea. Severe airflow obstruction causes significant hypoxemia and respiratory acidosis (pH less than 7.35 and Pco_2 greater than 42 mmHg), indicative of respiratory failure and the need for mechanical ventilation.

- *Skin testing* may be done to identify specific allergens if an allergic trigger is suspected for asthma attacks.

Disease Monitoring *Peak expiratory flow rate (PEFR)* is used on a day-to-day basis to evaluate the severity of bronchial hyperresponsiveness. Small, inexpensive meters to measure PEFR are available. Readings taken at varying times of day over several weeks are used to establish the client's personal best or normal PEFR. This value is then used to evaluate the severity of airway obstruction. Traffic signal colors are used for simplicity: *green* (80% to 100% of personal best) indicates asthma that is under control; *yellow* (50% to 80%) is caution, indicating a need for further medication or treatment; and *red* (50% or less) signals an immediate need for a bronchodilator and medical treatment if the level does not immediately return to the yellow range (Porth, 2002).

Preventive Measures

Asthma attacks often can be prevented by avoiding allergens and environmental triggers. Modifying the home environment by controlling dust, removing carpets, covering mattresses and pillows to reduce dust mite populations, and installing air filtering systems may be useful. Pets may need to be removed from the household. Eliminating all tobacco smoke in the home is vital. Wearing a mask that retains humidity and warm air while exercising in cold weather may help prevent attacks of exercise-induced asthma. Early treatment of respiratory infections is vital to prevent asthma exacerbations.

Medications

Medications are used to prevent and control asthma symptoms, reduce the frequency and severity of exacerbations, and reverse airway obstruction. Drugs used for long-term control of asthma are taken daily to maintain control of the disease. The primary drugs in this group are anti-inflammatory agents, long-acting bronchodilators, and leukotriene modifiers. Quick-relief medications provide prompt relief of bronchoconstriction and airflow obstruction with associated wheezing, cough, and chest tightness. Short-acting adrenergic stimulants (rapid-acting bronchodilators), anticholinergic drugs, and methylxanthines fall into this category.

Bronchodilators

Most asthmatics need bronchodilator therapy to control their symptoms. Inhalation of nebulized medication is the preferred means of administration. The primary bronchodilators used include adrenergic stimulants, methylxanthines, and anticholinergic agents.

Adrenergic stimulants affect receptors on smooth muscle cells of the respiratory tract, causing smooth muscle relaxation and bronchodilation. Long-acting adrenergic stimulants, such as inhaled salmeterol and oral sustained-release albuterol, are used in conjunction with anti-inflammatory drugs to control symptoms, but are not appropriate to treat an acute episode of asthma. Inhaled short-acting beta-adrenergic agonists such as albuterol, bitolterol, pirbuterol, and terbutaline, administered by metered-dose inhalers (MDIs), are the treatment of choice for quick relief. They act within minutes, but their duration generally is short, lasting only four to six hours. Tachycardia and muscle tremors, common side effects of adrenergic agonists, are minimal with inhalation therapy.

Anticholinergic medications prevent bronchoconstriction by blocking parasympathetic input to bronchial smooth muscle. Ipratropium bromide, an anticholinergic drug administered by metered-dose inhaler, is useful when asthma symptoms are poorly controlled by adrenergic stimulants alone. Anticholinergic drugs act more slowly than adrenergic stimulants, requiring up to 60 to 90 minutes to achieve maximal effect.

Theophylline is a methylxanthine used as adjunctive treatment for asthma. It relaxes bronchial smooth muscle and may also inhibit the release of chemical mediators of the inflammatory response. Monitoring of serum theophylline levels is necessary because of wide individual variations in metabolism and elimination of the drug and its toxic effects. Serum levels of 10 to 20 μg/mL or lower are recommended. Theophylline may be used as a long-term bronchodilator, given once or twice daily. A related drug, aminophylline, may be administered intravenously to treat an acute, severe exacerbation of the disease.

Anti-Inflammatory Agents

Corticosteroids and two nonsteroidal anti-inflammatory agents, cromolyn sodium and nedocromil, are used to suppress airway inflammation and reduce asthma symptoms.

Corticosteroids block the late response to inhaled allergens and reduce bronchial hyperresponsiveness. The preferred route of administration is by metered-dose inhaler to minimize systemic absorption and reduce the adverse effects of prolonged steroid use (cushingoid effects). For a severe acute attack, corticosteroids may be given systemically to alleviate symptoms and induce remission.

Cromolyn sodium and nedocromil are used to prevent acute episodes of asthma. They reduce airway hyperreactivity and inhibit the release of mediator substances. These drugs are used for long-term control of asthma, not quick relief. They have a wide margin of safety and few side effects.

Leukotriene Modifiers

Leukotriene modifiers, zafirlukast (Accolate) and zileuton (Zyflo Filmtab), are new oral medications that reduce the inflammatory response in asthma. They appear to improve lung function, diminish symptoms, and reduce the need for short-acting bronchodilators. These drugs affect the metabolism and excretion of other medications, such as warfarin and theophylline, and may cause liver toxicity.

Nursing implications for medications used to treat asthma are outlined in Table 15-4.

Complementary Therapies

A number of herbal preparations and other complementary therapies have been shown to be helpful in treating asthma. Herbal preparations may include atopa belladonna (the natural form of atropine) or ephedra (also called ma huang), an herb that contains ephedrine. These herbals have effects similar to those of drugs used to treat asthma, and should not be used in combination with sympathetic stimulants or anticholinergic preparations. The safety of ephedra is currently in question; advise clients to always check with a physician before using preparations containing ephedra. Capsaicin also may relieve acute asthma symptoms. Other herbal preparations include quercetin and grape seed extract. Refer clients interested in using natural preparations to a qualified herbalist, and emphasize the importance of talking to the physician before using these preparations along with conventional treatment.

In addition to herbals, other complementary therapies, such as biofeedback, yoga, breathing techniques, acupuncture, homeopathy, and massage, have been found to alleviate or help control asthma symptoms.

Table 15-4. Medication Administration — Asthma

Adrenergic Stimulants

Epinephrine
Isoproterenol (Isuprel)
Metaproterenol (Alupent, Metaprel)
Terbutaline (Brethaire, Brethine)

Continued on the next page

Table 15-4. Continued

Isoetharine (Bronkosol, Bronkometer)
Albuterol (Proventil, Ventolin)
Bitolterol (Tornalate)
Pirbuterol (Maxair)
Salmeterol (Serevent)

Adrenergic stimulants affect sympathetic receptors in the respiratory tract, resulting in smooth muscle relaxation and bronchodilation. Administered by metered-dose inhalers, these drugs are the treatment of choice for acute bronchial asthma. Oral forms may be used for prophylaxis, but are not effective in treating an acute attack because of their slow onset. When administered orally or parenterally, their effect on the sympathetic nervous system can produce undesirable side effects, such as nervousness, irritability, tachycardia, and cardiac dysrhythmias.

Nursing Responsibilities
• Use with caution in clients with hypertension, cardiovascular disease or dysrhythmias, hyperthyroidism, or diabetes.
• When given to a client who is hypoxemic and acidotic, these drugs may cause potentially dangerous cardiac stimulation.
• When given by MDI wait one to two minutes between puffs to allow airways to dilate, permitting the second dose to reach distal airways.
• Observe for desired effect of reduced dyspnea and wheezing. Central nervous system stimulation (anxiety, irritability, and insomnia) and tremor are common side effects.

Client and Family Teaching
• Use the prescribed inhaler or nebulizer as directed.
• If you are taking a bronchodilator along with another medication by inhalation, use the bronchodilator first to open airways and enhance the effectiveness of the second medication.
• Rinse the mouth after using inhalers to reduce systemic absorption of the medication.
• Keep a log to track your bronchodilator use. If the drug becomes less effective, or if you need a higher dosage or more frequent doses than prescribed, contact your physician.
• Report palpitations, irregular pulse, and other side effects to the physician.

Methylxanthines

Theophylline (Bronkotabs, Quibron, Slo-Phyllin Theolair, Theo-Dur, others)
Aminophylline (Somophyllin)

The methylxanthines are chemically related to caffeine. Once the drugs of choice for preventing and treating asthma attacks, they are now are used primarily to prevent nocturnal asthma in affected adult clients. Theophylline has a narrow margin of safety and high potential for toxicity. Because the metabolism and excretion of theophylline vary significantly from person to person—affected by such factors as age, smoking, genetic factors, alcoholism, and other chronic diseases—monitoring of serum levels is vital.

Nursing Responsibilities
• The therapeutic blood level for theophylline is 10 to 20 mg/mL.

Table 15-4. Continued

- Monitor for manifestations of toxicity. Anorexia, nausea, vomiting, restlessness, insomnia, cardiac dysrhythmias, and seizures are early manifestations. Other manifestations include epigastric pain, hematemesis, diarrhea, headache, irritability, muscle twitching, palpitations, tachycardia, flushing, and circulatory failure.
- Administer with meals or a full glass of water or milk to minimize gastric irritation.
- Monitor effect closely when administering concurrently with other medications, such as barbiturates, anticonvulsants, thyroid hormone, beta blockers, bronchodilators, and others.
- Aminophylline is incompatible with many other intravenous drugs. Use a separate line or flush the line with normal saline before and after administering any other preparation.

Client and Family Teaching
- Oral methylxanthines are ineffective to treat an acute asthma attack; do not delay other treatment by using these drugs.
- Check with the physician before taking any over-the-counter medications or other prescription drugs while on theophylline.
- Do not smoke while using this drug.
- Report adverse effects to the physician.

Anticholinergics

Atropine
Ipratropium bromide (Atrovent)

Anticholinergics are potent bronchodilators, blocking input from the parasympathetic nervous system. Atropine is used infrequently because of its tendency to dry secretions of the mucous membranes and other side effects. Ipratropium bromide is available as an inhaler and has fewer side effects than atropine.

Nursing Responsibilities
- Assess for possible contraindications to the drug, including hypersensitivity, glaucoma, prostatic hypertrophy, or bladder-neck obstruction.
- Assess for desired and/or adverse effects: improving or worsening symptoms; nausea, vomiting, abdominal cramping, anxiety, dizziness; headache.
- Provide ice chips, fluids, or hard candy to relieve dry mouth.

Client and Family Teaching
- To prevent overdose, take no more than the prescribed number of doses per day.
- If the drug becomes less effective over time, notify the physician; an adjustment in dosage may be needed.

Corticosteroids

Beclomethasone dipropionate (Vanceril, Beclovent)
Triamcinalone acetonide (Azmacort)
Flunisolide (AeroBid)
Dexamethasone sodium phosphate (Decadron Phosphate Respihaler)

Continued on the next page

Table 15-4. Continued

The anti-inflammatory effect of corticosteroids helps both prevent and treat acute episodes. Corticosteroids are used to reduce the frequency and severity of asthma attacks, and allow reduced dosages of other drugs. The cushingoid side effects of corticosteroids, always a major concern with their use, are minimized when they are inhaled.

Nursing Responsibilities
- Administer inhaler doses after bronchodilators to facilitate transit of the medication to distal airways.
- Assess for common side effects: sore throat; hoarseness; and oropharyngeal or laryngeal *Candida albicans* infection.
- Administer antifungal medications or gargles as ordered.

Client and Family Teaching
- Rinse the mouth after using the inhaler and maintain good oral hygiene to reduce the risk of fungal infections.
- These medications should not be used to alleviate the symptoms of an acute attack.
- Several weeks of continued therapy may be required before a beneficial effect is noticed.
- Notify the physician if you develop weight gain, fluid retention, muscle weakness, redistribution of fat, or mood changes.

Mast Cell Stabilizers

Cromolyn sodium (Intal, Nasalcrom)
Nedocromil (Tilade)

Cromolyn sodium and nedocromil inhibit inflammatory cells in the airway, blocking early and late responses to inhaled antigens. Both also prevent bronchoconstriction in response to inhaling cold air. They are administered by metered-dose inhaler, and have a wide margin of safety. Clients using nedocromil may complain of an unpleasant taste.

Nursing Responsibilities
- Evaluate for potential adverse effects of wheezing and bronchoconstriction.

Client and Family Teaching
- Gargling or sipping water can decrease the throat irritation associated with nebulizer treatment.
- Use appropriate technique. Inhale deeply with head tipped back to open airways, hold breath, and then exhale. Repeat until all of the drug has been inhaled.
- These drugs are used only to prevent asthma attacks; they are not effective in treating an acute attack.
- Several weeks may be required before a beneficial effect is noted.

Leukotriene Modifiers

Zafirlukast (Accolate)
Zileuton (Zyflo)

Leukotriene modifiers interfere with the inflammatory process in the airways, improving airflow, decreasing symptoms, and reducing the need for short-acting bronchodilators. They

Table 15-4. Continued

are used for maintenance therapy in adults and children over the age of 12 as an alternative to inhaled corticosteroid therapy. They are not used to treat an acute attack.

Nursing Responsibilities

• Administer at least one hour before or two hours after meals.

• These drugs inhibit some liver enzymes, affecting the metabolism of warfarin and possibly terfenadine and theophylline. Monitor prothrombin times and theophylline blood levels.

• Monitor liver enzymes, as these drugs may be toxic to the liver.

Client and Family Teaching

• Take the drugs as prescribed on an empty stomach.

• Notify the physician if a change in color of stools or urine is noted, or if jaundice develops.

Nursing Care

Nurses encounter clients with asthma both in the acute care setting, during an acute exacerbation and as outpatients or in homes. The priority nursing care needs differ with each setting.

Health Promotion

Although specific measures to prevent asthma have not yet been identified, the link between parental smoking and childhood asthma is strong. Discuss this link with young people and families with children. Encourage all clients to not start smoking, and if they are already smokers, to quit. Provide referrals to smoking cessation clinics, help groups, or a care provider for nicotine patches, as needed to facilitate quitting.

Assessment

Assessment of the client experiencing an acute asthma attack must be very focused and timely.

• *Health history:* current symptoms, including chest tightness, shortness of breath, dyspnea; duration of current attack; measures used to relieve symptoms and their effect; identified precipitating factors for the attack; frequency of attacks; current medications; known allergies.

• *Physical examination:* apparent level of distress; color; vital signs; respiratory rate and excursion, breath sounds throughout lung fields; apical pulse.

Nursing Diagnoses and Interventions

An acute asthma attack causes fear as breathing becomes increasingly difficult and hypoxemia develops. Anxiety in turn tends to increase the severity and manifestations of the attack. Priority nursing care needs during an acute attack focus on improving airway clearance and reducing fear and anxiety. Teaching about prevention of future attacks and home management must be postponed until adequate ventilation is restored.

Ineffective Airway Clearance

Bronchospasm and bronchoconstriction, increased mucus secretion, and airway edema narrow the airways and impair airflow during an acute attack of asthma. Both inspiratory and expiratory volume are affected, decreasing the oxygen available at the alveolus for the process of respiration. Narrowed air passages increase the work of breathing, increasing the metabolic rate and tissue demand for oxygen.

- Monitor skin color and temperature and level of consciousness. *Cyanosis, cool clammy skin, and changes in level of consciousness (agitation, lethargy, or confusion) indicate worsening hypoxia.*

- Assess arterial blood gas results and pulse oximetry readings; notify the physician of abnormal values or changes in status. *These values provide information about gas exchange and the adequacy of alveolar ventilation. A fall in oxygen saturation levels is an early indicator of impaired gas exchange.*

- Place in Fowler's, high-Fowler's, or orthopneic (with head and arms supported on the overbed table) position to facilitate breathing and lung expansion. *These positions reduce the work of breathing and increase lung expansion, especially of basilar areas.*

- Administer oxygen as ordered. If a mask is used, monitor closely for feelings of claustrophobia or suffocation. *Supplemental oxygen reduces hypoxemia. Although the mask is a very effective oxygen delivery system, it may increase anxiety.*

- Administer nebulizer treatments and provide humidification as ordered. *Nebulizer treatments are used to administer bronchodilators and other medications; humidity helps loosen secretions.*

- Initiate or assist with chest physiotherapy, including percussion and postural drainage. *Percussion and postural drainage facilitate the movement of secretions and airway clearance.*

- Increase fluid intake. *Increasing fluids helps keep secretions thin.*

- Provide endotracheal suctioning as needed. *Endotracheal suctioning may be necessary to remove secretions and improve ventilation if the client is unable to clear secretions by coughing.*

Ineffective Breathing Pattern

The physiologic changes in lung ventilation that occur during an acute asthma attack impair both lung expansion and emptying. Anxiety caused by hypoxia and dyspnea compounds the problem by increasing the respiratory rate. Collaborative and nursing interventions can help restore a more normal breathing pattern and adequate lung ventilation.

- Monitor vital signs and laboratory results. *Tachypnea, tachycardia, an elevated blood pressure, and increasing hypoxemia and hypercapnia are signs of compromised respiratory status.*

- Assist with ADLs as needed. *This conserves energy and reduces fatigue.*

- Provide rest periods between scheduled activities and treatments. *Scheduled rest is important to prevent fatigue and reduce oxygen demands.*

- Teach and assist to use techniques to control breathing pattern:
  a. Pursed-lip breathing
  b. Abdominal breathing
  c. Relaxation techniques including visualization, meditation, and others.

Pursed-lip breathing helps keep airways open by maintaining positive pressure, and abdominal breathing improves lung expansion. Relaxation techniques reduce anxiety and its effect on the respiratory rate.

- Administer medications, including bronchodilators and anti-inflammatory drugs, as ordered. Monitor for desired and possible adverse effects. *Medications are used to improve airway status and facilitate breathing.*

Anxiety

Acute exacerbations of asthma can produce significant anxiety. Fear of being unable to breathe and feelings of suffocation associated with acute asthma are significant. Financial or other concerns may cause the client to want to avoid hospitalization. Increasingly frequent and severe episodes may cause fear for the future. Hypoxia contributes to anxiety as well, stimulating the sympathetic nervous system and the fight-or-flight response.

- Assess level of anxiety. *Interventions for severe anxiety or panic differ from those for mild or moderate anxiety.*
- Assist to identify coping skills that have been successful in the past. *Successful coping helps the client regain control of the situation, reducing anxiety.*
- Listen actively to concerns; do not deny or negate the fear of dying or of being unable to breathe. *Active listening promotes trust and helps the client express concerns.*
- Include the client in care planning and decisions as appropriate, without making excessive demands. *Participating in decision making increases the client's sense of control. Because high levels of anxiety interfere with the ability to make decisions, it is important to avoid placing demands on the client that may further increase the level of anxiety.*
- Reduce excessive environmental stimuli, and maintain a calm demeanor. *This promotes rest.*
- Allow supportive family members to remain with the client. *Family members provide additional support and can help reduce anxiety.*
- Assist to use relaxation techniques, such as guided imagery, muscle relaxation, and meditation. *These techniques help restore psychologic balance and reduce sympathetic stimulation and responses.*

Ineffective Therapeutic Regimen Management

Once acute asthma is under control and effective respirations have been reestablished, it is important to help the client identify contributing factors to the attack. This helps the client prevent future episodes.

- Assess level of understanding about asthma and the prescribed treatment regimen. Provide additional information and teaching as indicated. *Assessment helps to identify and clarify misperceptions and difficulties with disease management.*
- Discuss the client's perception of the illness and its effect on his or her lifestyle. *Open discussion can help identify conflicts between lifestyle and the treatment regimen.*
- Assist the client and significant others to identify problems or difficulties integrating the treatment regimen into their lifestyle. *Asthma and its management may necessitate lifestyle modifications to prevent acute exacerbations. This can significantly impact family members, for example, eliminating cigarette smoking or pets from the household, removing carpets, or daily damp-dusting to remove dust mites.*
- Assess knowledge and understanding of prescribed medications and use of over-the-counter preparations. *This is important to determine misperceptions or possible misuse of medications.*
- Provide verbal and written instructions. *Written instructions reinforce teaching and allow future reference.*
- Refer to counseling, support groups, or self-help organizations. *Counseling, support groups, and self-help organizations can help the client and family adapt to living with asthma and the treatment regimen.*

Home Care

Asthma is a chronic disease that is best managed by the client with assistance from medical personnel. Teaching for home care focuses on promoting the highest level of wellness and preventing and managing acute episodes and exacerbations of the disease. Topics to include in teaching are as follows:

- Suggestions for lifestyle changes to avoid specific triggers for asthma attacks, for example:
    - Warm up slowly before exercising in cold weather; wear a special mask or scarf to retain air warmth and humidity while exercising.
    - Substitute indoor exercises during cold, dry weather.
    - Reduce the risk for respiratory infections (e.g., adequate rest, good nutrition, and stress management to maintain immune function, yearly influenza vaccines and immunization against pneumococcal pneumonia).
    - Use techniques to reduce or manage physical and psychologic stress.
    - Using PEFR meter to monitor airway status; how to manage the disease based on results
- Using prescribed medications, including:
    - Name, frequency, dose, and desired effect.
    - Potential adverse effects and their management, including effects to report to the physician.
    - Potential interactions with other drugs (including over-the-counter herbal preparations) or foods.
    - If tolerance is a potential risk, how to identify it and steps to take.

Provide referrals to local or regional resources for further teaching and support as needed. Consider the need for home health services, home respiratory care services, and others as needed.

The Client with Chronic Obstructive Pulmonary Disease

Clients with chronic airflow obstruction due to chronic bronchitis and/or emphysema are said to have **chronic obstructive pulmonary disease (COPD).**

In 2000, approximately 11.4 million Americans were affected by COPD. It is more common in whites than in blacks and affects men more frequently than women. It is the fourth leading cause of death in the United States. The death rate from COPD continues to rise, particularly among black males and females of all ethnic groups. In the year 2000, COPD and other chronic obstructive lung diseases accounted for over 123,500 deaths (NHLBI, 2002). In addition, COPD morbidity is significant. In people under age 65, COPD is second only to heart disease as a cause of disability, resulting in an estimated 250 million lost work hours yearly.

Obstructive lung disease typically affects middle-aged and older adults. Cigarette smoking is clearly implicated as the primary cause of COPD, even though it develops in only 10% to 15% of smokers. Cigarette smoke, and the irritants it contains impair ciliary movement, inhibit the function of alveolar macrophages, and cause mucus-secreting glands to hypertrophy. It also produces emphysema or airway destruction and constricts smooth muscle, increasing airway resistance. Other contributing factors include air pollution, occupational exposure to noxious dusts and gases, airway infection, and familial and genetic factors.

Pathophysiology and Manifestations

COPD is characterized by slowly progressive obstruction of the airways. The disease is one of periodic exacerbations, often related to respiratory infection, with increased symptoms of dyspnea and sputum production. Unlike acute processes in which lung tissues recover, airways and lung parenchyma do not return to normal following an exacerbation; instead, they demonstrate progressive destructive changes.

Although one or the other may predominate, COPD typically includes components of both chronic bronchitis and emphysema, two distinctly different processes. Chronic asthma is also often present. Through different mechanisms, these processes cause airways to narrow, resistance to airflow to increase, and expiration to become slow or difficult. The result is a mismatch between alveolar ventilation and blood flow or perfusion, leading to impaired gas exchange.

The clinical presentation of COPD varies from simple chronic bronchitis without disability to chronic respiratory failure and severe disability. Manifestations are typically absent or minor early in the disease. When the client finally seeks care, productive cough, dyspnea, and exercise intolerance have often been present for as long as ten years. The cough typically occurs in the mornings and often is attributed to "smoker's cough." Initially, dyspnea occurs only on extreme exertion; as the disease progresses, dyspnea becomes more severe and accompanies mild activity. Manifestations characteristic of chronic bronchitis and emphysema develop. The clinical features and manifestations of COPD are summarized in Table 15-5.

Chronic Bronchitis

Chronic bronchitis is a disorder of excessive bronchial mucus secretion. It is characterized by a productive cough lasting three or more months in two consecutive years (Porth, 2002). Cigarette smoke is the major factor implicated in the development of chronic bronchitis.

Inhaled irritants lead to a chronic inflammatory process with vasodilation, congestion, and edema of the bronchial mucosa. Thick, tenacious mucus is produced in increased amounts. Narrowed airways and excess secretions obstruct airflow; expiration is affected first, then inspiration. Because ciliary function is impaired, normal defense mechanisms are unable to clear the mucus and any inhaled pathogens. Recurrent infection is common in chronic bronchitis. An imbalance between ventilation and perfusion leads to hypoxemia, hypercapnia, and pulmonary hypertension. Pulmonary hypertension often leads to right-sided heart failure.

Manifestations of chronic bronchitis are a cough productive of copious amounts of thick, tenacious sputum, cyanosis, and evidence of right-sided heart failure, including distended neck veins, edema, liver engorgement, and an enlarged heart. Adventitious sounds, including loud rhonchi and possible wheezes, are prominent on auscultation.

Emphysema

Emphysema is characterized by destruction of the walls of the alveoli, with resulting enlargement of abnormal air spaces. As in chronic bronchitis, cigarette smoking is strongly implicated as a causative factor in most cases of emphysema. Deficiency of alpha$_1$-antitrypsin, an enzyme that normally inhibits the activity of proteolytic enzymes and tissue destruction in the lungs, leads to an early onset of emphysema, often before age 40 (Braunwald, et al., 2001).

Alveolar wall destruction causes alveoli and air spaces to enlarge with loss of corresponding portions of the pulmonary capillary bed. As a result, the surface area for alveolar-capillary diffusion is reduced, affecting gas exchange. Elastic recoil is lost, reducing the volume of air that is passively expired. The loss of support tissue also affects airways, increasing the risk of expiratory collapse and further air trapping. Anatomically, either respiratory bronchioles or alveoli may be the primary tissue involved.

Emphysema is insidious in onset. Dyspnea is the initial symptom. Initially occurring only with exertion, dyspnea may progress to become severe, even at rest. Cough is minimal or absent. Air trapping and hyperinflation increase the anterior-posterior chest diameter, causing *barrel chest*. The client often is thin, tachypneic, uses accessory muscles of respiration and often assumes a position of sitting and leaning forward. The expiratory phase of the respiratory cycle is prolonged. On auscultation, breath sounds are diminished, and the percussion tone is hyperresonant.

Table 15-5. Clinical Features and Manifestations of COPD

	Feature	Chronic Bronchitis	Emphysema
History	Onset	After age 35; recurrent respiratory infections	After age 50; insidious progressive dyspnea
	Smoking	Usual	Usual
	Cough	Persistent, productive of copious mucopurulent sputum	Absent or mild with scant clear sputum, if any
Physical Examination	Appearance	Often obese; edematous and cyanotic; distended neck veins and other symptoms of right-sided heart failure	Usually thin and cachectic; barrel chest; prominent accessory muscles of respiration
	Chest	Adventitious sounds with wheezing and rhonchi; normal percussion note	Distant or diminished breath sounds; hyperresonant percussion note
Other Features	Blood gases	Hypercapnia and hypoxemia; respiratory acidosis	Normal or mild hypoxemia; normal pH
	Pulmonary function studies	Normal or decreased total lung capacity; moderately increased residual volume	Increased total lung capacity; markedly increased residual volume
	Pulmonary hypertension	May be severe	Only when advanced

Collaborative Care

Although COPD can be prevented in most people, it cannot be cured. Smoking abstinence is the only certain way to prevent COPD and to slow its progression. To a certain extent, airway obstruction can be reversed and disability minimized early in the disease. Treatment generally focuses on relieving symptoms, minimizing obstruction, and slowing disability.

Diagnostic Tests

Diagnostic tests are used to help establish the diagnosis of chronic obstructive pulmonary disease and identify the predominant component, emphysema or chronic bronchitis. These procedures are also used to assess respiratory status and monitor treatment effectiveness.

- *Pulmonary function testing* is performed to establish the diagnosis and evaluate the extent and progress of COPD. Fasting is not required for this noninvasive test; however, tobacco products, bronchodilators, and eating a heavy meal should be avoided for four to six hours prior to testing. Results are based on calculated norms for each person by age, height, sex, and weight; note these, as well as all current medications on the requisition. In COPD, the total lung capacity and residual volume typically are increased. The forced expiratory volume (FEV_1) and forced vital capacity (FVC) are decreased due to narrowed airways and resistance to airflow.

- *Ventilation-perfusion scanning* may be performed to determine the extent of ventilation/perfusion mismatch—that is, the extent to which lung tissue is ventilated but not perfused (dead space), or perfused but inadequately ventilated (physiologic shunting). A radioisotope is injected or inhaled to illustrate areas of shunting and absent capillaries.

- *Serum alpha₁-antitrypsin levels* may be drawn to screen for deficiency, particularly in clients with a family history of obstructive airway disease, those with an early onset, women, and nonsmokers. Normal adult serum alpha1-antitrypsin levels range from 80 to 260 mg/dL. Fasting is not required prior to this test.

- *Arterial blood gases (ABGs)* are drawn to evaluate gas exchange, particularly during acute exacerbations of COPD. Clients with predominant emphysema often have mild hypoxemia and normal or low carbon dioxide tension. Respiratory alkalosis may be present due to an increased respiratory rate. Predominant chronic bronchitis and airway obstruction may cause marked hypoxemia and hypercapnia with respiratory acidosis. Oxygen saturation levels are low due to marked hypoxemia.

- **Pulse oximetry** is used to monitor oxygen saturation of the blood. Marked airway obstruction and hypoxemia often causes oxygen saturation levels less than 95%. Pulse oximetry may be continuously monitored to assess the need for supplemental oxygen.

- *Exhaled carbon dioxide (capnogram or $ETco_2$)* may be measured to evaluate alveolar ventilation. The normal $ETco_2$ reading is 35 to 45 mmHg; it is elevated when ventilation is inadequate, and decreased when pulmonary perfusion is impaired. $ETco_2$ monitoring can reduce the frequency of ABG determinations.

- *CBC with WBC differential* often shows increased RBCs and hematocrit (erythrocytosis) as chronic hypoxia stimulates increased erythropoiesis to increase the oxygen-carrying capacity of the blood. *Polycythemia,* increased numbers of all blood cells, may be evident. Increased WBC count and a higher percentage of immature WBCs (bands) are often indicative of bacterial infection.

- *Chest X-ray* may show flattening of the diaphragm due to hyperinflation and evidence of pulmonary infection if present.

Smoking Cessation

Smoking cessation can not only prevent COPD from developing, but also can improve lung function once the disease has been diagnosed. Forced expiratory volume (FEV$_1$) improves, and survival is prolonged, largely due to lower rates of lung cancer and heart disease. Sustained quitting is difficult; only 6% of smokers succeed in long-term abstinence from smoking (Braunwald, et al., 2001). Use of nicotine patches or gum and an antidepressant, such as bupropion (Wellbutrin, Zyban), improve the chances of success.

Medications

Immunization against pneumococcal pneumonia and yearly influenza vaccine are recommended to reduce the risk of respiratory infections. A broad-spectrum antibiotic is prescribed if infection is suspected. Recent studies indicate that clients with purulent sputum and increased dyspnea will likely benefit from antibiotic therapy, even if no other signs of infection are present. Prophylactic antibiotics may be ordered for clients who experience four or more disease exacerbations per year (Braunwald, et al., 2001).

Bronchodilators improve airflow and reduce air trapping in COPD, resulting in improved dyspnea and exercise tolerance. Bronchodilators may be given by metered-dose inhaler (MDI), by nebulizer, or orally. Oral administration may promote adherence, but is associated with much higher rates of adverse effects. A spacer or holding chamber may facilitate effective use of an MDI. Ipratropium bromide, an anticholinergic agent administered by MDI, is frequently prescribed. It has a longer duration of action than the short-acting b$_2$-adrenergic stimulant bronchodilators and few side effects. Salmeterol, a longer-acting b$_2$ agonist, may be used in combination therapy. Oral theophylline, a methylxanthine, is a weak bronchodilator and has a narrow therapeutic range, but is often prescribed for its other effects. Theophylline stimulates the respiratory drive, strengthens diaphragmatic contractions, and improves cardiac output. As a result, dyspnea, exercise tolerance, and quality of life improve for the client with COPD.

Corticosteroid therapy may be used when asthma is a major component of COPD. It also improves symptoms and exercise tolerance, and may reduce the severity of exacerbations and the need for hospitalization. Oral corticosteroids, such as prednisone, are used initially. If a beneficial response occurs, the amount is reduced to the lowest effective dose. Every-other-day dosing or administration by inhaler is preferred to minimize steroid side effects, such as cushingoid effects and an increased risk for osteoporosis and vertebral fractures.

Alpha$_1$-antitrypsin (a$_1$AT) replacement therapy is available for clients with emphysema due to a genetic deficiency of the enzyme. Although expensive and inconvenient (a$_1$AT is administered weekly by intravenous infusion), it has been shown to reduce the rate of airflow decline and mortality.

Treatments

In addition to refraining from smoking, exposure to other airway irritants and allergens should be avoided. The client should remain indoors during periods of significant air pollution to prevent exacerbations of the disease. Air filtering systems or air conditioning may be useful.

Pulmonary hygiene measures, including hydration, effective cough, percussion, and postural drainage, are used to improve clearance of airway secretions. Maintaining adequate systemic hydration is essential to keep secretions thin. Forceful coughing is often less effective than leaning forward and repeatedly "huffing," with relaxed breathing between huffs. Percussion and postural drainage may be necessary if the client is unable to clear secretions by usual means. Cough suppressants and sedatives generally are avoided as they may cause retention of secretions.

Unless disabling cardiac disease is present, a regular exercise program is beneficial in:

• Improving exercise tolerance.
• Enhancing ability to perform activities of daily living.
• Preventing deterioration of physical condition.

A program of regular aerobic exercise (e.g., walking for 20 minutes at least three times weekly) designed to gradually increase exercise tolerance is recommended. Activities that strengthen the muscles used for breathing and ADLs, such as swimming and golf, are also beneficial.

Breathing exercises are used to slow the respiratory rate and relieve accessory muscle fatigue. Pursed-lip breathing slows the respiratory rate and helps maintain open airways during exhalation by keeping positive pressure in the airways. Abdominal breathing relieves the work of accessory muscles of respiration.

Oxygen

Long-term oxygen therapy is used for severe and progressive hypoxemia. Oxygen therapy improves exercise tolerance, mental functioning, and quality of life in advanced COPD. It also reduces the rate of hospitalization and increases length of survival. Oxygen may be used intermittently, at night, or continuously. For severely hypoxemic clients, the greatest benefit is seen with continuous oxygen. Home oxygen may be supplied as liquid oxygen, compressed gas cylinders, or oxygen concentrators.

An acute exacerbation of COPD may necessitate oxygenation and inspiratory positive-pressure assistance with a face mask or intubation and mechanical ventilation. Oxygen administered without intubation and mechanical ventilation requires caution: Chronic elevated carbon dioxide levels in the blood inhibit this normal stimulus to breathe, leaving only the stimulus of low blood oxygen tension. Oxygen administered at high flow rates or a high percentage can reduce this stimulus, leading to respiratory insufficiency or arrest.

Surgery

When medical therapy is no longer effective, lung transplantation may be an option. Both single and bilateral transplants have been performed successfully, with a 2-year survival rate of 75%. Lung reduction surgery is an experimental surgical intervention for advanced diffuse emphysema and lung hyperinflation. The procedure reduces the overall volume of the lung, reshapes it, and improves elastic recoil. As a result, pulmonary function and exercise tolerance improve and dyspnea is reduced.

Complementary Therapies

Complementary therapies may be useful to help manage symptoms of COPD. Dietary measures, such as minimizing intake of dairy products and salt, may help reduce mucous production and to keep mucus more liquefied. Be sure to recommend measures to replace the protein and calcium in dairy products to help maintain nutritional balance.

Herbal teas made with peppermint and yarrow, coltsfoot, or comfrey may act as expectorants to help relieve chest congestion. Licorice root, which may be taken in several forms, also has expectorant and anti-inflammatory effects that may be beneficial. Licorice root can, however, cause toxicity when used for extended periods of time. Refer clients to a qualified herbalist for treatment.

Acupuncture may help the client with smoking cessation, and has also been used to treat asthma and other respiratory conditions. Hypnotherapy and guided imagery are used to assist with smoking cessation. These techniques can also help the client control anxiety and breathing patterns. Refer clients to a trained professional. Nurses, physicians, psychologists, counselors, social workers, and others can take professional training in hypnotherapy and guided imagery (Fontaine, 2000).

Nursing Care

Health Promotion

Avioding the habit of smoking is the best preventive measure for chronic obstructive pulmonary disease. Even in clients with COPD, smoking cessation improves lung function and increases survival. Educate all clients, including preschool and school-age children, about the risks of smoking. See upcoming section on smoking.

Assessment

Focused assessment for the client with chronic obstructive pulmonary disease includes:

- *Health history:* current symptoms, including cough, sputum production, shortness of breath or dyspnea, activity tolerance; frequency of respiratory infections and most recent episode; previous diagnosis of emphysema, chronic bronchitis, or asthma; current medications; smoking history (in pack years—packs per day times number of years smoked), history of exposure to secondhand smoke, occupational or other pollutants.
- *Physical examination:* general appearance, weight for height, mental status; vital signs including temperature; skin color and temperature; anterior-posterior:lateral chest diameter, use of accessory muscles, nasal flaring or pursed-lip breathing; respiratory excursion and diaphragmatic excursion; percussion tone; breath sounds throughout; neck veins, apical pulse and heart sounds, peripheral pulses, edema.

Nursing Diagnoses and Interventions

Clients with chronic obstructive pulmonary disease, whether hospitalized or in the community, have multiple nursing care needs. Because of the obstructive nature of the disease, airway clearance is a high priority. Nutritional deficit is common, particularly when emphysema is predominant. Because this chronic disease affects all functional health patterns, psychosocial issues are also of concern in planning nursing care.

Ineffective Airway Clearance

Both chronic bronchitis and emphysema affect the ability to maintain open airways. In chronic bronchitis, copious amounts of thick, tenacious mucus are produced. Ciliary action is impaired, making it difficult to clear mucus from the airways. The loss of supporting tissue caused by emphysema increases the the risk for airway collapse. In both cases, air is trapped distally, and less oxygen is available to the alveoli for diffusion. Normal respiratory defense mechanisms are impaired, and mucus-plugged airways provide an ideal environment for bacterial growth. Respiratory infection further impairs airway clearance, and is often the cause of an acute exacerbation.

- Assess respiratory status every one to two hours or as indicated. Assess rate and pattern; cough and secretions (color, amount, consistency, and odor); and breath sounds, both normal and adventitious. *Frequent assessment is vital to monitor current status and response to treatment. Adventitious sounds should decrease with effective intervention. Diminished or absent breath sounds may indicate increasing airway obstruction and possible atelectasis.*

- Monitor arterial blood gas results. *Increasing hypoxemia, hypercapnia, and respiratory acidosis may indicate increasing airway obstruction.*

- Weigh daily, monitor intake and output, and assess mucous membranes and skin turgor. *Dehydration causes respiratory secretions to become thicker, more tenacious, and difficult to expectorate; fluid overload can further compromise respiratory status.*

- Encourage a fluid intake of at least 2000 to 2500 mL per day unless contraindicated. *Adequate fluid intake helps keep mucous secretions thin.*

- Place in Fowler's, high-Fowler's, or orthopneic position; encourage movement and activity to tolerance. *Upright positions improve ventilation and reduce the work of breathing. Activity helps mobilize secretions and prevent them from pooling.*

- Assist with coughing and deep breathing at least every two hours while awake. Position seated upright, leaning forward during coughing. *The upright position promotes chest expansion, increasing the effectiveness of coughing and reducing the work involved.*

- Provide tissues and a paper bag to dispose of expectorated sputum. *This important infection control measure reduces the spread of respiratory organisms to other people.*

- Refer to a respiratory therapist, and assist with or perform percussion and postural drainage as needed. *Percussion helps loosen secretions in airways; postural drainage facilitates movement of these secretions out of the respiratory tract.*

- Provide rest periods between treatments and procedures. *The client with COPD fatigues easily; adequate rest is important to conserve energy and reduce fatigue.*

- Administer expectorant and bronchodilator medications as ordered. Correlate timing with respiratory treatments. *Using expectorants and bronchodilators prior to coughing, percussion, and postural drainage increases their effectiveness in clearing airways.*

- Provide supplemental oxygen as ordered. *Supplemental oxygen helps maintain adequate blood and tissue oxygenation.*

Imbalanced Nutrition: Less Than Body Requirements

With advanced COPD, minimal activity, including eating, can cause fatigue and dyspnea. The client may be unable to consume a full meal without resting. At the same time, the increased work of breathing increases metabolic demands, and more calories are required. The client may appear cachectic (thin and wasted). Poor nutritional status further impairs immune function and increases the risk of a complicating infection.

- Assess nutritional status, including diet history, weight for height (use reference tables of desired weights), and anthropometric (skinfold) measurements. *It is important to differentiate nutritional status from body type, rather than assume a nutritional impairment.*

- Observe and document food intake, including types, amounts, and caloric intake. *This information can provide direction for supplementation, if needed.*
- Monitor laboratory values, including serum albumin and electrolyte levels. *These values provide information about the adequacy of nutritional intake, including protein.*
- Consult with a dietitian to plan meals and nutritional supplements that meet caloric needs. *More concentrated sources of high-energy foods may be required to maintain caloric intake without excess fatigue. A diet high in proteins and fats without excess carbohydrates is recommended to minimize carbon dioxide production during metabolism (carbohydrates are metabolized to form CO_2 and water).*
- Provide frequent, small feedings with between-meal supplements. *Frequent, small meals help maintain intake and reduce fatigue associated with eating.*
- Place seated or in high-Fowler's position for meals. *An upright position promotes lung expansion and reduces dyspnea.*
- Assist to choose preferred foods from the menu; encourage family members to bring food from home if allowed. *Providing preferred foods encourages eating.*
- Keep snacks at the bedside. *Snacks provide additional caloric intake.*
- Provide mouth care prior to meals. *This helps enhance the appetite.*
- If unable to maintain oral intake, consult with the physician about enteral or parenteral feedings. *Maintenance of caloric and nutrient intake is vital to prevent catabolism.*

Compromised Family Coping

Chronic illness affects the entire family structure. Roles and relationships change; additional demands are placed on the family. Family members may blame the client for causing the illness or have distorted perceptions about it, even denying its existence. They may refuse to assist or participate in care. The client may develop an attitude of helplessness or dependence or may demonstrate anger, hostility, or aggression.

- Assess interactions between client and family. *Assessment helps identify desired and potential destructive behaviors.*
- Assess the effect of the illness on the family. *Assessment of family interactions, roles, and relationships assists in planning appropriate interventions.*
- Help the client and family identify strengths for coping with the situation. *Identifying personal and family strengths helps the family regain a sense of control.*
- Provide information and teaching about COPD. *Education helps the family gain an understanding of the client's condition and needs.*
- Encourage expression of feelings. Avoid judging feelings expressed or family members as "good" or "bad," "right" or "wrong." *It is important that the nurse remain objective to maintain the therapeutic relationship.*
- Help family members recognize behaviors and attitudes that may hinder effective treatment, such as continuing to smoke in the house. *Family members may be unaware of the effect of their behavior on the client's ability to change habits and cope with a disabling disease.*
- Encourage family members to participate in care. *This helps develop skills for use at home.*
- Initiate a care conference involving the client, family, and health care team members from a variety of disciplines. *A wide range of perspectives and areas of expertise aids in problem solving and facilitates communication.*

- If dysfunctional family relationships interfere with measures to enhance coping, advocate for the client, reaffirming his or her right to make decisions. *Dysfunctional family relationships are not likely to change simply because of illness. The nurse can better meet the client's needs by accepting his or her limitations in dealing with family members.*

- Refer the client and family to support groups and pulmonary rehabilitation programs, as available. *Support groups and structured rehabilitation programs enhance coping abilities.*

- Arrange a social services consultation. *This can help the client and family identify care and support service needs.*

- Refer community agencies or services, such as home health, homemaker services, or Meals-on-Wheels, as appropriate. *Agencies or community services can provide additional support beyond the family's means or capability.*

Decisional Conflict: Smoking

Smoking is more than a habit; it is an addiction. The client who must quit is facing a significant loss, not only of nicotine, but also of a lifestyle. Although the client may fully comprehend the consequences of continuing to smoke, the decision to give up a part of his or her life is not easy. This fear may be expressed in such concerns as "I'll gain weight," or "What will I do with my hands?" In addition to providing practical information, a plan, and assistance with nicotine withdrawal, the nurse must support the client's decision-making process to comply with an order to stop smoking.

- Assess knowledge and understanding of the choices involved and possible consequences of each. *The decision to quit smoking ultimately belongs to the client. He or she needs a full understanding of the consequences of quitting or continuing to smoke.*

- Acknowledge concerns, values, and beliefs; listen nonjudgmentally. *The nurse needs to avoid imposing his or her values and beliefs about smoking on the client.*

- Spend time with the client, encouraging expression of feelings. *This demonstrates acceptance of the client and his or her right to make the decision.*

- Help plan a course of action for quitting smoking and adapt it as necessary. *When the client develops the plan, he or she has more ownership in it and interest in making it work.*

- Demonstrate respect for decisions and the right to choose. *Respect supports self-esteem and the ability to cope.*

- Provide referral to a counselor or other professional as needed. *Counselors or other people trained to assist with smoking cessation can help with decision making.*

Home Care

As with any chronic disease, the client and family will have primary responsibility for disease management. Teaching is vital to promote optimal health and slow disease progression. Teaching for home care focuses on effective coughing and breathing techniques, preventing exacerbations, and managing prescribed therapies.

Pursed-lip and diaphragmatic breathing techniques help minimize air trapping and fatigue. Pursed-lip breathing helps maintain open airways by maintaining positive pressures longer during exhalation. Teach the client to:

1. Inhale through the nose with the mouth closed.
2. Exhale slowly through pursed lips, as though whistling or blowing out a candle, making exhalation twice as long as inhalation.

Diaphragmatic or abdominal breathing helps conserve energy by using the larger and more efficient muscles of respiration. Teach the client to:

1. Place one hand on the abdomen, the other on the chest.
2. Inhale, concentrating on pushing the abdominal hand outward while the chest hand remains still.
3. Exhale slowly, while the abdominal hand moves inward and the chest hand remains still.

Repeat these exercises as often as necessary, until the techniques become incorporated into normal breathing.

Several different coughing techniques may be useful. For controlled cough technique, teach the client to:

1. Following prescribed bronchodilator treatment, inhale deeply, and hold breath briefly.
2. Cough twice, the first time to loosen mucus, the second to expel secretions.
3. Inhale by sniffing to prevent mucus from moving back into deep airways.
4. Rest. Avoid prolonged coughing to prevent fatigue and hypoxemia.

For Huff Coughing, teach the client to:

1. Inhale deeply while leaning forward.
2. Exhale sharply with a "huff" sound, to help keep airways open while mobilizing secretions.

In addition, include the following topics when teaching for home care:

- Maintaining adequate fluid intake, at least 2.0 to 2.5 quarts of fluid daily.
- Avoiding respiratory irritants, including cigarette smoke, both primary and secondary, other smoke sources, dust, aerosol sprays, air pollution, and very cold dry air.
- Preventing exposure to infection, especially upper respiratory infections.
- Importance of pneumococcal vaccine and annual influenza immunization.
- Prescribed exercise program, maintaining ADLs, and balancing rest and exercise.
- Maintaining nutrient intake (e.g., eating small frequent meals and using nutritional supplements to provide adequate calories).
- Ways of reducing sodium intake if prescribed.
- Identifying early signs of an infection or exacerbation and the importance of seeking medical attention for the following: fever, increased sputum production, purulent (green or yellow) sputum, upper respiratory infection, increased shortness of breath or difficulty breathing, decreased activity tolerance or appetite, increased need for oxygen.
- Prescribed medications, including purpose, proper use, and expected effects.
- Avoiding use of over-the-counter medications unless approved by the physician.
- Other prescribed therapies, such as use of home oxygen, percussion, postural drainage, and nebulizer treatments.
- Use, cleaning, and maintenance of any required special equipment.
- Importance of wearing an identification band and carrying a list of medications at all times in case of an emergency.

Provide referrals to home care services, such as home health, assistance with ADLs as needed, home maintenance services, respiratory therapy, and home oxygen services, and other agencies, such as Meals-on-Wheels and senior services, as indicated.

16

Assessing Clients with Nutritional and Gastrointestinal Disorders

Nutrition is the process by which the body ingests, absorbs, transports, uses, and eliminates food. The digestive organs responsible for these processes are the gastrointestinal tract (also called the alimentary canal) and the accessory digestive organs. The gastrointestinal tract consists of the mouth, pharynx, esophagus, stomach, small intestine, and large intestine. The accessory digestive organs include the liver, gallbladder, and pancreas. This chapter discusses the assessment of these organs, except the large intestine. Assessment of the large intestine, which is primarily responsible for elimination, is discussed in Chapter 20.

Review of Anatomy and Physiology

The gastrointestinal (GI) tract is a continuous hollow tube, extending from the mouth to the anus. Once foods are ingested into the mouth, they are subjected to a variety of processes that move them and break them down into end products that can be absorbed from the lumen of the small intestine into the blood or lymph. These digestive processes are as follows:

- Ingestion of food
- Movement of food and wastes
- Secretion of mucus, water, and enzymes
- Mechanical digestion of food
- Chemical digestion of food
- Absorption of digested food.

The Mouth

The mouth, also called the oral or buccal cavity, is lined with mucous membranes and is enclosed by the lips, cheeks, palate, and tongue.

The lips and cheeks are skeletal muscle covered externally by skin. Their function is to keep food in the mouth during chewing. The palate consists of two regions: the hard palate and the soft palate. The hard palate covers bone and provides a hard surface against which the tongue forces food. The soft palate is primarily muscle; it ends at the back of the mouth as a fold called the uvula. When food is swallowed, the soft palate rises as a reflex to close off the oropharynx.

The tongue, composed of skeletal muscle and connective tissue, is located in the floor of the mouth. It contains mucous and serous glands, taste buds, and papillae. The tongue mixes food with saliva during chewing, forms the food into a mass (called a bolus), and initiates swallowing. Some papillae provide surface roughness to facilitate licking and moving food; other papillae house the taste buds.

Saliva moistens food so it can be made into a bolus, dissolves food chemicals so they can be tasted, and provides enzymes, such as amylase, that begin the chemical breakdown of starches. Saliva is produced by salivary glands, most of which lie superior or inferior to the mouth and drain into it. The salivary glands include the parotid, the submaxillary, and the sublingual glands.

The teeth chew (masticate) and grind food to break it down into smaller parts. As the food is masticated, it is mixed with saliva. Adults have 32 permanent teeth. The teeth are embedded in the gingiva (gums), with the crown of each tooth visible above the gingiva.

The Pharynx

The pharynx consists of the oropharynx and the laryngopharynx. Both structures provide passageways for food, fluids, and air. The pharynx is skeletal muscles and is lined with mucous membranes. The skeletal muscles move food to the esophagus via the pharynx through **peristalsis** (alternating waves of contraction and relaxation of involuntary muscle). The mucosa of the pharynx contains mucus-producing glands that provide fluid to facilitate the passage of the bolus of food as it is swallowed.

The Esophagus

The esophagus, a muscular tube about 10 inches (25 cm) long, serves as a passageway for food from the pharynx to the stomach. The epiglottis, a flap of cartilage over the top of the larynx, keeps food out of the larynx during swallowing. The esophagus descends through the thorax and diaphragm, entering the stomach at the cardiac orifice. The gastroesophageal sphincter surrounds this opening. This sphincter, along with the diaphragm, keeps the orifice closed when food is not being swallowed.

For most of its length, the esophagus is lined with stratified squamous epithelium; simple columnar epithelium lines the esophagus where it joins the stomach. The mucosa and submucosa of the esophagus lie in longitudinal folds when the esophagus is empty.

The Stomach

The stomach, located high on the left side of the abdominal cavity, is connected to the esophagus at the upper end and to the small intestine at the lower end. Normally about 10 inches (25 cm) long, the stomach is a distensible organ that can expand to hold up to 4 L of food and fluid. The concave surface of the stomach is called the lesser curvature; the convex surface is called the greater curvature. The stomach may be divided into regions extending from the distal end of the esophagus to the opening into the small intestine. These regions are the cardiac region, fundus, body, and pylorus. The pyloric sphincter controls emptying of the stomach into the duodenal portion of the small intestine. The stomach is a storage reservoir for food, continues the mechanical breakdown of food, begins the process of protein digestion, and mixes the food with gastric juices into a thick fluid called **chyme.**

The stomach is lined with columnar epithelial, mucus-producing cells. Millions of openings in the lining lead to gastric glands that can produce 4 to 5 L of gastric juice each day. The gastric glands contain a variety of secretory cells, including the following:

- Mucous cells produce alkaline mucus that clings to the lining of the stomach and protects it from gastric juice.
- Zymogenic cells produce pepsinogen (an inactive form of pepsin, a protein-digesting enzyme).
- Parietal cells secrete hydrochloric acid and intrinsic factor. Hydrochloric acid activates and increases the activity of protein-digesting cells and also is bactericidal. Intrinsic factor is necessary for the absorption of vitamin B12 in the small intestine.
- Enteroendocrine cells secrete gastrin, histamine, endorphins, serotonin, and somatostatin. These hormones or hormonelike substances diffuse into the blood. Gastrin is important in regulating secretion and motility of the stomach.

The secretion of gastric juice is under both neural and endocrine control. Stimulation of the parasympathetic vagus nerve increases secretory activity; in contrast, stimulation of sympathetic nerves decreases secretions. The three phases of secretory activity are the cephalic phase, the gastric phase, and the intestinal phase.

- The cephalic phase prepares for digestion and is triggered by the sight, odor, taste, or thought of food. During this initial phase, motor impulses are transmitted via the vagus nerve to the stomach.
- The gastric phase begins when food enters the stomach. Stomach distention (stimulating stretch receptors) and chemical stimuli from partially digested proteins initiate this phase. Gastrin-secreting cells produce gastrin, which in turn stimulates the gastric glands (especially the parietal cells) to produce more gastric juice. Histamine also stimulates hydrochloric acid secretion.
- The intestinal phase is initiated when partially digested food begins to enter the small intestine, stimulating mucous cells of the intestine to release a hormone that promotes continued gastric secretion.

Mechanical digestion in the stomach is accomplished by peristaltic movements that churn and mix the food with the gastric juices to form chyme. Gastric motility is enhanced or retarded by the same factors that affect secretion, namely, distention and the effect of gastrin. After a person eats a normal, well-balanced meal, the stomach empties completely in approximately four to six hours. Gastric emptying depends on the volume, chemical composition, and osmotic pressure of the gastric contents. The stomach empties large volumes of content more rapidly, while gastric emptying is slowed by solids and fats.

The Small Intestine

The small intestine begins at the pyloric sphincter and ends at the ileocecal junction at the entrance of the large intestine. The small intestine is about 20 ft (6 m) long but only about 1 inch (2.5 cm) in diameter. This long tube hangs in coils in the abdominal cavity, suspended by the mesentery and surrounded by the large intestine. The small intestine has three regions: the duodenum, the jejunum, and the ileum. The duodenum begins at the pyloric sphincter and extends around the head of the pancreas for about 10 inches (25 cm). Both pancreatic enzymes and bile from the liver enter the small intestine at the duodenum. The jejunum, the middle region of the small intestine, extends for about 8 ft (2.4 m). The ileum, the terminal end of the small intestine, is approximately 12 ft (3.6 m) long and meets the large intestine at the ileocecal valve.

Food is chemically digested, and most of it absorbed, as it moves through the small intestine. Circular folds (deep folds of the mucosa and submucosa layers), villi (fingerlike projections of the mucosa cells), and microvilli (tiny projections of the mucosa cells) increase the surface area of the small intestine to enhance absorption of food. Although up to 10 L of food, liquids, and secretions enter the GI tract each day, less than 1 L reaches the large intestine.

Enzymes in the small intestine break down carbohydrates, proteins, lipids, and nucleic acids. Pancreatic amylase acts on starches, converting them to maltose, dextrins, and oligosaccharides; the intestinal enzymes dextrinase, glucoamylase, maltase, sucrase, and lactase further break down these products into monosaccharides. Pancreatic enzymes (trypsin and chymotrypsin) and intestinal enzymes continue to break down proteins into peptides. Pancreatic lipases digest lipids in the small intestine. Triglycerides enter as fat globules and are coated by bile salts and emulsified. Nucleic acids are hydrolyzed by pancreatic enzymes and then broken apart by intestinal enzymes. Both pancreatic enzymes and bile are excreted into the duodenum in response to the secretion of secretin and cholecystokinin, hormones produced by the intestinal mucosa cells when chyme enters the small intestine.

Nutrients are absorbed through the mucosa of the intestinal villi into the blood or lymph by active transport, facilitated transport, and passive diffusion. Almost all food products and water, as well as vitamins and most electrolytes, are absorbed in the small intestine, leaving only indigestible fibers, some water, and bacteria to enter the large intestine.

The Accessory Digestive Organs

The Liver and Gallbladder

The liver is the largest gland in the body, weighing about 3 lb (1.4 kg) in the average-size adult. It is located in the right side of the abdomen, inferior to the diaphragm and anterior to the stomach. The liver has four lobes: right, left, caudate, and quadrate. A mesenteric ligament separates the right and left lobes and suspends the liver from the diaphragm and anterior abdominal wall. The liver is encased in a fibroelastic capsule.

Liver tissue consists of units called lobules, which are composed of plates of hepatocytes (liver cells). A branch of the hepatic artery, a branch of the hepatic portal vein, and a bile duct communicate with each lobule. Sinusoids, blood-filled spaces within the lobules, are lined with Kupffer cells. These phagocytic cells remove debris from the blood.

The liver performs the following digestive and metabolic functions:

- Secretes bile.
- Stores fat-soluble vitamins (A, D, E, and K).
- Metabolizes bilirubin.
- Stores blood and releases blood into the general circulation during hemorrhage.
- Synthesizes plasma proteins to maintain plasma oncotic pressure.
- Synthesizes prothrombin, fibrinogen, and factors I, II, VII, IX, and X, which are necessary for blood clotting.
- Synthesizes fats from carbohydrates and proteins to be either used for energy or stored as adipose tissue.

- Synthesizes phospholipids and cholesterol necessary for the production of bile salts, steroid hormones, and plasma membranes.
- Converts amino acids to carbohydrates through deamination.
- Releases glucose during times of hypoglycemia.
- Takes up glucose during times of hyperglycemia and stores it as glycogen or converts it to fat.
- Alters chemicals, foreign molecules, and hormones to make them less toxic.
- Stores iron as ferritin, which is released as needed for the production of red blood cells.

Bile production is the liver's primary digestive function. **Bile** is a greenish, watery solution containing bile salts, cholesterol, bilirubin, electrolytes, water, and phospholipids. These substances are necessary to emulsify and promote the absorption of fats. Liver cells make from 700 to 1200 mL of bile daily. When bile is not needed for digestion, the sphincter of Oddi (located at the point at which bile enters the duodenum) is closed, and the bile backs up the cystic duct into the gallbladder for storage.

Bile is concentrated and stored in the gallbladder, a small sac cupped in the inferior surface of the liver. When food containing fats enters the duodenum, hormones stimulate the gallbladder to secrete bile into the cystic duct. The cystic duct joins the hepatic duct to form the common bile duct, from which bile enters into the duodenum.

The Pancreas

The pancreas, a gland located between the stomach and small intestine, is the primary enzyme-producing organ of the digestive system. It is a triangular gland extending across the abdomen, with its tail next to the spleen and its head next to the duodenum. The body and tail of the pancreas are retroperitoneal, lying behind the greater curvature of the stomach. The pancreas is actually two organs in one, having both exocrine and endocrine structures and functions. The exocrine portion of the pancreas, through secretory units called acini, secretes alkaline pancreatic juice containing many different enzymes. The acini, clusters of secretory cells surrounding ducts, drain into the pancreatic duct. The pancreatic duct joins with the common bile duct just before it enters the duodenum (so that pancreatic juice and bile from the liver enter the small intestine together). The pancreas also has endocrine functions.

The pancreas produces from 1 to 1.5 L of pancreatic juice daily. Pancreatic juice is clear and has high bicarbonate content. This alkaline fluid neutralizes the acidic chyme as it enters the duodenum, optimizing the pH for intestinal and pancreatic enzyme activity. The secretion of pancreatic juice is controlled by the vagus nerve and the intestinal hormones secretin and cholecystokinin. Pancreatic juice contains enzymes that aid in the digestion of all categories of foods: lipase promotes fat breakdown and absorption; amylase completes starch digestion; and trypsin, chymotrypsin, and carboxypeptidase are responsible for half of all protein digestion. Nucleases break down nucleic acids.

Metabolism

After nutrients (carbohydrates, fats, and proteins) are ingested, digested, absorbed, and transported across cell membranes, they must be metabolized to produce and provide energy to maintain life. **Metabolism** is the complex of biochemical reactions occurring in the body's cells. Metabolic processes are either catabolic or anabolic. Catabolism involves the breakdown of complex structures into simpler forms; for example, the breakdown of carbohydrates to produce adenosine triphosphate (ATP), an energy molecule that fuels cellular activity. In the process of anabolism, simpler molecules combine to build more complex structures; for example, amino acids bond to form proteins.

The biochemical reactions of metabolism produce water, carbon dioxide, and ATP. The energy value of foods is measured in kilocalories (kcal). A kilocalorie is defined as the amount of heat energy needed to raise the temperature of 1 kilogram (kg) of water 1 degree centigrade.

Nutrients

Nutrients are substances found in food and are used by the body to promote growth, maintenance, and repair. The categories of nutrients are carbohydrates, proteins, fats, vitamins, minerals, and water.

Carbohydrates

The primary sources of carbohydrates (which include sugars and starches) are plant foods. Monosaccharides and disaccharides come from milk, sugar cane, sugar beets, honey, and fruits. Polysaccharide starch is found in grains, legumes, and root vegetables. Following ingestion, digestion, and metabolism, carbohydrates are converted primarily to glucose, the molecule body cells use to make ATP. Glucose is carefully regulated to maintain cellular functions. Excess glucose in the healthy person is converted to glycogen or fat. Glycogen is stored in the liver and muscles; fat is stored as adipose tissue.

Regardless of source, all carbohydrates supply 4 kcal per gram. The minimum necessary daily carbohydrate intake is unknown, but the recommended daily intake is 125 to 175 g, most of which should be complex carbohydrates, such as milk, potatoes, and whole grains. Excess intake of carbohydrates over time can result in obesity, dental caries, and elevated plasma triglycerides. Over extended periods of time, carbohydrate deficiencies lead to tissue wasting from protein breakdown and metabolic acidosis from an excess of ketones as a by-product of fat breakdown.

Proteins

Proteins are classified as either complete or incomplete. Complete proteins are found in animal products, such as eggs, milk, milk products, and meat. They contain the greatest amount of amino acids and meet the body's amino acid requirements for tissue growth and maintenance. Incomplete proteins are found in legumes, nuts, grains, cereals, and vegetables. These sources are low in or lack one or more of the amino acids essential for building complete proteins.

The body uses proteins to build many different structures, including skin keratin, the collagen and elastin in connective tissues, and muscles. They also are used to make enzymes, hemoglobin, plasma proteins, and some hormones.

Proteins provide 4 kcal per gram. The recommended daily intake of protein is 56 g for men and 45 g for women. Healthy people with adequate caloric intake have an equal rate of protein synthesis and protein breakdown and loss, reflected as nitrogen balance. If the breakdown and loss of proteins exceeds intake, a negative nitrogen balance results. This may be due to starvation, altered physical states (e.g., from injury or illness), and altered emotional states, such as depression or anxiety. A positive nitrogen balance, which results when protein intake exceeds breakdown, is normal during growth, tissue repair, and pregnancy. Anabolic steroids affect the rate of protein; for example, the adrenal corticosteroids are released in times of stress to increase protein breakdown and conversion of amino acids to glucose. Excessive intake of proteins may lead to obesity, whereas deficits cause weight loss and tissue wasting, edema, and anemia.

Fats (Lipids)

Fats, or lipids, include phospholipids; steroids, such as cholesterol; and neutral fats, more commonly known as triglycerides. Neutral fats are the most abundant fats in the diet. They may be either saturated or unsaturated. Saturated fats are found in animal products (milk and meats) and in some plant products, such as coconut. Unsaturated fats are found in seeds, nuts, and most vegetable oils. Sources of cholesterol include meats, milk products, and egg yolks.

Fats are a necessary part of the structure and function of the body. For example:

- Phospholipids are a part of all cell membranes.
- Triglycerides are the major energy source for hepatocytes and skeletal muscle cells.
- Adipose tissue serves as a protection around body organs, as a layer of insulation under the skin, and as a concentrated source of fuel for cellular energy.
- Dietary fats facilitate absorption of fat-soluble vitamins.
- Linoleic acid, an essential fatty acid, helps form prostaglandins, regulatory molecules that assist in smooth muscle contraction, maintenance of blood pressure, and control of inflammatory responses.
- Cholesterol is the essential component of bile salts, steroid hormones, and vitamin D. Fats supply 9 kcal per gram. The recommended intake of fats is 30% or less of the total daily caloric intake. Saturated fats should account for no more than 10% of the total daily caloric intake, and cholesterol intake should not exceed 250 mg per day. When a person consumes more than the body requires, the excess is stored as adipose tissue, increasing the risk of obesity and heart disease. A deficit of fats may cause excessive weight loss and skin lesions.

Vitamins

Vitamins are organic compounds that facilitate the body's use of carbohydrates, proteins, and fats. All of the vitamins, except vitamins D and K, must be ingested in foods or taken as supplements. Vitamin D is made by ultraviolet irradiation of cholesterol molecules in the skin, and vitamin K is synthesized by bacteria in the intestine. Vitamins are categorized as either fat soluble or water soluble. The fat-soluble vitamins (A, D, E, and K) bind to ingested fats and are absorbed as the fats are absorbed. Water-soluble vitamins (the B complex and C) are absorbed with water in the GI tract (however, vitamin B_{12} must become attached to intrinsic factor to be absorbed). Fat-soluble vitamins are stored in the body, and excesses may cause toxicity; water-soluble vitamins in excess of body requirements are excreted in the urine. The recommended amounts of vitamins, previously labeled recommended daily allowances (RDAs), are now labeled by the National Academy of Sciences as dietary reference intakes (DRIs) per day. DRIs are provided for each vitamin in the following discussion.

Fat-soluble vitamins:

- Vitamin A (retinol) is found in fish liver oils, egg yolk, liver, fortified milk, and margarine. Vitamin A is necessary to vision, skin and mucous membrane integrity, normal reproductive function, and cell membrane structure. The DRI is 1000 µg for men and 800 µg for women.
- Vitamin D is formed by the action of sunlight on cholesterol in the skin. Vitamin D is necessary for blood calcium homeostasis, which in turn is essential to normal blood clotting, bone formation, and neuromuscular function. The DRI is 7.5 µg.
- Vitamin E is found in vegetable oils, margarine, whole grains, and dark green leafy vegetables. Vitamin E is believed to be an antioxidant; that is, it helps prevent the oxidation of vitamins A and C in the intestine and decreases the oxidation of unsaturated fatty acids to facilitate cell membrane integrity. The DRI is 15 mg.
- Vitamin K is synthesized by coliform bacteria in the large intestine and is found in green leafy vegetables, cabbage, cauliflower, and pork. Vitamin K is essential for the formation of clotting proteins in the liver. The DRI is 2 g.

Water-soluble vitamins:

- Vitamin B_1 (thiamin) is found in lean meats, liver, eggs, green leafy vegetables, legumes, and whole grains. This B vitamin is an essential coenzyme for carbohydrate catabolism and use. It is essential for the healthy functioning of the nerves, muscles, and heart. The DRI is 1.5 mg for men and 1.1 mg for women.
- Vitamin B_2 (riboflavin) is found in liver, egg whites, whole grains, meat, poultry, and fish; a major source is milk. This B vitamin is involved in the catabolism and use of carbohydrates, fats, and proteins, and the use of other B vitamins. It is also important in the production of adrenal hormones. The DRI is 1.7 mg for men and 1.3 mg for women.
- Vitamin B_6 (pyridoxine) is found in meat, poultry, fish, potatoes, tomatoes, sweet potatoes, and spinach. This B vitamin is necessary for amino acid metabolism, formation of antibodies, and formation of hemoglobin. The DRI is 2.2 mg for men and 2 mg for women.
- Vitamin B_{12} (cyanocobalamin) is found in liver, meat, poultry, fish, dairy foods (except butter), and eggs. Vitamin B_{12} is not found in any plant foods, however. It is essential for the production of nucleic acids and of red blood cells in the bone marrow. It also plays an important role in the use of folic acid and carbohydrates, and in the healthy functioning of the nervous system. The DRI is 3 µg.
- Vitamin C (ascorbic acid) is found in citrus fruits, fresh potatoes, tomatoes, and green leafy vegetables. Vitamin C acts as an antioxidant and a vasoconstrictor. It also serves in the formation of connective tissue, in the conversion of cholesterol to bile salts, in iron absorption and use, and in the conversion of folic acid to its active form. The DRI is 90 mg for men and 75 mg for women.
- Niacin (nicotinamide) is found in meat, poultry, fish, liver, peanuts, and green leafy vegetables. Niacin plays an important role in the metabolism of carbohydrates and fats and inhibits cholesterol synthesis. It is important for the health of the integumentary, nervous, and digestive systems, and assists in the manufacture of reproductive hormones. The DRI is 19 mg for men and 14 mg for women.

- Biotin is found in liver, egg yolk, nuts, and legumes. Biotin is essential for the catabolism of fatty acids and carbohydrates. It also helps dispose of the waste products of protein catabolism. The DRI is 100 to 200 mg.

- Pantothenic acid is found in meats, whole grains, egg yolk, liver, yeast, and legumes. Pantothenic acid assists in the synthesis of steroids and the heme of hemoglobin. It is essential for the metabolism of carbohydrates and fats and for the manufacture of reproductive hormones. The DRI is 10 mg.

- Folic acid (folacin) is found in liver, dark green vegetables, lean beef, eggs, veal, and whole grains. Folic acid is also synthesized by bacteria in the intestine. Folic acid is the basis of a coenzyme necessary to the manufacture of nucleic acids, and therefore is essential for the formation of red blood cells, growth and development, and the health of the nervous system. The RDA is 0.4 mg. (DRI not available.)

Minerals

Minerals work with other nutrients to maintain the structure and function of the body. An adequate supply of calcium, phosphorus, potassium, sulfur, sodium, chloride, and magnesium—as well as other trace elements such as iron, iodine, copper, and zinc—is necessary to health. Most minerals in the body are found in body fluids or are bound to organic compounds. The best sources of minerals are vegetables, legumes, milk, and some meats. Dietary sources for minerals are discussed in Chapter 5. The recommended daily intake for each is as follows:

- Calcium: 1000 mg, although after menopause, women who do not take estrogen supplements should increase their uptake to 1200 mg
- Phosphorus: 700 mg
- Iron: 15 mg
- Zinc: 12 mg
- Iodine: 150 µg
- Fluoride: 3.1 mg
- Selenium: 55 µg
- Potassium: 2 g.

Assessing Nutritional Status and the Gastrointestinal System

The nurse conducts both a health assessment interview (to collect subjective data) and a physical assessment (to collect objective data) to assess the client's nutritional status and gastrointestinal function. Physical assessment of the integumentary system, nervous system, musculoskeletal system, cardiovascular system, and respiratory system may also reflect the client's nutritional status.

The Health Assessment Interview

This section provides guidelines for collecting subjective data through a health assessment interview specific to nutritional status, the gastrointestinal system, and the accessory digestive organs.

A health assessment interview to determine problems with nutrition and digestion may be conducted during a health screening, may focus on a chief complaint, such as nausea or unexplained weight loss, or may be part of a total health assessment. If the client has a health problem involving nutrition and digestion, analyze its onset, characteristics and course, severity, precipitating and relieving factors, and any associated symptoms, noting the timing and circumstances. For example, ask the client:

- Have you had any episodes of indigestion, nausea, vomiting, diarrhea, or constipation? If so, describe the appearance of what was vomited or the stools and anything that makes these problems better or worse. How long have you had these problems?
- What is your usual dietary intake pattern during a 24-hour period?
- Describe what you believe to be a "healthy" diet.

When collecting information about the client's current health status, ask about any changes in weight, appetite, and the ability to taste, chew, or swallow. What is the client's perception of the role of nutrition in maintaining health? Who buys and prepares the food? What medications (prescribed, over-the-counter, or vitamins) is the client currently taking? Does the client take any vitamins, herbal supplements, or other "health-food" items? Does the client consume alcohol (how much and type)? If the client has experienced nausea or vomiting, ask whether the vomitus contains bright red blood, dark (old) blood, bile, or fecal material. If the client is very thin, or verbalizes concerns about body size incongruent with the ratio of height to weight, ask whether the client induces vomiting or uses laxatives to control weight. Ask whether the client has appliances such as braces, bridges, or dentures, and what self-care measures are used for such appliances, as well as oral hygiene practices and frequency of dental visits.

Ask the client to describe any heartburn, indigestion, abdominal discomfort, or pain. Explore the location of the pain, the type of pain, the time it occurs, foods that aggravate or relieve it, and how it is relieved. Abdominal pain is often referred to other sites (see Chapter 38). For example, a client with a liver disorder may experience pain over the right shoulder (Kehr's sign). Epigastric (middle upper abdominal) pain is experienced in cases of acute gastritis, obstruction of the small intestine, and acute pancreatitis. Pain in the right upper quadrant is associated with cholecystitis. Pain in the left upper quadrant may be related to a gastric ulcer.

The health history should include questions about any prior surgeries or trauma of the gastrointestinal tract. Explore the past history of any medical condition that may affect the client's ingestion, digestion, and/or metabolism (for example, Crohn's disease, diabetes mellitus, irritable bowel syndrome, peptic ulcers, or pancreatitis). Other areas significant to assessment of nutritional status and the gastrointestinal system are food allergies (especially to milk, which is evidenced as lactose intolerance with abdominal cramping, excessive flatus, and loose stools) and a family history that may provide clues to increased risk for health problems.

Physical Assessment

Physical assessment of gastrointestinal and nutritional status may be performed as part of a total health assessment, in combination with assessment of the urinary and reproductive systems (problems which may cause clinical manifestations similar to those of the gastrointestinal system), or alone for clients with known or suspected health problems. The techniques of inspection, auscultation, percussion, and palpation are used. Palpation is the last method used in assessing the abdomen, because pressure on the abdominal wall and contents may interfere with bowel sounds and cause pain, ending the examination.

Collect objective data by obtaining **anthropometric measurements** (height, weight, triceps skinfolds, and midarm circumference) and by examining the mouth and abdomen. The equipment necessary for the assessment are a stethoscope, a scale, a tape measure, and skinfold calipers. Prior to the examination, collect all necessary equipment and explain techniques to the client to decrease anxiety. The client may be seated during assessment of the mouth, but is supine during the abdominal assessment.

Anthropometric Assessment with Abnormal Findings

- Weigh the client and compare the client's actual weight to ideal body weight (IBW).
  - ✓ A weight 10% to 20% less than ideal body weight indicates malnutrition.
  - ✓ A weight 10% above ideal body weight is considered overweight.
  - ✓ A weight 20% above ideal body weight is considered obese.
- Calculate the client's percentage of ideal body weight (%IBW).
- Calculate the client's percentage of usual body weight (%UBW) to determine weight change, using this formula:

$$\frac{\text{current weight}}{\text{usual weight}} \times 100$$

  - ✓ Using %IBW may result in overlooking malnutrition in a very obese client.
- Measure triceps skinfold thickness (TSF).
  - ✓ Find the midpoint between the client's olecranon and acromion processes.
  - ✓ Grasp the skin and fat, and pull it away from the muscle. Apply skinfold calipers for three seconds, and record reading.
  - ✓ Repeat three times, and average the three readings.
  - ✓ Compare the client's reading to the standard values for anthropometric measurement.
  - ✓ Triceps readings are 10% or more below standards in malnutrition and 10% or more above standards in obesity or overnutrition.
- Measure midarm circumference (MAC).
- Find the midpoint between the client's olecranon and acromion processes.
- Wind tape measure around arm. Compare the client's reading to the standard values for anthropometric measurement.
- MAC decreases with malnutrition and increases with obesity.
- Calculate midarm muscle circumference (MAMC).
  - ✓ Use the client's triceps skinfold measurement and midarm circumference readings to calculate the client's MAMC, using: MAMC = MAC − (0.314 ¥ TSF).
  - ✓ Compare the result to the standard values for anthropometric measurement.
- In mild malnutrition, the MAMC is 90% of the standard; in moderate malnutrition, 60% to 90%. In severe malnutrition (muscle wasting), the MAMC is less than 60% of the standard.

Oral Assessment with Abnormal Findings

Note: Wear gloves!

- Inspect and palpate the lips.
    - ✓ *Cheilosis* (painful lesions at corners of mouth) is seen with riboflavin and/or niacin deficiency.
    - ✓ Cold sores or clear vesicles with a red base are seen in herpes simplex I.
- Inspect and palpate the tongue.
    - ✓ Atrophic smooth glossitis is characterized by a bright red tongue. It is seen in B_{12}, folic acid, and iron deficiencies.
    - ✓ Vertical fissures are seen in dehydration.
    - ✓ A black, hairy tongue may be seen following antibiotic therapy.
- Inspect and palpate the buccal mucosa.
    - ✓ *Leukoplakia* (small white patches) may be a sign of a premalignant condition.
    - ✓ A reddened, dry, swollen mucosa may be seen in stomatitis.
    - ✓ *Candidiases* (white cheesy patches that bleed when scraped) may be seen in immune-suppressed clients receiving antibiotics or chemotherapy and in terminally ill clients.
- Inspect and palpate the teeth.
    - ✓ Cavities and excessive plaque are seen with poor nutrition and/or poor oral hygiene.
- Inspect and palpate the gums.
    - ✓ Swollen, red gums that bleed easily (*gingivitis*) are seen in periodontal disease, vitamin C deficiencies, or with hormonal changes.
- Inspect the throat and tonsils.
    - ✓ In acute infections, tonsils are red and swollen and may have white spots.
- Note the client's breath.
    - ✓ Sweet, fruity breath is noted in diabetic ketoacidosis.
    - ✓ Acetone breath may be a sign of uremia.
    - ✓ Foul breath may result from liver disease, respiratory infections, and poor oral hygiene.

Abdominal Assessment with Abnormal Findings

- Inspect abdominal contour, skin integrity, venous pattern, and aortic pulsation.
    - ✓ Generalized abdominal distention may be seen in gas retention or obesity.
    - ✓ Lower abdominal distention is seen in bladder distention, pregnancy, or ovarian mass.
    - ✓ General distention and an everted umbilicus is seen with ascites and/or tumors.
    - ✓ A scaphoid (sunken) abdomen is seen in malnutrition or when fat is replaced with muscle.
    - ✓ *Striae* (whitish-silver stretch marks) are seen in obesity and during or after pregnancy.

- ✓ Spider angiomas may be seen in liver disease.
- ✓ Dilated veins are prominent in cirrhosis of the liver, ascites, portal hypertension, or venocaval obstruction.
- ✓ Pulsation is increased in aortic aneurysm.
- Auscultate all four quadrants of the abdomen with the diaphragm of the stethoscope. Begin in the lower right quadrant, where bowel sounds are almost always present. Normal bowel sounds (gurgling or clicking) occur every 5 to 15 seconds. Listen for at least 5 minutes in each of the four quadrants to confirm the absence of bowel sounds.
  - ✓ *Borborygmus* (hyperactive high-pitched, tinkling, rushing, or growling bowel sounds) is heard in diarrhea or at the onset of bowel obstruction.
  - ✓ Bowel sounds may be absent later in bowel obstruction, with an inflamed peritoneum, and/or following surgery of the abdomen.
- Auscultate the abdomen for vascular sounds with the bell of the stethoscope.
  - ✓ *Bruits* (blowing sound due to restriction of blood flow through vessels) may be heard over constricted arteries. A bruit over the liver may be heard in hepatic carcinoma.
  - ✓ A venous hum (continuous medium-pitched sound) may be heard over a cirrhotic liver.
  - ✓ Friction rubs (rough grating sounds) may be heard over an inflamed liver or spleen.
- Percuss the abdomen in all four quadrants. Normally, tympany is heard over the stomach and gas-filled bowels.
  - ✓ Dullness is heard when the bowel is displaced with fluid or tumors or filled with a fecal mass.
- Percuss the liver.
  - ✓ In cirrhosis and/or hepatitis, the liver is greater than 6 to 10 cm in the MCL and greater than 4 to 8 cm in the midsternal line (MSL).
- Percuss the spleen for dullness posterior to the midaxilliary line at the level of the 6th to 11th rib.
  - ✓ A large area of dullness that extends to the left anterior axcillary line on inspiration is associated with an enlarged spleen and may be related to in trauma, infection, or mononucleosis.
- Percuss for shifting dullness.
  - ✓ In a client with ascites, the level of dullness increases when the client turns to the side.
- Palpate the abdomen in all four quadrants.
  - Use a circular motion to move the abdominal wall over underlying structures. Feel for masses and note any tenderness or pain the client may have during this part of the exam. Palpate lightly at first (0.5 to 0.75 inch), then deeply (1.5 to 2 inches) with caution.
- Never use deep palpation in a client who has had a pulsatile abdominal mass, renal transplant polycystic kidneys, or is at risk for hemorrhage.

✓ In cases of peritoneal inflammation, palpation causes abdominal pain and involuntary muscle spasms.

✓ Abnormal masses include aortic aneurysms, neoplastic tumors of the colon or uterus, and a distended bladder or distended bowel due to obstruction.

✓ A rigid, boardlike abdomen may be palpated when the client has a perforated duodenal ulcer.

✓ If a mass is palpated, ask the client to raise head and shoulders. A mass in the abdomen may become more prominent with this maneuver, as will a ventral abdominal wall hernia. If the mass is no longer palpable, it is deeper in the abdomen.

- Palpate for rebound tenderness.

  ✓ Press the fingers into the abdomen slowly and release the pressure quickly.

  ✓ In peritoneal inflammation, pain occurs when the fingers are withdrawn.

  ✓ Right upper quadrant pain occurs with acute cholecystitis.

  ✓ Upper middle abdominal pain occurs with acute pancreatitis.

  ✓ Right lower quadrant pain occurs with acute appendicitis.

  ✓ Left lower quadrant pain is seen in acute diverticulitis.

- Palpate the liver.

  ✓ An enlarged liver with a smooth, tender edge may indicate hepatitis or venous congestion.

  ✓ An enlarged, nontender liver may be felt in malignant condition.

  ✓ Note whether the client guards the abdomen or reports any sharp pain, especially on inspiration.

  ✓ The client with inflammation of the gallbladder feels sharp pain on inspiration and stops inspiring. This is called Murphy's sign.

17 Nursing Care of Clients with Nutritional Disorders

Obesity and malnutrition, the major nutritional disorders in the world today, affect many systems and organs. They often cause serious health problems, such as hypertension, heart disease, fluid and electrolyte imbalances, disability, and even death.

Clients with nutritional disorders require complex, skilled nursing care. Developmental, sociocultural, psychologic, and physiologic factors may play a role in these disorders: A holistic approach to nursing care is vital. Nursing care focuses on identifying causes, meeting nutritional and physiologic needs, providing client education, and meeting the psychologic needs of clients and families.

The Client with Obesity

Obesity, an excess of adipose tissue, is one of the most prevalent, preventable health problems in the United States. While obesity is often defined by weight, it is more accurately defined by amount of body fat, or adipose tissue. Adipose tissue is created when energy consumption exceeds energy expenditure. Obesity has serious physiologic and psychologic consequences, and is associated with increased morbidity and mortality.

Incidence and Prevalence

Up to one-third of the population in the United States is obese. The incidence of obesity is higher in women, African-Americans, and economically disadvantaged people of all races (Braunwald, et al., 2001; Tierney, et al., 2001). Of particular concern is the increasing incidence of obesity in children and young adults.

Overview of Normal Physiology

All body activities require energy, including activities of daily living, as well as those necessary to maintain cell and tissue function. Nutrients in food (or enteral or parenteral feedings) provide this energy and the building blocks for growth and tissue repair. The body stores excess nutrients and energy (measured as kilocalories) to meet the body's needs when required nutrients are unavailable. This ability to store and release energy is important to maintaining body function.

Energy is primarily stored as fat in adipose tissue. Although mature fat cells (adipocytes) do not multiply, the immature cells in adipose tissue can multiply, particularly when exposed to estrogen during puberty, in late adolescence, during breastfeeding, and in middle-aged adults who are overweight. Fat cells store excess energy as **triglycerides,** formed from dietary fats and carbohydrates. The body breaks down the triglycerides in fat cells when needed to provide energy (Porth, 2002).

Pathophysiology

Obesity occurs when excess calories are stored as fat. It can result from excess energy intake, decreased energy expenditure, or a combination of both.

Appetite, which affects food intake, is regulated by the central nervous system and by emotional factors. The hunger center in the hypothalamus stimulates appetite in response to stimuli, such as hypoglycemia. As nutrient levels rise, the satiety center (also in the hypothalamus) sends the message to stop eating. Gastrointestinal filling and hormonal factors also signal *satiety* (a sensation of fullness). Appetite may have little relationship to hunger: People may eat to relieve depression or anxiety.

Several hormones are involved in regulating obesity, including thyroid hormone, insulin, and leptin (a peptide produced by fatty tissue that suppresses appetite and increases energy expenditure). Some studies suggest that leptin resistance is a cause of obesity. Insulin is associated with body fat distribution (Bullock & Henze, 2000). The two major types of body fat distribution are upper body and lower body obesity.

Upper body obesity (also called central obesity) is identified by a waist/hip ratio of greater than 1 in men or 0.8 in women. People with upper body obesity tend to have more intra-abdominal fat and higher levels of circulating free fatty acids (Porth, 2002). As a result, upper body obesity is associated with a greater risk of complications, such as hypertension, abnormal blood lipid levels, heart disease, stroke, and elevated insulin levels. Men tend to have more intra-abdominal fat than women, although women develop a central fat distribution pattern after menopause.

Lower body obesity (also known as peripheral obesity), in which the waist/hip ratio is less than 0.8, is more commonly seen in women. The risk for hyperinsulinemia, abnormal lipids, and heart disease is lower in people with lower body obesity than in those with upper body obesity. Lower body obesity may be more difficult to treat, however.

Risk Factors

Many factors contribute to obesity, including genetic, physiologic, psychologic, environmental, and sociocultural factors. There is a strong link between heredity and obesity. A person with one obese parent has a 40% chance of becoming obese; one with two obese parents, an 80% chance. Researchers have reported a strong correlation between the weight of adopted children and their biologic parents.

Physical inactivity is probably the most important factor contributing to obesity. Inactive people may consume fewer calories than active people and continue to gain weight due to lack of energy expenditure.

Environmental influences, such as an abundant and readily accessible food supply, fast-food restaurants, advertising, and vending machines, contribute to increased food intake.

Sociocultural influences that contribute to obesity include overeating at family meals, rewarding behavior with food, religious and family gatherings that promote food intake, and sedentary lifestyles.

Psychologic factors, such as low self-esteem, also play a role in obesity. Low self-esteem may precipitate unhealthy eating behaviors, and the resulting weight gain in turn may diminish self-image even further. A person may overeat as a result of anxiety, depression, guilt, boredom, or as a means of getting attention. Some experts characterize overeating as a food addiction, and as a coping mechanism for stressful life events.

Complications of Obesity

As obesity increases, adverse consequences of obesity increase. Individuals with **morbid obesity** (those whose weight is more than 100% over ideal body weight) have a risk of dying that is 12 times that of people who are not obese (Braunwald et al., 2001). Obesity increases the risk of insulin resistance and type 2 diabetes. It affects reproductive function in both men and women. Androgen (male sex hormone) levels are reduced in obese men; menstrual irregularities and polycystic ovarian syndrome (PCOS) are more common in obese women. Obesity is a significant risk factor for cardiovascular disease, including hypertension, coronary heart disease, and heart failure.

Collaborative Care

Because obesity has many contributing factors, its treatment is far more complex than just reducing the amount of food consumed. Treatment is an ongoing process requiring a number of strategies. Most experts recommend an individualized program of exercise, diet, and behavior modification designed to meet the client's specific needs.

Diagnostic Tests

Although body weight may be used to identify obesity, measures of body fat are more accurate. Males at ideal body weight have 10% to 20% body fat, whereas females at ideal body weight have 20% to 30% body fat.

*   *Body mass index (BMI)* is used to identify excess adipose tissue. BMI is calculated by dividing the weight (in kilograms) by the height in meters squared (m^2).
*   *Anthropometry,* skinfold or fatfold measurements, uses calipers to measure skinfold thickness at various sites on the body.
*   *Underwater weighing (hydrodensitometry)* is considered the most accurate way to determine body fat. This technique involves submerging the whole body and then measuring the amount of displaced water.
*   *Bioelectrical impedance* uses a low-energy electrical impulse to determine the percentage of body fat by measuring the electrical resistance of the body.

Other diagnostic tests may be done to help identify a physiologic cause of obesity, as well as complications of obesity.

*   A *thyroid profile,* including a T_3, T_4, and TSH, is done to rule out thyroid disease.
*   *Serum glucose* is measured to identify coexisting diabetes mellitus.
*   *Serum cholesterol* is measured to assess for elevated levels.

- *A lipid profile* is ordered; high-density lipoprotein (HDL) levels are reduced in obese clients, whereas low-density lipoprotein (LDL) levels are elevated.
- *An electrocardiogram (ECG)* is performed to detect effects of obesity on the heart, such as rate or rhythm disruptions, myocardial infarction, or heart enlargement.

Treatments

Treatment of obesity focuses on changing both eating and exercise habits. A pound of body fat is equivalent to 3500 kcal. To lose one pound, therefore, a person must reduce daily caloric intake by 250 kcal for 14 days or increase activity enough to burn the equivalent kcal.

Exercise

Exercise is a critical element in weight loss and maintenance. Physical activity increases energy consumption and promotes weight loss while preserving lean body mass. Physical activity improves physical fitness, decreases appetite, promotes selfesteem, and increases the basal metabolic rate. An exercise or activity program should reflect the client's physical condition, interest, lifestyle, and abilities. Evaluation by a health care practitioner is important before beginning an exercise program. The practitioner instructs the client to increase the duration and intensity of activity and to stop exercising and report symptoms if chest pain or shortness of breath occurs. An aerobic exercise program of 30 minutes of exercise 3 to 5 days a week promotes weight loss while reducing adipose tissue, increasing lean body mass, and promoting long-term weight control.

Dietary Management

The diet should be low in kilocalories and fat and contain adequate nutrients, minerals, and fiber. The client should eat regular meals with small servings. A gradual, slow weight loss of no more than one to two pounds per week is recommended. For most people, this means a diet of 1000 to 1500 kcal per day. Fewer than 1200 kcal each day may lead to loss of lean tissue and nutritional deficiencies. The recommended diet generally is low in fat and high in dietary fiber. Excessive calorie restrictions can lead to failure to follow the prescribed diet, feelings of guilt, and overeating. "Yo-yo" dieting (repeated cycles of weight loss and gain) may lead to a metabolic deficiency that makes subsequent weight loss efforts increasingly difficult. Therefore, it is critical that dieters take any weight loss effort seriously and include plans for long-term maintenance. The best approach is to modify dietary intake without severe restrictions, eating a well-balanced, low-fat diet and developing improved eating habits.

Very low calorie diets (VLCD) are generally reserved for clients who are more than 35% overweight. This type of program offers a protein-sparing modified fast (400 to 800 kcal/day or less) under close medical supervision. In a typical program, the client observes a 12-week fast, ingesting only a liquid protein supplement. This initial fast is followed by a 12-week refeeding program with nutrition and behavior modification counseling. The client generally experiences a dramatic and rapid weight loss while maintaining lean body mass. This type of program is indicated for short-term use only and requires very close medical supervision.

Behavior Modification

Behavior modification is a critical component of successful weight management. Strategies, such as keeping food records, eliminating cues that precipitate eating, and changing the act of eating, are often helpful.

Recording food intake, amount, location of eating, and situations that induce eating often help the dieter gain self-control. These strategies are often most effective when used in combination with other behavior modification approaches.

Researchers have found that most overweight people are stimulated to eat by external cues, such as the proximity to food and the time of day. In contrast, hunger and satiety are the cues that regulate eating in adults of normal weight. Strategies to control food cues include keeping food out of view, eliminating snack foods, and eating only in designated areas.

Other behavior modification approaches focus on helping clients examine factors that affect eating behaviors. Examining lifestyle, personality, and environment helps the client understand eating behaviors and their consequences. The goal is to empower the person who is stimulated to eat to choose activities that are not related to food.

Social support and group programs such as Weight Watchers, Overeaters Anonymous, and Take Off Pounds Sensibly (TOPS) promote weight loss success through peer support. Most organized programs require participants to pay a fee, which may improve compliance.

Medications

Many prescription and over-the-counter drugs have been used to help people lose weight. When used in combination with diet and exercise, drugs can help promote weight loss. Their long-term efficacy, however, is questionable. In addition, tolerance, addiction, and side effects may occur. These products are usually recommended only as an adjunct to therapy and only when traditional therapies have been unsuccessful.

Amphetamines (which have a high potential for abuse) and nonamphetamine appetite suppressants, such as phenteramine, may be used for a short time to promote weight loss. Sibutramine (Meridia) is an appetite suppressant that acts on the CNS. Sibutramine also may increase the metabolic rate, promoting weight loss. It has the additional benefit of lowering cholesterol and triglyceride levels. Orlistat (Xenical) has a different mechanism of action: It inhibits fat absorption from the GI tract, leading to weight loss. It has the added benefit of lowering blood glucose and cholesterol.

Over-the-counter products, such as phenylpropanolamine, benzocaine, and bulk-forming agents, are commonly used in weight management efforts. Phenylpropanolamine (Acutrim, Dexatrim) is an adrenergic agent that suppresses appetite. This product is contraindicated in clients with hypertension, coronary heart disease, diabetes mellitus, and thyroid disease. Methylcellulose and other bulk-forming products may decrease appetite by producing a sensation of fullness. Clients taking these products may experience flatulence or diarrhea and may need to increase fluid intake.

Surgery

Surgical treatment of obesity generally is limited to morbidly obese clients (BMI of over 40 kg/m² or 100% over ideal body weight). In addition, clients must be able to tolerate surgery and be free of addiction to alcohol or other drugs. A thorough psychologic evaluation is done before surgery.

The most common surgical procedures used in the United States to treat obesity are the vertical banded gastroplasty and Roux-en-Y gastric bypass. These procedures reduce stomach capacity. Although the risk for postoperative complications is high, the mortality rate for these procedures is low. Possible postoperative complications include anastomosis leak with peritonitis, abdominal wall hernia, wound infections, deep vein thrombosis, nutritional deficiencies, and gastrointestinal symptoms (Tierney, et al., 2001). Clients may lose as much as half their initial body weight following surgery.

Maintaining Weight Loss

Losing weight and maintaining that loss are two separate but related issues. Most experts agree that the majority of dieters regain lost weight within a 2-year period. The potential risks associated with regaining weight make maintenance a critical issue. Clients are encouraged to continue exercise, self-monitoring, and treatment support. Long-term weight loss and maintenance mean a lifelong commitment to significant lifestyle changes, including food and eating habits, activity and exercise routines, and behavior modification.

Nursing Care

Health Promotion

Maintaining a healthy weight throughout the life span begins in childhood. Obese children and teenagers become obese adults. Promote healthy eating, including a diet rich in whole grains, fruits, and vegetables and low in fat. Encourage all children and adults to maintain an active lifestyle, engaging in at least 30 minutes of aerobic activity daily. Encourage parents to limit time children spend watching television, using the computer, and playing video games. Discuss the effect of smoking and excess alcohol use on nutrition and activity.

Adults commonly gain about 20 pounds between early and middle adulthood. Encourage clients to reduce the amount of calories consumed as energy needs change.

Assessment

Collect the following data through the health history and physical examination:

- *Health history:* risk factors; current and usual weight; recent weight gains or losses; perception of weight and effect on health; usual diet and food intake; exercise/activity patterns; prior weight-loss efforts; current medications; coexisting disorders, such as cardiovascular disease and diabetes.
- *Physical examination:* vital signs; weight and height; skinfold measurements; waist/hip ratio; BMI.

Nursing Diagnoses and Interventions

Nursing care for overweight and obese clients is community based and holistic, focusing on both physiologic and psychologic responses to weight and appearance.

Imbalanced Nutrition: More Than Body Requirements

Although many factors contribute to obesity, it always involves an imbalance of kcal consumption to energy expenditure.

- Encourage the client to identify the factors that contribute to excess food intake. *Identification of cues to eating helps the client eliminate or reduce these cues.*
- Establish realistic weight-loss goals and exercise/activity objectives. *Small, reasonable goals, such as loss of one to two pounds per week, increase the likelihood of success.*

- Assess the client's knowledge and discuss well-balanced diet plans. Provide necessary teaching about diet. *Knowledge empowers the client to participate and make appropriate diet choices.*
- Discuss behavior modification strategies, such as self-monitoring and environmental management. *Behavior modification, diet, and exercise are critical to promoting successful, long-term weight loss.*

Activity Intolerance

Obese clients may experience excess fatigue, tachycardia, and shortness of breath with activity due to the physiologic effects of excess weight as well as a sedentary lifestyle. A medical evaluation may be needed before beginning an exercise program.

- Assess current activity level and tolerance of that activity. Assess vital signs. *This provides baseline information to plan an activity program and assess response to that activity.*
- After medical clearance, plan with the client a program of regular, gradually increasing exercise. Consider a consultation with an exercise physiologist. *An individualized exercise program promotes activities within the client's physical capabilities.*

Ineffective Therapeutic Regimen Management

Most overweight or obese clients experience some difficulty integrating all the components of a weight-loss program into a daily routine. For a weight loss and maintenance program to be successful, the overweight client must modify dietary intake in a world of daily temptations. There may be many obstacles to exercise, including a busy schedule, activity intolerance, impaired physical mobility, lack of equipment, and the embarrassment of being fat.

- Discuss ability and willingness to incorporate changes into daily patterns of diet, exercise, and lifestyle. *This provides data from which to set realistic goals with the client.*
- Help the client identify behavior modification strategies and support systems for weight loss and maintenance. *Weight loss and maintenance are most successful if the client establishes lifestyle patterns that promote interest and motivation and thus exercise and diet management. Family and social support is critical to successful adherence to the therapeutic regime.*
- Have the client establish strategies for dealing with "stress" eating or interruptions in the therapeutic regime. *A sense of failure associated with overeating or lack of exercise can lead to further overeating. Identifying positive strategies to deal with these situations promotes self-acceptance and limits self-punishment through overeating.*

Chronic Low Self-Esteem

Although many obese clients may have accepted their weight and body appearance on some level, most overweight and obese individuals verbalize the experience of "fat prejudice" in their family, workplace, or community. Obese clients may experience ridicule, prejudice, and health problems attributed to being "fat." These experiences, coupled with day-to-day problems, such as finding attractive clothing or a chair large enough to sit on, can affect self-esteem. Many clients report that "fat" jokes or comments contribute to a sense of negative self-worth.

- Encourage the client to verbalize the experience of being overweight, and validate the client's experience. *This provides baseline data to use in developing individualized interventions to addresses self-esteem issues.*

- Set small goals with the client and offer positive feedback and encouragement. *Small goals provide more opportunities for success. Positive feedback and encouragement provide a comfortable environment in which to develop self-esteem.*
- Refer for counseling as appropriate. *Many clients benefit from counseling for issues related to self-esteem.*

Home Care

Weight reduction usually occurs in community-based settings. Weight loss and maintenance requires a long-term commitment by the client, family, and support systems. Address the following topics with the client and family:

- Lifestyle changes are more effective than diets. Fad diets promote rapid weight loss, but often are not nutritionally sound, or may be difficult to maintain for a lifetime.
- All household members should consume a diet that is nutritionally sound, low in fat, and high in fiber.
- Establish realistic weight loss goals and a system of nonfood rewards for achieving each goal.
- Identify an "exercise buddy" or support system to promote continued physical activity.
- Expect occasional failures. Resume prescribed diet and exercise routine as soon as possible; the goal is long-term weight management.
- Community resources, such as Weight Watchers, TOPS, or health care–based programs, provide information, strategies, and support for successful weight management.

The Client with an Eating Disorder

Eating disorders are characterized by severely disturbed eating behavior and weight management. Eating disorders are more common in affluent societies where food is plentiful. Women are much more commonly affected than men. **Anorexia nervosa** is characterized by a body weight less than 85% of expected for age and height, and an intense fear of gaining weight. Anorexia nervosa affects about 0.5% to 1% of women in the United States. **Bulimia nervosa,** which affects 1% to 3% of women in the United States, is characterized by recurring episodes of binge eating followed by purge behaviors, such as self-induced vomiting, use of laxatives or diuretics, fasting, or excessive exercise.

Anorexia Nervosa

Anorexia nervosa typically begins during adolescence. Clients with anorexia nervosa have a distorted body image and irrational fear of gaining weight. They maintain weight loss by restricted calorie intake, often accompanied by excessive exercise. Some clients may exhibit binge–purge behavior. A number of risk factors, both biologic and psychosocial, have been identified for anorexia nervosa. Abnormal levels of neurotransmitters and other hormones may play a role. Women who develop anorexia nervosa tend to be obsessive and perfectionistic. Family, social, or occupational (e.g., a career in modeling or ballet) pressures to maintain low body weight also contribute.

Bulimia Nervosa

Bulimia nervosa develops in late adolescence or early adulthood, often following a diet. The client with bulimia typically reports binge eating followed by purging five to ten times per week (Braunwald, et al., 2001). Foods consumed during a binge often are high calorie, high fat, and sweet. After binge eating, the client induces vomiting (usually by stimulating the gag reflex), or may take excessive quantities of laxatives or diuretics. In contrast to anorexia, the client's weight often is normal. Fluid and electrolyte balance, in contrast, may be severely disrupted by loss of fluid and gastrointestinal secretions. The complications of bulimia nervosa primarily result from the purging behavior.

Collaborative Care

Eating disorders, anorexia nervosa in particular, are difficult to effectively treat. Because of the intense fear of weight gain and the distorted body image of clients with anorexia, they strongly resist increasing food intake. A combination of nutritional, behavioral, and psychologic treatment is necessary.

Clients with anorexia nervosa may require hospitalization, particularly if their weight is less than 75% of normal. Refeeding is gradually introduced to avoid complications, such as heart failure. Meals must be supervised and a firm but empathetic attitude conveyed about the importance of adequate food intake. Psychologic treatment focuses on providing emotional support during weight gain and helping the client base their self-esteem on factors other than weight (e.g., personal relationships, satisfaction with achieving occupational goals; Braunwald, et al., 2001).

An antidepressant drug, such as fluoxetine (Prozac), may benefit the client with bulimia nervosa. Cognitive behavioral therapy is also used to treat bulimia, focusing on excessive concerns about weight, persistent dieting, and binge–purge behaviors.

Nursing Care

Nurses can be instrumental in identifying clients with anorexia nervosa or bulimia nervosa and referring them for treatment. It is particularly important to identify these disorders early to prevent adverse effects on growth and increase the success of treatment.

The nurse is an integral part of the eating disorders treatment team. Although *Imbalanced nutrition: Less than body requirements* is a primary nursing diagnosis for clients with anorexia or bulimia, the following nursing diagnoses also should be considered:

- *Ineffective sexuality patterns*
- *Chronic low self-esteem*
- *Disturbed body image*
- *Ineffective family therapeutic regimen management.*

When planning and implementing care, consider the following nursing activities:

- Regularly monitor weight, using standard conditions. *Weight gain or loss provides information about the effectiveness of care, as well as the client's risk for complications.*

- Monitor food intake during meals, recording percentage of meal and snack consumed. Maintain close observation for at least one hour following meals; do not allow client alone in bathroom. *Observing the client during and after meals helps prevent disposal of food and purging behavior after eating. Recording actual food intake allows accurate calculation of calorie intake.*

- Serve balanced meals, including all nutrient groups. Increase serving size gradually. *The client may find "normal" food servings overwheming, reducing the desire to eat. Calorie intake is initially limited to prevent complications associated with refeeding, then gradually increased.*

- Serve frequent, small feedings of cold or room temperature foods. *Cool foods reduce sensations of early satiety, promoting greater food intake at a meal or snack.*

- Administer a multivitamin and mineral supplement to replace losses.

Clients with anorexia nervosa or bulimia nervosa require extended treatment of the disorder. Involvement of the family and social support persons is vital to success. Encourage family members to participate in teaching and diet counseling sessions. Discuss the value of family therapy to address issues that have contributed to the disorder. Emphasize the need to provide consistent messages of support for healthy eating habits. Discuss using rewards for food and calorie intake rather than weight gain. Provide referrals to a dietitian, nutritional support team, counseling, and support groups for people with eating disorders.

18 Nursing Care of Clients with Upper Gastrointestinal Disorders

The upper gastrointestinal tract includes the mouth, esophagus, stomach, and proximal small intestine. Food and fluids, ingested through the mouth, move through the esophagus to the stomach. The stomach and upper intestinal tract (duodenum and jejunum) are responsible for the majority of food digestion. When an acute or chronic disease process interferes with the function of this portion of the gastrointestinal (GI) tract, nutritional status can be affected and the client may experience symptoms that interfere with lifestyle.

Nurses provide both acute care for the hospitalized client and teaching about the skills and knowledge needed to manage these conditions at home.

Disorders of the Mouth

Inflammations, infections, and neoplastic lesions of the mouth affect food ingestion and nutrition. Oral lesions may have a variety of causes, including infection, mechanical trauma, irritants, such as alcohol, and hypersensitivity. Appropriate treatment of the disorder, any underlying factors, and associated symptoms is essential.

The Client with Stomatitis
Stomatitis, inflammation of the oral mucosa, is a common disorder of the mouth. It may be caused by viral (herpes simplex) or fungal (Candida albicans) infections, mechanical trauma (e.g., cheek biting), and irritants, such as tobacco or chemotherapeutic agents.

Pathophysiology

The oral mucosa, which lines the oral cavity, is a relatively thin, fragile layer of stratified squamous epithelial cells. The blood supply to the oral mucosa is rich. Frequent exposure to the environment, a rich blood supply, and the oral mucosa's delicate nature increase the risk of infection or inflammation, reaction to toxins, and trauma. The clinical manifestations of stomatitis vary according to its cause.

Collaborative Care

Stomatitis is diagnosed by direct physical examination and, if indicated, cultures, smears, and evaluation for systemic illness. Treatment addresses both the underlying cause and any coexisting illnesses. An undiagnosed oral lesion present for more than one week and that does not respond to therapy must be evaluated for malignancy.

Direct smears and cultures of lesions may be obtained to identify causative organisms. If systemic illness is suspected, a variety of diagnostic tests may be ordered to identify the underlying cause.

General treatment measures include using a topical anesthetic, such as 2% viscous lidocaine, as an oral rinse. This solution is not swallowed to avoid impairment of the swallowing mechanism. Orabase, a protective paste, may be applied to oral ulcers to promote comfort. Triamcinolone acetonide may be mixed in Orabase to reduce inflammation and promote healing. Sodium bicarbonate mouthwashes may provide relief and promote cleansing, whereas alcohol-based mouthwashes may cause pain and burning.

Fungal infections often are treated with a nystatin oral suspension; clients "swish and swallow" the solution. Clotrimazole lozenges also treat oral fungal infections. If the infection does not resolve, oral antifungal medications, such as fluconazole or ketoconazole, may be used. Antifungals are usually continued for at least three days after symptoms disappear.

Herpetic lesions may be treated with topical or oral acyclovir. Acyclovir ointment provides comfort and lubrication while limiting the spread of the virus. Acyclovir capsules reduce the severity of symptoms and the duration of the lesions.

Bacterial infections are treated with antibiotics based on cultures and smears. Oral penicillin is the treatment of choice if the client is not allergic and the cultured bacteria is sensitive. Nursing implications for selected drugs used to treat stomatitis are outlined below.

Nursing Care

Nursing care for the client with stomatitis focuses not only on the oral inflammation, but also on any underlying systemic diseases and the effects of the condition on the client's comfort and nutrition.

Nursing Diagnoses and Interventions

Impaired Oral Mucous Membrane   Stomatitis disrupts the integrity of the oral mucous membrane. Regardless of cause, the pain and symptoms of stomatitis must be relieved to promote comfort as well as food and fluid intake.

- Assess and document oral mucous membranes and the character of any lesions every four to eight hours. *Baseline and ongoing assessment data provide the basis for evaluation.*
- Assist with thorough mouth care after meals, at bedtime, and every two to four hours while awake. If unable to tolerate a toothbrush, offer sponge or gauze toothettes. Avoid using alcohol-based mouthwashes. *Mouth care promotes hygiene, comfort, and healing. Alcohol-based mouthwashes may be irritating to mucous membranes, causing pain and further tissue damage.*
- Assess knowledge and teach about condition, mouth care, and treatments. Instruct client to avoid alcohol, tobacco, and spicy or irritating foods. *Knowledge promotes client*

participation in the plan of care and compliance. Alcohol, tobacco, and hot, spicy rough foods may injure the inflamed mucous membranes.

Imbalanced Nutrition: Less Than Body Requirements   Oral lesions and pain may limit oral intake, which may in turn lead to nutritional deficits. Anorexia and general malaise may also contribute to decreased intake.

- Assess food intake as well as the client's ability to chew and swallow. Weigh daily. Provide appropriate assistive devices, such as straws or feeding syringes. *Adequate nutrition is essential for healing. Daily weights allow monitoring of the adequacy of food intake. Assistive devices may allow food intake while avoiding irritation of ulcerations or lesions.*

- Encourage a high-calorie, high-protein diet considerate of food preferences. Offer soft, lukewarm, or cool foods or liquids, such as eggnogs, milk shakes, nutritional supplements, popsicles, and puddings, frequently in small amounts. Obtain nutritional consultation. *Oral intake may be limited, and enriched foods and liquids enhance nutrition. A nutritional consultation can help ensure an adequate diet and assist in meeting nutritional needs.*

Table 18-1. Medication Administration — Drugs Used to Treat Stomatitis

Topical Oral Anesthetics

Orajel
Anbesol
Viscous lidocaine
Triamcinolone acetonide

These drugs reduce the pain associated with mucous membrane lesions or stomatitis. They provide temporary relief of pain. Any oral lesion that persists longer than one week should be evaluated by an oral surgeon.

Nursing Responsibilities
- Instruct the client to seek medical attention for any oral lesion that does not heal within one week.
- Monitor for local hypersensitivity reactions, and discontinue use if they occur.

Client and Family Teaching
- Apply every one to two hours as needed.
- Perform oral hygiene after meals and at bedtime.

Topical Antifungal Agents

Clotrimazole
Nystatin

These products help in the topical treatment of candidiasis. Their effects are primarily local rather than systemic.

Continued on the next page

Table 18-1. Continued

Nursing Responsibilities
- Instruct the client to dissolve lozenges in the mouth.
- Instruct the client to rinse mouth with oral suspension, for at least two minutes, and expectorate or swallow as directed.
- These drugs are contraindicated in pregnancy.

Client and Family Teaching
- Take medication as prescribed.
- Do not eat or drink 30 minutes after medication.
- Contact physician if symptoms worsen.
- Perform good oral hygiene after meals and at bedtime; remove dentures at bedtime.

Antiviral Agent

Acyclovir (Zovirax)
Acyclovir is useful in the treatment of oral herpes simplex virus. It helps reduce the severity and frequency of infections. It interferes with the DNA synthesis of herpes simplex virus.

Nursing Responsibilities
- Start therapy with acyclovir as soon as herpetic lesions are noted.
- Administer with food or on an empty stomach.

Client and Family Teaching
- The virus remains latent and can recur during stressful events, fever, trauma, sunlight exposure, and treatment with immunosuppressive drugs.
- Take the medication as ordered, and contact the physician if symptoms worsen.

Home Care

Clients with stomatitis generally provide self-care. Include the following topics in teaching for home care:

- Managing any underlying health conditions and ongoing treatments such as chemotherapy
- The recommended diet and oral hygiene regime
- Nutritional supplements to help meet nutritional requirements
- Prescribed medication, its route, side effects, frequency of administration, and signs and symptoms to report
- The importance of completing the full course of antibiotic, antiviral, or antifungal treatment
- Manifestations to report and the importance of follow-up care.

Disorders of the Esophagus

The esophagus plays an essential role in the ingestion of food and liquids. Disorders of the esophagus can be inflammatory, mechanical, or cancerous. Because of its location and neighboring organs, the symptoms of esophageal disorders may mimic those of a variety of other illnesses.

The Client with Gastroesophageal Reflux Disease

Gastroesophageal reflux is the backward flowing of gastric contents into the esophagus. When this occurs, the client experiences heartburn. Many people with gastroesophageal reflux have few symptoms, while others develop inflammatory esophagitis as a result of exposure to gastric juices.

Gastroesophageal reflux disease (GERD) is a common gastrointestinal disorder that affects 15% to 20% of adults. As many as 10% of people experience daily symptoms such as heartburn and indigestion (Braunwald, et al., 2001; Mattonen, 2001; Tierney, et al., 2001).

Pathophysiology

Normally, the lower esophageal sphincter remains closed except during swallowing. Reflux (backflow) of gastric contents into the esophagus is prevented by pressure differences between the stomach and the lower esophagus. The diaphragm, the lower esophageal sphincter, and the location of the gastroesophageal junction below the diaphragm help maintain this pressure difference.

Gastroesophageal reflux may result from transient relaxation of the lower esophageal sphincter, an incompetent lower esophageal sphincter, and/or increased pressure within the stomach. Factors contributing to gastroesophageal reflux include increased gastric volume (e.g., after meals), positioning that allows gastric contents to remain close to the gastroesophageal junction (e.g., bending over, lying down), and increased gastric pressure (e.g., obesity or wearing tight clothing). A hiatal hernia may contribute to GERD.

Gastric juices contain acid, pepsin, and bile, which are corrosive substances. Esophageal peristalsis and bicarbonate in salivary secretions normally clear and neutralize gastric juices in the esophagus. During sleep, however, and in clients with impaired esophageal peristalsis or salivation, the esophageal mucosa is damaged by gastric juices, causing an inflammatory response. With prolonged exposure, esophagitis develops. Superficial ulcers develop, and the mucosa becomes red, friable (easily torn), and may bleed. If untreated, scarring and esophageal stricture may develop.

Manifestations and Complications

GERD causes heartburn, usually after meals, with bending over, or when reclining. Regurgitation of sour material into the mouth, or difficulty and pain with swallowing may develop. Other manifestations may include atypical chest pain, sore throat, and hoarseness. Aspiration of gastric contents can cause hoarseness or respiratory symptoms.

Complications include esophageal strictures and Barrett's esophagus. Strictures can lead to dysphagia. Barrett's esophagus is characterized by changes in the cells lining the esophagus and an increased risk of developing esophageal cancer (Porth, 2002).

Collaborative Care

Often the diagnosis of GERD is made by the history of symptoms and predisposing factors. Collaborative care focuses on lifestyle changes, diet modification, and for more severe cases, drug therapy. Surgery is reserved for clients who develop serious complications.

Diagnostic Tests

Diagnostic tests that may be ordered for clients with manifestations of GERD include:

- *Barium swallow* to evaluate the esophagus, stomach, and upper small intestine.
- *Upper endoscopy* to permit direct visualization of the esophagus. Tissue may be obtained for biopsy to establish the diagnosis and rule out malignancy.
- *24-hour ambulatory pH monitoring* may be performed to establish the diagnosis of GERD. For this test, a small tube with a pH electrode is inserted through the nose into the esophagus. The electrode is attached to a small box worn on the belt which records the data. The data are later analyzed by computer.
- *Esophageal manometry* measures pressures of the esophageal sphincters and esophageal peristalsis.

Medications

Antacids, such as Mylanta or Maalox, relieve mild or moderate symptoms by neutralizing stomach acid. Gaviscon, which forms a floating barrier between the gastric contents and the esophageal mucosa when the client is upright, may also be used.

Table 18-2. Nursing Implications for Diagnostic Tests: Upper Endoscopy

Client Preparation

- Schedule at least two days after barium swallow or upper gastrointestinal series.
- Ensure the informed consent is signed prior to premedication.
- Encourage questions, and provide answers and support.
- Withhold food and fluids for six to eight hours before the procedure.
- Remove dentures and eyewear. Provide mouth care.

Client and Family Teaching

- Do not eat or drink anything for six to eight hours before the procedure.
- The procedure is somewhat uncomfortable but requires only 20 to 30 minutes to complete.
- A local anesthetic will be used in your throat and you will be given a sedative during the procedure.
- After the procedure, you will be allowed to eat and drink as soon as your gag reflex returns and you are able to swallow.
- You may experience mild bloating, belching, or flatulence following the procedure.
- Contact your physician immediately if you develop any of the following: difficulty swallowing; epigastric, substernal or shoulder pain; vomiting blood or black tarry stools; or fever.

Histamine$_2$-receptor (H$_2$-receptor) blockers reduce gastric acid production and are effective in treating GERD symptoms. When treating GERD, H$_2$-receptor blockers are usually given twice a day or more frequently for a prolonged period of time. Cimetidine, ranitidine, famotidine, and nizatidine are all approved by the FDA for the treatment of GERD and are available over the counter.

Omeprazole (Prilosec), lansoprazole (Prevacid), pantoprazole (Protonix), and rabeprazole (Aciphex) are proton-pump inhibitors (PPIs) that reduce gastric secretions. PPIs promote healing of erosive esophagitis, as well as relieve symptoms. An 8-week course of treatment is initially prescribed, although some clients may require three to six months of therapy.

A promotility agent, such as metoclopramide (Reglan), may be ordered to enhance esophageal clearance and gastric emptying. Metoclopramide is used to treat clients with regurgitation, symptoms of indigestion, and nighttime symptoms. However, it is not recommended for long-time use. See the Table 18-3 below for the nursing implications of drugs used to treat GERD.

Table 18-3. Medication Administration — Drugs Used to Treat GERD, Gastritis, and Peptic Ulcer Disease

Antacids

Maalox	Gaviscon
Gelusil	Tums
Mylanta	Aludrox
Riopan	Amphojel

Antacids buffer or neutralize gastric acid, usually acting locally. Antacids are used in GERD, gastritis, and peptic ulcer disease to relieve pain and prevent further damage to esophageal and gastric mucosa.

Nursing Responsibilities
- Antacids interfere with the absorption of many drugs given orally; separate administration times by at least two hours.
- Monitor for constipation or diarrhea resulting from antacid therapy. Notify the physician should either develop; a different antacid may be ordered.
- Although most antacids have little systemic effect, electrolyte imbalances can develop. Monitor serum electrolytes, particularly sodium, calcium, and magnesium levels.

Client and Family Teaching
- Take your antacid frequently as prescribed, one to three hours after meals and at bedtime. To be effective, the antacid must be in your stomach.
- Avoid taking an antacid for approximately two hours before and one hour after taking another medication.
- Shake suspensions well prior to administration.
- Chew tablets thoroughly, and follow with four to six ounces of water.
- Report worsening symptoms, diarrhea, or constipation to your primary care provider.
- Continue taking the antacid for the duration prescribed. While pain and discomfort often are relieved soon after treatment begins, healing takes six to eight weeks.

Continued on the next page

Table 18-3. Continued

H₂-Receptor Blockers

Cimetidine (Tagamet)   Ranitidine (Zantac)
Famotidine (Pepcid)   Nizatidine (Axid)

H_2-receptor blockers reduce acidity of gastric juices by blocking the ability of histamine to stimulate acid secretion by the gastric parietal cells. As a result, both the volume and concentration of hydrochloric acid in gastric juice is reduced. H_2-receptor blockers are given orally or intravenously. Both prescription and over-the-counter preparations are available.

Nursing Responsibilities
- To ensure absorption, do not give an antacid within one hour before or after giving an H_2-receptor blocker.
- When administered intravenously, do not mix with other drugs. Administer in 20 to 100 mL of solution over 15 to 30 minutes. Rapid intravenous injection as a bolus may cause dysrhythmias and hypotension.
- Monitor for interaction with such drugs as oral anticoagulants, beta blockers, benzodiazepines, tricyclic antidepressants, and others. H_2-receptor blockers may inhibit the metabolism of other drugs, increasing the risk of toxicity.

Client and Family Teaching
- Take the drug as directed, even if pain and gastric discomfort are relieved early in the course of therapy.
- Take at bedtime if once-a-day dosing is ordered. If spaced through the day, take before meals. Avoid taking antacids for one hour before and one hour after taking this drug.
- To promote healing, avoid cigarette smoking (which increases gastric acid secretion) and gastric mucosal irritants, such as alcohol, aspirin, and NSAIDs.
- Long-term use of these drugs can lead to gynecomastia (breast enlargement) and impotence in men and breast tenderness in women. Discontinuing the drug will reverse these effects.
- Report possible adverse effects, such as diarrhea, confusion, rash, fatigue, malaise, or bruising, to your care provider.

Proton-Pump Inhibitors

Lansoprazole (Prevacid)
Omeprazole (Prilosec)
Pantoprazole (Protonix)
Rabeprazole (Aciphex)

Proton-pump inhibitors (PPIs) are the drugs of choice for severe GERD. PPIs inhibit the hydrogen-potassium-ATP pump, reducing gastric acid secretion. Initially, the PPI may be given twice a day, with the dose reduced to once daily (at bedtime) after eight weeks.

Nursing Responsibilities
- Administer before breakfast and at bedtime if ordered twice a day; at bedtime if once a day.
- Do not crush tablets.
- Monitor liver function tests for possible abnormal values, including increased AST, ALT, alkaline phosphatase, and bilirubin levels.

Table 18-3. Continued

Client and Family Teaching

- Take the drug as ordered for the full course of therapy, even if symptoms are relieved.
- Do not crush, break, or chew tablets.
- Avoid cigarette smoking, alcohol, aspirin, and NSAIDs while taking this drug as these substances may interfere with healing.
- Report black tarry stools, diarrhea, or abdominal pain to your primary care provider.

Anti-Ulcer Agent

Sucralfate (Carafate)

Sucralfate reacts with gastric acid to form a thick paste which adheres to damaged gastric mucosal tissue. It protects gastric mucosa and promotes healing through this local action.

Nursing Responsibilities

- Administer on an empty stomach, one hour before meals and at bedtime.
- Do not crush tablets.
- Separate administration time from antacids by at least 30 minutes.

Client and Family Teaching

- Take as directed, even after symptoms have been relieved.
- Do not crush or chew tablets; shake suspension well.
- Increase your intake of fluids and dietary fiber to prevent constipation.

Promotility Agent

Metoclopramide (Reglan)

By acting on the central nervous system, metoclopramide stimulates upper gastrointestinal motility and gastric emptying. As a result, nausea, vomiting, and symptoms of GERD are reduced.

Nursing Implications

- Do not administer this drug to clients with possible gastrointestinal obstruction or bleeding, or a history of seizure disorders, pheochromocytoma, or Parkinson's disease.
- Monitor for extrapyramidal side effects (e.g., difficulty speaking or swallowing, loss of balance, gait disruptions, twitching or twisting movements, weakness of arms or legs) or manifestations of tardive dyskinesia (uncontrolled rhythmic facial movement, lip-smacking, tongue rolling). Report immediately.
- Give oral doses 30 minutes before meals and at bedtime.
- May be given by direct intravenous push over 1 to 2 minutes, or diluted by slow infusion over 15 to 30 minutes.

Client and Family Teaching

- Take this drug as directed. If you miss a dose, take as soon as you remember unless it is close to time for the next dose.
- Do not drive or engage in other activities that require alertness if this drug makes you drowsy.
- Avoid using alcohol or other CNS depressants while you are taking this drug.
- Immediately contact your health care provider if you develop involuntary movements of your eyes, face, or limbs.

Dietary and Lifestyle Management

GERD is a chronic condition. Dietary and lifestyle changes are important to reduce symptoms and long-term effects of the disorder. Acidic foods, such as tomato products, citrus fruits, spicy foods, and coffee, are eliminated from the diet. Fatty foods, chocolate, peppermint, and alcohol relax the lower esophageal sphincter or delay gastric emptying, so should be avoided. The client is advised to maintain ideal body weight, eat smaller meals, refrain from eating for three hours before bedtime, and stay upright for two hours after meals. Elevating the head of the bed on 6- to 8-inch blocks often is beneficial. Stopping smoking is a necessary lifestyle change. Avoiding tight clothing and avoiding bending may help to relieve symptoms.

Surgery

Surgery may be used for clients who do not respond to pharmacologic and lifestyle management. Antireflux surgeries increase pressure in the lower esophagus, inhibiting gastric content reflux. Laparoscopic procedures for GERD include tightening the lower esophageal sphincter with an endoscopic suturing system or burning spots on the muscle surrounding the lower esophageal sphincter to create scar tissue (Mattonen, 2001). An open surgical procedure known as Nissen fundoplication may also be done.

Nursing Care

Assessment

Assessment data related to GERD include the following:

- *Health history:* manifestations, such as frequent heartburn; intolerance of foods that are acidic, spicy, or fatty; regurgitation of acidic gastric juice; increased symptoms when bending over, lying down, or wearing tight clothing; difficulty swallowing.
- *Physical assessment:* Epigastric tenderness.

Nursing Diagnoses and Interventions

Pain   The epigastric pain associated with GERD can be severe, interfering with rest and causing anxiety.

- Provide small, frequent meals. Restrict intake of fat, acidic foods, coffee, and alcohol. *Limiting the size of meals reduces pressure in the stomach, reducing esophageal reflux. Fatty, acidic foods, coffee, and alcohol increase gastric acidity and interfere with gastric emptying, increasing the incidence of gastroesophageal reflux.*
- Instruct client to stop smoking. Refer to a smoking cessation clinic or program as needed. *Cigarette smoking increases gastric acidity and interferes with healing of damaged mucosa.*
- Administer antacids, H_2-receptor blockers, and proton-pump inhibitors as ordered. Instruct client to continue therapy as prescribed, even after symptoms have been relieved. *These drugs neutralize or reduce gastric acid secretion, relieving symptoms and promoting healing.*
- Discuss the long-term nature of GERD and its management. *Lifestyle changes need to be continued after healing and symptom relief to manage the long-term effects of GERD.*

Home Care

GERD is a lifelong condition best managed by the client. Teach the client and family about continuing management strategies, including dietary changes, remaining upright after meals, and avoiding eating for at least three hours before bedtime. Suggest elevating the head of the bed on 6- to 8-inch wooden blocks placed under the legs. Discuss the need for continued gastric acid reduction using antacids, H_2-receptor blockers, or proton-pump inhibitors. All are effective to reduce the acidity of gastric juices. Antacids, the most cost-effective measure, require frequent doses to neutralize gastric acid. H_2-receptor blockers, also available over the counter, are a cost-effective management strategy that require only twice-a-day dosing.

The Client with Hiatal Hernia

A **hiatal hernia** occurs when part of the stomach protrudes through the esophageal hiatus of the diaphragm into the thoracic cavity. While hiatal hernia is thought to be a common problem, most affected individuals are asymptomatic. The incidence of hiatal hernia increases with age.

In a *sliding hiatal hernia,* the gastroesophageal junction and the fundus of the stomach slide upward through the esophageal hiatus. Several factors may contribute to a sliding hiatal hernia, including weakened gastroesophageal-diaphragmatic anchors, shortening of the esophagus, or increased intra-abdominal pressure. Small sliding hiatal hernias produce few symptoms.

In a *paraesophageal hiatal hernia,* the junction between the esophagus and stomach remains in its normal position below the diaphragm, while a part of the stomach herniates through the esophageal hiatus. A paraesophageal hernia can become incarcerated (constricted) and strangulate, impairing blood flow to the herniated tissue. Clients with paraesophageal hernia may develop gastritis, or chronic or acute gastrointestinal bleeding.

A barium swallow or an upper endoscopy may be done to diagnose hiatal hernia. Many clients with hiatal hernia require no treatment. If symptoms are present, treatment measures such as those for clients with GERD, may be ordered. If medical management is ineffective or the hernia becomes incarcerated, surgery may be required. The most common surgical procedure is the Nissen fundoplication. This surgery prevents the gastroesophageal junction from slipping into the thoracic cavity.

Nursing care for the client with a hiatal hernia is similar to that for the client with GERD.

The Client with Impaired Esophageal Motility

Disorders of esophageal motility can cause dysphagia or chest pain. **Achalasia,** a disorder of unknown etiology, is characterized by impaired peristalsis of the smooth muscle of the esophagus and impaired relaxation of the lower esophageal sphincter. The client experiences gradually increasing dysphagia with both solid foods and liquids. Fullness in the chest during meals, chest pain, and nighttime cough are additional manifestations. Other clients may experience **diffuse esophageal spasm** that causes nonperistaltic contraction of esophageal smooth muscle. This disorder causes chest pain and/or dysphagia. The chest pain can be severe, and usually occurs at rest.

Treatment of achalasia may include endoscopically guided injection of botulinum toxin into the lower esophageal sphincter or balloon dilation of the LES. Botulinum toxin injection lowers LES pressure, but may need to be repeated every six to nine months. Balloon dilation tears muscle fibers in the LES, reducing its pressure. A laparoscopic myotomy (incision into the circular muscle layer of the LES) also reduces pressure and relieves symptoms.

Disorders of the Stomach and Duodenum

The stomach and upper small intestine (duodenum and jejunum) are responsible for the majority of food digestion. The major disorders that affect digestion are gastritis, peptic ulcer disease, and cancer of the stomach. Nursing roles in managing these disorders include both acute care for the hospitalized client and teaching to give the client the skills and knowledge to manage these conditions at home.

Overview of Normal Physiology

Normally, the stomach is protected from the digestive substances it secretes—namely hydrochloric acid and pepsin—by the **gastric mucosal barrier**. The gastric mucosal barrier includes:

- An impermeable hydrophobic lipid layer that covers gastric epithelial cells. This lipid layer prevents diffusion of water-soluble molecules, but substances such as aspirin and alcohol can diffuse through it.

- Bicarbonate ions secreted in response to hydrochloric acid secretion by the parietal cells of the stomach. When bicarbonate (HCO_3-) secretion is equal to hydrogen ion ($H+$) secretion, the gastric mucosa remains intact. Prostaglandins, chemical messengers involved in the inflammatory response, support bicarbonate production and blood flow to the gastric mucosa.

- Mucus gel that protects the surface of the stomach lining from the damaging effects of pepsin and traps bicarbonate to neutralize hydrochloric acid. This gel also acts as a lubricant, preventing mechanical damage to the stomach lining from its contents.

When an acute or chronic irritant disrupts the mucosal barrier, or when disease alters the processes that maintain the barrier, the gastric mucosa becomes irritated and inflamed. Lipid-soluble substances, such as aspirin and alcohol, penetrate the gastric mucosal barrier, leading to irritation and possible inflammation. Bile acids also break down the lipids in the mucosal barrier, increasing the potential for irritation (Porth, 2002). In addition, aspirin and other nonsteroidal anti-inflammatory drugs (NSAIDs) inhibit prostaglandins. Aspirin and NSAIDs also alter the nature of gastric mucus, affecting its protective function.

The Client with Gastritis

Gastritis, inflammation of the stomach lining, results from irritation of the gastric mucosa. Gastritis is common, and may be caused by a variety of factors. The most common form of gastritis, **acute gastritis,** is generally a benign, self-limiting disorder associated with the ingestion of gastric irritants, such as aspirin, alcohol, caffeine, or foods contaminated with certain bacteria. Manifestations of acute gastritis may range from asymptomatic to mild heartburn to severe gastric distress, vomiting, and bleeding with **hematemesis** (vomiting blood).

Chronic gastritis is a separate group of disorders characterized by progressive and irreversible changes in the gastric mucosa (Porth, 2002). Chronic gastritis is more common in the elderly, chronic alcoholics, and cigarette smokers. When symptoms of chronic gastritis occur, they are often vague, ranging from a feeling of heaviness in the epigastric region after meals to gnawing, burning, ulcerlike epigastric pain unrelieved by antacids.

Pathophysiology

Acute Gastritis

Acute gastritis is characterized by disruption of the mucosal barrier by a local irritant. This disruption allows hydrochloric acid and pepsin to come into contact with the gastric tissue, resulting in irritation, inflammation, and superficial erosions. The gastric mucosa rapidly regenerates, generally making acute gastritis a self-limiting disorder, with resolution and healing occurring within several days.

The ingestion of aspirin or other NSAIDS, corticosteroids, alcohol, and caffeine is commonly associated with the development of acute gastritis. Accidental or purposeful ingestion of a corrosive alkali, such as ammonia, lye, Lysol, and other cleaning agents, or acid leads to severe inflammation and possible necrosis of the stomach. Gastric perforation, hemorrhage, and peritonitis are possible results. Iatrogenic causes of acute gastritis include radiation therapy and administration of certain chemotherapeutic agents.

Erosive Gastritis A severe form of acute gastritis, **erosive** or **stress-induced gastritis,** occurs as a complication of other life-threatening conditions, such as shock, severe trauma, major surgery, sepsis, burns, or head injury. When these erosions follow a major burn, they are called **Curling's ulcers,** after Thomas Curling, a British physician, who first described them in 1842. When stress ulcers occur following head injury or central nervous system surgery, they are referred to as **Cushing's ulcers,** after Harvey Cushing, a U.S. surgeon.

The primary mechanisms leading to erosive gastritis appear to be ischemia of the gastric mucosa resulting from sympathetic vasoconstriction, and tissue injury due to gastric acid. As a result, multiple superficial erosions of the gastric mucosa develop. Maintaining the gastric pH at greater than 3.5 and inhibiting gastric acid secretion with medications help prevent erosive gastritis.

Manifestations The client with acute gastritis may have mild symptoms such as **anorexia** (loss of appetite), or mild epigastric discomfort relieved by belching or defecating. More severe manifestations include abdominal pain, nausea, and vomiting. Gastric bleeding may occur, with hematemesis or **melena** (black, tarry stool that contains blood). Erosive gastritis is not typically associated with pain. The initial symptom often is painless gastric bleeding occurring two or more days after the initial stressor. Bleeding typically is minimal, but can be massive. Corrosive gastritis can cause severe bleeding, signs of shock, and an *acute abdomen* (severely painful, rigid, boardlike abdomen) if perforation occurs.

Chronic Gastritis

Unrelated to acute gastritis, chronic gastritis is a progressive disorder that begins with superficial inflammation and gradually leads to atrophy of gastric tissues. The initial stage is characterized by superficial changes in the gastric mucosa and a decrease in mucus. As the disease evolves, glands of the gastric mucosa are disrupted and destroyed. The inflammatory process involves deep portions of the mucosa, which thins and atrophies. There appear to be at least two different forms of chronic gastritis, classified as type A and type B.

Type A gastritis, the less common form of chronic gastritis, usually affects people of Northern European heritage. This type of gastritis is thought to have an autoimmune component. In type A or autoimmune gastritis, the body produces antibodies to parietal cells and to intrinsic factor. These antibodies destroy gastric mucosal cells, resulting in tissue atrophy and the loss of hydrochloric acid and pepsin secretion. Because intrinsic factor is required for the absorption of vitamin B_{12}, this immune response also results in pernicious anemia. For further discussion of pernicious anemia, see Chapter 11.

Type B gastritis is the more common form of chronic gastritis. Its incidence increases with age, reaching nearly 100% in people over the age of 70. Type B gastritis is caused by chronic infection of the gastric mucosa by *Helicobacter pylori* (*H. pylori*), a gram-negative spiral bacterium. *H. pylori* infection causes inflammation of the gastric mucosa, with infiltration by neutrophils and lymphocytes. The outermost layer of gastric mucosa thins and atrophies, providing a less effective barrier against the autodigestive properties of hydrochloric acid and pepsin.

Infection with *H. pylori* also is associated with an increased risk for peptic ulcer disease. *H. pylori* infection significantly increases the risk of developing gastric cancer. See the sections that follow for more information about these disorders.

Manifestations Chronic gastritis is often asymptomatic until atrophy is sufficiently advanced to interfere with digestion and gastric emptying. The client may complain of vague gastric distress, epigastric heaviness after meals, or ulcerlike symptoms. These symptoms typically are not relieved by antacids. In addition, the client may experience fatigue and other symptoms of anemia. If intrinsic factor is lacking, paresthesias and other neurologic manifestations of vitamin B_{12} deficiency may be present.

Collaborative Care

Acute gastritis is usually diagnosed by the history and clinical presentation. In contrast, the vague symptoms of chronic gastritis may require more extensive diagnostic testing.

Clients with acute and chronic gastritis are generally managed in community settings. The client requires acute care only when nausea and vomiting are severe enough to interfere with normal fluid and electrolyte balance and nutritional status. If hemorrhage results, surgical intervention may be required.

Diagnostic Tests

Diagnostic tests that may be ordered for the client with gastritis include the following:

- *Gastric analysis* to assess hydrochloric acid secretion. A nasogastric tube is passed into the stomach, and pentagastrin is injected subcutaneously to stimulate gastric secretion of hydrochloric acid. Secretion may be decreased in clients with chronic gastritis.

- *Hemoglobin, hematocrit,* and *red blood cell indices* are evaluated for evidence of anemia. The client with gastritis may develop pernicious anemia because of parietal cell destruction, or iron-deficiency anemia because of chronic blood loss.

- *Serum vitamin B_{12} levels* are measured to evaluate for possible pernicious anemia. Normal values for vitamin B12 are 200 to 1000 pg/mL, with lower levels seen in older adults.

- *Upper endoscopy* may be done to inspect the gastric mucosa for changes, identify areas of bleeding, and obtain tissue for biopsy. Bleeding sites may be treated with electro- or laser coagulation or injected with a sclerosing agent during the procedure.

Medications

Drugs such as a proton-pump inhibitor (PPI), histamine$_2$ (H$_2$)-receptor blocker, or sucralfate may be ordered to prevent or treat acute stress gastritis. PPIs and H$_2$-receptor blockers reduce the amount or effects of hydrochloric acid on the gastric mucosa. Lansoprazole (Prevacid) and omeprazole (Prilosec) are examples of PPIs. H$_2$-receptor blockers include cimetidine (Tagamet), ranitidine (Zantac), famotidine (Pepcid), and nizatidine (Axid). These drugs also are available in nonprescription strength. Sucralfate (Carafate) works locally to prevent the damaging effects of acid and pepsin on gastric tissue. It does not neutralize or reduce acid secretion. Nursing implications for drugs commonly used in managing gastritis are included in Table 18-3.

The client with type B chronic gastritis may be treated to eradicate the *H. pylori* infection. This generally involves combination therapy consisting of two antibiotics, such as metronidazole and clarithromycin or tetracycline, and a PPI. In some cases, eradication of the infection is not warranted, and the client is treated symptomatically.

Treatments

In acute gastritis, gastrointestinal tract rest is provided by 6 to 12 hours of NPO status, then slow reintroduction of clear liquids (broth, tea, gelatin, carbonated beverages), followed by ingestion of heavier liquids (cream soups, puddings, milk) and finally a gradual reintroduction of solid food.

If nausea and vomiting threaten fluid and electrolyte balance, intravenous fluids and electrolytes are ordered.

Gastric Lavage Acute gastritis resulting from ingestion of a poisonous or corrosive substance (acid or strong alkali), is treated with immediate dilution and removal of the substance. Vomiting is not induced because it might further damage the esophagus and possibly the trachea; instead, **gastric lavage,** washing out of the stomach contents, is performed.

Nursing Care

Health Promotion

Teach all clients and community members about measures to prevent acute gastritis. Food contaminated with bacteria is a significant cause of acute gastritis. Discuss food safety measures, such as fully cooking meats and egg products, and promptly refrigerating foods after cooking to avoid bacterial growth. Stress that food contaminated with potential pathogens often looks, smells, and tastes good, making it difficult to identify. Teach clients to abstain from eating or drinking anything during an acute episode of vomiting, then reintroduce clear liquids gradually once vomiting has stopped (two to four hours after the last episode of vomiting). Suggest using liquids such as Pedialyte or sport drinks to replace lost electrolytes and fluid. Instruct clients to avoid milk and milk products until they easily tolerate clear liquids and solid foods, such as dry toast or saltine crackers.

Assessment

Assessment data to collect for clients with acute or chronic gastritis include the following:

- *Health history:* current symptoms and their duration; relieving and aggravating factors; history of ingestion of toxins, contaminated food, alcohol, aspirin, or NSAIDs; other medications.
- *Physical examination:* vital signs including orthostatic vitals if indicated; peripheral pulses; general appearance; abdominal assessment including appearance, bowel sounds, and tenderness.

Nursing Diagnoses and Interventions

In planning and implementing nursing care for the client with acute or chronic gastritis, consider both the direct effects of the disorder on the gastrointestinal system and nutritional status as well as its effects on lifestyle and psychosocial integrity. This section focuses on problems of fluid balance and nutrition.

Deficient Fluid Volume   Nausea, vomiting, and abdominal distress are the primary manifestations of acute gastritis. The risk for fluid and electrolyte imbalance is high because of inadequate intake of food and fluids, and abnormal losses of fluids and electrolytes with vomiting.

- Monitor and record vital signs at least every two hours until stable, then every 4 hours. Check for orthostatic hypotension.
- Weigh daily. Monitor and record intake and output; record urine output every one to four hours as indicated. *Daily weights are an accurate indicator of fluid volume. Urine output of less than 30 mL per hour indicates decreased cardiac output and a need for prompt fluid replacement.*
- Monitor skin turgor, color, and condition and status of oral mucous membranes frequently. Provide skin and mouth care frequently. *Skin turgor and mucous membrane assessments indicate hydration status. Good skin and mouth care are necessary to maintain skin and mucous membrane integrity.*
- Monitor laboratory values for electrolytes and acid-base balance. Report significant changes or deviations from normal. *Electrolytes are lost through vomiting, increasing the risk of electrolyte and acid-base imbalances. These imbalances, in turn, affect multiple body systems.*
- Administer oral or parenteral fluids as ordered. *Oral fluids may be withheld until vomiting has ceased, then gradually reintroduced. Intravenous fluids restore or maintain hydration until adequate oral intake is resumed.*
- Administer antiemetic and other drugs as ordered to relieve vomiting and facilitate oral feeding. Encourage fluids as soon as feasible. *The oral route is preferred for fluid and nutrient intake; medications may be used to allow earlier resumption of feeding.*

Imbalanced Nutrition: Less Than Body Requirements   Manifestations of chronic gastritis may lead to reduced food intake and malnutrition. The client often associates these unpleasant sensations with eating, and may gradually reduce food intake. Associated anorexia also contributes to poor food intake.

- Monitor and record food and fluid intake and any abnormal losses, such as vomiting. *Careful monitoring can help in developing a dietary plan to meet the caloric needs of the client.*

- Monitor weight and laboratory studies, such as serum albumin, hemoglobin, and red blood cell indices. *Weights and laboratory values provide data regarding nutritional status and the effectiveness of interventions.*

- Arrange for dietary consultation to determine caloric and nutrient needs and develop a dietary plan. Consider food preferences and tolerances in menu planning. *A diet high in protein, vitamins, and minerals may be prescribed to meet nutritional needs of the client with chronic gastritis. In addition, specific food intolerances may need to be considered. Planning to include preferred foods in the diet helps ensure consumption of the prescribed diet.*

- Provide nutritional supplements between meals or frequent small feedings as needed. *Many clients with chronic gastritis tolerate small, frequent feedings better than three large meals per day.*

- Maintain tube feedings or parenteral nutrition as ordered. Refer to Chapter 17 for further information on enteral and parenteral feedings.

Home Care

Because acute or chronic gastritis is usually managed in community-based settings, teaching is vital. For the client with acute gastritis, teaching focuses on managing acute symptoms, reintroducing fluids and solid foods, indicators of possible complications (e.g., continued vomiting, signs of fluid and electrolyte imbalance), and preventing future episodes.

Provide the following information for clients with chronic gastritis:

- Maintaining optimal nutrition
- Helpful dietary modifications
- Using prescribed medications
- Avoiding known gastric irritants, such as aspirin, alcohol, and cigarette smoking.

Referral to smoking-cessation classes or programs to treat alcohol abuse may be necessary.

The Client with Peptic Ulcer Disease

Peptic ulcer disease (PUD), a break in the mucous lining of the gastrointestinal tract where it comes in contact with gastric juice, is a chronic health problem. PUD affects approximately 10% of the population or 4 million people in the United States every year (Braunwald, et al., 2001; Tierney, et al., 2001).

Peptic ulcers occur in any area of the gastrointestinal tract exposed to acid-pepsin secretions, including the esophagus, stomach, or duodenum. **Duodenal ulcers** are the most common. They usually develop between the ages of 30 and 55, and are more common in men than women. **Gastric ulcers** more often affect older clients, between the ages of 55 and 70. Ulcers are more common in people who smoke and who are chronic users of NSAIDs. Alcohol and dietary intake do not seem to cause PUD, and the role of stress is uncertain. Although the incidence of PUD has dramatically decreased, the incidence of gastric ulcers is increasing, believed due to the widespread use of NSAIDs (Tierney, et al., 2001).

Risk Factors

Chronic *H. pylori* infection and use of aspirin and NSAIDs are the major risk factors for PUD. Overall, an estimated one in six clients infected with *H. pylori* develop PUD. Of the NSAIDs, aspirin is the most ulcerogenic. A strong familial pattern suggests a genetic factor in the development of PUD. Cigarette smoking is a significant risk factor, doubling the risk of PUD. Cigarette smoking inhibits the secretion of bicarbonate by the pancreas and possibly causes more rapid transit of gastric acid into the duodenum.

Pathophysiology

The innermost layer of the stomach wall, the gastric mucosa, consists of columnar epithelial cells, supported by a middle layer of blood vessels and glands, and a thin outer layer of smooth muscle. The mucosal barrier of the stomach, a thin coating of mucous gel and bicarbonate, protects the gastric mucosa. The mucosal barrier is maintained by bicarbonate secreted by the epithelial cells, by mucus gel production stimulated by prostaglandins, and by an adequate blood supply to the mucosa.

An **ulcer,** or break in the gastrointestinal mucosa, develops when the mucosal barrier is unable to protect the mucosa from damage by hydrochloric acid and pepsin, the gastric digestive juices.

H. pylori infection, found in about 70% of people who have PUD, is unique in colonizing the stomach. It is spread person to person (oral–oral or fecal–oral), and contributes to ulcer formation in several ways. The bacteria produce enzymes that reduce the efficacy of mucus gel in protecting the gastric mucosa. In addition, the host's inflammatory response to *H. pylori* contributes to gastric epithelial cell damage without producing immunity to the infection. Although the gastric mucosa is the usual site for *H. pylori* infection, this infection also contributes to duodenal ulcers. This is possibly related to increased gastric acid production associated with *H. pylori* infection.

NSAIDs contribute to PUD through both systemic and topical mechanisms. Prostaglandins are necessary for maintaining the gastric mucosal barrier. NSAIDs interrupt prostaglandin synthesis by disrupting the action of the enzyme cyclooxygenase (COX). The two forms of this enzyme are COX-1 and COX-2. The COX-1 enzyme is necessary to maintain the integrity of the gastric mucosa, but the anti-inflammatory effects of NSAIDs are due to their ability to inhibit the COX-2 enzyme. The COX-2 selective NSAIDs are less damaging to the gastric mucosa because they have less effect on the COX-1 enzyme. In addition to their systemic effect, aspirin and many NSAIDs cross the lipid membranes of gastric epithelial cells, damaging the cells themselves.

The ulcers of PUD may affect the esophagus, stomach, or duodenum. They may be superficial or deep, affecting all layers of the mucosa. Duodenal ulcers, the most common, usually develop in the proximal portion of the duodenum, close to the pyloris. They are sharply demarcated and usually less than 1 cm in diameter. Gastric ulcers often are found on the lesser curvature and the area immediately proximal to the pylorus. Gastric ulcers are associated with an increased incidence of gastric cancer.

Peptic ulcer disease may be chronic, with spontaneous remissions and exacerbations. Exacerbations of the disease may be associated with trauma, infection, or other physical or psychologic stressors.

Manifestations

Pain is the classic symptom of peptic ulcer disease. The pain is typically described as gnawing, burning, aching, or hungerlike and is experienced in the epigastric region, sometimes radiating to the back. The pain occurs when the stomach is empty (two to three hours after meals and in the middle of the night) and is relieved by eating with a classic "pain-food-relief" pattern. The client may complain of heartburn or regurgitation and may vomit.

The presentation of peptic ulcer disease in the older adult is often less clear, with vague and poorly localized discomfort, perhaps chest pain or dysphagia, weight loss, or anemia. In the older adult, a complication of PUD, such as upper GI hemorrhage or perforation of the stomach or duodenum, may be the presenting symptom.

Complications

The complications associated with peptic ulcers include hemorrhage, obstruction, and perforation.

Among people with PUD, 10% to 20% experience **hemorrhage** as a result of ulceration and erosion into the blood vessels of the gastric mucosa. In the older adult, bleeding is the most frequent complication. When small blood vessels erode, blood loss may be slow and insidious, with occult blood in the stool the only initial sign. If bleeding continues, the client becomes anemic and experiences symptoms of weakness, fatigue, dizziness, and orthostatic hypotension. Erosion into a larger vessel can lead to sudden and severe bleeding with hematemesis, melena, or **hematochezia** (blood in the stool), and signs of hypovolemic shock.

Gastric outlet obstruction may result from edema surrounding the ulcer, smooth muscle spasm, or scar tissue. Generally, obstruction is a gradual rather than an acute process. Symptoms include a feeling of epigastric fullness, accentuated ulcer symptoms, and nausea. If the obstruction becomes complete, vomiting occurs. Hydrochloric acid, sodium, and potassium are lost in vomitus, potentially leading to fluid and electrolyte imbalance and metabolic alkalosis.

The most lethal complication of PUD is **perforation** of the ulcer through the mucosal wall. When perforation occurs, gastric or duodenal contents enter the peritoneum, causing an inflammatory process and peritonitis. Chemical peritonitis from the hydrochloric acid, pepsin, bile, and pancreatic fluid is immediate; bacterial peritonitis follows within 6 to 12 hours from gastric contaminants entering the normally sterile peritoneal cavity. When an ulcer perforates, the client has immediate, severe upper abdominal pain, radiating throughout the abdomen and possibly to the shoulder. The abdomen becomes rigid and boardlike, with absent bowel sounds. Signs of shock may be present, including diaphoresis, tachycardia, and rapid, shallow respirations. Classic symptoms of perforation may not be present in an older adult. The older adult may instead present with mental confusion and other nonspecific symptoms. This atypical presentation can lead to delays in diagnosis and treatment, increasing the associated mortality rate.

Zollinger-Ellison Syndrome

Zollinger-Ellison syndrome is peptic ulcer disease caused by a gastrinoma, or gastrin-secreting tumor of the pancreas, stomach, or intestines. Gastrinomas may be benign, although 50% to 70% are malignant tumors. Gastrin is a hormone that stimulates the secretion of pepsin and hydrochloric acid. The increased gastrin levels associated with these tumors result in hypersecretion of gastric acid, which in turn causes mucosal ulceration.

The peptic ulcers of Zollinger-Ellison syndrome may affect any portion of the stomach or duodenum, as well as the esophagus or jejunum. Characteristic ulcerlike pain is common. The high levels of hydrochloric acid entering the duodenum may also cause diarrhea and **steatorrhea** (excess fat in the feces), from impaired fat digestion and absorption. Complications of bleeding and perforation are often seen with Zollinger-Ellison syndrome. Fluid and electrolyte imbalances may also result from persistent diarrhea with resultant losses of potassium and sodium, in particular.

Collaborative Care

Treatment for PUD focuses on eradicating *H. pylori* infection and treating or preventing ulcers related to use of NSAIDs.

Diagnostic Tests

*   *Upper GI series* using barium as a contrast medium can detect 80% to 90% of peptic ulcers. It commonly is the diagnostic procedure chosen first; it is less costly and less invasive than gastroscopy. Small or very superficial ulcers may be missed, however.

*   *Gastroscopy* allows visualization of the esophageal, gastric, and duodenal mucosa and direct inspection of ulcers. Tissue can also be obtained for biopsy.

*   Biopsy specimens obtained during a gastroscopy can be tested for the presence of *H. pylori* using several different methods. In the biopsy urease test, the specimen is put into a gel containing urea. If *H. pylori* is present, the urease that it produces changes the color of the gel, often within minutes. Biopsy specimen cells also can be microscopically examined or cultured for evidence of *H. pylori*.

*   Noninvasive methods of detecting *H. pylori* infection include *serologic testing* (to detect IgG antibodies through ELISA) and the *urea breath test*. In this test, radiolabeled urea is given orally. The urease produced by *H. pylori* bacteria converts the urea to ammonia and radiolabeled carbon dioxide, which can then be measured as the client exhales. This test also can be used to evaluate the effectiveness of treatment to eradicate *H. pylori*.

*   If Zollinger-Ellison syndrome is suspected, *gastric analysis* may be performed to evaluate gastric acid secretion. Stomach contents are aspirated through a nasogastric tube and analyzed. In Zollinger-Ellison syndrome, gastric acid levels are very high.

Medications

The medications used to treat PUD include agents to eradicate *H. pylori,* drugs to decrease gastric acid content, and agents that protect the mucosa. Nursing responsibilities related to selected drugs to treat GERD, gastritis, and PUD are found in Table 18-3.

Eradication of *H. pylori* is often difficult. Combination therapies that use two antibiotics with either bismuth or proton-pump inhibitors (e.g., a combination of omeprazole, metronidazole, and clarithromycin or bismuth subsalicylate, tetracycline, and metronidazole) are necessary. With complete eradication of *H. pylori,* reinfection rates are less than 0.5% per year.

In clients who have NSAID-induced ulcers, the NSAID in use should be discontinued if at all possible. If this is not possible, twice-daily PPIs enable ulcer healing.

Medications that decrease gastric acid content include proton-pump inhibitors and the H_2-receptor antagonists.

- Proton pump inhibitors bind the acid-secreting enzyme (H+, K+ ATPase) that functions as the proton pump, disabling it for up to 24 hours. These drugs are very effective, resulting in over 90% ulcer healing after four weeks. Compared to the H_2-receptor blockers, the proton-pump inhibitors provide faster pain relief and more rapid ulcer healing.

- Histamine$_2$-receptor blockers inhibit histamine binding to the receptors on the gastric parietal cells to reduce acid secretion. These drugs are very well tolerated and have few serious side effects; however, drug interactions can occur. These drugs must be continued for eight weeks or longer for ulcer healing.

Agents that protect the mucosa include sucralfate, bismuth, antacids, and prostaglandin analogs.

- Sucralfate binds to proteins in the ulcer base, forming a protective barrier against acid, bile, and pepsin. Sucralfate also stimulates the secretion of mucus, bicarbonate, and prostaglandin.

- Bismuth compounds (Pepto-Bismol) stimulate mucosal bicarbonate and prostaglandin production to promote ulcer healing. In addition, bismuth has an antibacterial action against *H. pylori*. There are very few side effects, other than a harmless darkening of stools.

- Prostaglandin analogs (misoprostol) promote ulcer healing by stimulating mucus and bicarbonate secretions and by inhibiting acid secretion. Although not as effective as the other drugs discussed, misoprostol is used to prevent NSAID-induced ulcers.

- Antacids stimulate gastric mucosal defenses, thereby aiding in ulcer healing. They provide rapid relief of ulcer symptoms, and are often used as needed to supplement other antiulcer medications. Antacids are inexpensive, but clients often have difficulty with a regular regimen because the drugs must be taken frequently and may cause either constipation (from the aluminum-type antacids) or diarrhea (from the magnesium-based antacids). Antacids also interfere with the absorption of iron, digoxin, some antibiotics, and other drugs.

Treatments

Dietary Management In addition to pharmacologic treatment, clients are encouraged to maintain good nutrition, consuming balanced meals at regular intervals. It is important to teach clients that bland or restrictive diets are no longer necessary. Mild alcohol intake is not harmful. Smoking should be discouraged, as it slows the rate of healing and increases the frequency of relapses.

Surgery The identification of *H. pylori* as a cause of PUD and the availability of drugs to treat the infection and heal peptic ulcers has all but eliminated surgery as a treatment option for peptic ulcer disease. Older clients, however, may have undergone gastric resection surgery for PUD, and may have long-term complications related to the surgery. See the section on gastric cancer for more information about gastric surgery and its potential complications.

Treatment of Complications The client hospitalized with a complication of PUD, such as bleeding, gastrointestinal obstruction, or perforation and peritonitis, requires additional interventions to restore homeostasis.

In hemorrhage associated with PUD, initial interventions focus on restoring and maintaining circulation. Normal saline, lactated Ringer's, or other balanced electrolyte solutions are administered intravenously to restore intravascular volume if signs of shock (tachycardia, hypotension, pallor, low urine output, and anxiety) are present. Whole blood or packed red blood cells may be administered to restore hemoglobin and hematocrit levels.

Gastroscopy with direct injection of a clotting or sclerosing agent into the bleeding vessel may be performed. Laser photocoagulation, using light energy, or electrocoagulation, which uses electric current to generate heat, can also be done via gastroscopy to seal bleeding vessels.

The client is kept NPO until bleeding is controlled. Antacids are administered hourly via the nasogastric tube to protect the bleeding ulcer from gastric acid and to prevent acid reflux. H$_2$-receptor blockers, such as cimetidine, ranitidine, and famotidine, are administered intravenously until the client can resume oral intake. Surgery may be necessary if medical measures are ineffective in controlling bleeding. Older adults who experience bleeding as a complication of PUD are more likely to rebleed or require surgery to control the hemorrhage.

Repeated inflammation, healing, scarring, edema, and muscle spasm can lead to gastric outlet (pyloric) obstruction. Initial treatment includes gastric decompression with nasogastric suction and administration of intravenous normal saline and potassium chloride to correct fluid and electrolyte imbalance. H$_2$-receptor blockers are given intravenously as well. Balloon dilation of the gastric outlet may be done via upper endoscopy. If these measures are unsuccessful in relieving obstruction, surgery may be required.

Gastric or duodenal perforation resulting in contamination of the peritoneum with gastrointestinal contents often requires immediate intervention to restore homeostasis and minimize peritonitis. Intravenous fluids maintain fluid and electrolyte balance. Nasogastric suction removes gastric contents and minimizes peritoneal contamination. Placing the client in Fowler's or semi-Fowler's position allows peritoneal contaminants to pool in the pelvis. Intravenous antibiotics aggressively treat bacterial infection from intestinal flora. Laparoscopic surgery or an open laparotomy may close the perforation.

Nursing Care

Health Promotion
Although it is difficult to predict which clients will develop peptic ulcer disease, promote health by advising clients to avoid risk factors, such as excessive aspirin or NSAID use and cigarette smoking. In addition, encourage clients to seek treatment for manifestations of gastroesophageal reflux disease (GERD) or chronic gastritis, both of which also are associated with *H. pylori* infection.

Assessment
Collect the following subjective and objective data when assessing the client with peptic ulcer disease:

* *Health history:* complaints of epigastric or left upper quadrant pain, heartburn, or discomfort; its character, severity, timing and relationship to eating, measures used for relief; nausea or vomiting, presence of bright blood or "coffee-ground" appearing material in vomitus; current medications, including use of aspirin or other NSAIDs; cigarette smoking and use of alcohol or other drugs.

- *Physical examination:* general appearance, including height and weight relationship; vital signs, including orthostatic measurements; abdominal examination, including shape and contour, bowel sounds, and tenderness to palpation; presence of obvious or occult blood in vomitus and stool.

Nursing Diagnoses and Interventions

Pain   The pain of peptic ulcer disease is often predictable and preventable. Pain is typically experienced two to four hours after eating, as high levels of gastric acid and pepsin irritate the exposed mucosa. Measures to neutralize the acid, minimize its production, or protect the mucosa often relieve this pain, minimizing the need for analgesics.

- Assess pain, including location, type, severity, frequency, and duration, and its relationship to food intake or other contributing factors.
- Administer proton-pump inhibitors, H_2-receptor antagonists, antacids, or mucosal protective agents as ordered. Monitor for effectiveness and side effects or adverse reactions. *The pain associated with PUD is generally caused by the effect of gastric juices on exposed mucosal tissue. These medications reduce pain and promote healing by reducing acid production, neutralizing acid, or providing a barrier for the damaged mucosa.*
- Teach relaxation, stress-reduction, and lifestyle management techniques. Refer client for stress management counseling or classes as indicated. *Although there is no clear relationship between stress and PUD, measures to relieve stress and promote physical and emotional rest help reduce the perception of pain and may reduce ulcer genesis.*

Sleep Pattern Disturbance   Nighttime ulcer pain, which typically occurs between 1:00 and 3:00 A.M., may disrupt the sleep cycle and result in inadequate rest. Anticipation of pain may lead to insomnia or other sleep disruptions.

- Stress the importance of taking medications as prescribed. *The bedtime dose of proton-pump inhibitor or H_2-receptor blocker minimizes hydrochloric acid production during the night, reducing nighttime pain.*
- Instruct to limit food intake after the evening meal, eliminating any bedtime snack. *Eating before bed can stimulate the production of gastric acid and pepsin, increasing the likelihood of nighttime pain.*
- Encourage use of relaxation techniques and comfort measures, such as soft music, as needed to promote sleep. *Once the pain associated with PUD has been controlled, these measures help reduce anxiety and reestablish a normal sleep pattern.*

Imbalanced Nutrition: Less Than Body Requirements   In an attempt to avoid discomfort, the client with peptic ulcer disease may gradually reduce food intake, sometimes jeopardizing nutritional status. Anorexia and early satiety are additional problems associated with PUD.

- Assess current diet, including pattern of food intake, eating schedule, and foods that precipitate pain or are being avoided in anticipation of pain. *The client may not realize the extent of self-imposed dietary limitations, especially if symptoms have persisted for an extended time. Assessment increases awareness and also helps identify the adequacy of nutrient intake.*
- Refer to a dietitian for meal planning to minimize PUD symptoms and meet nutritional needs. Consider normal eating patterns and preferences in meal planning. *Although no specific diet is recommended for PUD, clients should avoid foods that increase pain. Six small meals per day often help increase food tolerance and decrease postprandial discomfort.*

- Monitor for complaints of anorexia, fullness, nausea, and vomiting. Adjust dietary intake or medication schedule as indicated. *PUD and resultant scarring can lead to impaired gastric emptying, necessitating a treatment change.*

- Monitor laboratory values for indications of anemia or other nutritional deficits. Monitor for therapeutic and side effects of treatment measures, such as oral iron replacement. Instruct the client taking oral iron replacement to avoid using an antacid within one to two hours of taking the iron preparation. *Anemia can result from poor nutrient absorption or chronic blood loss in clients with PUD. Oral iron supplements may cause GI distress, nausea, and vomiting; if these side effects are intolerable, notify the physician for a possible change of therapy. Antacids bind with oral iron preparations, blocking absorption.*

Deficient Fluid Volume   Erosion of a blood vessel with resultant hemorrhage is a significant risk for the client with peptic ulcer disease. Acute bleeding can lead to hypovolemia and fluid volume deficit, which can lead to a decrease in cardiac output and impaired tissue perfusion.

- Monitor stools and gastric drainage for overt and occult blood. Assess gastric drainage (vomitus or from a nasogastric tube) to estimate the amount and rapidity of hemorrhage. *Drainage is bright red with possible clots in acute hemorrhage; dark red or the color of coffee grounds when blood has been in the stomach for a period of time. Hematochezia (stool containing red blood and clots) is present in acute hemorrhage; melena (black, tarry stool) is an indicator of less acute bleeding. When small vessels are disrupted, bleeding may be slow and not overtly evident. With chronic or slow gastrointestinal bleeding, the risk of a fluid volume deficit is minimal; anemia and activity intolerance are more likely.*

- Maintain intravenous therapy with fluid volume and electrolyte replacement solutions; administer whole blood or packed cells as ordered. *Both fluids and electrolytes are lost through vomiting, nasogastric drainage, and diarrhea in an episode of acute bleeding. To prevent shock, it is essential to maintain a blood volume and cardiac output sufficient to perfuse body tissues. Whole blood and packed cells replace both blood volume and red blood cells, providing additional oxygen-carrying capacity to meet cell needs.*

- Insert a nasogastric tube and maintain its position and patency; if ordered, irrigate with sterile normal saline until returns are clear. Initially, measure and record gastric output every hour (be sure to subtract the volume of irrigant), then every four to eight hours. *Nasogastric suction removes blood from the gastrointestinal tract, preventing vomiting and possible aspiration. Irrigation with sterile saline solution at room temperature has a vasoconstrictive effect, slowing active bleeding. Water is not used as an irrigant to avoid water intoxication. Sterile solution is used because of the possibility of perforation. Gastric output is replaced milliliter for milliliter with a balanced electrolyte solution to maintain homeostasis.*

- Monitor hemoglobin and hematocrit, serum electrolytes, BUN, and creatinine values. Report abnormal findings. *Hemoglobin and hematocrit are lower than normal with acute or chronic GI bleeding. In acute hemorrhage, initial results may be within normal range because both cells and plasma are lost. Loss of fluids and electrolytes with gastric drainage and diarrhea will alter normal levels. Digestion and absorption of blood in the GI tract may result in elevated BUN and creatinine levels.*

- Assess abdomen, including bowel sounds, distention, girth, and tenderness every four hours and record findings. *Borborygmi or hyperactive bowel sounds with abdominal tenderness are common with acute GI bleeding. Increased distention, increasing abdominal girth, absent bowel sounds, or extreme tenderness with a rigid, boardlike abdomen may indicate perforation.*

- Maintain bed rest with the head of the bed elevated. Ensure safety. *Loss of blood volume may cause orthostatic hypotension with resultant syncope or dizziness upon standing.*

Home Care

Peptic ulcer disease is managed in home and community-based settings; only its complications typically require treatment in an acute care setting. Provide the following information when preparing the client for home care:

- Prescribed medication regimen, including desired and potential adverse effects.
- Importance of continuing therapy even when symptoms are relieved.
- Relationship between peptic ulcers and factors, such as NSAID use and smoking. If indicated, refer to a smoking-cessation clinic or program.
- Importance of avoiding aspirin and other NSAIDs; stress the necessity of reading the labels of over-the-counter medications for possible aspirin content.
- Manifestations of complications that should be reported to the care provider, including increased abdominal pain or distention, vomiting, black or tarry stools, lightheadedness, or fainting.
- Stress and lifestyle management techniques that may help prevent exacerbation. Refer to resources for stress management, such as classes, counseling, and formal or informal groups.

Table 18-4. Nursing Care of the Client with a Gastrostomy or Jejunostomy Tube

---

Clients who have had extensive gastric surgery or who require long-term enteral feedings to maintain nutrition may have a gastrostomy or jejunostomy tube inserted.

Procedure

Gastrostomy tubes are surgically placed in the stomach, with the stoma in the epigastric region of the abdomen. Jejunostomy tubes are placed in the proximal jejunum. Immediately following the procedure, the tube may be connected to low suction or plugged. If the client has been receiving tube feedings, these may be reinitiated shortly after tube placement.

Nursing Care

- Assess tube placement by aspirating stomach contents and checking the pH of aspirate to determine gastric or intestinal placement. A pH of 5 or less indicates gastric placement; the pH is generally 7 or higher with intestinal placement. *Recent studies show auscultation to be ineffective in determining feeding tube placement. Measuring the pH of aspirate from the tube is more reliable as a means of determining tube placement.*
- Inspect the skin surrounding the insertion site for healing, redness, swelling, and the presence of any drainage. If drainage is present, note the color, amount, consistency, and odor. *Changes in the insertion site, drainage, or lack of healing may indicate an infection.*

Continued on the next page

Table 18-4. Continued

- Assess the abdomen for distention, bowel sounds, and tenderness *to evaluate functioning of the gastrointestinal tract.*

- Until the stoma is well healed, use sterile technique for dressing changes and site care. Clean technique is appropriate for use once healing is complete. *Sterile technique reduces the risk of wound contamination by pathogens that can lead to infection. Once healing has occurred, clean technique is acceptable because the gastrointestinal tract is not a sterile body cavity.*

- Wearing clean gloves, remove old dressing. Cleanse the site with saline or soap and water, and rinse as appropriate. A well-healed stoma may be cleansed in the shower with the tube clamped or plugged. Pat dry with 4X4 gauze pads, and allow to air dry. Apply Stomadhesive, karaya, or other protective agents around tube as needed to protect the skin. *Gastric acid and other wound drainage is irritating to the skin. Meticulous care is important to maintain the integrity of the skin surrounding the stoma.*

- Redress the wound using a stoma dressing or folded 4X4 gauze pads. *Do not cut gauze pads, because threads may enter the wound, causing irritation and increasing the risk of inflammation.*

- Irrigate the tube with 30 to 50 mL of water, and clean the tube inside and out as indicated or ordered. Soft gastric tubes may require cleaning of the inner lumen with a special brush to maintain patency. *Tube feeding formulas may coat the inside of the gastrostomy tube and eventually cause it to become occluded. Regular irrigation with water and brushing as indicated maintain tube patency.*

- Provide mouth care or remind the client to do so. *When feedings are not being taken orally, the usual stimulus to do mouth care is lost. In addition, salivary fluids may not be as abundant, and oral mucous membranes may become dry and cracked.*

- If indicated, teach the client and family how to care for the tube and feedings. Refer client to a home health agency or visiting nurse for support and reinforcement of learning. *Gastrostomy tubes are often in place long term. When the client and family are able to assume care, independence and self-image are enhanced.*

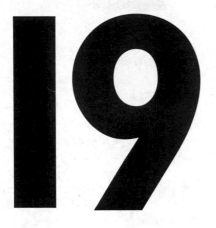

Nursing Care of Clients with Gallbladder, Liver, and Pancreatic Disorders

Gallbladder, liver, and exocrine pancreatic disorders may occur as primary disorders, or develop secondarily to other disease processes. One organ's functioning frequently affects that of another. Duct inflammation or obstruction, and changes in the multiple functions of these organs, can cause significant health effects.

Clients with a gallbladder, liver, or pancreatic disorder may experience pain, multiple metabolic and nutritional disturbances, and altered body image. Nursing care addresses physiologic and psychosocial needs of the client and family.

Gallbladder Disorders

Altered bile flow through the hepatic, cystic, or common bile duct is a common problem. It often leads to inflammation and other complications. Gallstones are the most common cause of obstructed flow. Tumors and abscesses also can obstruct bile flow.

The Client with Cholelithiasis and Cholecystitis

Cholelithiasis is the formation of stones (*calculi*) within the gallbladder or biliary duct system. Cholelithiasis is a common problem in the United States, affecting more than 10% of men and 20% of women by age 65 (Tierney, et al., 2001).

Physiology Review

Normally, bile is formed by the liver and stored in the gallbladder. Bile contains bile salts, bilirubin, water, electrolytes, cholesterol, fatty acids, and lecithin. In the gallbladder, some of the water and electrolytes are absorbed, further concentrating the bile. Food entering the intestine stimulates the gallbladder to contract and release bile through the common bile duct and sphincter of Oddi into the intestine. The bile salts in bile increase the solubility and absorption of dietary fats.

Pathophysiology and Manifestations

Cholelithiasis

Gallstones form when several factors interact: abnormal bile composition, biliary stasis, and inflammation of the gallbladder. Most gallstones (80%) consist primarily of cholesterol; the rest contain a mixture of bile components. Excess cholesterol in bile is associated with obesity, a high-calorie, high-cholesterol diet, and drugs that lower serum cholesterol levels. When bile is supersaturated with cholesterol, it can precipitate out to form stones. Biliary stasis, or slowed emptying of the gallbladder, contributes to cholelithiasis. Stones do not form when the gallbladder empties completely in response to hormonal stimulation. Slowed or incomplete emptying allows cholesterol to concentrate and increases the risk of stone formation. Finally, inflammation of the gallbladder allows excess water and bile salt reabsoprtion, increasing the risk for lithiasis.

Most gallstones are formed in the gallbladder. They may then migrate into the ducts, leading to *cholangitis* (duct inflammation). Although some people with cholelithiasis are asymptomatic, many develop manifestations. Early manifestations of gallstones may be vague: epigastric fullness or mild gastric distress after eating a large or fatty meal. Stones that obstruct the cystic duct or common bile duct lead to distention and increased pressure behind the stone. This causes **biliary colic,** a severe, steady pain in the epigastric region or right upper quadrant of the abdomen. The pain may radiate to the back, right scapula, or shoulder. The pain often begins suddenly following a meal, and may last as long as five hours. It often is accompanied by nausea and vomiting.

Obstruction of the common bile duct may cause bile reflux into the liver, leading to jaundice, pain, and possible liver damage. If the common duct is obstructed, pancreatitis is a potential complication.

Cholecystitis

Cholecystitis is inflammation of the gallbladder. *Acute cholecystitis* usually follows obstruction of the cystic duct by a stone. The obstruction increases pressure within the gallbladder, leading to ischemia of the gallbladder wall and mucosa. Chemical and bacterial inflammation often follow. The ischemia can lead to necrosis and perforation of the gallbladder wall.

Acute cholecystitis usually begins with an attack of biliary colic. The pain involves the entire right upper quadrant (RUQ), and may radiate to the back, right scapula, or shoulder. Movement or deep breathing may aggravate the pain. The pain usually lasts longer than biliary colic, continuing for 12 to 18 hours. Anorexia, nausea, and vomiting are common. Fever often is present, and may be accompanied by chills. The RUQ is tender to palpation.

Chronic cholecystitis may result from repeated bouts of acute cholecystitis or from persistent irritation of the gallbladder wall by stones. Bacteria may be present in the bile as well. Chronic cholecystitis often is asymptomatic.

Complications of cholecystitis include *empyema,* a collection of infected fluid within the gallbladder; gangrene and perforation with resulting peritonitis or abscess formation; formation of a fistula into an adjacent organ, such as the duodenum, colon, or stomach; or obstruction of the small intestine by a large gallstone (*gallstone ilius*). Table 19-1 compares the manifestations and complications of acute cholelithiasis with those of cholecystitis.

Collaborative Care

Treatment of the client with cholelithiasis or cholecystitis depends of the acuity of the condition and the client's overall health status. When gallstones are present but asymptomatic and the client has a low risk for complications, conservative treatment is indicated. However, when the client experiences frequent symptoms, has acute cholecystitis, or has very large stones, the gallbladder and stones are usually surgically removed.

Diagnostic Tests

Diagnostic tests are ordered to identify the presence and location of stones, identify possible complications, and help differentiate gallbladder disease from other disorders.

- *Serum bilirubin* is measured. Elevated direct (conjugated) bilirubin may indicate obstructed bile flow in the biliary duct system (see Table 19-2).
- *Complete blood count (CBC)* may indicate infection and inflammation if the WBC is elevated.
- *Serum amylase* and *lipase* are measured to identify possible pancreatitis related to common duct obstruction.
- *Abdominal X-ray* (flat plate of the abdomen) may show gallstones with a high calcium content.
- *Ultrasonography of the gallbladder* is a noninvasive exam that can accurately diagnose cholelithiasis. It also can be used to assess emptying of the gallbladder.
- *Oral cholecystogram* is performed using a dye administered orally to assess the gallbladder's ability to concentrate and excrete bile.
- *Gallbladder scans* use an intravenous radioactive solution that is rapidly extracted from the blood and excreted into the biliary tree to diagnose cystic duct obstruction and acute or chronic cholecystitis.

Table 19-1.   Manifestations and Complications of Cholelithiasis and Cholecystitis

Manifestations	Cholelithiasis	Cholecystitis
Pain	• Abrupt onset • Severe, steady • Localized to epigastrium and RUQ of abdomen • May radiate to back, right scapula, and shoulder • Lasts 30 minutes to 5 hours	• Abrupt onset • Severe, steady • Generalized in RUQ of abdomen • May radiate to back, right scapula, and shoulder • Lasts 12 to 18 hours • Aggravated by movement, breathing
Associated symptoms	• Nausea, vomiting	• Anorexia, nausea, vomiting • RUQ tenderness and guarding • Chills and fever

Continued on the next page

Table 19-1. Continued

| Complications | • Cholecystitis
• Common bile duct obstruction with possible jaundice and liver damage
• Common duct obstruction with pancreatitis | • Gangrene and perforation with peritonitis
• Chronic cholecystitis
• Empyema
• Fistula formation
• Gallstone ilius |

Medications

Clients who refuse surgery, or for whom surgery is inappropriate, may be treated with a drug to dissolve the gallstones. Ursodiol (Actigall) and chenodiol (Chenix) reduce the cholesterol content of gallstones, leading to their gradual dissolution. These drugs are most effective in treating stones with high cholesterol content. They are less effective in treating radiopaque stones with high calcium salt content. Ursodiol is generally well tolerated with few side effects, while chenodiol has a high incidence of diarrhea at therapeutic doses. It also is hepatotoxic, so periodic liver function studies are required during therapy.

The primary disadvantages of pharmacologic treatment for gallstones include its cost, long duration (2 years or more), and the high incidence of recurrent stone formation when treatment is discontinued. If infection is suspected, antibiotics may be ordered to cure the infection and reduce associated inflammation and edema. Clients with pruritus (itching) due to severe obstructive jaundice and an accumulation of bile salts on the skin may be given cholestyramine (Questran). This drug binds with bile salts to promote their excretion in the feces. A narcotic analgesic such as morphine may be required for pain relief during an acute attack of cholecystitis.

Table 19-2. Sorting Out Total, Direct, and Indirect Bilirubin Levels

When serum bilirubin levels are drawn, the results usually are reported as the total bilirubin, direct bilirubin, and indirect bilirubin levels. Most bilirubin is formed from hemoglobin, as aging or abnormal RBCs are removed from circulation and destroyed. It is then bound to protein and transported to the liver. This protein-bound bilirubin is called *indirect* or *unconjugated* bilirubin. Once in the liver, bilirubin is separated from the protein and converted to a soluble form, *direct* or *conjugated* bilirubin. Conjugated bilirubin is then excreted in the bile.

<   **Total** (serum) **bilirubin,** the total bilirubin in the blood, includes both indirect and direct forms. In adults, the normal total bilirubin is 0.3 to 1.2 mg/dL or SI 5 to 21 µmol/L. Total bilirubin levels increase when more is being produced (e.g., RBC hemolysis), or when its metabolism or excretion are impaired (e.g., liver disease or biliary obstruction).

<   **Direct** (conjugated) **bilirubin** levels, normally 0 to 0.2 mg/dL or SI <3.4 µmo/L in adults, rise when its excretion is impaired by obstruction within the liver (e.g., in cirrhosis, hepatitis, exposure to hepatotoxins) or in the biliary system.

<   **Indirect** (unconjugated) **bilirubin** levels, normally <1.1 mg/dL or SI <19 µmol/L in adults, rise in RBC hemolysis (e.g., sickle cell disease or transfusion reaction).

Treatments

Surgery **Laparoscopic cholecystectomy** (removal of the gallbladder) is the treatment of choice for symptomatic cholelithiasis or cholecystitis. This minimally invasive procedure has a low risk of complications and generally requires a hospital stay of less than 24 hours. Not all clients are candidates for laparoscopic cholecystectomy, and there is a risk that a laparoscopic cholecystectomy may be converted to a *laparotomy* (surgical opening into the abdomen) during the procedure.

When stones are lodged within the ducts, a **cholecystectomy** with common bile duct exploration may be done. A T-tube is inserted to maintain patency of the duct and promote bile passage while the edema decreases. Excess bile is collected in a drainage bag secured below the surgical site. If it is suspected that a stone has been retained following surgery, a postoperative cholangiogram via the T-tube or direct visualization of the duct with an endoscope may be performed.

Some clients who are poor surgical risks, and for whom laparoscopic cholecystectomy is inappropriate, may have either a *cholecystostomy* to drain the gallbladder, or a *choledochostomy* to remove stones and position a T-tube in the common bile duct.

Dietary Management

Food intake may be eliminated during an acute attack of cholecystitis, and a nasogastric tube inserted to relieve nausea and vomiting. Dietary fat intake may be limited, especially if the client is obese. If bile flow is obstructed, fat-soluble vitamins (A, D, E, and K) and bile salts may need to be administered.

Other Therapies

In some cases, shock wave lithotripsy may be used with drug therapy to dissolve large gallstones. In *extracorporeal shock wave lithotripsy (ESWL),* ultrasound is used to align the stones with the source of shock waves and the computerized lithotripter. Positioning is of prime importance throughout the procedure, which usually takes an hour. Mild sedation may be given during the procedure. Postprocedure nursing care includes monitoring for biliary colic that may result from the gallbladder contracting to remove stone fragments, nausea, and transient hematuria. *Percutaneous cholecystostomy,* ultrasound-guided drainage of the gallbladder, may be done in high-risk clients to postpone or even eliminate the need for surgery.

Complementary Therapies

The herb goldenseal has been used in treating cholecystitis. One of the active ingredients in goldenseal, berberine, stimulates secretion of bile and bilirubin. It also inhibits the growth of many common pathogens, including those known to infect the gallbladder. A study of the effectiveness of berberine in clients with cholecystitis demonstrated relief of all symptoms. Goldenseal can stimulate the uterus, so it is contraindicated for use during pregnancy. It also should not be used by nursing mothers.

Nursing Care

Health Promotion

While most risk factors for cholelithiasis cannot be controlled or modified, several can. Modifiable risk factors include obestity, hyperlipidemia, extreme low-calorie diets, and diets high in cholesterol. Encourage clients who are obese to increase their activity level and follow a low-carbohydrate, low-fat, low-cholesterol diet to promote weight loss and reduce their risk for developing gallstones. Discuss the dangers of "yo-yo" dieting, with cycles of weight loss followed by weight gain, and of extremely low calorie diets. Encourage clients with high serum cholesterol levels to discuss using cholesterol-lowering drugs with their primary care provider.

Assessment

Assessment data related to cholelithiasis and cholecystitis include the following:

- *Health history:* current manifestations, including RUQ pain, its character and relationship to meals, duration, and radiation, nausea and vomiting or other symptoms; duration of symptoms; risk factors or previous history of symptoms; chronic diseases, such as diabetes, cirrhosis, or inflammatory bowel disease; current diet; use of oral contraceptives or possibility of pregnancy.
- *Physical assessment:* current weight; color of skin and sclera; abdominal assessment, including light palpation for tenderness; color of urine and stool.

Nursing Diagnoses and Interventions

Priority nursing diagnoses for the client with cholelithiasis or cholecystitis often include pain related to biliary colic or surgery, imbalanced nutrition related to the effects of altered bile flow and to nausea and anorexia, and risk for infection related to potential rupture of an acutely inflamed gallbladder. Nursing interventions for the client who has undergone a laparoscopic or open cholecystectomy are similar to those for other clients having abdominal surgery.

Pain

The pain associated with cholelithiasis can be severe. Sometimes a combination of interventions is indicated.

- Discuss the relationship between fat intake and the pain. Teach ways to reduce fat intake. *Fat entering the duodenum initiates gallbladder contractions, causing pain when gallstones are present in the ducts.*
- Withhold oral food and fluids during episodes of acute pain. Insert nasogastric tube and connect to low suction if ordered. *Emptying the stomach reduces the amount of chyme entering the duodenum and the stimulus for gallbladder contractions, thus reducing pain.*
- For severe pain, administer meperidine or other narcotic analgesia as ordered. *Recent research indicates that morphine is no more likely to cause spasms of the sphincter of Oddi than meperidine.*
- Place in Fowler's position. *Fowler's position decreases pressure on the inflamed gallbladder.*
- Monitor vital signs, including temperature, at least every four hours. *Bacterial infection often is present in acute cholecystitis, and may cause an elevated temperature and respiratory rate.*

Imbalanced Nutrition: Less Than Body Requirements

The client with severe gallbladder disease may develop nutritional imbalances related to anorexia, pain and nausea following meals, and impaired bile flow that alters absorption of fat and fat-soluble vitamins (A, D, E, K) from the gut.

- Assess nutritional status, including diet history, height and weight, and skinfold measurements (see Chapters 16 and 17). *Even though they are often obese, clients with gallbladder disease may have an imbalanced diet or may have specific vitamin deficiencies, particularly of the fat-soluble vitamins.*

- Evaluate laboratory results, including serum bilirubin, albumin, glucose, and cholesterol levels. Report abnormal results to the primary care provider. *Elevated serum bilirubin may indicate impaired bilirubin excretion due to obstructed bile flow. A low serum albumin may indicate poor nutritional status. Glucose intolerance and hypercholesterolemia are risk factors for cholelithiasis.*

- Refer to a dietitian or nutritionist for diet counseling to promote healthy weight loss and reduce pain episodes. *A low-carbohydrate, low-fat, higher-protein diet reduces symptoms of cholecystitis. While fasting and very-low-calorie diets are contraindicated, a moderate reduction in calorie intake and increased activity levels promote weight loss.*

- Administer vitamin supplements as ordered. *Clients who do not absorb fat well due to obstructed bile flow may require supplements of the fat-soluble vitamins.*

Risk for Infection

An acutely inflamed gallbladder may become necrotic and rupture, releasing its contents into the abdominal cavity. While the resulting infection often remains localized, peritonitis can result from chemical irritation and bacterial contamination of the peritoneal cavity.

Following open cholecystectomy (*laparotomy*), the risk for pulmonary infection is significant due to the high abdominal incision.

- Monitor vital signs including temperature every four hours. Promptly report vital sign changes or temperature elevation. *Tachycardia, increased respiratory rate, or an elevated temperature may indicate an infectious process.*

- Assess abdomen every four hours and as indicated (e.g., when pain level changes abruptly). *Increasing abdominal tenderness or a rigid, boardlike abdomen may indicate rupture of the gallbladder with peritonitis.*

- Assist to cough and deep breathe or use incentive spirometer every one to two hours while awake. Splint abdominal incision with a blanket or pillow during coughing. *The high abdominal incision of an open cholecystectomy interferes with effective coughing and deep breathing, increasing the risk of atelectasis and respiratory infections, such as pneumonia.*

- Place in Fowler's position and encourage ambulation as allowed. *Fowler's position and ambulating promote lung expansion and airway clearance, reducing the risk of respiratory infections.*

- Administer antibiotics as ordered. *Antibiotics may be given preoperatively to reduce the risk of infection from infected gallbladder contents, and may be continued postoperatively to prevent infection.*

Home Care

Teaching varies, depending on the choice of treatment options for cholelithiasis and cholecystitis. If surgery is not an option, teach about medications that dissolve stones, their use and adverse effects (diarrhea is a common side effect), and maintaining a low-fat, low-carbohydate diet if indicated. Include an explanation about the role of bile and the function of the gallbladder in terms that the client and family can understand.

Provide appropriate preoperative teaching for the planned procedure. Discuss the possibility of open cholecystectomy, even when a laparoscopic procedure is planned. Teach postoperative self-care measures to manage pain and prevent complications. If the client will be discharged with a T-tube, provide instructions about its care. Discuss manifestations of complications to report to the physician. Stress the importance of follow-up appointments.

Following cholecystectomy, a low-fat diet may be initially recommended. Refer the client and food preparer to a dietitian to review low-fat foods. Higher fat foods may be gradually added to the diet as tolerated.

The Client with Cancer of the Gallbladder

Gallbladder cancer is rare, primarily affecting people over age 65. Women are more likely to develop the disorder. Manifestations of gallbladder cancer include intense pain and a palpable mass in the RUQ of the abdomen. Jaundice and weight loss are common. Gallbladder cancers spread by direct extension to the liver, and metastasize via the blood and lymph system.

At the time of diagnosis, the cancer usually is too advanced to treat surgically. Ninety-five percent of clients with primary cancer of the gallbladder die within one year. Radical and extensive surgical interventions may be performed, but the prognosis is poor regardless of treatment (Tierney, et al., 2001). Nursing care is palliative, focusing on maintaining comfort and independence to the extent possible.

Liver Disorders

The liver is a complex organ with multiple metabolic and regulatory functions. Optimal liver function is essential to health. Because of the significant amount of blood in the liver at all times, it is exposed to the effects of pathogens, drugs, toxins, and possibly malignant cells. As a result, liver cells may become inflamed or damaged, or cancerous tumors may develop.

The Client with Hepatitis

Hepatitis is inflammation of the liver. It is usually caused by a virus, although it may result from exposure to alcohol, drugs and toxins, or other pathogens. Hepatitis may be acute or chronic in nature. Cirrhosis, discussed in the next section, is a potential consequence of severe hepatocellular damage.

Pathophysiology and Manifestations

The essential functions of the liver are multiple. One of its primary functions is the metabolism and elimination of bilirubin. Bilirubin is a breakdown product of hemoglobin, released when RBCs are broken down and destroyed. This insoluble form of bilirubin (unconjugated bilirubin) is metabolized by the liver into a soluble form (conjugated bilirubin), which is then eliminated in bile. The liver also metabolizes carbohydrates, proteins, and fats. Most drugs are metabolized in the liver, and substances, such as alcohol and many toxins, are detoxified. These metabolic functions and bile elimination are disrupted by the inflammation of hepatitis.

Viral Hepatitis

At least five viruses are known to cause hepatitis: hepatitis A virus (HAV), hepatitis B virus (HBV), hepatitis C virus (HCV), the hepatitis B-associated delta virus (HDV), and hepatitis E virus (HEV). These viruses differ from one another in mode of transmission, incubation period, the severity and type of liver damage they cause, and their ability to become chronic or develop a carrier (asymptomatic) state. Table 19-3 identifies unique features of the primary hepatitis viruses. Two additional viruses, hepatitis F and hepatitis G, have recently been identified. Their characteristics are yet to be defined.

Hepatitis viruses replicate in the liver, damaging liver cells (hepatocytes). The viruses provoke an immune response that causes inflammation and necrosis of hepatocytes as well. Although the extent of damage and the immune response vary among the different hepatitis viruses, the disease itself usually follows a predictable pattern.

No manifestations are present during the incubation period after exposure to the virus. The *prodromal* or *preicteric* (before jaundice) *phase* may begin abruptly or insidiously, with general malaise, anorexia, fatigue, and muscle and body aches. These manifestations often are mistaken for the flu. Nausea, vomiting, diarrhea, or constipation may develop, as well as mild RUQ abdominal pain. Chills and fever may be present.

The *icteric* (jaundiced) *phase* usually begins five to ten days after the onset of symptoms. It is heralded by jaundice of the sclera, skin, and mucous membranes. Inflammation of the liver and bile ducts prevents bilirubin from being excreted into the small intestine. As a result, the serum bilirubin levels are elevated, causing yellowing of the skin and mucous membranes. Pruritus may develop due to deposition of bile salts on the skin. The stools are light brown or clay colored because bile pigment is not excreted through the normal fecal pathway. Instead, the pigment is excreted by the kidneys, causing the urine to turn brown.

During the icteric phase, the initial prodromal manifestations usually diminish, even though the serum bilirubin increases. The appetite increases, and the temperature returns to normal. When uncomplicated, spontaneous recovery usually begins within two weeks of the onset of jaundice.

The *convalescent phase* follows jaundice and lasts several weeks. During this time, manifestations gradually improve: Serum enzymes decrease, liver pain decreases, and gastrointestinal symptoms and weakness subside.

Table 19-3. Comparison of Types of Viral Hepatitis

Virus	Hepatitis A (HAV)	Hepatitis B (HBV)	Hepatitis C (HCV)	Hepatitis D (HDV)	Hepatitis E (HEV)
Mode of transmission	Fecal–oral	Blood & body fluids; perinatal	Blood & body fluids	Blood & body fluids; perinatal	Fecal–oral
Incubation (in weeks)	2–6	6–24	5–12	3–13	3–6
Onset	Abrupt	Slow	Slow	Abrupt	Abrupt
Carrier state	No	Yes	Yes	Yes	Yes

Continued on the next page

Table 19-3. Continued

Possible complications	Rare	Chronic hepatitis Cirrhosis Liver cancer	Chronic hepatitis Cirrhosis Liver cancer	Chronic hepatitis Cirrhosis Fulminant hepatitis	May be severe in pregnant women
Laboratory findings	Anti-HAV antibodies present	Positive HBsAg (HBV surface antigen); anti-HBV antibodies present	Anti-HCV antibodies present	Positive HDVAg (delta antigen) early; anti-HDV antibodies later	Anti-HEV antibodies present

Hepatitis A

Hepatitis A, or *infectious hepatitis,* often occurs in either sporadic attacks or mild epidemics. It is transmitted by the fecal–oral route via contaminated food, water, shellfish, and direct contact with an infected person. The virus is in the stool of infected persons up to two weeks before symptoms develop. Although hepatitis A usually has an abrupt onset, it is typically a benign and self-limited disease with few long-term consequences. Symptoms last up to two months.

Hepatitis B

Hepatitis B can cause acute hepatitis, chronic hepatitis, fulminant hepatitis, or a carrier state. This virus is spread through contact with infected blood and body fluids. Health care workers are at risk through exposure to blood and needle-stick injuries. Other high-risk groups for hepatitis B include injection drug users, people with multiple sex partners, men who have sex with other men, and people frequently exposed to blood products, such as people on hemodialysis. Hepatitis B is a major risk factor for primary liver cancer.

In hepatitis B, liver cells are damaged by the immune response to this antigen. Damage may affect only portions or the majority of the liver. The liver shows evidence of injury and scarring, regeneration, and proliferation of inflammatory cells (Bullock & Henze, 2000).

Hepatitis C

Hepatitis C, formerly known as non-A, non-B hepatitis, is the primary worldwide cause of chronic hepatitis, cirrhosis, and liver cancer (Porth, 2002). It is transmitted through infected blood and body fluids. Injection drug use is the primary risk factor for HCV infection. The initial manifestations of this type of hepatitis often are mild and nonspecific. The disease is often recognized long after exposure occurred, when secondary effects of the disease, such as chronic hepatitis or cirrhosis, develop.

Hepatitis Delta

Hepatitis delta (HDV) only causes infection in people who are also infected with hepatitis B. It can cause acute or chronic infection, and can increase the severity of HBV infection (Porth, 2002). It is transmitted in the same manner as HBV.

Hepatitis E

Hepatitis E is rare in the United States. It is transmitted by fecal contamination of water supplies in developing areas, such as southeast Asia, parts of Africa, and Central America. It primarily affects young adults. It can cause fulminant, fatal hepatitis in pregnant women.

Chronic Hepatitis

Chronic hepatitis is chronic infection of the liver. While it may cause few symptoms, it is the primary cause of liver damage leading to cirrhosis, liver cancer, and liver transplantation. Three of the known hepatitis viruses cause chronic hepatitis: HBV, HCV, and HDV. Manifestations of chronic hepatitis include malaise, fatigue, and hepatomegaly. Occasional icteric (jaundiced) periods may occur. Liver enzymes, particularly serum aminotransferase levels, typically are elevated.

Fulminant Hepatitis

Fulminant hepatitis is a rapidly progressive disease, with liver failure developing within two to three weeks after the onset of symptoms. Although uncommon, it is usually related to HBV with concurrent HDV infection.

Toxic Hepatitis

Many substances, including alcohol, certain drugs, and other toxins, can directly damage liver cells. Alcoholic hepatitis can result from chronic alcohol abuse or from an acute toxic reaction to alcohol. Alcoholic hepatitis causes necrosis of hepatocytes and inflammation of the liver parenchyma (functional tissue). Unless alcohol intake is avoided, progression to cirrhosis is common.

Other potential hepatotoxins include acetaminophen, benzene, carbon tetrachloride, halothane, chloroform, and poisonous mushrooms. These substances directly damage liver cells, leading to necrosis. The degree of damage often depends on age and the extent of exposure (dose) to the hepatoxin. Acetaminophen is a common cause of hepatocellular damage.

Hepatobiliary Hepatitis

Hepatobiliary hepatitis is due to cholestasis, the interruption of the normal flow of bile. Cholestasis may result from obstruction of the hepatic duct with stones or inflammation secondary to cholelithiasis. Other agents, such as oral contraceptives and allopurinol (a drug used to lower uric acid levels), can also cause cholestasis. When bile flow is disrupted, the liver parenchyma may become inflamed. Reestablishing bile flow by removing the stone or other causative agent is the treatment for hepatobiliary hepatitis.

Collaborative Care

Management of hepatitis focuses on determining its cause, providing appropriate treatment and support, and teaching strategies to prevent further liver damage. Effective management begins with thorough assessment of diagnostic and laboratory data.

Diagnostic Tests

Liver function tests, such as blood levels of bilirubin and enzymes commonly released when liver cells are damaged, are obtained. These include the following:

- *Alanine aminotransferase (ALT)* is an enzyme contained within each liver cell. When liver cells are damaged, it is released into the blood. Levels may exceed 1000 IU/L or more in acute hepatitis.

- *Aspartate aminotransferase (AST)* is an enzyme found predominantly in heart and liver cells. AST levels rise when liver cells are damaged; with severe damage, blood levels may be 20 to 100 times normal values (Malarkey & McMorrow, 2000).

- *Alkaline phosphatase (ALP)* is an enzyme present in liver cells and bone. Serum ALP levels often are elevated in hepatitis.

- *Gamma-glutamyltransferase (GGT)* is an enzyme present in cell membranes. Its blood levels rise in hepatitis and obstructive biliary disease, and remain elevated until function is restored.

- *Lactic dehydrogenase (LDH)*, an enzyme present in many body tissues, is a nonspecific indicator of tissue damage. Its isoenzyme, LDH5, is a specific indicator of liver damage.

- *Serum bilirubin* levels, including *conjugated* and *unconjugated*, are elevated in viral hepatitis due to impaired bilirubin metabolism and obstruction of the hepatobiliary ducts by inflammation and edema. The bilirubin level decreases as inflammation and edema subside.

- Laboratory tests for viral antigens and their specific antibodies may be done to identify the infecting virus and its state of activity.

- A *liver biopsy* may be done to detect and evaluate chronic hepatitis.

Medications

Prevention

Hepatitis A and hepatitis B are preventable diseases. Vaccines are available, as are preparations to prevent the disease following known or suspected exposure.

VACCINES. Hepatitis A vaccine provides long-term protection against HAV infection. It is an inactivated whole virus vaccine available in pediatric and adult formulations. Although more than 95% of adults achieve immunity after one dose of the vaccine, two doses are recommended for full protection.

Three doses of hepatitis B vaccine provide immunity to HBV infection in 90% of healthy adults. Hepatitis B vaccine is a recombinant vaccine. Vaccines produced by different manufacturers may be used interchangeably, although their dosages differ. Older adults are less likely to achieve immunity than younger adults. Clients on hemodialysis and people who are immunocompromised may need larger or more doses of the vaccine to achieve adequate protection. Serologic testing for immunity is recommended on completion of the series for people in these high-risk groups.

POSTEXPOSURE PROPHYLAXIS. Postexposure prophylaxis may be recommended for household or sexual contacts of people with HAV or HBV and other people who are known to have been exposed to these viruses. It is not necessary if the exposed person has been vaccinated and is known to be immune.

Hepatitis A prophylaxis is provided by a single dose of immune globulin (IG) given within two weeks after exposure. IG is recommended for all people with household or sexual contact with a person known to be infected with hepatitis A.

Hepatitis B postexposure prophylaxis is indicated for people exposed to the hepatitis B virus. Hepatitis B immune globulin (HBIG) is given to provide for short-term immunity. HBV vaccine may be given concurrently. Candidates for postexposure prophylaxis include those with known or suspected percutaneous or permucosal contact with infected blood, sexual partners of clients with acute HBV or who are HBV carriers, and household contacts of clients with acute HBV infection (Atkinson, et al., 2000).

Treatment

In most cases of acute viral hepatitis, pharmacologic treatment of the infection is not indicated. Acute hepatitis C may be treated with interferon alpha, an antiviral agent, to reduce the risk of chronic hepatitis C.

Interferon alpha is used to treat both chronic hepatitis B and chronic hepatitis C. Interferon alpha interferes with viral replication, reducing the viral load. It is given by intramuscular or subcutaneous injection. Virtually all clients treated with interferon alpha develop a flulike syndrome with fever, fatigue, muscle aches, headache, and chills. Acetaminophen helps alleviate some of these adverse effects. Depression also is a common adverse effect of this drug.

An alternate drug for treating chronic hepatitis B is lamivudine (Epivir HBV), an antiviral drug that can reduce liver inflammation and fibrosis. Although it has minimal side effects, clients may become resistant to the beneficial effects of lamivudine.

The treatment of choice for chronic hepatitis C is combination therapy of interferon alpha with ribavirin (Rebetol), an oral antiviral drug. This combination therapy improves the response rate over either drug used alone. Ribavirin has two major adverse effects: hemolytic anemia and birth defects. Blood counts are obtained before and during treatment to detect early signs of hemolytic anemia. Because of the risk for birth defects, this drug is contraindicated for use during pregnancy, and two reliable methods of birth control must be used by women taking the drug and female sexual partners of men taking the drug.

Treatments

Treatment of acute hepatitis also includes as-needed bed rest, adequate nutrition as tolerated, and avoidance of strenuous activity, alcohol, and agents that are toxic to the liver. In most cases, clinical recovery takes 3 to 16 weeks.

Complementary Therapies

Milk thistle, with its active ingredient silymarin, has been used by herbalists to treat liver disease for over 2000 years. Clinical studies have demonstrated that treatment with silymarin promotes recovery and reduces complications in clients with viral hepatitis. It is also beneficial for clients who have liver damage due to toxins, cirrhosis, and alcoholic liver disease. Silymarin's beneficial effects are attributed to its ability to promote liver cell growth, block toxins from entering and damaging liver cells, and reduce liver inflammation. It also is a powerful antioxidant.

Herbalists may also use licorice root to treat hepatitis. It has both antiviral and anti-inflammatory effects. Long-term use of licorice root, however, can lead to hypertension and affect fluid and electrolyte balance.

Herbal preparations may also be used to relieve the adverse effects of interferon alpha. Ginger can help relieve nausea, and St. John's wort is used for the depression associated with interferon alpha.

Nursing Care

Health Promotion

Nurses play an instrumental role in preventing the spread of hepatitis. Stress the importance of hygiene measures, such as handwashing after toileting and before all food handling. Discuss the dangers of injection drug use, and, with drug users, of sharing needles or other equipment. Encourage all sexually active clients to use safer sexual practices, such as abstinence, mutual monogamy, and barrier protection (e.g., male or female condoms).

Discuss recommendations for hepatitis A and hepatitis B vaccine with people in high or moderate risk groups for these infections. Encourage all people with known or probable exposure to HAV or HBV to obtain postexposure prophylaxis.

Assessment

Collect assessment data related to hepatitis, such as the following:

- *Health history:* current manifestations, including anorexia, nausea, vomiting, abdominal discomfort, changes in bowel elimination or color of stools; muscle or joint pain, fatigue; changes in color of skin or sclera; duration of symptoms; known exposure to hepatitis; high-risk behaviors, such as injection drug use or multiple sexual partners; previous history of liver disorders; current medications, prescription and over the counter.

- *Physical assessment:* vital signs including temperature; color of sclera and mucous membranes; skin color and condition; abdominal contour and tenderness; color of stool and urine.

Nursing Diagnoses and Interventions

Clients with acute or chronic hepatitis usually are treated in community settings; rarely is hospitalization required. Nursing care focuses on preventing spread of the infection to others and promoting the client's comfort and ability to provide self-care.

Risk for Infection (Transmission)

An important goal when caring for clients with acute viral hepatitis is preventing spread of the infection.

- Use standard precautions. Practice meticulous handwashing. *The hepatitis viruses are spread by direct contact with feces or blood and body fluids. Standard precautions and good handwashing protect both health care workers and other clients from exposure to the virus.*

- For clients with HAV or HEV, use standard precautions and contact isolation if fecal incontinence is present. *The fecal–oral route is the primary mode of transmission of these viruses. Other hepatitis viruses are transmitted through blood and other body fluids.*

- Encourage prophylactic treatment of all members of household and intimate sexual contacts. *Prophylactic treatment of people in close contact with the client decreases their risk of contacting the disease, or if already infected, the severity of the disease.*

Fatigue

Fatigue, and possible weakness, is common in acute hepatitis. Although bed rest is rarely indicated, adequate rest periods and limitation of activities may be necessary. Many clients with acute hepatitis may be unable to resume normal activity levels for four or more weeks.

- Encourage planned rest periods throughout the day. *Adequate rest is necessary for optimal immune function.*
- Assist to identify essential activities and those that can be deferred or delegated to others. *Identifying essential and nonessential activities promotes the client's sense of control.*
- Suggest using level of fatigue to determine activity level, with gradual resumption of activities as fatigue and sense of well-being improves. *Fatigue associated with activity is an indicator of appropriate and inappropriate activity levels. As recovery progresses, increasing activity levels are tolerated with less fatigue.*

Imbalanced Nutrition: Less Than Body Requirements

Adequate nutrition is important for immune function and healing in clients with acute or chronic hepatitis.

- Help plan a diet of appealing foods that provides a high kilocaloric intake of approximately 16 carbohydrate kilocalories per kilogram of ideal body weight. *Sufficient energy is required for healing; adequate carbohydrate intake can spare protein.*
- Encourage planning food intake according to symptoms of the disease. Discuss eating smaller meals and using between-meal snacks to maintain nutrient and calorie intake. *Clients with acute hepatitis often are more anorexic and nauseated in the afternoon and evening; planning the majority of calorie intake in the morning helps maintain adequate intake. Limiting fat intake and the size of meals may reduce the incidence of nausea.*
- Instruct client to avoid alcohol intake and diet drinks. *Alcohol avoidance is vital to prevent further liver damage and promote healing. Diet drinks (e.g. diet sodas or juice drinks) provide few calories when an increased calorie intake is needed for healing.*
- Encourage use of nutritional supplements such as Ensure or Instant Breakfast drinks, to maintain calorie and nutrient intake. *Nutritional supplement drinks are an additional source of concentrated calories and nutrients.*

Disturbed Body Image

Jaundice and associated rashes and itching can affect the client's body image. Nursing measures to prevent skin breakdown and address body image are discussed in the following section on cirrhosis.

Home Care

Provide discharge teaching to clients and their families for home care. Include the following topics:

- Recommended prophylactic treatment
- Infection control measures, such as frequent handwashing, not sharing eating utensils, avoiding food handling or preparation activities by the client with hepatitis A; abstaining from sexual relations during acute infection and using barrier protection if a carrier or for chronic infection.
- Managing fatigue and limited activity

- Promoting nutrient intake
- Avoiding hepatic toxins, such as alcohol, acetaminophen, and selected other drugs; encourage to alert all care providers to presence of infection
- Recommended follow-up.

If chronic hepatitis B or C is being treated with medications, teach the client how to administer the drug, its dosing schedule, precautions, and management of adverse effects. Stress the importance of keeping follow-up appointments, including recommended laboratory testing.

The Client with Liver Trauma

Blunt or penetrating trauma to the abdomen can damage the liver. Liver trauma is frequently seen in combination with injuries to other abdominal organs. Motor vehicle crashes, stab or gunshot wounds, and iatrogenic sources, such as liver biopsy, are among the causes of these injuries.

Pathophysiology

Liver trauma generally causes bleeding due to the vascularity of the organ. Liver injury may cause a surface hematoma, hematoma within the liver parenchyma, laceration of liver tissue, or disruption of vessels leading to or from the liver. Severe bleeding can rapidly disrupt hemodynamic stability and lead to shock.

Collaborative Care

Diagnostic peritoneal lavage is often used along with CT scan to diagnose liver trauma. The procedure is performed by making a small abdominal incision into the peritoneum (after the bladder has been emptied), and inserting a small catheter into the peritoneal cavity. If blood is immediately detected, the client is taken directly to surgery for abdominal exploration. If frank bleeding is not apparent, a liter of isotonic fluid is instilled into the abdomen, then drained and sent for laboratory analysis.

Intravenous fluids, fresh frozen plasma, platelets, and other clotting factors are administered to restore blood volume and promote hemostasis. Hemodynamic status is closely monitored; continued instability may indicate a need for surgical intervention to control hemorrhage. Postoperative nursing care focuses on preventing pulmonary complications, such as atelectasis, and detecting and preventing infection.

Nursing Care

Nursing care of the client with liver trauma focuses on fluid management and other supportive care related to shock. Keeping family members informed is an important aspect of care, especially during the period of client instability. Diagnoses include the following:

- *Deficient fluid volume* related to hemorrhage
- *Risk for infection* related to wound or abdominal contamination
- *Ineffective protection* related to impaired coagulation.

The Client with Liver Abscess

Liver abscesses usually are bacterial or amebic (protozoal) in origin. Bacterial abscesses may follow trauma or surgical procedures, including biopsy. Multiple or single abscesses occur most commonly in the right lobe. Amebic abscesses most frequently occur following infestation of the liver by *Entamoeba histolytica*. Amebic infestation is associated with poor hygiene, unsafe sexual practices, or travel in areas where drinking water is contaminated.

Pathophysiology

Following bacterial or amebic invasion of the liver, healthy tissue is destroyed, leaving an area of necrosis, inflammatory exudate, and blood. This damaged region becomes walled off from the healthy liver tissue. Pyogenic (bacterial) liver abscess may be caused by cholangitis, or distant or intra-abdominal infections, such as peritonitis or diverticulitis. *Escherichia coli* is the most frequently identified causative organism. The onset of pyogenic abscess is usually sudden, causing acute symptoms, such as fever, malaise, vomiting, hyperbilirubinemia, and pain in the right upper abdomen.

The infection pathway for amebic hepatic abscesses is usually the portal venous circulation from the right colon. Generally, the onset of amebic abscess is insidious.

Collaborative Care

Hepatic abscess is diagnosed through biopsy, hepatic aspirate, blood and fecal cultures, and CT scan and ultrasound studies. Therapy is based on identifying the causative organism through laboratory cultures. Pyogenic abscesses are treated with antibiotics to which the causitive organism is sensitive.

Pharmacologic agents used for amebic hepatic abscess are the same as those used for intestinal amebic infestation (see Chapter 21); combination therapy is commonly used. Two commonly used drugs for treating amebic liver abscesses are metronidazole (Flagyl) and iodoquinol (Diquinol). Both medications can cause gastrointestinal symptoms. Bone marrow suppression is a risk with metronidazole.

If the abscess does not respond to antibiotic therapy, percutaneous aspiration or surgical drainage may be done. In these procedures, a *percutaneous closed-catheter drain* is placed in the abscess to promote drainage of purulent material.

Nursing Care

A major aspect of nursing care is prevention; teaching clients to avoid contaminated water and foods is especially important. Nursing interventions include teaching hikers to treat water and food handlers to wash hands thoroughly.

Clients who have a liver abscess require supportive care to prevent dehydration from the accompanying fever, nausea, vomiting, and anorexia. Careful monitoring of fluid and electrolyte status is indicated, as are comfort measures for abdominal pain. Possible nursing diagnoses include the following:

- *Risk for deficient fluid volume,* related to effects of prolonged fever and vomiting
- *Deficient knowledge* about transmission of amebic abscess
- *Activity intolerance,* related to pain and weakness.

Exocrine Pancreas Disorders

The pancreas is both an exocrine and an endocrine gland. It is made up of two basic cell types, each having different functions. The exocrine cells produce enzymes that empty through ducts into the small intestine, whereas the endocrine cells produce hormones that enter the bloodstream directly. Disorders of the exocrine pancreas affect the secretion and glandular control of digestive enzymes, whereas disorders of the endocrine pancreas affect the production of hormones necessary for normal carbohydrate, protein, and fat metabolism. Disorders of the exocrine pancreas are discussed in this section of the chapter; diabetes mellitus, a disorder of the endocrine pancreas, is discussed in Chapter 27.

The Client with Pancreatitis

Pancreatitis, or inflammation of the pancreas, is characterized by release of pancreatic enzymes into the tissue of the pancreas itself, leading to hemorrhage and necrosis. Pancreatitis may be either acute or chronic. About 5000 new cases of acute pancreatitis are diagnosed every year in the United States. It is a serious disease, with a mortality rate of approximately 10% (Braunwald, et al., 2001). Alcoholism and gallstones are the primary risk factors for acute pancreatitis.

The incidence of chronic pancreatitis is less clear, because many people with chronic pancreatitis do not have classic manifestations of the disease. Clients with pancreatitis may have long-term effects of the disease, with chronic changes in enzyme and hormone production.

Physiology Review

Knowledge of the normal structure and functions of the exocrine pancreas is important to understand how inflammation affects it and the client. The exocrine pancreas consists of lobules of acinar cells. The acinar cells secrete digestive enzymes and fluids (pancreatic juices) into ducts that empty into the main pancreatic duct (the duct of Wirsung). The pancreatic duct joins the common bile duct and empties into the duodenum through the ampulla of Vater (in some people the main pancreatic duct empties directly into the duodenum). The epithelial lining of the pancreatic ducts secretes water and bicarbonate to modify the composition of the pancreatic secretions. Pancreatic enzymes are secreted primarily in an inactive form and are activated in the intestine, a modification that prevents digestion of pancreatic tissue by its own enzymes (Porth, 2002). The pancreatic enzymes, with related functions, are as follows:

- Proteolytic enzymes, including trypsin, chymotrypsin, carboxypolypeptidase, ribonuclease, and deoxyribonuclease, which break down dietary proteins
- Pancreatic amylase, which breaks down starch
- Lipase, which breaks down fats into glycerol and fatty acids.

Pathophysiology

Acute Pancreatitis

Acute pancreatitis is an inflammatory disorder that involves self-destruction of the pancreas by its own enzymes through autodigestion. The milder form of acute pancreatitis, *interstitial edematous pancreatitis,* leads to inflammation and edema of pancreatic tissue. It often is self-limiting. The more severe form, *necrotizing pancreatitis,* is characterized by inflammation, hemorrhage, and ultimately necrosis of pancreatic tissue. Acute pancreatitis is more common in middle adults; its incidence is higher in men than in women. Acute pancreatitis is usually associated with gallstones in women and with alcoholism in men. Some clients recover completely, others experience recurring attacks, and still others develop chronic pancreatitis. The mortality and symptoms depend on the severity and type of pancreatitis: With mild pancreatic edema, mortality is low (6%); with severe necrotic pancreatitis, the mortality rate is high (23%) (Porth, 2002).

Although the exact cause of pancreatitis is not known, the following factors may activate pancreatic enzymes within the pancreas, leading to autodigestion, inflammation, edema, and/or necrosis.

- Gallstones may obstruct the pancreatic duct or cause bile reflux, activating pancreatic enzymes in the pancreatic duct system.
- Alcohol causes duodenal edema, and may increase pressure and spasm in the sphincter of Oddi, obstructing pancreatic outflow. It also stimulates pancreatic enzyme production, thus raising pressure within the pancreas.

Other factors associated with acute pancreatitis include tissue ischemia or anoxia, trauma or surgery, pancreatic tumors, third-trimester pregnancy, infectious agents (viral, bacterial, or parasitic), elevated calcium levels, and hyperlipidemia. Some medications have been linked with this disorder, including thiazide diuretics, estrogen, steroids, salicylates, and nonsteroidal anti-inflammatory drugs (NSAIDs). Regardless of the precipitating factor, the pathophysiologic process begins with the release of activated pancreatic enzymes into pancreatic tissue. Activated proteolytic enzymes, trypsin in particular, digest pancreatic tissue and activate other enzymes, such as phospholipase A, which digests cell membrane phospholipids, and elastase, which digests the elastic tissue of blood vessel walls. This leads to proteolysis, edema, vascular damage and hemorrhage, and necrosis of parenchymal cells. Cellular damage and necrosis releases activated enzymes and vasoactive substances that produce vasodilation, increase vascular permeability, and cause edema. A large volume of fluid may shift from circulating blood into the retroperitoneal space, the peripancreatic spaces, and the abdominal cavity.

Manifestations

Acute pancreatitis develops suddenly, with an abrupt onset of continuous severe epigastric and abdominal pain. This pain commonly radiates to the back and is relieved somewhat by sitting up and leaning forward. The pain often is initiated by a fatty meal or excessive alcohol intake.

Other manifestations include nausea and vomiting; abdominal distention and rigidity; decreased bowel sounds; tachycardia; hypotension; elevated temperature; and cold, clammy skin. Within 24 hours, mild jaundice may appear. Retroperitoneal bleeding may occur three to six days after the onset of acute pancreatitis; signs of bleeding include bruising in the flanks (Turner's sign) or around the umbilicus (Cullen's sign).

Complications

Systemic complications of acute pancreatitis include intravascular volume depletion with acute tubular necrosis and renal failure (see Chapter 24 for more information about acute renal failure), and acute respiratory distress syndrome (ARDS). Acute renal failure usually develops within 24 hours after the onset of acute pancreatitis. Manifestations of ARDS may be seen three to seven days after its onset, particularly in clients who have experienced severe volume depletion. See Chapter 15 for more information about ARDS.

Localized complications include pancreatic necrosis, abscess, pseudocysts, and pancreatic ascites. Pancreatic necrosis causes an inflammatory mass which may be infected. It may lead to shock and multiple organ failure. A pancreatic abscess may form late in the course of the disease (6 or more weeks after its onset), causing an epigastric mass and tenderness (Tierney, et al., 2001). Pancreatic pseudocysts, encapsulated collections of fluid, may develop both within the pancreas itself and in the abdominal cavity. They may impinge on other structures, or may rupture, causing generalized peritonitis. Rupture of a pseudocyst or of the pancreatic duct can lead to pancreatic ascites. Pancreatic ascites is recognized by gradually increasing abdominal girth and persistent elevation of the serum amylase level without abdominal pain.

Chronic Pancreatitis

Chronic pancreatitis is characterized by gradual destruction of functional pancreatic tissue. In contrast to acute pancreatitis, which may completely resolve with no long-term effects, chronic pancreatitis is an irreversible process that eventually leads to pancreatic insufficiency. Alcoholism is the primary risk factor for chronic pancreatitis in the United States. Malnutrition is a major worldwide risk factor. About 10% to 20% of chronic pancreatitis is idiopathic, with no identified cause. A genetic mutation on a gene associated with cystic fibrosis may play a role in these cases. Children or young adults with cystic fibrosis may develop chronic pancreatitis as well.

In chronic pancreatitis related to alcoholism, pancreatic secretions have an increased concentration of insoluble proteins. These proteins calcify, forming plugs that block pancreatic ducts and the flow of pancreatic juices. This blockage leads to inflammation and fibrosis of pancreatic tissue. In other cases, a stricture or stone may block pancreatic outflow, causing chronic obstructive pancreatitis. In chronic pancreatitis, recurrent episodes of inflammation eventually lead to fibrotic changes in the parenchyma of the pancreas, with loss of exocrine function. This leads to malabsorption from pancreatic insufficiency. If endocrine function is disrupted as well, clinical diabetes mellitus may develop.

Manifestations and Complications

Chronic pancreatitis typically causes recurrent episodes of epigastric and left upper abdominal pain that radiates to the back. This pain may last for days to weeks. As the disease progresses, the interval between episodes of pain becomes shorter. Other manifestations include anorexia, nausea and vomiting, weight loss, flatulence, constipation, and **steatorrhea** (fatty, frothy, foul-smelling stools caused by a decrease in pancreatic enzyme secretion).

Complications of chronic pancreatitis include malabsorption, malnutrition, and possible peptic ulcer disease. Pancreatic pseudocyst or abscess may form, or stricture of the common bile duct may develop. Diabetes mellitus may develop, and there is an increased risk for pancreatic cancer. Narcotic addiction related to frequent, severe pain episodes is common.

Collaborative Care

Acute pancreatitis often is a mild, self-limiting disease. Treatment focuses on reducing pancreatic secretions and providing supportive care. Treatment to eliminate the causative factor is begun after the acute inflammatory process resolves. Severe necrotizing pancreatitis may require intensive care management. Treatment for chronic pancreatitis often focuses on managing pain and treating malabsorption and malnutrition.

Diagnostic Tests

The laboratory tests that may be ordered when pancreatitis is suspected are summarized in Table 19-4. Diagnostic studies include the following:

- *Ultrasonography* can identify gallstones, a pancreatic mass, or pseudocyst.
- *Computed tomography (CT) scan* may be ordered to identify pancreatic enlargement, fluid collections in or around the pancreas, and perfusion deficits in areas of necrosis.
- *Endoscopic retrograde cholangiopancreatography (ERCP)* may be performed to diagnose chronic pancreatitis and to differentiate inflammation and fibrosis from carcinoma.
- *Endoscopic ultrasonography* can detect changes indicative of chronic pancreatitis in the pancreatic duct and parenchyma.
- **Percutaneous fine-needle aspiration biopsy** may be performed to differentiate chronic pancreatitis from cancer of the pancreas; the cells that are aspirated are examined for malignancy.

Medications

The treatment of acute pancreatitis is largely supportive. Narcotic analgesics such as morphine sulfate are used to control pain. Antibiotics often are prescribed to prevent or treat infection.

Clients with chronic pancreatitis also require analgesics, but are closely monitored to prevent drug dependence. Narcotics are avoided when possible. Pancreatic enzyme supplements are given to reduce steatorrhea. H_2 blockers such as cimetidine (Tagamet) and ranitidine (Zantac), and proton-pump inhibitors, such as omeprazole (Prilosec), may be given to neutralize or decrease gastric secretions. Octreotide (Sandostatin), a synthetic hormone, suppresses pancreatic enzyme secretion and may be used to relieve pain in chronic pancreatitis.

Fluid and Dietary Management

Oral food and fluids are withheld during acute episodes of pancreatitis to reduce pancreatic secretions and promote rest of the organ. A nasogastric tube may be inserted and connected to suction. Intravenous fluids are administered to maintain vascular volume, and total parenteral nutrition (TPN) is initiated. Oral food and fluids are begun once the serum amylase levels have returned to normal, bowel sounds are present, and pain disappears. A low-fat diet is ordered, and alcohol intake is strictly prohibited.

Table 19-4.   *Laboratory Tests in Exocrine Pancreatic Disorders*

Test	Normal Value	Significance
Serum amylase	25 to 125 U/L	Rises within 2 to 12 hours of onset of acute pancreatitis to 2 to 3 times normal. Returns to normal in 3 to 4 days.
Serum lipase	<200 U/L	Levels rise in acute pancreatitis; remains elevated for 7 to 14 days.
Serum trypsinogen	<80 µg/L	Elevated in acute pancreatitis; may be decreased in chronic pancreatitis.
Urine amylase	4 to 37 U/L/2h	Urine amylase levels rise in acute pancreatitis.
Serum glucose	70 to 110 mg/dL	May be transient elevation in acute pancreatitis.
Serum bilirubin	0.1 to 1.0 mg/dL	Compression of the common duct may increase bilirubin levels in acute pancreatitis.
Serum alkaline phosphatase	30 to 95 U/L	Compression of the common duct may increase levels in acute pancreatitis.
Serum calcium	8.9 to 10.3 mg/dL or 4.5 to 5.5 mEq/L	Hypocalcemia develops in up to 25% of clients with acute pancreatitis.
White blood cells	4500/mm³ to 10,000/mm³	Leukocytosis indicates inflammation and is usually present in acute pancreatitis.

Surgery

If the pancreatitis is the result of a gallstone lodged in the sphincter of Oddi, an *endoscopic transduodenal sphincterotomy* may be performed to remove the stone. When cholelithiasis is identified as a causative factor, a cholecystectomy is performed once the acute pancreatitis has resolved. Surgical procedures to promote drainage of pancreatic enzymes into the duodenum or resection of all or part of the pancreas may be done to provide pain relief in clients with chronic pancreatitis. Large pancreatic pseudocysts may be drained endoscopically or surgically.

Complementary Therapies

Several complementary therapies may be used in conjunction with traditional treatments for clients with acute or chronic pancreatitis. Fasting or use of low-salt, low-fat vegetarian diets may reduce episodes of recurrent pain. Qigong, a system of gentle exercise, meditation, and controlled breathing, is believed to balance the flow of qi (a vital life force) through the body. Qigong lowers the metabolic rate, and may reduce the stimulation of pancreatic enzyme secretion. Magnetic field therapy may also be employed for clients with pancreatitis. All complementary therapies should be prescribed by a trained and competent practitioner.

Nursing Care

Health Promotion

Teach clients who abuse alcohol about the risk for developing pancreatitis. Advise abstinence to reduce this risk, and refer to an alcohol treatment program or Alcoholics Anonymous.

Assessment

Assessment data related to acute or chronic pancreatitis include the following:

- *Health history:* current manifestations; abdominal pain (location, nature, onset and duration, identified precipitating factors); anorexia, nausea or vomiting; flatulence, diarrhea, constipation, or stool changes; recent weight loss; history of previous episodes or gallstones; alcohol use (extent and duration); current medications.
- *Physical assessment:* vital signs including orthostatic vitals and peripheral pulses; temperature; skin temperature and color, presence of any flank or periumbilical ecchymoses; abdominal assessment including bowel sounds, presence of distention, tenderness, or guarding.

Nursing Diagnoses and Interventions

Nursing care for the client with acute pancreatitis focuses on managing pain, nutrition, and maintaining fluid balance.

Pain

Obstruction of pancreatic ducts and inflammation, edema, and swelling of the pancreas caused by pancreatic autodigestion cause severe epigastric, left upper abdominal, or midscapular back pain. The pain often is accompanied by nausea and vomiting, abdominal tenderness, and muscle guarding.

- Using a standard pain scale (see Chapter 38), assess pain, including location, radiation, duration, and character. Note nonverbal cues of pain: restlessness or remaining rigidly still; tense facial features; clenched fists; rapid, shallow respirations; tachycardia; and diaphoresis. Administer analgesics on a regular schedule. *Pain assessment before and after analgesic administration measures its effectiveness. Administering analgesics on a regular schedule prevents pain from becoming established, severe, and difficult to control. Unrelieved pain has negative consequences; for example, pain, anxiety, and restlessness may increase pancreatic enzyme secretion.*
- Maintain nothing by mouth (NPO) status and nasogastric tube patency as ordered. *Gastric secretions stimulate hormones that stimulate pancreatic secretion, aggravating pain. Eliminating oral intake and maintaining gastric suction reduces gastric secretions. Nasogastric suction also decreases nausea, vomiting, and intestinal distention.*
- Maintain bed rest in a calm, quiet environment. Encourage use of nonpharmacologic pain management techniques, such as meditation and guided imagery. *Decreasing physical movement and mental stimulation decreases metabolic rate, gastrointestinal secretion, pancreatic secretions, and resulting pain. Adjunctive pain relief measures enhance the effectiveness of analgesics (see Chapter 38).*

- Assist to a comfortable position, such as a side-lying position with knees flexed and head elevated 45 degrees. *Sitting up, leaning forward, or lying in a fetal position tend to decrease pain caused by stretching of the peritoneum by edema and swelling.*

- Remind family and visitors to avoid bringing food into the client's room. *The sight or smell of food may stimulate secretory activity of the pancreas through the cephalic phase of digestion.*

Imbalanced Nutrition: Less Than Body Requirements

The effects of pancreatitis and its treatment may result in malnutrition. Inflammation increases metabolic demand and frequently causes nausea, vomiting, and diarrhea. At a time of increased metabolic demand, NPO status and gastric suction further decrease available nutrients. In the client with chronic pancreatitis, loss of digestive enzymes affects the digestion and use of nutrients.

- Monitor laboratory values: serum albumin, serum transferrin, hemoglobin, and hematocrit. *Serum albumin, serum transferrin (which transports iron in the blood), hemoglobin, and hematocrit levels are decreased in malnutrition. Decreased pancreatic enzymes affect protein catabolism and absorption; decreased transferrin affects iron absorption and transport, thereby decreasing hematocrit and hemoglobin levels.*

- Weigh daily or every other day. *Short-term weight changes (over hours to days) accurately reflect fluid balance, whereas weight changes over days to weeks reflect nutritional status.*

- Maintain stool chart; note frequency, color, odor, and consistency of stools. *Protein and fat metabolism are impaired in pancreatitis; undigested fats are excreted in the stool. Steatorrhea indicates impaired digestion and, possibly, an increase in the severity of pancreatitis.*

- Monitor bowel sounds. *The return of bowel sounds indicates return of peristalsis; nasogastric suction usually is discontinued within 24 to 48 hours thereafter.*

- Administer prescribed intravenous fluids and/or TPN. *Intravenous fluids are given to maintain hydration. TPN is used to provide fluids, electrolytes, and kilocalories when fasting is prolonged (more than two to three days).*

- Provide oral and nasal care every one to two hours. *Fasting and nasogastric suction increase the risk for mucous membrane irritation and breakdown.*

- When oral intake resumes, offer small, frequent feedings. Provide oral hygiene before and after meals. *Oral hygiene decreases oral microorganisms that can cause foul odor and taste, decreasing appetite. Small, frequent feedings reduce pancreatic enzyme secretion and are more easily digested and absorbed.*

Risk for Deficient Fluid Volume

Acute pancreatitis can lead to a fluid shift from the intravascular space into the abdominal cavity (third spacing). Third spacing of fluid may cause hypovolemic shock, affecting cardiovascular function, respiratory function, renal function, and mental status.

- Assess cardiovascular status every four hours or as indicated, including vital signs, cardiac rhythm, hemodynamic parameters (central venous and pulmonary artery pressures); peripheral pulses and capillary refill; skin color, temperature, moisture, and turgor. *These measurements are indicative of fluid volume status and are used to monitor response to treatment. Stable values are as follows: heart rate less than 100; blood pressure within 10 mmHg of baseline; central venous pressure 0 to 8 mmHg; pulmonary wedge pressure 8 to 12 mmHg; cardiac output approximately 5 L/min; and skin warm, dry, with good turgor and color. (See Chapter 40 for a full discussion of hypovolemic shock.)*

- Monitor renal function. Obtain hourly urine output; report if less than 30 mL per hour. Weigh daily. *Urine output of less than 30 mL per hour indicates decreased renal perfusion or acute renal failure, a major complication of acute pancreatitis. Weight changes are an effective indicator of fluid volume status.*

- Monitor neurologic function, including mental status, level of consciousness, and behavior. *Hypotension and hypoxemia may decrease cerebral perfusion, causing changes in mental status, decreased level of consciousness, and changes in behavior. In addition, alcohol withdrawal is a risk in the client with acute pancreatitis.*

Home Care

The client with pancreatitis is often acutely ill and, along with family members, needs information about both hospital procedures and self-care at home following discharge. During the acute stage, keep explanations brief and simple.

Prior to discharge, teach the client and family about the disease and how to prevent further attacks of inflammation. Include the following topics as appropriate:

- Alcohol can cause stones to form, blocking pancreatic ducts and the outflow of pancreatic juice. Continued alcohol intake is likely to cause further inflammation and destruction of the pancreas. Avoid alcohol entirely.

- Smoking and stress stimulate the pancreas and should be avoided.

- If pancreatic function has been severely impaired, discuss appropriate use of pancreatic enzymes, including timing, dose, potential side effects, and monitoring of effectiveness.

- A low-fat diet is recommended. Provide a list of high-fat foods to avoid. Crash dieting and binge eating should also be avoided as they may sometimes precipitate attacks. Spicy foods, coffee, tea, or colas, and gas-forming foods, stimulate gastric and pancreatic secretions and may precipitate pain. Avoid them if this occurs.

- Report symptoms of infection (fever of 102°F (38.8°C) or more, pain, rapid pulse, malaise) as a pancreatic abscess may develop after initial recovery.

Refer to a dietitian or nutritionist for diet teaching as needed. If appropriate, refer to community agencies, such as Alcoholics Anonymous, or to an alcohol treatment program. Provide referrals to community or home health agencies as needed for continued monitoring and teaching at home.

20

Assessing Clients with Bowel Elimination Disorders

After foods are eaten and broken down into usable elements, nutrients are absorbed and indigestible materials are eliminated. Bowel elimination is the end process in digestion. This chapter describes the structure and function of the large intestine, including the rectosigmoid region and the anus, as well as the assessment of bowel function. The anatomy and physiology of the small intestine are discussed more fully in Chapter 16; the information in this chapter is provided as a base for understanding health problems from altered bowel function. In addition, this chapter discusses the function of the small intestine in the absorption of digested end products. Malabsorption (impaired absorption of nutrients) is discussed fully in Chapter 21.

Review of Anatomy and Physiology

The Small Intestine

The small intestine begins at the pyloric sphincter and ends at the ileocecal junction at the entrance of the large intestine. The small intestine is about 20 feet (6 m) long, but only about 1 inch (2.5 cm) in diameter. This long tube hangs in coils in the abdominal cavity, suspended by the mesentery and surrounded by the large intestine.

The small intestine has three regions: the duodenum, the jejunum, and the ileum. The duodenum begins at the pyloric sphincter and extends around the head of the pancreas for about 10 inches (25 cm). Both pancreatic enzymes and bile from the liver enter the small intestine at the duodenum. The jejunum is the middle region of the small intestine. It extends for about 8 feet (2.4 m). The ileum, the terminal end of the small intestine, is approximately 12 feet (3.6 m) long and meets the large intestine at the ileocecal valve.

Food is chemically digested and mostly absorbed as it moves through the small intestine. Circular folds (deep folds of the mucosa and submucosa layers), villi (fingerlike projections of the mucosa cells), and microvilli (tiny projections of the mucosa cells) all increase the surface area of the small intestine to enhance absorption of food. Although up to 10 L of food, liquids, and secretions enter the gastrointestinal tract each day, most is digested and absorbed in the small intestine; less than 1 L reaches the large intestine.

Enzymes in the small intestine break down carbohydrates, proteins, lipids, and nucleic acids.

- Pancreatic amylase acts on starches, converting them to maltose, dextrins, and oligosaccharides; the intestinal enzymes dextrinase, glucoamylase, maltase, sucrase, and lactase further break down these products into monosaccharides.
- Proteins are broken down into peptides by the pancreatic enzymes trypsin and chymotrypsin and by intestinal enzymes. Pancreatic enzymes (trypsin and chymotrypsin) and intestinal enzymes continue to break down proteins into peptides.
- Pancreatic lipases break down lipids in the small intestine.
- Triglycerides enter as fat globules, and are then coated by bile salts and emulsified.
- Nucleic acids are hydrolyzed by pancreatic enzymes, then broken apart by intestinal enzymes.

Both pancreatic enzymes and bile are excreted into the duodenum in response to the secretion of secretin and cholecystokinin, hormones produced by the intestinal mucosa cells when chyme enters the small intestine.

Nutrients are absorbed through the mucosa of the intestinal villi into the blood or lymph by active transport, facilitated transport, and passive diffusion. Almost all food products and water, as well as vitamins and most electrolytes, are absorbed in the small intestine, leaving only indigestible fibers, some water, and bacteria to enter the large intestine.

The Large Intestine

The large intestine, or colon, begins at the ileocecal valve and terminates at the anus. It is about 5 feet (1.5 m) long. The large intestine frames the small intestine on three sides and includes the cecum, the appendix, the colon, the rectum, and the anal canal.

The first section of the large intestine is the cecum. The appendix is attached to its surface as an extension. The appendix, a twisted structure in which bacteria can accumulate, may become inflamed.

The colon is divided into ascending, transverse, and descending segments. The ascending colon extends along the right side of the abdomen to the hepatic flexure, where it makes a right-angle turn. The next segment, called the transverse colon, crosses the abdomen to the splenic flexure. At this juncture, the descending colon descends down the left side of the abdomen and ends at the S-shaped sigmoid colon. The sigmoid colon terminates at the rectum.

The rectum is a mucosa-lined tube approximately 12 cm in length. The rectum has three transverse folds (*valves of Houston*) that retain feces yet allow flatus to be passed through the anus. The rectum ends at the anal canal, which terminates at the anus.

The anus, a hairless, dark-skinned area, is the end of the digestive tract. It has both an internal involuntary sphincter and an external voluntary sphincter. The sphincters are usually open only during defecation. The anorectal junction separates the rectum from the anal canal and may be the site of internal hemorrhoids (clusters of dilated veins in swollen anal tissue).

The major function of the large intestine is to eliminate indigestible food residue from the body. The large intestine absorbs water, salts, and vitamins formed by the food residue and bacteria. The semiliquid chyme that passes through the ileocecal valve is formed into feces as it moves through the large intestine. Feces are moved along the intestine by peristalsis, waves of alternating contraction and relaxation. Goblet cells lining the large intestine secrete mucus that facilitates the lubrication and passage of feces.

The defecation reflex is initiated when feces enter the rectum and stretch the rectal wall. This spinal cord reflex causes the walls of the sigmoid colon to contract and the anal sphincters to relax. This reflex can be suppressed by voluntary control of the external sphincter. Closing the glottis and contracting the diaphragm and abdominal muscles to increase intra-abdominal pressure facilitates expulsion of feces; this movement is called *Valsalva's maneuver*. Prolonged suppression of defecation can result in a weakened reflex that may, in turn, lead to *constipation* (infrequent and often uncomfortable passage of hard, dry stool). Frequent bouts of constipation may lead to external hemorrhoids at the area of the external hemorrhoidal plexus.

Assessing Bowel Function

The nurse conducts both a health assessment interview (to collect subjective data) and a physical assessment (to collect objective data).

Health Assessment Interview

This section provides guidelines for collecting subjective data through a health assessment interview specific to bowel function. Problems with bowel elimination may be assessed as part of a health screening, may focus on a chief complaint, such as abdominal pain or change in bowel patterns, or may be part of a total health assessment. The assessment of bowel sounds is a common part of routine assessments.

Clients may feel embarrassed and hesitant to provide information about bowel elimination patterns. To promote effective rapport, remain nonjudgmental and ask for less personal information first.

If the client has a health problem involving bowel function, analyze its onset, characteristics and course, severity, precipitating and relieving factors, and any associated symptoms, noting the timing and circumstances. For example, ask the client:

- Can you describe the type of cramping and abdominal pain you are experiencing?
- Have you ever had bleeding from your rectum?
- Have you noticed increased constipation since your surgery?

Begin the interview by inquiring about any medical conditions that may influence the client's bowel elimination pattern, such as a stroke or spinal cord impairment, inflammatory gastrointestinal diseases, endocrine disorders, and allergies. Note any recent travel to other countries. Information about the client's psychosocial history is also important. Assess the client's lifestyle for any patterns of psychologic stress and/or depression, which may alter bowel elimination patterns. Depression may be associated with constipation, whereas *diarrhea* (frequent passage of loose, watery stools) may occur in situations of high stress and anxiety. Explore the client's activities of daily living, including exercise, sleep-rest patterns, and dietary and fluid intake. Changes in activities of daily living can influence bowel elimination patterns.

Determine whether the client has had any lower abdominal pain or rectal pain, which may be associated with a distended colon filled with gas or fluid. Crampy, colicky pains occur with diarrhea and/or constipation. Sudden onset of lower abdominal cramping occurs in obstruction of the colon. Left lower abdominal pain is associated with diverticulitis. Rectal pain may occur with stool retention and/or hemorrhoids.

Ask the client to describe the frequency and character of the stools. Ask about any history of diarrhea, constipation, or bleeding from the rectum, and collect information about the use of laxatives, suppositories, or enemas. Anticholinergic drugs, antihistamines, tranquilizers, or narcotics may cause constipation.

If the client has an **ostomy** (surgical opening into the bowel), ask about skin care problems, consistency of stool, foods that cause problems, the number of times that the client empties the appliance bag each day, and irrigation habits. Finally, explore the client's feelings about the appliance.

To obtain information about the client's nutritional status, ask about changes in weight, appetite, food preferences, food intolerances, special diets, and any cultural or ethnic influences on dietary intake. Ask whether the client is experiencing nausea and vomiting; if so, determine any relation to food intake, and ask the client to describe character of the emesis. In addition, ask about indigestion, the use of antacids or other over-the-counter medications, herbal preparations, and episodes of diarrhea and its character.

Explore any family history of colon cancer, colitis, gallbladder disease, or malabsorption syndromes, such as lactose intolerance and celiac sprue. Assess the client's risk factors for cancer, including age greater than 50; family member with colon cancer; history of endometrial, ovarian, or breast cancer; and previous diagnoses of colon inflammation, polyps, or cancer.

Physical Assessment

The function of the bowels is assessed through a rectal examination, an anal examination, and examination of the client's stool. A complete assessment also includes inspection of the abdomen and auscultation of bowel sounds. Guidelines for abdominal assessment and assessment of bowel sounds are outlined in Chapter 16.

Physical assessment of the abdomen may be performed as part of a total health assessment, in combination with assessment of the urinary and reproductive systems (problems which may cause clinical manifestations similar to those of the gastrointestinal system), or alone for clients with known or suspected health problems. The techniques of inspection, auscultation, percussion, and palpation are used. Palpation is the last method used in assessing the abdomen, because pressure on the abdominal wall and contents may interfere with bowel sounds and cause pain, ending the examination.

Necessary equipment includes water-soluble lubricant, material for testing the stool, and disposable gloves for the examiner. Ask the client to empty the bladder before the examination and lie in the supine position. Have the client turn to the left lateral (Sims') position for the rectal examination. The older client or the client with limited mobility may need assistance in assuming this position.

Explain what will happen during the examination, and encourage the client to take deep, regular breaths to increase relaxation. Explain that during the examination, it may feel as though the client is about to have a bowel movement and that sometimes flatus (gas) is passed. Assure the client that this is normal. Ensure that the examination area is private and the client is draped properly to prevent unnecessary exposure.

Abdominal Assessment with Abnormal Findings (✓)

- Inspect the abdomen.
    - ✓ Retention of flatus (gas) or stool may cause generalized abdominal distention.
    - ✓ Malnutrition causes a scaphoid (concave) abdomen.
- Auscultate the four quadrants of the abdomen with the diaphragm of the stethoscope. Begin in the lower right quadrant, where bowel sounds are almost always present. Normal bowel sounds (gurgling or clicking) occur every 5 to 15 seconds. Listen for at least five minutes in each of the four quadrants to confirm the absence of bowel sounds.
    - ✓ High-pitched, tinkling, rushing, or growling bowel sounds may be heard in the client who has diarrhea or who is experiencing the onset of a bowel obstruction.
    - ✓ Bowel sounds may be absent in later stages of a bowel obstruction or after surgery of the abdominal organs.

Perianal Assessment with Abnormal Findings(✓)

- Inspect the perianal area. Wearing gloves, spread the client's buttocks apart. Observe the area, and ask client to bear down as if they were trying to have a bowel movement.
    - ✓ Swollen, painful, longitudinal breaks in the anal area may appear in clients with anal fissures. (These are caused by the passing of large, hard stools, or by diarrhea.)
    - ✓ Dilated anal veins appear with hemorrhoids.
    - ✓ A red mass may appear with prolapsed internal hemorrhoids.
    - ✓ Doughnut-shaped red tissue at the anal area may appear with a prolapsed rectum.
- Palpate the anus and rectum. Lubricate the gloved index finger and ask the client to bear down. Touch the tip of your finger to the client's anal opening. Flex the index finger, and slowly insert it into the anus, pointing the finger towards the umbilicus. Rotate the finger in both directions to palpate any lesions or masses.
    - ✓ Movable, soft masses may be polyps.
    - ✓ Hard, firm, irregular embedded masses may indicate carcinoma.

Fecal Assessment with Abnormal Findings (✓)

- Inspect the client's feces. After palpating the rectum, withdraw your finger gently. Inspect any feces on the glove. Note color and/or presence of blood. Also use gloved fingers to note consistency.
- Test the feces for occult blood. Use a commercial testing kit.
    - ✓ A positive occult blood test requires further testing for colon cancer or gastrointestinal bleeding due to peptic ulcers, ulcerative colitis, or diverticulosis.
- Note the odor of the feces.
    - ✓ Distinctly foul odors may be noted with stools containing blood or extra fat or in cases of colon cancer.

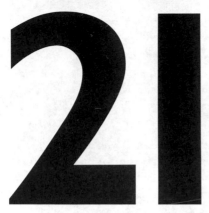

Nursing Care of Clients with Bowel Disorders

Disorders of intestinal absorption and bowel elimination can affect health, comfort, and well-being. Bowel function can be affected by inflammations, infections, tumors, obstructions, or changes in structure.

Clients with intestinal disorders often face extensive diagnostic testing, surgery, and permanent changes in physical appearance and lifestyle. Nursing care is directed toward meeting the client's physiologic needs, providing emotional support, and educating the client to adapt to changes in lifestyle.

Disorders of Intestinal Motility

Few body functions respond as readily to internal and external influences as the process of defecation. Factors affecting the gastrointestinal (GI) tract directly, such as food intake and bacterial population, affect the number and consistency of stools. Indirect factors, such as psychologic stress or voluntary postponement of defecation, also affect elimination.

In modern society, "normal" bowel elimination patterns vary widely. For some clients, two to three stools per day is the usual pattern. Others may normally have as few as three stools per week. It is important to evaluate each client's elimination pattern against his or her own normal pattern.

The Client with Diarrhea

Diarrhea is an increase in the frequency, volume, and fluid content of the stool. In diarrhea, the water content of feces is increased, usually due to either malabsorption or water secretion in the bowel. It is a symptom rather than a primary disorder.

Diarrhea may be acute or chronic. Acute diarrhea, which usually lasts less than a week, is usually due to an infectious agent. Chronic diarrhea (diarrhea that persists longer than three to four weeks) may be caused by inflammatory bowel disorders, malabsorption, or even endocrine disorders.

Pathophysiology

About 1500 mL of digested material enters the large intestine daily. Most of the water and some of the solutes are reabsorbed in the bowel, leaving only about 200 mL of feces to be eliminated.

Large volume diarrhea, characterized by both increased numbers and volume of stools, is caused by increased water content of the stool. This increased water content may result from either osmotic or secretory processes. Water may be pulled into the bowel lumen by osmosis when the feces contains osmotically active molecules. Some stool softeners and laxatives work on this principle. When the lactose in milk is not broken down and absorbed, the lactose molecules exert an osmotic draw, causing diarrhea. The diarrhea associated with cholera and *Escherichia coli* infection is caused by increased water secretion in the small and large intestines. Unabsorbed dietary fat, some cathartics and other drugs, and other factors can cause secretory diarrhea.

Small volume diarrhea, characterized by frequent small stools, is usually caused by inflammation or disease of the colon. Diseases that affect the intestinal mucosa, such as inflammatory bowel disease, cause an exudative diarrhea. The mucosal inflammation causes plasma, serum proteins, blood, and mucus to accumulate in the bowel, increasing fecal bulk and fluidity. An increased rate of propulsion within the bowel can also decrease the amount of water normally absorbed from the chyme, leading to diarrhea. For this reason, laxatives that increase bowel motility and bowel resection or bypass can lead to diarrhea.

Manifestations and Complications

The manifestations of diarrhea depend on its cause, duration, and severity, as well as the area of bowel affected and the client's general health. Diarrhea can present as several large, watery stools daily, or very frequent small stools that contain blood, mucus, or exudate.

Diarrhea can have devastating effects. Water and electrolytes are lost in diarrheal stool. This can lead to dehydration, particularly in the very young, the older adult, or the debilitated client unable to respond to thirst. With severe diarrhea, vascular collapse and hypovolemic shock may occur. Potassium and magnesium are lost, potentially leading to hypokalemia and hypomagnesemia. The loss of bicarbonate in the stool can lead to metabolic acidosis. See Chapter 39 for further discussion of the effects of these imbalances.

Collaborative Care

Management of diarrhea focuses on identifying and treating the underlying cause. In addition, the diarrhea itself may need to be treated to promote comfort and to prevent complications. The history (including the onset and associated circumstances of the diarrhea) and physical examination often provide enough information to identify its cause.

Diagnostic Tests

The following laboratory and diagnostic tests may be ordered to help identify the cause of diarrhea.

- *Stool specimen* is obtained for gross and microscopic examination. Gross examination includes volume and water content, and the presence of any blood, pus, mucus, or excess fat. Microscopic examination evaluates the presence of WBCs, unabsorbed fat, and parasites. WBCs in the stool may indicate a bacterial infection or mucosal ulceration. Because parasites, ova, or larvae may not be continuously present in stool, a series of three specimens, spaced 2 to 3 days apart, is obtained when parasitic infection is suspected.
- *Stool culture* is ordered when an enteric pathogen is suspected (e.g., for persistent or bloody diarrhea accompanied by fever and/or recent travel out of the country).
- *Serum electrolytes, serum osmolality,* and *arterial blood gases* may be ordered to assess for adverse effects of diarrhea. Increased serum osmolality indicates water loss and dehydration. Other potential imbalances include hypokalemia, hypomagnesemia, and metabolic acidosis as a result of diarrhea. The serum sodium may be increased or decreased, depending on the type of diarrhea.
- *Sigmoidoscopy* allows direct examination of the bowel mucosa. Stool may also be obtained during sigmoidoscopy for microscopic examination.
- *Tissue biopsy* may be performed to identify chronic inflammatory processes, infection, and other causes of diarrhea. For biopsy, a small section of tissue (which may include the mucosal and muscle layers) is removed and examined for gross microscopic and histologic (cell character) changes.

Medications

Antidiarrheal medications are used sparingly or not at all until the cause of diarrhea has been identified. In diarrhea associated with botulism or bacillary dysentery, giving an antidiarrheal agent can worsen or prolong the disease by slowing elimination of the toxin from the bowel. Once the underlying cause for diarrhea has been established, specific medications may be ordered to treat the underlying cause. Antibiotics are used with caution because they alter the normal bacterial population of the bowel and may actually worsen diarrhea. A balanced electrolyte solution may be required to replace fluid losses. Intravenous or oral potassium preparations may also be prescribed.

Opium and some of its derivatives, anticholinergics, absorbants, and demulcents are commonly used as antidiarrheal preparations. Specific preparations, their method of action, and the nursing implications for these medications are outlined in Table 21-1.

Table 21-1. Medication Administration – Antidiarrheal Preparations

---

Absorbants and Protectants

Kaolin and pectin (Kaopectate, Donnagel-MB)
Charcoal
Bismuth subsalicylate (Pepto-Bismol)

Absorbant preparations act locally in the intestines to bind substances that can cause diarrhea. Absorbants are safe and are generally available over the counter. Their efficacy has not been proved, although bismuth subsalicylate has been shown to be somewhat effective in preventing and managing traveler's diarrhea, usually related to contaminated water supplies. Bismuth salts also have a protective and antimicrobial effect.

Continued on the next page

Table 21-1. Continued

Nursing Responsibilities

- Assess for contraindications to antidiarrheal therapy, such as some infections or chronic inflammatory bowel disease, including ulcerative colitis.
- If fever is present, check with physician before giving the medication.
- Administer these medications at least one hour before or two hours after other oral medications; they may interfere with the absorption of other drugs.
- Observe the client's response to the medication. Constipation is a potential problem.

Client and Family Teaching

- Take the recommended dosage at the onset of diarrhea and after each loose stool.
- Do not take any of these preparations for more than 48 hours. If diarrhea persists, notify the physician.
- Do not give antidiarrheal medications to debilitated older clients without physician supervision.
- Chew bismuth subsalicylate tablets, rather than swallowing them whole, for maximal effectiveness. This medication may cause harmless darkening of the tongue and stool.
- If you are allergic to aspirin, use bismuth subsalicylate with caution; as a general rule, avoid taking aspirin while taking bismuth subsalicylate.

Opium and Opium Derivatives

Camphorated tincture of opium (Paregoric)
Tincture of opium (laudanum, opium tincture)
Difenoxin (Motofen)
Diphenoxylate (Lomotil, Lotrol, others)
Loperamide hydrochloride (Imodium)

Opium and its derivatives act on the central nervous system (CNS) to decrease the motility of the ileum and colon, slowing transit time and promoting more water absorption. They also decrease the sensation of a full rectum and increase anal sphincter tone. Paregoric and tincture of opium have a greater potential for abuse and are prescription drugs subject to controls under the federal Controlled Substance Act of 1970. Difenoxin, diphenoxylate, and loperamide are derivatives of opium with few analgesic, euphoric, or abuse-promoting effects and are in more common use today.

Nursing Responsibilities

- Assess for contraindications to antidiarrheal or narcotic medications prior to giving these drugs.
- Administer paregoric undiluted with water.
- Do not administer difenoxin and diphenoxylate to clients receiving monoamine oxidase inhibitors (MAOI); hypertensive crises may occur.
- Observe closely for increased effects of other CNS depressants, such as alcohol, narcotic analgesics, or barbiturate sedatives.
- Observe for abdominal distention; toxic megacolon may occur if these drugs are given to the client with ulcerative colitis.

Table 21-1. Continued

Client and Family Teaching
- Take the medication as recommended at the onset of diarrhea and after each loose stool.
- These drugs may be habit forming, use for no more than 48 hours.
- Avoid using alcohol and over-the-counter cold preparations while taking these drugs.
- These preparations may cause drowsiness, avoid driving or operating machinery while taking them.

Anticholinergics

Atropine
Belladonna alkaloids (Donnagel, Donnatal)

Anticholinergic medications reduce bowel spasticity and acid secretion in the stomach. They are used to treat diarrhea that is associated with peptic ulcer disease and irritable bowel syndrome. These are nonspecific drugs; their systemic effects are their major drawback.

Nursing Responsibilities
- Assess for contraindications to atropine and other anticholinergic medications: glaucoma, prostatic hypertrophy, and gastrointestinal or genitourinary obstruction.
- Observe for side effects, such as eye pain, impaired urination, or constipation.

Client and Family Teaching
- Take only as directed, stop the drug and notify the physician if you develop eye pain, impaired urination, constipation.
- Do not operate machinery while taking this medication; drowsiness may occur.
- Hard candies help relieve oral dryness associated with these preparations.

Dietary Management

Fluid replacement is of primary importance in managing the client with diarrhea. If the client is able to tolerate oral fluids (i.e., if the client is not experiencing nausea and vomiting), an oral glucose/balanced electrolyte solution provides the best fluid replacement. Commercial preparations, such as Gatorade and other sports drinks, are available, as are pediatric solutions (e.g., Pedialyte), which can be used for adults as well as children. A solution of 5 mL (1 teaspoon) each of table salt and baking soda and 4 teaspoons (20 mL) of granulated sugar added with desired flavoring (such as lemon extract or juice) to 1 quart (1 L) of water can be made at home to replace water and electrolytes.

Solid food is withheld in the first 24 hours of acute diarrhea to rest the bowel. After that time, frequent, small, soft feedings can be added. Milk and milk products are added last, because the lactose they contain frequently aggravates the diarrhea. Raw fruits and vegetables, fried foods, bran, whole-grain cereals, condiments, spices, coffee, and alcoholic beverages are avoided during the recovery period.

Clients with chronic diarrhea may benefit by eliminating specific foods from the diet. The diet should be high in calories and nutritional value. Vitamin supplements may be necessary, particularly the fat-soluble vitamins (A, D, E, and K). Clients with severe chronic diarrhea may require parenteral nutrition (see Chapter 17).

Complementary Therapies

Herbal or homeopathic therapies may be used to help relieve diarrhea. Herbal treatments may include a strong tea of black pepper, chamomile, coriander, rosemary, sandalwood, or thyme. Homeopathic practitioners may use podophyllum tablets to treat diarrhea (Fontaine, 2000). Refer the client to a qualified practitioner for more information about using complementary therapies to treat diarrhea.

Nursing Care

Health Promotion

Teach all clients about the importance of handwashing as a measure to prevent the spread of infectious diseases, including those that cause diarrhea. Teach safe food handling techniques to prevent bacterial contamination, and discuss measures to ensure safe drinking water. For clients planning to travel outside the United States or to wilderness areas, teach measures to purify water for drinking and cooking.

Assessment

The nursing assessment can help identify the cause of the client's diarrhea, as well as early signs of complications. Collect the following assessment data:

- *Health history:* duration and extent of diarrhea; associated symptoms; dietary intake; recent travel out of the country or to wilderness areas; previous history of diarrhea; chronic diseases; prescription and nonprescription medications.
- *Physical examination:* vital signs (including orthostatic vitals); peripheral pulses; skin temperature, moisture, turgor; color and moisture of mucous membranes; abdominal contour and girth; bowel sounds; stool for obvious or occult blood, pus, mucus, or steatorrhea (bulky, foul-smelling stool).

Nursing Diagnoses and Interventions

Nursing care of the client with diarrhea focuses on identifying the cause, relieving the symptoms, preventing complications, and preventing the potential spread of infection to others.

Diarrhea

Nursing interventions for diarrhea focus helping the client recover a normal elimination pattern without adverse consequences.

- Monitor and record the frequency and characteristics of bowel movements *to provide a measure of the effectiveness of treatment.*
- Measure abdominal girth and auscultate bowel sounds every eight hours as indicated. *Loud, rushing bowel sounds (borborygmi) indicates increased peristalsis, and may be heard in clients with acute diarrhea. Diminished or absent bowel sounds may indicate a complication of treatment, such as constipation or toxic megacolon.*
- Use standard precautions, including gloves and handwashing. *Standard precautions help prevent the spread of infection to others.*
- Provide ready access to bathroom, commode, or bedpan. *The client may have little warning of the need to defecate. Easily accessed toileting facilities reduce the risk for soiling or injury.*

- Administer antidiarrheal medications as prescribed, *to promote comfort and prevent excess fluid loss.*
- Limit food intake if the diarrhea is acute, reintroducing solid foods slowly, in small amounts, *to allow the bowel to rest and mucosa to heal in acute diarrhea states.*

Risk for Deficient Fluid Volume

The increased water content of diarrheal stool places the client at risk for fluid deficit.

- Record intake and output; weigh daily; assess skin turgor, mucous membranes, and urine specific gravity every eight hours. *These assessments help monitor fluid volume status.*
- Monitor vital signs, including orthostatic blood pressures. *Orthostatic hypotension is identified by a drop in BP of more than 10 mmHg and pulse increase of 10 BPM when changing from a lying to a sitting position or from a sitting to a standing position. It is an indicator of fluid volume deficit.*
- Provide fluid and electrolyte replacement solutions as indicated. Ensure ready access to fluids; assist the debilitated client with fluid intake. Notify the care provider if the client is unable to tolerate oral fluids. *Oral fluids are encouraged as tolerated to prevent dehydration. Intravenous fluids are necessary if oral fluids are not tolerated. An intake of 3000 mL per day or more is often needed to replace fluid losses.*

Risk for Impaired Skin Integrity

Decreased extracellular fluid volume and the irritating effects of diarrheal stool increase the risk for skin breakdown.

- Assist with cleaning the perianal area as needed. Use warm water, a gentle cleanser, and soft cloths. *Cleansing removes irritating substances in the stool. Gentle cleansing helps maintain integrity of dehydrated skin.*
- Apply protective ointment to the perianal area. *Moisture-barrier ointments or creams protect the skin from excoriation and help prevent tissue breakdown.*

Home Care

Acute and chronic diarrhea generally are managed by the client in the home. Teach the client and family members about the following subjects:

- Causes of diarrhea (as directed by the diagnosis)
- Importance of handwashing and hygiene measures
- Importance of maintaining adequate fluid intake to replace lost water and electrolytes
- Use of a balanced electrolyte solution, such as Gatorade or a similar product (purchased or home prepared), for fluid replacement
- Recommendations to limit food intake during acute diarrhea, and resume gradually with small feedings of foods that have a constipating effect: applesauce, bananas, crackers, rice, potatoes
- To avoid foods high in fiber, milk products, and caffeine
- Ways to maintain nutrition if chronic diarrhea is a problem: frequent small meals, nutritional supplements, vitamin supplements
- Precautions and limitations of antidiarrheal preparations
- Importance of seeking medical intervention if diarrhea continues or recurs.

The Client with Constipation

Constipation is defined as the infrequent (two or fewer bowel movements weekly) or difficult passage of stools. Constipation affects older adults more frequently than younger people. Recent studies indicate that approximately 20% to 35% of people over age 65 report recurrent constipation and laxative use. Although fecal transit in the large intestine slows with aging, the increased incidence of constipation is thought to relate more to impaired general health status, increased medication use, and decreased physical activity in the older adult.

Pathophysiology and Manifestations

Constipation may be a primary problem or a symptom of another disease or condition. Acute constipation, a definite change in the bowel elimination pattern, often is caused by an organic process. A change in bowel patterns that persists or becomes more frequent or severe may be due to a tumor or other partial bowel obstruction. With chronic constipation, functional causes that impair storage, transport, and evacuation mechanisms impede the normal passage of stools.

Psychogenic factors are the most frequent causes of chronic constipation. These factors include postponing defecation when the urge is felt, and the perception of satisfaction with defecation. Clients often abuse the use of laxatives and enemas to stimulate a bowel movement when constipation is perceived. Overuse of these measures can lead to real intestinal problems that worsen the condition. For example, *cathartic colon,* impaired colonic motility and changes in bowel structure, mimics ulcerative colitis in that the normal pouchlike or saccular appearance of the colon is lost. *Melanosis coli* is a brownish-black discoloration of the colon mucosa. Both conditions may be caused by long-term laxative use.

With significant constipation or long-term dependence on laxatives or enemas, *fecal impaction* may develop. Impaction may also occur following barium administration for radiologic exam. The impaction is felt as a rock-hard or puttylike mass of feces in the rectum. Abdominal cramping and a full sensation in the rectal area may be manifestations of impaction. Watery mucus or liquid stool may be passed around the impaction, causing the client to complain of diarrhea.

Collaborative Care

Initial evaluation of constipation is based on the history and physical examination. The abdomen may appear somewhat distended, and bowel sounds may be reduced. If an impaction is present, digital examination of the rectum reveals a palpable hard or puttylike fecal mass.

Simple or chronic constipation is treated with education (a daily bowel movement is not necessary for health), and modification of diet and exercise routines. If the problem is acute or does not resolve, further diagnostic examination may be ordered.

Diagnostic Tests
* *Serum electrolytes* and *thyroid function tests* may be done to identify metabolic and endocrine problems that may contribute to constipation.

- *Barium enema* may be ordered to evaluate bowel structure and to identify tumors or diverticular disease. Barium is instilled into the large intestine and X-rays are taken.
- *Sigmoidoscopy* or *colonoscopy* may also be used to evaluate constipation, particularly when the problem is acute and a tumor or obstruction is suspected. A flexible endoscope is used to inspect bowel mucosa and structure. Suspicious lesions may be biopsied at the time of the scope.

Medications

Laxative and cathartic preparations to promote stool evacuation were among the earliest drugs. Milder preparations are generally known as laxatives; cathartics have a stronger effect. Most laxatives are appropriate only for short-term use. Cathartics and enemas interfere with normal bowel reflexes and should not be used for simple constipation. Laxatives should never be given if a bowel obstruction or impaction is suspected, nor to people with abdominal pain of undetermined origin (Tierney, et al., 2001). When the bowel is obstructed, laxatives or cathartics may cause serious mechanical damage and perforate the bowel.

The only laxatives that are appropriate and safe for long-term use are bulking agents, such as psyllium seed, calcium polycarbophil, and methylcellulose. These agents act by increasing the bulk of the feces and drawing water into the bowel to soften it. Commonly prescribed laxatives and cathartics are discussed in Table 21-2.

Table 21-2. Medication Administration – Laxatives and Cathartics

Bulk-Forming Agents

Bran
Calcium polycarbophil (Fibercon)
Methylcellulose (Citrucel)
Psyllium hydrophilic mucilloid (Metamucil, Effer-Syllium)

Bulk-forming agents are the only safe laxatives for long-term use. They contain vegetable fiber, which is not digested or absorbed in the gut. This natural fiber creates bulk and draws water into the intestine, softening the stool mass.

Nursing Responsibilities
- Mix the agent with a full glass of cool liquid just prior to administering.
- Do not administer to clients with possible stool impaction or bowel obstruction.

Client and Family Teaching
- Drink at least six to eight full glasses of nonalcoholic fluid per day. Adequate hydration is necessary to produce the drugs laxative effect.
- These agents may be mixed with water, milk, or fruit juice.
- Take the drug in the morning or with meals. To reduce the risk of impaction, do not take at bedtime.
- Because of the increased risk of impaction, check with the physician before increasing dietary fiber while you are taking these agents.

Continued on the next page

Table 21-2. Continued

Wetting Agents

Docusate (Colace, Surfak, Doxidan, others)

Wetting agents reduce stool surface tension and form an emulsion of fat and water, softening the stool. They are used primarily to prevent straining and reduce the discomfort of expelling hard stools.

Nursing Responsibilities
- Administer with ample fluids to promote softening effect.
- Wetting agents may alter the absorption of other drugs. Do not administer within one hour of other oral medications.
- Do not attempt to crush or open caplets; a liquid form is available for clients who cannot swallow pills or capsules.

Client and Family Teaching
- Do not use for more than one week or less unless specifically recommended by the physician.
- Take the medication in the morning or evening, but avoid taking it with other medications.
- Adequate fluid is necessary to obtain the beneficial effect of the drug. Drink six to eight glasses of nonalcoholic fluid per day.

Osmotic and Saline Laxatives/Cathartics

Lactulose (Rhodialose)
Sorbitol
Magnesium hydroxide (Milk of Magnesia)
Magnesium citrate
Polyethylene glycol (Klean-Prep)

Laxatives in this group contain poorly absorbed salts or carbohydrates that remain in the bowel, increasing osmotic pressure and drawing water into the intestine. Stool volume increases, consistency decreases, and peristalsis is stimulated. Many of these agents also have an irritant effect on the bowel, further stimulating peristalsis. They are used to stimulate rapid or complete bowel evacuation to relieve constipation and to prepare the bowel for diagnostic and surgical procedures. They should be limited to acute, short-term use; chronic use may suppress normal bowel reflexes.

Nursing Responsibilities
- Assess for possible contraindications to osmotic or saline laxatives, including bowel ulceration or obstruction, dehydration, electrolyte imbalances, heart failure (which may be aggravated by the sodium content), or renal failure.
- Administer with a full glass of liquid, preferably in the morning to avoid sleep disturbance.
- Monitor fluid and electrolyte status: skin turgor, mucous membranes, intake and output; daily weight, and laboratory studies, such as hemoglobin and hematocrit levels, serum osmolality and electrolytes, and urine specific gravity.

Table 21-2. Continued

Client and Family Teaching

- Do not use these agents on a routine basis to treat or prevent constipation.
- Chill the solution to increase its palatability.
- Expect some abdominal cramping.
- Use only as directed. Increase fluid intake to at least six to eight glasses of nonalcoholic fluid.
- Notify the physician if adverse effects occur, including abdominal pain, bloody stool, excessive skin or mucous membrane dryness, rapid weight loss, dizziness, or other unusual symptoms.
- These agents work in three to six hours; take them in the morning or early evening to avoid sleep disturbance.

Irritant or Stimulant Laxatives

Bisacodyl (Dulcolax, Bisco-Lax, Carter's Liver Pills, Codylax, others)
Phenolphthalein (Evac-U-Gen, Evac-U-Lax, Feen-A-Mint, Phenolax, others)
Cascara sagrada
Senna (Senna laxative, Fletcher's Castoria)
Castor oil

Stimulant laxatives work by stimulating the motility and secretion of intestinal mucosa. Their use results in watery stool, often accompanied by abdominal cramping and pain. They are used to relieve constipation, although they should not be used as the initial treatment. Stimulant laxatives are also used for preparing the bowel for diagnostic testing.

Nursing Responsibilities

- Assess for potential contraindications to these laxatives, including abdominal pain and cramping, nausea and vomiting, anal or rectal fissures.
- Administer on an empty stomach to minimize the effects of food on its dissolution and absorption.
- Do not crush enteric-coated bisacodyl tablets or administer with alkaline products. This may hasten their dissolution in the stomach, leading to gastric distress.

Client and Family Teaching

- Discourage the use of this type of laxative, even in overthe-counter preparations, for the initial or continuing relief of constipation.
- Do not use the laxative for more than one week; chronic use can be habit forming and may suppress normal bowel reflexes.
- These laxatives are excreted in breast milk and should not be used by lactating women.
- Phenolphthalein-containing products may discolor the urine pink or red. Report possible hypersensitivity manifestations, such as difficulty breathing, dizziness or lightheadedness, or skin rashes, to the primary care provider, and stop taking the medication.

Continued on the next page

Table 21-2. Continued

Lubricants

Mineral oil

Mineral oil is the only lubricant laxative available. It acts by forming an oily coat on the fecal mass, preventing the reabsorption of water, and resulting in softer stool. Problems associated with the use of mineral oil as a laxative include reduced absorption of the fat-soluble vitamins A, D, E, and K; possible damage to the liver and spleen due to systemic absorption, and potential pneumonitis from aspiration of oil droplets into the lungs.

Nursing Responsibilities
- Assess for possible contraindications to use of mineral oil, including advanced age, preexisting lung disease, and hemorrhoids or other rectal lesions.
- Do not give mineral oil concurrently with wetting agents or stool softeners, because these increase the potential for systemic absorption and increase the effects of the mineral oil.
- Administer mineral oil in the evening before bedtime to reduce the effect on the absorption of fat-soluble vitamins and minimize the risk of aspiration.
- Assess for manifestations of vitamin deficiency. Monitor the client taking oral anticoagulants for evidence of increased bleeding, such as bleeding gums, easy bruising, or melena.

Client and Family Teaching
- Long-term use of mineral oil is not recommended because of its risks and adverse effects.
- Do not use mineral oil if hemorrhoids or rectal lesions are present, leakage of the oil through the anal sphincter may cause itching and interfere with healing.
- Suck on a lemon or orange slice after taking oral mineral oil to reduce the oily aftertaste.

Dietary Management

Foods that have a high fiber content are recommended. Vegetable fiber is largely indigestible and unabsorbable, so it increases stool bulk. Fiber also helps draw water into the fecal mass, softening the stool and making defecation easier. Raw fruits and vegetables are good sources of dietary fiber, as is cereal bran. Use two to three teaspoons of unprocessed bran with meals (sprinkled on fruit or cereal) or up to 1/4 cup daily to supply adequate fiber.

Fluids are also important to maintain bowel motility and soft stools. The client should drink six to eight glasses of fluid per day.

In older adults, constipation may be due to inadquate food intake. Carefully evaluate diet history and usual daily intake.

Enemas
Significant or chronic constipation or a fecal impaction may require the administration of an enema. As a general rule, enemas should be used only in acute situations and only on a short-term basis. They may also be ordered to prepare the bowel for diagnostic testing or examination. The following types of enemas may be prescribed:
- A saline enema using 500 to 2000 mL of warmed physiologic saline solution is the least irritating to the bowel.

- Tap-water enemas use 500 to 1000 mL of water to soften feces and irritate the bowel mucosa, stimulating peristalsis and evacuation.
- Soap-suds enemas consist of a tap-water solution to which soap is added as a further irritant.
- Phosphate enemas (e.g., Fleet) use a hypertonic saline solution to draw fluid into the bowel and irritate the mucosa, leading to evacuation.
- Oil retention enemas instill mineral or vegetable oil into the bowel to soften the fecal mass. The instilled oil is retained overnight or for several hours before evacuation.

The repeated use of enemas can lead not only to impaired bowel function, but also to fluid and electrolyte imbalances. Tap-water and phosphate enemas are particularly likely to cause these problems. In acute conditions with risk of bowel obstruction, perforation, ulceration, or other problem, enemas should not be administered until their safe use can be established.

Nursing Care

Health Promotion

Education can prevent constipation. Teach clients the importance of maintaining a diet high in natural fiber. Foods such as fresh fruits, vegetables, whole-grain products, and bran, provide natural fiber. Encourage reducing consumption of meats and refined foods, which are low in fiber and can be constipating. Emphasize the need to maintain a high fluid intake every day, particularly during hot weather and exercise. Discuss the relationship between exercise and bowel regularity. Encourage clients to engage in some form of exercise, such as walking daily.

Discuss normal bowel habits, and explain that a daily bowel movement is not the norm for all people. Encourage clients to respond to the urge to defecate when it occurs. Suggest setting aside a time, usually following a meal, for elimination.

Assessment

To assess the client with real or perceived constipation, collect the following data:

- *Health history:* usual and current pattern of defecation, including time of day, amount, and stool consistency; usual diet, fluid intake, and activity pattern; possible contributing factors, such as narcotic analgesics, activity limitations, painful hemorrhoids, perianal surgery; chronic diseases, such as endocrine or neurologic disorders; prescribed and nonprescription medications.
- *Physical examination:* abdominal girth and shape, bowel sounds, tenderness, and percussion tone; digital exam of the rectum if impaction is suspected.

Nursing Diagnoses and Interventions
Nursing interventions for the client with constipation focus chiefly on education.

Constipation
Whether real or perceived, constipation is disruptive to the client's activities of daily living (ADLs) and life satisfaction.

- Monitor pattern of defecation and stool consistency. *This information helps establish the client's usual pattern of defecation and differentiate between actual and perceived constipation.*
- Provide additional fluids to maintain an intake of at least 2500 mL per day. *A generous fluid intake helps maintain soft stool consistency and promote intestinal motility.*

- Encourage drinking a glass of warm water before breakfast. Provide time and privacy following breakfast for bowel elimination. *This helps develop a pattern of natural elimination; the warm water provides mild stimulation of bowel peristalsis.*

- Consult with the dietitian to provide a diet high in natural fiber unless contraindicated. Provide foods, such as natural bran, prunes, or prune juice. *Natural fiber adds bulk to the stool and has a mild stimulant effect.*

- Encourage activities, such as ambulation or chair exercises (range of motion, stretching, wheelchair lifts, etc.), as tolerated. *Activity stimulates peristalsis and strengthens abdominal muscles, facilitating elimination.*

- If indicated, consult with primary care provider about the use of bulk laxatives, stool softeners, or other laxatives as needed. *Laxatives may be necessary to relieve acute constipation. Clients with long-term activity or diet restrictions or impaired abdominal muscle strength may need a bulk-forming laxative to maintain normal elimination patterns and prevent constipation.*

Home Care

Include the following topics when teaching for home care measures to prevent and treat constipation:

- Increasing dietary fiber intake by including fresh fruits and vegetables, whole grains, high-fiber breakfast cereals, and unprocessed bran in the diet. (Bran can be sprinkled on cereals, mixed into bread or muffin recipes, or mixed with fruit juice to increase its palatability.)

- Maintaining fluid intake of six to eight glasses of water per day (unless contraindicated)

- Suggestions for remaining physically active to promote bowel function and maintain muscle tone.

- Responding to the urge to defecate when perceived.

- Appropriate use of laxatives:
  a. Do not use laxatives, suppositories, or enemas on a regular basis.
  b. Bulk-forming agents provide insoluble fiber, and are safe for long-term use; it is important to drink at least six to eight glasses of water daily when using these (or any) laxatives.

- Other laxatives such as milk of magnesia, docusate (Colase, DSS, others), bisacodyl (Dulcolax, others), cascara, or castor oil should be used only occasionally to relieve constipation.

- The need to report any change in bowel habits such as new or persistent constipation or diarrhea, abdominal pain, black or bloody stools, nausea or anorexia, weakness, or unexplained weight loss, to the primary care provider.

The Client with Irritable Bowel Syndrome

Irritable bowel syndrome (IBS), also known as spastic bowel or functional colitis, is a motility disorder of the gastrointestinal tract. It is a functional disorder with no identifiable organic cause. IBS is often characterized by abdominal pain with constipation, diarrhea, or both.

Irritable bowel syndrome is common, affecting up to 20% of people in Western civilization. It usually affects young people, although may also be prevalent in older adults. Women are affected two to three times more frequently than men (Braunwald, et al., 2001).

Pathophysiology

In IBS, it appears that central nervous system (CNS) regulation of the motor and sensory functions of the bowel are altered. Clients with IBS often experience increased motor reactivity of the small bowel and colon in response to stimuli, such as food intake, hormonal influences, and physiologic or psychologic stress. Sensory responses from the gut are also exaggerated in response to the movement of chime through the bowel (Braunwald, et al., 2001). Hypersecretion of colonic mucus is a common feature of the syndrome.

A lower visceral pain threshold is often found in clients with IBS. Clients may complain of pain, bloating, and distention when intestinal gas levels are normal.

Psychologic factors, such as depression or anxiety, have been linked to IBS; however, they have not been identified as causes of the disorder. Clients with underlying psychologic factors may be more likely to seek medical attention for symptoms, but normal psychologic profiles are noted in clients with the disorder who do not seek medical attention (Tierney, et al., 2001). Recent research does indicate a correlation between emotional, physical, and sexual abuse and IBS. Again, however, causation could not be established.

Manifestations

Irritable bowel syndrome is characterized by abdominal pain that often is relieved by defecation and a change in bowel habits. The pain may be either colicky, occurring in spasms, or dull and continuous. Altered patterns of defecation may include:

- A change in frequency
- Abnormal stool form (hard or lumpy, loose or watery)
- Altered stool passage (straining, urgency, or a sensation of incomplete evacuation)
- Passage of mucus.

The client may also complain of abdominal bloating and excess gas. Other manifestations include nausea, vomiting, and anorexia; fatigue, headache, depression, or anxiety. The abdomen is often tender to palpation, particularly over the sigmoid colon.

Collaborative Care

Irritable bowel syndrome is diagnosed based on the presence of abdominal pain or discomfort that has two of the following three characteristics: (1) relieved by defecation; (2) associated with a change in frequency of elimination; (3) associated with a change in stool form (Tierney, et al., 2001). Management is directed toward relieving manifestations and reducing or eliminating precipitating factors. Stress reduction measures, exercises, or counseling may benefit the client.

Diagnostic Tests

The primary purpose of diagnostic testing is to rule out other causes of abdominal pain and altered fecal elimination.

- *Stool* may be examined for *occult blood, ova* and *parasites,* and *culture.* A stool smear for WBCs may also be done; an elevated WBC count may indicate an inflammatory or infectious process.

- *Complete blood count (CBC) with differential and erythrocyte sedimentation rate (ESR)* are evaluated. Anemia may indicate blood loss and a possible tumor, polyps, or other organic problem. An elevated WBC may indicate bacterial infection, and an elevated ESR is seen with many inflammatory processes.
- *Sigmoidoscopy* or *colonoscopy* may be ordered to visually examine bowel mucosa, measure intraluminal pressures, and biopsy suspicious lesions. In IBS, the bowel appears normal, with increased mucus, marked spasm, and possible hyperemia (increased redness), but no suspicious lesions. Intraluminal pressures are often increased. The procedure itself may stimulate manifestations of the syndrome.
- *Small bowel series (upper GI series with small bowel follow-through)* and *barium enema* may be ordered. For the small bowel series, an oral barium preparation is administered, and the small intestine is examined under fluoroscopy. With IBS, the entire GI tract may show increased motility.

Medications

Although not curative, medications may be prescribed to manage the symptoms of IBS. Bulk-forming laxatives, such as bran, methylcellulose, or psyllium, may help reduce bowel spasm and normalize the number and form of bowel movements. An anticholinergic drug, such as dicyclomine (Antispas, Bentyl, others) or hyoscyamine (Anaspaz, others), may be ordered to inhibit bowel motility by interfering with parasympathetic stimulation of the gastrointestinal tract. It relieves postprandial abdominal pain when given 30 to 60 minutes before meals. In clients with diarrhea, loperamide (Imodium) or diphenoxylate (Lomotil) may be used prophylactically to prevent diarrhea in selected situations.

New drugs that affect GI motility by altering serotonin receptors in the GI tract are being researched. The initial approved drug, alosetron, was later withdrawn from the market due to severe complications associated with its use.

Antidepressant drugs, including tricyclics and selective serotonin reuptake inhibitors (SSRIs), may help relieve abdominal pain associated with IBS. While the anticholinergic side effects of the tricyclics, such as desipramine (Norpramin) and imipramine (Tofranil), may help decrease diarrhea, they have more adverse effects than SSRIs such as sertraline (Zoloft) and fluoxetine (Prozac).

Dietary Management

Many clients with IBS benefit from additional dietary fiber. Adding bran to meals provides added bulk and water content to the stool, reducing the incidence of both loose diarrheal stools and hard, constipated stools. Other dietary changes are specific to individual triggers for IBS symptoms. Some clients may benefit from limiting lactose, fructose, or sorbitol intake. When excess gas and flatulence is a problem, reducing the intake of gas-forming foods, such as beans, cabbage, apple and grape juices, nuts, and raisins, may be helpful. Caffeinated drinks, such as coffee, tea, and soft drinks, act as gastrointestinal stimulants; limiting intake of these fluids may also prove beneficial.

Complementary Therapies

Herbal preparations may provide some benefit for clients with IBS. Herbs with an antispasmotic effect, such as anise, chamomile, peppermint, and sage, may be used to reduce the manifestations of IBS. Refer the client to a certified herbologist or naturopathic physician for treatment.

Nursing Care

Clients with irritable bowel syndrome rarely require acute care for IBS as a primary problem. However, nurses frequently interact with these clients in clinics and other outpatient settings.

Assessment

Careful assessment is important to help identify the effects of IBS on the client. Collect the following assessment data:

- *Health history:* current symptoms, their onset and duration; current treatment measures; effect of symptoms on lifestyle; careful exploration of history of emotional, physical, or sexual abuse.
- *Physical examination:* apparent general state of health; abdominal shape and contour, bowel sounds, tenderness.

Nursing Diagnoses and Interventions

The primary nursing responsibility is education; providing referrals and counseling are additional nursing responsibilities to clients who have irritable bowel syndrome.

The following nursing diagnoses may be appropriate for clients with IBS:

- *Constipation* related to altered gastrointestinal motility
- *Diarrhea* related to altered gastrointestinal motility and excess mucous secretion
- *Anxiety* related to situational stress
- *Ineffective coping* related to effects of disorder on lifestyle.

Refer to the previous sections on diarrhea and constipation for selected nursing interventions.

Home Care

Include the following topics in teaching the client with irritable bowel syndrome:

- The nature of the disorder and the reality of the client's symptoms
- The relationship between irritable bowel syndrome and stress, anxiety, and depression
- Stress- and anxiety-reduction techniques, such as meditation, visualization, exercise, "time out," and progressive relaxation
- Dietary influences that may contribute to IBS and suggested dietary changes, such as additional fiber and water intake
- The use and role of prescribed medications, their adverse effects, and when to contact the physician
- The importance of routine follow-up appointments and of notifying the primary care provider if manifestations change, such as blood in the stool, significant constipation or diarrhea, increasing abdominal pain, or weight loss.

Refer the client to a counselor or other mental health professional for assistance in dealing with psychologic factors.

Chronic Inflammatory Bowel Disease

The Client with Inflammatory Bowel Disease

Chronic inflammatory bowel disease (IBD) includes two separate, but closely related, conditions: ulcerative colitis and Crohn's disease. These conditions have a number of similarities. The etiology of both illnesses is unknown, but both have a geographic distribution and a genetic component. IBD occurs more frequently in the United States and northern European nations than it does in southern Europe and countries in the Southern Hemisphere. IBD is two to four times more prevalent in Jewish populations of the United States and Europe than it is in non-Jewish Caucasians, African Americans, Hispanics, and Asians (Braunwald, et al., 2001). It tends to run in families. Other studies suggest that factors, such as an infectious agents and altered immune responses, play a role in the development of IBD. Autoimmunity is thought to play a role (see Chapter 42). Lifestyle factors, such as smoking, may also affect its development.

The peak incidence of IBD is in young adults between the ages of 15 and 35 years. A second peak occurs between age 60 and 80 (Braunwald et al., 2001). IBD is a chronic and recurrent disease process. Responses to physiologic or psychologic stresses do not cause IBD, but often play a role in exacerbations of the disease.

Despite the similarities, ulcerative colitis and Crohn's disease have distinct differences. Ulcerative colitis primarily affects the large bowel in a continuous pattern, progressing distally to proximally. In Crohn's disease, a patchy pattern of involvement is seen, affecting primarily the small intestine. Ulcerative colitis shows mainly mucosal involvement; in Crohn's disease, the submucosal layers of the bowel are affected.

Ulcerative Colitis

Ulcerative colitis is a chronic inflammatory bowel disorder that affects the mucosa and submucosa of the colon and rectum. Its annual incidence in the United States is about 11 per 100,000 people (Braunwald, et al., 2001).

Chronic intermittent colitis (recurrent ulcerative colitis) is the most common form of the disease. Its onset is insidious, with attacks that last one to three months occurring at intervals of months to years. Typically, only the distal colon is affected, with few systemic manifestations of the disease. Approximately 15% of people with ulcerative colitis develop *fulminant colitis,* with involvement of the entire colon, severe bloody diarrhea, acute abdominal pain, and fever. Clients with fulminant disease are at high risk for complications.

Physiology Review

The wall of the colon has three layers: the mucosa, the submucosa, and the muscularis externa. The mucosal layer contains an abundance of goblet cells and glands which secrete lubricating mucus to facilitate the movement of feces. The colon wall forms a series of pouches, or *haustra.* These pouches allow the colon to expand and contract. Feces moves through the colon by both peristaltic waves and by segmentation movements that mix the contents of adjacent haustra. As feces moves, water and other substances, such as bile salts, are reabsorbed.

Pathophysiology

The inflammatory process of ulcerative colitis begins at the rectosigmoid area of the anal canal and progresses proximally. In most clients, the disease is confined to the rectum and sigmoid colon. It may progress to involve the entire colon, stopping at the ileocecal junction.

Ulcerative colitis begins with inflammation at the base of the crypts of Lieberkühn in the distal large intestine and rectum. Microscopic, pinpoint mucosal hemorrhages occur, and crypt abscesses develop. These abscesses penetrate the superficial submucosa and spread laterally, leading to necrosis and sloughing of bowel mucosa. Further tissue damage is caused by inflammatory exudates and the release of inflammatory mediators, such as prostaglandins and other cytokines (see Chapter 41 for further discussion of the inflammatory process). The mucosa is red and edematous due to vascular congestion, friable (easily broken), and ulcerated. It bleeds easily, and hemorrhage is common. Edema creates a granular appearance. Pseudopolyps, tonguelike projections of bowel mucosa into the lumen, may develop as the epithelial lining of the bowel regenerates. Chronic inflammation leads to atrophy, narrowing, and shortening of the colon, with loss of its normal haustra.

Manifestations

Diarrhea is the predominant symptom of ulcerative colitis. Stools contain both blood and mucus. Nocturnal diarrhea may occur. Mild ulcerative colitis is characterized by fewer than five stools per day, intermittent rectal bleeding and mucus, and few constitutional symptoms. Severe ulcerative colitis can lead to more than 6 to 10 bloody stools per day, extensive colon involvement, anemia, hypovolemia, and malnutrition. Rectal inflammation causes fecal urgency and tenesmus. Left lower quadrant cramping relieved by defecation is common. Other systemic manifestations include fatigue, anorexia, and weakness.

Clients with severe disease may also have systemic manifestations, such as arthritis involving one or several joints, skin and mucous membrane lesions, or *uveitis* (inflammation of the uvea, the vascular layer of the eye, which may also involve the sclera and cornea). Some clients develop thromboemboli, with blood vessel obstruction due to clots carried from the site of their formation. Sclerosing cholangitis (inflammation and scarring of the bile ducts) may occur (Tierney, et al., 2001).

Complications

Acute complications of ulcerative colitis include hemorrhage, toxic megacolon, and colon perforation. Massive hemorrhage may occur with severe attacks of the disease. **Toxic megacolon,** a condition characterized by acute motor paralysis and dilation of the colon to greater than 6 cm, may affect part or all of the colon. The transverse segment of the bowel is most often affected. Toxic megacolon may be triggered by electrolyte imbalances or narcotic administration (Braunwald, et al., 2001). Manifestations of toxic megacolon include fever, tachycardia, hypotension, dehydration, abdominal tenderness and cramping, and a change in the number of stools per day. Perforation is rare, but the risk of this dangerous complication is increased with toxic megacolon. Perforation leads to peritonitis, and has a mortality rate of about 15% (Braunwald, et al., 2001).

The risk for colorectal cancer is increased in clients with ulcerative colitis. When the entire colon is involved by ulcerative colitis, the risk is 20 to 30 times greater than for the general public (Porth, 2002). Beginning 8 to 10 years after the diagnosis, yearly colonoscopies with biopsy to detect masses or cell dysplasia are recommended for clients who have extensive ulcerative colitis (Tierney, et al., 2001).

Crohn's Disease

Like ulcerative colitis, **Crohn's disease,** also known as regional enteritis, is a chronic, relapsing inflammatory disorder affecting the gastrointestinal tract. The overall incidence of Crohn's disease in the United States is approximately 7 per 100,000 people (Braunwald, et al., 2001).

Crohn's disease can affect any portion of the GI tract from the mouth to the anus, but usually affects the terminal ileum and ascending colon. Only the small bowel is involved in about 30% to 40% of clients with Crohn's disease. The disease is limited to the colon only in 15% to 20% of those affected. Both the small and large intestine are involved in the majority (Braunwald, et al., 2001).

Pathophysiology

Crohn's disease typically begins as a small inflammatory *aphthoid lesion* (shallow ulcers with a white base and elevated margin, similar to a canker sore) of the mucosa and submucosa of the bowel. These initial lesions may regress, or the inflammatory process can progress to involve all layers of the intestinal wall. Deeper ulcerations, granulomatous lesions, and fissures (knifelike clefts that extend deeply into the bowel wall) develop. The inflammatory process involves the entire bowel wall (transmural).

The lumen of the affected bowel assumes a "cobblestone appearance" as fissures and ulcers surround islands of intact mucosa over edematous submucosa. The inflammatory lesions of Crohn's disease are not continuous; rather, they often occur as "skip" lesions with intervening areas of normal-appearing bowel. Some evidence suggests that despite its normal appearance, the entire bowel is affected by this disorder.

As the disease progresses, fibrotic changes in the bowel wall cause it to thicken and lose flexibility, taking on an appearance that has been likened to a rubber hose. The inflammation, edema, and fibrosis can lead to local obstruction, abscess development, and the formation of fistulas between loops of bowel or bowel and other organs. Fistulas between loops of bowel are known as enteroenteric fistulas; those that occur between bowel and bladder are known as enterovesical fistulas; and fistulas that occur between bowel and skin are known as enterocutaneous fistulas. Perineal fistulas are relatively common, originating in the ileum.

Depending on the severity and extent of the disease, malabsorption and malnutrition may develop as the ulcers prevent absorption of nutrients. When the jejunum and ileum are affected, the absorption of multiple nutrients may be impaired, including carbohydrates, proteins, fats, vitamins, and folate. Disease in the terminal ileum can lead to vitamin B_{12} malabsorption and bile salt reabsorption. The ulcerations can also lead to protein loss and chronic, slow blood loss with consequent anemia.

Manifestations

Because the GI system involvement in Crohn's disease can be so diverse, manifestations may vary among clients. The majority of people with Crohn's disease experience continuous or episodic diarrhea. Stools are liquid or semiformed and typically do not contain blood, although blood may be passed if the colon is involved. Abdominal pain and tenderness is also common. The pain may be located in the right lower quadrant and relieved by defecation. A palpable right lower quadrant mass is often present. Systemic manifestations, such as fever, fatigue, malaise, weight loss, and anemia, are common. Anorectal lesions, such as fissures, ulcers, fistulas, and abscesses, are also common and may occur years before intestinal disease is apparent. If the stomach and duodenum are involved, nausea, vomiting, and epigastric pain may occur.

Complications

Certain complications of Crohn's disease (e.g., intestinal obstruction, abscess, and fistula) are so common that they are considered part of the disease process. For many clients, the disease initially presents with one of these complications. Intestinal obstruction is a common complication caused by repeated inflammation and scarring of the bowel that leads to fibrosis and stricture. Obstruction of the bowel lumen causes abdominal distention, cramping pain, and borborygmi. Nausea and vomiting may occur.

Fistulas may be asymptomatic, particularly if they occur between loops of small bowel. When fistulization causes an abscess, chills and fever, a tender abdominal mass, and leukocytosis develop. A fistula between the small bowel and colon may exacerbate diarrhea, weight loss, and malnutrition. When the bladder is involved, recurrent urinary tract infections occur.

Perforation of the bowel is uncommon, but can lead to generalized peritonitis. Massive hemorrhage is also an uncommon complication of Crohn's disease. Long-standing Crohn's disease increases the risk of cancer of the small intestine or colon by five to six times. This cancer risk, however, is significantly lower than the risk associated with ulcerative colitis.

Collaborative Care

Collaborative care for inflammatory bowel disease begins by establishing the diagnosis and the extent and severity of the disease. Treatment is supportive, including medications and dietary measures to decrease inflammation, promote intestinal rest and healing, and reduce intestinal motility. Many clients with IBD require surgery at some point to manage the disease or its complications.

Diagnostic Tests

Diagnostic testing is used to establish the diagnosis of IBD, assess the extent of the disease, and evaluate the effects of the disorder.

- *Sigmoidoscopy* or *colonoscopy* is performed to inspect the bowel mucosa for characteristic changes of IBD: edema, inflammation, mucus and pus, mucosal ulcers or abscesses, and either a continuous or segmental pattern of involvement. Biopsy of bowel mucosa may differentiate ulcerative colitis or Crohn's disease from cancer and other inflammatory bowel disorders. There is a small risk of bowel perforation during these exams, particularly if the disease is severe.
- *Radiologic examination* of the entire gastrointestinal tract includes an upper GI series with small bowel follow-through and a barium enema. These studies can show the characteristic small and large bowel changes of IBD, such as ulcerations, strictures, fistulas, shortening and loss of colon haustra, or complications, such as a dilated colon in toxic megacolon.

- *Stool examination* for blood and mucus and *stool cultures* are done to rule out infectious causes of bowel inflammation and diarrhea.
- *CBC with hemoglobin* and *hematocrit* shows anemia from chronic inflammation, blood loss, and malnutrition; and leukocytosis due to inflammation and possible abscess formation. The sedimentation rate is typically elevated during periods of acute inflammation.
- *Serum albumin* may be decreased because of malabsorption, malnutrition, protein loss through intestinal lesions, and chronic inflammation.
- *Folic acid and serum levels* of most vitamins, including A, B complex, C, and the fat-soluble vitamins, often are decreased due to malabsorption.
- *Liver function tests* may show elevated liver enzymes, such as ALT, alkaline phosphatase, AST, GGTP, and LDH, and bilirubin levels if sclerosing cholangitis is present.

Medications

The ultimate goal of care is to terminate acute attacks as quickly as possible and reduce the incidence of relapse. Drug therapy plays a key role in achieving this goal. Locally acting and systemic anti-inflammatory drugs are the primary medications used to manage mild to moderate IBD. Drugs to suppress the immune response may be used to treat clients with severe disease.

Sulfasalazine (Azulfidine) is a sulfonamide antibiotic that is poorly absorbed from the gastrointestinal tract and acts topically on the colonic mucosa to inhibit the inflammatory process. The active anti-inflammatory ingredient in sulfasalazine, 5-aminosalicylic acid, also is available in preparations that do not contain sulfa, such as olsalazine and mesalamine. They have the advantage of causing fewer adverse effects than sulfasalazine.

Table 21-3. Medication Administration – Inflammatory Bowel Disease

Sulfasalazine (Azulfidine)

Sulfasalazine is an anti-inflammatory drug used for its local effect on the intestinal mucosa in inflammatory bowel disease. The active part of the drug is 5-aminosalicylic acid, which inhibits prostaglandin production in the bowel. Prostaglandin is an important mediator of the inflammatory process; blocking its production reduces inflammation.

Nursing Responsibilities

- Assess for contraindications, including pregnancy or a history of hypersensitivity to sulfonamides or salicylates.
- Assess baseline values for renal function tests (serum creatinine, BUN, urinalysis), liver function tests, and CBC.
- Administer as ordered. Suppositories or retention enemas may be administered at bedtime. Administer oral forms with a full glass of water.
- Have resuscitation equipment available; anaphylactic responses may occur.
- Evaluate for therapeutic response, including reduced number of stools, reduced mucus and blood, and improved stool consistency.
- Monitor for possible adverse responses:
  - a. Skin rash, dermatitis, urticaria, or pruritus
  - b. Evidence of blood dyscrasias, such as bleeding, easy bruising, fever
  - c. Leukopenia, thrombocytopenia, hemolytic anemia, or angranulocytosis

---

Table 21-3. Continued

    d.   Changes in urinary output or renal function studies

    e.   Evidence of hepatitis or myocarditis.

Client and Family Teaching
- Take oral preparations after meals to decrease gastric distress.
- Drink at least two quarts of fluid per day to reduce the risk of kidney damage.
- Use sunscreen to prevent burns; this drug increases sensitivity to sun.
- Do not take aspirin, vitamin C, or any other over-the-counter medications containing aspirin or vitamin C without consulting your doctor.
- This medication may interfere with the effectiveness of oral contraceptives; use alternative methods of contraception.
- Notify your doctor if you develop skin rash or hives, sore throat or mouth, bleeding gums, joint pain, easy bruising, or fever.

Mesalamine (Asacol Rowasa) and Olsalazine (Dipentum)

Mesalamine and olsalazine contain the same active ingredient, 5-aminosalicylic acid, as sulfasalazine, but cause fewer adverse effects. Their mechanism of action is the same as that of sulfasalazine. These drugs are available as suppositories, suspension for enema, or oral tablets.

Nursing Responsibilities
- Assess for possible contraindications such as pregnancy, lactation, or hypersensitivity to these drugs or aspirin.
- Administer as ordered. If more than one dose per day is ordered, space doses evenly over the 24-hour period.
- Evaluate for desired effects (as for sulfasalazine) and potential adverse effects.
  - a.   Nausea, diarrhea, abdominal cramps, or flatulence
  - b.   CNS effects including headache, dizziness, insomnia, weakness, or fatigue
  - c.   Rash or itching
  - d.   Flulike symptoms, general malaise.

Client and Family Teaching
- Teach the recommended method of administration, including how to insert rectal suppositories or administer a retention enema.
- Shake suspension forms well prior to using.
- Diarrhea is the most common side effect of these drugs. Notify your doctor if adverse effects occur.

Corticosteroids

Methylprednisolone (Medrol, Solu-Medrol)
Prednisolone (Delta-Cortel)
Prednisone

Glucocorticoids are hormones produced by the adrenal cortex. These hormones are necessary for the stress response. Cortisol, the main glucocorticoid, has potent anti-inflammatory

Continued on the next page

Table 21-3. Continued

effects. Corticosteroids are used to treat acute episodes of IBD. Because of their multiple and significant side effects, they are not used to maintain remission.

Nursing Responsibilities

- Assess for conditions that may be adversely affected by corticosteroid drugs: peptic ulcer disease, glaucoma or cataracts, diabetes, or psychiatric disorders.
- Obtain baseline vital signs and weight; monitor both routinely during therapy. Hypertension and weight gain may result from salt and water retention.
- Monitor for edema.
- Administer as ordered. For daily or alternate-day dosing, administer in the morning, when physiologic glucocorticoid levels are highest, to reduce adrenal cortisone suppression.
- Administer oral preparations with food to decrease gastrointestinal side effects. Antacids or histamine H_2-receptor blocking agents, such as cimetidine (Tagamet), may be prescribed during corticosteroid therapy.
- Monitor for desired effects reduced diarrhea, less blood and mucus in the stool, and less abdominal cramping.
- Monitor for adverse effects:
  a. Increased susceptibility to infection and masking of early signs of infection
  b. Hyperglycemia
  c. Hypokalemia, as manifested by muscle weakness, nausea, vomiting, and cardiac rhythm disturbances
  d. Edema, hypertension, and signs of heart failure
  e. Peptic ulcer formation and possible gastrointestinal hemorrhage (abdominal pain, black or tarry stools, and signs of bleeding)
  f. Changes in mental status, including depression, euphoria, aggression, and behavioral changes.
  g. With long-term use, Cushingoid effects, such as abnormal fat deposits in the face (moon faces) and trunk (buffalo hump), muscle wasting and thin extremities, thinning of the skin, and osteoporosis.

Client and Family Teaching

- Take as prescribed; do not change the dose or time of day. Do not stop the medication abruptly. The dose will be tapered down gradually when the drug is discontinued.
- Notify the physician if adverse or Cushingoid effects occur.
- Take with food or at mealtimes to decrease the gastrointestinal effects.
- Monitor weight. If a gain of more than five pounds is noted notify the physician.
- Moderate salt intake and avoid foods and snacks high in sodium, such as processed meats and potato chips. Increase intake of foods high in potassium, such as fruits, vegetables, and lean meats.
- Carry a card or wear a bracelet or tag at all times identifying corticosteroid use.

For acute exacerbations of IBD, corticosteroids are given to reduce inflammation and induce remission. For ulcerative colitis, the drug may be administered by enema for its local effect and to minimize systemic effects. Hydrocortisone can be administered by enema. Intravenous corticosteroids may be required to treat severe disease; oral preparations are used for less severe manifestations and long-term therapy. Many clients are unable to withdraw from steroid therapy without experiencing relapse and may need chronic low-dose therapy.

Mercaptopurine (6-MP, Purinethol) and other immunosuppressive agents, such as azathioprine (Imuran) and cyclosporine (Sandimmune) may be used to treat clients who have not responded to other treatments or who require chronic steroid therapy. These drugs may allow withdrawal from corticosteroids, maintain remission, and facilitate healing. Long-term therapy may be required to produce a beneficial effect. For more information about immunosuppressive drugs, see Chapter 42.

Newer treatments for IBD employ other immune response modifiers, such as monoclonal antibodies to suppress tumor necrosis factor (TNF, an inflammatory mediator substance), and natural anti-inflammatory cyctokines, such as interleukins (Braunwald, et al., 2001).

Although antibiotic therapy generally is not indicated in IBD, metronidazole (Flagyl) has active anti-inflammatory effects. It may be prescribed to help prevent remission after ileal resection in Crohn's disease.

Antidiarrheal agents, such as loperamide and diphenoxylate, may be given to slow gastrointestinal motility and reduce diarrhea. These drugs are safe for clients with mild, chronic symptoms, but they are not given during acute attacks because they may precipitate toxic dilation of the colon.

Dietary Management

Antigens in the diet may stimulate the immune response in the bowel, exacerbating IBD. As a result, dietary management for inflammatory bowel disease is individualized. Some clients benefit from eliminating all milk and milk products from the diet. Increased dietary fiber may help reduce diarrhea and relieve rectal symptoms, but is contraindicated for clients with intestinal strictures caused by repeated inflammation and scarring.

All food is withheld to promote bowel rest during an acute exacerbation of Crohn's disease. Nutritional status is maintained using enteral or total parenteral nutrition (TPN). (See Chapter 20 for more information about enteral feedings and TPN.) TPN carries a higher risk of complications than does enteral nutrition. An elemental diet, such as Ensure, which contains all essential nutrients in a residue-free formula, may be prescribed. Enteral diets provide essential nutrients to the small intestine to support cell growth, but are not always palatable.

Surgery

Surgical interventions for IBD differ, depending on the primary disease process and the portion of the bowel affected. Generally, surgery is performed only when necessitated by complications of the disease or failure of conservative treatment measures.

Bowel obstruction is the leading indication for surgery in Crohn's disease. Other complications that may require surgical intervention include perforation, internal or external fistula, abscess, and perianal complications. Resection of the affected portion of bowel with an end-to-end anastomosis to preserve as much bowel as possible is the usual treatment. The disease process tends to recur in other areas following removal of affected bowel segments. There is an increased risk of fistula formation following surgery. Bowel strictures may be treated with a strictureplasty. In this procedure, longitudinal incisions are made in the narrowed segment to relieve the stricture while preserving bowel.

Clients with extensive chronic ulcerative colitis may require a **total colectomy** (surgical removal of the colon) to treat the disease itself, for complications, such as toxic megacolon, perforation, or hemorrhage, or as a prophylactic measure due to the high colon cancer risk associated with extensive ulcerative colitis. The surgical procedure of choice for extensive ulcerative colitis is a *total colectomy with an ileal pouch-anal anastomosis (IPAA)*. In this procedure, the entire colon and rectum are removed; a pouch is formed from the terminal ileum; and the pouch is brought into the pelvis and anastomosed to the anal canal. A temporary or loop ileostomy (described below) is generally performed at the same time and is maintained for two to three months to allow the anal anastomosis to heal. When the healing is complete, the ileostomy is closed, and the client has six to eight daily bowel movements through the anus.

Advanced age, obesity, or other factors may preclude an IPAA. For these clients, a permanent ileostomy or continent ileostomy may be created.

An intestinal **ostomy** is a surgically created opening between the intestine and the abdominal wall which allows the passage of fecal material. The surface opening is called a **stoma**.

The precise name of the ostomy depends on the location of the stoma. An **ileostomy** is an ostomy made in the ileum of the small intestine. In an ileostomy, the colon, rectum, and anus are usually completely removed (*total proctocolectomy with permanent ileostomy*). The anal canal is closed, and the end of the terminal ileum is brought to the body surface through the right abdominal wall to form the stoma. A temporary or *loop ileostomy* may be formed to eliminate feces and allow tissue healing for two to three months following an IPAA. A loop of ileum is brought to the body surface to form a stoma and allow stool drainage into an external pouch. When the ileostomy is no longer necessary, a second surgery is performed to close the stoma and repair the bowel, restoring fecal elimination through the anus.

In a *continent* (or *Kock's*) *ileostomy*, an intra-abdominal reservoir is constructed and a nipple valve formed (the ileum folded back on itself) from the terminal ileum, before it is brought to the surface of the abdominal wall. Stool collects in the internal pouch; the nipple valve prevents it from leaking through the stoma. A catheter is inserted into the pouch to drain the stool.

Table 21-4.   Low-Residue Diet

Food Group	Allowed	Avoid
Beverages	Coffee, teas, juices, carbonated beverages; milk limited to 2 cups per day	Alcohol, prune juice
Breads and cereals	Products made from refined flours (white bread, crackers) or finely milled grains (e.g., corn flakes, crisp rice cereal, puffed wheat)	Whole-grain breads, rolls, or cereal; breads or rolls with seeds, nuts, or bran
Desserts	Gelatins, tapioca, plain custards, or puddings; angel-food or sponge cake; ice cream or frozen desserts without fruit or nuts	Any desserts containing dried fruits, nuts, seeds, or coconut; rich pastries, pies

Table 21-4. Continued

Fruits	Fruit juices and strained fruits; cooked or canned apples, apricots, cherries, peaches, pears; bananas	All other raw or cooked fruits
Meats and other protein sources	Roasted, baked, or broiled tender or ground beef, veal, pork, lamb, poultry, or fish; smooth peanut butter; cottage, cream, American, or mild chedder cheeses in small amounts	Tough or spiced meats and those prepared by frying; highly flavored cheeses; nuts
Potatoes, rice, and pasta	Peeled potatoes; white rice; most pasta products	Potato skins, potato chips, or fried potatoes; brown rice; whole-grain pasta products
Sweets	Sugar, honey, jelly, hard candy and gumdrops, plain chocolates	Jam, marmalade; candy made with seeds, nuts, coconut
Vegetables	Vegetable juices and strained vegetables; cooked or canned vegetables	Raw or whole cooked vegetables
Other	Salt, ground seasonings; cream sauce and plain gravy	Chili sauce, horseradish; popcorn, seeds of any kind; whole spices, olives, vinegar

Complementary Therapies

The chronic nature of inflammatory bowel disease and adverse effects of many prescribed treatments lead many clients with IBD to seek or use complementary therapies. Chiropractic care, megavitamin therapy, dietary supplements, and herbal medicine have been reported as common complementary therapies for IBD (Heuschkel et al., 2002; Verhoef, et al., 2002). A study by Langmead et al (2002) concluded that herbal remedies such as slippery elm, fenugreek, devil's claw, Mexican yam, termentil and wei tong ning have antioxidant effects and may provide an effect similar to that of 5-aminosalicylic acid preparations. Many complementary therapies for IBD may interact with prescribed medications; instruct the client to discuss all potential therapies with the primary care provider.

Nursing Care

Health Promotion

Although inflammatory bowel disease cannot, at this time, be predicted or prevented, effective management may help the client avoid complications of the disease. Stress the importance of complying with the prescribed treatment regimen and promptly reporting manifestations of exacerbations to the physician.

Assessment

Assessment data related to inflammatory bowel disease includes the following subjective and objective data:

- *Health history:* current manifestations, including onset, duration, severity (number of stools per day, presence of blood or mucus in stool, abdominal pain or cramping, tenasmus); usual diet, ability to maintain weight and nutrition, food intolerances; associated manifestations, such as arthralgias, fatigue, malaise; current medications; previous treatment and diagnostic tests.

- *Physical examination:* general appearance; weight; vital signs including orthostatic vitals and temperature; abdominal assessment including shape, contour, bowel sounds, palpation for tenderness and masses, presence of stoma or scars.

Nursing Diagnoses and Interventions

When planning nursing care for the client with inflammatory bowel disease, it is vital to consider the chronic, recurrent nature of the disorder. Teaching is a major aspect of care. Diarrhea and disturbed body image are significant nursing care problems for the client with IBD. With severe disease, impaired nutrition must be considered a priority problem as well.

Diarrhea

During an acute exacerbation of IBD, diarrhea can be frequent and painful. The frequency of defecation and associated abdominal pain and cramping may interfere with ADLs and increase the risk for fluid volume deficit and impaired skin integrity.

- Record the frequency, amount, and color of stools using a stool chart. Measure and record liquid stool as output. *The severity of diarrhea is an indicator of the severity of the disease and helps determine the need for fluid replacement.*

- Assess vital signs every four hours. *Tachycardia, tachypnea, and fever may be indicators of fluid volume deficit.*

- Weigh daily and record. *Rapid weight loss (over days to a week) usually indicates fluid loss, whereas weight loss over weeks to months may indicate malnutrition.*

- Assess for other indications of fluid deficit: warm, dry skin, poor skin turgor, dry shiny mucous membranes, weakness, lethargy, complaints of thirst. *The extent of fluid loss may not be readily evident with diarrhea, particularly if the client uses the bathroom without assistance. Systemic manifestations of fluid volume deficit may be the first indicators of the problem.*

- Maintain bowel rest by keeping NPO or limiting oral intake to elemental feedings as indicated. *Bowel rest during an acute exacerbation of IBD promotes healing and reduces diarrhea and other symptoms.*

- Administer prescribed anti-inflammatory and antidiarrheal medications as indicated. *Anti-inflammatory medications reduce the extent of bowel inflammation and diarrhea. Unless contraindicated, antidiarrheal medications help reduce fluid loss and increase comfort.*

- Maintain fluid intake by mouth or intravenously as indicated. *The client with IBD requires fluid to replace ongoing losses, as well as fluid to meet the usual daily needs of the body. If an elemental diet or total parenteral nutrition is prescribed, additional fluids may be required to meet fluid intake needs.*

- Provide good skin care. *Fluid deficit and tissue dehydration increase the risk for skin excoriations or breakdown.*

- Assess perianal area for irritation or denuded skin from the diarrhea. Use gentle cleansing agents, such as Periwash or Tucks, or cottonballs saturated with witch hazel. Apply a protective cream, such as zinc oxide–based preparations, to protect skin from the irritating effects of diarrheal stool. *Digestive enzymes in the stool are very corrosive, increasing the risk of skin breakdown where exposed to diarrheal stool.*

Disturbed Body Image

The client with IBD may experience frustration at not being able to control, or even predict, fecal elimination, particularly when the disease is severe. Diarrhea can interfere with the ability to complete tasks, maintain employment or engage in social activities, and even meet basic needs, such as eating, sleeping, and sexual activity. Body image can suffer as a result. Treatment of IBD, be it total colectomy with ileal pouch-anal anastomosis, ileostomy, or chronic corticosteroid therapy, can also affect the view of self.

- Accept feelings and perception of self. *Negating or denying the reality of the client's perception impairs trust.*

- Encourage discussion of physical changes and their consequences as they relate to self-concept. *This demonstrates acceptance and provides an opportunity to express the impact of the disease and its treatment on the client's life.*

- Encourage discussion about concerns regarding the effect of the disease or treatment on close personal relationships. *This demonstrates understanding and provides an opportunity for the client to express feelings about the impact of the disease on relationships and significant others.*

- Encourage the client to make choices and decisions regarding care. *This increases the client's sense of control over the disease and his or her future.*

- Discuss possible treatment options and their effects openly and honestly. *Open discussion allows more informed decisions.*

- Involve the client in care, teaching and demonstrating as needed. *This encourages and facilitates independence and decision making.*

- Provide care in an accepting, nonjudgmental manner. *Acceptance of the client despite potential embarrassment about odors or diarrhea enhances self-esteem.*

- Arrange for interaction with other clients or groups of people with IBD or ostomies. *The client may feel that no one who has not experienced a similar problem can understand his or her feelings.*

- Teach coping strategies (odor control, dietary modifications, and so on), and support their use. *This facilitates healthy adaptation to the disease.*

Imbalanced Nutrition: Less Than Body Requirements

Crohn's disease can significantly alter the bowel's ability to absorb nutrients. In both forms of IBD, blood and protein-rich fluid may be lost in diarrheal stools. With malabsorption and continuing nutrient losses, multiple nutrient deficits can develop, affecting growth and development, healing, muscle mass, bone density, and electrolyte balances.

- Monitor laboratory results, including hemoglobin and hematocrit, serum electrolytes, and total serum protein and albumin levels. *These studies provide an indicator of nutritional status.*

- Provide the prescribed diet: high-kcal, high-protein, low-fat diet with restricted milk and milk products if lactose intolerance is present. *Calories and protein are important to replace lost nutrients. Fat restriction helps reduce diarrhea and nutrient loss, particularly when significant portions of the terminal ileum have been resected.*

- Provide parenteral nutrition as necessary if the client is unable to absorb enteral nutrients. *Parenteral nutrition can help reverse nutritional deficits and promote weight gain and healing in the client with acute symptoms.*

- Arrange for dietary consultation. Consider food preferences as allowed. *Providing preferred foods in the prescribed diet increases intake and supports nutritional status.*

- Provide or administer elemental enteral nutrition and supplements as ordered. *Elemental enteral nutritional supplements support healing while providing for bowel rest. They can replace losses and improve nutritional status more rapidly than diet alone.*

- Include family members, the primary food preparer in particular, in teaching and dietary discussions. *Families can reinforce teaching and help the client maintain required restrictions or kcal intake.*

Home Care

Inflammatory bowel disease is a chronic condition for which the client needs to provide daily self-management. For this reason, teaching is a vital component of care. Teach the client and family about the following topics:

- The type of inflammatory bowel disease affecting the client, including the disease process, short- and long-term effects, the relationship of stress to disease exacerbations, and the manifestations of complications

- Prescribed medications, including drug names, desired effects, schedules for tapering the doses if ordered (as with corticosteroids), and possible side effects or adverse reactions and their management

- The recommended diet and the rationale for any specific restrictions

- Use of nutritional supplements, such as Ensure, to maintain weight and nutritional status

- Indicators of malabsorption and impaired nutrition; recommendations for self-care and when to seek medical intervention

- If discharged with a central catheter and home parenteral nutrition, written and verbal instructions on catheter care, troubleshooting, and TPN administration. (Have the client and a family member demonstrate catheter care and TPN maintenance.)

- The importance of maintaining a fluid intake of at least two to three quarts per day, increasing fluid intake during warm weather, exercise or strenuous work, and when fever is present

- The increased risk for colorectal cancer and importance of regular bowel exams

- Risks and benefits of various treatment options.

If surgery is planned or has been done, include the following topics in home care instructions:

- Ileal pouch-anal anastomosis or ileostomy care as indicated

- Where to obtain ostomy supplies

- Use of nonprescription drugs, such as enteric-coated and timed-release capsules, that may not be adequately absorbed before elimination through the ileostomy
- Community and national ostomy support groups.

The Client with Colorectal Cancer

Colorectal cancer, malignancy of the colon or rectum, is the third most common cancer diagnosed in the United States. In the United States, about 148,300 new cases of colorectal cancer were diagnosed in 2002, and over 56,000 people died from this disease (American Cancer Society [ACS], 2002). Earlier diagnosis and improved treatment have improved the survival rate for colorectal cancer. Its incidence, which is nearly equal among men and women, is declining in the United States. Colorectal cancer occurs most frequently after age 50. The incidence continues to rise with increasing age. With early diagnosis and treatment, the 5-year survival rate for colorectal cancer is 90%; however, less than half of colorectal cancers are diagnosed at this early stage. The 5-year survival rate drops to 65% when it has spread locally at the time of diagnosis, and 8% when distant sites are involved (ACS, 2002).

Although the specific cause of colorectal cancer is unknown, a number of risk factors have been identified. Genetic factors are strongly linked to the risk for colorectal cancer. Up to 25% of people who develop colorectal cancer have a family history of the disease (Braunwald, et al., 2001). Persons with familial adenomatous polyposis inevitably will develop colon cancer unless the colon is removed (Tierney et al., 2001). Hereditary nonpolyposis colorectal cancer (also known as Lynch syndrome) is an autosomal dominant disorder that significantly increases the risk for developing colorectal and other cancers. Tumors associated with Lynch syndrome often affect the ascending colon, and tend to occur at an earlier age (Braunwald, et al., 2001). Inflammatory bowel disease (ulcerative colitis and Crohn's disease) also increases the risk of colorectal cancer.

Diet plays a role in the development of colorectal cancer. The disease is prevalent in economically prosperous countries where people consume diets high in calories, meat proteins, and fats. This dietary pattern, common in the United States, is thought to increase the population of anaerobic bacteria in the gut. These anaerobes convert bile acids into carcinogens (Braunwald, et al., 2001). Diets high in fruits and vegetables, folic acid, and calcium appear to reduce the risk of colorectal cancer. Cereal fiber, once thought to reduce colorectal cancer risk, does not now appear to play a role either way in its development. Other factors that may reduce the risk of colorectal cancer include use of aspirin and other NSAIDs and hormone replacement therapy in post menopausal women (Tierney, et al., 2001).

Pathophysiology

Nearly all colorectal malignancies are adenocarcinomas that begin as adenomatous polyps. Most tumors develop in the rectum and sigmoid colon, although any portion of the colon may be affected. The tumor typically grows undetected, producing few symptoms. By the time symptoms occur, the disease may have spread into deeper layers of the bowel tissue and adjacent organs. Colorectal cancer spreads by direct extension to involve the entire bowel circumference, the submucosa, and outer bowel wall layers. Neighboring structures, such as the liver, greater curvature of the stomach, duodenum, small intestine, pancreas, spleen, genitourinary tract, and abdominal wall, may also be involved by direct extension. Metastasis to regional lymph nodes is the most common form of tumor spread. This is not always an orderly process; distal nodes may contain cancer cells while regional nodes remain normal. Cancerous cells from the primary tumor may also spread by way of the lymphatic system or circulatory system to secondary sites, such as the liver, lungs, brain, bones, and kidneys. "Seeding" of the tumor to other areas of the peritoneal cavity can occur when the tumor extends through the serosa or during surgical resection.

Manifestations and Complications

As noted earlier, bowel cancer often produces no symptoms until it is advanced. Because it grows slowly, 5 to 15 years of growth may occur before symptoms develop. The manifestations depend on its location, type and extent, and complications. Bleeding is often the initial manifestation that prompts clients to seek medical care. Other common early symptoms include a change in bowel habits, either diarrhea or constipation. Pain, anorexia, and weight loss are characteristic in advanced disease. A palpable abdominal or rectal mass may be present. Occasionally the client presents with anemia from occult bleeding.

The primary complications associated with colorectal cancer: (1) bowel obstruction due to narrowing of the bowel lumen by the lesion; (2) perforation of the bowel wall by the tumor, allowing contamination of the peritoneal cavity by bowel contents; and (3) direct extension of the tumor to involve adjacent organs.

Most recurrences of colorectal cancer after tumor removal occur within the first four years. The size of the primary tumor does not necessarily relate to long-term survival. The number of involved lymph nodes, penetration of the tumor through the bowel wall, and tumor adherence to adjacent organs are better predictors of the prognosis for the disease (Braunwald, et al., 2001).

Collaborative Care

The focus of collaborative care for colorectal cancer is early detection and intervention. Colorectal cancer is always treated by surgical resection, with chemotherapy and radiation therapy used as adjuncts.

Screening

The American Cancer Society recommends annual digital rectal examination beginning at age 40, with annual fecal occult blood testing beginning at age 50. Because colorectal tumors bleed intermittently, several fecal occult blood specimens typically are collected over a period of several days. Debate exists regarding recommendations for periodic (every three to five years) flexible sigmoidoscopy or colonoscopy for everyone over age 50.

Diagnostic Tests

*   *CBC* is ordered to detect anemia resulting from chronic blood loss and tumor growth.
*   *Fecal occult blood* (by guaiac or hemoccult testing) is ordered to detect blood in the feces, because nearly all colorectal cancers bleed intermittently.
*   *Carcinoembryonic antigen (CEA)* is a tumor marker that can be detected in the blood of clients with colorectal cancer. CEA levels are used to estimate prognosis, monitor treatment, and detect cancer recurrence. Because this test is not specific for colorectal

cancer and does not always detect early-stage cancer, it is not used as a screening measure (Malarkey & McMorrow, 2000).

- *Sigmoidoscopy* or *colonoscopy* is the primary diagnostic test used to detect and visualize tumors. It also allows tissue collection for biopsy. While flexible sigmoidoscopy can detect 50% to 65% of colorectal cancers, many clinicians recommend colonoscopy, endoscopic examination of the entire colon. Tumors typically appear as raised, red, centrally ulcerated, bleeding lesions.

- *Chest X-ray* is obtained to detect tumor metastasis to the lung.

- *Computed tomography (CT) scan, magnetic resonance imaging (MRI), or ultrasonic examination* may be used to assess tumor depth and involvement of other organs by direct extension or metastasis.

- *Tissue biopsy* is obtained at the time of endoscopy to confirm cancerous tissue and evaluate cell differentiation.

Surgery

Surgical resection of the tumor, adjacent colon, and regional lymph nodes is the treatment of choice for colorectal cancer. Options for surgical treatment vary from destruction of the tumor by laser photocoagulation performed during endoscopy to abdominoperineal resection with permanent colostomy. When possible, the anal sphincter is preserved and colostomy avoided.

Laser photocoagulation uses a very small, intense beam of light to generate heat in tissues toward which it is directed. The heat generated by the laser beam can be used to destroy small tumors. It is also used for palliative surgery of advanced tumors to remove obstruction. Laser photocoagulation can be performed endoscopically and is useful for clients who cannot tolerate major surgery.

Other surgical treatment options for small, localized tumors include local excision and fulguration. These procedures also may be performed during endoscopy, eliminating the need for abdominal surgery. Local excision may be used to remove a disk of rectum containing the tumor in clients with a small, well-differentiated, mobile polypoid lesion. *Fulguration* or electrocoagulation is used to reduce the size of some large tumors for clients who are poor surgical risks. This procedure requires general anesthesia and may need to be repeated at intervals.

Most clients with colorectal cancer undergo surgical resection of the colon with anastomosis of remaining bowel as a curative procedure. The distribution of regional lymph nodes determines the extent of resection as these may contain metastatic lesions. Most tumors of the ascending, transverse, descending, and sigmoid colon can be resected.

Tumors of the rectum usually are treated with an abdominoperineal resection in which the sigmoid colon, rectum, and anus are removed through both abdominal and perineal incisions. A permanent sigmoid colostomy is performed to provide for elimination of feces.

Colostomies Surgical resection of the bowel may be accompanied by a colostomy for diversion of fecal contents. A **colostomy** is an ostomy made in the colon. It may be created if the bowel is obstructed by the tumor, as a temporary measure to promote healing of anastomoses, or as a permanent means of fecal evacuation when the distal colon and rectum are removed. Colostomies take the name of the portion of the colon from which they are formed: ascending colostomy, transverse colostomy, descending colostomy, and sigmoid colostomy.

A *sigmoid colostomy* is the most common permanent colostomy performed, particularly for cancer of the rectum. It is usually created during an abdominoperineal resection. This procedure involves the removal of the sigmoid colon, rectum, and anus through abdominal and perineal incisions. The anal canal is closed, and a stoma formed from the proximal sigmoid colon. The stoma usually is located on the lower left quadrant of the abdomen.

When a *double-barrel colostomy* is performed, two separate stomas are created. The distal colon is not removed, but bypassed. The proximal stoma, which is functional, diverts feces to the abdominal wall. The distal stoma, also called the mucus fistula, expels mucus from the distal colon. It may be pouched or dressed with a 4X4 gauge dressing. A double-barrel colostomy may be created for cases of trauma, tumor, or inflammation, and it may be temporary or permanent.

An emergency procedure used to relieve an intestinal obstruction or perforation is called a *transverse loop colostomy*. During this procedure, a loop of the transverse colon is brought out from the abdominal wall and suspended over a plastic rod or bridge, which prevents the loop from slipping back into the abdominal cavity. The loop stoma may be opened at the time of surgery or a few days later at the client's bedside. The bridge may be removed in one to two weeks. Transverse loop colostomies are typically temporary.

In a *Hartmann procedure,* a common temporary colostomy procedure, the distal portion of the colon is left in place and is oversewn for closure. A temporary colostomy may be done to allow bowel rest or healing, such as following tumor resection or inflammation of the bowel. It may also be created following traumatic injury to the colon, such as a gunshot wound. Anastomosis of the severed portions of the colon is delayed because bacterial colonization of the colon would prevent proper healing of the anastomosis. About three to six months following a temporary colostomy, the colostomy is closed and the colon is reconnected. Clients with temporary colostomies require the same care as clients with permanent colostomies. See Table 21-5.

Radiation Therapy

While radiation therapy is not used as a primary treatment for colon cancer, it is used along with surgical resection for treating rectal tumors. Small rectal cancers may be treated with intracavitary, external, or implantation radiation. Rectal cancer has a high rate of regional recurrence following complete surgical resection, particularly when the tumor has invaded tissues outside the bowel wall or regional lymph nodes. Pre- or postoperative radiation therapy reduces the recurrence of pelvic tumors, although the effect of radiation therapy on long-term survival is less clear. Radiation therapy is also used preoperatively to shrink large rectal tumors enough to permit surgical removal of the tumor (Braunwald, et al., 2001).

Chemotherapy

Chemotherapeutic agents, such as intravenous fluorouracil (5-FU) and folinic acid (leucovorin), are also used postoperatively as adjunctive therapy for colorectal cancer. When combined with radiation therapy, chemotherapy reduces the rate of tumor recurrence and prolongs survival for clients with stage II and stage III rectal tumors. The benefit for colon cancers is less clear, but chemotherapy may be used to reduce its spread to the liver and prevent recurrence. Irinotecan (CPT-11) or oxaliplatin also may be used in chemotherapy regimens for colorectal cancer.

Table 21-5. Nursing Care of the Client with a Colostomy

- Assess the location of the stoma and the type of colostomy performed. *Stoma location is an indicator of the section of bowel in which it is located and a predictor of the type of fecal drainage to expect.*

- Assess stoma appearance and surrounding skin condition frequently. *Assessment of stoma and skin condition is particularly important in the early postoperative period, when complications are most likely to occur and most treatable.*

- Position a collection bag or drainable pouch over the stoma. *Initial drainage may contain more mucus and serosanguineous fluid than fecal material. As the bowel starts to resume function, drainage becomes fecal in nature. The consistency of drainage depends on the stoma location in the bowel.*

- If ordered, irrigate the colostomy, instilling water into the colon similar to an enema procedure. *The water stimulates the colon to empty.*

- When a colostomy irrigation is ordered for a client with a double-barrel or loop colostomy, irrigate the proximal stoma. Digital assessment of the bowel direction from the stoma can assist in determining which is the proximal stoma. *The distal bowel carries no fecal contents and does not need irrigation. It may be irrigated for cleansing just prior to reanastomosis.*

- Empty a drainable pouch or replace the colostomy bag as needed or when it is no more than one-third full. *If the pouch is allowed to overfill, its weight may impair the seal and cause leakage.*

- Provide stomal and skin care for the client with a colostomy as for the client with an ileostomy. *Good skin and stoma care is important to maintain skin integrity and function as the first line of defense against infection.*

- Use caulking agents, such as Stomahesive or karaya paste, and a skin barrier wafer as needed to maintain a secure ostomy pouch. This may be particularly important for the client with a loop colostomy. *The main challenge for a client with a transverse loop colostomy is to maintain a secure ostomy pouch over the plastic bridge.*

- A small needle hole high on the colostomy pouch will allow flatus to escape. This hole may be closed with a Band-Aid and opened only while the client is in the bathroom for odor control. *Ostomy bags may "balloon" out, disrupting the skin seal, if excess gas collects.*

Client and Family Teaching

- Prior to discharge, provide written, verbal, and psychomotor instruction on colostomy care, pouch management, skin care, and irrigation for the client. *Whether the colostomy is temporary or permanent, the client will be responsible for its management. Good understanding of procedures and care enhances the ability to provide self-care, as well as self-esteem and control.*

- Allow ample time for the client (and family, if necessary) to practice changing the pouch, either on the client or a model. *Practice of psychomotor skills improves learning and confidence.*

- If an abdominoperineal resection has been performed, emphasize the importance of using no rectal suppositories, rectal temperatures, or enemas. Suggest that the client carry medical identification or a MedicAlert tag or bracelet. *These measures are important to prevent trauma to the tissues when the rectum has been removed.*

- The diet for a client with a colostomy is individualized and may require no alteration from that consumed preoperatively. Dietary teaching should, however, include information on foods that cause stool odor and gas and foods that thicken and loosen stools. Foods that cause these effects on ostomy output are listed below.

Continued on the next page

Table 21-5. Continued

Foods That Increase Stool Odor

- Asparagus
- Beans
- Cabbage
- Eggs
- Fish
- Garlic
- Onions
- Some spices

Foods That Increase Intestinal Gas

- Beer
- Broccoli
- Brussels sprouts
- Cabbage
- Carbonated drinks
- Cauliflower
- Corn
- Cucumbers
- Dairy products
- Dried beans
- Peas
- Radishes
- Spinach

Foods That Thicken Stools

- Applesauce
- Bananas
- Bread
- Cheese
- Yogurt
- Pasta
- Pretzels
- Rice
- Tapioca
- Creamy peanut butter

Foods That Loosen Stools

- Chocolate
- Dried beans
- Fried foods
- Greasy foods
- Highly spiced foods
- Leafy green vegetables
- Raw fruits and juices
- Raw vegetables

Foods That Color Stools

- Beets
- Red gelatin

Nursing Care

Health Promotion

Primary prevention of colorectal cancer is a significant nursing care issue. Teach clients about dietary recommendations provided by the American Cancer Society for the prevention of colorectal cancer. These recommendations include decreasing the amount of fat, refined sugar, and red meats in the diet while increasing intake of dietary fiber. Foods that contain high amounts of fiber include raw fruits and vegetables, legumes, and whole-grain products.

Stress the importance of regular health examinations, including digital rectal exams. Discuss recommendations for regular hemoccult testing of stool after age 40. Include the importance of seeking medical treatment if blood is noted in or on the stool. Teach clients the warning signs for cancer, including those specific to bowel cancer, such as a change in bowel habits.

Assessment

- *Health history:* usual bowel patterns and any recent changes; weight loss, fatigue, decreased activity tolerance; presence of blood in the stool; pain with defecation, abdominal discomfort, perineal pain; usual diet; family history of colon cancer, other specific risk factors, such as inflammatory bowel disease or colon polyps.
- *Physical examination:* general appearance; weight; abdominal shape, contour; bowel sounds, abdominal tenderness; stool hemoccult or guaiac.

Nursing Diagnoses and Interventions

In planning and implementing care, consider both physical care needs and emotional response to the diagnosis. Because colorectal cancer is often advanced at the time of diagnosis, the prognosis, even with treatment, may be poor. Denial and anger are common. Extensive abdominal surgery and, potentially, a colostomy may be necessary, and the effects of chemotherapy and radiation therapy can leave the client fatigued and discouraged.

Nursing care includes providing emotional support, teaching, and direct care, before and after diagnostic procedures and surgery, and during adjunctive treatments. Priority nursing diagnoses include *pain, imbalanced nutrition,* and *anticipatory grieving. Risk for sexual dysfunction* should be considered as a priority diagnosis if a colostomy has been created.

Pain

The client with colorectal cancer may experience pain related to preparatory procedures, diagnostic examinations, and surgery. Following an abdominoperineal resection, "phantom" rectal pain related to severing nerves during the wide excision of the rectum may develop. Finally, the primary tumor itself and, potentially, metastatic tumors may impinge on nerves and other organs, causing pain. In the early postoperative period, an epidural infusion or patient-controlled analgesia (PCA) often is used to manage pain. PCA, routine administration of ordered analgesics, or a continuous analgesia delivery (CAD) system may also be used for pain management when the tumor is far enough advanced to preclude surgical resection. See Chapter 38 for more information on caring for clients with pain.

- Assess frequently for adequate pain relief. Use subjective and objective information, including the location, intensity, and character of the pain, as well as nonverbal signs, such as grimacing; muscle tension; apparent dozing; changes in pulse or blood pressure; rapid, shallow respirations. *The client may assume that pain is to be expected or tolerated or may fear becoming addicted to analgesic medications. Careful questioning and assessment can provide accurate information about pain status, allowing better control of discomfort.*
- Ask client to rate pain using a pain scale. Document the level of pain. *Pain is a subjective experience. Clients perceive and respond to pain differently. Religion and ethnic background may affect the response to pain.*
- Assess analgesic effectiveness 30 minutes after administration. Monitor for pain relief and adverse effects. *The method of delivery, dosage, or medication itself may need to be adjusted to provide adequate pain relief.*
- Assess the incision for inflammation or swelling; assess drainage catheters and tubes for patency. *Poorly controlled pain or pain that changes may be related to organ distention from an obstructed nasogastric tube, urinary catheter, or wound drain, or may indicate an infection.*

- Assess the abdomen for distention, tenderness, and bowel sounds. *Intra-abdominal bleeding, peritonitis, or paralytic ileus can cause pain that may be confused with incisional pain.*
- Administer analgesia prior to an activity or procedure. *Adequate pain relief reduces muscle tension, allowing for more comfortable participation in activities.*
- Assist with adjunctive relief measures, such as positioning, diversional activities, management of environmental stimuli, guided imagery, and teaching relaxation techniques. *These measures enhance the effects of analgesia by reducing muscle tension.*
- Splint incision with a pillow, and teach the client how to self-splint when coughing and deep breathing, *to prevent respiratory complications related to fear of pain.*

Imbalanced Nutrition: Less Than Body Requirements

Bowel preparation for diagnostic procedures and surgery, surgery, radiation therapy, and chemotherapy place the client with colorectal cancer at risk for nutritional deficiencies. Fluid and electrolyte replacement is provided following surgery, along with possible total parenteral nutrition (see Chapter 20). Adequate kcal and nutrient intake is necessary for healing after surgery. Additionally, if the tumor is advanced, metabolic needs may be increased and the appetite decreased.

- Assess nutritional status, using data such as height and weight, skinfold measurements, body mass index (BMI) calculation (see Chapter 17), and laboratory data including serum albumin level. Refer to dietitian or nutritionist for dietary management. *The client who is malnourished before beginning aggressive cancer treatment requires more vigorous nutrition management to promote healing.*
- Assess readiness for resumption of oral intake after surgery or procedures using data, such as statements of hunger, presence of bowel sounds, passage of flatus, and minimal abdominal distention. *Manipulation of the bowel interrupts peristalsis of the GI tract. It is important to ensure that peristalsis has resumed prior to resumption of oral intake.*
- Monitor and document food and fluid intake. *Documentation helps determine the adequacy of kilocalories and other nutrient intake.*
- Weigh daily. *Weight fluctuation may indicate adequate or inadequate dietary intake.*
- Maintain total parenteral nutrition and central intravenous lines as ordered. *Parenteral nutrition prevents tissue catabolism and promotes healing when food intake is disrupted for more than two to three days.*
- When oral intake resumes, help the client develop a meal plan that incorporates food preferences and considers the client's schedule and environment. *Consideration of likes, dislikes, and circumstances in meal planning promotes an adequate intake.*

Anticipatory Grieving

When a bowel resection is performed for colorectal cancer, the client needs to adjust to the loss of a major body part as well as to the diagnosis of cancer. Even when the prognosis for recovery is good, many people perceive cancer as fatal. Supporting the client and family during the initial stages of grieving can improve physical recovery as well as psychologic coping and eventual adaptation.

- Work to develop a trusting relationship with the client and family. *This increases the nurse's effectiveness in helping them work through the grieving process.*

- Listen actively, encouraging the client and family to express their fears and concerns. Assist to identify strengths, past experiences, and support systems.
  a. Demonstrate respect for cultural, spiritual, and religious values and beliefs; encourage use of these resources to cope with losses.
  b. Encourage discussion of the potential impact of loss on individual family members, family structure, and family function. Assist family members to share concerns with one another.
  c. Refer to cancer support groups, social services, or counseling as appropriate. *These resources can be used throughout the grieving process.*

Risk for Sexual Dysfunction

Colorectal cancer and ostomy surgery increase the risk for sexual dysfunction, defined as a change in sexual function, so that it becomes unsatisfying, unrewarding, inadequate (NANDA, 2001). Physical factors that can lead to sexual dysfunction include disruption of nerves and blood vessels that supply the genitals, radiation therapy, chemotherapy, and other medications prescribed after surgery.

- Psychologically, an *ostomate* (client with an ostomy), experiences an altered body image and may develop low selfesteem. The client may feel undesirable and fear rejection. He or she may be concerned about odors or pouch leakage during sexual activity. This emotional stress can also contribute to sexual dysfunction.
- Provide opportunities for the client and family to express feelings about the cancer diagnosis, ostomy, and effects of other treatments. *Encouraging verbalization of feelings about the diagnosis, ostomy, and treatments provides an opportunity to validate that feelings of anger and depression are normal responses to the diagnosis and change in body function.*
- Provide consistent colostomy care. *An accepting attitude and consistent care that provides a secure appliance and controls odor and leakage instills a sense of confidence in the client.*
- Encourage expression of sexual concerns. Provide privacy and caregivers who have established trust with the client and family and are comfortable in discussions about sexual concerns. *Sexuality is a very private concern to most people. The client and family are not likely to express their concerns openly unless trust has been established.*
- Reassure the client and significant other that the effect of physical illness and prescribed interventions on sexuality usually is temporary. *The client and partner may misinterpret an initial decrease in libido as evidence that sexual activity will not be possible or resume following recovery.*
- Refer the client and partner to social services or a family counselor for further interventions. *Clients are often discharged from acute care settings well before concerns about sexual activity surface. Ongoing counseling provides a continuing resource.*
- Arrange for a visit from a member of the United Ostomy Association. *People who are living and coping with an ostomy can provide information and support, helping the new ostomate overcome feelings of isolation and rejection.*

Home Care

During the diagnostic and preoperative periods, provide instruction about the following topics:

- Tests to be performed and preparatory procedures, including dietary restrictions, laxatives, enemas, and food and fluid restrictions just prior to the procedure
- Recommended postprocedure care and potential adverse effects to report
- Preoperative care, such as intestinal preparation and food and fluid restrictions.

If a colostomy is planned, refer to an enterostomal therapist for stoma placement and initial teaching.

Once treatment has been initiated, include the following topics (as appropriate) in teaching for home care:

- Pain management
- Skin care and management of potential adverse effects of radiation therapy and/or chemotherapy
- Incision and ostomy care
- Recommended diet
- Follow-up appointments and care.

If the tumor is inoperable or a cure is not anticipated, provide information about pain and symptom management. Discuss the hospice philosophy and available services. Provide a referral to a local hospice or home health department.

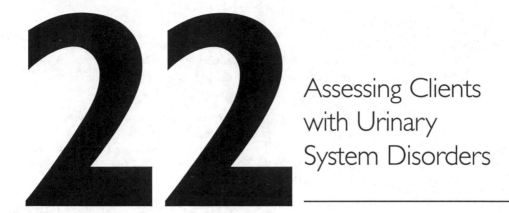

Assessing Clients with Urinary System Disorders

The functions of the renal system are to regulate body fluids, to filter metabolic wastes from the bloodstream, to reabsorb needed substances and water into the bloodstream, and to eliminate metabolic wastes and water as urine. Any alteration in the structure or function of the renal system affects the whole body. In turn, healthy urinary system function depends on the health of other body systems, especially the circulatory, endocrine, and nervous systems.

Review of Anatomy and Physiology

The organs of the urinary system are the paired kidneys, the paired ureters, the urinary bladder, and the urethra. Each structure is essential to the total functioning of the urinary system.

The Kidneys

The two kidneys are located outside the peritoneal cavity and on either side of the vertebral column at the levels of T12 through L3. These highly vascular, bean-shaped organs are approximately 4.5 inches (11.4 cm) long and 2.5 inches (6.4 cm) wide. The lateral surface of the kidney is convex; the medial surface is concave and forms a vertical cleft, the hilum. The ureter, renal artery, renal vein, lymphatic vessels, and nerves enter or exit the kidney at the level of the hilum.

The kidney is supported by three layers of connective tissue: the outer renal fascia, the middle adipose capsule, and the inner renal capsule. The renal fascia, made up of dense connective tissue, surrounds the kidney (and the adrenal gland, a discrete organ that sits on top of each kidney) and anchors it to surrounding structures. The middle adipose capsule is a fatty mass that holds the kidney in place and also cushions it against trauma. The inner renal capsule provides a barrier against infection and helps protect the kidney from trauma.

The functions of the kidney are to:

- Balance solute and water transport.
- Excrete metabolic waste products.
- Conserve nutrients.
- Regulate acid-base balance.
- Secrete hormones to help regulate blood pressure, erythrocyte production, and calcium metabolism.
- Form urine.

Internally, each kidney has three distinct regions: the cortex, medulla, and pelvis. The outer region, or renal cortex, is light in color and has a granular appearance. This region of the kidney contains the glomeruli, small clusters of capillaries. The glomeruli bring blood to and carry waste products from the nephrons, the functional units of the kidney.

The renal medulla, just below the cortex, contains cone-shaped tissue masses called renal pyramids, formed almost entirely of bundles of collecting tubules. Areas of lighter-colored tissue called renal columns are actually extensions of the cortex and serve to separate the pyramids. The collecting tubules that make up the pyramids channel urine into the innermost region, the renal pelvis.

The renal pelvis is continuous with the ureter as it leaves the hilum. Branches of the pelvis known as the major and minor calyces extend toward the medulla and serve to collect urine and empty it into the pelvis. From the pelvis, urine is channeled through the ureter and into the bladder for storage. The walls of the calyces, the renal pelvis, and the ureter contain smooth muscle that moves urine along by peristalsis.

Each kidney contains approximately 1 million nephrons, which process the blood to make urine. Each nephron contains a tuft of capillaries called the glomerulus, which is completely surrounded by the glomerular capsule (or Bowman's space). Together, the glomerulus and its surrounding capsule are called the renal corpuscle. The endothelium of the glomerulus allows capillaries to be extremely porous. Thus, large amounts of solute-rich fluid pass from the capillaries into the capsule. This fluid, called the filtrate, is the raw material of urine. Filtrate leaves the capsule and is channeled into the proximal convoluted tubule (PCT) of the nephron. Microvilli on the tubular cells increase the surface area for reabsorption of substances from the filtrate into plasma in the peritubular capillaries. Substances moved by active transport include glucose, sodium, potassium, amino acids, proteins, and vitamins. About 70% of the water in the filtrate, as well as chloride and bicarbonate, are reabsorbed by passive transport. The filtrate then moves into the U-shaped loop of Henle and is concentrated. The descending limb of the U is relatively thin and freely permeable to water, whereas the ascending segment is thick and thereby less permeable. The distal convoluted tubule (DCT) receives filtrate from the loop of Henle. Although this segment is structurally similar to the PCT, it lacks microvilli and is more involved with secreting solutes into the filtrate than in reabsorbing substances from it. The collecting duct receives the newly formed urine from many nephrons and channels urine through the minor and major calyces of the renal pelvis and into the ureter.

The Ureters

The ureters are bilateral tubes approximately 10 to 12 inches (25 to 30 cm) long. They transport urine from the kidney to the bladder through peristaltic waves originating in the renal pelvis. The wall of the ureter has three layers: an inner epithelial mucosa, a middle layer of smooth muscle, and an outer layer of fibrous connective tissue.

The Urinary Bladder

The urinary bladder is posterior to the symphysis pubis and serves as a storage site for urine. In males, the bladder lies immediately in front of the rectum; in females, the bladder lies next to the vagina and the uterus. Openings for the ureters and the urethra are inside the bladder: the trigone is the smooth triangular portion of the base of the bladder outlined by these three openings.

The layers of the bladder wall (from internal to external) are the epithelial mucosa lining the inside, the connective tissue submucosa, the smooth muscle layer, and the fibrous outer layer. The muscle layer, called the detrusor muscle, consists of fibers arranged in inner and outer longitudinal layers and in a middle circular layer. This arrangement allows the bladder to expand or contract according to the amount of urine it holds.

The size of the bladder varies with the amount of urine it contains. In healthy adults, the bladder holds about 300 to 500 mL of urine before internal pressure rises and signals the need to empty the bladder through **micturition** (also called *urination* or voiding). However, the bladder can hold more than twice that amount if necessary. The bladder has an internal urethral sphincter that relaxes in response to a full bladder and signals the need to urinate. A second external urethral sphincter is formed by skeletal muscle and is under voluntary control.

The Urethra

The urethra is a thin-walled muscular tube that channels urine to the outside of the body. It extends from the base of the bladder to the external urinary meatus. In females, the urethra is approximately 1.5 inches (3 to 5 cm) long, and the urinary meatus is anterior to the vaginal orifice. In males, the urethra is approximately 8 inches (20 cm) long and serves as a channel for semen as well as urine. The prostate gland encircles the urethra at the base of the bladder in males. The male urinary meatus is located at the end of the glans penis.

Formation of Urine

The complex structures of the kidneys process about 180 L (47 gal) of blood-derived fluid each day. Of this amount, only 1% is excreted as urine; the rest is returned to the circulation. (The normal characteristics of urine on laboratory analysis are listed in Table 22-1.) Urine formation is accomplished entirely by the nephron through three processes: glomerular filtration, tubular reabsorption, and tubular secretion.

Glomerular Filtration

Glomerular filtration is a passive, nonselective process in which hydrostatic pressure forces fluid and solutes through a membrane. The amount of fluid filtered from the blood into the capsule per minute is called the **glomerular filtration rate (GFR).** Three factors influence this rate: the total surface area available for filtration, the permeability of the filtration membrane, and the net filtration pressure.

Table 22-1.	Characteristics of Normal Urine
Color	Pale to deep yellow, clear
Odor	Aromatic
Specific gravity	1.001–1.030
pH	4.5–8.0
Protein	Negative to trace
Glucose	Negative
Ketones	Negative
WBCs	0–5/high power field (hpf)
RBCs	0–5/hpf
Casts	Negative to occasional

The glomerulus is a far more efficient filter than most capillary beds, because the filtration membrane of the glomerulus is much more permeable to water and solutes than are other capillary membranes. In addition, the glomerular blood pressure is much higher, resulting in higher net filtration pressure.

Net filtration pressure is responsible for the formation of filtrate and is determined by two forces: hydrostatic pressure ("push") and osmotic pressure ("pull"). The glomerular hydrostatic pressure pushes water and solutes across the membrane. This pressure is opposed by the osmotic pressure in the glomerulus (primarily the colloid osmotic pressure of plasma proteins in the glomerular blood) and the capsular hydrostatic pressure exerted by fluids within the glomerular capsule. The difference between these forces determines the net filtration pressure, which is directly proportional to the GFR.

The normal GFR in both kidneys is 120 to 125 mL/min in adults. This rate is held constant under normal conditions by intrinsic controls (or renal autoregulation). The myogenic mechanism, which responds to pressure changes in the renal blood vessels, controls the diameter of the afferent arterioles, thereby achieving autoregulation. An increase in systemic blood pressure causes the renal vessels to constrict, whereas a decline in blood pressure causes the afferent arterioles to dilate. These changes adjust the glomerular hydrostatic pressure and, indirectly, maintain the glomerular filtration rate.

Another intrinsic control of the GFR is the result of the **renin-angiotensin mechanism** at work in the kidneys. Special cells known as the juxtaglomerular apparatus are located in the distal tubules and respond to slow filtrate flow by releasing chemicals that cause intense vasodilation of the afferent arterioles. Conversely, an increase in the flow of filtrate promotes vasoconstriction, decreasing the GFR. A drop in systemic blood pressure often triggers the juxtaglomerular cells to release renin. Renin acts on a plasma globulin, angiotensinogen, to release angiotensin I, which is in turn converted to angiotensin II. As a vasoconstrictor, angiotensin II activates vascular smooth muscle throughout the body, causing systemic blood pressure to rise. Thus, the renin-angiotensin mechanism is a factor in renal autoregulation, even though its main purpose is the control of systemic blood pressure.

Glomerular filtration is also under an extrinsic control mechanism through the sympathetic nervous system. During periods of extreme stress or emergency, sympathetic nervous system stimulation causes strong constriction of the afferent arterioles and inhibits filtrate formation. The sympathetic nervous system also stimulates the juxtaglomerular cells to release renin, increasing systemic blood pressure.

Tubular Reabsorption

Tubular reabsorption is a transepithelial process that begins as the filtrate enters the proximal tubules. In healthy kidneys, virtually all organic nutrients such as glucose and amino acids are reabsorbed. However, the tubules constantly regulate and adjust the rate and degree of water and ion reabsorption in response to hormonal signals. Reabsorption may be active or passive. Substances reclaimed through active tubular reabsorption are usually moving against electrical and/or chemical gradients. These substances, including glucose, amino acids, lactate, vitamins, and most ions, require an ATP-dependent carrier to be transported into the interstitial space. In passive tubular reabsorption, which includes diffusion and osmosis, substances move along their gradient without expenditure of energy.

Tubular Secretion

The final process in urine formation is tubular secretion, which is essentially reabsorption in reverse. Substances, such as hydrogen and potassium ions, creatinine, ammonia, and organic acids, move from the blood of the peritubular capillaries into the tubules themselves as filtrate. Thus, urine consists of both filtered and secreted substances. Tubular secretion is important for disposing of substances not already in the filtrate, such as medications. This process eliminates undesirable substances that have been reabsorbed by passive processes and rids the body of excessive potassium ions. It is also a vital force in the regulation of blood pH.

Maintaining Normal Composition and Volume of Urine

Maintaining the normal composition and volume of urine involves a countercurrent exchange system. In this system, fluid flows in opposite directions through the parallel tubes of the loop of Henle and the vasa recta, tiny capillaries that run along the loop of Henle. Fluid is exchanged across these parallel membranes in response to a concentration gradient. When the filtrate enters the proximal convoluted tubule, its osmolality (at 300 mOsm/kg) is essentially the same as that of the plasma and the interstitial fluid of the renal cortex. Note the following steps in the process.

1. The descending loop of Henle is highly permeable to water and allows chloride and sodium to enter the loop through diffusion. The hyperosmotic interstitium causes water to move out of the descending loop, so that the remaining filtrate becomes increasingly concentrated.

2. The lumen of the ascending loop of Henle is impermeable to water but allows chloride and sodium to move out into the interstitium of the medulla. As a result, the filtrate in the ascending loop becomes hypo-osmotic, and the medullary interstitium becomes hyperosmotic.

3. As the filtrate progresses through the ascending limb of the loop of Henle and enters the distal convoluted tubule, sodium and chloride are removed and water is retained. Thus, the filtrate becomes more dilute.

4. As the filtrate passes through the deep medullary regions, urea (an end product of protein metabolism and, along with water, the main constituent of urine) begins to diffuse out from the collecting tubules into the interstitial space and establishes a concentration gradient to facilitate water movement.

5. Some urea enters the ascending loop of Henle. Urea entering the vasa recta typically diffuses out again.

The dilution or concentration of urine is largely determined by the action of antidiuretic hormone (ADH), which is secreted by the posterior pituitary gland. ADH causes the pores of the collecting tubules to enlarge, so that increased amounts of water move into the interstitial space. As the end result, water is reabsorbed and urine is more highly concentrated. When ADH is not secreted, the filtrate passes through the system without further water reabsorption, so that the urine is more dilute.

Urine is composed, by volume, of about 95% water and 5% solutes. The largest component of urine by weight is urea. Other solutes normally excreted in the urine include sodium, potassium, phosphate, sulfate, creatinine, uric acid, calcium, magnesium, and bicarbonate.

Clearance of Waste Products

The kidneys excrete water-soluble waste products and other chemicals or substances from the body. This process is called renal plasma clearance, which refers to the ability of the kidneys to clear (cleanse) a given amount of plasma of a particular substance in a given time (usually 1 minute). The kidneys clear 25 to 30 g of urea (a nitrogenous waste product formed in the liver from the breakdown of amino acids) each day. They also clear creatinine (an end product of creatine phosphate, found in skeletal muscle), uric acid (a metabolite of nucleic acid metabolism), and ammonia, as well as bacterial toxins and water-soluble drugs. Tests of renal clearance are often used to determine the GFR and glomerular damage.

Renal Hormones

Hormones either activated or synthesized by the kidneys include the active form of vitamin D, erythropoietin, and natriuretic hormone.

Vitamin D is necessary for the absorption of calcium and phosphate by the small intestine. In an inactive form, vitamin D enters the body either by dietary intake or through the action of ultraviolet rays on cholesterol in the skin. Activation occurs in two steps, the first in the liver and the second in the kidneys. The renal step is stimulated by parathyroid hormone, which in turn responds to a decreased plasma calcium level.

Erythropoietin stimulates the bone marrow to produce red blood cells in response to tissue hypoxia. The stimulus for the production of erythropoietin by the kidneys is decreased oxygen delivery to kidney cells.

The right atria of the heart releases natriuretic hormone in response to increased volume and stretch, as occurs in increased extracellular volume. This hormone inhibits ADH secretion, so that the collecting tubules are less porous and a large amount of dilute urine is produced.

Assessing Urinary System Function

The nurse conducts both a health assessment interview (to collect subjective data) and a physical assessment (to collect objective data) to assess the function of the urinary system.

The Health Assessment Interview

This section provides guidelines for collecting subjective data through a health assessment interview specific to urinary elimination. Problems with urinary elimination may be assessed as part of the total health assessment, or may be part of a focused interview if the client has problems specific to the urinary system.

Current urinary status should include the following data:

- Color, odor, and amount of urine
- Difficulty initiating a stream of urine
- Frequency of urination
- Painful urination (**dysuria**)
- Excessive urination at night (**nocturia**)
- Blood in the urine (**hematuria**)

- Voiding scant amounts of urine (**oliguria**)
- Voiding excessive amounts of urine (**polyuria**)
- Discharge
- Flank pain.

If you identify a problem with urinary elimination, analyze its onset, characteristics and course, severity, precipitating and relieving factors, and any associated symptoms, noting the timing and circumstances. For example, you may ask the following questions:

- Have you noticed any burning when you urinate?
- Do you have difficulty starting to urinate?
- When did you first notice that you were unable to control the loss of urine from your bladder?

Further explore any abnormalities in the client's current urinary status. Focus questions on changes in patterns of urination, changes in the urine, and pain.

Assess changes in patterns of urination by asking the client these questions: How many times a day do you urinate? Do you feel that you empty your bladder each time? How many times do you get up at night to urinate? Do you experience a very strong desire to urinate and feel that you just cannot wait? Have you noticed that you urinate small amounts of dark, strong-smelling urine?

Changes in the urine that should be explored include the presence of blood or a cloudy appearance of the urine. If the client has noticed blood, explore the use of medications, such as anticoagulants or dye-containing drugs, and other bleeding problems. Women may not understand that blood in the toilet after urination is normal during menstruation. Cloudy, foul-smelling urine often indicates infection (**pyuria**); ask the client about temperature elevations, chills, and general malaise. Cloudy urine in men may result from retrograde ejaculation (when semen is discharged into the bladder instead of from the penis) during intercourse.

If the client reports pain, explore its location, duration, and intensity. Kidney pain is experienced in the back and the costovertebral angle (the angle between the lower ribs and adjacent vertebrae) and may spread toward the umbilicus. Renal colic is severe, sharp, stabbing, and excruciating; often it is felt in the flank, bladder, urethra, testes, or ovaries. Bladder and urethral pain is usually dull and continuous, but may be experienced as spasms. The client with a distended bladder experiences constant pain increased by any pressure over the bladder.

Information about surgeries or other treatment of previous urinary problems is essential to the health history, as is a family history of altered structure or function. A family history of renal problems may be the first clue to abnormalities in the client's urinary function. Explore information regarding family occurrence of end-stage renal disease, renal calculi, and frequent infections, as well as related problems, such as hypertension and diabetes mellitus.

Questions about lifestyle, diet, and work history should explore cigarette smoking, exposure to toxic chemicals, usual fluid intake, type of fluid intake, and self-care measures to replace fluids lost during work or physical activity in hot temperatures.

Physical Assessment

Physical assessment of the urinary system may be performed as part of a total health assessment, as part of an abdominal assessment, or as part of the back examination (for the kidneys). For clients with known or suspected problems of this system, assessment requires the techniques of inspection, palpation, percussion, and auscultation. Auscultate immediately after inspection because percussion or palpation may increase bowel motility and interfere with sound transmission during auscultation.

The equipment necessary to assess the urinary system is a urine specimen cup and disposable gloves. At the beginning of the assessment, the client may be sitting or lying supine. Prior to the examination, collect all necessary equipment and explain the techniques to the client to decrease anxiety.

Before beginning the assessment, ask the client to provide you with a clean-catch urine specimen and give the client a specimen cup. Assess the specimen for color, odor, and clarity before you send it to the laboratory.

Because the examination involves exposure of the genital area, give the client a gown and drape the client appropriately to minimize exposure.

Skin Assessment with Abnormal Findings (✓)

- Inspect the skin and mucous membranes, noting color, turgor, and excretions.

  ✓ Pallor of the skin and mucous membranes may indicate kidney disease with resultant anemia.
  ✓ Decreased turgor of the skin may indicate dehydration.
  ✓ Edema may indicate fluid volume excess.

(Either change in turgor may indicate renal insufficiency with either excess fluid loss or retention.)

  ✓ An accumulation of uric acid crystals, called *uremic frost*, may be seen on the skin of the client with untreated renal failure.

Abdominal Assessment with Abnormal Findings (✓)

- Inspect the abdomen, noting size, symmetry, masses or lumps, swelling, prominent veins, distention, glistening, or skin tightness.

  ✓ Enlargements or asymmetry may indicate a hernia or superficial mass.
  ✓ Prominent veins may indicate renal dysfunction.
  ✓ Distention, glistening, or skin tightness may be associated with fluid retention.
  ✓ Ascites is an accumulation of fluid in the peritoneal cavity.

Urinary Meatus Assessment with Abnormal Findings (✓)

(This technique is not part of a routine assessment, but it is an important component in clients with health problems of the urinary system.)

- For the male client: With the client in a sitting or standing position, compress the tip of the glans penis with your gloved hand to open the urinary meatus.
- For the female client: With the client in the dorsal lithotomy position, spread the labia with your gloved hand to expose the urinary meatus.

✓ Increased redness, swelling, or discharge may indicate infection or sexually transmitted disease.

✓ Ulceration may indicate a sexually transmitted disease.

✓ In male clients, a deviation of the meatus from the midline may suggest a congenital defect.

Kidney Assessment with Abnormal Findings (✓)

• Auscultate the renal arteries by placing the bell of the stethoscope lightly in the areas of the renal arteries, located in the left and right upper abdominal quadrants.

✓ Systolic bruits ("whooshing" sounds) may indicate renal artery stenosis.

• Percuss the kidneys for tenderness or pain.

✓ Tenderness and pain on percussion of the costovertebral angle suggest glomerulonephritis or glomerulonephrosis.

• Palpate the kidneys.

✓ A mass or lump may indicate a tumor or cyst.

✓ Tenderness or pain on palpation may suggest an inflammatory process.

✓ A soft kidney that feels spongy may indicate chronic renal disease.

✓ Bilaterally enlarged kidneys may suggest polycystic kidney disease.

✓ Unequal kidney size may indicate hydronephrosis.

Bladder Assessment with Abnormal Findings (✓)

• Percuss the bladder for tone and position.

✓ A dull percussion tone over the bladder of a client who has just urinated may indicate urinary retention.

• Palpate the bladder (over the symphysis pubis and abdomen) for distention.

✓ A distended bladder may be palpated at any point from the symphysis pubis to the umbilicus and is felt as a firm, rounded organ.

23 Nursing Care of Clients with Urinary Tract Disorders

The urinary system includes the kidneys, ureters, urinary bladder, and urethra. This organ system can be affected by a variety of disorders, including congenital malformations, infections, obstructions, trauma, tumors, and neurologic conditions. Any portion of the system—from the kidney through the urethra—can be affected with serious or even life-threatening consequences unless the problem is appropriately diagnosed and treated. Kidney disorders can affect urine production and waste elimination directly, and are discussed in the next chapter. Disorders of the **urinary drainage system** (the kidney pelvis, ureters, bladder, and urethra) may obstruct urine flow or spread to the kidneys, affecting urine production and elimination. The anatomy and physiology and nursing assessment related to the urinary tract is presented in Chapter 22.

When caring for clients with urinary tract disorders, it is important to consider the client's modesty in voiding, possible difficulty in discussing the genitals, embarrassment about being exposed for examination and testing, and fear of changes in body image or function. These psychosocial issues may interfere with the client's willingness to seek help, discuss treatment, and learn about preventive measures.

Nursing interventions for clients with urinary tract disorders are directed toward primary prevention, early detection, and management of the disorder through health teaching and nursing care.

The Client with a Urinary Tract Infection

Bacterial infections of the urinary tract are a common reason for seeking health services, second only to upper respiratory infections. More than 8 million people are treated annually for urinary tract infection (UTI) (Porth, 2002). Community-acquired UTIs are common in young women, and unusual in men under the age of 50.

Most community-acquired UTIs are caused by *Escherichia coli*, a common gram-negative enteral bacteria. About 10% to 15% of symptomatic UTIs are caused by *Staphylococcus saprophyticus*, a gram-positive organism. Catheter-associated UTIs often involve other gram-negative bacteria, such as *Proteus, Klebsiella, Seratia,* and *Pseudomonas.*

Physiology Review

The urinary tract is normally sterile above the urethra. Adequate urine volume, a free flow from the kidneys through the urinary meatus, and complete bladder emptying are the most important mechanisms maintaining sterility. Pathogens that enter and contaminate the distal urethra are washed out during voiding. Other defenses for maintaining sterile urine include its normal acidity and bacteriostatic properties of the bladder and urethral cells. The peristaltic activity of the ureters and a competent ureterovesical junction help maintain sterility of the upper urinary tract. As the ureter enters the bladder, its distal portion tunnels between the mucosa and muscle layers of the bladder wall. During voiding, increased *intravesicular* (within the bladder) pressure compresses the ureter, preventing **reflux,** or backflow of urine toward the kidneys. In males, a long urethra and the antibacterial effect of zinc in prostatic fluid also help prevent contamination of this normally sterile environment.

Pathophysiology and Manifestations

Pathogens usually enter the urinary tract by ascending from the mucous membranes of the perineal area into the lower urinary tract. Bacteria that have colonized the urethra, vagina, or perineal tissues are the usual source of infection (Porth, 2002). From the bladder, bacteria may continue to ascend the urinary tract, eventually infecting the *parenchyma* (functional tissue) of the kidneys (Braunwald, et al., 2001). Hematogenous spread of infection to the urinary tract is rare. Infections introduced in this manner are usually associated with previous damage or scarring of the urinary tract. Bacteria introduced into the urinary tract may cause asymptomatic bacteriuria or in an inflammatory response with manifestations of UTI.

Urinary tract infections can be categorized in several ways. Anatomically, UTIs may affect the lower or the upper urinary tract. Lower urinary tract infections include *urethritis*, inflammation of the urethra; *prostatitis,* inflammation of the prostate gland; and **cystitis,** inflammation of the urinary bladder. The most common upper urinary tract infection is **pyelonephritis,** inflammation of the kidney and renal pelvis. The infection may involve superficial tissues, such as the bladder mucosa, or may invade other tissues, such as prostate or renal tissues. Epidemiologically, UTIs are identified as community acquired or nosocomial, associated with catheterization.

Clients can be predisposed to UTI by a variety of factors. Some risk factors cannot be changed (e.g., aging and the short urethra of the female). In women, sexual activity increases the risk for UTI, as bacteria are introduced into the bladder via the urethra during sexual intercourse. Use of spermicidal compounds with a diaphragm, cervical cap, or condom alters the normal bacterial flora of the vagina and perineal tissues, and further increases the risk for UTI. Some females lack a normally protective mucosal enzyme and have decreased levels of cervicovaginal antibodies to enterobacteria, further increasing their risk. Prostatic hypertrophy and bacterial prostatitis are risk factors among males. Circumcision appears to have a protective effect. Anal intercourse is also a risk factor for men. Congenital or acquired factors contributing to the risk of infection include urinary tract obstruction by tumors or calculi, structural abnormalities, such as strictures, impaired bladder innervation, bowel incontinence, and chronic diseases, such as diabetes mellitus. Instrumentation of the urinary tract (e.g., catheterization or cystoscopy) is a major risk factor for UTI. Even when performed under strict aseptic conditions, catheterization can result in bladder infection. The placement of the catheter prevents the flushing action of voiding, and bacteria may ascend to the bladder either through the catheter lumen or via exudate between the urethral mucosa and the catheter.

Older clients have an increased incidence of UTI. The greatest degree of increase is seen in men, as the ratio of female to male UTI in older adults changes from 50:1 to less than 5:1. An increased risk of urinary stasis, chronic disease states, such as diabetes mellitus, and an impaired immune response contribute to the higher incidence of UTI in the older adult. In men, the prostate typically hypertrophies with aging, potentially resulting in urinary retention as the urethra narrows. Prostatic secretions are lessened, diminishing their protective, antibacterial effect. In older women, loss of tissue elasticity and weakening of perineal muscles often contribute to the development of a cystocele or rectocele. Resulting changes in bladder and urethral position increase the risk of incomplete bladder emptying.

Cystitis

Cystitis, inflammation of the urinary bladder, is the most common UTI. The infection tends to remain superficial, involving the bladder mucosa. The mucosa becomes hyperemic (red) and may hemorrhage. The inflammatory response causes pus to form. This process causes the classic manifestations associated with cystitis. Typical presenting symptoms of cystitis include **dysuria** (painful or difficult urination), urinary frequency and **urgency** (a sudden, compelling need to urinate), and **nocturia** (voiding two or more times at night). In addition, the urine may have a foul odor and appear cloudy (*pyuria*) or bloody (**hematuria**) because of mucus, excess white cells in the urine, and bleeding of the inflamed bladder wall. Suprapubic pain and tenderness may also be present.

Older clients may not experience the classic symptoms of cystitis. Instead, they often present with nonspecific manifestations, such as nocturia, incontinence, confusion, behavior change, lethargy, anorexia, or "just not feeling right." Fever may be present; however, hypothermia may also develop in an older adult.

Cystitis occurs most frequently in adult females, usually because of colonization of the bladder by bacteria normally found in the lower gastrointestinal tract. These bacteria gain entry by ascending the short, straight female urethra. Personal hygiene practices and voluntary urinary retention can also contribute to the risk for UTI in women.

Although the bacteriostatic effect of prostatic fluid and a longer urethra provide an effective barrier to bladder infection for adult males, prostatic hypertrophy commonly associated with aging increases the risk of cystitis in elderly males. An enlarged prostate can impede urine flow, leading to incomplete bladder emptying and urinary stasis. Bacteria are not completely flushed with voiding, allowing colonization of the bladder.

Cystitis is usually uncomplicated and readily responds to treatment. When left untreated, the infection can ascend to involve the kidneys. Severe or prolonged infection may lead to sloughing of bladder mucosa and ulcer formation. Chronic cystitis can lead to bladder stones.

Catheter-Associated UTI

At least 10% to 15% of hospitalized clients with indwelling urinary catheters develop bacteriuria. The longer the catheter remains in place, the greater the risk for infection. Bacteria, including *E. coli, Proteus, Pseudomonas, Klebsiella,* and others, reach the bladder by either migrating through the column of urine within the catheter or by moving up the mucous sheath of the urethra outside the catheter (Braunwald, et al., 2001). Bacteria enter the catheter system at the connection between the catheter and drainage system or through the emptying tube of the drainage bag. Colonization of perineal skin by bowel flora is a common source of infection in catheterized women.

Catheter-associated UTIs often are asymptomatic. Gram-negative bacteremia is the most significant complication associated with these UTIs. Most catheter-associated UTIs resolve quickly when the catheter is removed and a short course of antibiotic is administered. Intermittent catheterization carries a lower risk of infection than does an indwelling catheter, and is preferred for clients who are unable to empty their bladder by voiding.

Pyelonephritis

Pyelonephritis is inflammation of the renal pelvis and *parenchyma*, the functional kidney tissue. *Acute pyelonephritis* is a bacterial infection of the kidney; *chronic pyelonephritis* is associated with nonbacterial infections and inflammatory processes that may be metabolic, chemical, or immunologic in origin.

Acute Pyelonephritis

Acute pyelonephritis usually results from an infection that ascends to the kidney from the lower urinary tract. Asymptomatic bacteriuria or cystitis can lead to acute pyelonephritis. Risk factors include pregnancy (because of slowed ureteral peristalsis), urinary tract obstruction, and congenital malformation. Urinary tract trauma, scarring, calculi (stones), kidney disorders such as polycystic or hypertensive kidney disease, and chronic diseases, such as diabetes may also contribute to pyelonephritis. *Vesicoureteral reflux,* a condition in which urine moves from the bladder back toward the kidney, is a common risk factor in children who develop pyelonephritis and is also seen in adults when bladder outflow is obstructed.

The infection spreads from the renal pelvis to the renal cortex. The pelvis, calyces, and medulla of the kidney are primarily affected, with white blood cell infiltration and inflammation. The kidney becomes grossly edematous. Localized abscesses may develop on the cortical surface of the kidney (Bullock & Henze, 2000). As with cystitis, *E. coli* is the organism responsible for 85% of the cases of acute pyelonephritis. Other organisms commonly found include *Proteus* and *Klebsiella,* bacteria that normally inhabit the intestinal tract.

The onset of acute pyelonephritis is typically rapid, with chills and fever, malaise, vomiting, flank pain, costovertebral tenderness, urinary frequency, and dysuria. Symptoms of cystitis may also be present. The older adult may experience a change in behavior, acute confusion, incontinence, or a general deterioration in condition.

Chronic Pyelonephritis

Chronic pyelonephritis involves chronic inflammation and scarring of the tubules and interstitial tissues of the kidney (Bullock & Henze, 2000). It is a common cause of chronic renal failure. It may develop as a result of UTIs or other conditions that damage the kidneys, such as hypertension or vascular conditions, severe vesicoureteral reflux, or obstruction of the urinary tract.

The client with chronic pyelonephritis may be asymptomatic or have mild manifestations, such as urinary frequency, dysuria, and flank pain. Hypertension can develop as kidney tissue is destroyed.

Collaborative Care

Treatment of UTI focuses on eliminating the causative organism, preventing relapse or reinfection, and identifying and correcting any contributing factors. Drug treatment with antibiotics and urinary anti-infectives is commonly used. In some cases, surgery may be indicated to correct contributing factors.

Diagnostic Tests

Laboratory testing for UTI includes:

- *Urinalysis* to assess for pyuria, bacteria, and blood cells in the urine. A bacteria count greater than 100,000 (10^5) per milliliter is indicative of infection. Rapid tests for bacteria in the urine include using a *nitrite dipstick* (which turns pink in the presence of bacteria) and the *leukocyte esterase test,* an indirect method of detecting bacteria by identifying lysed or intact white blood cells (WBCs) in the urine.

Urine should be a midstream clean-catch specimen; if necessary, straight catheterization or "mini-cath," with strict aseptic technique may be used. Catheterization is avoided if possible to reduce the risk of further infection.

- *Gram stain of the urine* may be done to identify the infecting organism by shape and characteristic (Gram positive or negative).
- *Urine culture and sensitivity* tests may be ordered to identify the infecting organism and the most effective antibiotic. Culture requires 24 to 72 hours, so treatment to eliminate the most common organisms is often initiated without culture.
- *WBC with differential* may be done to detect typical changes associated with infection, such as *leukocytosis* (elevated WBC) and increased numbers of neutrophils.

In men and in adult women with recurrent infections or persistent bacteriuria, additional diagnostic testing may be ordered to evaluate for structural abnormalities and other contributing factors.

- *Intravenous pyelography (IVP),* also known as *excretory urography,* is used to evaluate the structure and excretory function of the kidneys, ureters, and bladder. As the kidneys clear an intravenously injected contrast medium from the blood, the size and shape of the kidneys, their calices and pelvises, the ureters, and the bladder can be evaluated, and structural or functional abnormalities, such as vesicoureteral reflux, may be detected.
- *Voiding cystourethrography* involves instilling contrast medium into the bladder, then using X-rays to assess the bladder and urethra when filled and during voiding. This study can detect structural or functional abnormalities of the bladder and urethral strictures. This test has a lower risk of allergic response to the contrast dye than IVP.
- *Cystoscopy,* direct visualization of the urethra and bladder through a cystoscope, may be used to diagnose conditions, such as prostatic hypertrophy, urethral strictures, bladder calculi, tumors, polyps or diverticula, and congenital abnormalities. A tissue biopsy may be obtained during the procedure, and other interventions performed (e.g., stone removal or stricture dilation).
- *Manual pelvic or prostate examinations* are done to assess for structural changes of the genitourinary tract, such as prostatic enlargement, cystocele, or rectocele.

Medications

Most uncomplicated infections of the lower urinary tract can be treated with a short course of antibiotic therapy. Upper urinary tract infections, in contrast, usually require longer treatment (two or more weeks) to eradicate the infecting organism.

Short-course therapy (either a single antibiotic dose or a 3-day course of treatment) reduces treatment cost, increases compliance, and has a lower rate of side effects. Single dose therapy is associated with a higher rate of recurrent infection and continued vaginal colonization with *E. coli,* making a 3-day course of treatment the preferred option for uncomplicated cystitis. Oral trimethoprim-sulfamethoxazole (TMP-SMZ), TMP, or a quinolone antibiotic such as ciprofloxacin (Cipro) or enoxacin (Penetrex) may be ordered.

Men and women with pyelonephritis, urinary tract abnormalities or stones, or a history of previous infections with antibiotic-resistant infections require a 7 to 10 day course of TMP-SMZ, ciprofloxacin, ofloxacin (Floxin), or an alternate antibiotic. The client with severe illness may need hospitalization. Intravenous ciprofloxacin, gentamicin, ceftriaxone (Rocephin), or ampicillin may be prescribed for severe illness or sepsis associated with UTI. See Chapter 41 for the nursing implications for antibiotic therapy.

The outcome of treatment for UTI is determined by follow-up urinalysis and culture. *Cure,* as evidenced by no pathogens present in the urine, is the desired outcome. When therapy fails to eradicate bacteria in the urine, it is known as *unresolved bacteriuria. Persistent bacteriuria* or *relapse* occurs when a persistent source of infection causes repeated infection after initial cure. *Reinfection* is the development of a new infection with a different pathogen following successful UTI treatment (Tierney, et al., 2001).

Clients who experience frequent symptomatic UTIs may be treated with prophylactic antibiotic therapy with a drug such as TMP-SMZ, TMP, or nitrofurantoin (Furadantin, Nitrofan). TMP and nitrofurantoin do not achieve effective plasma concentrations at recommended doses, but do reach effective concentrations in the urine. Nitrofurantoin also may be used to treat UTI in pregnant women. Nursing implications for these urinary anti-infectives and for phenazopyridine (Pyridium), a urinary analgesic, are outlined in Table 23-1.

Antibiotics and urinary anti-infectives are not generally recommended to treat asymptomatic bacteriuria in catheterized clients. The preferred treatment for catheter-associated UTI is removal of the indwelling catheter followed by a 10 to 14 day course of antibiotic therapy to eliminate the infection.

Surgery

Surgery may be indicated for recurrent UTI if diagnostic testing indicates calculi, structural anomalies, or strictures that contribute to the risk of infection.

Table 23-1. Medication Administration – Urinary Anti-Infectives and Analgesics

Urinary Anti-Infectives

Nitrofurantoin (Furadantin; Macrodantin)
Trimethoprim (Proloprim, Trimpex)

Table 23-1. Continued

Urinary anti-infectives are usually used prophylactically to prevent recurrence of UTI in clients with frequent symptomatic infections. Nitrofurantoin may also be used to treat UTI in pregnant women.

Nursing Responsibilities
- Ensure adequate fluid intake (1500 to 2000 mL per day) to maintain a urine output of at least 1500 mL of urine per 24 hours. Do not overhydrate.
- Administer with meals to minimize GI side effects, such as nausea, gastric upset, and abdominal cramping.
- Trimethoprim is contraindicated for use in clients with renal or hepatic impairment; nitrofurantoin is contraindicated for clients with impaired renal function. Report abnormal laboratory values, such as elevated creatinine or BUN, bilirubin, alanine aminotransferase (ALT), aspartate aminotransferase (AST), and lactic dehydrogenase (LDH).
- Use with caution in older or chronically ill clients. Monitor closely for adverse effects.
- Do not administer trimethoprim to pregnant women because of possible adverse effects on the fetus.
- Monitor the client taking nitrofurantoin for an acute or chronic pulmonary reaction with manifestations of dyspnea, cough, chills, fever, and chest pain. Discontinue the drug and notify the physician.
- Nitrofurantoin may cause peripheral neuropathy, especially in older clients and adult diabetics. Notify the physician if symptoms develop.
- Nitrofurantoin oral suspension may stain the teeth; have the client rinse the mouth thoroughly after administering.
- Monitor for signs of phenytoin toxicity (sedation, ataxia, and increased blood levels) if trimethoprim is given concurrently. Phenytoin doses may need to be reduced.

Client and Family Teaching
- These drugs are used along with hygiene practices to prevent recurrent UTI. Take as directed, even when no symptoms are present.
- Drink six to eight glasses of water or fluid per day while taking these drugs.
- Take the drug with meals or food to reduce gastric effects; however, avoid milk products because they may interfere with absorption.
- Trimethoprim should not be taken during pregnancy. Contact your physician before attempting to become pregnant.
- Contact your doctor if you develop any of the following: chest pain, difficulty breathing, cough, chills, and fever; numbness and tingling or weakness of the extremities; rash or pruritus (itching).
- If you are taking an oral suspension of nitrofurantoin, rinse your mouth thoroughly after each dose to avoid staining the teeth.
- Nitrofurantoin turns the urine brown. This is not harmful and subsides when the drug is discontinued.
- If you are taking trimethoprim along with phenytoin (Dilantin) or a related anticonvulsant, contact your doctor if you become sedated or begin to stagger.

Continued on the next page

Table 23-1. Continued

Urinary Analgesic

Phenazopyridine (Pyridium)

Phenazopyridine is a urinary tract analgesic that may be used for symptomatic relief of the pain, burning, frequency, and urgency associated with UTI during the first 24 to 48 hours of therapy. Its use is somewhat controversial, because it does not treat the infection and may delay effective treatment in the client with recurrent UTI who saves a dose or two "for the next time."

Nursing Responsibilities
- Monitor renal function (urine output, weight, serum creatinine, and BUN) during treatment; report changes.
- Stop the drug and contact the physician if sclera or skin become yellow-tinged. This may indicate reduced excretion and toxicity.

Client and Family Teaching
- Take with meals to minimize gastric upset.
- This drug turns urine orange or red. Protect your clothing from staining.
- Promptly contact your doctor if symptoms of UTI recur; do not take phenazopyridine before you seek medical treatment.
- If you notice a yellow tinge to your skin or eyes, stop taking the drug and notify the physician.

Stones, or *calculi,* in the renal pelvis or in the bladder are an irritant and provide a matrix for bacterial colonization. Treatment may include surgical removal of a large calculus from the renal pelvis or cystoscopic removal of bladder calculi. *Percutaneous ultrasonic pyelolithotomy* or *extracorporeal shock wave lithotripsy (ESWL)* may be used instead of surgery to crush and remove stones.

Ureteroplasty, surgical repair of a ureter, may be indicated for structural abnormality or stricture of a ureter. This may be combined with a ureteral reimplantation if vesicoureteral reflux is present. The client returns from these surgeries with an indwelling urinary catheter (Foley or suprapubic) and a **ureteral stent** (a thin catheter inserted into the ureter to provide for urine flow and ureteral support), which remains in place for three to five days.

Complementary Therapies

Complementary therapies, such as aromatherapy or herbal preparations, may be used in conjunction with antibiotics to treat UTI. Adding bergamot, sandalwood, lavender, or juniper oil to bath water helps relieve the discomfort of UTI. Herbal supplements, such as saw palmetto, have a urinary antiseptic effect, and may be beneficial in treating or preventing UTI. Consult a qualified herbologist for recommended doses and appropriate use.

Nursing Care

Health Promotion

Teach measures to prevent UTI to all clients, particularly to young, sexually active women. Encourage clients to maintain a generous fluid intake of 2.0 to 2.5 quarts per day, increasing intake during hot weather or strenuous activity. Discuss the need to avoid voluntary urinary retention, emptying the bladder every three to four hours. Instruct women to cleanse the perineal area from front to back after voiding and defecating. Teach client to void before and after sexual intercourse to flush out bacteria introduced into the urethra and bladder. Teach measures to maintain the integrity of perineal tissues: Avoid bubble baths, feminine hygiene sprays, and vaginal douches; wear cotton briefs, avoid synthetic materials; if postmenopausal, use hormone replacement therapy or estrogen cream. Unless contraindicated, suggest measures to maintain acid urine: Drink two glasses of cranberry juice daily; take ascorbic acid (vitamin C), and avoid excess intake of milk and milk products, other fruit juices, and sodium bicarbonate (baking soda).

Assessment

Focused assessment data for the client with a UTI includes the following:

- *Health history:* current symptoms, including frequency, urgency, burning on urination, voidings per night; color, clarity, and odor of urine; other manifestations, such as lower abdominal, back, or flank pain, nausea or vomiting, fever; duration of symptoms and any treatment attempted; history of previous UTIs and their frequency; possibility of pregnancy and type of birth control used; chronic diseases, such as diabetes; current medications and any known allergies.
- *Physical examination:* general health; vital signs including temperature; abdominal shape, contour, tenderness to palpation (especially suprapubic); percuss for costovertebral tenderness (see Table 22-1).

See Chapter 22 for complete nursing assessment of the urinary system.

Nursing Diagnoses and Interventions

The client's general health, abilities for self-care, and risk factors that may contribute to UTI are considered when planning and implementing nursing care for the client with a UTI. Priority nursing diagnoses focus on comfort, urinary elimination, and teaching/learning needs.

Pain

Pain is a common manifestation of both lower and upper UTI. Urinary tract pain is caused primarily by distention and increased pressure within the tract. The severity of the pain is related to the rate at which inflammation and distention develop, not their degree.

In cystitis, inflammation causes a sensation of fullness; dull, constant suprapubic pain; and possibly low back pain. The inflamed bladder wall and urethra cause dysuria, pain, and burning on urination. Bladder spasms may develop, causing periodic severe, stabbing discomfort. Pain associated with pyelonephritis is often steady and dull, localized to the outer abdomen or flank region. Urologic disorders rarely cause central abdominal pain.

- Assess pain: timing, quality, intensity, location, duration, and aggravating and alleviating factors. *A change in the nature, location, or intensity of the pain could indicate an extension of the infection or a related but separate problem.*

- Teach or provide comfort measures, such as warm sitz baths, warm packs or heating pads, balanced rest and activity. Systemic analgesics, urinary analgesics, or antispasmodic medication may be used as ordered. *Warmth relaxes muscles, relieves spasms, and increases local blood supply. Because pain can stimulate a stress response and delay healing, it should be relieved when possible.*

- Increase fluid intake unless contraindicated. *Increased fluid dilutes urine, reducing irritation of the inflamed bladder and urethral mucosa.*

Impaired Urinary Elimination

Inflammation of the bladder and urethral mucosa affects the normal process and patterns of voiding, causing frequency, urgency, and burning on urination, as well as nocturia. Urine may be blood-tinged, cloudy, and malodorous. The client with short- or long-term urinary retention requires additional measures to assess for and prevent UTI.

- Monitor (or instruct the client to monitor) color, clarity, and odor of urine. *Urine should return to clear yellow within 48 hours, unless drug therapy causes a change in the color of urine. If clarity does not return, further investigation may be necessary.*

- Instruct to avoid caffeinated drinks, including coffee, tea, and cola; citrus juices, drinks containing artificial sweeteners; and alcoholic beverages. *Caffeine, citrus juices, and artificial sweeteners irritate bladder mucosa and the detrusor muscle, and can increase urgency and bladder spasms.*

- Use strict aseptic technique and a closed urinary drainage system when inserting a straight or indwelling urinary catheter. *Bacteria colonizing the perineal tissues or on the nurse's hands can be introduced into the bladder during catheterization. Aseptic technique reduces this risk.*

- When possible, use intermittent straight catheterization to relieve urinary retention. Remove indwelling urinary catheters as soon as possible. *Using intermittent straight catheterization allows the bladder to fill and completely empty in a more normal manner, maintaining physiologic function. The risk of infection associated with an indwelling catheter is about 3% to 5% per day of catheterization* (Braunwald, et al., 2001).

- Maintain the closed urinary drainage system, and use aseptic technique when emptying catheter drainage bag. Maintain gravity flow, preventing reflux of urine into the bladder from the drainage system. *Bacteria can enter the drainage system when its integrity is interrupted (e.g., disconnecting the catheter from the drainage system) or during emptying of the drainage bag. These bacteria can ascend the column of urine to the bladder, causing UTI.*

- Provide perineal care on a regular basis and following defecation. Use antiseptic preparations only as ordered. *Regular cleansing of perineal tissues reduces the risk of colonization by bowel or other bacteria. While antiseptic solutions may be ordered for catheter care, they can dry perineal tissues and reduce normal flora, increasing the risk of colonization by pathogens, and should not routinely be used.*

Ineffective Health Maintenance

The client with a urinary tract infection is at an increased risk for future UTI and needs to understand the disease process, risk factors, measures to prevent recurrent infection, diagnostic procedures, and home care. In addition, once the manifestations of UTI are relieved, motivation to continue the treatment plan declines. Failure to complete the full course of therapy and recommended follow-up can lead to continued bacteriuria and recurrent infections.

- Teach client how to obtain a midstream clean-catch urine specimen. *Cleansing of the urinary meatus and perineal area reduces contamination of the specimen by external cells and bacteria. 90% of urethral bacteria are cleared in the first 10 mL of voided urine; a midstream specimen is representative of urine in the bladder.*

- Assess knowledge about the disease process, risk factors, and preventive measures. *The client may have little understanding of UTI, its causes, and contributing factors.*

- Discuss the prescribed treatment plan and the importance of taking all prescribed antibiotics.

- Help the client develop a plan for taking medications, such as taking them with meals (unless contraindicated) or setting out all doses for the day in the morning. *Missed doses of antibiotic can result in subtherapeutic blood levels and reduced effectiveness. Taking medication in association with a regular daily activity such as meals helps clients remember doses.*

- Instruct to keep appointments for follow-up and urine culture. *Follow-up urine culture, often scheduled 7 to 14 days after completion of antibiotic therapy, is vital to ensure complete eradication of bacteria and prevent relapse or recurrence.*

- Teach measures to prevent future UTI (see the preceding Health Promotion section). *Keeping urine dilute and acidic, and voiding regularly flush bacteria out of the bladder and urethra. The proximity of the female urethral meatus to the vagina and anus increases the risk of bacterial contamination, especially during intercourse. Bubble baths, feminine hygiene sprays, synthetic fibers, and douches may dry and irritate perineal tissues, promoting bacterial growth.*

Home Care

Because both upper and lower urinary tract infections are usually managed in the community, teaching is the most important nursing intervention. Provide instruction on the following topics:

- Risk factors for UTI and how to minimize or eliminate these factors through increased fluid intake, regular elimination, and personal hygiene measures

- Early manifestations of UTI and the importance of seeking medical intervention promptly

- Maintaining optimal immune system function by attending to physical and psychosocial stressors, such as lack of adequate rest, poor nutrition, and high levels of emotional stress

- The importance of completing the prescribed treatment and keeping follow-up appointments

- Minimizing the risk of UTI when an indwelling urinary catheter is necessary:
  1. Use alternatives to an indwelling catheter when possible. For urinary incontinence, try scheduled toileting, incontinence pads or diapers, and external catheters if possible. For urinary retention, teach the client or a family member to perform straight catheterization every three to four hours using clean technique.
  2. Teach care measures such as perineal care, managing and emptying the collection chamber, maintaining a closed system, and bladder irrigation or flushing if ordered when an indwelling catheter is necessary.

The Client with Urinary Incontinence

The most common manifestation of impaired bladder control is **urinary incontinence,** or involuntary urination. Incontinence can have significant impact, leading to physical problems, such as skin breakdown, infection, and rashes. Psychosocial consequences include embarrassment, isolation and withdrawal, feelings of worthlessness and helplessness, and depression.

Approximately 13 million people in the United States have some degree of urinary incontinence. The estimated cost of managing incontinence is $10 billion yearly. Urinary incontinence is especially common among older clients. Up to 30% of older women living in the community experience urinary incontinence. In long-term care, foster care, and homebound populations, the incidence is about 50% (Gallo, et al., 1999; Tierney, et al., 2001). The actual prevalence of urinary incontinence is nearly impossible to determine. Embarrassment and the availability of products to protect clothing and prevent detection contribute to clients not seeking evaluation of and treatment for incontinence.

Pathophysiology

Urinary continence requires a bladder able to expand and contract and sphincters that can maintain a urethral pressure higher than that in the bladder. Incontinence results when the pressure within the urinary bladder exceeds urethral resistance, allowing urine to escape. Any condition causing higher than normal bladder pressures or reduced urethral resistance can potentially result in incontinence. Relaxation of the pelvic musculature, disruption of cerebral and nervous system control, and disturbances of the bladder and its musculature are common contributing factors.

Incontinence may be an acute, self-limited disorder, or it may be chronic. The causes may be congenital or acquired, reversible or irreversible. Congenital disorders associated with incontinence include *epispadias* (absence of the upper wall of the urethra), and *meningomyelocele* (a neural tube defect in which a portion of the spinal cord and its surrounding meninges protrude through the vertebral column). Central nervous system or spinal cord trauma, stroke, and chronic neurologic disorders, such as multiple sclerosis and Parkinson's disease, are examples of acquired, irreversible causes of incontinence. Reversible causes include acute confusion, medications, such as diuretics or sedatives, prostatic enlargement, vaginal and urethral atrophy, UTI, and fecal impaction.

Incontinence is commonly categorized as stress incontinence, urge incontinence (also known as overactive bladder), overflow incontinence, and functional incontinence. Table 23-2 summarizes each type with its physiologic cause and associated factors. *Mixed incontinence,* with elements of both stress and urge incontinence, is common. *Total incontinence* is loss of all voluntary control over urination, with urine loss occurring without stimulus, and in all positions.

Incontinence is associated with an increased risk for falls, fractures, pressure ulcers, urinary tract infection, and depression. It contributes to the stress of caregivers, and may be a factor in institutionalizing the client.

Collaborative Care

Urinary incontinence management is directed at identifying and correcting the cause if possible. If the underlying disorder cannot be corrected, techniques to manage urine output can often be taught.

Table 23-2. Types of Urinary Incontinence

	Description	Pathophysiology	Contributing Factors
Stress	Loss of urine associated with increased intra-abdominal pressure during sneezing, coughing, lifting. Quantity of urine lost is usually small.	Relaxation of pelvic musculature and weakness of urethra and surrounding muscles and tissues leads to decreased urethral resistance	• Multiple pregnancies • Decreased estrogen levels • Short urethra, change in angle between bladder and urethra • Abdominal wall weakness • Prostate surgery • Increased intra-abdominal pressure due to tumor, ascites, obesity
Urge	Involuntary loss of urine associated with a strong urge to void	Hypertonic or over-active detrusor muscle leads to increased pressure within bladder and inability to inhibit voiding	• Neurologic disorders, such as stroke, Parkinson's disease, multiple sclerosis; peripheral nervous system disorders • Detrusor muscle overactivity associated with bladder outlet obstruction, aging, or disorders, such as diabetes
Overflow	Inability to empty bladder, resulting in overdistention and frequent loss of small amounts of urine	Outlet obstruction or lack of normal detrusor activity leads to over-filling of bladder and increased pressure	• Spinal cord injuries below S2 • Diabetic neuropathy • Prostatic hypertrophy • Fecal impaction • Drugs, especially those with anticholinergic effect
Functional	Incontinence resulting from physical, environ-mental, or psycho-social causes	Ability to respond to the need to urinate is impaired	• Confusion or dementia • Physical disability or impaired mobility • Diuretic therapy or sedation • Depression • Regression

Evaluation for incontinence begins with a complete history, including the duration, frequency, volume, and associated circumstances of urine loss. A voiding diary is often used to collect detailed information. The history also includes information about chronic or acute illnesses, previous surgeries, and current medication use, both prescription and over the counter.

Physical assessment includes abdominal, rectal, and pelvic assessment, as well as evaluation of mental and neurologic status, mobility, and dexterity. Findings often associated with incontinence in women include weak abdominal and pelvic muscle tone, cystocele or urethrocele, and atrophic vaginitis. In men, an enlarged prostate gland is the physical finding most commonly associated with incontinence.

Diagnostic Tests

- *Urinalysis and urine culture* using a clean-catch specimen are done to rule out infection and other acute causes of incontinence.

- *Postvoiding residual (PVR) volume* is measured to determine how completely the bladder empties with voiding. Less than 50 mL PVR is expected; when 100 mL or more is obtained, further testing is indicated.

- *Cystometrography* is used to assess neuromuscular function of the bladder by evaluating detrusor muscle function, pressure within the bladder, and the filling pattern of the bladder. The client describes sensations and any urge to void as sterile water or saline is instilled into the bladder. Normally, the urge to void is perceived at 150 to 450 mL, and the bladder feels full at 300 to 500 mL. Bladder pressure and volume are recorded on a graph. When the bladder is full, the client voids, and intravesical pressure is noted during voiding.

- *Uroflowmetry* is a noninvasive test used to evaluate voiding patterns. The uroflowmeter, contained in a funnel, measures the rate of urine flow, the continuous flow time, and the total voiding time.

- *Intravenous pyelography* may be ordered to evaluate structure and function of the upper and lower urinary tract.

- *Cystoscopy or ultrasonography* may be ordered to identify structural disorders contributing to incontinence, such as an enlarged prostate or a tumor.

Medications

Both stress and urge incontinence may improve with drug treatment.

Drugs that contract the smooth muscles of the bladder neck may reduce episodes of mild stress incontinence. Phenylpropanolamine (Acutrim, Allerest, Contac, others), a commonly used decongestant and nonprescription diet aid, is an effective preparation. Adverse effects, such as hypertension, palpitations, and nervousness, may limit its use.

When incontinence is associated with postmenopausal atrophic vaginitis, estrogen therapy may be effective. Both systemic estrogens and local creams are used.

Clients with urge incontinence may be treated with preparations that increase bladder capacity. The primary drugs used to inhibit detrusor muscle contractions and increase bladder capacity include oxybutinin (Ditropan), an anticholinergic drug, and tolterodine (Detrol), a more specific antimuscarinic agent. These drugs can be taken once or twice a day, and have fewer side effects than less specific anticholinergic drugs. Drugs with anticholinergic effects are contraindicated for the client with acute glaucoma. Urinary retention is a potential side effect that must be considered when these drugs are used.

Surgery

Surgery may be used to treat stress incontinence associated with cystocele or urethrocele and overflow incontinence associated with an enlarged prostate gland.

Suspension of the bladder neck, a technique that brings the angle between the bladder and urethra closer to normal, is effective in treating stress incontinence associated with urethrocele in 80% to 95% of clients. A laparoscopic, vaginal, or abdominal approach may be used to perform this surgery.

Prostatectomy, using either the transurethral or suprapubic approach, is indicated for the client who is experiencing overflow incontinence as a result of an enlarged prostate gland and urethral obstruction.

Other surgical procedures of potential benefit in the treatment of incontinence include implantation of an artificial sphincter, formation of a urethral sling to elevate and compress the urethra, and augmentation of the bladder with bowel segments to increase bladder capacity.

Complementary Therapies

Biofeedback and relaxation techniques may help reduce episodes of urinary incontinence. Biofeedback uses electronic monitors to teach conscious control over physiologic responses of which the individual is not normally aware. Developing awareness of perceptible information allows the client to gain voluntary control over urination. Biofeedback is widely used to manage urinary incontinence.

Nursing Care

Health Promotion

Although urinary incontinence rarely causes serious physical effects, it frequently has significant psychosocial effects, and can lead to lowered self-esteem, social isolation, and even institutionalization. Get the word out—inform all clients that UI is not a normal consequence of aging and that treatments are available. To reduce the incidence of UI, teach all women to perform pelvic floor exercises to improve perineal muscle tone. Advise women to seek advice from their women's health care or primary care practitioner about using topical or systemic hormone therapy during menopause to maintain perineal tissue integrity. Advise older men to have routine prostate examinations to prevent urethral obstruction and overflow incontinence.

Assessment

Nursing assessment for the client with urinary incontinence includes both subjective and objective data.

*   *Health history:* voiding diary; frequency of incontinent episodes, amount of urine loss and activities associated with incontinence; methods used to deal with incontinence; use of Kegel exercises or medications; any chronic diseases, related surgeries, etc.; effects of incontinence on usual activities, including social activities.
*   *Physical examination:* physical and mental status, including any physical limitations or impaired cognition; inspect, palpate, and percuss abdomen for bladder distention; inspect perineal tissues for redness, irritation, or tissue breakdown; observe for bulging of bladder into vagina when bearing down; assess pelvic muscle tone as indicated.

Nursing Diagnoses and Interventions

In planning nursing care, consider the client's mental status, mobility, and motivation. Behavioral techniques can be effective, but require long-term commitment and the physical and mental capability to use them.

Nursing care and modification of routines can restore continence fully or partially even in the institutionalized client. Scheduled toileting, bladder training, and prompted voiding combined with positive reinforcement, such as praise, can reduce the need for diapers, incontinence pads, and indwelling catheters.

Urinary Incontinence: Stress and/or Urge

Exercises to strengthen pelvic floor muscles, dietary modifications, and bladder training programs are often effective to help restore and maintain continence.

- Instruct client to keep a voiding diary, recording the time and amount of all fluid intake and urinary output, status at the time of voiding (dry or wet) and on arising from sleep, and activities. *Voiding diaries provide valuable information for identifying the type of incontinence and possible measures to reduce or eliminate incontinent episodes.*

- Teach pelvic floor muscle exercises. Instruct to consciously tighten pelvic muscles when the need to void is perceived and to relax the abdomen while walking to the bathroom. *Improved pelvic muscle strength helps retain urine and prevent stress incontinence by increasing urethral pressure. Exercises also decrease abnormal detrusor muscle contractions, decreasing pressure within the bladder.*

- Using the client's voiding diary, suggest dietary and fluid intake modifications to reduce stress and urge incontinence. Include limiting caffeine, alcohol, citrus juice, and artificial sweetener consumption; limiting fluid intake to no less than 1.5 to 2.0 L per day; and limiting evening fluid intake. *Caffeine, alcohol, and citrus juices are bladder irritants and tend to promote detrusor instability, increasing the risk of urge incontinence. Artificial sweeteners may also irritate the bladder. Fluid intake of 1.5 to 2.0 L per day is adequate to maintain health for most clients; excess fluid may increase stress incontinence if bathroom facilities are not readily available.*

Self-Care Deficit: Toileting

Functional incontinence may be the predominant problem in an institutionalized older adult. Limited mobility, impaired vision, dementia, lack of access to facilities and privacy, and tight staffing patterns increase the risk for incontinence in previously continent residents. The primary problem in functional incontinence is an outside factor that interferes with the ability to respond normally to the urge to void. An immobilized client may wet the bed if a call light is not within reach; a client with Alzheimer's disease may perceive the urge to void but be unable to interpret its meaning or respond by seeking a bathroom. For these clients, self-care deficit in toileting is a primary problem.

- Assess physical and mental abilities and limitations, usual voiding pattern, and ability to assist with toileting. *A thorough assessment allows planned interventions to address specific needs and promote independence.*

- Provide assistive devices as needed to facilitate independence, such as raised toilet seats, grab bars, a bedside commode, or night lights. *Fostering independence in toileting bolsters self-concept and maintains a positive body image.*

- Plan a toileting schedule based on the client's normal elimination patterns to achieve approximately 300 mL of urine output with each voiding. *Allowing the bladder to fill to a point at which the urge to void is experienced and then emptying it completely helps maintain normal bladder capacity and bacteriostatic functions.*

- Position for ease of voiding—sitting for females, standing for males—and provide privacy. *Normal positioning, usual toileting facilities, and privacy enhance the ability to void on schedule and empty the bladder completely.*

- Adjust fluid intake so that the majority of fluids are consumed during times of day when the client is most able to remain continent. Unless fluids are restricted, maintain a fluid intake of at least 1.5 to 2.0 L per day. *An adequate fluid intake is vital to promote hydration and urinary function. Overly concentrated urine can irritate the bladder, increasing incontinence.*

- Assist with clothing that is easily removed (e.g., elastic-waisted pants or loose dresses). Velcro and zipper fasteners may be easier to use than snaps and buttons. *Clothing that is difficult to remove can increase the risk of incontinence in the client with mobility problems or impaired dexterity.*

Social Isolation

Urinary incontinence increases the risk for social isolation due to embarrassment, fear of not having ready access to a bathroom, body odor, or other factors. Social isolation, in turn, can increase problems of incontinence, because normal cues and relationships are lost, and the need to remain dry is less strongly felt.

- Assess reasons for and extent of social isolation. Verify the degree of social isolation with the client or significant other. *Do not assume that social isolation is only related to urinary incontinence. Other problems frequently associated with aging, such as a hearing loss, may be primary or contributing factors.*

- Refer client for urologic examination and incontinence evaluation. *Clients who assume that urinary incontinence is a normal part of the aging may not be aware of treatment options.*

- Explore alternative coping strategies with client, significant other, staff, and other health team members. *Protective pads or shields, good perineal hygiene, scheduled voiding, and clothing that does not interfere with toileting can enhance continence.*

Home Care

Because urinary incontinence is a contributing factor in the institutionalization of many older people, client and family teaching can have a significant impact on maintaining independence and residence in the community. Address possible causes of incontinence and appropriate treatment measures. Refer for urologic examination if not already completed. Discuss fluid intake management, perineal care, and products for clothing protection.

24 Nursing Care of Clients with Kidney Disorders

The internal environment of the body normally remains in a relatively constant or *homeostatic* state. The kidneys help maintain homeostasis by regulating the composition and volume of extracellular fluid. They excrete excess water and solutes and can also conserve water and solutes when deficits occur. In addition, the kidneys help regulate acid-base balance and they excrete metabolic wastes. Regulation of blood pressure is also a key function of the kidneys.

Both primary kidney disorders, such as glomerulonephritis, and systemic diseases, such as diabetes mellitus, can affect renal function. In North America, more than 20 million people are affected by kidney and urinary tract diseases. Every year, approximately 1 in every 1000 people in the United States develops end-stage renal disease (ESRD), the final phase of chronic renal failure in which little or no kidney function remains. Chronic renal disease accounts for about 80,000 deaths per year and is a major cause of lost work time and wages. Ironically, the increased prevalence of chronic renal disease in recent years is partially related to the success of dialysis and transplantation.

Age-Related Changes in Kidney Function

Glomeruli in the renal cortex (see Chapter 22 for a review of normal kidney structure and function) are lost with aging, reducing kidney mass. Because of the large functional reserve of the kidneys, however, renal function remains adequate unless additional stressors affect the renal system. The **glomerular filtration rate (GFR),** the amount of filtrate made by the kidneys per minute, declines due to age-related factors affecting the renovascular system, such as arteriosclerosis, decreased renal vascularity, and decreased cardiac output. By age 80, the GFR may be less than half of what it was at age 30.

Age-related changes in renal function have significant implications. The kidneys are less able to concentrate urine and compensate for increased or decreased salt intake. When combined with diminished effectiveness of antidiuretic hormone (ADH) and a reduced thirst response, both common in aging, this decreased ability to concentrate urine increases the risk for dehydration. Potassium excretion may be decreased because of lower aldosterone levels. As a result, fluid and electrolyte imbalances are more common and potentially critical in the older client.

Decreased GFR in the older adult also reduces the clearance of drugs excreted through the kidneys. This reduced clearance prolongs the half-life of drugs and may necessitate lower drug doses and longer dosing intervals. Common medications affected by decreased GFR include:

- Cardiac drugs: digoxin, procainamide
- Antibiotics: aminoglycosides, tetracyclines, cephalosporins
- Histamine H_2 antagonists: cimetidine
- Antidiabetic agents: chlorpropamide.

When caring for older adults, it is especially important to monitor drugs that are toxic to the renal tubules. Radiologic dyes and aminoglycoside, tetracycline, and the cephalosporin antibiotics are part of this group.

The Client with a Congenital Kidney Malformation

Congenital kidney disorders can affect the form and/or function of the kidney. Functional congenital kidney disorders are usually identified in childhood or adolescence. If function is not affected, congenital malformations may be detected only coincidentally. Malformations include agenesis, hypoplasia, alterations in kidney position, and horseshoe kidney.

Agenesis, absence of the kidney, and *hypoplasia,* underdevelopment of the kidney, typically affect only one of these paired organs. Renal function remains normal unless the unaffected kidney is compromised. Abnormal kidney position affects the ureters and urine flow, potentially leading to urinary stasis, increased risk of urinary tract infection (UTI), and lithiasis, or stone formation (see Chapter 23).

One in every 500 to 1000 people has *horseshoe kidney,* making it one of the most common renal malformations (Porth, 2002). Failure of the embryonic kidneys to ascend normally can result in a single, horseshoe-shaped organ. The two kidneys are fused at either the upper or lower pole (usually the lower). This malformation does not typically affect renal function; however, because the ureters cross the fused poles, there is an increased risk for *hydronephrosis,* or distention of the renal pelvis and calyces with urine (see Chapter 23). Recurrent UTI and renal calculi are also common in clients with horseshoe kidney.

Renal ultrasonography and intravenous pyelography are used to diagnose horseshoe kidney. Correction of the abnormality is rarely necessary, although surgical resection of the isthmus (connection between the kidneys) may be done to relieve ureteral obstruction or allow access to the abdominal aorta, which lies behind it.

Nursing care for clients with horseshoe kidney or other congenital malformations is primarily educational. Because abnormal kidney shape or position increases the risk of infection and stone formation, teach the client to maintain a fluid intake of at least 2500 mL per day. Emphasize the importance of avoiding dehydration by increasing fluids during hot weather and strenuous exercise. Teach hygiene practices, such as perineal cleansing and voiding before and after intercourse, to help prevent UTI. Teach the early manifestations of UTI and instruct to seek treatment promptly to prevent infection of the kidney. (See Chapter 23.)

The Client with Polycystic Kidney Disease

Polycystic kidney disease, a hereditary disease characterized by cyst formation and massive kidney enlargement, affects both children and adults. This disease has two forms: The autosomal dominant form affects adults; the autosomal recessive form is present at birth (Bullock & Henze, 2000; Porth, 2002). Autosomal recessive polycystic kidney disease is rare. It usually is diagnosed prenatally or in infancy. Renal failure generally develops during childhood, necessitating kidney transplant or dialysis. Autosomal dominant polycystic kidney disease is relatively common, affecting 1 in every 300 to 1000 people and accounting for approximately 10% of clients with ESRD in the United States (Braunwald, et al., 2001). This section focuses on autosomal dominant polycystic kidney disease, the more common, adult form of the disorder.

Pathophysiology

Renal cysts are fluid-filled sacs affecting the nephron, the functional unit of the kidneys. They develop in the tubular epithelium of the nephron, filling with straw-colored glomerular filtrate. The cysts may range in size from microscopic to several centimeters in diameter and affect the renal cortex and medulla of both kidneys. As the cysts fill, enlarge, and multiply, the kidneys also enlarge. Renal blood vessels and nephrons are compressed and obstructed, and functional tissue destroyed. The renal parenchyma atrophies and becomes fibrotic and scarred (Braunwald, et al., 2001).

People affected by polycystic kidney disease often develop cysts elsewhere in the body, including the liver, spleen, pancreas, and other organs. Up to 10% of people affected experience subarachnoid hemorrhage from a type of congenital intracranial aneurysm. People with polycystic kidney disease also have an increased incidence of incompetent or "floppy" cardiac valves.

Manifestations

Polycystic kidney disease is slowly progressive. Symptoms usually develop by age 40 to 50. Common manifestations include flank pain, microscopic or gross **hematuria** (blood in the urine), **proteinuria** (proteins in the urine), and *polyuria* and *nocturia,* as the concentrating ability of the kidney is impaired. Urinary tract infection and renal calculi are common, as cysts interfere with normal urine drainage. Most clients develop hypertension from disruption of renal vessels. The kidneys become palpable, enlarged, and knobby. Symptoms of renal insufficiency and chronic renal failure typically develop by age 60 to 70.

Collaborative Care

Diagnostic tests used to determine the extent of polycystic kidney disease include the following:

- *Renal ultrasonography* is the diagnostic procedure of choice for polycystic kidney disease. Reflected sound waves are used to assess kidney size and to identify, locate, and differentiate renal masses, such as cysts, tumors, and calculi.

- *Intravenous pyelography (IVP)*, a radiologic examination, is used to evaluate the structure and excretory function of the kidneys, ureters, and bladder. An intravenously injected contrast medium illuminates kidney size and shape, the calyces and pelvis, the ureters, and the bladder as it is cleared from the blood. Cysts can be detected and sized, and the extent of kidney involvement determined.

- *Computed tomography (CT scan)* of the kidney uses X-rays passed through the kidneys at many angles to create a detailed picture of renal tissue densities and composition. CT may be done with or without contrast media. Kidney CT is used to detect and differentiate renal masses such as cystic disease or tumors.

Management of adult polycystic kidney disease is largely supportive. Care is taken to avoid further renal damage by nephrotoxic substances, UTI, obstruction, or hypertension. A fluid intake of 2000 to 2500 mL per day is encouraged to help prevent UTI and lithiasis. Hypertension associated with polycystic disease is generally controlled using angiotensinconverting enzyme (ACE) inhibitors or other antihypertensive agents (see Chapter 12). Ultimately, dialysis or renal transplantation is required. Clients with polycystic kidney disease are typically good candidates for transplantation because of the absence of associated systemic disease.

Nursing Care

For those with adult polycystic kidney disease, an autosomal dominant disorder, discuss genetic counseling and screening of family members for evidence of the disease. This is particularly important if renal transplantation is contemplated and family members are potential donors. Consider the following nursing diagnoses when planning care for the client with polycystic kidney disease:

- *Excess fluid volume* related to impaired renal function
- *Anticipatory grieving* related to potential loss of kidney function
- *Deficient knowledge* regarding measures to help preserve kidney function
- *Risk for ineffective coping* related to potential genetic transmission of the disorder
  to offspring.

Teach the client with polycystic kidney disease about the disease, its genetic nature, and usual course. Discuss measures to maintain optimal renal function. Instruct client to maintain a fluid intake of at least 2500 mL per day. Include additional information about preventing UTI, such as hygiene measures, and early manifestations of UTI. Stress the importance of seeking treatment to prevent further kidney damage. Advise to avoid drugs that are potentially toxic to the kidneys and to check with primary care provider before taking any new drug.

The Client with a Glomerular Disorder

Disorders and diseases involving the glomerulus are the leading cause of chronic renal failure in the United States. They are the underlying disease process for half of those people needing dialysis and result in 12,000 deaths per year.

Glomerular disorders may be either primary, involving mainly the kidney, or secondary to a multisystem disease or hereditary condition. Primary glomerular disease is often immunologic or idiopathic in origin. Diabetes mellitus, systemic lupus erythematosus (SLE), and Goodpasture's syndrome are frequently implicated in secondary glomerular disorders.

Physiology Review

The glomerulus is a tuft of capillaries surrounded by a thin, double-walled capsule (Bowman's capsule). About 20% of the resting cardiac output flows through the glomeruli of the kidneys, forming approximately 180 L of plasma ultrafiltrate. More than 99% of this filtrate is reabsorbed in the renal tubules. The rate of glomerular filtration (GFR) is controlled by opposing forces: The pressure and amount of blood flowing through the glomeruli promote filtration, and the pressure in Bowman's capsule and colloid osmotic pressure of the blood oppose it. The total surface area of glomerular capillaries also affects the GFR. The glomerular capillary membrane has three layers: the capillary endothelial layer, the basement membrane, and the capsule epithelial layer. Water and the smallest solutes, such as electrolytes, pass freely across this membrane, while larger molecules, such as plasma proteins, are retained in the blood.

Pathophysiology

Glomerular disease affects both the structure and function of the glomerulus, disrupting glomerular filtration. The capillary membrane becomes more permeable to plasma proteins and blood cells. This increased permeability in the glomerulus causes the manifestations common to glomerular disorders: hematuria, proteinuria, and edema. The GFR falls, leading to **azotemia** (increased blood levels of nitrogenous waste products), and hypertension. Glomerular involvement may be diffuse, involving all glomeruli, or focal, involving some glomeruli while others remain essentially normal.

Both hematuria and proteinuria are caused by glomerular capillary membrane damage, which allows blood cells and proteins to escape from the blood into the glomerular filtrate. Hematuria may be either gross or microscopic. Proteinuria is considered to be the most important indicator of glomerular injury, because it increases progressively with increased glomerular damage. Loss of plasma proteins leads to *hypoalbuminemia* (low serum albumin levels), which in turn reduces the plasma oncotic pressure (osmotic pressure created by plasma proteins), leading to edema.

As plasma proteins are lost, the forces opposing filtration diminish, and the amount of filtrate increases. The increased flow of filtrate stimulates the renin-angiotensin-aldosterone mechanism (see Chapter 22), producing vasoconstriction and a fall in GFR. Increased aldosterone production causes salt and water retention which further contribute to edema. As the GFR falls, filtration and elimination of nitrogenous wastes, including urea, decreases, causing azotemia. **Oliguria,** urine output of less than 400 mL in 24 hours, may result from the decreased GFR. Hypertension results from fluid retention and disruption of the renin-angiotensin system, a key regulator of blood pressure.

The major primary glomerular disorders include acute glomerulonephritis, rapidly progressive glomerulonephritis, chronic glomerulonephritis, and nephrotic syndrome. Diabetic nephropathy and lupus nephritis are the most common secondary forms of glomerular disease.

Acute Glomerulonephritis

Glomerulonephritis is inflammation of the glomerular capillary membrane. Acute glomerulonephritis can result from systemic diseases or primary glomerular diseases, but acute poststreptococcal glomerulonephritis (also known as acute proliferative glomerulonephritis) is the most common form. Infection of the pharynx or skin with group A β-hemolytic streptococcus is the usual initiating event for this disorder. Staphylococcal or viral infections, such as hepatitis B, mumps, or varicella (chickenpox), can lead to a similar postinfectious acute glomerulonephritis (Porth, 2002). This primarily childhood disease can also affect adults.

In acute glomerulonephritis, circulating antigen-antibody immune complexes formed during the primary infection become trapped in the glomerular membrane, leading to an inflammatory response. The complement system is activated, and vasoactive substances and inflammatory mediators are released. Endothelial cells proliferate, and the glomerular membrane swells and becomes permeable to plasma proteins and blood cells. Renal involvement is diffuse, spread throughout the kidneys.

Manifestations and Complications

Acute glomerulonephritis is characterized by an abrupt onset of hematuria, proteinuria, salt and water retention, and evidence of azotemia occurring 10 to 14 days after the initial infection. The urine often appears brown or cola-colored. Salt and water retention increase extracellular fluid volume, leading to hypertension and edema. The edema is primarily noted in the face, particularly around the eyes (*periorbital* edema). Dependent edema, affecting the hands and upper extremities in particular, may also be noted. Other manifestations may include fatigue, anorexia, nausea and vomiting, and headache.

The older adult may have less apparent symptoms. Nausea, malaise, arthralgias, and proteinuria are common manifestations; hypertension and edema are seen less often. Pulmonary infiltrates may occur early in the disorder, often due to worsening of a preexisting condition, such as heart failure.

The prognosis for adults with acute glomerulonephritis is less favorable than it is for children. The symptoms may resolve spontaneously within 10 to 14 days. Full recovery is usual in children, whereas 60% or more affected adults recover completely. The remainder have persistent symptoms, and some have permanent kidney damage (Porth, 2002).

Rapidly Progressive Glomerulonephritis

Rapidly progressive glomerulonephritis (RPGN) is characterized by manifestations of severe glomerular injury without a specific, identifiable cause. This type of glomerulonephritis often progresses to renal failure within months. It may be idiopathic (primary), or secondary to a systemic disorder such as SLE or Goodpasture's syndrome. It affects people of all ages.

In RPGN, glomerular cells proliferate and, together with macrophages, form crescent-shaped lesions that obliterate Bowman's space (Porth, 2002). Glomerular damage is diffuse, leading to a rapid, progressive decline in renal function. Irreversible renal failure often develops over weeks to months (Braunwald, et al., 2001; Bullock & Henze, 2000).

Clients with RPGN typically present with complaints of weakness, nausea, and vomiting. Some may relate a history of a flulike illness preceding the onset of the glomerulonephritis. Other symptoms include oliguria and abdominal or flank pain. Moderate hypertension may develop. On urinalysis, hematuria and massive proteinuria are noted.

Goodpasture's Syndrome

Goodpasture's syndrome is a rare autoimmune disorder of unknown etiology. It is characterized by formation of antibodies to the glomerular basement membrane. These antibodies also may bind to alveolar basement membranes, damaging alveoli and causing pulmonary hemorrhage. Goodpasture's syndrome usually affects young men between 18 and 35, although it can occur at any age and affect women as well.

Although the glomeruli may be nearly normal in appearance and function in Goodpasture's syndrome, extensive cell proliferation and crescent formation characteristic of rapidly progressive glomerulonephritis are more common. Renal manifestations include hematuria, proteinuria, and edema. Rapid progression to renal failure may occur. Alveolar membrane damage can lead to mild or life-threatening pulmonary hemorrhage. Cough, shortness of breath, and hemoptysis (bloody sputum) are early respiratory manifestations.

Chronic Glomerulonephritis

Chronic glomerulonephritis is typically the end stage of other glomerular disorders, such as RPGN, lupus nephritis, or diabetic nephropathy. In many cases, however, no previous glomerular disease has been identified.

Slow, progressive destruction of the glomeruli and a gradual decline in renal function are characteristic of chronic glomerulonephritis. The kidneys decrease in size symmetrically, and their surfaces become granular or roughened. Eventually, entire nephrons are lost.

Symptoms develop insidiously, and the disease is often not recognized until signs of renal failure develop. Chronic glomerulonephritis may also be diagnosed when hypertension and impaired renal function are found coincidentally during a routine physical examination or treatment for an unrelated disorder. Viral or bacterial infectious diseases can exacerbate the disorder, prompting its diagnosis.

The course of chronic glomerulonephritis varies, with years to decades between the diagnosis and the development of end-stage renal failure.

Nephrotic Syndrome

Nephrotic syndrome is a group of clinical findings as opposed to a specific disorder. It is characterized by massive proteinuria, hypoalbuminemia, hyperlipidemia, and edema. A number of disorders can affect the glomerular capillary membrane, changing its porosity and allowing plasma proteins to escape into the urine. *Minimal change disease (MCD) is* the most common cause of nephrotic syndrome in children and accounts for 20% of adults with nephrotic syndrome (Braunwald, et al., 2001). In MCD, the size and form of glomeruli appear normal by light microscopy. The prognosis for MCD is good. In adults, *membranous glomerulonephropathy* is the most common cause of idiopathic nephrotic syndrome. The glomerular basement membrane thickens, although no inflammation is present. This form of nephrotic syndrome also occurs with some systemic diseases, such as SLE and hepatitis B, and with drugs such as gold or penicillamine. *Focal sclerosis,* in which scarring (sclerosis) of glomeruli occurs, and *membranoproliferative glomerulonephritis,* caused by thickening and proliferation of glomerular basement membrane cells, are additional forms of nephrotic syndrome.

With plasma protein loss in the urine and resulting hypoalbuminemia, the oncotic pressure of the plasma falls. Fluid shifts from the vascular compartment to interstitial spaces, causing the edema characteristic of nephrotic syndrome. Salt and water retention, possibly due to activation of the renin-angiotensin system, contribute to the edema. Edema may be severe, affecting the face and periorbital area, as well as dependent tissues.

Loss of plasma proteins stimulates the liver to increase albumin production and lipoprotein synthesis. As a result, serum triglyceride and low-density lipoprotein (LDL) levels increase, as do urine lipids (*lipiduria*). Hyperlipidemia increases the risk for atherosclerosis in clients with nephrotic syndrome.

Thromboemboli (mobilized blood clots) are a relatively common complication of nephrotic syndrome. Loss of clotting and anticlotting factors, along with plasma proteins, are thought to disrupt the coagulation system, increasing the risk for renal vein thrombosis, deep vein thrombosis, and pulmonary embolism. Renal vein thrombosis can cause flank or groin pain on one or both sides, gross hematuria, and a reduced GFR (Porth, 2002).

Nephrotic syndrome usually resolves without long-term effects in children. The prognosis for adults is less optimistic. Less than 50% of adults recover completely. Many have persistent proteinuria and may develop progressive renal impairment. As many as 30% of adults with nephrotic syndrome develop end-stage renal failure.

Diabetic Nephropathy

Diabetic nephropathy, kidney disease common in the later stages of diabetes mellitus (DM), is the leading cause of end-stage renal disease in North America. Thirty percent of clients with type 1 DM and about 20% of type 2 diabetic clients develop nephropathy. ESRD resulting from diabetic nephropathy is seen more frequently in blacks with type 2 DM, and in whites with type 1 DM (Braunwald, et al., 2001).

Initial evidence of microproteinuria indicating renal damage is typically seen within 10 to 15 years after the onset of diabetes. Overt proteinuria and nephropathy generally develop within 15 to 20 years of the initial diagnosis.

The characteristic lesion of diabetic nephropathy is glomerulosclerosis and thickening of the glomerular basement membrane. Arteriosclerosis, a common feature of long-term diabetes and hypertension, contributes to the disease, as do nephritis and tubular lesions. Pyelonephritis, inflammation of the kidney, is also implicated in the development of diabetic nephropathy. A further discussion is found in Chapter 27.

Lupus Nephritis

Systemic lupus erythematosus (SLE) is an inflammatory autoimmune disorder affecting the connective tissue of the body. Between 40% and 85% of clients with SLE develop manifestations of nephritis (Braunwald, et al., 2001). Immune complexes that form within the glomerular capillary wall are the usual trigger for glomerular injury in SLE. Manifestations of lupus nephritis range from microscopic hematuria to massive proteinuria. Its progession may be slow and chronic or *fulminant,* with a sudden onset and the rapid development of renal failure. Most clients with minimal or mild lesions survive for at least ten years. Improved management of the underlying disease, immunotherapy, dialysis, and renal transplantation have significantly improved the prognosis in recent years.

Collaborative Care

Management of all types of glomerulonephritis, acute and chronic, primary and secondary, focuses on identifying the underlying disease process and preserving kidney function. In most glomerular disorders, there is no specific treatment to achieve a cure. Treatment goals are to maintain renal function, prevent complications, and support the healing process.

Diagnostic Tests

Laboratory and diagnostic testing are valuable to identify the cause of glomerulonephritis and evaluate kidney function.

The following studies may be ordered to help identify the underlying cause or etiology:

- *Throat or skin cultures* detect infection by group A β-hemolytic streptococci. Although poststreptococcal glomerulonephritis typically follows the acute infection by one to two weeks, treatment to eradicate any remaining organisms is initiated to minimize antibody production.

- *Antistreptolysin O (ASO) titer* and other tests detect streptococcal exoenzymes (bacterial enzymes that stimulate the immune response in acute poststreptococcal glomerulonephritis). Other titers, such as antistreptokinase (ASK) or antideoxyribonuclease B (ADNAase B), may be obtained as well.

- *Erythrocyte sedimentation rate (ESR)* is a general indicator of inflammatory response. It may be elevated in acute poststreptococcal glomerulonephritis and in lupus nephritis.

- *KUB* (kidney, ureter, bladder) *abdominal X-ray* may be done to evaluate kidney size and rule out other causes of the client's manifestations. The kidneys may be enlarged in acute glomerulonephritis, whereas bilateral small kidneys are typical of late chronic glomerulonephritis.

- *Kidney scan,* a nuclear medicine procedure, allows visualization of the kidney after intravenous administration of a radioisotope. In glomerular diseases, the uptake and excretion of the radioactive material are delayed.

- *Biopsy,* microscopic examination of kidney tissue, is the most reliable diagnostic procedure for glomerular disorders. Biopsy helps determine the type of glomerulonephritis, the prognosis, and appropriate treatment. Renal biopsy is usually done percutaneously, by inserting a biopsy needle through the skin into the kidney to obtain a tissue sample. Open biopsy, which requires surgery, may also be done.

The following studies are used to evaluate kidney function:

- *Blood urea nitrogen (BUN)* measures urea nitrogen, the end product of protein metabolism. It is created by the breakdown and metabolism of both dietary and body proteins. Urea is eliminated from the body by filtration in the glomerulus; minimal amounts are reabsorbed in the renal tubules. Glomerular diseases interfere with filtration and elimination of urea nitrogen, causing blood levels to rise. Increased protein catabolism (destruction), which may occur with GI bleeding or tissue breakdown, can also raise the BUN. Normal BUN values are listed in Table 24-1. Levels up to 50 mg/dL or 17.7 mmol/L indicate mild azotemia, and levels higher than 100 mg/dL or 35.7 mmol/L indicate severe renal impairment.

- *Serum creatinine* measures the amount of creatinine in the blood. Creatinine is also a metabolic by-product, produced in relatively constant amounts by skeletal muscles. It is excreted entirely by the kidneys, making the serum creatinine a good indicator of kidney function. Normal values (see Table 24–1) are lower in the older adult, because of decreased muscle mass. Levels greater than 4 mg/dL indicate serious impairment of renal function.

- *Urine creatinine* is also an indicator of renal function and the GFR. Urine creatinine levels decrease when renal function is impaired as it is not effectively eliminated from the body.

- *Creatinine clearance* is a specific indicator of renal function used to evaluate the GFR. The clearance, or amount of blood cleared of creatinine in one minute, depends on the amount and pressure of blood being filtered and the filtering ability of the glomeruli. Levels normally decline with aging as the GFR decreases in the older adult. Disorders, such as glomerulonephritis, affect glomerular filtration, decreasing the creatinine clearance.

- *Serum electrolytes* are evaluated because impaired kidney function alters their excretion. Monitoring serum electrolytes is particularly important to prevent complications associated with imbalances.

- *Urinalysis* often shows red blood cells and proteins in the urine of clients with a glomerular disorder. These substances, normally too large to enter glomerular filtrate, escape due to increased porosity of glomerular capillaries in glomerular disorders. A 24-hour urine specimen is used to determine the amount of protein in the urine.

Medications

Although no drugs are available to cure glomerular disorders, medications are used to treat underlying disorders, reduce inflammation, and manage the symptoms.

Antibiotics are prescribed for the client with poststreptococcal glomerulonephritis to eradicate any remaining bacteria, removing the stimulus for antibody production. Nephrotoxic antibiotics, such as the aminoglycoside antibiotics, streptomycin, and some cephalosporins, are avoided.

Table 24-1 Changes in Laboratory Values Associated with Kidney Disease

Test	Normal Value	Value in Renal Disease
Blood urea nitrogen (BUN)	5–20 mg/dL Slightly higher in older adult	20–50 mg/dL or higher
Creatinine, serum	Female: 0.5–1.1 mg/dL Male: 0.6–1.2 mg/dL Slightly lower in older adult	Elevated; levels >4 mg/dL indicate severe impairment of renal function
Creatinine clearance	Female: 88–128 mL/min Male: 97–137 mL/min Values decline in older adult	Reduced renal reserve: 32.5–90.0 mL/min Renal insufficiency: 6.5–32.5 mL/min Renal failure: >6.5 mL/min
Serum albumin	3.2–5 g/dL; 3.2–4.8 g/dL in older adult	Decreased in nephrotic syndrome

Table 24-1. Continued

Serum electrolytes	Potassium: 3.5–5.0 mEq/L Sodium: 136–145 mEq/L Calcium: 4.5–5.5 mEq/L or 8.2–10.5 mg/dL Phosphorus: 3.0–4.5 mg/dL	Increased in renal insufficiency Decreased in nephrotic syndrome Decreased in renal failure Increased in renal failure
Red blood cell count	Female: 4.0–5.5 million/mm³ Male: 4.5–6.2 million/mm³	Decreased in chronic renal failure
Urine creatinine	Female: 600–1800 mg/24 hours Male: 800–2000 mg/24 hours	Decreased in disorders of impaired renal function
Urine protein	Resting: 50–80 mg/24 hours Ambulatory: <150–250 mg/ 24 hours	Increased in disorders of impaired renal function
Urine red blood cells	<2–3/HPF; no RBC casts	Present in glomerular disorders

Aggressive immunosuppressive therapy is used to treat acute inflammatory processes, such as rapidly progressive glomerulonephritis, Goodpasture's syndrome, and exacerbations of SLE. When begun early, immunosuppressive therapy significantly reduces the risk of end-stage renal disease and renal failure. Prednisone, a glucocorticoid, is prescribed in relatively large doses of 1 mg per kilogram of body weight per day (e.g., a 160-pound man would receive 70 to 75 mg per day). Other immunosuppressive agents such as cyclophosphamide (Cytoxan) or azathioprine (Imuran), are prescribed in conjunction with corticosteroids. Corticosteroid use in poststreptococcal glomerulonephritis may actually worsen the condition, so it should be avoided.

Oral glucocorticoids, such as prednisone, are also used in high doses to induce remission of nephrotic syndrome. When glucocorticoids alone are ineffective, other immunosuppressive agents, such as cyclophosphamide or chlorambucil (Leukeran), may be used to induce or maintain remission. See Chapter 42 for more information about corticosteroids and other immunosuppressive drugs.

ACE inhibitors may be ordered to reduce protein loss associated with nephrotic syndrome. These drugs reduce proteinuria and slow the progression of renal failure. They have a protective effect on the kidney in clients with diabetic nephropathy. Nonsteroidal anti-inflammatory drugs (NSAIDs) also reduce proteinuria in some clients, but can increase salt and water retention (Braunwald, et al., 2001).

Antihypertensives may be prescribed to maintain the blood pressure within normal levels. Blood pressure management is important because systemic and renal hypertension are associated with a poorer prognosis in clients with glomerular disorders.

Treatments

Bed rest may be ordered during the acute phase of poststreptococcal glomerulonephritis. When the edema of nephrotic syndrome is significant or the client is hypertensive, sodium intake may be restricted to 1 to 2 g per day. Dietary protein may be restricted if azotemia is present. When proteins are restricted, those included in the diet should be complete or high-value proteins. Complete proteins supply the essential amino acids required for growth and tissue maintenance.

Plasma exchange therapy (**plasmapheresis**), a procedure to remove damaging antibodies from the plasma, is used in conjunction with immunosuppressive therapy to treat RPGN and Goodpasture's syndrome. Plasma and glomerular-damaging antibodies are removed using a blood cell separator. The red blood cells are then returned to the client along with albumin or human plasma to replace the plasma removed. This procedure is usually done in a series of treatments. It is not without risk, and informed consent is required. Potential complications of plasma exchange therapy include those associated with intravenous catheters, fluid volume shifts, and altered coagulation.

Renal failure resulting from a glomerular disorder may necessitate dialysis to restore fluid and electrolyte balance and remove waste products from the body.

Nursing Care

Health Promotion

Discuss the importance of effectively treating streptococcal infections in all age groups to help reduce the risk for acute glomerulonephritis. Stress the importance of completing the full course of antibiotic therapy to eradicate the infecting bacteria. Teach clients with diabetes mellitus and SLE about potential renal effects of their disease. Discuss measures to reduce the risk of associated nephritis, such as effectively managing the disease, treating hypertension, and avoiding drugs and substances that are potentially toxic to the kidneys.

Assessment

Review Chapter 22 for complete assessment of the renal and urinary systems. Focused assessment data related to glomerular disorders includes the following:

- *Health history:* complaints of facial or peripheral edema or weight gain, fatigue, nausea and vomiting, headache, general malaise, abdominal or flank pain; cough or shortness of breath; changes in amount, color, or character of urine (e.g., frothy urine); history of skin or pharyngeal streptococcal infection, diabetes, SLE, or kidney disease; current medications.
- *Physical examination:* General appearance; vital signs; weight; presence of periorbital, facial, or peripheral edema; skin for lesions, infection; inspect throat, obtain culture as indicated; urine specimen for color, character, odor.

Nursing Diagnoses and Interventions

Nursing care is supportive and educational. Monitoring renal function and fluid volume status are key components of care, as is protecting the client from infection. Both manifestations of glomerular disorders and their treatment can interfere with a client's ability to maintain usual roles and responsibilities.

Excess Fluid Volume

Excess fluid volume and resulting edema are common manifestations of glomerular disorders. When proteins are lost in the urine, the oncotic pressure of plasma falls, and fluid shifts into the interstitial spaces. The body responds to this fluid shift by retaining sodium and water to maintain intravascular volume, leading to excess fluid volume.

- Monitor vital signs, including blood pressure, apical pulse, respirations, and breath sounds, at least every four hours. Report significant changes. *Excess fluid increases the cardiac workload and the blood pressure. Tachycardia may result. Associated electrolyte imbalances can cause dysrhythmias. Increased pulmonary vascular pressure can lead to pulmonary edema, tachypnea, dyspnea, and crackles (rales) in the lungs.*
- Record intake and output every four to eight hours, or more frequently as indicated. *Accurate intake and output records help determine fluid volume status.*
- Monitor serum electrolytes, hemoglobin and hematocrit, BUN, and creatinine. *Glomerular disorders affect fluid balance and may alter electrolyte balance as well, potentially leading to complications such as cardiac dysrhythmias (see Chapter 39). Increased intravascular volume can result in low hemoglobin and hematocrit values. BUN and creatinine provide information about renal function.*
- Maintain fluid restriction as ordered. Offer ice chips (in limited and measured amounts) and frequent mouth care to relieve thirst. With the client, develop a fluid intake schedule. *Fluids may be restricted to reduce fluid overload, edema, and hypertension. Ice chips and frequent mouth care moisten mucous membranes and help relieve thirst while maintaining oral tissue integrity. Including the client in planning fluid intake promotes a sense of control and understanding of the treatment regimen.*
- Arrange dietary consultation regarding sodium or protein-restricted diets. *Including the client and dietitian in planning allows individualization of the diet to client preferences. The glomerular disorder may reduce appetite; considering food preferences can help maintain adequate nutrition.*
- Monitor for desired and adverse effects of prescribed medications. *Diuretic therapy helps reduce excess fluid volume; however, glomerular disorders can affect the client's response to treatment. In addition, diuretics can exacerbate electrolyte imbalances and muscle weakness often associated with glomerular disorders.*
- Provide frequent position changes and good skin care. *Perfusion may be altered by tissue edema, increasing the risk of breakdown.*

Fatigue

Fatigue is a common manifestation of glomerular disorders. Anemia, loss of plasma proteins, headache, anorexia, and nausea compound this fatigue. The ability to maintain usual physical and mental activities may be impaired.

- Document energy level. *As glomerular function improves, fatigue begins to resolve, and energy increases.*
- Schedule activities and procedures to provide adequate rest and energy conservation. Prevent unnecessary fatigue. *Adequate rest and energy conservation reduce fatigue and improve the client's ability to tolerate and cope with required treatments and activities.*
- Assist with ADLs as needed. *The goal is to conserve limited energy reserves.*
- Discuss the relationship between fatigue and the disease process with client and family. *Understanding the nature of the disease and associated fatigue helps the client and family cope with reduced energy and comply with prescribed rest.*

- Reduce energy demands with frequent, small meals and short periods of activity. Limit the number of visitors and visit length. *Small, frequent meals reduce the energy needed for eating and digestion. Limiting visitors and visit length helps conserve energy. In addition, nurses can assist the fatigued client who may be reluctant to ask visitors to leave.*

Ineffective Protection

The effects of both the glomerular disorder and treatment with anti-inflammatory and cytotoxic drugs can depress the immune system, increasing the risk for infection. The anti-inflammatory effect of corticosteroids may also mask early manifestations of infection.

- Assess frequently for other signs of infection such as purulent wound drainage, productive cough, adventitious breath sounds, and red or inflamed lesions. Monitor for manifestations of UTI, such as dysuria, frequency and urgency, and cloudy, foul-smelling urine. *Early identification and treatment of infection is important to prevent systemic complications in the susceptible client.*

- Monitor CBC, focusing on the WBC and differential. *An elevated WBC and increased numbers of immature WBCs in the blood (left shift) may be early indicators of infection.*

- Use good handwashing technique. Protect from crossinfection by providing a private room and restricting ill visitors. *Clients with decreased resistance to infection need increased protection.*

- Avoid or minimize invasive procedures. *Maintaining the protective skin barrier is especially important for the client with altered immune status.*

- If catheterization is required, use sterile intermittent straight catheterization or maintain a closed drainage system for an indwelling catheter. Prevent urine reflux from the drainage system to the bladder or the bladder to the kidneys by ensuring a patent, gravity system. *The urinary tract is a frequent entry point for infection, particularly in the hospitalized or institutionalized client. Maintaining strict asepsis during catheterization is vital. Intermittent catheterization is associated with a lower risk of UTI than an indwelling catheter.*

- Provide a nutritionally sound diet with complete proteins. *A well-balanced, nutritionally sound diet is important to maintain nutritional status and support immune function.*

- Teach measures to prevent infection. *Care often is provided in the home, requiring the client and family to use appropriate infection control measures.*

Ineffective Role Performance

The manifestations and treatment of glomerular disorders can affect the ability to maintain usual roles and activities. Fatigue and muscle weakness may limit physical and social activities. Bed rest or activity limitations may be ordered to minimize the degree of proteinuria. If azotemia is present, malaise, nausea, and mental status changes can interfere with role function. Facial and periorbital edema affect the client's self-esteem and may lead to isolation.

- Establish a strong therapeutic relationship. *It is important to gain the client's trust and confidence.*

- Encourage self-care and participation in decision making. *Increased autonomy helps restore self-confidence and reduce powerlessness.*

- Provide for time for verbalization of thoughts and feelings; listen actively, acknowledging and accepting fears and concerns. *Adequate time and active listening encourage expression of concerns and the affect of the disease or treatments on daily life. This helps the client deal with the illness, its treatment, and associated losses.*

- Support coping skills, helping the client identify personal strengths. *This support helps the client gain confidence.*

- When possible, enlist the support of family, other clients, and friends. *These people can provide physical, psychologic, emotional, and social support.*

- Discuss the effect of the disease and treatments on roles and relationships, helping identify potential changes in roles, relationships, and lifestyle. Help the client and family develop a plan for alternative behaviors and relationships, encouraging the client to maintain usual roles to the extent possible. *Developing a plan helps reduce the strain of role changes and maintain a sense of dignity and control.*

- Provide accurate and optimistic information about the disorder and its short- and long-term effects. *The client and family need accurate information to plan for the future.*

- Evaluate the need for additional support and social services for the client and family. Provide referrals as indicated. *Depending on client and family strengths, the severity of the disorder, and its treatment and prognosis, ongoing social support services may be necessary to facilitate coping and adaptation.*

Renal Failure

Renal failure is a condition in which the kidneys are unable to remove accumulated metabolites from the blood, leading to altered fluid, electrolyte, and acid-base balance. The cause may be a primary kidney disorder, or renal failure may be secondary to a systemic disease or other urologic defects. Renal failure may be either acute or chronic. **Acute renal failure** has an abrupt onset and with prompt intervention is often reversible. **Chronic renal failure** is a silent disease, developing slowly and insidiously, with few symptoms until the kidneys are severely damaged and unable to meet the excretory needs of the body. Both forms of renal failure are characterized by azotemia, increased levels of nitrogenous wastes in the blood.

Renal failure is common and costly. In 1999, approximately 89,000 new clients began receiving treatment for **end-stage renal disease (ESRD).** Annually, more than 243,000 clients with ESRD undergo dialysis, about 13,500 have kidney transplants, and another 53,000 are awaiting kidney transplants. The annual cost of ESRD treatment (in 1999 dollars) is $17.87 billion. The cost is also measured in lives and lifestyle. The 5-year survival rate for clients undergoing dialysis is 31.3 % (National Kidney and Urologic Diseases Information Clearinghouse [NKUDIC], 2001). Although many clients report satisfaction with their quality of life, often clients on dialysis are unable to work, and the family structure may disintegrate under the strain of treatment.

The Client with Acute Renal Failure

Acute renal failure (ARF) is a rapid decline in renal function with azotemia and fluid and electrolyte imbalances. Approximately 5% of all hospitalized clients develop ARF; the incidence jumps to as much as 30% in critical and special care units (Braunwald, et al., 2001). The mortality rate for ARF in seriously ill clients is up to 88%. This high death rate is probably more related to the populations affected by ARF—older clients and the critically ill—than to the disorder itself (Porth, 2002).

Major trauma or surgery, infection, hemorrhage, severe heart failure, severe liver disease, and lower urinary tract obstruction are risk factors for ARF. Drugs and radiologic contrast media that are toxic to the kidney (*nephrotoxic*) also increase the risk for ARF. Older adults develop ARF more frequently due to their higher incidence of serious illness, hypotension, major surgeries, diagnostic procedures, and treatment with nephrotoxic drugs. The older adult may also have some degree of preexisting renal insufficiency associated with aging.

The most common causes of acute renal failure are ischemia and nephrotoxins. The kidney is particularly vulnerable to both because of the amount of blood that passes through it. A fall in blood pressure or volume can cause ischemia of kidney tissues. Nephrotoxins in the blood damage renal tissue directly.

Physiology Review

The functional unit of the kidneys, the nephron, produces urine through three processes: glomerular filtration, tubular reabsorption, and tubular secretion. In the *glomerulus,* a filtrate of water and small solutes is formed. The solute concentration of this filtrate is equal to that of plasma, with the exception of large molecules, such as plasma proteins and blood cells. The glomerular filtration rate (GFR), the amount of filtrate formed per minute, is affected by blood volume and pressure, the autonomic nervous system, and other factors. From the glomerulus, the filtrate flows into the *tubules,* where its composition is changed by the processes of *tubular reabsorption* and *tubular secretion.* Most water and many filtered solutes, such as electrolytes and glucose, are reabsorbed. Metabolic waste products, such as urea, hydrogen ion, ammonia, and some creatinine, are secreted into the tubule for elimination. By the time urine exits the collecting duct into the renal pelvis, 99% of the filtrate has been reabsorbed.

Pathophysiology

The causes of acute renal failure are commonly categorized as prerenal, intrarenal, and postrenal. Prerenal causes account for 55% to 60% of ARF, intrarenal for 35% to 40%, and postrenal for less than 5%.

Prerenal ARF

Prerenal causes of ARF affect renal blood flow and perfusion. Any condition that significantly decreases vascular volume, cardiac output, or systemic vascular resistance can affect renal blood flow. The kidneys normally receive 20% to 25% of the cardiac output to maintain the GFR. A drop in renal blood flow to less than 20% of normal causes ischemic changes in kidney tissue and a fall in GFR. If renal perfusion is rapidly restored, these changes are reversible. Continued ischemia can lead to tubular cell necrosis and significant nephron damage (Porth, 2002). Intrarenal ARF may result.

Intrarenal ARF

Intrarenal failure is characterized by acute damage to the renal parenchyma and nephrons. Intrarenal causes include diseases of the kidney itself and acute tubular necrosis, the most common intrarenal cause of ARF.

In acute glomerulonephritis, glomerular inflammation can reduce renal blood flow and cause ARF. Vascular disorders affecting the kidney, such as vasculitis (inflammation of the blood vessels), malignant hypertension, and arterial or venous occlusion, can damage nephrons sufficiently to result in acute renal failure.

Acute Tubular Necrosis

Nephrons are especially susceptible to injury from ischemia or exposure to nephrotoxins. **Acute tubular necrosis (ATN),** destruction of tubular epithelial cells, causes an abrupt and progressive decline of renal function. Prolonged ischemia is the primary cause of ATN. When ischemia and nephrotoxin exposure occur concurrently, the risk for ATN and tubular dysfunction is especially high. Risk factors for ischemic ATN include major surgery, severe hypovolemia, sepsis, trauma, and burns. The impact of ischemia resulting from vasodilation and fluid loss in sepsis, trauma, and burns often is compounded by toxins released by bacteria or from damaged tissue.

Ischemia lasting more than two hours causes severe and irreversible damage to kidney tubules with patchy cellular necrosis and sloughing. The GFR is significantly reduced as a result of (1) ischemia, (2) activation of the renin-angiotensin system, and (3) tubular obstruction by cellular debris, which raises the pressure in the glomerular capsule.

Common nephrotoxins associated with ATN include the aminoglycoside antibiotics and radiologic contrast media. Many other drugs (e.g., nonsteroidal anti-inflammatory drugs and some chemotherapy drugs), heavy metals, such as mercury and gold, and some common chemicals, such as ethylene glycol (antifreeze), are also potentially toxic to the renal tubule. The risk for ATN is higher when nephrotoxic drugs are given to older clients or clients with preexisting renal insufficiency, and when used in combination with other nephrotoxins. Dehydration increases the risk by increasing the toxin concentration in nephrons.

Nephrotoxins destroy tubular cells by both direct and indirect effects. As tubular cells are damaged and lost through necrosis and sloughing, the tubule becomes more permeable. This increased permeability results in filtrate reabsorption, further reducing the ability of the nephron to eliminate wastes.

Rhabdomyolysis may cause up to 25% of all cases of ARF (Wallace, 2001). It is caused by release of excess myoglobin from injured skeletal muscles. Myoglobin is a protein that acts as the oxygen reservoir for muscle fibers, much as hemoglobin does for the blood. Muscle trauma, strenuous exercise, hyperthermia or hypothermia, drug overdose, infection, and other factors can precipitate rhabdomyolysis. The myoglobin clogs renal tubules causing ischemic injury, and contains an iron pigment that directly damages the tubules. *Hemolysis,* red blood cell destruction, releases hemoglobin into the circulation, with much the same effect as rhabdomyolysis.

Postrenal ARF

Obstructive causes of acute renal failure are classified as postrenal. Any condition that prevents urine excretion can lead to postrenal ARF. Benign prostatic hypertrophy is the most common precipitating factor. Others include renal or urinary tract calculi and tumors. See Chapter 25 for further discussion of urinary tract obstruction.

Course and Manifestations

The course of acute renal failure typically includes three phases: initiation, maintenance, and recovery.

Initiation Phase

The *initiation phase* may last hours to days. It begins with the initiating event (e.g., hemorrhage) and ends when tubular injury occurs. If ARF is recognized and the initiating event is effectively treated during this phase, the prognosis is good. The initiation phase of ARF has few manifestations; in fact, it is often identified only when manifestations of the maintenance phase develop.

Maintenance Phase

The *maintenance phase* of ARF is characterized by a significant fall in GFR and tubular necrosis. Oliguria may develop, although many clients continue to produce normal or near normal amounts of urine (nonoliguric ARF). Even though urine may be produced, the kidney cannot efficiently eliminate metabolic wastes, water, electrolytes, and acids from the body during the maintenance phase of ARF. Azotemia, fluid retention, electrolyte imbalances, and metabolic acidosis develop. These abnormalities are more severe in the oliguric client than in the nonoliguric one, leading to a poorer prognosis with oliguria.

During the maintenance phase, salt and water retention cause edema, increasing the risk for heart failure and pulmonary edema. Impaired potassium excretion leads to hyperkalemia. When the serum potassium level is greater than 6.0 to 6.5 mEq/L, manifestations of its effect on neuromuscular function develop. These include muscle weakness, nausea and diarrhea, electrocardiographic changes, and possible cardiac arrest. Other electrolyte imbalances include hyperphosphatemia and hypocalcemia. Metabolic acidosis results from impaired hydrogen ion elimination by the kidneys.

Anemia develops after several days of ARF due to suppressed erythropoietin secretion by the kidneys. Immune function may be impaired, increasing the risk for infection. Other manifestations of the maintenance phase include:

- Edema and hypertension due to salt and water retention.
- Confusion, disorientation, agitation or lethargy, hyperreflexia, and possible seizures or coma due to azotemia, electrolyte and acid-base imbalances.
- Anorexia, nausea, vomiting, and decreased or absent bowel sounds.
- Uremic syndrome if ARF is prolonged (see the section on chronic renal failure that follows).

Recovery Phase

The recovery phase of ARF is characterized by a process of tubule cell repair and regeneration and gradual return of the GFR to normal or pre-ARF levels. Diuresis may occur as the nephrons and GFR recover, and retained salt, water, and solutes are excreted. Serum creatinine, BUN, potassium, and phosphate levels remain high and may continue to rise in spite of increasing urine output. Renal function improves rapidly during the first 5 to 25 days of the recovery phase, and continues to improve for up to 1 year.

Collaborative Care

Preventing acute renal failure is a goal in caring for all clients, especially those in high-risk groups. Maintaining an adequate vascular volume, cardiac output, and blood pressure is vital to preserve kidney perfusion. Nephrotoxic drugs are avoided if possible. When a nephrotoxic drug or substance must be used, the risk of ARF can be reduced by using the minimum effective dose, maintaining hydration, and eliminating other known nephrotoxins from the medication regimen.

Treatment goals for acute renal failure are to (1) identify and correct the underlying cause, (2) prevent additional kidney damage, (3) restore the urine output and kidney function, and (4) compensate for renal impairment until kidney function is restored. Fluid and electrolyte balance is a key component in managing ARF.

The client's history and physical assessment can provide clues about the initiating event for ARF. Impaired perfusion for as few as 30 minutes may cause significant renal ischemia.

Diagnostic Tests

Diagnostic tests are used to identify the cause of acute renal failure and monitor its effects on homeostasis.

- *Urinalysis* often shows the following abnormal findings in acute renal failure.
  a. A fixed specific gravity of 1.010 (equal to the specific gravity of plasma) as the tubules are unable to concentrate the filtrate
  b. Proteinuria if glomerular damage is the cause of ARF
  c. The presence of red blood cells (due to glomerular dysfunction), white blood cells (related to inflammation), and renal tubular epithelial cells (indicating ATN)
  d. Cell casts, which are protein and cellular debris molded in the shape of the tubular lumen. (In ARF, RBC, WBC, and renal tubular epithelial casts may be present. Brownish pigmented casts and positive tests for occult blood indicate hemoglobinuria or myoglobinuria.)
- *Serum creatinine* and *BUN* are used to evaluate renal function. In ARF, serum creatinine levels increase rapidly, within 24 to 48 hours of the onset. Creatinine levels generally peak within 5 to 10 days. Creatinine and BUN levels tend to increase more slowly when urine output is maintained. The onset of recovery is marked by a halt in the rise of the serum creatinine and BUN.
- *Serum electrolytes* are monitored to evaluate the fluid and electrolyte status. The serum potassium rises at a moderate rate and is often used to indicate the need for dialysis. Hyponatremia is common, due to the water excess associated with ARF.
- *Arterial blood gases* often show a metabolic acidosis due to the kidneys' inability to adequately eliminate metabolic wastes and hydrogen ions (see Chapter 39).
- *Complete blood count* shows reduced RBCs, moderate anemia, and a low hematocrit. ARF affects erythropoietin secretion and RBC production. Iron and folate absorption may also be impaired, further contributing to anemia.

Laboratory findings associated with kidney disease are summarized in Table 24-1.

- *Renal ultrasonography* is used to identify obstructive causes of renal failure, and to differentiate acute renal failure from end-stage chronic renal failure. In ARF, the kidneys may be enlarged, whereas they typically appear small and shrunken in chronic renal failure.
- *Computed tomography (CT)* scan also may be done to evaluate kidney size and identify possible obstructions.
- *Intravenous pyelography (IVP), retrograde pyelography,* or *antegrade pyelography* may also be used to evaluate kidney structure and function. Radiologic contrast media are used

with extreme caution because of their potential nephrotoxicity. Retrograde pyelography, in which contrast dye is injected into the ureters, and antegrade pyelography, in which the contrast medium is injected percutaneously into the renal pelvis, are preferred because they have fewer nephrotoxic effects than IVP.

• *Renal biopsy* may be necessary to differentiate between acute and chronic renal failure

Medications

The primary focus in drug management for acute renal failure is to restore and maintain renal perfusion and to eliminate drugs that are nephrotoxic from the treatment regimen.

Intravenous fluids and blood volume expanders are given as needed to restore renal perfusion. Dopamine (Intropin), administered in low doses by intravenous infusion, increases renal blood flow. Dopamine is a sympathetic neurotransmitter that improves cardiac output and dilates blood vessels of the mesentery and kidneys when given in low therapeutic doses.

If restoration of renal blood flow does not improve urinary output, a potent loop diuretic, such as furosemide (Lasix), or an osmotic diuretic, such as mannitol, may be given with intravenous fluids. The purpose is twofold. First, if nephrotoxins are present, the combination of fluids and potent diuretics may, in effect, "wash out" the nephrons, reducing toxin concentration. Second, establishing urine output may prevent oliguria, and reduce the degree of azotemia and fluid and electrolyte imbalances. Furosemide may also be used to manage salt and water retention associated with ARF.

Aggressive hypertension management limits renal injury when ARF is associated with disorders, such as toxemia and pregnancy-induced hypertension. ACE inhibitors or other antihypertensive medications are used to control arterial pressures.

All drugs that are either directly nephrotoxic, or that may interfere with renal perfusion, such as potent vasoconstrictors, are discontinued. NSAIDs, nephrotoxic antibiotics, and other potentially harmful drugs are avoided throughout the course of acute renal failure.

The client in acute renal failure has an increased risk of gastrointestinal bleeding, probably related to the stress response and impaired platelet function. Regular doses of antacids, histamine H_2-receptor antagonists (e.g., famotidine or ranitidine), or a proton-pump inhibitor, such as omeprazole (Prilosec) are often ordered to prevent GI hemorrhage.

Hyperkalemia may require active intervention as well as restricted potassium intake. Serum levels of greater than 6.5 mEq/L are treated to prevent cardiac effects of hyperkalemia. With significant hyperkalemia, calcium chloride, bicarbonate, and insulin and glucose may be given intravenously to reduce serum potassium levels by moving potassium into the cells. A potassium-binding exchange resin, such as sodium polystyrene sulfonate (Kayexalate, SPS Suspension), may be given orally or by enema. This agent removes potassium from the body by exchanging sodium for potassium, primarily in the large intestine. When given orally, it is often combined with sorbitol to prevent constipation. Rectally, it is instilled as a retention enema, allowed to remain in the bowel for approximately 30 to 60 minutes, and then irrigated out using a tap-water enema.

Aluminum hydroxide (AlternaGEL, Amphojel, Nephrox), an antacid, is used to control hyperphosphatemia in renal failure. It binds with phosphates in the GI tract, which are then excreted in the feces.

Because many drugs are eliminated from the body by the kidney, drug dosages may need to be adjusted. Doses within the usual range can lead to potentially toxic blood levels, because their elimination is slowed and half-life prolonged. Nursing implications for medications commonly prescribed for the client in ARF are summarized in Table 24-2.

Table 24-2. Medication Administration – The Client with Acute Renal Failure

Loop Diuretics

Bumetanide (Bumex)
Ethacrynic acid (Edecrin)
Furosemide (Lasix)
Torsemide (Demadex)

The loop diuretics, named for their primary site of action in the loop of Henle, are *high-ceiling diuretics:* The response increases with increasing doses. These are highly effective diuretics used in early ARF to reestablish urine flow and convert oliguric renal failure to nonoliguric renal failure. Loop diuretics may be given with intravenous dopamine to promote renal blood flow. In ATN due to a nephrotoxin, loop diuretics are used to clear the toxin from the nephrons more rapidly. Loop diuretics cause potassium wasting, which is generally not a concern in ARF, because renal failure impairs normal potassium elimination.

Nursing Responsibilities
- Assess weight and vital signs for baseline data.
- Monitor intake and output, daily weight (or more frequently as ordered), vital signs, skin turgor, and other indicators of fluid volume status frequently.
- Assess for orthostatic hypotension as these potent diuretics can lead to hypovolemia.
- Monitor laboratory results, especially serum electrolyte, glucose, BUN, and creatinine levels.
- Administer by mouth or, if ordered, by intravenous injection:
  a. Furosemide undiluted at a rate of no more than 20 mg per minute.
  b. Ethacrynic acid 50 mg diluted with 50 mL of normal saline at a rate of no more than 10 mg per minute.
  c. Bumetanide undiluted over at least one minute or diluted in lactated Ringer's solution, normal saline, or 5% dextrose in water for infusion.
  d. Torsemide undiluted over at least two minutes.
- Assess response. Urine output typically increases within ten minutes after intravenous administration.
- Monitor hearing and for complaints, such as tinnitus. High doses of loop diuretics increase the risk of ototoxicity especially with ethacrynic acid. These effects may be reversible if detected early and the drug is discontinued.
- Avoid administering concurrently with other ototoxic agents, such as aminoglycoside antibiotics and cisplatin.

Client and Family Teaching
- Unless contraindicated, maintain a fluid intake of two to three quarts per day.
- Rise slowly from lying or sitting positions, because a fall in blood pressure may cause lightheadedness.

Continued on the next page

Table 24-2. Continued

- Take in the morning and, if ordered twice a day, late afternoon to avoid sleep disturbance.
- Take with food or milk to prevent gastric distress.
- Nonsteroidal anti-inflammatory drugs (NSAIDs) interfere with the effectiveness of loop diuretics and should be avoided.

Osmotic Diuretics

Mannitol (Osmitrol, Isotol)
Urea (Ureaphil)

The osmotic diuretics act by increasing the osmotic draw in the blood and urine. In the blood, the effect is to pull extracellular water into the vascular system, increasing the GFR. These substances are then freely filtered in the glomerulus and increase the osmotic draw of the urine, inhibiting water reabsorption. The effect is to increase urine volume and flow. In addition, osmotic diuretics dilute waste products in the urine, decreasing the risk of renal damage due to excess concentrations.

Nursing Responsibilities
- Assess urine output. Osmotic diuretics are used in early renal failure to maintain urine output, but are contraindicated in anuria. A test dose may be administered; urine output of 30 mL per hour following the test dose shows an adequate response.
- Do not give these diuretics to clients who have heart failure, or who are severely dehydrated. They increase vascular volume and may worsen heart failure. These drugs are not effective unless extracellular volume is adequate.
- Administer mannitol intravenously, diluting before use if indicated. Check solution for crystallization. Dissolve crystals by warming the solution slightly. Infuse 15% to 25% mannitol solutions through a filter over 30 to 90 minutes.
- Administer urea intravenously, diluting in 100 mL of 5% or 10% dextrose in water for every 30 g of urea. Administer no faster than 4 mL per minute through a filter.
- Monitor vital signs, breath sounds, and urinary output.
- Discontinue the drug if signs of heart failure or pulmonary edema develop, or if renal function continues to decline.

Client and Family Teaching
- Report shortness of breath, headache, chest pain, or dizziness immediately.

Electrolytes and Electrolyte Modifiers

Calcium chloride
Calcium gluconate
Sodium bicarbonate
Sodium polystyrene sulfonate (Kayexalate)

Calcium chloride or gluconate and sodium bicarbonate are administered intravenously in the initial management of hyperkalemia. Calcium is also administered to correct hypocalcemia and reduce hyperphosphatemia (calcium and phosphate have a reciprocal relationship in the body; as the level of one rises, the level of the other falls). Sodium bicarbonate helps correct acidosis and move potassium back into the intracellular space. Sodium polystyrene sulfonate

Table 24-2. Continued

is not used to replace an electrolyte, but to remove excess potassium from the body by exchanging sodium for potassium in the large intestine.

Nursing Responsibilities
* Assess serum electrolyte levels prior to and during therapy. Report rapid shifts or adverse responses to the physician.
* Administer as appropriate:
  a. Intravenous calcium choride at less than 1 mL per minute; intravenous calcium gluconate at 0.5 mL per minute. Inject into a large vein through a small-bore needle; avoid infiltration because extravasation of intravenous solution will cause tissue necrosis.
  b. Intravenous sodium bicarbonate infusion over four to eight hours; oral tablets as prescribed.
  c. Sodium polystyrene sulfonate as an oral solution mixed with sorbitol to prevent constipation, or as a retention enema mixed with warm water. Leave in the bowel for 30 to 60 minutes, irrigate using a small tap-water enema.
* Monitor for adverse reactions, such as dysrhythmias, electrolyte imbalances, and metabolic alkalosis.

Client and Family Teaching
* Intravenous calcium may make you lightheaded; remain in bed for at least 30 minutes after administration.
* Chew sodium bicarbonate tablets and follow with eight ounces of water. Do not take with milk.
* Retain the sodium polystyrene sulfonate enema as long as possible.

Fluid Management

Once vascular volume and renal perfusion are restored, fluid intake is usually restricted. The allowed daily fluid intake is calculated by allowing 500 mL for insensible losses (respiration, perspiration, bowel losses) and adding the amount excreted as urine (or lost in vomitus) during the previous 24 hours. For example, if a client with ARF excretes 325 mL of urine in 24 hours, the client is allowed a fluid intake (including oral and intravenous fluids) of 825 mL for the next 24 hours. Fluid balance is carefully monitored, using accurate weight measurements and the serum sodium as the primary indicators.

Dietary Management

Renal insufficiency and the underlying disease process increase the rate of *catabolism* (the breakdown of body proteins) and decrease the rate of *anabolism* (body tissue repair). The client with ARF needs adequate nutrients and calories to prevent catabolism. Proteins are limited to 0.6 g per kilogram of body weight per day to minimize the degree of azotemia. Dietary proteins should be of high biologic value (rich in essential amino acids). Carbohydrates are increased to maintain adequate calorie intake and provide a protein-sparing effect.

Parenteral nutrition providing amino acids, concentrated carbohydrates, and fats may be instituted when the client cannot consume an adequate diet (e.g., due to nausea, vomiting, or underlying critical illness). The disadvantages of parenteral nutrition in the client with ARF are the high volume of fluid required and the risk for infection through the venous line.

Dialysis

Manifestations of uremia, severe fluid overload, hyperkalemia, or metabolic acidosis in a client with renal failure indicate a need to replace renal function. **Dialysis** is the diffusion of solute molecules across a semipermeable membrane from an area of higher solute concentration to one of lower concentration. It is used to remove excess fluid and metabolic waste products in renal failure. Early use of dialysis can reduce the rate of complications. Dialysis may also be used to rapidly remove nephrotoxins in acute tubular necrosis. While dialysis compensates for lost renal elimination functions, it does not replace lost erythropoietin production. Anemia is a continuing problem for the client receiving dialysis.

In dialysis, blood is separated from a dialysis solution (**dialysate**) by a semipermeable membrane. Either **hemodialysis,** a procedure in which blood passes through a semipermeable membrane filter outside the body, or **peritoneal dialysis,** which uses the peritoneum surrounding the abdominal cavity as the dialyzing membrane, may be used for the client with ARF. **Continuous renal replacement therapy (CRRT),** in which blood is continuously circulated through a highly porous hemofilter from artery to vein, or vein to vein, is a newer form of dialysis that may be used to treat ARF.

Hemodialysis   Hemodialysis uses the principles of diffusion and ultrafiltration to remove electrolytes, waste products, and excess water from the body. Blood is taken from the client via a vascular access and pumped to the dialyzer. The porous membranes of the dialyzer unit allow small molecules, such as water, glucose, and electrolytes, to pass through, but block larger molecules, such as serum proteins and blood cells. The dialysate, a solution of approximately the same composition and temperature as normal extracellular fluid, passes along the other side of the membrane. Small solute molecules move freely across the membrane by diffusion. The direction of movement for any substance is determined by the concentrations of that substance in the blood and the dialysate. Electrolytes and waste products, such as urea and creatinine, diffuse from the blood into the dialysate. If it is necessary to add something to the blood, such as calcium to replace depleted stores, it can be added to the dialysate to diffuse into the blood. Excess water is removed by creating a higher hydrostatic pressure of the blood moving through the dialyzer than of the dialysate, which flows in the opposite direction. This process is known as **ultrafiltration.**

Initially, clients with ARF typically undergo daily hemodialysis, then three to four sessions per week as indicated. Hemodialysis is not used if the client is hemodynamically unstable (e.g., with hypotension or low cardiac output). Following are complications associated with hemodialysis:

- Hypotension, the most frequent complication during hemodialysis, is related to changes in serum osmolality, rapid removal of fluid from the vascular compartment, vasodilation, and other factors.
- Bleeding is related to altered platelet function associated with uremia and the use of heparin during dialysis.
- Infection (local or systemic) is related to WBC damage and immune system suppression. *Staphylococcus aureus* septicemia is commonly associated with contamination of the vascular access site. Clients on chronic hemodialysis have higher rates of hepatitis B, hepatitis C, cytomegalovirus, and HIV infection than the general population.

Continuous Renal Replacement Therapy

Clients with acute renal failure may be unable to tolerate hemodialysis and rapid fluid removal if their cardiovascular status is unstable (e.g., due to trauma, major surgery, heart failure). Continuous renal replacement therapy (CRRT), which allows more gradual fluid and solute removal, is often used for these clients. In CRRT, blood is continuously circulated from an artery to a vein, or a vein to a vein, through a highly porous hemofilter for a period of 12 or more hours. Excess water and solutes, such as electrolyes, urea, creatinine, uric acid, and glucose, drain into a collection device. Fluid may be replaced with normal saline or a balanced electrolyte solution as needed during CRRT. This slower process helps maintain hemodynamic stability and avoid complications associated with rapid changes in ECF composition.

CRRT is typically performed in an intensive care unit or specialized nephrology unit. Both arterial and venous lines are required for some types of CRRT; for others, a double-lumen venous catheter is used. Strict aseptic technique is vital in caring for vascular access sites to reduce the risk of infection.

Vascular Access

Acute or temporary vascular access for hemodialysis or CRRT is usually gained by inserting a double-lumen catheter into the subclavian, jugular, or femoral vein. The double-lumen catheter has a central partition separating the blood withdrawal side of the catheter from the return side. Blood is drawn into the catheter through small openings in the proximal portion of the catheter, and returned to the circulation through an opening in the distal end of the catheter to avoid withdrawing the blood that has just been dialyzed.

For longer-term vascular access, an *arteriovenous (AV) fistula* is created. In preparation for fistula formation, the nondominant arm is not used for venipuncture or blood pressure measurement during renal failure. The fistula is created by surgical anastomosis of an artery and vein, usually the radial artery and cephalic vein. It takes about a month for the fistula to mature so that it can be used for taking and replacing blood during dialysis. A functional AV fistula has a palpable pulsation and a bruit on auscultation. Venipunctures and blood pressures are avoided on the arm with the fistula.

In chronic renal failure, an *arteriovenous graft* is most often used for vascular access. The graft, a tube made of Gortex, is surgically implanted and connects the artery and the vein. Blood flows through the graft from the artery to the vein. Occasionally, an *external AV shunt* connecting a peripheral artery with a peripheral vein is used for vascular access.

Localized AV fistula, graft, or shunt problems can occur. Infection and clotting or thrombosis are the most common shunt problems. Aneurysms may also develop. Both infection and thrombosis can lead to systemic manifestations, such as septicemia and embolization. These local complications may cause the fistula or graft to fail, necessitating development of a new site. The psychologic impact of AV fistula or graft failure is significant, often causing depression and low self-esteem.

Peritoneal Dialysis

In peritoneal dialysis, the highly vascular peritoneal membrane serves as the dialyzing surface. Warmed sterile dialysate is instilled into the peritoneal cavity through a catheter inserted into the peritoneal cavity. Metabolic waste products and excess electrolytes diffuse into the dialysate while it remains in the abdomen. Water movement is controlled using dextrose as an osmotic agent to draw it into the dialysate. The fluid is then drained by gravity out of the peritoneal cavity into a sterile bag. This process of dialysate infusion, dwell time of the solution in the abdomen, and drainage is repeated at prescribed intervals.

Because excess fluid and solutes are removed more gradually in peritoneal dialysis, it poses less risk for the unstable client; however, this slower rate of metabolite removal can be a disadvantage in ARF. Peritoneal dialysis increases the risk for developing peritonitis. It is contraindicated for clients who have had recent abdominal surgery, significant lung disease, or peritonitis.

Nursing Care

Health Promotion

Acute renal failure often can be prevented by measures that maintain fluid volume and cardiac output and reduce the risk of exposure to nephrotoxins. Carefully monitor critically ill, postoperative, and other at-risk clients for early signs of hypovolemia (low urine output, altered mental status, changes in vital signs, skin color or temperature). Promptly report a fall in urine output to less than 30 mL per hour and other evidence of decreased cardiac output. Maintain intravenous fluids as ordered. Alert the physician if the client is receiving more than one nephrotoxic drug or if a nephrotoxic drug is ordered for a dehydrated client. Closely observe clients receiving blood or blood cells for early signs of transfusion reaction and intervene appropriately.

Assessment

Both subjective and objective data are useful when assessing the client with acute renal failure.

* *Health history:* complaints of anorexia, nausea, weight gain, or edema; recent exposure to a nephrotoxin, such as an aminoglycoside antibiotic or radiologic procedure using an injected contrast medium; previous transfusion reaction; chronic diseases, such as diabetes, heart failure, or kidney disease.

* *Physical examination:* vital signs including temperature; urine output (amount, color, clarity, specific gravity, presence of blood cells or protein); weight; skin color, peripheral pulses; presence of edema (periorbial or dependent); lung sounds, heart sounds, and bowel tones.

Nursing Diagnoses and Interventions

The client with acute renal failure has numerous nursing care needs related not only to the renal failure, but also to the underlying condition that precipitated it. Priority nursing care needs relate to fluid volume alterations, appetite and nutrition, and teaching/learning.

Excess Fluid Volume

In acute renal failure, the kidneys often cannot excrete adequate urine to maintain a normal extracellular fluid balance. Fluid retention is greater in oliguric renal failure than in nonoliguric failure. Rapid weight gain and edema indicate fluid retention. In addition, heart failure and pulmonary edema may develop. In the older adult or severely debilitated client, fluid retention can present a significant management problem.

* Maintain hourly intake and output records. *Accurate intake and output records help guide therapy, especially fluid restrictions.*

- Weigh daily or more frequently, as ordered. Use standard technique (same scale, clothing, or coverings) to ensure accuracy. *Rapid weight changes are an accurate indicator of fluid volume status, particularly in the oliguric client.*
- Assess vital signs at least every four hours. *Hypertension, tachycardia, and tachypnea may indicate excess fluid volume.*

Table 24-3. Nursing Care of the Client Undergoing Peritoneal Dialysis

Predialysis Care

- Document vital signs including temperature, orthostatic blood pressures (lying, sitting, and standing), apical pulse, respirations, and lung sounds. *These baseline data help assess fluid volume status and tolerance of the dialysis procedure. Hypertension, abnormal heart or lung sounds, or dyspnea may indicate excess fluid volume. Poor respiratory function may affect the ability to tolerate peritoneal dialysis. Temperature measurement is vital, because infection is the most common complication of peritoneal dialysis.*
- Weigh daily or between dialysis runs as indicated. *Weight is an accurate indicator of fluid volume status.*
- Note BUN, serum electrolyte, creatinine, pH, and hematocrit levels prior to peritoneal dialysis and periodically during the procedure. *These values are used to assess the efficacy of treatment.*
- Measure and record abdominal girth. *Increasing abdominal girth may indicate retained dialysate, excess fluid volume, or early peritonitis.*
- Maintain fluid and dietary restrictions as ordered. *Fluid and diet restrictions help reduce hypervolemia and control azotemia.*
- Have the client empty the bladder prior to catheter insertion. *Emptying the bladder reduces the risk of inadvertent puncture.*
- Warm the prescribed dialysate solution to body temperature (98.6°F or 37°C) using a warm water bath or heating pad on low setting. *Dialysate is warmed to prevent hypothermia.*
- Explain all procedures and expected sensations. *Knowledge helps reduce anxiety and elicit cooperation.*

Intradialysis Care

- Use strict aseptic technique during the dialysis procedure and when caring for the peritoneal catheter. *Peritonitis is a common complication of peritoneal dialysis; sterile technique reduces the risk.*
- Add prescribed medications to the dialysate; prime the tubing with solution and connect it to the peritoneal catheter, taping connections securely and avoiding kinks. *This allows dialysate to flow freely into the abdominal cavity and prevents leaking or contamination.*
- Instill dialysate into the abdominal cavity over a period of approximately ten minutes. Clamp tubing and allow the dialysate to remain in the abdomen for the prescribed dwell time. Keep drainage tubing clamped at all times during instillation and dwell time. *Dialysate should flow freely into the abdomen if the peritoneal catheter is patent. Dialysis, the exchange of solutes and water between the blood and dialysate, occurs across the peritoneal membrane during the dwell time.*

Continued on the next page

Table 24-3. Continued

- During instillation and dwell time, observe closely for signs of respiratory distress, such as dyspnea, tachypnea, or crackles. Place in Fowler's or semi-Fowler's position and slow the rate of instillation slightly to relieve respiratory distress if it develops. *Respiratory compromise may result from overly rapid filling or overfilling of the abdomen or from a diaphragmatic defect that allows fluid to enter the thoracic cavity.*

- After prescribed dwell time, open drainage tubing clamps and allow dialysate to drain by gravity into a sterile container. Note the clarity, color, and odor of returned dialysate. *Blood or feces in the dialysate may indicate organ or bowel perforation; cloudy or malodorous dialysate may indicate an infection.*

- Accurately record amount and type of dialysate instilled (including any added medications), dwell time, and amount and character of the drainage. *When more dialysate drains than has been instilled, excess fluid has been lost (output). If less dialysate is returned than has been instilled, a fluid gain has occurred (intake).*

- Monitor BUN, serum electrolyte, and creatinine levels. *These values are used to assess the effectiveness of dialysis.*

- Troubleshoot for possible problems during dialysis.

  a. Slow dialysate instillation. Increase the height of the container and reposition the client. Check tubing and catheter for kinks. Check abdominal dressing for wetness, indicating leakage around the catheter. *Slow dialysate flow may be related to a partially obstructed tube or catheter.*

  b. Excess dwell time. *Prolonged dwell time may lead to water depletion or hyperglycemia.*

  c. Poor dialysate drainage. Lower the drainage container, reposition, check for tubing kinks. Check abdominal dressing. *Tubing or catheter obstruction can also interfere with dialysate drainage.*

Postdialysis Care

- Assess vital signs, including temperature. *Comparison of pre- and postdialysis vital signs helps identify beneficial and adverse effects of the procedure.*

- Time meals to correspond with dialysis outflow. *Scheduling meals while the abdomen is empty of dialysate enhances intake and reduces nausea.*

- Teach the client and family about the procedure. *The client may elect to use peritoneal dialysis at home to manage end-stage renal disease and prevent uremia.*

- If not contraindicated, place in semi-Fowler's position, *to enhance cardiac and respiratory function.*

- Report abnormal serum electrolyte values and manifestations of electrolyte imbalance. The client with ARF is at particular risk for the following electrolyte imbalances:

  a. *Hyperkalemia* due to impaired potassium excretion. Manifestations include irritability, nausea, diarrhea, abdominal cramping, cardiac dysrhythmias, and ECG changes.

  b. *Hyponatremia* due to water retention. Manifestations include nausea, vomiting, and headache, with possible CNS manifestations of lethargy, confusion, seizures, and coma.

  c. *Hyperphosphatemia* due to decreased phosphate excretion. Manifestations include hyperreflexia, paresthesias, and possible tetany.

Table 24-3. Continued

ARF impairs electrolyte and water excretion, causing multiple electrolyte imbalances.

- Restrict fluids as ordered. Provide frequent mouth care and encourage using hard candies to decrease thirst. If ice chips are allowed, include the water content (approximately one-half of the total volume) as intake. *Fluids are restricted to minimize fluid retention and complications of fluid volume excess.*
- Administer medications with meals. *Giving oral medications with meals minimizes ingestion of excess fluids.*

Imbalanced Nutrition: Less Than Body Requirements

Anorexia and nausea associated with renal failure often interfere with food intake and nutrition. In addition, the disease process leading to ARF may contribute to increased nutritional needs for healing and decreased food intake.

- Monitor and record food intake, including the amount and type of food consumed. *A detailed intake record helps guide decisions about nutritional status and necessary supplements.*
- Weigh daily. *Weight changes over time (days to weeks) reflect nutritional status, while rapid weight changes are more reflective of fluid volume status. In ARF, weight may remain stable or increase due to fluid retention even though tissue mass is being lost.*
- Arrange for dietary consultation to plan meals within prescribed limitations that consider the client's food preferences. *Diets restricted in protein, salt, and potassium can be unpalatable; including preferred foods as allowed increases intake.*
- Engage the client in planning daily menus. *Participation in meal planning increases the client's sense of control and autonomy.*
- Allow family members to prepare meals within dietary restrictions. Encourage family members to eat with the client. *Familiar foods and social interaction encourage eating and increase enjoyment of meals.*
- Provide frequent, small meals or between-meal snacks. *These measures promote food intake in the fatigued or anorectic client.*
- Administer antiemetics as ordered and provide mouth care prior to meals. *Nausea and a metallic taste in the mouth, common manifestations of uremia, can decrease food intake.*
- Administer parenteral nutrition as ordered if the client is unable to eat or tolerate enteral nutrition. *Preventing or slowing tissue catabolism is important for the client with ARF.*

Deficient Knowledge

The client with ARF has multiple learning needs. These include information about ARF, diagnostic and laboratory studies, management strategies, and implications for the recovery period.

- Assess anxiety level and ability to comprehend instruction. Tailor information and presentation to developmental level and physical, mental, and emotional status. *The client with ARF may be critically ill or have uremic effects that hinder learning. During the initial stages of ARF it may be necessary to limit information to immediate concerns.*
- Assess knowledge and understanding. *To enhance understanding and retention, relate information presented to previous learning.*

- Teach about diagnostic tests and therapeutic procedures. *Teaching reduces anxiety and improves understanding and cooperation.*
- Discuss dietary and fluid restrictions. *These measures may be continued after discharge.*
- If the client is discharged prior to the recovery phase of ARF, teach the signs and symptoms of complications, such as fluid volume excess or deficit, heart failure, and electrolyte imbalances. *As kidney function returns, urine output increases, but the concentrating ability of the nephrons and electrolyte excretion remain impaired. This impaired function increases the risk of excess fluid loss, possible dehydration, orthostatic hypotension, and electrolyte imbalance.*
- Teach how to monitor weight, blood pressure, and pulse. *These are important means of assessing fluid status.*
- Instruct to avoid nephrotoxic drugs and chemicals for up to one year following an episode of ARF. *During recovery, nephrons are vulnerable to damage by nephrotoxins, such as NSAIDs, some antibiotics, radiologic contrast media, and heavy metals. Because alcohol can increase the nephrotoxicity of some materials, discourage alcohol ingestion.*

Home Care

Often the client is critically ill when ARF develops. Critical illness and the resulting state of client and family crisis can impair learning and retention of information. Include family members in teaching during the initial stages to promote understanding of what is happening and the reasons for specific treatment measures. Inclusion of the family reduces their anxiety, and provides a valuable resource for reinforcing client teaching about care after discharge.

Client teaching needs for home care include:

- Avoiding exposure to nephrotoxins, particularly those in over-the-counter products.
- Preventing infection and other major stressors that can slow healing.
- Monitoring weight, blood pressure, and pulse.
- Manifestations of relapse.
- Continuing dietary restrictions.
- Knowing when to contact the physician.

25 Assessing Clients with Endocrine Disorders

The endocrine system is an essential regulator of the body's internal environment. Through hormones secreted by its glands, the endocrine system regulates such varied functions as growth, reproduction, metabolism, fluid and electrolyte balance, and gender differentiation. It also helps the body adapt to constant alterations in the internal and external environment.

Review of Anatomy and Physiology

The major endocrine organs are the pituitary gland, thyroid gland, parathyroid glands, adrenal glands, pancreas, and gonads (reproductive glands). Table 25-1 summarizes the role of the endocrine organs and their hormones.

Pituitary Gland

The pituitary gland (or *hypophysis*) is located in the skull beneath the hypothalamus of the brain. It often is called the "master gland" because its hormones regulate many body functions. The pituitary gland has two parts: the anterior pituitary (or adenohypophysis) and the posterior pituitary (or neurohypophysis). The anterior pituitary is glandular tissue, whereas the posterior pituitary is actually an extension of the hypothalamus.

Anterior Pituitary

The *anterior pituitary* has several types of endocrine cells and secretes at least six major hormones.

- Somatotropic cells secrete growth hormone (GH), also called somatotropin. GH stimulates growth of the body by signaling cells to increase protein production and by stimulating the epiphyseal plates of the long bones.
- Lactotropic cells secrete prolactin (PRL). Prolactin stimulates the production of breast milk.
- Thyrotropic cells secrete thyroid-stimulating hormone (TSH). TSH stimulates the synthesis and release of thyroid hormones from the thyroid gland.
- Corticotropic cells secrete adrenocorticotropic hormone (ACTH). ACTH stimulates release of hormones, especially the *glucocorticoids*, from the adrenal cortex.
- Gonadotropic cells secrete the gonadotropin hormones, follicle-stimulating hormone (FSH), and luteinizing hormone (LH). These hormones stimulate the ovaries and testes

(the gonads). In women, FSH stimulates the development of ovarian follicles and induces the secretion of estrogenic female sex hormones. In men, FSH is involved in the development and maturation of sperm. In women, increasing levels of LH work together with FSH to lead to ovulation and the formation of the corpus luteum from an ovarian follicle. In men, LH is called interstitial cell–stimulating hormone (ICSH). This hormone stimulates the interstitial cells of the testes to produce male sex hormones.

Posterior Pituitary

The *posterior pituitary* is made of nervous tissue. Its primary function is to store and release two hormones produced in the hypothalamus:

- Antidiuretic hormone (ADH), also called *vasopressin,* inhibits urine production by causing the renal tubules to reabsorb water from the urine and return it to the circulating blood.
- Oxytocin induces contraction of the smooth muscles in the reproductive organs. In women, oxytocin stimulates the myometrium of the uterus to contract during labor. It also induces milk ejection from the breasts.

Thyroid Gland

The thyroid gland is anterior to the upper part of the trachea and just inferior to the larynx. This butterfly-shaped gland has two lobes connected by a structure called the isthmus.

The glandular tissue consists of follicles filled with a jellylike colloid substance called thyroglobin, a glycoprotein-iodine complex. Cells within the follicles secrete thyroid hormone (TH), a general name for two similar hormones: *thyroxine* (T_4) and *triiodothyronine* (T_3). The primary role of thyroid hormones is to increase metabolism; they are also responsible for growth and development in children. TH secretion is initiated by the release of TSH by the pituitary gland and is dependent on an adequate supply of iodine.

The thyroid gland also secretes calcitonin, a hormone that decreases excessive levels of calcium in the blood by slowing the calcium-releasing activity of bone cells.

Table 25-1. Organs, Hormones, Functions, and Feedback Mechanisms of the Endocrine System

Endocrine Organ	Hormone Secreted	Target Organ and Feedback Mechanism
Thyroid gland	Thyroid hormone (TH): thyroxine (T_4) is the major hormone secreted by the thyroid gland. It is converted to triiodothyronine (T_3) at the target tissues.	Maintains metabolic rate and growth and development of all tissues. T_3 and T_4 are secreted in response to thyroid-stimulating hormone (TSH).
	Calcitonin	Maintains serum calcium levels by decreasing bone resorption and decreasing resorption of calcium in the kidneys whenever levels of plasma calcium are elevated.

Table 25-1. Continued

Parathyroid gland	Parathyroid hormone (PTH)	Maintains serum calcium levels by stimulating bone resorption and formation and by stimulating kidney resorption of calcium in response to falling levels of plasma calcium.
Adrenal cortex	Mineralocorticoids (e.g., aldosterone)	Promote kidney tubule reabsorption of sodium and water and excretion of potassium in response to elevated levels of potassium and low levels of sodium, thereby increasing blood pressure and blood volume.
	Glucocorticoids (e.g., cortisol)	Help regulate metabolism of carbohydrates, fats, and proteins. Activate anti-inflammatory responses to stressors. Low cortisol levels stimulate hypothalamic secretion of corticotropin-releasing hormone (CRH), which stimulates the anterior pituitary gland to release ACTH, which in turn stimulates the adrenal cortex to secrete cortisol.
	Gonadocorticoids (androgens and small amounts of estrogen and progesterone)	The quantity of sex hormones produced here is small, and the mechanism is not well understood.
Adrenal medulla	Catecholamines (epinephrine and norepinephrine)	Stimulate the heart, constrict blood vessels, inhibit visceral muscles, dilate bronchioles, increase respiration and metabolism, promote hyperglycemia. Secreted in response to physical or psychologic stress.
Anterior pituitary (adenohypophysis)	Growth hormone (GH)	Promotes growth of body tissues by enhancing protein synthesis and promoting use of fat for energy and thus conserving glucose. Release is stimulated by growth hormone releasing hormone (GHRH) in response to low GH levels, hypoglycemia, increased amino acids, low fatty acids, and stress.

Parathyroid Glands

The parathyroid glands (usually four to six) are embedded on the posterior surface of the lobes of the thyroid gland. They secrete parathyroid hormone (PTH), or *parathormone*. When calcium levels in the plasma fall, PTH secretion increases. PTH also controls phosphate metabolism. It acts primarily by increasing renal excretion of phosphate in the urine, by decreasing the excretion of calcium, and by increasing bone reabsorption to cause the release of calcium from bones. Normal levels of vitamin D are necessary for PTH to exert these effects on bone and kidneys.

Adrenal Glands

The two adrenal glands are pyramid-shaped organs that sit on top of the kidneys. Each gland consists of two parts, which are distinct organs: an inner medulla and an outer cortex.

Adrenal Medulla

The adrenal medulla produces two hormones (also called catecholamines): epinephrine (also called *adrenaline*) and norepinephrine (or *noradrenaline*.) These hormones are similar to substances released by the sympathetic nervous system and, thus, are not essential to life. Epinephrine increases blood glucose levels and stimulates the release of ACTH from the pituitary; ACTH in turn stimulates the adrenal cortex to release glucocorticoids. Epinephrine also increases the rate and force of cardiac contractions; constricts blood vessels in the skin, mucous membranes, and kidneys; and dilates blood vessels in the skeletal muscles, coronary arteries, and pulmonary arteries.

Norepinephrine increases both heart rate and the force of cardiac contractions. It also vasoconstricts blood vessels throughout the body.

Adrenal Cortex

The adrenal cortex secretes several hormones, all corticosteroids. They are classified into two groups: mineralocorticoids and glucocorticoids. These hormones are essential to life. The release of the mineralocorticoids is controlled primarily by an enzyme called renin. When a decrease in blood pressure or sodium is detected, specialized kidney cells release renin to act on a substance called angiotensinogen, manufactured by the liver. Angiotensinogen is modified by renin and other enzymes to become angiotensin, which stimulates the release of aldosterone from the adrenal cortex. Aldosterone prompts the distal tubules of the kidneys to release increased amounts of water and sodium back into the circulating blood to increase volume and pressure. The glucocorticoids include cortisol and cortisone. These hormones affect carbohydrate metabolism by regulating glucose use in body tissues, mobilizing fatty acids from fatty tissue, and shifting the source of energy for muscle cells from glucose to fatty acids. Glucocorticoids are released in times of stress. An excess of glucocorticoids in the body depresses the inflammatory response and inhibits the effectiveness of the immune system.

Pancreas

The pancreas, located behind the stomach between the spleen and the duodenum, is both an endocrine gland (producing hormones) and an exocrine gland (producing digestive enzymes). The endocrine cells of the pancreas produce hormones that regulate carbohydrate metabolism. They are clustered in bodies called pancreatic islets (or islets of Langerhans) scattered throughout the gland. Pancreatic islets have at least four different cell types:

- Alpha cells produce glucagon, which decreases glucose oxidation and promotes an increase in the blood glucose level by signaling the liver to release glucose from glycogen stores.

- Beta cells produce insulin, which facilitates the uptake and use of glucose by cells and prevents an excessive breakdown of glycogen in the liver and muscle. In this way, insulin decreases blood glucose levels. Insulin also facilitates lipid formation, inhibits the breakdown and mobilization of stored fat, and helps amino acids move into cells to promote protein synthesis. In general, the actions of glucagon and insulin oppose one another, helping to maintain a stable blood glucose level.

- Delta cells secrete somatostatin, which inhibits the secretion of glucagon and insulin by the alpha and beta cells.

- F cells secrete pancreatic polypeptide, which is believed to inhibit the exocrine activity of the pancreas.

Gonads

The gonads are the testes in men and the ovaries in women. These organs are the primary source of steroid sex hormones in the body. The hormones of the gonads are important in regulating body growth and promoting the onset of puberty.

In men, androgens (primarily testosterone) produced by the testes maintain reproductive functioning and secondary sex characteristics. Androgens also promote the production of sperm. In women, the ovaries secrete estrogens and progesterone to maintain reproductive functioning and secondary sex characteristics. Progesterone also promotes the growth of the lining of the uterus to prepare for implantation of a fertilized ovum.

An Overview of Hormones

Hormones are chemical messengers secreted by the endocrine organs and transported throughout the body, where they exert their action on specific cells called target cells. Hormones do not cause reactions directly but rather regulate tissue responses. They may produce either generalized or local effects.

Hormones are transported from endocrine gland cells to target cells in the body in one of four ways:

- Endocrine glands release most hormones, including TH, insulin, and others, into the bloodstream. Some require a protein carrier.

- Neurons release some hormones, such as epinephrine, into the bloodstream. This is called the neuroendocrine route.

- The hypothalamus releases its hormones directly to target cells in the posterior pituitary by nerve cell extension.

- With the paracrine method, released messengers diffuse through the interstitial fluid. This method of transport involves a number of hormonal peptides that are released throughout various organs and cells and act locally. An example is endorphins, which act to relieve pain.

Hormones act by binding to specific receptor sites located on the surfaces of the target cells. These receptors recognize a specific hormone and translate the message into a cellular response. The receptor sites are structured so that they respond only to a specific hormone; in other words, receptors in the thyroid gland are responsive to TSH but not to LH.

Hormone levels are controlled by the pituitary gland and by feedback mechanisms. Although most feedback mechanisms are negative, a few are positive. Negative feedback is controlled much as the thermostat in a house regulates temperature. Sensors in the endocrine system detect changes in hormone levels and adjust hormone secretion to maintain normal body levels. When the sensors detect a decrease in hormone levels, they begin actions to cause an increase in hormone levels; when hormone levels rise above normal, the sensors cause a decrease in hormone production and release. For example, when the hypothalamus or anterior pituitary gland senses increased blood levels of TH, it releases hormones causing a reduction in the secretion of TSH, which in turn prompts a decrease in the output of TH by the thyroid gland.

With positive feedback mechanisms, increasing levels of one hormone cause another gland to release a hormone. For example, the increased production of estradiol (a female ovarian hormone) during the follicular stage of the menstrual cycle in turn stimulates increased FSH production by the anterior pituitary gland. Estradiol levels continue to increase until the ovarian follicle disappears, eliminating the source of the stimulation for FSH, which then decreases. Stimuli for hormone release may also be classified as hormonal, humoral, or neural. In hormonal release, hypothalamic hormones stimulate the anterior pituitary to release hormones. Fluctuations in the serum level of these hormones in turn prompt other endocrine glands to release hormones. In humoral release, fluctuations in the serum levels of certain ions and nutrients stimulate specific endocrine glands to release hormones to bring these levels back to normal. In neural release, nerve fibers stimulate the release of hormones.

Assessing Endocrine Function

Function of the endocrine glands is assessed both by a health assessment interview to collect subjective data and a physical assessment to collect objective data. Hormones affect all body tissues and organs, and manifestations of dysfunction are often nonspecific, making assessment of endocrine function often more difficult than assessment of other body systems.

Health Assessment Interview

A health assessment interview to determine problems with the endocrine system may be part of a health screening or total health assessment, or it may focus on a chief complaint, such as increased urination or changes in energy levels. If the client has a problem with endocrine function, the nurse analyzes its onset, characteristics and course, severity, precipitating and relieving factors, and any associated symptoms, noting the timing and circumstances. For example, the nurse may ask the client:

- Describe the swelling you noticed in the front of your neck. When did it begin? Have you noticed any changes in your energy level?
- When did you first notice that your hands and feet were getting larger?
- Have you noticed that your appetite has increased even though you have lost weight?

The health history includes information about the client's medical history, family history, and social and personal history. Ask the client about any changes in normal growth and development, as well as in height and weight. Changes in the size of extremities can often be detected by asking whether the client has had to have rings enlarged or to buy increasingly larger gloves and shoes. Enlargement of the neck may be identified by asking whether the client has difficulty finding shirts or blouses with a collar that fits. Also explore changes including difficulty swallowing; increased or decreased thirst, appetite, and/or urination; visual changes; sleep disturbances; altered patterns of hair distribution, such as increased facial hair in women; changes in menstruation; changes in memory or ability to concentrate; and changes in hair and skin texture. Ask the client about any blow to the head, as well as previous hospitalizations, chemotherapy, radiation (especially to the neck), and the use of medications (especially hormones or steroids).

Because many endocrine disorders have a familial tendency, ask the client about a family history of such diseases as diabetes mellitus, diabetes insipidus, thyroid disorders, hypertension, tumors, autoimmune disorders, and obesity. Ask women about problems with pregnancy, menstruation, and/or menopause.

The nurse should also ask about the client's occupational and social history. Include questions about the client's satisfaction with occupation, personal relationships, and lifestyle. Other areas of assessment include the client's usual means of coping; use of alcohol, smoking, or drugs; diet; exercise patterns; and sleep patterns. Although the client may not recognize changes in behavior, family members may be able to provide important information.

Physical Assessment

Physical assessment of the endocrine system may be performed as part of a total health assessment, or it may be a focused assessment of clients with known or suspected problems with endocrine function.

The only endocrine organ that can be palpated is the thyroid gland; however, other assessments that provide information about endocrine problems include inspection of the skin, hair and nails, facial appearance, reflexes, and musculoskeletal system. Measurement of height and weight as well as vital signs also provides clues to altered endocrine system function.

The client may sit during the examination. A reflex hammer is used to test deep-tendon reflexes. Prior to the examination, the nurse collects the necessary equipment and explains the techniques to the client to decrease anxiety. Additional techniques for assessing hypocalcemic tetany, a complication of endocrine disorders or surgery, are included in the examination sequence.

Skin Assessments with Abnormal Findings

- Inspect skin color.
    - ✓ Hyperpigmentation may be seen in clients with Addison's disease or Cushing's syndrome.
    - ✓ Hypopigmentation may be seen in diabetes mellitus, hyperthyroidism, or hypothyroidism.
    - ✓ A yellowish cast to the skin might indicate hypothyroidism.
    - ✓ Purple striae over the abdomen and bruising may be present in the client with Cushing's syndrome.
- Palpate the skin, assessing texture, moisture, and the presence of lesions.
    - ✓ Rough, dry skin is often seen in clients with hypothyroidism, whereas smooth and flushed skin can be a sign of hyperthyroidism.
    - ✓ Lesions on the lower extremities might indicate diabetes mellitus.

Nails and Hair Assessment with Abnormal Findings

- Assess texture and condition of nails and hair.
  - ✓ Increased pigmentation of the nails is often seen in clients with Addison's disease.
  - ✓ Dry, thick, brittle nails and hair may be apparent in hypothyroidism; thin, brittle nails and thin, soft hair may be apparent in hyperthyroidism.
  - ✓ Hirsutism (excessive facial, chest, or abdominal hair) may be seen in Cushing's syndrome.

Facial Assessments with Abnormal Findings

- Inspect the symmetry and form of the face.

- Inspect position of eyes.

  - ✓ Variations of form and structure may indicate growth abnormalities such as acromegaly.

Thyroid Gland Assessment with Abnormal Findings

- Palpate the thyroid gland for size and consistency.
  - ✓ Stand behind the client, and place your fingers on either side of the trachea below the thyroid cartilage. Ask the client to tilt the head to the right. Now ask the client to swallow. As the client swallows, displace the left lobe while palpating the right lobe. Repeat to palpate the left lobe.
  - ✓ Exophthalmos (protruding eyes) may be seen in hyperthyroidism.
  - ✓ The thyroid may be enlarged in clients with Graves' disease or a goiter.
  - ✓ Multiple nodules may be seen in metabolic disorders, whereas the presence of only one nodule may indicate a cyst or a benign or malignant tumor.
  - ✓ One enlarged nodule suggests malignancy.

Motor Function Assessment with Abnormal Findings

- Assess the deep-tendon reflexes. See Chapter 31 for guidelines on assessment.
  - ✓ Increased reflexes may be seen in hyperthyroidism; decreased reflexes may be seen in hypothyroidism.

Sensory Function Assessment with Abnormal Findings

- Test the client's sensitivity to pain, temperature, vibration, light touch, and stereognosis (the ability to identify an object merely by touch). Compare symmetric areas on both sides of the body, and compare the distal to the proximal regions of the extremities.

Ask the client to close his or her eyes.

- To test pain, use the blunt and sharp ends of a new safety pin. Discard the pin after use.
- To test temperature, use cups or other containers of cold and hot water.
- To test vibration, use a tuning fork over one of the client's finger or toe joints.
- To test light touch, use a cotton wisp.
- To test stereognosis, place in the client's hand a simple, familiar object, such as a rubber band, cotton ball, or button. Ask the client to identify the object.

✓ Peripheral neuropathy and paresthesias (altered sensations) may occur in diabetes, hypothyroidism, or acromegaly.

Musculoskeletal Assessment with Abnormal Findings

• Inspect the size and proportions of the client's body structure.

✓ Extremely short stature may indicate dwarfism, which is caused by insufficient growth hormone.

✓ Extremely large bones may indicate acromegaly, which is caused by excessive growth hormone.

Assessing for Hypocalcemic Tetany

• Assess for **Trousseau's sign:** Inflate pressure cuff above antecubital space to occlude blood supply to the arm.

✓ Decreased calcium levels cause the client's hand and fingers to contract (*carpal spasm*).

• Assess for **Chvostek's sign:** Tap your finger in front of the client's ear at the angle of the jaw.

✓ Decreased calcium levels cause the client's lateral facial muscles to contract.

26 Nursing Care of Clients with Endocrine Disorders

The thyroid, parathyroid, adrenal, and pituitary glands are part of the endocrine system. Disorders of the structure and function of these glands alter normal hormone levels and the way body tissues use those hormones. When hormone production increases or decreases, people experience alterations in health.

Clients with disorders of the glands discussed in this chapter require nursing care for multiple problems. They often face exhausting diagnostic tests, changes in physical appearance and emotional responses, and permanent alterations in lifestyle. Nursing care is directed toward meeting physiologic needs, providing education, and ensuring psychologic support for the client and family. A holistic approach to the complex needs of clients with these endocrine disorders is an essential component of nursing care.

Disorders of the Thyroid Gland

Altered thyroid hormone (TH) production or use affects all major organ systems. In the adult, TH changes primarily affect metabolism, cardiovascular function, gastrointestinal function, and neuromuscular function. Thyroid disorders—both hyperthyroidism and hypothyroidism—are among the most common endocrine disorders.

The Client with Hyperthyroidism

Hyperthyroidism (also called **thyrotoxicosis**) is a disorder caused by excessive delivery of TH to the peripheral tissues. Because the primary effect of TH is to increase metabolism and protein synthesis, hyperthyroidism affects all major organ systems of the body. The increase in metabolic rate and the alterations in cardiac output, peripheral blood flow, oxygen consumption, and body temperature are similar to those found in increased sympathetic nervous system activity (Porth, 2002).

The effects of hyperthyroidism are the result of increased circulating levels of TH. This hormonal excess increases the metabolic rate and heightens the sympathetic nervous system's physiologic response to stimulation. The sensitizing effect of abnormally elevated TH levels increases the cardiac rate and stroke volume. As a result, cardiac output and peripheral blood flow increase. Elevated TH levels also increase carbohydrate, protein, and lipid metabolism. Lipids are depleted, and glucose tolerance decreases. Protein degradation increases, resulting in a negative nitrogen balance. Over time, the hypermetabolic effects of excess TH result in caloric and nutritional deficiencies.

Pathophysiology and Manifestations

Hyperthyroidism results from many different factors, including autoimmune reactions (as in Graves' disease), excess secretion of thyroid-stimulating hormone (TSH) by the pituitary gland, thyroiditis, neoplasms, such as toxic multinodular goiter, and an excessive intake of thyroid medications. The most common etiologies of hyperthyroidism are Graves' disease and toxic multinodular goiter.

The client with hyperthyroidism typically has an increased appetite, yet loses weight and may have hypermotile bowels and diarrhea. Additional manifestations related to hypermetabolism include heat intolerance and increased sweating. The client's hair is fine, and the skin is smooth and warm. Emotional lability is common.

Graves' Disease

Graves' disease, the most common cause of hyperthyroidism, is an autoimmune disorder. The serum of more than 90% of clients with Graves' disease contains TSH-R (stim) Ab, an antibody directed against the TSH receptor site in the thyroid follicles (Tierney, et al., 2001). When this antibody binds to the TSH receptors, it stimulates hormone synthesis and secretion. The cause is unknown, but there is a hereditary link. Other factors associated with Graves' disease include an immune response against a viral antigen, a defect of the lymphocyte T helper cells, and the presence of other autoimmune disorders, such as myasthenia gravis and pernicious anemia, (Porth, 2002).

Graves' disease is seen five times more often in women than in men and occurs most frequently between the ages of 20 and 40. It is seen worldwide, with the incidence often correlated with the amount of iodine in the diet. Increased iodine intake, such as from radiocontrast dyes used in diagnostic tests or from ingestion of kelp tablets, has been associated with an increased frequency of hyperthyroidism.

Clients with Graves' disease have an enlarged thyroid gland (**goiter**) and manifestations of hyperthyroidism (See Table 26-1). The hypertrophy of the gland can result from excess TSH stimulation (when the amount of circulating TH is deficient), growth-stimulating immunoglobulins, or substances that inhibit TH synthesis. A goiter may be present in hyperthyroidism or hypothyroidism.

Table 26-1. *Laboratory Findings in Hyperthyroidism*

Test	Normal Values	Findings
Serum TA	Negative to 1:20	Increased
Serum TSH (Sensitive assay)	>1.0 mμ/L	Decreased in primary hyperthyroidism
Serum T_4	5 to 12 mμ/dL	Increased
Serum T_3	80 to 200 ng/dL	Increased
T_3 uptake (T_3RU)	25 to 35 relative percentage	Increased
Thyroid suppression		Increased RAI uptake and T_4 levels

Proptosis (forward displacement) of the eye occurs in about one-third of cases (Porth, 2002). The forward protrusion of the eyeballs (also called **exophthalmos**) results from an accumulation of fat deposits and inflammation by-products in the retro-orbital tissues. Often the sclera is visible above the iris. The upper lids are often retracted, and the person has a characteristic unblinking stare. Proptosis is usually bilateral, but it may involve only one eye. The client may experience blurred vision, diplopia, eye pain, lacrimation, and photophobia. The inability to close the eyelids completely over the protruding eyeballs increases the risk of corneal dryness, irritation, infection, and ulceration. The treatment of Graves' disease does not reverse these changes in the eyes.

Other manifestations include fatigue, difficulty sleeping, hand tremors, and changes in menstruation ranging from decreased flow to amenorrhea. Older clients may experience atrial fibrillation, angina, or congestive heart failure.

Toxic Multinodular Goiter

Toxic multinodular goiter is characterized by small, discrete, independently functioning nodules in the thyroid gland tissue that secrete excessive amounts of TH. It is not known how these nodules grow or become independent, but a genetic mutation of follicle cells is suspected. Elevated TH levels result in manifestations of hyperthyroidism; however, they are slower to develop and differ somewhat from those of Graves' disease. The client with this type of hyperthyroidism is usually a woman in her 60s or 70s who has had a goiter for a number of years.

Excess TSH Stimulation

Overproduction of TSH by the pituitary usually stimulates the thyroid gland to produce excess TH. The elevation in TSH secretion often results from a pituitary adenoma. This secondary form of hyperthyroidism is rare.

Thyroiditis

Thyroiditis (inflammation of the thyroid gland) is most often the result of a viral infection of the thyroid gland. The symptoms of thyroiditis are those of acute inflammation and the effects of increased TH. Thyroiditis is an acute disorder that may become chronic, resulting in a hypothyroid state as repeated infections destroy gland tissue. See the discussion of Hashimoto's thyroiditis later in this chapter.

Thyroid Crisis

Thyroid crisis (also called **thyroid storm**) is an extreme state of hyperthyroidism that is rare today because of improved diagnosis and treatment methods (Porth, 2002). When it does occur, those affected are usually people with untreated hyperthyroidism (most often Graves' disease) and people with hyperthyroidism who have experienced a stressor, such as an infection, trauma, untreated diabetic ketoacidosis, or manipulation of the thyroid gland during surgery. Thyroid crisis is a life-threatening condition.

The rapid increase in metabolic rate that results from the excessive TH causes the manifestations of thyroid crisis. The manifestations include hyperthermia, with body temperatures ranging from 102°F (39°C) to 106°F (41°C); tachycardia; systolic hypertension; and gastrointestinal symptoms (abdominal pain, vomiting, diarrhea). Agitation, restlessness, and tremors are common, progressing to confusion, psychosis, delirium, and seizures. The mortality rate is high. Rapid treatment of thyroid crisis is essential to preserve life. Treatment includes relieving respiratory distress, stabilizing cardiovascular function, and reducing TH synthesis and secretion.

Collaborative Care

Treatment of hyperthyroidism focuses on reducing the production of TH by the thyroid gland, thus establishing a **euthyroid** (normal thyroid) state, and preventing or treating complications. Depending on the client's age and physical status, either medications, radioactive iodine therapy, or surgery may be used.

Diagnostic Tests

Hyperthyroidism is diagnosed according to the manifestations of the specific disorders causing excessive TH, and by diagnostic test results. Elevated levels of TH (both T_3 and T_4) and increased radioactive iodine (RAI) uptake are diagnostic criteria of hyperthyroidism. Laboratory findings in hyperthyroidism are shown in Table 26-1.

The following diagnostic tests may be ordered:

- *TA test.* Serum thyroid antibodies (TA) are measured to determine whether a thyroid autoimmune disease is causing the client's symptoms. TA is elevated in Graves' disease.

- *TSH test (sensitive assay).* Serum TSH levels are measured and compared with thyroxine (T_4) levels to differentiate pituitary from thyroid dysfunction. The best indicator of primary hyperthyroidism, such as in Graves' disease, is suppression of TSH below 0.1 µg/mL. When the sensitive TSH is not suppressed, the hyperthyroidism is caused by a TSH-secreting pituitary tumor.

- *T_4 test.* Serum thyroxine (T_4) levels are measured to determine TH concentration and to test thyroid gland function. T_4 levels are elevated in hyperthyroidism and in acute thyroiditis.

- *T_3 test.* Serum triiodothyronine (T_3) is measured by radioimmunoassay (T_3RIA), which measures bound and free forms of this hormone. This test is effective for the diagnosis of hyperthyroidism. T_3 levels may also be elevated in thyroiditis.

- *T_3 uptake test.* T_3 uptake (T_3RU) is measured by an in vitro test in which the client's blood is mixed with radioactive T_3; the results are elevated in hyperthyroidism.

- *RAI uptake test.* A radioactive iodine (RAI) uptake test (thyroid scan) measures the absorption of ^{131}I or ^{123}I by the thyroid gland. A calculated dose of radioactive iodine is given orally or intravenously, and the thyroid is then scanned (often after 24 hours). The distribution of radioactivity in the gland is recorded (increased uptake of radioactive iodine is seen in Graves' disease). In addition, the scan reveals the size and shape of the gland.

- *Thyroid suppression test.* RAI and T_4 levels are measured first. The client then takes TH for seven to ten days, after which the tests are repeated. Failure of hormone therapy to suppress RAI and T_4 indicates hyperthyroidism.

Medications

Hyperthyroidism is treated by administering antithyroid medications that reduce TH production. Because these drugs do not affect the release or activity of hormone that is already formed, therapeutic effects may not be seen for several weeks. Some commonly prescribed drugs, their actions, and nursing implications are shown in Table 26-2.

Radioactive Iodine Therapy

Because the thyroid gland takes up iodine in any form, radioactive iodine (^{131}I) concentrates in the thyroid gland and damages or destroys thyroid cells so that they produce less TH. Radioactive iodine is given orally. Results typically occur in six to eight weeks. In most instances, the client is not hospitalized during treatment and does not require radiation precautions. This type of therapy is contraindicated in pregnant women because radioactive iodine crosses the placenta and can have negative effects on the developing fetal thyroid gland. Because the amount of gland destroyed is not readily controllable, the client may become hypothyroid and require lifelong TH replacement.

Table 26-2. Medication Administration – Hyperthyroidism

Iodine Sources

Potassium iodide (SSKI, Thyro-Block)
Potassium iodide (Pima)

Large doses of iodine inhibit TH synthesis and release. Iodine also makes the hyperplastic thyroid less vascular prior to surgery and hastens the ability of other antithyroid drugs to reduce natural hormone output.

Nursing Responsibilities
- Assess for hypersensitivity to iodine before giving medication; for example, ask client about allergies to shellfish.
- Dilute liquid iodine sources in water or orange juice to disguise bitter taste.
- Monitor for increased bleeding tendencies if the client is also taking anticoagulants; iodine increases their effect.

Client and Family Teaching
- The maximum effect of iodine in large doses usually occurs in one to two weeks.
- Long-term iodine therapy is not effective in controlling hyperthyroidism.

Antithyroid Drugs

Methimazole (Tapazole)
Propylthiouracil (PTU, Propyl-Thracil)

Antithyroid drugs inhibit TH production. They do not affect already formed hormones; thus, several weeks may elapse before the client experiences therapeutic effects.

Nursing Responsibilities
- Monitor for side effects: pruritus, rash, elevated temperature, (for iodides) swelling of the eyelids, anorexia, loss of taste, changes in menstruation.
- Administer drugs at the same time each day to maintain stable blood levels.
- Monitor for symptoms of hypothyroidism: fatigue, weight gain.

Continued on the next page

Table 26-2. Continued

Client and Family Teaching

- Watch for unusual bleeding, nausea, loss of taste, or epigastric pain. Report any such symptoms to the physician.
- If you are also taking anticoagulants, report any signs of bleeding.
- If you are taking lithium, be aware of symptoms of hypothyroidism.
- It may take up to twelve weeks before you experience the full effects of the drugs. Take the medication regularly and exactly as prescribed.

Surgery

Some hyperthyroid clients have such enlarged thyroid glands that pressure on the esophagus or trachea causes breathing or swallowing problems. In these cases, removal of all or part of the gland is indicated. A *subtotal thyroidectomy* is usually performed. This procedure leaves enough of the gland in place to produce an adequate amount of TH. A total **thyroidectomy** is performed to treat cancer of the thyroid; the client then requires lifelong hormone replacement.

Before surgery, the client should be in as nearly a euthyroid state as possible. The client may be given antithyroid drugs to reduce hormone levels and iodine preparations to decrease the vascularity and size of the gland, which also reduces the risk of hemorrhage during and after surgery.

Nursing Care

Health Promotion

Although hyperthyroidism is not preventable, it is important to teach clients the importance of regular health care provider visits and medication intake.

Assessment

The following data are collected through the health history and physical examination (see Chapter 25). Further focused assessments are described with nursing interventions.

- *Health history:* other diseases, family history of thyroid disease, when symptoms began, severity of symptoms, intake of thyroid medications, menstrual history, changes in weight, bowel elimination.
- *Physical assessment:* muscle strength, tremors, vital signs, cardiovascular and peripheral vascular systems, integument, size of thyroid, presence of bruit over thyroid, eyes and vision.

Nursing Diagnoses and Interventions

In planning and implementing nursing care for the client with hyperthyroidism, the nurse considers the client's responses to the systemic effects of the disorder. Although each client may have different needs, nursing diagnoses discussed in this section focus on the most common problems: cardiovascular problems, visual deficits, altered nutrition, and body image disturbance.

Risk for Decreased Cardiac Output

The client with hyperthyroidism is at risk for alterations in cardiac output. Excess TH directly affects the heart, resulting in increased rate and stroke volume. Increases in the metabolic demands and oxygen requirements of peripheral tissues increase the demands on the heart, and systolic hypertension, angina, arrhythmias, or cardiac failure may occur. The client often has palpitations and shortness of breath and is easily fatigued. The risk of complications is greater in clients with preexisting cardiovascular disorders.

- Monitor blood pressure, pulse rate and rhythm, respiratory rate, and breath sounds. Assess for peripheral edema, jugular vein distention, and increased activity intolerance. *Increased TH increases cardiac rate, stroke volume, and tissue demand for oxygen, causing stress on the heart. This may result in hypertension, arrhythmias, tachycardia, and congestive heart failure.*

- Suggest keeping the environment as cool and free of distraction as possible. Decrease stress by explaining interventions and teaching relaxation procedures. *A physically comfortable and psychologically calm environment can reduce stimuli and stressors. Stress increases circulating catecholamines, which further increase cardiac workload.*

- Encourage the client to balance activity with rest periods. *Rest periods decrease energy expenditure and tissue requirements for oxygen, decreasing demands on the heart by decreasing cardiac workload.*

Disturbed Sensory Perception: Visual

Visual changes that occur in clients with hyperthyroidism include difficulty in focusing, diplopia (double vision), or visual loss. If the client is unable to close the eyelids because of exophthalmos, the risk of corneal dryness with resultant infection or injury increases. Visual deficits may also result from pressure on the optic nerve from retro-orbital edema and the shortening of eye muscles. Although treatment of hyperthyroidism may stop the progression of eye changes, not all symptoms are reversible.

- Monitor visual acuity, photophobia, integrity of the cornea, and lid closure. *The cornea is at risk for dryness, injury, conjunctivitis, and corneal infections. Injury and infection of the cornea can result in further loss of visual acuity.*

- Teach measures for protecting the eye from injury and maintaining visual acuity:
  1. Use tinted glasses or shields as protection.
  2. Use artificial tears to moisten the eyes.
  3. Use cool, moist compresses to relieve irritation.
  4. Promptly report any pain or changes in vision.

The measures outlined decrease the risk of injury, provide comfort, decrease periorbital edema that can further compromise vision, and ensure immediate care for problems, thereby minimizing the risk of further visual loss.

Imbalanced Nutrition: Less Than Body Requirements

The hypermetabolic state that occurs in hyperthyroidism causes gastrointestinal hypermotility, with nausea, vomiting, diarrhea, and abdominal pain. Although the client may have an increased appetite and eat more than usual, weight loss continues.

- Ask the client to weigh daily (at the same time each day), and keep a record of results. *The inability to meet metabolic demands results in loss of body weight. Regular monitoring detects continued weight loss.*

- In collaboration with a dietitian, teach the client the need for a diet high in carbohydrates and protein, including between-meal snacks. Six small meals a day may be more desirable than three large meals. Caloric intake may need to be increased to 4000 kcal per day if weight loss exceeds 10% to 17% for height and frame. *Increased nutrients as part of a well-balanced diet are necessary to meet metabolic demands. Clients are often better able to increase food intake by eating frequent, small meals. A 1-lb weight gain requires approximately 3500 extra kcal.*

- Monitor nutritional status through results of laboratory data. Serum albumin, transferrin, and total lymphocyte counts are commonly lower than normal in nutritional deficits. *A negative nitrogen balance signifies a catabolic state in which protein is lost and metabolic demands are not being met.*

Disturbed Body Image

Physical changes common in hyperthyroidism include exophthalmos, goiter, tremors, hair loss, increased perspiration, loss of strength, fatigue, weight loss, and changes in reproductive and sexual function (amenorrhea in women, impotence in men, and increased libido in both men and women). In addition, the client often has mood changes and insomnia and is constantly nervous and anxious. There may even be periods of psychosis. These changes are frightening, not only for the client, but also for family members.

- Establish a trusting relationship; encourage the client to verbalize feelings about self and to ask questions about the illness and treatment. Provide reliable information, and clarify misconceptions. *Establishing trust facilitates open sharing of feelings and perceptions.*

Home Care

Clients with hyperthyroidism primarily provide self-care at home. Teaching is individualized to meet the client's needs. Address the following topics:

- The client taking oral medications must understand the need for lifelong treatment.
- The client who has a thyroidectomy requires information about postoperative wound care.
- The client having radioactive iodine therapy needs to know the symptoms of hypothyroidism.
- Depending on the age of the client and the support systems available, referral to community health care agencies may be necessary.
- In addition, suggest the following resources:
  1. American Thyroid Association
  2. Thyroid Foundation of Canada
  3. Endocrine Society.

The Client with Hypothyroidism

Hypothyroidism is a disorder that results when the thyroid gland produces an insufficient amount of TH. Because a decrease in TH levels decreases metabolic rate and heat production, hypothyroidism affects all body systems. Hypothyroidism is more common in women between ages 30 and 60; the incidence rises after age 50. However, the disorder can occur at any stage of life. Careful evaluation of symptoms is important in the older adult because manifestations of hypothyroidism are often thought to be the result of aging instead of a pathologic process.

The hypothyroid state in adults is sometimes called **myxedema.** The term reflects the characteristic accumulation of nonpitting edema in the connective tissues throughout the body. The edema is the result of water retention in mucoprotein (hydrophilic proteoglycans) deposits in the interstitial spaces. The face of a client with myxedema appears puffy, and the tongue is enlarged (Porth, 2002).

Pathophysiology and Manifestations

Hypothyroidism may be either primary or secondary. Primary hypothyroidism, which is more common, may be caused by congenital defects in the gland, loss of thyroid tissue following treatment for hyperthyroidism with surgery or radiation, antithyroid medications, thyroiditis, or endemic iodine deficiency. The cardiac drug, amiodarone (Cordarone), which contains 75 mg of iodine per 200 mg tablet, is increasingly being implicated in causing thyroid problems (Porth, 2002). Secondary hypothyroidism may result from pituitary TSH deficiency or peripheral resistance to thyroid hormones. Hypothyroidism has a slow onset, with manifestations occurring over months or even years. With treatment, the mental and physical symptoms rapidly reverse in clients of all ages.

When TH production decreases, the thyroid gland enlarges in a compensatory attempt to produce more hormone. The goiter that results is usually a simple or nontoxic form. People living in certain areas of the world where the soil is deficient in iodine, the substance necessary for TH synthesis and secretion, are more prone to become hypothyroid and develop simple goiter. (Iodine deficiency is discussed later in this chapter.)

Hypothyroid clients characteristically have the manifestations of goiter, fluid retention and edema, decreased appetite, weight gain, constipation, dry skin, dyspnea, pallor, hoarseness, and muscle stiffness. Many clients have a decreased sense of taste and smell, menstrual disorders, anemias, and cardiac enlargement. The pulse is typically slow. Deficient amounts of TH cause abnormalities in lipid metabolism, with elevated serum cholesterol and triglyceride levels. As a result, the client is at increased risk for atherosclerosis and cardiac disorders. Decreased renal blood flow and glomerular filtration rate reduces the kidney's ability to excrete water, which may cause hyponatremia. Sleep apnea is more common in clients with hypothyroidism. Factors that result in decreased TH, in addition to those described, include iodine deficiency and Hashimoto's thyroiditis. A severe state of hypothyroidism is called *myxedema coma.*

Iodine Deficiency

Iodine is necessary for TH synthesis and secretion. Iodine deficiency may result from certain goitrogenic drugs (which block TH synthesis); lithium carbonate, used to treat bipolar mental disorders; and antithyroid drugs. Goitrogenic compounds in foods, such as turnips, rutabagas, and soybeans, may also block TH synthesis if consumed in sufficient quantities. In areas of the world where the soil is deficient in iodine, dietary intake of iodine may be inadequate. However, the use of iodized salt has reduced this risk in the United States.

Hashimoto's Thyroiditis

Hashimoto's thyroiditis is the most common cause of primary hypothyroidism. In this autoimmune disorder, antibodies develop that destroy thyroid tissue. Functional thyroid tissue is replaced with fibrous tissue, and TH levels decrease. In addition, decreasing levels of TH in the early stages of the disease prompt the gland to enlarge to compensate, causing a goiter. However, as the disease progresses, the thyroid gland becomes smaller. This disorder is more common in women and has a familial link.

Myxedema Coma

Myxedema coma is a life-threatening complication of long-standing, untreated hypothyroidism. It is characterized by severe metabolic disorders (hyponatremia, hypoglycemia, lactic acidosis), hypothermia, cardiovascular collapse, and coma. Myxedema coma, although rare, most commonly occurs during the winter months in older women with long-standing chronic hypothyroidism (Porth, 2002).

Myxedema coma may be precipitated by trauma, infection, failure to take thyroid replacement medications, the use of central nervous system depressants, and exposure to cold temperatures (Porth, 2002). The treatment of myxedema coma addresses the precipitating factors and manifestations and involves maintaining a patent airway; maintaining fluid, electrolyte, and acid-base balance; maintaining cardiovascular status; increasing body temperature; and increasing TH levels. If untreated, the mortality rate is high (Tierney et al., 2001).

Collaborative Care

The treatment of the client with hypothyroidism focuses on diagnosis, prevention or treatment of complications, and replacement of the deficient TH. With early and continued treatment, both appearance and mental function return to normal.

Diagnostic Tests

Hypothyroidism is diagnosed by the manifestations and by a decrease in TH, especially T_4. TSH concentration often is increased, because the negative hormonal feedback from TH is lost. The same laboratory and diagnostic tests used to diagnose hyperthyroidism are also used to diagnose hypothyroidism, with opposite results in most cases (see Table 26-3).

Medications

Hypothyroidism is treated with medications that replace TH. Levothyroxine (thyroxine, T_4) is the treatment of choice (Tierney, et al., 2001). Medications commonly used to treat hypothyroidism and their nursing implications are shown in Table 26-4.

Table 26-3.   Laboratory Findings in Hypothyroidism

Test	Normal Values	Findings
Serum TA	None to 1:20	Normal
Serum TSH	>1.0 mµ/L	Increased in primary hypothyroidism
Serum T_4	5 to 12 µg/dL	Decreased
Serum T_3	80 to 200 ng/dL	Decreased
T_3 uptake (T_3RU)	25 to 35 relative percentage	Decreased
Thyroid suppression		No change in RAI uptake or T_4 levels

Surgery

If the hypothyroid client has a goiter large enough to cause respiratory difficulties or dysphagia, a subtotal thyroidectomy may be performed.

Table 26-4. Medication Administration — Hypothyroidism

Thyroid Preparations

Levothyroxine sodium (T_4) (Levoxyl, Levothroid, Synthroid)
Liothyronine sodium (T_3) (Cytomel)
Liotrix ($T_3 - T_4$) (Euthroid, Thyrolar)

Thyroid preparations increase blood levels of TH, thus raising the client's metabolic rate. As a result, cardiac output, oxygen consumption, and body temperature increase. The dosage depends on the drug chosen and the client's degree of thyroid dysfunction, sensitivity to TH, age, body size, and health. The older adult may require lower doses.

Nursing Responsibilities

- Give one hour before meals or two hours after meals for best absorption.
- Thyroid preparations potentiate the effect of anticoagulant drugs. If the client is also receiving an anticoagulant, monitor for bruising, bleeding gums, and blood in the urine.
- Thyroid medications potentiate the effect of digitalis. If the client is also receiving a digitalis preparation, monitor for signs of digitalis toxicity.
- Monitor for symptoms of coronary insufficiency: chest pain, dyspnea, tachycardia.
- If the client has insulin-dependent diabetes, monitor the effects of insulin. The effect of the insulin may change as thyroid function increases.
- During dose adjustment, take pulse before administering drug. Report pulse >100.

Client and Family Teaching

- Do not substitute brands of drugs or use generic equivalents without the physician's approval.
- The medications must be taken for the rest of one's life.
- Report symptoms of excess thyroid hormone to the physician: excess weight loss, palpitations, leg cramps, nervousness, or insomnia.
- If you have diabetes and use insulin, monitor blood glucose levels closely; the thyroid medications may alter the amount of insulin required.
- Thyroid preparations increase the risk of iodine toxicity. Do not use iodized salt or over-the-counter drugs containing iodine.
- If you are also taking an anticoagulant, report any signs of bleeding.
- Report any changes in menstrual periods.
- Take the thyroid preparation each morning to decrease the possibility of insomnia.
- Closely monitor blood pressure and pulse (older clients).
- Avoid excessive intake of foods that are known to inhibit TH utilization, such as turnips, cabbage, carrots, spinach, and peaches.

Nursing Care

Health Promotion

One of the most critical factors in preventing hypothyroidism is education of the public about the necessity of an adequate dietary intake of iodine. The use of iodized salt meets the requirements for hormone production. It is important to teach clients the importance of regular health care provider visits and medication intake.

Assessment

Collect the following data through the health history and physical examination (see Chapter 25). Further focused assessments are described with nursing interventions below:

- *Health history:* pituitary diseases, when symptoms began, severity of symptoms, treatment of hyperthyroidism with medications or radioactive iodine, thyroid surgery, treatment of head or neck cancer with radiation, diet, use of iodized salt, bowel elimination, respiratory difficulties.
- *Physical assessment:* muscle strength, deep tendon reflexes, vital signs, cardiovascular and peripheral vascular systems, integument, thyroid gland, weight.

Nursing Diagnoses and Interventions

In planning and implementing care for clients with hypothyroidism, the nurse takes into account that the disorder affects all organ systems. Although many nursing diagnoses might be valid, this section focuses on client problems with cardiovascular function, elimination, and skin integrity.

Decreased Cardiac Output

A TH deficit causes a reduction in heart rate and stroke volume, resulting in decreased cardiac output. There may also be an accumulation of fluid in the pericardial sac (from the edema characteristic of hypothyroidism), and coronary artery disease may be present, further compromising cardiac function.

- Monitor blood pressure, rate and rhythm of apical and peripheral pulses, respiratory rate, and breath sounds. *Hypotension indicates decreasing peripheral blood. Fluid in the pericardial sac restricts cardiac function. Monopolysaccharide deposits in the respiratory system decrease vital capacity and cause hypoventilation.*
- Suggest the client avoid cold air; increase room temperature, use additional bed covers, and avoid drafts. *Cold air increases metabolic rate and puts increased stress on the heart.*
- Explain the need to alternate activity with rest periods. Ask the client to report any breathing difficulties, chest pain, heart palpitations, or dizziness. *Activity increases demands on the heart and should be balanced with rest. Symptoms of cardiac stress include dyspnea, chest pain, palpitations, and dizziness.*

Constipation

The hypothyroid client is likely to have a reduced appetite and decreased food intake, a diminished activity level because of muscle aches and weakness, and reduced peristalsis to the point that fecal impactions may occur.

- Encourage a fluid intake of up to 2000 mL per day. Discuss preferred liquids and the best times of day to drink fluids. If kcal intake is restricted, ensure that liquids have no kcal or are low in kcal. *Sufficient fluid intake is necessary to promote proper stool consistency.*

- Discuss ways to maintain a high-fiber diet. *Diets high in fiber and fluid produce soft stools. Fiber that is not digested absorbs water, which adds bulk to the stool and assists in the movement of fecal material through the intestines.*

- Encourage activity as tolerated. *Activity influences bowel elimination by improving muscle tone and stimulating peristalsis.*

Risk for Impaired Skin Integrity

The client with hypothyroidism is at risk for impaired skin integrity related to the accumulation of fluid in the interstitial spaces and to dry, rough skin. Decreased peripheral circulation, decreased activity levels, and slow wound healing further increase the risk. These interventions are outlined for the older client who is hospitalized for surgery or severe hypothyroidism.

- Monitor skin surfaces for redness or lesions, especially if the client's activity is greatly reduced. Use a pressure ulcer risk assessment scale to identify clients at risk. *Hypothyroidism causes dry, rough, edematous skin conditions that increase the risk of skin breakdown.*

- Provide or teach the immobile client measures to promote optimal circulation:
  1. Use a turning schedule if the client is on bed rest, or teach the client to change position every two hours.
  2. Limit the time for sitting in one position; shift weight or lift the body using arm rests every 20 to 30 minutes.
  3. Use pillows, pads, or sheepskin or foam cushions for bed and/or chair.
  4. Teach and implement a schedule of range-of-motion exercises.

Prolonged pressure, especially in clients with edema and circulatory impairment, can occlude capillaries and cause hypoxic tissue damage.

- Provide or teach the client measures to maintain skin integrity:
  1. Take baths only as necessary; use warm (not hot) water.
  2. Use gentle motions when washing and drying skin.
  3. Use alcohol-free skin oils and lotions.

Dry skin and edema increase the risk of skin breakdown. Hot water, rough massage, and alcohol-based preparations may increase skin dryness, further impairing the body's ability to maintain skin integrity.

Home Care

Clients with hypothyroidism require lifelong care, primarily at home. Address the following topics:

- The need to take medications for the rest of one's life.
- The need for periodic dosage reassessments.
- If the client is older or does not have support system, helpful community resources.

- Additional resources:
  - American Thyroid Association
  - Thyroid Foundation of Canada
  - Endocrine Society

The Client with Cancer of the Thyroid

Thyroid cancer is relatively rare, with an estimated rate of 23,000 new cases annually. Thyroid cancer accounts for approximately 1300 cancer deaths a year (American Cancer Society, 2002). The most consistent risk factor is exposure to ionizing radiation to the head and neck during childhood. For example, many adults in their 50s and 60s received X-ray treatments for colds and sinus infections during childhood.

Of the several types of thyroid cancer, the most common types are listed here.

- Papillary thyroid carcinoma is the most common thyroid malignancy. It is usually detected as a single nodule, but may arise from a multinodular goiter. The average age of diagnosis is 42, with 70% of cases occurring in women. Risks for the development of this form are exposure to external X-ray treatments to the head or neck as a child, childhood exposure to radioactive isotopes of iodine in nuclear fallout, and a family history. Papillary thyroid carcinoma is the least aggressive type, but does metastasize to the local and regional lymph nodes and lungs.
- Follicular thyroid cancer is the second most common thyroid malignancy. The average age of diagnosis is 50, with 72% of cases occurring in women. This form is more aggressive, with metastasis commonly found in neck lymph nodes, bone, and lungs.

Thyroid cancer is manifested by a palpable, firm nontender nodule in the thyroid. If undetected, the tumor may grow and impinge on the esophagus or trachea, causing difficulty in swallowing or breathing. Most people with thyroid cancer do not have elevated thyroid hormone levels. The diagnosis is made by measuring thyroid hormones, performing thyroid scans, and by fine-needle biopsy of the nodule. The usual treatment is subtotal or total thyroidectomy. TSH suppression therapy with levothyroxine may be conducted prior to surgery. Radioactive iodine therapy (I^{131}) and chemotherapy are additional therapeutic options. The 5-year survival rate, if the tumor has not metastasized, is 95% (American Cancer Society, 2002).

Disorders of the Parathyroid Glands

Disorders of the parathyroid glands, hyperparathyroidism and hypoparathyroidism, are not as common as those of the thyroid gland. Hypercalcemia and hypocalcemia (the primary results of alterations in parathyroid function) are discussed in Chapter 39.

The Client with Hyperparathyroidism

Hyperparathyroidism results from an increase in the secretion of parathyroid hormone (PTH), which regulates normal serum levels of calcium. The increase in PTH affects the kidneys and bones, resulting in the following pathophysiologic changes:

- Increased resorption of calcium and excretion of phosphate by the kidneys, which increases the risk of hypercalcemia and hypophosphatemia.
- Increased bicarbonate excretion and decreased acid excretion by the kidneys, which increases the risk of metabolic acidosis and hypokalemia.
- Increased release of calcium and phosphorus by bones, with resultant bone decalcification.
- Deposits of calcium in soft tissues and the formation of renal calculi.

Pathophysiology and Manifestations

Hyperparathyroidism occurs more often in older adults and is three times more common in women. The disorder itself is not common. The three types of hyperparathyroidism are as follows:

- Primary hyperparathyroidism occurs when there is hyperplasia or an adenoma in one of the parathyroid glands. These disorders interrupt the normal regulatory mechanism between serum calcium levels and PTH secretion and increase the absorption of calcium through the gastrointestinal tract.
- Secondary hyperparathyroidism is a compensatory response by the parathyroid glands to chronic hypocalcemia. It is characterized by an increased secretion of PTH.
- Tertiary hyperparathyroidism results from hyperplasia of the parathyroid glands and a loss of response to serum calcium levels. This disorder is most often seen in clients with chronic renal failure.

Many clients with hyperparathyroidism are asymptomatic. When symptoms occur, they are related to hypercalcemia and various musculoskeletal, renal, and gastrointestinal manifestations. Bone reabsorption results in pathologic fractures, while elevated calcium levels alter neural and muscular activity, leading to muscle weakness and atrophy. Proximal renal tubule function is altered, and metabolic acidosis, renal calculi formation, and polyuria occur.

Manifestations of the effect of hypercalcemia on the gastrointestinal tract include abdominal pain, constipation, anorexia, and peptic ulcer formation. Hypercalcemia also affects the cardiovascular system, causing arrhythmias, hypertension, and increased sensitivity to cardiotonic glycosides (e.g., digitalis preparations).

Collaborative Care

Hyperparathyroidism is diagnosed by excluding all other possible causes of hypercalcemia; by at least a 6-month history of symptoms; by laboratory analysis of levels of calcium, phosphorus, magnesium, bicarbonate, and chloride; and by bone X-ray studies and scans (Tierney, et al., 2002).

Treatment of hyperparathyroidism focuses on decreasing the elevated serum calcium levels. Clients with mild hypercalcemia are urged to drink fluids and keep active. They should avoid immobilization, thiazide diuretics, large doses of vitamins A and D, antacids containing calcium, and calcium supplements. Severe hypercalcemia requires hospitalization and intensive treatment with intravenous saline. Medications to inhibit bone reabsorption and reduce hypercalcemia, such as pamidronate (Aredia) and alendronate (Fosamax), are administered.

Surgical removal of the parathyroid glands affected by hyperplasia or adenoma treats primary hyperparathyroidism. The preoperative and postoperative nursing care of the client having surgery of the parathyroids is essentially the same as that for the client having a thyroidectomy.

Nursing Care

Nursing care of the client with hypercalcemia is discussed in Chapter 39.

The Client with Hypoparathyroidism

Hypoparathyroidism results from abnormally low PTH levels. The most common cause is damage to or removal of the parathyroid glands during thyroidectomy. The lack of circulating PTH causes hypocalcemia and an elevated blood phosphate level.

Pathophysiology and Manifestations

Reduced levels of PTH result in impaired renal tubular regulation of calcium and phosphate. In addition, decreased activation of vitamin D results in decreased absorption of calcium by the intestines. The low calcium levels cause changes in neuromuscular activity, affecting peripheral motor and sensory nerves. Hypocalcemia lowers the threshold for nerve and muscle excitability; a slight stimulus anywhere along a nerve or muscle fiber initiates an impulse.

The neuromuscular manifestations that result include numbness and tingling around the mouth and in the fingertips, muscle spasms of the hands and feet, convulsions, and laryngeal spasms. Tetany, a continuous spasm of muscles, is the primary symptom of hypocalcemia. In severe cases of tetany, death may occur. Assessments for **tetany** include Chvostek's sign and Trousseau's sign (see Chapter 25).

Collaborative Care

Hypoparathyroidism is diagnosed by low serum calcium levels and high phosphorus levels in the absence of renal failure, an absorption disorder, or a nutritional disorder.

Treatment of hypoparathyroidism focuses on increasing calcium levels. Intravenous calcium gluconate is given immediately to reduce tetany. Long-term therapy includes supplemental calcium, increased dietary calcium, and vitamin D therapy.

Nursing Care

Nursing care for the client with hypocalcemia is discussed in Chapter 39.

Disorders of the Adrenal Glands

Disorders of the adrenal cortex or adrenal medulla result in changes in the production of adrenocorticotropic hormone (ACTH). Hormones of the adrenal cortex are essential to life. They maintain homeostasis in response to stressors. Disorders of the adrenal cortex result in complex physical, psychologic, and metabolic alterations that are potentially life threatening.

Hormones of the adrenal medulla are not essential to life, because the sympathetic nervous system produces similar body responses. The disorders that occur are hyperfunction and hypofunction of the adrenal cortex and hyperfunction of the adrenal medulla.

The Client with Hypercortisolism (Cushing's Syndrome)

Cushing's syndrome is a chronic disorder in which hyperfunction of the adrenal cortex produces excessive amounts of circulating cortisol or ACTH. Cushing's syndrome is more common in women, with the average age of onset between 30 and 50 years. However, the disorder may occur at any age, especially as the result of pharmacologic therapy. People who take steroids for long periods of time (e.g., for the treatment of arthritis, after an organ transplant, or as an adjunct to chemotherapy) are at increased risk for developing the disorder.

Pathophysiology

Cushing's syndrome may be the result of various causes. The most common etiologies of the disorder are (Porth, 2002):

- The pituitary form, with ACTH hypersecretion by a tumor of the pituitary (called *Cushing's disease*). This is most commonly caused by a small pituitary adenoma, with persistent but disorderly and random overproduction of ACTH.

- The ectopic form, caused by ACTH-secreting tumors, such as small-cell lung cancer. In this form, the ACTH is also random and episodic, but greater than in Cushing's disease.

- The adrenal form, resulting from excessive cortisol secretion by a benign or malignant adrenal tumor. The excess secretion suppresses pituitary ACTH production, resulting in atrophy of the uninvolved adrenal cortex.

- Iatrogenic Cushing's syndrome, resulting from long-term therapy with potent pharmacologic glucocorticoid preparations.

Manifestations

The manifestations of Cushing's syndrome result from the ACTH or cortisol excess, and manifest as exaggerated cortisol actions. Obesity and a redistribution of body fat result in fat deposits in the abdominal region (central obesity), fat pads under the clavicle, a "buffalo hump" over the upper back, and a round "moon" face. Changes in protein metabolism cause muscle weakness and wasting, especially in the extremities. Glucocorticoid excess inhibits fibroblasts, resulting in loss of collagen and connective tissue. Thinning of skin, abdominal striae (reddish purple "stretch marks"), easy bruising, poor wound healing, and frequent skin infections result. Glucose metabolism is altered in the majority of clients, and diabetes mellitus may occur. Electrolyte imbalances also occur with the increased hormone levels. Changes in calcium absorption result in osteoporosis, compression fractures of the vertebrae, fractures of the ribs, and renal calculi. Hypokalemia and hypertension occur as potassium is lost and sodium is retained. Inhibited immune responses increase the risk of infection, and increased gastric acid secretion increases the risk of peptic ulcers. Emotional changes range from depression to psychosis. In women, increasing androgen levels cause hirsutism (excessive facial hair in particular), acne, and menstrual irregularities.

The complications of untreated Cushing's syndrome include electrolyte imbalances (hyperglycemia, hypernatremia, and hypokalemia), hypertension, and emotional disturbances. Increased susceptibility to infections is also a factor. Compression fractures from osteoporosis and aseptic necrosis of the femoral head may result in serious disability. If the client undergoes a bilateral adrenalectomy as a treatment for Cushing's syndrome, an acute deficit of cortisol (addisonian crisis) may result.

Collaborative Care

The treatment of Cushing's syndrome includes medications, radiation therapy, or surgery, depending on the etiologic origin of the disorder.

Table 26-5. Laboratory Findings in Cushing's Syndrome

	Test	Normal Values	Findings
Serum	Cortisol	8 a.m. to 10 a.m.: 5 to 23 µg/dL 4 p.m. to 6 p.m.: 3 to 13 µg/dL	Increased
	Blood urea nitrogen (BUN)	5 to 25 mg/dL	Normal
	Sodium	135 to 145 mEq/L	Increased
	Potassium	3.5 to 5.0 mEq/L	Decreased
	Glucose (serum)	70 to 100 mg/dL	Increased
Urine	17-KS	Male: 5 to 25 mg/24h Female: 5 to 15 mg/24h >65: 4 to 8 mg/24h	Increased

Diagnostic Tests

Cushing's syndrome is diagnosed through a variety of diagnostic tests. Findings are shown in Table 26-5.

- *Plasma cortisol levels* are measured. If Cushing's disease is present, test results show a loss of the normal diurnal variations of higher levels in the morning and lower levels in the afternoon.
- *Plasma ACTH levels* are measured to determine the etiology of the syndrome. Normally, plasma ACTH levels are highest from 7 a.m. to 10 a.m. and lowest from 7 p.m. to 10 p.m. In secondary Cushing's syndrome, ACTH is elevated; in primary Cushing's syndrome, ACTH is decreased.

- *24-hour urine tests (17-ketosteroids* and *17-hydroxycorticosteroids)* are conducted to measure free cortisol and androgens; these hormones are increased in Cushing's syndrome.

- *Serum potassium, calcium, and glucose levels* are measured to identify electrolyte imbalances.

- *ACTH suppression* test may be conducted to identify the cause of the disorder. A synthetic cortisol (dexamethasone) is given to suppress the production of ACTH, and plasma cortisol levels are measured. If an extremely high dose of cortisol is necessary to suppress ACTH, the primary disorder is adrenal cortex hyperplasia. If ACTH is not suppressed with the synthetic cortisol, an adrenal tumor is suspected.

Medications

Cushing's syndrome that results from a pituitary tumor is treated by medications as an adjunct to surgery or radiation. Medications are also used for clients with inoperable pituitary or adrenal malignancies. Although the drugs control symptoms, they do not effect a cure. Examples of some commonly prescribed drugs include the following:

- Mitotane directly suppresses activity of the adrenal cortex and decreases peripheral metabolism of corticosteroids. It is used to treat metastatic adrenal cancer.

- Metyrapone or ketoconazole (or both) inhibit cortisol synthesis by the adrenal cortex and may be administered to clients with ectopic ACTH-secreting tumors that cannot be surgically removed.

- Somatostatis analog (octreotide) suppresses ACTH secretion in some clients.

Surgery

When Cushing's syndrome is caused by an adrenal cortex tumor, an adrenalectomy may be performed to remove the tumor. Only one adrenal gland is usually involved; however, if an ACTH-producing ectopic tumor is involved, a bilateral adrenalectomy is performed. Lifelong hormone replacement is necessary if both adrenal glands are removed.

Surgical removal of the pituitary gland (hypophysectomy) is indicated when Cushing's syndrome is the result of a pituitary disorder. The gland is removed either by a transphenoidal route or by a craniotomy. Nursing care for the client having cranial surgery is discussed in Chapter 33.

Nursing Care

Health Promotion

Stress the risk of developing Cushing's syndrome for clients taking long-term steroids. The risk of abruptly discontinuing the medications is an essential component of teaching.

Assessment

Collect the following data through the health history and physical examination (see Chapter 16). Further focused assessments are described with nursing interventions below:

- *Health history:* history of pituitary, adrenal, pancreatic, or pulmonary tumor; frequent infections; gastrointestinal bleeding; stress fractures; pain, changes in weight distribution; change in height; fatigue; weakness; change in appearance; bruising; skin infections; menstrual history; sexual function.

- *Physical assessment:* vital signs, behavior, appearance, fat distribution, face, skin, hair quantity and distribution, muscle size and strength, gait.

Nursing Diagnoses and Interventions

The nurse caring for the client with Cushing's syndrome must take a holistic approach to plan and implement interventions for a wide variety of responses, including problems related to fluid and electrolyte balance, injury, infection, and body image. For additional information about clients with alterations in fluid and electrolyte balance, see Chapter 39.

Fluid Volume Excess

The excess cortisol secretion associated with Cushing's syndrome results in sodium and water reabsorption, causing fluid volume excess. The client will have weight gain, edema, and hypertension.

- Ask the client to weigh at the same time each day, and maintain a record of results. *Body weight is an accurate indicator of fluid status. One liter of fluid retention corresponds to about 2 lb (0.9 kg) of body weight.*

- Monitor blood pressure, rate and rhythm of pulse, respiratory rate, and breath sounds. Assess for peripheral edema and jugular vein distention. *Extracellular fluid volume excess resulting from sodium and water retention is manifested by hypertension and a bounding, rapid pulse. There may also be crackles and wheezes, dependent edema, and venous distention.*

- Teach the client and family the reasons for restricting fluid and the importance of limiting fluids if ordered. *Restricting fluid can help decrease the risk of fluid volume excess. Involving the client and family in the plan of care and teaching the rationale for interventions helps achieve goals.*

Risk for Injury

The client with Cushing's syndrome is at risk for injury from several causes. Excess cortisol causes increased absorption of calcium and demineralization of bones, resulting in risk of pathologic fractures. Muscle weakness and fatigue are common, increasing the potential for accidental falls. Teach the client and family to maintain a safe environment:

- Keep unnecessary clutter and equipment out of the way and off the floor.
- Ensure adequate lighting, especially at night.
- Encourage the use of assistive devices for ambulation or to ask for help if needed.
- If the client wears corrective lenses, be sure they are available and clean.
- Encourage the use of nonskid slippers or shoes.
- Monitor for signs of fatigue (increased pulse and respirations); plan rest periods.

A well-lighted environment free of clutter decreases the risk of falls and injury. Sensory and motor deficits increase the risk of falls; corrective lenses, assistive devices, and nonslip footwear can decrease this risk. Rest relieves fatigue. To reduce energy expenditure, include alternating periods of rest and activity in daily schedules.

Risk for infection elevated cortisol levels impair the immune response and put the client with Cushing's syndrome at increased risk for infection. Increased cortisol also affects protein synthesis, causing delayed wound healing, and inhibits collagen formation, which results in epidermal atrophy, further inhibiting resistance to infection. In addition, impaired blood flow to edematous tissue results in altered cellular nutrition, which increases the potential for infection. The following interventions are outlined for the client with Cushing's syndrome who is hospitalized:

- Place in a private room, and limit visitors. *The client must avoid exposure to environmental infection.*
- Monitor vital signs and verbalizations of subjective manifestations (e.g., the client's response to "How do you feel?") every four hours. *Increased body temperature and pulse are systemic indicators of infection; however, because Cushing's syndrome impairs the normal inflammatory response, the usual indicators of inflammation may not be present.*
- Use principles of medical and sterile asepsis when caring for the client, conducting procedures, or providing wound care. *Impaired skin and tissues make aseptic techniques even more necessary to decrease the risk of infection. Intact skin is the first line of defense against infection; if invasive procedures are performed or a wound is present, this defense is lost.*
- If wounds are present, assess the color, odor, and consistency of wound drainage, and look for increased pain in and around the wound. *Cortisol excess delays wound healing and closure.*
- Teach the importance of increasing intake of protein and vitamins C and A. *Protein, vitamin C, and vitamin A are necessary to collagen formation; collagen helps support and repair body tissues.*

Disturbed Body Image

The client with Cushing's syndrome has obvious physical changes in appearance. The abnormal fat distribution, moon face, buffalo hump, striae, acne, and facial hair (in women) all contribute to disruptions in the way clients with this disorder perceive themselves.

- Encourage clients to express feelings and to ask questions about the disorder and its treatment. *The loss of one's normal body image may prompt feelings of hopelessness, powerlessness, anger, and depression. Understanding the disease and adapting to changes from that disease are the first steps in regaining control of one's own body.*
- Discuss strengths and previous coping strategies. Enlist the support of family or significant others in reaffirming the client's worth. *Disturbances in body image are often accompanied by low self-esteem. Self-esteem derives from one's perception of competence and from appraisals of others.*
- Discuss signs of progress in controlling symptoms; for example, decreased facial edema or increased activity tolerance. *Many physical changes from cortisol excess disappear with treatment. Clearly communicate this fact, because the client may believe changes are permanent.*

Home Care

The client with Cushing's syndrome requires education about self-care at home specific to the type of treatment given. Address the following topics:

- Safety measures to prevent falls if fatigue, weakness, and osteoporosis are present
- Taking medications as prescribed, with information about side effects. Clients often require medications for the rest of their lives, and dosage changes are highly likely.
- Having regular health assessments

- Wearing a medical ID indicating the client has Cushing's syndrome
- Helping the older client with referrals to social services or community health services because of the complexity of the treatment and care required
- Providing helpful resources:
  1. American Association of Clinical Endocrinologists
  2. Endocrine Society.

The Client with Chronic Adrenocortical Insufficiency (Addison's Disease)

Addison's disease is a disorder resulting from destruction or dysfunction of the adrenal cortex. The result is chronic deficiency of cortisol, aldosterone, and adrenal androgens, accompanied by skin pigmentation. It can occur at any age, although it is more common in adults under the age of 60. Like many endocrine disorders, Addison's disease is more common in women.

Pathophysiology

There are many possible causes of Addison's disease. The etiologies include:

- Autoimmune destruction of the adrenals. This is the most common cause, accounting for about 80% of spontaneous cases (Tierney, et al., 2001). It may occur alone, or as part of a polyglandular autoimmune syndrome (PGA). Type 2 PGA is seen in adults, often associated with autoimmune thyroid disease (usually hypothyroidism), type 1 diabetes, primary ovarian or testicular failure, and pernicious anemia.
- Clients who are taking anticoagulants, have major trauma, or are having open heart surgery. Such clients may have bilateral adrenal hemorrhage.
- Adrenoleukodystrophy, an X-linked disorder characterized by an accumulation of very long chain fatty acids in the adrenal cortex, testes, brain, and spinal cord.
- ACTH deficit, resulting from pituitary tumors, pituitary surgery or irradiation, and the use of exogenous steroids.
- Clients who are abruptly withdrawn from long-term, high-dose steroid therapy. Other clients at risk are those with tuberculosis or acquired immune deficiency syndrome (AIDS); the pathogens responsible for either disease can infiltrate and destroy adrenal tissue.

Adrenocortical destruction initially causes a decrease in adrenal glucocorticoid reserve. Basal glucocorticoid secretion is normal, but does not increase in response to stress and surgery. Trauma or infection can precipitate an adrenal crisis. As the destruction of the adrenal cortex continues, even basal secretion of glucocorticoids and mineralocorticoids is deficient. Decreasing plasma cortisol reduces the feedback inhibition of pituitary ACTH and plasma ACTH rises.

Secondary adrenocortical insufficiency occurs when large doses of glucocorticoids are given for their anti-inflammatory and immunosuppressive effects to treat diseases, such as arthritis and asthma. Treatment that extends for longer than four to five weeks suppresses ACTH and cortisol secretion. If the steroid medications are suddenly discontinued, the hypothalamus and pituitary cannot respond normally to the reduced level of circulating glucocorticoids. The client may develop manifestations of chronic adrenocortical insufficiency or, if subjected to stress, adrenal crisis (Tierney, et al., 2001).

Manifestations

The onset of Addison's disease is slow; the client experiences symptoms after about 90% of the function of the gland is lost. The primary manifestations are the result of elevated ACTH levels and decreased aldosterone and cortisol. Aldosterone deficiency affects the ability of the distal tubules of the nephron to conserve sodium. Sodium is lost, potassium is retained, extracellular fluid is depleted, and the blood volume is decreased. Postural hypotension and syncope are common, and hypovolemic shock may occur. Hyponatremia causes dizziness, confusion, and neuromuscular irritability. Hyperkalemia causes cardiac arrhythmias.

Cortisol insufficiency also causes decreased hepatic glyconeogenesis with hypoglycemia. The client tolerates stress poorly and experiences lethargy, weakness, anorexia, nausea, vomiting, and diarrhea. The increased ACTH levels stimulate hyperpigmentation in about 98% of clients with Addison's disease (Porth, 2002). In Caucasian clients, the skin looks deeply suntanned or bronzed in both exposed and unexposed areas.

Addisonian Crisis

Addisonian crisis is a life-threatening response to acute adrenal insufficiency. This response can occur in any person with Addison's disease; however, it is most commonly precipitated by major stressors, especially if the disease is poorly controlled. Addisonian crisis may also occur in clients who are abruptly withdrawn from glucocorticoid medications or who have hemorrhage into the adrenal glands from either septicemia or anticoagulant therapy.

The client with addisonian crisis may have any of the manifestations of Addison's disease, but the primary symptoms are a high fever, weakness, abdominal pain, severe hypotension, circulatory collapse, shock, and coma. Treatment of the crisis is rapid intravenous replacement of fluids and glucocorticoids. Fluid balance is usually restored in four to six hours.

Collaborative Care

The client with Addison's disease requires early diagnosis and treatment. Medical treatment includes cortisol replacement therapy.

Diagnostic Tests

Addison's disease is diagnosed through findings of decreased levels of cortisol, aldosterone, and urinary 17-ketosteroids. Dehydration may result in increased hematocrit and blood urea nitrogen (BUN). Blood glucose levels are decreased, and potassium is increased. A list of laboratory findings in Addison's disease is shown in Table 26-6. The following diagnostic tests are used:

- *Serum cortisol levels,* which are decreased in adrenal insufficiency
- *Blood glucose levels,* which are decreased in adrenal insufficiency
- *Serum sodium levels,* which are decreased in adrenal insufficiency

- *Serum potassium levels,* which are increased in adrenal insufficiency
- *Blood urea nitrogen (BUN) levels,* which are increased in adrenal insufficiency
- *Urinary 17-hydroxycorticoids* and *17-ketosteroids (17-KS) levels,* which are decreased in adrenal insufficiency
- *Plasma ACTH levels,* which are increased in primary adrenal insufficiency but decreased in secondary adrenal insufficiency
- *Possibly ACTH stimulation test,* cortisol levels rise with pituitary deficiency but do not rise in primary adrenal insufficiency
- *CT scans* of the head, which identify any intracranial lesion impinging on the pituitary gland.

Medications

The primary medical treatment of Addison's disease is replacement of corticosteroids and mineralocorticoids, accompanied by increased sodium in the diet. Hydrocortisone is given orally to replace cortisol; fludrocortisone (Florinef) is given orally to replace mineralocorticoids.

Table 26-6. Laboratory Findings in Addison's Disease

	Test	Normal Values	Findings
Serum	Cortisol	8 a.m. to 10 a.m.: 5 to 23 µg/dL 4 p.m. to 6 p.m.: 3 to 13 µg/dL	Decreased
	Blood urea nitrogen (BUN)	5 to 25 mg/dL	Increased
	Sodium	135 to 145 mEq/L	Decreased
	Potassium	3.5 to 5.0 mEq/L	Increased
	Glucose	70 to 100 mg/dL	Decreased
Urine	(serum) 17-KS	Male: 5 to 25 mg/24h Female: 5 to 15 mg/24h >65: 4 to 8 mg/24h	Low/Absent

Nursing Care

Health Promotion

Health promotion interventions for the client with or at risk for Addison's disease focus on careful assessments during anticoagulant therapy, open heart surgery, and trauma treatment. If the disease is present, teaching to prevent or treat an addisonian crisis is essential.

Assessment

Collect the following data through the health history and physical examination (see Chapter 25). Further focused assessments are described with nursing interventions below:

- *Health history:* weight loss, changes in skin color, nausea and vomiting, anorexia, diarrhea, abdominal pain, weakness, amenorrhea, changes in sexual desire, confusion, intolerance of stress.
- *Physical assessment:* height and weight, vital signs, skin, hair quality and distribution, muscle size and strength.

Nursing Diagnoses and Interventions

The client with Addison's disease requires nursing care for a wide variety of responses to the decrease in cortisol levels. Nursing diagnoses discussed in this section are directed toward problems with fluid and electrolyte balance and compliance with lifelong self-care.

Deficient Fluid Volume

Fluid volume deficit in the client with Addison's disease results from loss of water and sodium, as well as from vomiting and diarrhea. Extracellular fluid volume deficit, decreased cardiac output, hypotension, and hypovolemic shock may occur, especially in crisis situations. Interventions for this diagnosis are outlined for the client who is hospitalized.

- Monitor intake and output, and assess for signs of dehydration: dry mucous membranes; thirst; poor skin turgor; sunken eyeballs; scanty, dark urine; increased urine specific gravity; weight loss; and increased hemoconcentration (increased hematocrit and BUN).

Glucocorticoid and mineralocorticoid depletion causes fluid volume deficit. Fluid volume deficit may reach crisis levels if undetected, causing altered tissue perfusion and hypovolemic shock.

- Monitor cardiovascular status: Take and record vital signs, assess character of pulses, monitor potassium levels and ECGs. *Fluid volume deficit may lead to hypotension and a rapid, weak, or thready pulse. As aldosterone levels fall, renal excretion of potassium decreases, increasing blood levels of potassium.*
- Weigh the client daily at the same time and in the same clothing. *Dehydration is manifested by weight loss.*
- Encourage an oral fluid intake of 3000 mL per day and an increased salt intake. *Cortisol deficiency increases fluid loss, leading to extracellular fluid volume depletion. Oral fluid replacement is necessary to balance this loss. An increase in dietary sodium can decrease the hyponatremia characteristic of adrenal insufficiency.*
- Teach to sit and stand slowly, and provide assistance as necessary. *Extracellular fluid volume deficit causes orthostatic hypotension, dizziness, and possible loss of consciousness. These manifestations increase the risk of injury from falls.*

Risk for Ineffective Therapeutic Regimen Management

Clients with Addison's disease must learn to provide lifelong self-care that involves varied components: medications, diet, and recognizing and responding to responses to stress. Changes in lifestyle are difficult to maintain permanently.

- Teach the effects of illness and treatment. Discuss client and family concerns. *Lack of knowledge about the illness, as well as the possibility of complications from disregarding or altering the treatment, can negatively affect compliance.*

Include the following in the teaching plan:

- Self-administration of steroids
- The importance of carrying at all times an emergency kit containing parenteral cortisone and a syringe/needle
- Wearing a MedicAlert bracelet that says "Adrenal insufficiency—takes hydrocortisone"
- Increasing oral fluid intake
- Maintaining a diet high in sodium and low in potassium
- The necessity of altering the medication dose when experiencing emotional or physical stressors
- The importance of continuing health care.

One of the most important components of caring for the client with Addison's disease is teaching both the client and family to provide care. The length of treatment and the side effects of medications can discourage compliance.

Home Care

The client with Addison's disease provides self-care at home. One of the most important components of caring for the client with Addison's disease is teaching both the client and family to provide care. Family stability, an awareness of the serious nature of the disease, and the effectiveness of treatment all promote compliance. The length of treatment and the side effects of medications, however, can discourage compliance. In addition to the information in the teaching plans mentioned in the nursing diagnoses and interventions, include the following topics:

- The importance of continuing health care
- Referral to social worker, if appropriate
- Referral to community agencies for continued education and support
- Helpful resources:
  1. National Institute of Diabetes and Digestive and Kidney Diseases (Addison's disease)
  2. Endocrine Society
  3. American Association of Clinical Endocrinologists.

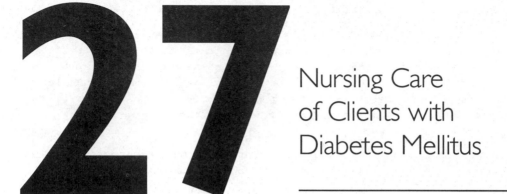

27

Nursing Care of Clients with Diabetes Mellitus

Diabetes mellitus (DM) is a common chronic disease of adults. However, depending on the type of diabetes and the age of the client, both client needs and nursing care may vary greatly. Consider the following examples:

- Cheryl Draheim is a 45-year-old schoolteacher. She developed diabetes at age 34 after an automobile accident caused severe pancreatic injuries. Cheryl has always been very careful about taking her insulin, following her diet, and exercising regularly. However, she is beginning to notice that her vision is getting worse and that she is having increasing pain in her legs, especially after standing for long periods of time. Cheryl says that sometimes she believes the disease controls her more than she controls it.

- Tom Chang is 53 years old. Early in his 40s, Tom was diagnosed with type 2 diabetes. Although Tom was taught about the disease and the importance of taking his oral medications, following his diet plan, and getting exercise, he rarely did more than take the medication. Five years ago, he was hospitalized for hyperglycemia and started taking insulin. Last year Tom had a stroke, leaving him unable to walk. He has now been admitted to the hospital for treatment of gangrene of the large toe on his left foot.

- Grace Staples is an independent 82-year-old woman who lives alone and happily takes care of her two cats. She is slightly overweight. Last year, during Grace's annual eye examination, eye changes typical for diabetes were found. She was referred to her family doctor, who diagnosed type 2 diabetes and started her on oral medications. Grace sticks to her diet, walks a mile every day, and plans to live to be 100.

As illustrated in these examples, diabetes mellitus is not a single disorder, but a group of chronic disorders of the endocrine pancreas, all categorized under a broad diagnostic label. The condition is characterized by inappropriate hyperglycemia caused by a relative or absolute deficiency of insulin or by a cellular resistance to the action of insulin. Of the several classifications of diabetes, this chapter will focus on the two major types, type 1 and type 2. **Type 1 DM** is the result of pancreatic islet cell destruction and a total deficit of circulating insulin; **type 2 DM** results from insulin resistance with a defect in compensatory insulin secretion.

Diabetes mellitus has been recognized as a disease for centuries. Diabetes derives from a Greek word meaning "to siphon," referring to the increased output of urine. Mellitus derives from a Latin word meaning "sweet." The two words together identify the disease as an outpouring of sweet urine. It was not until 1921 that techniques were developed for extracting insulin from pancreatic tissue and for measuring blood glucose. At the same time, researchers discovered that insulin, when injected, produces a dramatic drop in blood glucose. This meant that diabetes was no longer a terminal illness because hyperglycemia could now be controlled. Since that time, oral hypoglycemic drugs, human insulin products, insulin pumps, home blood glucose monitoring, and transplantation of the pancreas or of pancreatic islet or beta cells have advanced the treatment and care of people with diabetes.

Clients with DM face lifelong changes in lifestyle and health status. Nursing care is provided in many settings for the diagnosis and care of the disease and treatment of complications. A major role of the nurse is that of educator in both hospital and community settings.

Incidence and Prevalence

Approximately 1 million new cases of DM are diagnosed each year in the United States. This chronic illness affects an estimated 17 million people; of that number, 11.1 million have been diagnosed and an estimated 5.9 million are undiagnosed (National Institutes of Health [NIH], 2002, 1999). There is an increased prevalence of diabetes (especially type 2 diabetes) among older adults and in minority populations.

Diabetes is the sixth leading cause of death by disease in the United States, primarily because of the widespread cardiovascular effects that result in atherosclerosis, coronary artery disease, and stroke. People with diabetes are two to four times more likely to have heart disease, and two to six times more likely to have a stroke than people who do not have diabetes. Diabetes is the leading cause of end-stage renal disease (kidney failure), and the major cause of newly diagnosed blindness in people ages 20 to 74. Diabetes is also the most frequent cause of nontraumatic amputations.

Americans with diabetes use a disproportionate share of the nation's health care services. They visit outpatient services and physicians' offices more often than people who do not have the disease, and they require more frequent hospitalizations with longer days of in-hospital treatment. The cost of illness and resulting loss of productivity for people with diabetes exceeds $98 billion per year, according to an estimate by the National Institute for Diabetes and Kidney Disease.

Pathophysiology

Overview of Endocrine Pancreatic Hormones and Glucose Homeostasis

Hormones

The endocrine pancreas produces hormones necessary for the metabolism and cellular utilization of carbohydrates, proteins, and fats. The cells that produce these hormones are clustered in groups of cells called the islets of Langerhans. These islets have three different types of cells:

- Alpha cells produce the hormone *glucagon,* which stimulates the breakdown of glycogen in the liver, the formation of carbohydrates in the liver, and the breakdown of lipids in both the liver and adipose tissue. The primary function of glucagon is to decrease glucose oxidation and to increase blood glucose levels. Through *glycogenolysis* (the breakdown of liver glycogen) and *gluconeogenesis* (the formation of glucose from fats and proteins), glucagon prevents blood glucose from decreasing below a certain level when the body is fasting or in between meals. The action of glucagon is initiated in most people when blood glucose falls below about 70 mg/dL.

- Beta cells secrete the hormone *insulin*, which facilitates the movement of glucose across cell membranes into cells, decreasing blood glucose levels. Insulin prevents the excessive breakdown of glycogen in the liver and in muscle, facilitates lipid formation while inhibiting the breakdown of stored fats, and helps move amino acids into cells for protein synthesis. After secretion by the beta cells, insulin enters the portal circulation, travels directly to the liver, and is then released into the general circulation. Circulating insulin is rapidly bound to receptor sites on peripheral tissues (especially muscle and fat cells) or is destroyed by the liver or kidneys. Insulin release is regulated by blood glucose; it increases when blood glucose levels increase, and it decreases when blood glucose levels decrease. When a person eats food, insulin levels begin to rise in minutes, peak in 30 to 60 minutes, and return to baseline in 2 to 3 hours.

- Delta cells produce *somatostatin,* which is believed to be a neurotransmitter that inhibits the production of both glucagon and insulin.

Blood Glucose Homeostasis

All body tissues and organs require a constant supply of glucose; however, not all tissues require insulin for glucose uptake. The brain, liver, intestines, and renal tubules do not require insulin to transfer glucose into their cells. Skeletal muscle, cardiac muscle, and adipose tissue do require insulin for glucose movement into the cells.

Normal blood glucose is maintained in healthy people primarily through the actions of insulin and glucagon. Increased blood glucose levels, amino acids, and fatty acids stimulate pancreatic beta cells to produce insulin. As cells of cardiac muscle, skeletal muscle, and adipose tissue take up glucose, plasma levels of nutrients decrease, suppressing the stimulus to produce insulin. If blood glucose falls, glucagon is released to raise glucose levels. Epinephrine, growth hormone, thyroxine, and glucocorticoids (often referred to as glucose counterregulatory hormones) also stimulate an increase in glucose in times of hypoglycemia, stress, growth, or increased metabolic demand.

Pathophysiology of Diabetes

DM is a group of metabolic diseases characterized by hyperglycemia resulting from defects in the secretion of insulin, the action of insulin, or both. There are four major types of DM. Type I diabetes (5% to 10% of diagnosed cases) was formerly called juvenile-onset diabetes or insulin-dependent diabetes mellitus (IDDM). Type 2 diabetes (90% to 95% of diagnosed cases) was formerly labeled non-insulin-dependent diabetes mellitus (NIDDM) or adult-onset diabetes. The other major types are gestational diabetes (2% to 5% of all pregnancies) and other specific types of diabetes (1% to 2% of diagnosed cases). The classification and characteristics of the four types are described in Table 27-1.

Table 27-1.   Classification and Characteristics of Diabetes

	Classification	Characteristics
I. Type 1 diabetes	A. Immune-mediated	Beta cells are destroyed, usually leading to absolute insulindeficiency. Markers to the immune destruction of the beta cells include islet cell autoantibodies (ICAs) and insulin autoantibodies (IAAs). The rate of beta cell destruction is variable, usually more rapid in infants and children and slower in adults. Destruction of the beta cells has genetic predispositions and is also related to environmental factors as yet undefined.
	B. Idiopathic	Has no known etiologic causes. Most clients are of African or Asian descent. Is strongly inherited. Need for insulin may be intermittent.
II. Type 2 diabetes		May range from predominantly insulin resistance with relativeinsulin deficiency to a predominantly secretory defect with insulin resistance. There is no immune destruction of beta cells. Initially, and, in some cases, for the client's entire life, insulin is not necessary. Most people with this form are obese, or have an increased amount of abdominal fat. Risks for development include increasing age, obesity, and a sedentary lifestyle. Occurs more frequently in women who have had gestational diabetes, and in people with lipid disorders or hypertension. There is a strong genetic predisposition.
III. Other specific types	A. Genetic defects of beta cell	Hyperglycemia occurs at an early age (usually before age 25). This type is referred to as maturity-onset diabetes of the young (MODY).
	B. Genetic defects in insulin action	Are genetically determined. Dysfunctions may range fromhyperinsulinemia to severe diabetes.
	C. Diseases of the exocrine pancreas	Acquired processes causing diabetes include pancreatitis,trauma, infection, pancreatectomy, and pancreatic cancer. Severe forms of cystic fibrosis and hemochromatosis may also damage beta cells and impair insulin secretion.
	D. Endocrine disorders	Excess amount of hormones (e.g., growth hormone, cortisol, glucagon, and epinephrine) impair insulin secretion, resulting in diabetes in people with Cushing's syndrome, acromegaly, and pheochromocytoma.

Table 27-1. Continued

	E. Drug or chemical induced	Many drugs impair insulin secretion, precipitating diabetes in people with predisposing insulin resistance. Examples are nicotinic acid, glucocorticoids, thyroid hormone, thiazides, and dilantin.
	F. Infections	Certain viruses may cause beta cell destruction, including congenital measles, cytomegalovirus, adenovirus, and mumps.
IV. Gestational diabetes mellitus (GDM)		Any degree of glucose intolerance with onset or first recognition during pregnancy.

Type 1 Diabetes

Type 1 diabetes most often occurs in childhood and adolescence, but it may occur at any age, even in the 80s and 90s. This disorder is characterized by **hyperglycemia** (elevated blood glucose levels), a breakdown of body fats and proteins, and the development of **ketosis** (an accumulation of ketone bodies produced during the oxidation of fatty acids). Type 1 DM is the result of the destruction of the beta cells of the islets of Langerhans in the pancreas. When beta cells are destroyed, insulin is no longer produced. Although type 1 DM may be classified as either an autoimmune or idiopathic disorder, 90% of the cases are immune mediated. The disorder begins with insulinitis, a chronic inflammatory process that occurs in response to the autoimmune destruction of islet cells. This process slowly destroys beta cell production of insulin, with the onset of hyperglycemia occurring when 80% to 90% of beta cell function is lost. This process usually occurs over a long preclinical period. It is believed that both alpha-cell and beta-cell functions are abnormal, with a lack of insulin and a relative excess of glucagon resulting in hyperglycemia.

Risk Factors. Genetic predisposition plays a role in the development of type 1 DM. Although the risk in the general population ranges from 1 in 400 to 1 in 1000, the child of a person with diabetes has a 1 in 20 to 1 in 50 risk. Genetic markers that determine immune responses—specifically, DR3 and DR4 antigens on chromosome 6 of the human leukocyte antigen (HLA) system—have been found in 95% of people diagnosed with type 1 DM. (HLAs are cell surface proteins, controlled by genes on chromosome 6.) Although the presence of these markers does not guarantee that the person will develop type 1 DM, they do indicate increased susceptibility (Haire-Joshu, 1996).

Environmental factors are believed to trigger the development of type 1 DM. The trigger can be a viral infection (mumps, rubella, or coxsackievirus B4) or a chemical toxin, such as those found in smoked and cured meats. As a result of exposure to the virus or chemical, an abnormal autoimmune response occurs in which antibodies respond to normal islet beta cells as though they were foreign substances, destroying them. The manifestations of type 1 DM appear when approximately 90% of the beta cells are destroyed. However, manifestations may appear at any time during the loss of beta cells if an acute illness or stress increases the demand for insulin beyond the reserves of the damaged cells. The actual cause and exact sequence are not completely understood, but research continues to identify the genetic markers of this disorder and to investigate ways of altering the immune response to prevent or cure type 1 DM.

Manifestations. The manifestations of type 1 DM are the result of a lack of insulin to transport glucose across the cell membrane into the cells. Glucose molecules accumulate in the circulating blood, resulting in **hyperglycemia.** Hyperglycemia causes serum hyperosmolality, drawing water from the intracellular spaces into the general circulation. The increased blood volume increases renal blood flow, and the hyperglycemia acts as an osmotic diuretic. The resulting osmotic diuresis increases urine output. This condition is called **polyuria.** When the blood glucose level exceeds the renal threshold for glucose—usually about 180 mg/dL—glucose is excreted in the urine, a condition called **glucosuria.** The decrease in intracellular volume and the increased urinary output cause dehydration. The mouth becomes dry and thirst sensors are activated, causing the person to drink increased amounts of fluid (**polydipsia**).

Because glucose cannot enter the cell without insulin, energy production decreases. This decrease in energy stimulates hunger, and the person eats more food (**polyphagia**). Despite increased food intake, the person loses weight as the body loses water and breaks down proteins and fats in an attempt to restore energy sources. Malaise and fatigue accompany the decrease in energy. Blurred vision is also common, resulting from osmotic effects that cause swelling of the lenses of the eyes.

Thus, the classic manifestations are polyuria, polydipsia, and polyphagia, accompanied by weight loss, malaise, and fatigue. Depending on the degree of insulin lack, the manifestations vary from slight to severe. People with type 1 DM require an exogenous source of insulin to maintain life.

Diabetic Ketoacidosis. As the pathophysiology of untreated type 1 DM continues, the insulin deficit causes fat stores to break down, resulting in continued hyperglycemia and mobilization of fatty acids with a subsequent ketosis. **Diabetic ketoacidosis (DKA)** develops when there is an absolute deficiency of insulin and an increase in the insulin counterregulatory hormones. Glucose production by the liver increases, peripheral glucose use decreases, fat mobilization increases, and ketogenesis (ketone formation) is stimulated. Increased glucagon levels activate the gluconeogenic and ketogenic pathways in the liver. In the presence of insulin deficiency, hepatic overproduction of beta-hydroxybutyrate and acetoacetic acids (ketone bodies) causes increased ketone concentrations and an increased release of free fatty acids. As a result of a loss of bicarbonate (which occurs when the ketone is formed), bicarbonate buffering does not occur, and a metabolic acidosis occurs, called DKA. Depression of the central nervous system (CNS) from the accumulation of ketones and the resulting acidosis may cause coma and death if left untreated.

DKA also may occur in a person with diagnosed diabetes when energy requirements increase during physical or emotional stress. Stress states initiate the release of gluconeogenic hormones, resulting in the formation of carbohydrates from protein or fat. The person who is sick, has an infection, or who decreases or omits insulin doses is at a greatly increased risk for developing DKA.

DKA involves four metabolic problems:

- Hyperosmolarity from hyperglycemia and dehydration
- Metabolic acidosis from an accumulation of ketoacids
- Extracellular volume depletion from osmotic diuresis
- Electrolyte imbalances (such as loss of potassium and sodium) from osmotic diuresis.

Manifestations of DKA result from severe dehydration and acidosis. Laboratory findings include the following:

- Blood glucose levels higher than 250 mg/dL
- Plasma pH less than 7.3
- Plasma bicarbonate less than 15 mEq/L
- Presence of serum ketones
- Presence of urine ketones and glucose
- Abnormal levels of serum sodium, potassium, and chloride.

Type 2 Diabetes

Type 2 DM is a condition of fasting hyperglycemia that occurs despite the availability of endogenous insulin (Porth, 2002). Type 2 DM can occur at any age, but it is usually seen in middle-age and older people. Heredity plays a role in its transmission. Although the exact cause of type 2 DM is unknown, several theories have been suggested. These theories include limited beta-cell response to hyperglycemia, peripheral insulin resistance, and insulin-receptor or postreceptor abnormalities. Whatever the cause, there is sufficient insulin production to prevent the breakdown of fats with resultant ketosis; thus, type 2 DM is characterized as a nonketotic form of diabetes. However, the amount of insulin available is not sufficient to lower blood glucose levels through the uptake of glucose by muscle and fat cells.

A major factor in the development of type 2 DM is cellular resistance to the effect of insulin. This resistance is increased by obesity, inactivity, illnesses, medications, and increasing age. In obesity, insulin has a decreased ability to influence glucose metabolism and uptake by the liver, skeletal muscles, and adipose tissue. Although the exact reason for this is not clear, it is known that weight loss may improve the mechanism responsible for insulin receptor-binding or postreceptor activity (McCance & Huether, 2002).

Risk Factors. The major risk factors for type 2 DM are:

- History of diabetes in parents or siblings. Although there is no identified HLA linkage, the children of a person with type 2 DM have a 15% chance of developing type 2 DM and a 30% risk of developing a glucose intolerance (the inability to metabolize carbohydrate normally).
- Obesity, defined as being at least 20% over desired body weight or having a body mass index (BMI) of at least 27 kg/m². Obesity, especially of the upper body, decreases the number of available insulin receptor sites in cells of skeletal muscles and adipose tissues, a process called peripheral insulin resistance. In addition, obesity impairs the ability of the beta cells to release insulin in response to increasing glucose levels.
- Physical inactivity.
- Race/ethnicity (see Table 27-2).
- In women, a history of gestational DM, polycystic ovary syndrome, or delivering a baby weighing more than 9 lb.
- Hypertension (≥130/85 in adults), HDL cholesterol of ≥35 mg/dL and/or a triglyceride level of ≥250 mg/dL.

Manifestations. The person with type 2 DM experiences a slow onset of manifestations and is often unaware of the disease until seeking health care for some other problem. The hyperglycemia in type 2 is usually not as severe as in type 1, but similar symptoms occur, especially polyuria and polydipsia. Polyphagia is not often seen, and weight loss is uncommon. Other manifestations are also the result of hyperglycemia: blurred vision, fatigue, paresthesias, and skin infections. If available insulin decreases, especially in times of physical or emotional stress, the person with type 2 DM may develop DKA, but this occurrence is uncommon.

Hyperosmolar Hyperglycemic State. The metabolic problem called **hyperosmolar hyperglycemic state (HHS)** occurs in people who have type 2 DM. HHS is characterized by a plasma osmolarity of 340 mOsm/L or greater (the normal range is 280 to 300 mOsm/L), greatly elevated blood glucose levels (over 600 mg/dL and often 1000 to 2000 mg/dL), and altered levels of consciousness. HHS is a serious, life-threatening medical emergency and has a higher mortality rate than DKA. Mortality is high not only because the metabolic changes are serious but also because people with diabetes are usually older and have other medical problems that either cause or are caused by HHS. The precipitating factors associated with HHS include infection, therapeutic agents, therapeutic procedures, acute illness, and chronic illness (Table 27–2). The most common precipitating factor is infection. The manifestations of this disorder may be slow to appear, with onset ranging from 24 hours to 2 weeks. The manifestations are initiated by hyperglycemia, which causes increased urine output. With increased output, plasma volume decreases and glomerular filtration rate (GFR) drops. As a result, glucose is retained and water is lost. Glucose and sodium accumulate in the blood and increase serum osmolarity.

Table 27-2. Factors Associated with Hyperosmolar Hyperglycemic State (HHS)

Therapeutic Agents	**Therapeutic Procedures**
< Glucocorticoids	< Peritoneal dialysis
< Diuretics	< Hemodialysis
< Beta-adrenergic blocking agents	< Hyperosmolar alimentation (oral or parenteral)
< Immunosuppressants	< Surgery
< Chlorpromazine	
< Diazoxide	
Acute Illness	**Chronic Illness**
< Infection	< Renal disease
< Gangrene	< Cardiac disease
< Urinary infection	< Hypertension
< Burns	< Previous stroke
< Gastrointestinal bleeding	< Alcoholism
< Myocardial infarction	
< Pancreatitis	
< Stroke	

Serum hyperosmolarity results in severe dehydration, reducing intracellular water in all tissues, including the brain. The person has dry skin and mucous membranes, extreme thirst, and altered levels of consciousness (progressing from lethargy to coma). Neurologic deficits may include hyperthermia, motor and sensory impairment, positive Babinski's sign, and seizures. Treatment is directed toward correcting fluid and electrolyte imbalances, lowering blood glucose levels with insulin, and treating underlying conditions.

Complications of Diabetes

The person with DM, regardless of type, is at increased risk for complications involving many different body systems. Alterations in blood glucose levels, alterations in the cardiovascular system, neuropathies, an increased susceptibility to infection, and periodontal disease are common. In addition, the interaction of several complications can cause problems of the feet.

Alterations in Blood Glucose Levels

The following discussion provides additional information about hyperglycemia and hypoglycemia. Table 27-3 compares DKA, HHS, and hypoglycemia.

Hyperglycemia

The major problems resulting from hyperglycemia in the person with diabetes are DKA and HHS. Two other problems are the dawn phenomenon and the Somogyi phenomenon.

The **dawn phenomenon** is a rise in blood glucose between 4 A.M. and 8 A.M. that is not a response to hypoglycemia. This condition occurs in people with both type 1 and type 2 DM. The exact cause is unknown, but is believed to be related to nocturnal increases in growth hormone, which decreases peripheral uptake of glucose. The **Somogyi phenomena** is a combination of hypoglycemia during the night with a rebound morning rise in blood glucose to hyperglycemic levels. The hyperglycemia stimulates the counterregulatory hormones, which stimulate gluconeogenesis and glycogenolysis and also inhibit peripheral glucose use. This may cause insulin resistance for 12 to 48 hours (McCance & Huether, 2002).

Hypoglycemia

Hypoglycemia (low blood glucose levels) is common in people with type 1 DM, and occasionally occurs in people with type 2 DM who are treated with oral hypoglycemic agents. This condition is often called insulin shock, **insulin reaction,** or "the lows" in clients with type 1 DM. Hypoglycemia results primarily from a mismatch between insulin intake (e.g., an error in insulin dose), physical activity, and carbohydrate availability (e.g., omitting a meal). The intake of alcohol and drugs such as chloramphenicol (Chloromycetin), coumadin, monoamine oxidase (MAO) inhibitors, probenecid (Benemid), salicylates, and sulfonamides, can also cause hypoglycemia.

The manifestations of hypoglycemia result from a compensatory autonomic nervous system (ANS) response and from impaired cerebral function due to a decrease in glucose available for use by the brain. The manifestations vary, particularly in older adults. The onset is sudden, and blood glucose is usually less than 45 to 60 mg/dL. Severe hypoglycemia may cause death.

Table 27-3. DKA, HHS, and Hypoglycemia Compared

		DKA	HHS	Hypoglycemia
Diabetes Type		Primary Type 1	Type 2	Both
Onset		Slow	Slow	Rapid
Cause		↓ Insulin	↓ Insulin	↑ Insulin
		Infection	Older age	Omitted meal/snack
				Error in insulin dose
Risk Factors		Surgery	Surgery	Surgery
		Trauma	Trauma	Trauma
		Illness	Illness	Illness
		Omitted insulin	Dehydration	Exercise
		Stress	Medications	Medications
			Dialysis	Lipodystrophy
			Hyperalimentation	Renal failure
				Alcohol intake
Assessments	Skin	Flushed; dry; warm	Flushed; dry; warm	Pallor; moist; cool
	Perspiration	None	None	Profuse
	Thirst	Increased	Increased	Normal
	Breath	Fruity	Normal	Normal
	Vital signs	BP ↓	BP ↓	BP ↓
		P ↑	P ↑	P ↑
		R Kussmaul's	R normal	R normal
	Mental status	Confused	Lethargic	Anxious; restless
	Thirst	Increased	Increased	Normal
	Fluid intake	Increased	Increased	Normal
	Gastrointestinal effects	Nausea/vomiting; abdominal pain	Nausea/vomiting; abdominal pain	Hunger
	Level of consciousness	Decreasing	Decreasing	Decreasing
	Energy level	Weak	Weak	Fatigue
	Other	Weight loss	Weight loss	Headache
		Blurred vision	Malaise	Altered vision
			Extreme thirst	Mood changes
			Seizures	Seizures

Table 27-3. Continued

		DKA	HHS	Hypoglycemia
Laboratory	Blood glucose	>300 mg/dL	>600 mg/dL	<50 mg/dL
Findings	Plasma ketones	Increased	Normal	Normal
	Urine glucose	Increased	Increased	Normal
	Urine ketones	Increased	Normal	Normal
	Serum potassium	Abnormal	Abnormal	Normal
	Serum sodium	Abnormal	Abnormal	Normal
	Serum chloride	Abnormal	Abnormal	Normal
	Plasma pH	<7.3	Normal	Normal
	Osmolality	>340 mOsm/L	>340 mOsm/L	Normal
Treatment		Insulin	Insulin	Glucagon
		Treatment	Intravenous fluids	Rapid-acting carbohydrate
		Intravenous fluids	Electrolytes	Intravenous solution of 50% glucose
		Electrolytes		

People who have type 1 DM for four or five years fail to secrete glucagon in response to a decrease in blood glucose. They then depend on epinephrine to serve as a counterregulatory response to hypoglycemia. However, this compensatory response can become absent or blunted. The person then develops a syndrome called *hypoglycemia unawareness.* The person does not experience symptoms of hypoglycemia, even though it is present. Because treatment is not initiated in the absence of symptoms, the person is likely to have episodes of severe hypoglycemia.

Alterations in the Cardiovascular System

The macrocirculation (large blood vessels) in people with diabetes undergoes changes due to atherosclerosis; abnormalities in platelets, red blood cells, and clotting factors; and changes in arterial walls. It has been established that atherosclerosis has an increased incidence and earlier age of onset in people with diabetes (although the reason is unknown). Other risk factors that contribute to the development of macrovascular disease of diabetes are hypertension, hyperlipidemia, cigarette smoking, and obesity. Alterations in the vascular system increase the risk of the long-term complications of coronary artery disease, cerebral vascular disease, and peripheral vascular disease.

Alterations in the microcirculation in the person with diabetes involve structural defects in the basement membrane of smaller blood vessels and capillaries. (The basement membrane is the structure that supports and serves as the boundary around the space occupied by epithelial cells.) These defects cause the capillary basement membrane to thicken, eventually resulting in decreased tissue perfusion. Changes in basement membranes are believed to be due to one or more of the following: the presence of increased amounts of sorbitol (a substance formed as an intermediate step in the conversion of glucose to fructose), the formation of abnormal glycoproteins, or problems in the release of oxygen from hemoglobin (Porth, 2002). The effects of alterations in the microcirculation affect all body tissues, but are seen primarily in the eyes and the kidneys.

Coronary Artery Disease

Coronary artery disease is a major risk factor in the development of myocardial infarction in people with diabetes, especially in the middle to older adult with type 2 DM. Coronary artery disease is the most common cause of death in people with diabetes, accounting for 40% to 60% of all cases of mortality (Haire-Joshu, 1996). People with diabetes who have myocardial infarction are more prone to develop congestive heart failure as a complication of the infarction, and are also less likely to survive in the period immediately following the infarction. (Myocardial infarction is fully discussed in Chapter 8.)

Hypertension

Hypertension (blood pressure ≥140/90 mmHg) is a common complication of DM. It affects 20% to 60% of all people with diabetes, and is a major risk factor for cardiovascular disease and microvascular complications, such as retinopathy and nephropathy. Hypertension may be reduced by weight loss, exercise, and decreasing sodium intake and alcohol consumption. If these methods are not effective, treatment with antihypertensive medications is necessary.

Stroke (Cerebrovascular Accident)

People with diabetes, especially older adults with type 2 DM, are two to six times more likely to have a stroke. Although the exact relationship between diabetes and cerebral vascular disease is unknown, hypertension (a risk factor for stroke) is a common health problem in those who have diabetes. In addition, atherosclerosis of the cerebral vessels develops at an earlier age and is more extensive in people with diabetes (Porth, 1998).

The manifestations of impaired cerebral circulation (see Chapter 32) are often similar to those of hypoglycemia or HHS: blurred vision, slurred speech, weakness, and dizziness. People with these manifestations have potentially life-threatening health problems and require constant medical attention.

Peripheral Vascular Disease

Peripheral vascular disease of the lower extremities accompanies both types of DM, but the incidence is greater in people with type 2 DM. Atherosclerosis of vessels in the legs of people with diabetes begins at an earlier age, advances more rapidly, and is equally common in both men and women. Impaired peripheral vascular circulation leads to peripheral vascular insufficiency with intermittent claudication (pain) in the lower legs and ulcerations of the feet. Occlusion and thrombosis of large vessels and small arteries and arterioles, as well as alterations in neurologic function and infection, result in gangrene (necrosis, or the death of tissue). Gangrene from diabetes is the most common cause of nontraumatic amputations of the lower leg. In people with diabetes, dry gangrene is most common, manifested by cold, dry, shriveled, and black tissues of the toes and feet. The gangrene usually begins in the toes and moves proximally into the foot.

Diabetic Retinopathy

Diabetic retinopathy is the name for the changes in the retina that occur in the person with diabetes. The retinal capillary structure undergoes alterations in blood flow, leading to retinal ischemia and a breakdown in the blood-retinal barrier. Diabetic retinopathy is the leading cause of blindness in people between ages 25 and 74. Retinopathy has three stages:

- *Stage I:* Nonproliferative retinopathy. Dilated veins, microaneurysms, edema of the macula, and the presence of exudates characterize this stage.

- *Stage II:* Preproliferative retinopathy. Retinal ischemia causes infarcts of the nerve fiber layer, with characteristic "cotton wool" patches on the retina. Shunts form between occluded and patent vessels.

- *Stage III:* Proliferative retinopathy. As fibrous tissue and new vessels form in the retina or optic disc, traction on the vitreous humor may cause hemorrhage or retinal detachment.

After 20 years of diabetes, almost all clients with type 1 DM and more than 60% of clients with type 2 DM will have some degree of retinopathy (American Diabetes Association [ADA], 2002). If exudate, edema, hemorrhage, or ischemia occurs near the fovea, the person experiences visual impairment at any stage. In addition, the person with diabetes is at increased risk for developing cataracts (opacity of the lens) as a result of increased glucose levels within the lens itself. Screening for retinopathy is important, as laser photocoagulation surgery has proven beneficial in preventing loss of vision.

Diabetic Nephropathy

Diabetic nephropathy is a disease of the kidneys characterized by the presence of albumin in the urine, hypertension, edema, and progressive renal insufficiency. This disorder is the most common cause of renal failure requiring dialysis or transplantation in the United States. Nephropathy occurs in 20% to 40% of people with diabetes (ADA, 2002).

Despite research, the exact pathologic origin of diabetic nephropathy is unknown; it has been established, however, that thickening of the basement membrane of the glomeruli eventually impairs renal function. It is suggested that an increased intracellular concentration of glucose supports the formation of abnormal glycoproteins in the basement membrane. The accumulation of these large proteins stimulates glomerulosclerosis (fibrosis of the glomerular tissue). Glomerulosclerosis severely impairs the filtering function of the glomerulus, and protein is lost in the urine. *Kimmelstiel-Wilson syndrome* is a type of glomerulosclerosis found only in people with diabetes. In advanced nephropathy, tubular atrophy occurs, and end-stage renal disease results. (Renal failure is discussed in Chapter 24.)

The first indication of nephropathy is **microalbuminuria,** a low but abnormal level of albumin in the urine. Without specific interventions, people with type 1 DM with sustained microalbuminuria will develop overt nephropathy, accompanied by hypertension, over a period of 10 to 15 years. People with type 2 DM often have microalbuminuria and overt nephropathy shortly after diagnosis, because the diabetes has often been present but undiagnosed for many years. Because the hypertension accelerates the progress of diabetic nephropathy, aggressive antihypertensive management should be instituted. Management includes control of hypertension with ACE inhibitors, such as captopril (Capoten), weight loss, reduced salt intake, and exercise.

Alterations in the Peripheral and Autonomic Nervous Systems

Peripheral and visceral neuropathies are disorders of the peripheral nerves and the autonomic nervous system. In people with diabetes, these disorders are often called **diabetic neuropathies.** The etiology of diabetic neuropathies involves (1) a thickening of the walls of the blood vessels that supply nerves, causing a decrease in nutrients; (2) demyelinization of the Schwann cells that surround and insulate nerves, slowing nerve conduction; and (3) the formation and accumulation of sorbitol within the Schwann cells, impairing nerve conduction. The manifestations depend on the locations of the lesions.

Peripheral Neuropathies

The peripheral neuropathies (also called *somatic neuropathies*) include polyneuropathies and mononeuropathies. *Polyneuropathies,* the most common type of neuropathy associated with diabetes, are bilateral sensory disorders. The manifestations appear first in the toes and feet and progress upward. The fingers and hands may also be involved, but usually only in later stages of diabetes. The manifestations of polyneuropathy depend on the nerve fibers involved.

The person with polyneuropathy commonly has distal paresthesias (a subjective feeling of a change in sensation, such as numbness or tingling); pain described as aching, burning, or shooting; and feelings of cold feet. Other manifestations may include impaired sensations of pain, temperature, light touch, two-point discrimination, and vibration. There is no specific treatment for polyneuropathy.

Mononeuropathies are isolated peripheral neuropathies that affect a single nerve. Depending on the nerve involved, manifestations may include the following:

- Palsy of the third cranial (oculomotor) nerve, with headache, eye pain, and an inability to move the eye up, down, or medially

- Radiculopathy, with pain over a dermatome and loss of cutaneous sensation, most often located in the chest

- Diabetic femoral neuropathy, with motor and sensory deficits (pain, weakness, areflexia) in the anterior thigh and medial calf

- Entrapment or compression of the medial nerve at the wrist, resulting in carpal tunnel syndrome with pain and weakness of the hand; the ulnar nerve at the elbow, with weakness and loss of sensation over the palmar surface of the fourth and fifth fingers; and the peroneal nerve at the head of the fibula, with foot drop.

Visceral Neuropathies

The visceral neuropathies (also called *autonomic neuropathies*) cause various manifestations, depending on the area of the ANS involved. These neuropathies may include the following:

- Sweating dysfunction, with an absence of sweating *(anhydrosis)* on the hands and feet and increased sweating on the face or trunk

- Abnormal pupillary function, most commonly seen as constricted pupils that dilate slowly in the dark

- Cardiovascular dysfunction, resulting in such abnormalities as a fixed cardiac rate that does not change with exercise, postural hypotension, and a failure to increase cardiac output or vascular tone with exercise

- Gastrointestinal dysfunction, with changes in upper gastrointestinal motility *(gastroparesis)* resulting in dysphagia, anorexia, heartburn, nausea, and vomiting and altered blood glucose control. Constipation is one of the most common gastrointestinal symptoms associated with diabetes, possibly a result of hypomotility of the bowel. Diabetic diarrhea is not as common, but it does occur and is often associated with fecal incontinence during sleep due to a defect in internal sphincter function.

- Genitourinary dysfunction, resulting in changes in bladder function and sexual function. Bladder function changes include an inability to empty the bladder completely, loss of sensation of bladder fullness, and an increased risk of urinary tract infections. Sexual dysfunctions in men include ejaculatory changes and impotence. Sexual dysfunctions in women include changes in arousal patterns, vaginal lubrication, and orgasm. Alterations in sexual function in people with diabetes are the result of both neurologic and vascular changes.

Increased Susceptibility to Infection

The person with diabetes has an increased risk of developing infections. The exact relationship between infection and diabetes is not clear, but many dysfunctions that result from diabetic complications predispose the person to develop an infection. Vascular and neurologic impairments, hyperglycemia, and altered neutrophil function are believed to be responsible (Porth, 2002).

The person with diabetes may have sensory deficits resulting in inattention to trauma, and vascular deficits that decrease circulation to the injured area; as a result, the normal inflammatory response is diminished and healing is slowed. Nephrosclerosis and inadequate bladder emptying with retention of urine predispose the person with diabetes to pyelonephritis and urinary tract infections. Bacterial and fungal infections of the skin, nails, and mucous membranes are common. Tuberculosis is more prevalent in people with diabetes than in the general population.

Periodontal Disease

Although periodontal disease does not occur more often in people with diabetes, it does progress more rapidly, especially if the diabetes is poorly controlled. It is believed to be caused by microangiopathy, with changes in vascularization of the gums. As a result, gingivitis (inflammation of the gums) and periodontitis (inflammation of the bone underlying the gums) occur.

Complications Involving the Feet

The high incidence of both amputations and problems with the feet in people with diabetes is the result of angiopathy, neuropathy, and infection. People with diabetes are at high risk for amputation of a lower extremity, with increased risk in those who have had DM for more than ten years, are male, have poor glucose control, or have cardiovascular, retinal, or renal complications.

Vascular changes in the lower extremities of the person with diabetes result in arteriosclerosis. Diabetes-induced arteriosclerosis tends to occur at an earlier age, occurs equally in men and women, is usually bilateral, and progresses more rapidly. The blood vessels most often affected are located below the knee. Blockages form in the large, medium, and small arteries of the lower legs and feet. Multiple occlusions with decreased blood flow result in the manifestations of peripheral vascular disease. Peripheral vascular disease is discussed in Chapter 12.

Diabetic neuropathy of the foot produces multiple problems. Because the sense of touch and perception of pain is absent, the person with diabetes may have some type of foot trauma without being aware of it. The person thus is at increased risk for trauma to tissues of the feet, leading to ulcer development. Infections commonly occur in traumatized or ulcerated tissue.

Despite the many potential sources of foot trauma in the person with diabetes, the most common are cracks and fissures caused by dry skin or infections, such as athlete's foot, blisters caused by improperly fitting shoes, pressure from stockings or shoes, ingrown toenails, and direct trauma (cuts, bruises, or burns). It is important to remember that the person with diabetic neuropathy who has lost the perception of pain may not be aware that these injuries have occurred. In addition, when a part of the body loses sensation, the person tends to dissociate from or ignore the part, so that an injury may go unattended for days or weeks. The injury may even be forgotten entirely.

Foot lesions usually begin as a superficial skin ulcer. In time, the ulcer extends deeper into muscles and bone, leading to abscess or osteomyelitis. Gangrene can develop on one or more toes; if untreated, the whole foot eventually becomes gangrenous.

Diabetes in the Older Adult

Although the older adult may have either type 1 or type 2 DM, most have type 2. The National Institute of Diabetes and Kidney Disease estimates that nearly 11% of the U.S. population between the ages of 65 and 74 have diabetes. The prevalence of diabetes becomes greater with age, increasing from 8.2% with diagnosed diabetes in those age 20 years or older to 18.4% for those equal to or older than age 65 (ADA, 2002). It is predicted that the number of older adults with diabetes will continue to increase, because the incidence of the disease increases with age and because the number of people over 65 is increasing.

Although most older adults with diabetes have type 2 DM, the improved survival rates for people with diabetes have resulted in an increased number of older adults with type 1. The picture is complicated by the fact that blood glucose levels increase with age, beginning in the 50s. For this reason, it is more difficult to diagnose diabetes in the older adult; conversely, the older adult may be mistakenly diagnosed with the disease simply for exhibiting essentially normal age-related changes in glucose. The relationship between normal increases in glucose levels and the presence of diabetes is not yet understood.

The older adult with diabetes has multiple, complex health care problems and needs. The normal physiologic changes of aging may mask manifestations of the onset of diabetes and may also increase the potential for complications. The older adult with diabetes also has a longer recovery period after surgery or serious illness, often requiring insulin to maintain blood glucose levels.

Collaborative Care

The results of a 10-year Diabetes Control and Complications Trial (DCCT), sponsored by the National Institutes of Health (NIH), have significant implications for the management of type 1 DM. People in the study who kept their blood glucose levels close to normal by frequent monitoring, several daily insulin injections, and lifestyle changes that included exercise and a healthier diet reduced by 60% their risk for the development and progression of complications involving the eyes, the kidneys, and the nervous system. Treatment of the client with diabetes focuses on maintaining blood glucose at levels as nearly normal as possible through medications, dietary management, and exercise. Treatment of the acute complications of diabetes (hypoglycemia, DKA, and HHS) is also included in this section.

Diagnostic Tests

Diagnostic tests are conducted for screening purposes to diagnose diabetes, and ongoing laboratory tests are conducted to evaluate the effectiveness of diabetic management.

Definitions of normal blood glucose levels vary in clinical practice, depending on the laboratory that performs the assay.

Diagnostic Screening

Three diagnostic tests may be used to diagnose DM, and each must be confirmed, on a subsequent day, with one of the three tests. The diagnostic criteria recommended by the ADA (2002) are:

1. Symptoms of diabetes plus causal plasma glucose (PG) concentration >200 mg/dL (11.1 mmol/L). Causal is defined as any time of day without regard to time since last meal.

2. Fasting plasma glucose (FPG) >126 mg/dL (7.0 mmol/L). Fasting is defined as no caloric intake for eight hours.

3. Two-hour PG >200 mg/dL (11.1 mmol/L) during an oral glucose tolerance test (OGTT). The test should be performed with a glucose load containing the equivalent of 75 anhydrous glucose dissolved in water.

When using these criteria, the following levels are used for the FPG:

*   Normal fasting glucose = 110 mg/dL (6.1 mmol/L)
*   Impaired fasting glucose = >110 (6.1 mmol/L) and <126 mg/dL (7.0 mmol/L)
*   Diagnosis of diabetes = >126 mg/dL (7.0 mmol/L).

When using these criteria, the following levels are used for the OGTT:

*   Normal glucose tolerance = 2-hr PG: <140 mg/dL (7.8 mmol/L)
*   Impaired glucose tolerance = 2-hr PG: ≥140 (7.8 mmol/L) and <200 mg/dL (11.1 mmol/L)
*   Diagnosis of diabetes = 2-hr PG: ≥200 mg/dL (11.1 mmol/L).

Note that although either method may be used to diagnose diabetes, the FPG is the recommended screening test for nonpregnant adults in a clinical setting (ADA, 2002).

Diagnostic Tests to Monitor Diabetes Management

The following diagnostic tests may be used to monitor diabetes management:

*   *Fasting blood glucose (FBG).* This test is often ordered, especially if the client is experiencing symptoms of hypoglycemia or hyperglycemia. In most people, the normal range is 70 to 110 mg/dL.

*   *Glycosylated hemoglobin (c) (A1C).* This test determines the average blood glucose level over approximately the previous two to three months. When glucose is elevated or control of glucose is erratic, glucose attaches to the hemoglobin molecule and remains attached for the life of the hemoglobin, which is about 120 days. The normal level depends on the type of assay done, but values above 7% to 9% are considered elevated. The ADA recommends that A1C be performed at the initial assessment, and then at regular intervals, individualized to the medical regimen used.

*   *Urine glucose and ketone levels.* These are not as accurate in monitoring changes in blood glucose as blood levels. The presence of glucose in the urine indicates hyperglycemia. Most people have a renal threshold for glucose of 180 mg/dL; that is, when the blood glucose exceeds 180 mg/dL, glucose is not reabsorbed by the kidney

and spills over into the urine. This number varies highly, however. Ketonuria (the presence of ketones in the urine) occurs with the breakdown of fats and is an indicator of DKA; however, fat breakdown and ketonuria occur also in states of less than normal nutrition.

- *Urine test* for the presence of protein as albumin *(albuminuria)*. If albuminuria is present, a 24-hour urine test for creatinine clearance is used to detect the early onset of nephropathy.

- *Serum cholesterol and triglyceride levels.* These are indicators of atherosclerosis and an increased risk of cardiovascular impairments. The ADA (2002) recommends treatment goals to lower LDL cholesterol to <100 mg/dL, raise HDL cholesterol to >45 mg/dL, and lower triglycerides to <150 mg/dL.

- *Serum electrolytes.* Levels are measured in clients who have DKA or HHS to determine imbalances.

Monitoring Blood Glucose

People with diabetes must monitor their condition daily by testing glucose levels. Two types of tests are available. The first type, long used prior to the development of devices to directly measure blood glucose, is urine testing for glucose and ketones. Urine testing is less commonly used today. The second type, direct measurement of blood glucose, is widely used in all types of health care settings and in the home.

Urine Testing for Ketones and Glucose

Urine testing for glucose and ketones was at one time the only available method for evaluating the management of diabetes. An inexpensive and noninvasive test, it has unpredictable results and cannot be used to detect or measure hypoglycemia. Urine testing is recommended to monitor hyperglycemia and ketoacidosis in people with type 1 DM who have unexplained hyperglycemia during illness or pregnancy. Urine testing may also be used by people who choose not to self-monitor blood glucose by other methods.

Self-Monitoring of Blood Glucose

Self-monitoring of blood glucose (SMBG) allows the person with diabetes to monitor and achieve metabolic control and decrease the danger of hypoglycemia. The ADA recommends that all clients with diabetes must be taught some method of monitoring glycemic control. The timing of SMBG is highly individualized, depending on the person's diagnosis, general disease control, and physical state. SMBG is recommended three or more times a day for clients with type 1 DM. When adding or modifying therapy, clients with both types of DM should test more often than usual. SMBG is also useful when the person is ill or pregnant, or has symptoms of hypoglycemia or hyperglycemia.

The ADA annually publishes a comprehensive list of currently available blood glucose monitoring machines and strips with approximate prices in *Diabetes Forecast*. Most medical insurance policies cover the cost of these machines.

Following is the equipment needed for SMBG.

- Some type of lancet device to perform a finger-stick for obtaining a drop of blood, such as an Autolet, Penlet, or Soft Touch

- Chemically impregnated test strips that change color when they come into contact with glucose or that can be read by machine (e.g., Glucostix and Chemstrip bG). The strip may also be read by comparing its color with a color chart on the side of the container or on an insert.
- A blood glucose monitor (e.g., the Glucometer, the AccuChek, or the One Touch) if the most accurate measurement is desired or recommended. The manufacturer's instructions must be followed carefully. If the timing of the blood on the strip is not exact, the test will not be accurate. In addition, the machine must be cleaned according to the manufacturer's directions to ensure accuracy. Monitors that use no-wipe technology improve the accuracy of glucose measurement. Other monitors are computerized and/or include a memory of previous glucose readings to show a pattern of control.

Factors that may alter blood glucose results when testing with a monitor (Passaniza, 2001) are as follows:

- Increased triglyceride levels, which can interfere with the way light is reflected in light reflectance monitors, such as the AccuChek
- Insufficient amounts of blood on the testing strip, outdated strips, and exposure of the strips to air and humidity
- Both increased and decreased hematocrits, with blood glucose values varying as much as 30% for every 10% change in hematocrit
- High altitudes, which cause a decrease in blood oxygen
- High doses of acetaminophen (Tylenol), ascorbic acid (vitamin C), ibuprofen (Motrin, Advil), salicylates (Aspirin), and tetracycline.

Medications

The pharmacologic treatment for diabetes mellitus depends on the type of diabetes. People with type 1 must have insulin; those with type 2 are usually able to control glucose levels with an oral hypoglycemic medication, but they may require insulin if control is inadequate.

Insulin

The person with type 1 DM requires a lifelong exogenous source of the insulin hormone to maintain life. Insulin is not a cure for diabetes; rather, it is a means of controlling hyperglycemia. Insulin is also necessary in other situations, such as:

- People with diabetes who are unable to control glucose levels with oral antidiabetic drugs and/or diet. Approximately 40% of people with type 2 diabetes require insulin (NIH, 2002).
- People with diabetes who are experiencing physical stress, such as an infection or surgery, or who are taking corticosteroids.
- Women with gestational diabetes who are unable to control glucose with diet.
- People with DKA or HHS.
- People who are receiving high-calorie tube feedings or parenteral nutrition.

Sources of Insulin. Preparations of insulin are derived from animal (pork pancreas) or synthesized in the laboratory from either an alteration of pork insulin or recombinant DNA technology, using strains of *E. coli* to form a biosynthetic human insulin. Insulin analogs have been developed by modifying the amino acid sequence of the insulin molecule. Although different types are prescribed on an individualized basis, it is standard practice to prescribe human insulin.

Insulin Preparations. Insulins are available in rapid-acting, short-acting, intermediate-acting, and long-acting preparations. The trade names and times of onset, peak, and duration of action are listed in Table 27-4.

Table 27-4.   Insulin Preparations

Preparation	Name	Onset (h)	Peak (h)	Duration (h)
Rapid acting	Lispro	0.25	1–1.5	3–4
Short acting	Regular Regular Humulin (R) Regular Iletin II Velosulin	0.5–1.0	2–3	4–6
Intermediate acting	Lente Humulin (L) Lente Iletin II NPH Humulin (N) NPH Iletin II NPH	2	6–8	12–16
Long acting	Ultralente (U) Lantus	2 (onset and peak not defined)	16–20	24+ 24
Combinations	Humulin 50/50 Humulin 70/30 Novolin 70/30	0.5 0.5 0.5	3 4–8 4–8	22–24 24 24

Insulin lispro (Humalog) is a human insulin analog that is derived from genetically altered *E. coli* that includes the gene for insulin lispro. It is classified as a rapid-acting or ultra-short-acting insulin. Compared to regular insulin, insulin lispro has a more rapid onset (<15 minutes), an earlier peak of glucose lowering (30 to 60 minutes), and a shorter duration of activity (3 to 4 hours). This means that lispro should be administered 15 minutes before a meal, rather than 30 to 60 minutes before as recommended for regular insulin. Clients with type 1 DM usually also require concurrent use of a longer-acting insulin product. Lispro is much less likely than regular insulin to cause tissue changes and may lower the risk of nocturnal hypoglycemia in clients with type 1 DM.

Regular insulin is unmodified crystalline insulin, classified as a short-actin insulin. Regular insulin is clear in appearance and can be given by the intravenous route; the other types are suspensions and could be harmful if given by this route. Regular insulin is also used to treat DKA, to initiate treatment for newly diagnosed type 1 DM, and in combination with intermediate-acting insulins to provide better glucose control.

The onset and peak and duration of action of insulin can be changed by adding zinc, acetate buffers, and protamine. Zinc is added to make lente insulin, and zinc and protamine are added to NPH insulin to prolong their action, and they are classified as intermediate- or long-acting insulins. These preparations appear cloudy when properly mixed prior to injection. Protamine and zinc are foreign substances and may cause hypersensitivity reactions.

Insulin glargine (Lantus) is a 24-hour long-acting rDNA human insulin analog that is given subcutaneously once a day at bedtime to treat clients with both type 1 and type 2 diabetes. It has a relatively constant effect (meaning it does not have a peak time of effect). It may be used in combination with intermediate-acting or long-acting insulins.

Concentrations of Insulin. Insulin is dispensed as 100 U/mL (U-100) and 500 U/mL (U-500) in the United States. U-100 is the standard insulin concentration used. U-500 insulin is only used in rare cases of insulin resistance when clients require very large doses. U-500 and the insulin analog lispro are the only insulins that require a prescription.

Insulin Administration. Nursing implications for administering insulin are outlined in the Table 27-5 and further discussion follows in the chapter. The considerations for administering insulin include routes of administration, syringe and needle selection, preparing the injection, sites of injection, mixing insulins, and insulin regimens.

Routes of Administration. All insulins are given parenterally, although current research is investigating the development of a nasal spray and an oral preparation of insulin. Only regular insulin is given by both subcutaneous and intravenous routes; all others are given only subcutaneously. If the intravenous route is not available, regular insulin may also be administered intramuscularly in an emergency situation.

Table 27-5. Medication Administration – Insulin

Nursing Responsibilities

- Discard vials of insulin that have been open for several weeks or whose expiration date has passed.
- Refrigerate extra insulin vials not currently in use, but do not freeze them.
- Store insulin in a cool place, and avoid exposure to temperature extremes or sunlight.
- Store compatible mixtures of insulin for no longer than one month at room temperature or three months at 36° to 46°F (2° to 8°C).
- Discard any vials with discoloration, clumping, granules, or solid deposits on the sides.
- If breakfast is delayed, also delay the administration of rapid-acting insulin.
- Monitor and maintain a record of blood glucose readings 30 minutes before each meal and bedtime (or as prescribed).
- Monitor food intake, and notify the physician if food is not being consumed.
- Monitor electrolytes (especially potassium), blood urea nitrogen (BUN) levels, and creatinine.
- Observe injection sites for manifestations of hypersensitivity, lipodystrophy, and lipoatrophy.
- If symptoms of hypoglycemia occur, confirm by testing blood glucose level, and administer an oral source of a fast-acting carbohydrate, such as juice, milk, or crackers.

Continued on the next page

Table 27-5. Continued

Hypoglycemic symptoms may vary but commonly include feelings of shakiness, hunger, and/or nervousness accompanied by sweating, tachycardia, or palpitations.

- If symptoms of hyperglycemia occur, confirm by testing blood glucose level, and notify the physician.

Client and Family Teaching

- The manifestations of diabetes mellitus.
- Self-administration of insulin, with a return demonstration.
  - a. Wash hands carefully.
  - b. Have a vial of insulin, the insulin syringe with needle, and alcohol pads ready to use.
  - c. Remove the cover from the needle.
  - d. Fill the syringe with an amount of air equal to the number of units of insulin, and insert the needle into the vial.
  - e. Push air into the vial, invert the vial, and withdraw the prescribed units of insulin.
  - f. Replace the cover over the needle.
  - g. Wipe the selected site with alcohol. The injection is less likely to be painful if the alcohol is allowed to dry.
  - h. Pinch up a fold of skin, and insert the needle into the tissue at the recommended angle.
  - i. Insert the insulin.
  - j. Withdraw the needle; if desired, apply firm pressure to the site for a few seconds.
  - k. Recap the needle. Many people with diabetes reuse disposable syringes with attached needles without adverse effects. The primary reason for discarding after several uses is that the needle becomes dull and makes the injection painful.
- Follow instructions for mixing insulins.
- Always keep an extra vial of insulin available.
- Always have a vial of regular insulin available for emergencies.
- Be aware of the signs of hypersensitivity responses, hypoglycemia, and hyperglycemia.
- Keep candy or a sugar source available at all times to treat hypoglycemia, if it occurs.
- Vision may be blurred during the first six to eight weeks of insulin therapy; this is the result of fluid changes in the eye and should clear up in eight weeks.
- Avoid alcoholic beverages, which may cause hypoglycemia.
- Follow these guidelines for sick days:
  - a. Never omit insulin.
  - b. Always monitor blood glucose and/or urine ketones at least every two to four hours.
  - c. Always drink plenty of fluids, try to drink at least one glass of water or other calorie-free, caffeine-free liquid each hour.
  - d. Get as much rest as possible.
  - e. Contact the physician if there is persistent fever, vomiting, shortness of breath, severe pain in the abdomen, dehydration, loss of vision, chest pain, persistent diarrhea, blood glucose levels above 250, or ketones in the urine.
- Establish a plan for rotating injection sites, and observe closely for changes in tissues such as hardness, dimpling, or sunken areas.

Continuous Subcutaneous Insulin Infusion. Regular insulin is also used in continuous subcutaneous insulin infusion (CSII) devices, often called *insulin pumps* (e.g., Minimed and Disetronic pumps). CSII devices have a small pump that holds a syringe of insulin, connected to a subcutaneous needle by tubing. The pump is about the size of a pager and can be worn on a belt or tucked into a pocket. The needle is placed in the skin, usually in the abdomen. This device delivers a constant amount of programmed insulin throughout each 24-hour period. It also can be used to deliver a bolus of insulin manually (e.g., before meals).

Programming the amount of insulin to be delivered is determined by frequent blood glucose monitoring. Several different pumps are available, and each has rechargeable batteries, a syringe, a programmable computer, and a motor and drive mechanism. The rapid-acting insulin analog lispro is an appropriate insulin for insulin pumps, and short-acting regular insulin may also be used. Lispro is not approved for use during pregnancy (Tierney, et al., 2001).

Many people with diabetes believe the pump allows more normal regulation of blood glucose and provides greater lifestyle flexibility. Pumps are as safe as multiple-injection therapy when recommended procedures are followed. A potential complication is an undetected interruption in insulin delivery, which may result in a rapid onset of DKA. The needle site must be kept clean and changed on a regular basis (usually every 2 to 3 days) to prevent inflammation and infection. Although the client who chooses an insulin pump has more to learn, many are very satisfied with having more normal glucose control.

Syringe and Needle Selection. Insulin is administered in sterile, single-use, disposable insulin syringes, calibrated in units per milliliter. This means that in U-100 insulin, there are 100 U of insulin in 1 mL. Syringes for administering U-100 insulin can be purchased in either 0.3 mL (30 U), 0.5 mL (50 U), or 1.0 mL (100 U) size. The advantage of the 0.3 mL and 0.5 mL sizes is that the distance between unit markings is greater, making it easier to measure the dose accurately.

Most insulin syringes are manufactured with the needle permanently attached in a 25 to 27 gauge, 0.5 inch size. If this type of syringe is not available, an insulin syringe and a 25 gauge, 0.5 inch, or 0.75 inch needle should be used.

Other special injection products are available for people with physical handicaps. These products include automatic injectors and jet spray injectors. Prefilled syringes are useful for people who are visually impaired or traveling. Prefilled syringes are stable for up to 30 days if stored in the refrigerator.

Preparing the Injection. The vial of insulin in use may be kept at room temperature for up to four weeks. Stored vials should be kept in the refrigerator and brought to room temperature prior to administration.

Regular insulin does not require mixing. If the solution is cloudy or discolored, the vial should be discarded. The other types of insulin must be mixed to disperse the particles evenly throughout the solution. Mix the vial by gently rolling it between the hands; vigorous shaking causes bubble formation and frothing, which makes the dose inaccurate. It is critical that no air bubbles remain in the prepared dose, because even a small bubble can displace several units of insulin.

Sites of Injection. Although, in theory, any area of the body with subcutaneous tissue may be used for injections of insulin, certain sites are recommended. The rate of absorption and peak of action of insulin differs according to the site. The site that allows the most rapid absorption is the abdomen, followed by the deltoid muscle, then the thigh, and then the hip. Because of the rapid absorption, the abdomen is the recommended site.

When administering insulin, gently pinch a fold of skin and inject the needle at a 90-degree angle. If the person is very thin, a 45-degree angle may be required to avoid injecting into muscle. Routine aspiration to check for blood is not necessary. Do not massage the site after administering the injection, because this may interfere with absorption; pressure, however, may be applied for about one minute. Rotation of injection sites is recommended for clients using pork insulin; rotation within sites is recommended for those using human or purified pork insulin. The distance between injections should be about one inch (avoiding the area within a 2-inch radius around the umbilicus). Insulin should not be injected into an area to be exercised, such as the thigh before a vigorous walk, or to which heat will be applied; exercise or heat may increase the rate of absorption and cause a more rapid onset and peak of action.

Lipodystrophy. Lipodystrophy (hypertrophy of subcutaneous tissue) or **lipoatrophy** (atrophy of subcutaneous tissue) may result if the same injection sites are used repeatedly, especially with pork and beef insulins. The tissues become hardened and have an orange-peel appearance. The use of refrigerated insulin may trigger the development of tissue atrophy or hypertrophy. These problems rarely occur with the use of human insulins. Lipodystrophy and lipoatrophy alter insulin absorption, delaying its onset or retaining the insulin in the tissue for a period of time instead of allowing it to be absorbed into the body. Lipodystrophy usually resolves if the area is unused for a minimum of six months.

Mixing Insulins. When a person with diabetes requires more than one type of insulin, mixing is recommended to avoid administering two injections per dose. Two different concentrations are administered, because a single dose of intermediate-acting or long-acting insulin rarely provides adequate control of blood glucose levels. Following are some general guidelines:

- Commercially mixed insulins are recommended if the insulin ratio is appropriate for the requirements of the client.
- Regular insulin may be mixed with all other types of insulin; it may be injected immediately after mixing or stored for future use.
- NPH insulin and PZI insulin may be mixed only with regular insulin.
- Lente insulin preparations may be mixed with each other; mixing with regular insulin or with PZI and NPH insulin is not recommended.
- Do not mix human and animal insulins.
- Always withdraw regular insulin first to avoid contaminating the regular insulin with intermediate-acting insulin.

Insulin Regimens. The appropriate insulin dosage is individualized by achieving a balance among insulin, diet, and exercise. For most people with diabetes, the timing of insulin action requires two or more injections each day, often a mixture of rapid-acting and intermediate-acting insulins. Timing of the injections depends on blood glucose levels, food consumption, exercise, and types of insulin used. The objective is to avoid daytime hypoglycemia while achieving adequate blood glucose control overnight.

Hypersensitivity Responses. When injected, insulin may cause local and systemic hypersensitivity responses. Manifestations of local reactions are a hardening and reddening of the area that develops over several hours. Local reactions result from a contaminant in the insulin and are more likely to occur when less purified insulin products are used.

Systemic reactions occur rapidly and are characterized by widespread red, intensely pruritic welts. Respiratory difficulty may occur if the respiratory system is involved. Systemic responses are due to an allergy to the insulin itself and are most common with beef insulin. The client can be desensitized by administering small doses of purified pork or human insulin, followed by progressively larger doses.

Oral Hypoglycemic Agents

Oral hypoglycemic agents are used to treat people with type 2 DM. Nursing implications for this category of drugs are discussed in Table 27-5.

Aspirin Therapy

People with diabetes are up to four times more likely to die from cardiovascular disease. It is recommended that a once daily dose of 75 to 325 mg of enteric-coated aspirin be given to reduce atherosclerosis in clients with vascular disease or increased cardiovascular risk factors. Aspirin therapy is contraindicated for clients with aspirin allergy, bleeding tendency, recent gastrointestinal bleeding, or active liver disease.

Diet Therapy

The management of diabetes requires a careful balance between the intake of nutrients, the expenditure of energy, and the dose and timing of insulin or oral antidiabetic agents. Although everyone has the same need for basic nutrition, the person with diabetes must eat a more structured diet to prevent hyperglycemia. The goals for dietary management for adults with diabetes, based on guidelines established by the ADA (2002), are as follows:

Maintain as near normal blood glucose levels as possible by balancing food intake with insulin or oral glucose.

* Achieve optimal serum lipid levels.
* Provide adequate calories to maintain or attain reasonable weights, and to recover from catabolic illness.

Table 27-6. Medication Administration – Oral Hypoglycemic Agents

Sulfonylureas

Glimepiride (Amaryl)
Glipizide (Glucotrol, Glucotrol XL)
Glyburide (Diabeta, Micronase)
Tolazamide (Tolinase)
Tolbutamide (Orinase)

These drugs are used primarily to treat mild, nonketotic type 2 DM in people who are not obese. Glyburide, glipizide, and glimepiride are 100 to 200 times more potent than tolbutamide. These clients cannot control the symptoms by diet alone, but they do not require insulin. The drugs act by stimulating the pancreatic cells to secrete more insulin and by increasing the sensitivity of peripheral tissues to insulin. The most common side effect is hypoglycemia.

Continued on the next page

Table 27-6. Continued

Meglitinides

Repaglinide (Prandin)

This drug lowers blood glucose levels by stimulating release of insulin from the pancreatic islet cells.

Biguanides

Metformin (Glucophage)

Metformin reduces both the FBG and the degree of postprandial hyperglycemia in clients with type 2 DM. It primarily decreases the overproduction of glucose by the liver, and may also make insulin more effective in peripheral tissues. It is used as an adjunct to diet, especially in clients who are obese or not responding to the sufonylureas.

Alpha-Glucoside Inhibitors

Acarbose (Precose)
Miglitol (Glyset)

These drugs work locally in the small intestine to slow carbohydrate digestion and delay glucose absorption. As a result, postprandial glucose and glycosylated hemoglobin are better controlled, reducing the risk of long-term complications.

Thiazolidinediones

Rosiglitazone (Avandia)
Pioglitazone (Actos)

This class of drugs acts by sensitizing peripheral tissue to insulin. Both drugs can be used alone or in combination with sulfonylureas, metformin, and insulin.

D-phenylalanine (Amino Acid) Derivative

Netaglinide (Starlix)

This is the first in a new class of oral medications for treatment of type 2 diabetes. It stimulates rapid and short insulin secretion from the pancreatic beta cells to decrease spikes in glucose following meals, and also reduces the overall blood glucose level.

Nursing Responsibilities
- Assess clients taking oral hypoglycemic agents closely for the first seven days to determine therapeutic response.
- Administer the drug with food.
- Teach the client the importance of maintaining a prescribed diet and exercise program.
- Monitor for hypoglycemia if the client is also taking nonsteroidal anti-inflammatory agents (NSAIDs), sulfonamide antibiotics, ranitidine, cimetidine, or beta blockers; these drugs intensify the action of sulfonylureas.

Table 27-6. Continued

- Monitor for hyperglycemia if the client is also taking calcium channel blockers, oral contraceptives, glucocorticoids, phenothiazines, or thiazide diuretics; these drugs decrease the hypoglycemic responses to sulfonylureas.
- Do not administer these drugs to pregnant or lactating women.
- Assess for side effects: nausea, heartburn, diarrhea, dizziness, fever, headache, jaundice, skin rash, urticaria, photophobia, thrombocytopenia, leukopenia, or anemia.
- If the client is to have a thyroid test, determine whether the drug has been taken; sulfonylureas interfere with the uptake of radioactive iodine.
- Monitor for hypoglycemia with concurrent administration of an oral antidiabetic agent and insulin.
- Temporarily hold metformin for two days prior to injection of any radiocontrast agent to avoid potential lactic acidosis if renal failure occurs.
- Closely monitor liver function tests with administration of rosiglitazone and pioglitazone.

Client and Family Teaching
- Maintain prescribed diet and exercise regimen.
- You may need insulin if you have surgery, trauma, fever, or infection.
- Follow instructions to monitor blood glucose.
- Report illness or side effects to the health care provider.
- Undergo periodic laboratory evaluations as prescribed by your health care provider.
- Avoid alcohol intake, which may cause a reaction involving flushing, palpitations, and nausea.
- The medication interferes with the effectiveness of oral contraceptives; other birth control measures may be required.
- Mild symptoms of hyperglycemia may appear if a different agent is begun.
- Take medications as prescribed; for example, once a day at the same time each day. If you are taking acarbose, take the pill with the first bite of food at breakfast, lunch, and dinner.
- Prevent and treat the acute complications of insulin-treated DM, short-term illnesses, and exercise-related problems; or the long-term complications of diabetes.
- Improve overall health through optimal nutrition, using Dietary Guidelines for Americans and the food guide pyramid.

Carbohydrates
The ADA recommends that carbohydrates should be individualized to the client's needs, with the combination of carbohydrates and monosaturated fats constituting 60% to 70% of the daily diet. Carbohydrates contain 4 kcal per gram. This group of nutrients consists of plant foods (grains, fruits, vegetables), milk, and some dairy products. Carbohydrates can be divided into simple sugars and complex carbohydrates. Despite a long-held belief, research does not support that sugars are more rapidly digested and therefore aggravate hyperglycemia. Fruits and milk have a lower glycemic response than most starches, and the glycemic response of sucrose is similar to that of bread, rice, and potatoes (ADA, 2002)

The use of sucrose as part of the total carbohydrate content in the diet does not impair blood glucose control in people with diabetes. Sucrose and sucrose-containing foods must be substituted for other carbohydrates gram for gram. Dietary fructose (from fruits and vegetables or from fructose-sweetened foods) produces a smaller rise in plasma glucose than sucrose and most starches, so it may offer an advantage as a sweetening agent. However, large amounts of fructose have potentially adverse effects on serum cholesterol and LDL cholesterol, so amounts used should be controlled.

Protein

The recommended daily protein intake is 15% to 20% of total daily kcal intake. Protein has 4 kcal per gram. Sources of protein should be low in fat, low in saturated fat, and low in cholesterol. Although this amount of protein is much less than that which most people normally consume, it is recommended to help prevent or delay renal complications. To help the client accept the decrease in the amount of protein, the nurse may suggest a less severe restriction at diagnosis with a gradual decrease to take place over a period of years.

Fats

Dietary fats should be low in saturated fat and cholesterol. Saturated fats should be no higher than 10% of the total kcal allowed per day, with dietary cholesterol less than 300 mg per day. Fat has 9 kcal per gram. Sources of the different types of fat include:

- *Saturated fat.* Sources are animal meats (meat and butter fats, lard, bacon), cocoa butter, coconut oil, palm oil, and hydrogenated oils.
- *Polyunsaturated fat.* Sources are oils of corn, safflower, sunflower, soybean, sesame seed, and cottonseed.
- *Monosaturated fat.* Sources are peanut oil, olive oil, and canola oil.

Limiting fat and cholesterol intake may help prevent or delay the onset of atherosclerosis, a common complication of diabetes.

Fiber

Dietary fiber may be helpful in treating or preventing constipation and other gastrointestinal disorders, including colon cancer. It also helps provide a feeling of fullness, and large amounts of soluble fiber may be beneficial to serum lipids. Soluble fiber is found in dried beans, oats, barley, and in some vegetables and fruits (e.g., peas, corn, zucchini, cauliflower, broccoli, prunes, pears, apples, bananas, oranges). Insoluble fiber, which is found in wheat, corn, and in some vegetables and fruits (e.g., carrots, brussels sprouts, eggplant, green beans, pears, apples, strawberries), does facilitate intestinal motility and give a feeling of fullness.

The ideal level of fiber has not been determined, but an intake of 20 to 35 g per day is recommended. An increase in fiber may cause nausea, diarrhea or constipation, and increased flatulence, especially if the person does not also increase fluid intake. Fiber in the diet should therefore be increased gradually.

Sodium

Although the body requires sodium, most people consume much more than is needed each day, especially in processed foods. The recommended daily intake is 1000 mg of sodium per 1000 kcal, not to exceed 3000 mg. The primary concern with sodium is its association with hypertension, a common health problem in people with diabetes. It is suggested that table salt (which is 40% sodium) and processed foods high in sodium be avoided in the diabetes meal plan.

Sweeteners

The diet plan for people with diabetes restricts the amount of refined sugars. As a result, many people use noncaloric sweeteners and foods or drinks made with noncaloric sweeteners. Commercially produced nonnutritive sweeteners are approved for use by the Food and Drug Administration (FDA). Although questions have been raised about the safety of these substances in laboratory animal studies, they are considered safe for use by humans. Included in this category of sweeteners are saccharin (Sweet & Low), aspartame (Nutrasweet, Equal), and acesulfame potassium (Sunnette). The nonnutritive sweeteners have negligent amounts of or no kilocalories and produce very little or no changes in blood glucose levels.

People with diabetes also use nutritive sweeteners, including fructose, sorbitol, and xylitol. The kcal content of these substances is similar to that of table sugar (sucrose), but they cause less elevation in blood glucose. They are often included in foods labeled as "sugar free." Sorbitol may cause flatulence and diarrhea.

Researchers are continuing to study the safety and effectiveness of the sweeteners. In addition, the FDA recommends that the food industry label products with the amount of each ingredient in milligrams per serving and the number of servings per container. When teaching clients about diet, the nurse should include information about the kilocalorie content of sweeteners and the meaning of such words as "sugar free" and "dietetic" on labels.

Alcohol

Although drinking alcoholic beverages is not encouraged, neither is it totally prohibited for the client with diabetes. Alcohol consumption may potentiate the hypoglycemic effects of insulin and oral agents. The ADA recommends that men with diabetes consume no more than two drinks and women with diabetes no more than one drink per day. In the following list are guidelines for people who include alcohol in their diet plan.

- The signs of intoxication and hypoglycemia are similar; thus, the person with type 1 DM is at increased risk for an insulin reaction.
- Two oral hypoglycemic agents (chlorpropamide and tolbutamide) may interact with the alcohol, causing headache, flushing, and nausea.
- Liqueurs, sweet wines, wine coolers, and sweet mixes contain large amounts of carbohydrate.
- Light beer is the recommended alcoholic drink.
- Alcohol should be consumed with meals and added to the daily food intake. In most instances, the alcohol is substituted for fat in calculating the diet; a drink with 1.5 oz of alcohol is the equivalent of two fat exchanges (90 kcal). (Food exchanges are discussed below.)

Meal Planning

Several different systems for meal planning are available to the person with diabetes. These systems include a consistent-carbohydrate diabetes meal plan, exchange lists, point systems, food groups, and calorie counting. No matter what system is used, however, it must take into account the person's individualized eating habits, diet history, food values, and special needs. Altering foods and meal patterns are often one of the most difficult parts of diabetes management; careful consideration of individualized preferences enhances compliance with the diet. Although the ADA recommends that a registered dietitian provide the nutrition prescription, nurses must know what is prescribed and be able to reinforce teaching and answer questions.

The Consistent-Carbohydrate Diabetes Meal Plan. The consistent-carbohydrate diabetes meal plan, which is replacing the traditional exchange list plan, focuses on carbohydrate content. The client eats a similar amount of carbohydrates at each meal or snack each day, based on an individual diet prescription and the food guide pyramid. Carbohydrates in a meal have the most effect on postprandial (after meals) blood glucose levels. They also determine, to a greater extent than do proteins and fats, insulin requirements before meals. Clients should be taught to count carbohydrates so they can administer 1 unit of regular insulin or insulin lispro for each 10 or 15 g of carbohydrate eaten at a meal. This method provides a better connection between food, medications, and exercise.

The Exchange Lists. The exchange list diet is based on the person's ideal (or reasonable) weight, activity level, age, and occupation. These factors determine the total kilocalories that the person may consume each day. After the calories have been determined, the proportions of carbohydrates, proteins, and fats are calculated, using guidelines established by the American Diabetes Association and the American Dietetic Association.

The distribution of foods throughout the day is based on exchange lists. The name and quantity of food that make up one exchange (or serving) are listed; standard household measurements are used. One food portion on the list can be substituted ("exchanged") for another with very little difference in calories or amount of carbohydrates, proteins, and fats. The meal plan prescribes how many exchanges are allowed for each food group per meal and snacks.

Diet Plan for Type 1 Diabetes. Diet and insulin prescription must be integrated for optimal energy metabolism and the prevention of hyperglycemia or hypoglycemia. The goals of the diet plan are to achieve optimal glucose and lipid levels, improve overall health, and maintain reasonable body weight. To meet these goals, the following strategies must be implemented:

- Glucose regulation requires correlating eating patterns with insulin onset and peak of action.
- Meals, snacks, and insulin regimens should be based on the person's lifestyle.
- Meal planning depends on the specific insulin regimen prescribed.
- Snacks are an important consideration in relation to the amount and timing of exercise.
- The diet plan must consider the availability of foods, based on occupational, financial, religious, and ethnic constraints.
- Self-monitoring of blood glucose levels helps the client make adjustments for planned and unplanned changes in routines.

Diet Plan for Type 2 Diabetes. The goals of the diet plan are to improve blood glucose levels, improve overall health, prevent or delay complications, and attain or maintain reasonable body weight. Because the majority of these clients are overweight, weight loss is important and facilitates achieving the other goals.

There are no specific guidelines for the type 2 diet, but in addition to decreasing kilocalories, it is recommended that the client consume three meals of equal size, evenly spaced approximately four to five hours apart, with one or two snacks. The person with type 2 DM should also decrease fat intake. If the exchange list is difficult to use, calorie counting or designing the diet by grams of fat may be more useful.

Sick-Day Management

When the person with diabetes is sick or has surgery, blood glucose levels increase, even though food intake decreases. The person often mistakenly alters or omits the insulin dose, causing further problems. The guidelines for dietary management during illness focus on preventing dehydration and providing nutrition for promoting recovery. In general, sick-day management includes the following:

- Monitoring blood glucose at least four times a day throughout an illness
- Testing urine for ketones if blood glucose is greater than 240 mg/dL
- Continuing to take the usual insulin dose or oral hypoglycemic agent
- Sipping 8 to 12 oz of fluid each hour
- Substituting easily digested liquids or soft foods if solid foods are not tolerated. The substituted liquids and foods should be carbohydrate equivalents, for example, 1/2 cup sweetened gelatin, 1/2 cup fruit juice, one Popsicle, 1/4 cup sherbet, and 1/2 cup regular soft drink.
- Calling the health care provider if the client is unable to eat for more than 24 hours or if vomiting and diarrhea last for more than 6 hours.

Diet Plan for the Older Adult

The majority of older adults have type 2 DM and should follow the general guidelines for that diet plan. However, special considerations for the older adult are important if the diet plan is to be followed, including:

- Dietary likes and dislikes
- Who prepares the meals
- Age-related changes in taste perception
- Dental health
- Transportation to buy foods
- Available income.

Other factors to consider in planning the diet for the older adult include the age-related decline in kcal requirements, decline in physical activity due to age and/or chronic illnesses, and the onset or progression of other chronic illnesses. The older adult who is overweight should reduce kcal intake to ensure weight loss, but at the same time, careful monitoring for malnutrition is necessary. It is possible for the older adult to revert to normal glucose tolerance if ideal body weight is regained.

Exercise

The third component of diabetes management is a regular exercise program. The benefits of exercise are the same for everyone, with or without diabetes: improved physical fitness, improved emotional state, weight control, and improved work capacity. In people with diabetes, exercise increases the uptake of glucose by muscle cells, potentially reducing the need for insulin. Exercise also decreases cholesterol and triglycerides, reducing the risk of cardiovascular disorders. People with diabetes should consult their primary health care provider before beginning or changing an exercise program. The ability to maintain an exercise program is affected by many different factors, including fatigue and glucose levels. It is as important to assess the person's usual lifestyle before establishing an exercise program as it is before planning a diet. Factors to consider include the client's usual exercise habits, living environment, and community programs. The exercise that the person enjoys most is probably the one that he or she will continue throughout life.

All people with diabetes should follow the recommendations of the ADA when exercising: Use proper footwear, inspect the feet daily and after exercise, avoid exercise in extreme heat or cold, and avoid exercise during periods of poor glucose control. The ADA further recommends that people over age 35 have an exercise-stress electrocardiogram prior to beginning an exercise program.

Type 1 Diabetes

In the person with type 1 DM, glycemic responses to exercise vary according to the type, intensity, and duration of the exercise. Other factors that influence responses include the timing of exercise in relation to meals and insulin injections, and the time of day of the activity. Unless these factors are integrated into the exercise program, the person with type 1 DM has an increased risk of hypoglycemia and hyperglycemia. Following are general guidelines for an exercise program:

- People who have frequent hyperglycemia or hypoglycemia should avoid prolonged exercise until glucose control improves.
- The risk of exercise-induced hypoglycemia is lowest before breakfast, when free-insulin levels tend to be lower than they are before meals later in the day or at bedtime.
- Low-impact aerobic exercises are encouraged.
- Exercise should be moderate and regular; brief, intense exercise tends to cause mild hyperglycemia, and prolonged exercise can lead to hypoglycemia.
- Exercising at a peak insulin action time may lead to hypoglycemia.
- Self-monitoring of blood glucose levels is essential both before and after exercise.
- Food intake may need to be increased to compensate for the activity.
- Fluid intake, especially water, is essential.

Young adults may continue participating in sports with some modifications in diet and insulin dosage. Athletes should begin training slowly, extend activity over a prolonged period, take a carbohydrate source, such as a drink consisting of 5% to 10% carbohydrate after about one hour of exercise, and monitor blood glucose levels for possible adjustments. In addition, a snack should be available after the activity is completed. It may be necessary to omit the usual regular insulin dose prior to an athletic event; even if the athlete is hyperglycemic at the beginning of the event, blood glucose levels will fall to normal after the first 60 to 90 minutes of exercise.

Type 2 Diabetes

An exercise program for the person with type 2 DM is especially important. The benefits of regular exercise include weight loss in those who are overweight, improved glycemic control, increased well-being, socialization with others, and a reduction of cardiovascular risk factors. A combination of diet, exercise, and weight loss often decreases the need for oral hypoglycemic agents. This decrease is due to an increased sensitivity to insulin, increased kcal expenditure, and increased self-esteem. Regular exercise may prevent type 2 DM in high-risk individuals (ADA, 2002).

Following are general guidelines for an exercise program:

- Before beginning the program, have a medical screening for previously undiagnosed hypertension, neuropathy, retinopathy, nephropathy, and cardiac ischemia.
- Begin the program with mild exercises, and gradually increase intensity and duration.
- Self-monitor blood glucose before and after exercise.
- Exercise at least three times a week or every other day, for at least 20 to 30 minutes.
- Include muscle-strengthening and low-impact aerobic exercises in the program.

Treatments

Surgery

Surgical management of diabetes involves replacing or transplanting the pancreas, pancreatic cells, or beta cells. Although it is still in the investigative stage, many researchers believe that transplantation of the tail of the pancreas is the most promising technique for achieving long-term disease control. Islet cell transplantation has had moderate success, and research is continuing. Other research is being conducted in the use of an internally implanted artificial pancreas, or closed-loop artificial beta cell.

Surgery is a stressor that often alters self-management and glycemic control in people with diabetes. In response to stress, levels of catecholamines, cortisol, glucagon, and growth hormones increase, as does insulin resistance. Hyperglycemia occurs, and protein stores are decreased. In addition, diet and activity patterns change, and medication types and dosages vary. As a result, surgical clients who have diabetes are at increased risk for postoperative infection, delayed wound healing, fluid and electrolyte imbalances, hypoglycemia, and DKA.

Preoperatively, all clients should be in the best possible metabolic state. Screening for complications and regular blood glucose monitoring are part of preoperative preparation. Oral hypoglycemic agents may be withheld for one or two days before surgery, and regular insulin is often administered to the client with type 2 DM during the perioperative period. The client with type 1 DM follows a carefully prescribed insulin regimen individualized to specific needs.

The insulin regimen in the preoperative, intraoperative, and immediate postoperative periods is individualized and may involve any of the following:

- No intermediate- or long-acting insulin is given the day of surgery; regular insulin is given with intravenous glucose.
- Half of the usual intermediate- or long-acting insulin is given before surgery and the remaining half is given in the recovery room.
- The total daily dose of insulin is divided into four equal doses of regular insulin, and one dose is administered subcutaneously every six hours. An intravenous solution of 5% dextrose in 0.45% normal saline is administered for fluid replacement, and blood glucose monitoring precedes each insulin dose (Guthrie & Guthrie, 1997).

The surgical procedure should be scheduled for as early as possible in the morning to minimize the length of fasting. If there is no food intake after surgery, intravenous dextrose should be administered, accompanied by subcutaneous regular insulin every six hours. The dose can be adjusted to blood glucose levels. Although kcal intake is decreased postoperatively, stress can increase insulin requirements. Glucose control is also affected postoperatively by nausea and vomiting, anorexia, and gastrointestinal suction.

During the postoperative period, the client with type 2 DM may continue to require insulin or may resume oral medications, depending on glucose control. The client with type 1 DM may require reduced insulin as healing progresses and stress diminishes. Regular blood glucose monitoring is essential, as are assessments for hypoglycemia.

Treatment of Hypoglycemia

Mild Hypoglycemia. When mild hypoglycemia occurs, immediate treatment is necessary. People experiencing hypoglycemia should take about 15 g of a rapid-acting sugar. This amount of sugar is found, for example, in three glucose tablets, 1/2 cup of fruit juice or regular soda, 8 oz of skim milk, five Life Savers candies, three large marshmallows, or 3 tsp of sugar or honey. Sugar should not be added to fruit juice. Adding sugar to the fruit sugar already in the juice could cause a rapid rise in blood glucose, with persistent hyperglycemia.

If the manifestations continue, the 15/15 rule should be followed: Wait 15 minutes, monitor blood glucose, and, if it is low, eat another 15 g of carbohydrate. This procedure can be repeated until blood glucose levels return to normal (Haire-Joshu, 1996). People with diabetes should have some source of carbohydrate readily available at all times so that hypoglycemic symptoms can be quickly reversed. If hypoglycemia occurs more than two or three times a week, the diabetes management plan should be adjusted.

Severe Hypoglycemia. People with diabetes who have severe hypoglycemia are often hospitalized. The criteria for hospitalization are one or more of the following:

- Blood glucose is less than 50 mg/dL, and the prompt treatment of hypoglycemia has not resulted in recovery of sensorium.
- The client has coma, seizures, or altered behavior.
- The hypoglycemia has been treated, but a responsible adult cannot be with the client for the following 12 hours.
- The hypoglycemia was caused by a sulfonylurea drug.

If the client is conscious and alert, 10 to 15 g of an oral carbohydrate may be given. If the client has altered levels of consciousness, parenteral glucose or glucagon is administered.

Glucose is administered intravenously as a 25% to 50% solution, usually at a rate of 10 mL over one minute by intravenous push, followed by intravenous infusion of 5% dextrose in water (D5W) at 5 to 10 g/h (Haire-Joshu, 1996). This is the most rapid method of increasing blood glucose levels.

Glucagon is an antihypoglycemic agent that raises blood glucose by promoting the conversion of hepatic glycogen to glucose. It is used in severe insulin-induced hypoglycemia and may be given in the recommended dose of 1 mg by the subcutaneous, intramuscular, or intravenous route. Glucagon has a short period of action; an oral (if the client is conscious) or intravenous carbohydrate should be administered following the glucagon to prevent a recurrence of hypoglycemia. If the client has been unconscious, glucagon may cause vomiting when consciousness returns.

Treatment of DKA

DKA requires immediate medical attention. Admission to the hospital is appropriate when the person has a blood glucose of greater than 250 mg/dL, a decreasing pH, and ketones in the urine. If the client is alert and conscious, fluids may be replaced orally. However, alterations in levels of consciousness, vomiting, and acidosis are common, necessitating intravenous fluid replacement. The initial fluid replacement may be accomplished by administering 0.9% saline solution at a rate of 500 to 1000 mL/h. After two to three hours (or when blood pressure is returning to normal), the administration of 0.45% saline at 200 to 500 mL/h may continue for several more hours. When the blood glucose levels reach 250 mg/dL, dextrose is added to prevent rapid decreases in glucose; hypoglycemia could result in fatal cerebral edema.

Table 27-7. Medication Administration – Intravenous Insulin

General Guidelines

- Regular insulin may be given undiluted directly into the vein or through a Y-tube or three-way stopcock.
- Insulin is usually diluted in 0.9% saline or 0.45% saline solution for infusion.
- The glass or plastic infusion container and plastic tubing may reduce insulin potency by at least 20%, and possibly by up to 80%, before the insulin reaches the venous system.

Nursing Responsibilities

- Monitor blood glucose levels hourly.
- Infuse the insulin solution separately from the hydration solution.
- Flush the intravenous tubing with 50 mL of insulin mixed with normal saline solution to saturate binding sites on the tubing before administering the insulin to the client; this step increases the amount of insulin delivered over the first few hours.
- Do not discontinue the intravenous infusion until subcutaneous administration of insulin is resumed.
- Monitor for manifestations of hypoglycemia.
- Ensure that glucagon is readily available as an antidote for insulin overdose.

Regular insulin is used in the management of DKA and may be given by various routes, depending on the severity of the condition. Mild ketosis may be treated with subcutaneous insulin, whereas severe ketosis requires intravenous insulin infusion. Nursing responsibilities for the client receiving intravenous insulin are described in Table 27-7.

The electrolyte imbalance of primary concern is depletion of body stores of potassium. Initially, serum potassium levels may be normal, but they decrease during treatment. In DKA (and from rehydration), the body loses potassium from increased urinary output, acidosis, catabolic state, and vomiting or diarrhea. Potassium replacement is begun early in the course of treatment, usually by adding potassium to the rehydration fluids. Replacement is essential for preventing cardiac dysrhythmias secondary to hypokalemia. Cardiac rhythms and potassium levels must be monitored every two to four hours.

Treatment of HHS

HHS is a serious, life-threatening metabolic condition. The client admitted to the intensive care unit for treatment typically manifests blood glucose levels over 700 mg/dL, increased serum osmolarity, and altered levels of consciousness or seizures. Treatment is similar to that of DKA: correcting fluid and electrolyte imbalances and providing insulin to lower hyperglycemia. In general, treatment modalities include the following:

- Establishing and maintaining adequate ventilation.
- Correcting shock with adequate intravenous fluids.
- Instituting nasogastric suction if comatose to prevent aspiration.
- Maintaining fluid volume with intravenous isotonic or colloid solutions.
- Administering potassium intravenously to replace losses.
- Administering insulin to reduce blood glucose, usually discontinuing administration when blood glucose levels reach 250 mg/dL. (Because ketosis is not present, there is no need to continue insulin, as with DKA.)

Nursing Care

The responses of the person with diabetes to the illness are often complex and individual, involving multiple body systems. Assessments, planning, and implementation differ for the person with newly diagnosed diabetes, the person with long-term diabetes, and the person with acute complications of diabetes. The plan of care and content of teaching also differ according to the type of diabetes, the person's age and culture, and the person's intellectual, psychological, and social resources. However, nursing care often focuses on teaching the client to manage the illness.

Health Promotion

Health promotion activities primarily focus on preventing the complications of diabetes. The prevention of the disease has not been determined, although it is recommended that all people should prevent or decrease excess weight, follow a sensible and well-balanced diet, and maintain a regular physical exercise program. Blood glucose screening at 3-year intervals beginning at age 45 is recommended for those in the high-risk groups. These same activities, when combined with medications and self-monitoring, are also beneficial in reducing the onset of complications.

Assessment

The following data are collected through the health history and physical examination (see Chapter 25). Further focused assessments are described with nursing interventions below. When assessing the older client, be aware of normal aging changes in all body systems that may alter interpretation of findings.

- *Health history:* Family history of diabetes; history of hypertension or other cardiovascular problems; history of any change in vision (e.g. blurring) or speech, dizziness, numbness or tingling in hands or feet; pain when walking; frequent voiding; change in weight, appetite, infections, and healing; problems with gastrointestinal function or urination; or altered sexual function.
- *Physical assessment:* Height/weight ratio, vital signs, visual acuity, cranial nerves, sensory ability (touch, hot/cold, vibration) of extremities, peripheral pulses, skin and mucous membranes (hair loss, appearance, lesions, rash, itching, vaginal discharge).

Nursing Diagnoses and Interventions

Although many different nursing diagnoses are appropriate for the person with diabetes, those discussed in this section address problems with skin integrity, infection, injury, sexuality, coping, and health maintenance. The goals of care are to maintain function, prevent complications, and teach self-management.

Risk for Impaired Skin Integrity

The person with diabetes is at increased risk for altered skin integrity as a result of decreased or absent sensation from neuropathies, decreased tissue perfusion from cardiovascular complications, and infection. In addition, poor vision increases the risk of trauma, and an open lesion is more prone to infection and delayed healing. Impaired skin and tissue integrity, with resultant gangrene, is especially common in the feet and lower extremities. Conduct baseline and ongoing assessments of the feet, including:

- Musculoskeletal assessment that includes foot and ankle joint range of motion, bone abnormalities (bunions, hammertoes, overlapping digits), gait patterns, use of assistive devices for walking, and abnormal wear patterns on shoes.
- Neurologic assessment that includes sensations of touch and position, pain, and temperature.
- Vascular examination that includes assessment of lower-extremity pulses, capillary refill, color and temperature of skin, lesions, and edema.
- Hydration status, including dryness or excessive perspiration.
- Lesions, fissures between toes, corns, calluses, plantar warts, ingrown or overgrown toenails, redness over pressure points, blisters, cellulitis, or gangrene.

People with diabetes are at significant risk for lower-extremity gangrene. Peripheral neuropathies may result in alterations in the perception of pain, loss of deep tendon reflexes, loss of cutaneous pressure and position sensation, foot drop, changes in the shape of the foot, and changes in bones and joints. Peripheral vascular disease may cause intermittent claudication, absent pulses, delayed venous filling on elevation, dependent rubor, and gangrene. Injuries, lesions, and changes in skin hydration potentiate infections, delayed healing, and tissue loss in the person with diabetes mellitus.

- Teach foot hygiene. Wash the feet daily with lukewarm water and mild hand soap; pat dry, and dry well between the toes. Apply a very thin coat of lubricating cream if dryness is present (but not between the toes). *Proper hygiene decreases the chance of infection. Temperature receptors may be impaired, so the water should always be tested before use.*
- Discuss the importance of not smoking if client smokes. *Nicotine in tobacco causes vasoconstriction, further decreasing the blood supply to the feet.*

Risk for Infection

The person with diabetes is at increased risk for infection. The risk of infection is believed to be due to vascular insufficiency that limits the inflammatory response, neurologic abnormalities that limit the awareness of trauma, and a predisposition to bacterial and fungal infections.

- Use and teach meticulous handwashing. *Handwashing is the single most effective method for preventing the spread of infection.*
- Monitor for manifestations of infection: increased temperature, pain, malaise, swelling, redness, discharge, cough. *Early diagnosis and treatment of infections can control their severity and decrease complications.*

- Discuss the importance of skin care. Keep the skin clean and dry, using lukewarm water and mild soap. *People with diabetes are more prone to develop furuncles and carbuncles; the infection often increases the need for insulin. Clean, intact skin and mucous membranes are the first line of defense against infection.*

- Teach dental health measures:

  1. Obtain a dental examination every four to six months.
  2. Maintain careful oral hygiene, which includes brushing the teeth with a soft toothbrush and fluoridated toothpaste at least twice a day and flossing as recommended.
  3. Be aware of the symptoms requiring dental care: bad breath; unpleasant taste in the mouth; bleeding, red, or sore gums; and tooth pain.
  4. If dental surgery is necessary, monitor for need to make adjustments in insulin. *All people with diabetes need to be taught proper oral hygiene, the risk of periodontal disease, and the importance of obtaining dental care for symptoms of oral or dental problems.*

- Teach women with diabetes the symptoms and preventive measures for vaginitis caused by Candida albicans. The symptoms are an odorless, white or yellow cheeselike discharge and itching. Sexual transmission is unlikely, but discomfort may cause the client to avoid sexual activity. *Diabetes is a predisposing factor for* Candida albicans *vaginitis, the most common form of vaginitis. Poor personal hygiene and wearing clothing that keeps the vaginal area warm and moist increase the risk of vaginitis. The infection may spread to the urinary tract, resulting in urinary tract infections; preventing and treating vaginitis decrease this risk.*

Risk for Injury

The person with diabetes is at risk for injury from multiple factors. Neuropathies may alter sensation, gait, and muscle control. Cataracts or retinopathy may cause visual deficits. Hyperglycemia often causes osmotic changes in the lenses of the eye, resulting in blurred vision. In addition, changes in blood glucose alter levels of consciousness and may cause seizures. The impaired mobility, sensory deficits, and neurologic effects of complications of diabetes increase the risk of accidents, burns, falls, and trauma.

- Assess for the presence of contributing or causative factors that increase the risk of injury: blurred vision, cataracts, decreased adaptation to dark, decreased tactile sensitivity, hypoglycemia, hyperglycemia, hypovolemia, joint immobility, unstable gait. *A knowledge base is necessary to develop an individualized plan of care. The risk of injury increases with the number of factors identified.*

- Reduce environmental hazards in the health care facility, and teach the client about safety in the home and in the community.

In the Health Care Facility

- Orient the client to new surroundings on admission.
- Keep the bed at the lowest level.
- Keep the floors free of objects.
- Use a night light.
- Check the temperature of the bath or shower water before the client uses it.
- Instruct the client to wear shoes or slippers when out of bed.
- Monitor blood glucose levels regularly.
- Monitor for side effects of prescribed medications, such as dizziness or drowsiness.

In the Home and Community

- Use a night light, preferably one with a soft, nonglare bulb.
- Turn the head away when switching on a bright light.
- Avoid directly looking into headlights when driving at night.
- Test the temperature of the bath or shower water before use.
- Conduct a daily foot inspection.
- Wear shoes and slippers with nonskid soles.
- Do not use throw rugs.
- Install hand grips in the tub and shower and next to the toilet.
- Wear a seat belt when driving or riding in a car.

Strange environments and the presence of hazardous environmental factors increase the risk of falls or other accidents. Glare is often responsible for falls in people with visual deficits. The nurse can reduce factors that increase the risk of injury by implementing care and teaching safe practices during the activities of daily life.

- Monitor for, and teach the client and family to recognize and seek care for, the manifestations of DKA in the client with type 1 DM: hyperglycemia, thirst, headaches, nausea and vomiting, increased urine output, ketonuria, dehydration, and decreasing level of consciousness. *Blood glucose levels increase if the insulin need is unmet or insufficiently met; the cellular use of fats for fuel results in ketosis. Osmotic diuresis increases urinary output, resulting in thirst and dehydration.*

- Monitor for, and teach the client and family to recognize and seek care for, the manifestations of HHS in the client with type 2 DM: extreme hyperglycemia, increased urinary output, thirst, dehydration, hypotension, seizures, and decreasing level of consciousness. *HHS is a life-threatening condition requiring recognition and treatment.*

- Monitor for, and teach the client and family to recognize and treat, the manifestations of hypoglycemia: low blood glucose, anxiety, headache, uncoordinated movements, sweating, rapid pulse, drowsiness, and visual changes. Teach client and family to carry some form of rapid-acting sugar source at all times. *Severe hypoglycemia causes a decrease in the level of consciousness. The decrease in blood glucose most often results from too much insulin, too little food, or too much exercise.*

- Recommend that the client wear a MedicAlert bracelet or necklace identifying self as a person with diabetes. *In case of sudden, severe illness or accident, a MedicAlert bracelet can allow immediate medical attention for diabetes to be instituted.*

Sexual Dysfunction

Sexuality is a complex and inseparable part of every person. It involves not only physical sexual activities, but also a person's self-perception as male or female, roles and relationships, and attractiveness and desirability. Changes in sexual function and in sexuality have been identified in both men and women with diabetes.

Alterations in erectile ability occur in approximately 50% of all men with diabetes. The incidence of impotence increases with the duration of the diabetes, and is often associated with peripheral neuropathy. Libido is usually unaffected, even when impotence is present.

Women with diabetes also have alterations in sexual function, although the reason is less clear. The problems reported by women involve decreased desire and decreased vaginal lubrication.

Women with diabetes are also at increased risk for vaginitis and may avoid sexual intercourse in order to avoid pain.

- Include a sexual history as a part of the initial and ongoing assessment of the client with diabetes. A specific history form may be used that addresses sexual development, personal and family values, current sexual practices and concerns, and changes desired. Ask a nonthreatening, open-ended question to elicit information, such as, "Tell me about your experience with sexual function since you have been diagnosed with diabetes." *Obtaining accurate information to assess the sexual health of a client is necessary before counseling can begin or referrals can be made.*

- Provide information about the actual and potential physical effects of diabetes on sexual function. Include the effect of poor control of blood glucose on sexual function as part of any teaching plan. *Clients benefit from basic information about male and female anatomy and the sexual response cycle, and how diabetes can affect this part of the body. Changes in blood glucose levels may not only cause changes in desire and physical response, but also may alter sexual responses as a result of depression, anxiety, and fatigue.*

- Provide counseling or make referrals as appropriate. The nurse is responsible for knowing about sexuality and sexual health throughout the life span and provides information based on knowledge of the effects of illness and treatment on sexual function. For example, men who are impotent may regain the ability to have sexual intercourse through penile implants, suction apparatus, the use of sildenafil citrate (Viagra), or injections of medications, such as yohimbine, an alpha-2 adrenergic blocker, that increase vascular blood flow into the corpus of the penis. Women with decreased vaginal lubrication can decrease painful intercourse by using vaginal lubricants, such as K-Y Jelly, or estrogen creams.

The nurse may make specific suggestions to facilitate positive sexual functioning, referring the client to the appropriate health care provider as necessary for intensive therapy.

Ineffective Coping

Coping is the process of responding to internal or environmental stressors or potential stressors. When coping responses are ineffective, the stressors exceed the individual's available resources for responding. The person diagnosed with diabetes is faced with lifelong changes in many parts of his or her life. Diet, exercise habits, and medications must be integrated into the person's lifestyle and be carefully controlled. Daily injections may be a reality. Fear of potential complications and of negative effects on the future is common.

If the person is unable to cope successfully with these changes, emotional stress can interfere with glycemic control. In addition, unsuccessful coping often results in noncompliance with prescribed treatment modalities, further impairing glycemic control and increasing the potential for acute and chronic complications.

- Assess the client's psychosocial resources, including emotional resources, support resources, lifestyle, and communication skills. *Chronic illness affects all dimensions of a person's life, as well as the lives of family members and significant others. A comprehensive assessment of strengths and weaknesses is the first step in developing an individualized plan of care to facilitate coping.*

- Explore with the client and family the effects (actual and perceived) of the diagnosis and treatment of diabetes on finances, occupation, energy levels, and relationships. *Common frustrations associated with diabetes are the disease itself, the treatment modalities, and the health care system. Effective coping involves maintaining a healthy self-concept and satisfying relationships, emotional balance, and handling emotional stress.*

- Teach constructive problem-solving techniques. *Problem-focused behaviors include setting attainable and realistic goals, learning about all aspects of the problem, learning new procedures or skills that increase self-esteem, and reaching out to others for support.*

- Provide information about support groups and resources, such as suppliers of products, journals, books, and cookbooks for people with diabetes. *Sharing with others who have similar problems provides opportunities for mutual support and problem solving. Using available resources improves the ability to cope.*

Home Care

Teaching the client and family to self-manage diabetes is a nursing responsibility. Even if a formal teaching plan is developed and implemented by advanced practice nurses, all nurses must be able to reinforce knowledge and answer questions. Teaching is necessary for both the person who is newly diagnosed and for the person who has had diabetes for years. In fact, the latter may need almost as much teaching as the newly diagnosed person (Guthrie & Guthrie, 1997).

The American Diabetes Association recommends that teaching be carried out on three levels. The first level focuses on survival skills, with the person learning basic knowledge and skills to be able to provide diabetes management for the first week or two while he or she adjusts to the idea of having the disease. The second level focuses on home management, emphasizing self-reliance and independence in the daily management of diabetes. The third level aims at improving lifestyle and educating clients to individualize self-management of the illness.

For the hospitalized client with diabetes, teaching should begin on admission. Prior to designing the teaching plan, the nurse makes an initial assessment of the client's and family's knowledge and learning needs, outlining past diabetes management practices and identifying physical, emotional, and sociocultural needs. Educational level, preferred learning methods and style, life experiences, and support systems are also assessed.

It is important that the nurse and client mutually establish goals based on the assessment data. It is equally important that family members understand that the responsibility for daily management lies with the client and that the primary role of the family is supportive. The client is the person with the disease, and it is the client who each day must take medications or inject insulin, test blood or urine, calculate and balance foods, exercise, adjust medications, inspect the body for injury, and determine whether and when medical assistance is needed. However, family members require the same knowledge so that they can provide emotional support as well as physical care if necessary.

The following should be included in teaching the client and family about care at home:

- Information about normal metabolism, diabetes mellitus, and how diabetes changes metabolism
- Diet plan: how diet helps keep blood glucose in normal range; number of kcal required and why; amount of carbohydrates, meats, and fats allowed and why; and how to calculate the diet, integrating personal food preferences
- Exercise: how it helps lower blood glucose; the importance of a regular program; types of exercise; integrating personal exercise preferences; how to handle increased activity
- Self-monitoring of blood glucose: how to perform the tests accurately, how to care for equipment, what to do for high or low blood glucose

- Medications:
  1. Insulin: type, dosage, mixing instructions (if necessary), times of onset and peak actions, how to get and care for equipment, how to give injections, where to give injections
  2. Oral agents: type, dosage, side effects, interaction with other drugs
- Manifestations of acute complications of hypoglycemia and hyperglycemia; what to do when they occur
- Hygiene: skin care, dental care, foot care
- Sick days: what to do about food, fluids, and medications
- Helpful resources:
  1. The American Diabetes Association
  2. The American Dietetic Association
  3. National Diabetes Information Clearinghouse
  4. Department of Veterans Affairs
  5. Indian Health Service
  6. National Council of La Raza.

Teaching may have to be adapted to the special needs of the older adult. Because 40% of all people with diabetes are over the age of 65, considering the special needs of this population is essential. Uncontrolled diabetes in the older adult increases the potential for functional loss, social disengagement, and increased morbidity and mortality. Education for self-care allows the older adult to be more actively involved in his or her diabetes management and decreases the potential for acute and long-term complications from the disease. Considerations for teaching the older adult with diabetes include the following:

- Changes in diet may be difficult to implement for many reasons. Favorite foods are difficult to give up. Balanced meals at regular intervals may not have been part of the client's lifestyle. Purchasing, storing, and preparing foods may be a problem. Dentures may not fit well. Changes in taste sensation often cause the client to increase the use of salt and sugar.
- Exercise of any type may not have been part of the activities of daily living. Exercise must be individualized for any physical limitations imposed by other chronic illnesses, such as arthritis, Parkinson's disease, chronic respiratory diseases, and/or cardiovascular diseases.
- The diagnosis of a chronic illness threatens independence and self-worth. After years of taking care of self, the older adult with diabetes may now have to depend on others for help in meeting self-care needs. This in turn often leads to withdrawal from social interactions with others.
- Money to purchase medications and supplies often must be taken out of a fixed income.
- Visual deficits make insulin administration difficult or impossible. Visual deficits also interfere with blood glucose monitoring, food preparation, exercises, and foot care.

28

Assessing Clients with Musculoskeletal Disorders

The tissues and structures of the musculoskeletal system perform many functions, including support, protection, and movement. The musculoskeletal system has two subsystems: the bones and joints of the skeleton, and the skeletal muscles. These subsystems work together to allow the body to perform both basic, simple movements, such as closing a door, and fine, complex movements, such as repairing a watch.

Review of Anatomy and Physiology

The Skeleton

The human skeleton is made up of 206 bones. The axial skeleton includes the bones of the skull, the ribs and sternum, and the vertebral column. The appendicular skeleton consists of all the bones of the limbs, the shoulder girdles, and the pelvic girdle.

Bones form the body's structure and provide support for soft tissues. They also protect vital organs from injury and serve to move body parts by providing points of attachment for muscles. Bones also store minerals and serve as a site for *hematopoiesis* (blood cell formation).

Bone cells include osteoblasts (cells that form bone), osteocytes (cells that maintain bone matrix), and osteoclasts (cells that resorb bone). Bone matrix is the extracellular element of bone tissue; it consists of collagen fibers, minerals (primarily calcium and phosphate), proteins, carbohydrates, and ground substance. Ground substance is a gelatinous material that facilitates diffusion of nutrients, wastes, and gases between the blood vessels and bone tissue. Bones are covered with **periosteum,** a double-layered connective tissue. The outer layer of the periosteum contains blood vessels and nerves; the inner layer is anchored to the bone.

Bones consist of a rigid connective tissue called osseous tissue, of which there are two types: Compact bone is smooth and dense; spongy bone contains spaces between meshworks of bone. Both types contain the same elements and are found in almost all bones of the body.

The basic structural unit of compact bone is the Haversian system (also called an osteon). The Haversian system consists of a central canal, called the Haversian canal; concentric layers of bone matrix, called lamellae; spaces between the lamellae, called lacunae; osteocytes within the lacunae; and small channels, called canaliculi.

Spongy bone has no Haversian systems. Instead, the lamellae are arranged in concentric layers called trabeculae which branch and join to form meshworks. The spongy sections of long bones and flat bones contain tissue for hematopoiesis. In the adult, these sections, called red marrow cavities, are present in the spongy center of flat bones (especially the sternum) and in only two long bones: the humerus and the head of the femur. This red marrow is active in hematopoiesis in adults.

Bones are classified by shape:

- Long bones are longer than they are wide. They have a midportion, or shaft, called a **diaphysis** and two broad ends, called **epiphyses.** The diaphysis is compact bone and contains the marrow cavity, which is lined with endosteum. Each epiphysis is spongy bone covered by a thin layer of compact bone. Long bones include the bones of the arms and legs, fingers, and toes.

- Short bones, also called cuboid bones, are spongy bone covered by compact bone. They include the bones of the wrist and ankle.

- Flat bones are thin and flat, and most are curved. Their disclike structure consists of a layer of spongy bone between two thin layers of compact bone. Flat bones include most bones of the skull, the sternum, and the ribs.

- Irregular bones are of various shapes and sizes and, like flat bones, are plates of compact bone with spongy bone between. Irregular bones include the vertebrae, the scapulae, and the bones of the pelvic girdle.

Bone Remodeling in Adults

Although the bones of adults do not normally increase in length and size, constant remodeling of bones, as well as repair of damaged bone tissue, occurs throughout life. In the bone remodeling process, bone resorption and bone deposit occur at all periosteal and endosteal surfaces. Hormones and forces that put stress on the bones regulate this process, which involves a combined action of the osteocytes, osteoclasts, and osteoblasts. Bones that are in use, and are therefore subjected to stress, increase their osteoblastic activity to increase ossification (the development of bone). Bones that are inactive undergo increased osteoclast activity and bone resorption.

The hormonal stimulus for bone remodeling is controlled by a negative feedback mechanism that regulates blood calcium levels. This stimulus involves the interaction of parathyroid hormone (PTH) from the parathyroid glands and calcitonin from the thyroid gland. When blood levels of calcium decrease, PTH is released; PTH then stimulates osteoclast activity and bone resorption so that calcium is released from the bone matrix. As a result, blood levels of calcium rise, and the stimulus for PTH release ends. Rising blood calcium levels stimulate the secretion of calcitonin, inhibit bone resorption, and cause the deposit of calcium salts in the bone matrix. Thus, bones regulate blood calcium levels. Calcium ions are necessary for the transmission of nerve impulses, the release of neurotransmitters, muscle contraction, blood clotting, glandular secretion, and cell division. Of the body's 1200 to 1400 g of calcium, over 99% is present as bone minerals.

Bone remodeling is also regulated by the response of bones to gravitational pull and to mechanical stress from the pull of muscles. Although the exact mechanism is not fully understood, it is known that bones that undergo increased stress are heavier and larger. This finding supports Wolff's law, which states that bone develops and remodels itself to resist the stresses placed on it.

The process of bone repair following a fracture is discussed in Chapter 29.

Joints, Ligaments, and Tendons

Joints, or **articulations,** are regions where two or more bones meet. Joints hold the bones of the skeleton together while allowing the body to move. Joints may be classified by function as synarthroses, amphiarthroses, or diarthroses.

Joints are also classified by structure as fibrous, cartilaginous, or synovial. Fibrous joints permit little or no movement, because the articulating bones are joined either by short connective tissue fibers that bind the bones together, as with the sutures of the skull, or by short cords of fibrous tissue called ligaments, which permit slight give but no true movement.

Some cartilaginous joints, such as the sternocostal joints of the rib cage, are composed of hyaline cartilage growths that fuse together the articulating bone ends. These joints are immobile. In other cartilaginous joints, such as the intervertebral discs, the hyaline cartilage fuses to an intervening plate of flexible fibrocartilage. This structural feature accounts for the flexibility of the vertebral column.

Bones in synovial joints are enclosed by a cavity that is filled with synovial fluid, a filtrate of blood plasma. These joints are freely movable. Synovial joints are found at all articulations of the limbs. They have several characteristics:

* The articular surfaces are covered with articular cartilage.
* The joint cavity is enclosed by a tough, fibrous, double-layered articular capsule; internally, the cavity is lined with a synovial membrane that covers all surfaces not covered by the articular cartilage.
* Synovial fluid fills the free spaces of the joint capsule, enhancing the smooth movement of the articulating bones.

Synovial joints allow many kinds of movements, listed and described in Table 28-1.

Table 28-1. Movements Allowed by Synovial Joints

Movement	Description
Abduction	Move limb away from body midline
Adduction	Move limb toward body midline
Extension	Straighten limbs at joint
Flexion	Bend limbs at joint
Dorsiflexion	Bend ankle to bring top of foot toward shin
Plantar flexion	Straighten ankle to point toes down
Pronation	Turn forearm to place palm down
Supination	Turn forearm to place palm up
Eversion	Turn out
Inversion	Turn in
Circumduction	Move in circle
Internal rotation	Move inward on a central axis
External rotation	Move outward on a central axis
Protraction	Move forward and parallel to ground
Retraction	Move backward and parallel to ground

The fibrous capsules that surround synovial joints are supported by ligaments, dense bands of connective tissue that connect bones to bones. Ligaments limit or enhance movement, provide joint stability, and enhance joint strength. Tendons are fibrous connective tissue bands that connect muscles to the periosteum of bones and enable the bones to move when skeletal muscles contract. When muscles contract, increased pressure causes the tendon to pull, push, or rotate the bone to which it is connected.

Bursae are small sacs of synovial fluid that cushion and protect bony areas that are at high risk for friction, such as the knee and the shoulder. Tendon sheaths are a form of bursae, but they are wrapped around tendons in high-friction areas.

Muscles

The three types of muscle tissue in the body are skeletal muscle, smooth muscle, and cardiac muscle. This discussion focuses on skeletal muscle, the only muscle that allows musculoskeletal function.

Skeletal muscle cells have typical functional properties:

- *Excitability:* the ability to receive and respond to a stimulus. The stimulus is usually a neurotransmitter released by a neuron, and the response is the generation and transmission of an action potential along the plasma membrane of the muscle cell. (Chapter 31 discusses action potentials.)

- *Contractibility:* the ability to respond to a stimulus by forcibly shortening.

- *Extensibility:* the ability to respond to a stimulus by extending and relaxing; muscle fibers shorten when they contract and extend when they relax.

- *Elasticity:* the ability to resume its resting length after it has shortened or lengthened.

Skeletal muscles are thick bundles of parallel multinucleated contractile cells called fibers. Each single muscle fiber is itself a bundle of smaller structures called myofibrils. The myofibrils have alternating light and dark bands that give skeletal muscle its striated (striped) appearance under an electron microscope. Myofibrils are strands of smaller repeating units called sarcomeres, which consist of thick filaments of myosin and thin filaments of actin, proteins that contribute to muscle contraction.

Skeletal muscle movement is triggered when motor neurons release acetylcholine, a neurotransmitter that alters the permeability of the muscle fiber. Sodium ions enter the fiber, producing an action potential that causes muscle contraction. The more fibers that contract, the stronger the contraction of the entire muscle.

Prolonged strenuous activity causes continuous nerve impulses and eventually results in a buildup of lactic acid and reduced energy in the muscle, or muscle fatigue. However, continuous nerve impulses are also responsible for maintaining muscle tone. Lack of use results in muscle atrophy, whereas regular exercise increases the size and strength of muscles.

Skeletal muscles attach to and cover the bones of the skeleton. Skeletal muscles promote body movement, help maintain posture, and produce body heat. They may be moved by conscious, voluntary control or by reflex activity. The body has approximately 600 skeletal muscles.

Assessing Musculoskeletal Function

The function of the musculoskeletal system is assessed by both a health assessment interview to collect subjective data and a physical assessment to collect objective data.

Health Assessment Interview

This section provides guidelines for collecting subjective data through a health assessment interview specific to musculoskeletal function. An assessment interview to determine problems with musculoskeletal function may be conducted as part of a health screening or as part of a total health assessment, or it may focus on a chief complaint, such as pain, swelling, or limited mobility. Health problems affecting the neurologic system may manifest as musculoskeletal function problems; an assessment of both systems may be necessary. (See Chapter 31 for assessment of the neurologic system.) If the client has a health problem involving the bones or muscles, analyze its onset, characteristics and course, severity, precipitating and relieving factors, and any associated manifestations, noting the timing and circumstances. For example, ask the client:

- Describe the pain you have had in your elbow. Does the pain increase with movement? Have you noticed any redness or swelling?
- Did you injure your ankle before you began to experience difficulty walking?
- Is your pain worse in the morning, or does it get worse through the day?

The primary manifestations of altered function of the musculoskeletal system are pain and limited mobility. Specific descriptors of the pain, its location, and its nature are important. Other significant information includes associated manifestations, such as fever, fatigue, changes in weight, rash, and/or swelling. Also collect information about the client's lifestyle: type of employment, ability to carry out activities of daily living (ADLs) and provide self-care, exercise or participation in sports, use of alcohol or drugs, and nutrition. Explore past injuries and measures to self-treat pain, such as over-the-counter medications, prescribed medications, application of heat or cold, splinting, wrapping, or rest.

Physical Assessment

Physical assessment of the musculoskeletal system is conducted through inspection, palpation, and measurement of muscle mass and range of motion. The client should be comfortably dressed in clothing that lets you see the movement of all joints clearly. The client may be standing, sitting, or lying down; the sequence of the examination should be such that the client does not have frequent position changes. An assessment of the older adult, the client in pain, or the client who is weak may take extra time.

The equipment necessary for assessing the musculoskeletal system is a tape measure to determine muscle size and a goniometer to measure joint range of motion (ROM). Prior to the examination, collect all equipment and explain the techniques to decrease the client's anxiety.

The general sequence for a musculoskeletal examination follows:

1. Begin the examination with an assessment of the client's gait and posture. Observe how the client walks, sits, and/or moves about in bed.
2. Inspect and palpate the client's bones for any obvious deformity or changes in size or shape. Palpation also will elicit tenderness or pain.

3. Measure the extremities for length and circumference. Before taking measurements, make sure the client is lying in a comfortable position. Remember to compare limbs bilaterally.

4. Assess muscle mass by first inspecting for obvious increase or decrease in size. Assess and document muscle strength on a scale of 0 to 5.

5. Assess joints for swelling, pain, redness, warmth, crepitus, and ROM. Only assess the ROM of every joint if the client has a specific musculoskeletal problem; however, assessing one or more joints is a common part of nursing care. Use a goniometer for precise measurements of joint ROM. This device has a pointer joined to a protractor at 0 degrees. These two arms are placed along articulating bones, and the angle of joint movement is recorded in degrees.

Gait and Body Posture Assessment with Abnormal Findings (✓)

- Inspect gait and body posture.
  - ✓ Joint stiffness, pain, deformities, and muscle weakness can cause changes in gait and posture.

- Inspect the spine for curvature. Ask the client to stand and bend back slowly as far as possible, bend slowly to the right and then to the left as far as possible, turn slowly to the right and left in a circular motion, and bend forward slowly and try to touch fingers to toes.
  - ✓ With herniated lumbar discs, the lumbar curve flattens and spinal mobility is decreased.
  - ✓ An increased lumbar curve, called **lordosis,** may be seen in obesity or pregnancy.
  - ✓ A lateral, S-shaped curvature of the spine is called **scoliosis.** Functional scoliosis usually is a compensatory response to painful paravertebral muscles, herniated discs, or discrepancy in leg length. It disappears with forward flexion. Structural scoliosis is often congenital and tends to appear during adolescence. It is accentuated with forward bending.
  - ✓ **Kyphosis** is an exaggerated thoracic curvature of the spine common in older adults.

Joint Assessment with Abnormal Findings (✓)

- Inspect the joints for deformity, swelling, and redness.
  - ✓ Diseases of the joints may be manifested by such deformities as tissue loss, tissue overgrowth, or contractures, irreversible shortenings of muscles and tendons.
  - ✓ Edema in a joint may cause obvious bulging.
  - ✓ Redness, swelling, and pain are evidence of an inflammation or infection in the joint.

- Palpate the joints for tenderness, warmth, crepitation, consistency, and muscle mass.
  - ✓ Inflammation and injury cause joint pain.
  - ✓ Arthritis, bursitis, tendonitis, and osteomyelitis (infection of a bone) result in painful, hot joints.
  - ✓ **Crepitation** (a grating sound) is present in a joint when the articulating surfaces have lost their cartilage, such as in arthritis.

Range-of-Motion Assessment with Abnormal Findings (✓)

Assess joint ROM by asking the client to perform activities specific to:

- *Temporomandibular joint:* "Open your mouth wide, and then close your mouth." (As the client opens and closes the mouth, palpate the temporomandibular joints with your index and middle fingers.)

  ✓ Clicking or popping noises, decreased ROM, pain, and swelling may indicate temporomandibular joint syndrome or, in rare cases, osteoarthritis.

- *Cervical spine:*

  45-degree flexion: "Touch your chin to your chest."

  55-degree extension: "Look at the ceiling."

  40-degree lateral bending: "Try to touch your right ear to your right shoulder." Repeat with the left side

  70-degree rotation: "Try to touch your chin to each shoulder."

  ✓ Neck pain and limited extension with lateral bending are seen with herniated cervical discs and in cervical spondylosis.

  ✓ An immobile neck with head and neck thrust forward is seen with ankylosing spondylitis.

- *Lumbar spine:*

  75- to 90-degree flexion: "Touch your toes with your fingers".

  30-degree extension: "Bend backward slowly."

  35-degree lateral bending: "Bend right and left".

  30-degree rotation: "Twist your shoulders right and left".

  ✓ Decreased movement or pain with movement may indicate an abnormal spinal curvature, arthritis, herniated disc, or spasm of paravertebral muscles.

- *Fingers:*

  Flexion: "Make a fist."

  Extension: "Open your hand."

  Abduction: "Spread your fingers."

  Adduction: "Close your fingers."

  ✓ Flexion and extension of fingers is decreased in arthritis.

  ✓ Heberden's nodes and Bouchard's nodes are hard, nontender nodules on the dorsolateral parts of the distal and proximal interphalangeal joints, respectively. They are common in osteoarthritis.

  ✓ Stiff, painful, swollen finger joints are seen in acute rheumatoid arthritis.

  ✓ Boutonnière and swan-neck deformities are seen in chronic rheumatoid arthritis.

  ✓ Swollen finger joints with a white chalky discharge may be seen in chronic gout.

- *Wrists:*

  90-degree flexion: "Bend wrist down."

  70-degree extension: "Bend wrist up."

55-degree ulnar deviation: "Bend wrist toward little finger."

20-degree radial deviation: "Bend wrist toward thumb."

✓ Bilateral chronic swelling in the wrist is seen in arthritis.

- *Elbows:*

160-degree flexion: "Touch your hands to your shoulders."

180-degree extension: "Straighten your elbows."

90-degree supination: "Bend your elbows 90 degrees, and turn hands palm up."

90-degree pronation: "Bend your elbows 90 degrees, and turn fists down."

✓ Swollen, tender, inflamed elbows are apparent in gouty arthritis and rheumatoid arthritis.

✓ Pain and tenderness at the lateral epicondyle occurs in tennis elbow.

- *Shoulders:*

180-degree flexion: "Hold your arms straight up and out."

50-degree hyperextension: "Put your straight arm behind your back."

90-degree internal rotation: "Put your forearm behind your lower back."

180-degree abduction: "Raise your straight arm up and out to your side."

50-degree adduction: "Put your straight arm across your chest."

✓ Pain and tenderness over the biceps tendon occurs with tendinitis (inflammation of a tendon).

✓ The arm cannot be abducted fully when the supraspinatus tendon of the shoulder is ruptured.

✓ Pain and limited abduction is also seen with bursitis (inflammation of a bursa) and calcium deposits in this area.

- *Toes:*

90-degree flexion: "Walk on your toes."

✓ The great toe is excessively abducted in hallux valgus.

✓ The joint above the great toe is swollen, inflamed, and painful in gouty arthritis.

✓ There is hyperextension of the metatarsophalangeal joint and flexion of the proximal interphalangeal joint with hammer toes.

- *Ankles:*

20-degree dorsiflexion: "Point your foot to the ceiling."

45-degree plantar flexion: "Point your foot to the floor."

30-degree inversion: "Walk on the outside of your feet."

20-degree eversion: "Walk on the inside of your feet."

✓ Contractures of the Achilles tendon may occur in clients with rheumatoid arthritis following prolonged bed rest.

- *Knees:*

  130-degree flexion: "Do a deep knee bend."

  180-degree extension: "Sit down and hold your legs straight out in front of you."

  ✓ Swelling over the suprapatellar pouch is seen with inflammation and fluid in the articular capsule of the knee. Synovitis is inflammation of the synovial membrane lining the articular capsule of a joint. It is common with knee trauma.

  ✓ Swelling over the patella is seen in bursitis.

- *Hips:* (The client is lying down.)

  120-degree flexion: "Bring bent knee up to your chest."

  30-degree hyperextension: "Lie on the abdomen, and lift up one leg at a time."

  45-degree abduction: "Hold your leg straight, and move it out to the side."

  40-degree internal rotation: "Bend your knee, and swing it toward your other leg."

  45-degree external rotation: "Bend your knee, and swing it out to the side."

  ✓ Movement of the hip is limited and/or painful in arthritis.

Special Assessments with Abnormal Findings (✓)

- Perform *Phalen's test.* Ask the client to hold the wrist in acute flexion for 60 seconds.

  ✓ Numbness and burning in the fingers during Phalen's test may indicate carpal tunnel syndrome.

- Check for small amounts of fluid on the knee by assessing for a "bulge sign." Milk upward on the medial side of the knee, and then tap the lateral side of the patella.

  ✓ A fluid bulge indicates increased fluid in the knee joint rather than soft tissue swelling.

- Check for larger amounts of fluid by assessing ballottement. Apply downward pressure on the knee with one hand while pushing the patella backward against the femur with the other hand.

  ✓ Increased fluid will cause a tapping sound as the patella displaces the fluid and hits the femur.

- Perform *McMurray's test.* While reclining, ask the client to turn the flexed knee toward the center of the body. Stabilize the knee with one hand, and apply pressure on the lower leg with the other hand.

  ✓ Pain, locking (inability to fully extend the knee), or a popping sound may indicate an injury to a meniscus, a disc of cartilaginous tissue in the knee.

- Perform the *Thomas test.* Ask the client to lie down and extend one leg while bringing the knee of the opposite leg to the chest.

  ✓ A hip flexion contracture will cause the extended leg to rise off the table.

29

Nursing Care of Clients with Musculoskeletal Trauma

Musculoskeletal trauma is an injury to muscle, bone, or soft tissue that results from excessive external force. The external source transmits more kinetic energy than the tissue can absorb, and injury results. The severity of the trauma depends not only on the amount of force but also on the location of the impact, because different parts of the body can withstand different amounts of force. A wide variety of external sources can cause trauma, and the force involved can vary in severity (e.g., a step off the curb, a fall, being tackled in a football game, and a motor vehicle crash). See Chapter 40 for a detailed discussion of the results of different forces and types of injury from trauma.

Musculoskeletal injuries resulting from trauma include blunt tissue trauma, alterations in tendons and ligaments, and fractures of bones. Various forces that cause musculoskeletal trauma are typical for a specific environment, activity, or age group. For example, motorcycle crashes resulting in fractures of the distal tibia, midshaft femur, and radius are common in young men. Sports injuries, resulting from either overuse or acute trauma, are seen more often in adolescents and young adults. Falls are the most common cause of injury in people age 65 or older, with fractures of the vertebrae, proximal humerus, and hip seen most often (Porth, 2002).

Musculoskeletal trauma can result in mild or severe injuries. A client may experience a soft-tissue injury, a fracture, and/or a complete amputation. In addition, trauma to one part of the musculoskeletal system often produces dysfunction in adjacent structures. For example, a fracture of the femur prevents the adjacent muscles from abducting and adducting. Nursing care helps minimize the effects of trauma, prevents complications, and hastens restoration of function. The injury may require rehabilitation and temporary or permanent changes in lifestyle. This chapter discusses fractures, amputations, soft-tissue injuries, dislocations, and repetitive use injuries.

Traumatic Injuries of the Muscles, Ligaments, and Joints

The Client with a Contusion, Strain, or Sprain

Contusion, strains, and sprains are among the most commonly reported injuries. They account for about 50% of work-related injuries, with lower back injuries the most commonly reported occupational injury. However, many sprains and strains are not work related, and often are not reported. The lower back and cervical region of the spine are the most common sites for muscle strains; the ankle is the most commonly sprained joint, usually caused by forced inversion of the foot.

Pathophysiology and Manifestations

A **contusion,** the least serious form of musculoskeletal injury, is bleeding into soft tissue that results from a blunt force, such as a kick or striking a body part against a hard object. The skin remains intact, but small blood vessels rupture and bleed into soft tissues. A contusion with a large amount of bleeding is referred to as a **hematoma.** The manifestations of a contusion include swelling and discoloration of the skin. The blood in the soft tissue initially results in a purple and blue color commonly referred to as a mark or bruise. As the blood begins to reabsorb, the mark becomes brown and then yellow, until it disappears.

A **strain** is a stretching injury to a muscle or a muscle-tendon unit caused by mechanical overloading. A muscle that is forced to extend past its elasticity will become strained. Lifting heavy objects without bending the knees, or a sudden acceleration-deceleration, as in a motor vehicle crash, can cause strains. The most common sites for a muscle strain are the lower back and cervical regions of the spine. The manifestations of a strain include a sharp or dull pain that increases with isometric contraction of the muscle, swelling, and stiffness.

A **sprain** is an injury to a ligament surrounding a joint. Forces going in opposite directions cause the ligament to overstretch and/or tear. The ligaments may be incompletely or completely torn. Although any joint may be involved, sprains of the ankle and knee are most common. Manifestations include joint instability, discoloration, heat, pain, edema, and rapid swelling. Motion increases the joint pain. A comparison of sprains and strains is presented in Table 29-1.

Table 29-1. Comparison of Sprains and Strains

Sprain

- < Defined as an injury to a ligament that results from a twisting motion.
- < Can cause joint instability.
- < Pain, edema, and swelling are present.
- < Motion increases the joint pain.

Strain

- < Defined as a microscopic tear in the muscle.
- < Sharp or dull pain is present.
- < Pain increases with isometric contraction of the muscle.
- < Swelling and local tenderness are present.

Collaborative Care

Soft-tissue trauma is treated with measures that decrease swelling and alleviate pain. Severe sprains may require surgical repair. A splint may be applied to rest the injured area. Ice is applied for the first 24 to 48 hours, after which heat can be applied. A compression dressing, such as an Ace bandage, may be applied. The injured extremity should be elevated to or above the level of the heart to increase venous return and decrease swelling. Ankle sprains may be immobilized with an air cast, with no limitations on weight bearing. A knee injury also requires a knee immobilizer. If the upper extremity is injured, a sling is provided. Physical therapy may be recommended during rehabilitation.

Diagnostic Tests

The following diagnostic tests may be ordered when soft-tissue trauma is suspected:

- X-rays rule out a fracture before making a diagnosis of soft-tissue injury.
- Magnetic resonance imaging (MRI) is used if further assessment is necessary.

Medications

Medications used to treat soft-tissue trauma include NSAIDs and analgesics.

Nursing Care

The nursing care of each client is individualized. A strain or sprain may not be as devastating to an attorney as it is to a professional athlete; therefore, the nurse should determine what the injury means to the particular client.

Nursing Diagnoses and Interventions

Nursing diagnoses focus on providing information about self-care to decrease pain and return physical mobility to preinjury levels.

Acute Pain

The pain that results from soft-tissue trauma is due primarily to the injury to the muscle or ligament, and secondarily to bleeding and edema at the injury site.

- Teach the client the acronym RICE (rest, ice, compression, elevation) to care for the injury:
  1. Rest the injured extremity. *Rest allows the injured muscle or ligament to heal.*
  2. Apply ice to the injured area. *Cold causes vasoconstriction and decreases the pooling of blood in the injured area. Ice may also numb the tender area.*
  3. Apply a compression dressing, such as an Ace bandage. *A compression dressing can decrease the formation of edema and thereby decrease pain.*
  4. Elevate the extremity above the heart. *Elevating the extremity promotes venous return and decreases edema, which will decrease pain.*
- If pain is still present after 24 to 48 hours of applying ice, instruct the client to apply heat. *Heat increases blood flow and venous return and thereby decreases edema and pain.*

Impaired Physical Mobility

Pain causes the client to avoid using or bearing weight with the injured extremity. Always observe the client's use of assistive devices; if the device is inappropriate, the client can face a greater risk of falling. The device may be appropriate, but the client may not be using it correctly or safely. As a person ages, muscle mass in the upper extremities declines. As a result, the older client with a sprained ankle may not be able to use crutches, because crutches require that the person distribute body weight along the upper extremities. Older clients may therefore find a walker more useful.

- Teach the correct use of crutches, walkers, canes, or slings if prescribed. *The correct technique increases safety and encourages use of these devices.*
- Encourage follow-up care. *Severe sprains may require further testing to determine if surgical intervention is indicated.*

The Client with a Joint Dislocation

A **dislocation** of a joint is the loss of articulation of the bone ends in the joint capsule. Dislocations usually follow severe trauma, with the bone ends displaced or separated from their normal position in the joint capsule. They occur most frequently in the shoulder and acromioclavicular joints. A **subluxation** is a partial dislocation in which the bone ends are still partially in contact with each other.

Pathophysiology and Manifestations

Dislocations may be congenital, traumatic, or pathologic. Congenital dislocations are present at birth and are seen in the hip and knee. Traumatic dislocations result from falls, blows, or rotational injuries. Pathologic dislocations result from disease of the joint, including infection, rheumatoid arthritis, paralysis, and neuromuscular diseases. The manifestations of a dislocation include pain, deformity, and limited motion.

Collaborative Care

Care of the client with a dislocation focuses on relieving pain, correcting the dislocation, and preventing complications. The dislocation is diagnosed by physical examination and X-rays. The joint is reduced by means of manual traction.

Shoulder joint dislocations are reduced and immobilized in a sling for three weeks, after which time rehabilitation can begin. A dislocated hip requires immediate reduction in the emergency room to prevent necrosis of the femoral head and injury to the sciatic and femoral nerves. After reduction, the client is placed on bed rest. In some cases, traction is needed for several weeks. If a hip dislocation is accompanied by a fracture, the client will undergo surgery to increase mobility, decrease complications, and rapidly stabilize the joint.

Nursing Care

Nursing care of the client with a dislocation or subluxation is individualized to the cause of injury, the type of dislocation, and the age of the client.

Nursing Diagnoses and Interventions

Nursing diagnoses focus on relieving pain (see previous section) and preventing complications.

Risk for Injury

The client with a dislocation requires frequent assessments to ensure that neurovascular compromise does not develop.

- Monitor neurovascular status by assessing pain, pulses, pallor, paralysis, and paresthesia. *Neurovascular compromise is indicated by increased pain, decreased or absent pulses, pale skin, inability to move a body part or extremity, and changes in sensation, such as "pins and needles" sensations, or loss of sense of sharp/dull touch.*
- Maintain immobilization after reduction. *Immobilization prevents the joint from dislocating again.*

Home Care

Joint dislocations often tend to be recurring injuries for clients actively participating in contact sports and other vigorous physical activities. Younger adults have a 60% to 80% recurrence rate for anterior shoulder dislocations. Prolonged immobilization (for several weeks after the injury) and aggressive rehabilitation following the initial dislocation can reduce the risk of recurrent dislocation. The following topics should be addressed in preparing the client for home care:

- Importance of complying with the prescribed length of immobilization
- Skin care and ways to prevent skin-to-skin contact, particularly in the axillary area
- Prescribed rehabilitation exercises that will strengthen muscles and other supportive structures in the shoulder, decreasing the risk of future dislocations
- Alternatives to activities that precipitate recurrent dislocations
- Instructions or referrals to physical therapy if needed for further teaching about using assistive devices
- Referrals to physical and occupational therapy and home health services as needed.

Traumatic Injuries of Bones

The Client with a Fracture

A **fracture** is any break in the continuity of a bone. Fractures vary in severity according to the location and the type of fracture. Although fractures occur in all age groups, they are more common in people who have sustained trauma and in older clients.

Pathophysiology

Any of the 206 bones in the body can sustain a fracture. A fracture occurs when the bone is subjected to more kinetic energy than it can absorb. Fractures may result from a direct blow, a crushing force (compression), a sudden twisting motion (torsion), a severe muscle contraction, or disease that has weakened the bone (called a **pathologic fracture**). Two basic mechanisms produce fractures: direct force and indirect force. With direct force, the kinetic energy is applied at or near the site of the fracture. The bone cannot withstand the force. With indirect force, the kinetic energy is transmitted from the point of impact to a site where the bone is weaker. The fracture occurs at the weaker point.

Fractures are classified in the following ways:

- If the skin is intact, the fracture is considered a **closed** (or **simple**) **fracture.** If the skin integrity is interrupted, the fracture is considered an **open** (or **compound**) **fracture.** An open fracture allows bacteria to enter the injured area and increases the risk of complications.

- The fracture line may be **oblique** (at a 45-degree angle to the bone) or **spiral** (curves around the bone). An **avulsed** fracture occurs when the fracture pulls bone and other tissues away from the point of attachment. It may also be described as **comminuted** (the bone breaks in many pieces), **compressed** (the bone is crushed), **impacted** (the broken bone ends are forced into each other), or **depressed** (the broken bone is forced inward).

- **Complete fractures** involve the entire width of the bone, whereas **incomplete fractures** do not involve the entire width of the bone.

- A **stable (nondisplaced) fracture** is one in which the bones maintain their anatomic alignment. An **unstable (displaced) fracture** occurs when the bones move out of correct anatomic alignment. If a fracture is displaced, immediate interventions are required to prevent further damage to soft tissue, muscle, and bone.

- Fractures may also be classified by point of reference on the bone, such as midshaft, middle third, and distal third. The point of reference may also be specific, such as intrarticular or diaphyseal.

Manifestations and Complications

Fractures are often accompanied by soft tissue injuries that involve muscles, arteries, veins, nerves, or skin. The degree of soft-tissue involvement depends on the amount of energy or force transmitted to the area. The section following fracture healing describes manifestations and complications, with related collaborative and nursing care, for fractures of specific bones.

Fracture Healing

Regardless of classification or type, fracture healing progresses over three phases: the inflammatory phase, the reparative phase, and the remodeling phase. The bleeding and inflammation that develop at the site of the fracture initiate the inflammatory phase. A hematoma forms between the fractured bone ends and around the bone surfaces. The osteocytes at the bone ends die as the hematoma clots, obstructing blood flow and depriving them of oxygen and nutrients. Necrosis of the cells heightens the inflammatory response, which in turn leads to vasodilation and edema. In addition, fibroblasts, lymphocytes, macrophages, and even osteoblasts from the bone migrate to the fracture site. Fibroblasts form a fibrin meshwork and promote the growth of granulation tissue and capillary buds. The lymphocytes and macrophages wall off the area, localizing and containing the inflammation. The capillary buds invade the fracture site and supply a source of nutrients to promote the formation of collagen. The collagen allows calcium to be deposited.

Once calcium is deposited, a callus begins to form. In this reparative phase, osteoblasts promote the formation of new bone, and osteoclasts destroy dead bone and assist in the synthesis of new bone. Collagen formation and calcium deposition continues. During the remodeling phase, excess callus is removed and new bone is laid down along the fracture line. Eventually, the fracture site is calcified, and the bone is reunited.

The age, physical condition of the client, and the type of fracture sustained influence the healing of fractures. Other factors influence bone healing either positively or negatively, and may be grouped according to their local or systemic influence. Healing time varies with the individual. An uncomplicated fracture of the arm or foot can heal in 6 to 8 weeks. A fractured vertebra will take at least 12 weeks to heal. A fractured hip may take from 12 to 16 weeks.

Collaborative Care

A fracture requires treatment involving stabilizing the fractured bone(s), maintaining bone immobilization, preventing complications, and restoring function. The diagnosis of a fracture is primarily based on physical assessments and X-rays.

Emergency Care

Emergency care of the client with a fracture includes immobilizing the fracture, maintaining tissue perfusion, and preventing infection. In the case of serious trauma, normal body alignment must be maintained and may involve cervical immobilization. Once the client is in a secure location, he or she is assessed for instability or deformity of the bone. If any deformity or instability is detected, the extremity is rapidly immobilized. Open wounds are covered with sterile dressings, and bleeding may be controlled with a pressure dressing. The extremities are assessed for the presence of pulses, movement, and sensation. The joint above and below the deformity is immobilized. Pulses, movement, and sensation are reevaluated after splinting.

The fracture is splinted to maintain normal anatomical alignment and prevent the fracture from dislocating. Splinting relieves pain and prevents further damage to the arteries, nerves, and bones. Splinting can be accomplished with air splints. If equipment is not available, the limb may be secured to the body. For example, an arm may be secured with a sling, or one leg may be strapped to the other leg.

Diagnostic Tests

Diagnosis of a fracture begins with the history and initial assessment and usually is confirmed by radiographic tests. The following tests may be ordered:

- *X-rays* are commonly used to assess bones for fractures.
- *Bone scan* may be necessary to determine if a fracture is present, indicated by an increased uptake, or a "hot spot."
- *Blood chemistry studies, complete blood count (CBC),* and *coagulation studies* may be used to assess blood loss, renal function, muscle breakdown, and the risk of excessive bleeding or clotting.

Medications

Most clients with a fracture require pharmacologic interventions. The first and foremost intervention focuses on relieving pain. In the case of multiple fractures or fractures of large bones, narcotics are administered initially. As healing progresses, the client begins to take oral medication for pain. Pain management for the client with a fracture is described in Table 29-2.

Stool softeners may be administered to decrease the risk of constipation secondary to narcotics and immobility. Clients who have sustained trauma are often placed on antiulcer medications or antacids. NSAIDs may continue to be prescribed to decrease inflammation. Antibiotics may be administered prophylactically, particularly to clients with open or complex fractures. Anticoagulants may be prescribed to prevent deep vein thrombosis.

Treatments

Surgery

Surgery is indicated in the client who has a fracture that requires direct visualization and repair, a fracture with common long-term complications, or a fracture that is severely comminuted and threatens vascular supply.

The simplest form of surgery is done by external fixation with an external fixator device. An external fixator consists of a frame connected to pins that are inserted perpendicular to the long axis of the bone. The number of pins inserted varies with the type and site of the fracture, but in all cases the same number of pins is inserted above and below the fracture line. The pins require care similar to that of skeletal traction pins. The client is monitored for infection, and frequent neurovascular assessment is performed. The fixator increases independence while maintaining immobilization.

Table 29-2. Pain Management in the Client with a Fracture

The client who has had musculoskeletal trauma from an accident or surgery experiences pain from many different causes:

- The interruption in the continuity of the bone itself.
- Damage to ligaments and tendons.
- Swelling of tissues around the trauma site.
- Muscle spasms.
- Tissue anoxia from swelling inside a cast, splint, or the muscle fascia sheath.
- Hematoma formation.
- Pressure over bony prominences from casts or splints.

The pain is often severe and may be described as sharp, aching, or burning. Carefully assess any complaint of pain; pain may be an indication of a serious complication, such as compartment syndrome, decreased tissue perfusion and neurovascular impairment, or pressure ulcers. Do not administer analgesics until the location, character, and duration of pain has been carefully assessed. After the cause of the pain has been identified, the following nursing interventions may be implemented:

1. Administer prescribed analgesics, which may include NSAIDs and narcotic analgesics. For serious fractures or following orthopedic surgery, PCA or epidural methods of providing pain relief may be used. If medications are used on an as-needed basis, tell the client to request the medication before the pain is severe; alternatively, offer the medications at regular intervals for the first 24 to 48 hours. Reassure the client that addiction does not result from taking medications to relieve fracture or surgical pain. Most clients require only oral analgesics by the third or fourth day after orthopedic surgery. Refer to Chapter 38 for information about narcotic and nonnarcotic pain medications.
2. Elevate the involved extremity, and apply cold (if prescribed) to help decrease swelling.

Table 29-2. Continued

3. Monitor and drain the accumulated fluids in any drainage devices to ensure patency and to decrease the possibility of hematoma formation.

4. Encourage the client to wiggle fingers and toes on an extremity in a cast or traction to improve venous return and decrease edema.

5. Assist the client to change positions to relieve pressure and use pillows to provide support.

6. Teach the client alternative methods of pain management, such as relaxation and guided imagery.

7. Notify the physician of unrelieved pain, which may indicate a serious complication, such as compartment syndrome or neurovascular impairment.

Internal fixation can be accomplished through a surgical procedure called an *open reduction and internal fixation (ORIF)*. In this procedure, the fracture is reduced (placed in correct anatomic alignment) and nails, screws, plates, or pins are inserted to hold the bones in place. Open fractures of the arms and legs are most commonly repaired in this way. Hip fractures in older clients are almost always repaired with ORIF to prevent complications and to allow early rehabilitation.

Traction

Muscle spasms usually accompany fractures and may pull bones out of alignment. Traction is the application of a straightening or pulling force to return or maintain the fractured bones in normal anatomic position. Weights are applied to maintain the necessary force. Types of traction are as follows:

*   In **manual traction,** the hand directly applies the pulling force. Other common types of traction include straight traction, balanced suspension traction, skin traction, and skeletal traction.

*   **Straight traction** is a pulling force applied in a straight line to the injured body part resting on the bed. The most common type of straight traction is Buck's traction, in which the lower portion of the injured extremity is placed in a cradlelike sleeve. This sleeve is harnessed to itself, and a weight is hung from the bottom of a traction frame. The result is a force that pulls straight away from the body. This traction exerts its grabbing and pulling force through the client's skin. Therefore, this traction may be considered straight skin traction. The advantage of skin traction is the relative ease of use and ability to maintain comfort. The disadvantage is that the weight required to maintain normal body alignment or fracture alignment cannot exceed the tolerance of the skin, about 6 lb. per extremity.

*   **Balanced suspension traction** involves more than one force of pull. Several forces work in unison to raise and support the client's injured extremity off the bed and pull it in a straight fashion away from the body. The advantage of this type of traction is that it increases mobility without threatening joint continuity. The disadvantage is that the increased use of multiple weights makes the client more likely to slide in the bed.

*   **Skeletal traction** is the application of a pulling force through placement of pins into the bone. The client receives local anesthetic, and the pin is inserted in a twisting

motion into the bone. This type of traction must be applied under sterile conditions because of the increased risk of infection. One or more pulling forces may be applied with skeletal traction. The advantage of this type of traction is that more weight can be used to maintain the proper anatomic alignment, if necessary. The disadvantages include increased anxiety, increased risk of infection, and increased discomfort. Nursing implications for clients receiving traction are presented in Table 29-3.

Casts

A **cast** is a rigid device applied to immobilize the injured bones and promote healing. The cast is applied to immobilize the joint above and the joint below the fractured bone so that the bone will not move during healing. A fracture is first reduced manually and a cast is then applied. Casts are applied on clients who have relatively stable fractures

The cast, which may be composed of plaster or fiberglass, is applied over a thin cushion of padding and molded to the normal contour of the body. The cast must be allowed to dry before any pressure is applied to it; simply palpating a wet cast with the fingertips will leave dents that may cause pressure sores. A plaster cast may require up to 48 hours to dry, whereas a fiberglass cast dries in less than 1 hour. The type of cast applied is determined by the location of the fracture. During follow-up appointments, the physician may X-ray the bone to assess alignment and healing, and possibly remove the cast for skin assessment.

Table 29-3. Nursing Implications for Clients Receiving Traction

- In skeletal traction, never remove the weights.
- In skin traction, remove weights only when intermittent skin traction has been ordered to alleviate muscle spasm.
- For traction to be successful, a countertraction is necessary. In most instances, the countertraction is the client's weight. Therefore, do not wedge the client's foot or place it flush with the foot-board of the bed.
- Maintain the line of pull:
  a. Center the client on the bed.
  b. Ensure that weights hang freely and do not touch the floor.
- Ensure that nothing is lying on or obstructing the ropes. Do not allow the knots at the end of the rope to come into contact with the pulley.
- If a problem is detected, assist in repositioning. The area of the fracture must be stabilized when the client is repositioned.
- In skin traction:
  a. Frequently assess skin for evidence of pressure, shearing, or pending breakdown.
  b. Protect pressure sites with padding and protective dressings as indicated.
- In skeletal traction:
  a. Frequent skin assessments should include pin care per policy.
  b. Report signs of infection at the pin sites, such as redness, drainage, and increased tenderness.
  c. The client may require more frequent analgesic administration.

Table 29-3. Continued

- Perform neurovascular assessments frequently.
- Assess for common complications of immobility, including formation of pressure ulcers, formation of renal calculi, deep vein thrombosis, pneumonia, paralytic ileus, and loss of appetite.
- Teach the client and family about the type and purpose of the traction.

Electrical Bone Stimulation

Electrical bone stimulation is the application of an electrical current at the fracture site. It is used to treat fractures that are not healing appropriately. The electrical stress increases the migration of osteoblasts and osteoclasts to the fracture site. Mineral deposition increases, promoting bone healing. Electrical bone stimulation can be accomplished invasively or noninvasively. In invasive stimulation, the surgeon inserts a cathode and a lead wire at the fracture site. The lead wire is attached to an internal or external generator, which delivers electricity through the lead wire to the cathode 24 hours a day. In noninvasive inductive stimulation, a treatment coil encircles the cast or skin directly over the fracture site. The coil is attached to an external generator that runs on batteries. The electricity goes through the skin to the fracture site. The time period for external stimulation can vary from 3 to 10 hours per day. The client may be taught to self-administer the noninvasive electrical stimulation. Electrical bone stimulation is contraindicated in the presence of infection.

Fracture Complications with Related Collaborative Care

Complications of musculoskeletal trauma are associated with pressure from edema and hemorrhage, development of fat emboli, deep vein thrombosis, infection, loss of skeletal integrity, or involvement of nerve fibers. Bone fragments may also result in further injury or complications.

Compartment Syndrome

A compartment is a space enclosed by a fibrous membrane or fascia. The fascia lines the compartment within the limbs and is nonexpandable. Compartments within the limbs may enclose and support bones, nerves, and blood vessels. **Compartment syndrome** occurs when excess pressure in a limited space constricts the structures within a compartment, reducing circulation to muscles and nerves. Acute compartment syndrome may result from hemorrhage and edema within the compartment following a fracture or from a crush injury, or from external compression of the limb by a cast that is too tight. Increased pressure within the confined space of the compartment results in entrapment of nerves, blood vessels, and muscles.

Entrapment of the blood vessels limits tissue perfusion, beginning a cycle of events that may result in the loss of the limb. Inadequate oxygen supply causes cellular acidosis, which intensifies as cellular energy requirements are met through anaerobic metabolism. The capillaries inside the compartment dilate in an attempt to increase the supply of blood and oxygen. Additional blood and oxygen are not available, and plasma proteins leak out into the interstitial tissues. The interstitial tissue then pulls fluid in to balance the protein load. As a result, edema within the compartment increases. The edema causes further compression of the vascular network, and the cycle continues. Uninterrupted, this cycle threatens the client's limb and increases the risk of sepsis. Compartment syndrome usually develops within the first 48 hours of injury, when edema is at its peak. It is important to note that arterial pulses may remain normal, even when pressure within the compartment is high enough to significantly impair tissue perfusion.

If compartment syndrome develops, interventions to alleviate pressure will be implemented; these may include removal of a tightly fitting cast. If the pressure is internal, a **fasciotomy,** a surgical intervention in which muscle fascia is cut to relieve pressure within the compartment, may be necessary. After a fasciotomy, the incision is left open, and passive ROM exercises are performed on the extremity.

Volkmann's contracture, a common complication of elbow fractures, can result from unresolved compartment syndrome. Arterial blood flow decreases, leading to ischemia, degeneration, and contracture of the muscle. Arm mobility is impaired, and the client is unable to completely extend the arm.

Fat Embolism Syndrome

Fat emboli occur when fat globules lodge in the pulmonary vascular bed or peripheral circulation. **Fat embolism syndrome (FES)** is characterized by neurologic dysfunction, pulmonary insufficiency, and a petechial rash on the chest, axilla, and upper arms. Long bone fractures and other major trauma are the principle risk factors for fat emboli; hip replacement surgery also poses a risk for FES.

When a bone is fractured, pressure within the bone marrow rises and exceeds capillary pressure; as a result, fat globules leave the bone marrow and enter the bloodstream. Another contributing factor may be the stress-induced release of catecholamine, which causes the rapid mobilization of fatty acids. Once the fat globules are released, they combine with platelets and travel to the brain, lungs, kidneys, and other organs, occluding small blood vessels and causing tissue ischemia.

Manifestations usually develop within a few hours to a week after injury. The manifestations result from the occlusion of the blood supply and the presence of fatty acids. Altered cerebral blood flow causes confusion and changes in level of consciousness. Pulmonary circulation may be disrupted, and free fatty acids damage the alveolar-capillary membrane. Pulmonary edema, impaired surfactant production, and atelectasis can result in significant respiratory insufficiency and manifestations of acute respiratory distress syndrome (ARDS) (see Chapter 15). Fat droplets activate the clotting cascade, causing thrombocytopenia. Petechiae (pin-sized purplish areas from bleeding under the skin) appearing on the skin, buccal membranes, and conjunctival sacs are thought to result from either microvascular clotting or the accompanying thrombocytopenia.

Early stabilization of long bone fractures is preventive for FES. Prompt identification and treatment of the syndrome are necessary to maintain adequate pulmonary function. In severe cases, the client may require intubation and mechanical ventilation to prevent hypoxemia. Fluid balance is closely monitored. Corticosteroids may be administered to decrease the inflammatory response of lung tissues, stabilize lipid membranes, and reduce bronchospasm (Porth, 2002).

Deep Vein Thrombosis

A **deep vein thrombosis (DVT)** is a blood clot that forms along the intimal lining of a large vein. Three precursors linked to DVT formation are (1) venous stasis, or decreased blood flow, (2) injury to blood vessel walls, and (3) altered blood coagulation (Table 29–4). Any or all of these precursors can cause a DVT to form. Damage to the lining of the vein causes the platelets to aggregate or clump together, forming the thrombus. Fibrin, WBCs, and RBCs begin to cling to the thrombus, and a tail forms. This tail or the entire thrombus may dislodge and move to the brain, lungs, or heart. Five percent of DVTs dislodge and enter the pulmonary circulation to form a pulmonary embolus. If the thrombus remains in the vein, venous insufficiency may result from scarring and valve damage.

The best treatment for DVT is prevention. Early immobilization of the fracture and early ambulation of the client are imperative. The extremity should be elevated above the level of the heart. Frequent assessments of the injured extremity may lead to early recognition of DVT and prevent the formation of pulmonary embolus. Prophylactic anticoagulant administration is also beneficial. Antiembolism stockings and compression boots also increase venous return and prevent stasis of blood. Constrictive clothing should be avoided.

Table 29-4. Precursors of Deep Vein Thrombosis

Precursor	Implications for Fractures
Decreased blood flow	Common in fracture clients, who are immobilized and less active. Bed rest alone can decrease venous flow by 50%.
Injury to blood vessel wall	May occur as a direct result of the force that caused the fracture or from surgical manipulation.
Altered blood coagulation	May result from active blood loss. The body's attempt to maintain homeostasis leads to increased production of platelets and clotting factor.

If a DVT is present, there may be swelling, leg pain, tenderness, or cramping. Not all clients experience manifestations, however. For this reason, diagnostic tests, such as a venogram or Doppler ultrasound of lower extremities, may be required. A venogram requires intravenous administration of dye in the radiology department, whereas a Doppler ultrasound study is noninvasive and can be performed at the client's bedside. Doppler ultrasonography uses sound waves to form an image on a computer screen.

The diagnosis of DVT requires rapid intervention. The client is placed on bed rest for five to seven days to prevent dislodgment of the clot. Thrombolytic agents, which dissolve the clot, may be administered. Heparin may be administered intravenously to prevent more clots from forming. A vena cava filter may be placed to prevent the existing clot from entering the pulmonary circulation and forming a pulmonary embolus. In extreme cases in which anticoagulation therapy is contraindicated, a thrombectomy (surgical removal of the clot) may be necessary. See Chapter 12 for further discussion of DVT.

Infection

Infection is more likely to occur in an open fracture than a closed fracture, but any complication that decreases blood supply increases the risk of infection. Infection may result from contamination at the time of injury or during surgery. *Pseudomonas, Staphylococcus,* or

Clostridium organisms may invade the wound or bone. *Clostridium* infection is particularly serious because it may lead to severe gas gangrene and cellulitis, but any infection may delay healing and result in **osteomyelitis**, infection within the bone that can lead to tissue death and necrosis. (See Chapter 30 for a discussion of osteomyelitis.)

Delayed Union and Nonunion

Delayed union is the prolonged healing of bones beyond the usual time period. Many factors may inhibit bone healing, including poor nutrition, inadequate immobilization, prolonged reduction time, infection, necrosis, age, immunosuppression, and severe bone trauma resulting in multiple fragments. Delayed union is diagnosed by means of serial X-ray studies. It is important to note that X-ray findings may lag one to two weeks behind the healing process; for example, a client may be completely healed by week 13, but this fact may not be apparent on the X-ray until week 14.

Delayed union may lead to **nonunion**, which can cause persistent pain and movement at the fracture site. Nonunion may require surgical interventions, such as internal fixation and bone grafting. If infection is present, the bones are surgically debrided. Electrical stimulation of the fracture site may be as effective as bone grafting.

Reflex Sympathetic Dystrophy

Reflex sympathetic dystrophy may occur after musculoskeletal or nerve trauma. This term refers to a group of poorly understood posttraumatic conditions involving persistent pain, hyperesthesias, swelling, changes in skin color and texture, changes in temperature, and decreased motion. Diagnosis is made by the client's history and physical examination. X-rays may demonstrate spotty osteoporosis, and bone scans may reveal increased uptake of radionucleide. Treatment with a sympathetic nervous system blocking agent often alleviates the symptoms.

Fractures of Specific Bones or Bony Areas

Fracture of the Skull

The skull may be fractured as a result of either a fall or a direct blow. The client must be assessed for neurologic damage and any loss of consciousness must be documented. A complete neurologic assessment is conducted: Pupillary reaction to light, movement and strength of all extremities, complaints of nausea and vomiting, level of consciousness and orientation to person, place, and time are noted. A displaced skull fracture, which is referred to as depressed, may press on the brain and cause neurologic damage. Brain injuries related to skull fractures are discussed in Chapter 33.

Fracture of the Face

Fracture of the facial bones may result from a direct blow. The client experiences hematomas, pain, edema, and bony deformity. Nondisplaced fractures are monitored to ensure the airway is not compromised. The client is observed for any neurologic deficits. Severely displaced or multiple facial fractures are treated with open reduction and internal fixation with wires or plates.

Nursing care focuses on maintaining the airway by helping the client clear secretions from the oropharynx. The nurse monitors the client's breathing for increased effort or tachypnea and notifies the physician immediately if these findings are noted. Pain is treated with analgesics, and body image disturbances are addressed. If the client asks to see his or her face, the nurse should plan to stay with the client and answer questions while the client looks in a mirror.

Fracture of the Spine

The spine can be injured in many ways, including sports injuries, falls, and motor vehicle crashes. The spine can be fractured in the cervical, thoracic, lumbar, or sacral area. The most severe complication of spine fracture is injury to the spinal cord. A fracture to the vertebrae may cause the bones to become displaced and apply pressure on the spinal cord. This pressure on the spinal cord may result in permanent paralysis.

A nondisplaced cervical spinal fracture may be treated with a cervical collar or a halo immobilizing brace. The displaced cervical fracture is reduced by manual or skeletal traction and, eventually, application of a brace and/or surgical stabilization of the bones with plates and screws. Immobilization after a spinal fracture may last as long as six months. Chapter 32 discusses spinal fractures and spinal cord injury.

Fracture of the Clavicle

A fracture of the clavicle commonly results from a direct blow or a fall. The most common location is midclavicular. A person with a midclavicular fracture typically assumes a protective slumping position to immobilize the arm and prevent shoulder movement. A less common fracture occurs along the distal third of the clavicle. This type of fracture may be associated with ligament damage. Injuries to the clavicle may be associated with skull or cervical fractures. The fractured bone, if displaced, may lacerate the subclavian vessels and result in hemorrhage. The fractured bone may also puncture the lung, resulting in a pneumothorax. Malunion may occur at the fracture site and result in asymmetry of the clavicles. Injury to the brachial plexus may result in numbness and decreased movement of the arm on the affected side.

A deformity may be observed or palpated along the clavicle. Treatment focuses on immobilizing the fractured bone in normal anatomic position by applying a clavicular strap, or a surgical repair may be necessary.

Fracture of the Humerus

The exact location of the fracture, the presence of displacement, and the results of the neurovascular examination determine the severity of a fracture of the humerus and the appropriate interventions. Treatment focuses on immobilizing the fractured bone in normal anatomic position. Common complications of humeral fracture include nerve and ligament damage, frozen or stiff joints, and malunion. Early interventions and follow-up may prevent permanent damage.

Fractures of the proximal humerus are common in older adults. A simple nondisplaced fracture of the proximal humerus (near the humeral head) with a normal neurovascular assessment can be safely treated with immobilization. A more complicated displaced fracture of the proximal humerus with bone fragmentation requires surgical intervention. The more severe the fracture and damage to soft tissue, the more likely the range of motion of the shoulder will be impaired. Rehabilitative measures focus on increasing ROM.

The humerus may also fracture along the shaft, usually as a direct result of trauma. If the humeral shaft fracture is simple and nondisplaced, a hanging arm cast is applied. This cast maintains alignment of the fracture by using the pulling force of gravity; therefore, the client must be instructed not to rest the cast on anything to alleviate the weight. If the client is on bed rest, a hanging arm cast is not applied, because the arm would not be able to hang freely. Instead, the fracture is immobilized with external skeletal traction. This traction places the injured arm in an upright position over the face, and weights are hung off the distal portion of the humerus.

Fracture of the Elbow

The most common location of an elbow fracture is the distal humerus. Elbow fractures usually result from a fall or direct blow to the elbow. The client guards the injured extremity, holding the arm rigidly in a flexed position or an extended position. Because the radius, ulna, or humerus may be involved in the elbow fracture, all three bones must be visualized by X-ray.

Complications of an elbow fracture include nerve or artery damage and **hemarthrosis**, a collection of blood in the elbow joint. The most serious complication of an elbow fracture is **Volkmann's contracture**, which results from arterial occlusion and muscle ischemia. The client complains of forearm pain, impaired sensation, and loss of motor function. Rapid interventions are aimed at relieving pressure on the brachial artery and nerve and preventing muscle atrophy.

Nondisplaced elbow fractures are treated by immobilizing the fracture with a posterior splint or cast. The displaced fracture is first reduced and then immobilized. Nursing interventions focus on alleviating pain, maintaining immobilization, and educating clients in neurovascular assessments.

Fracture of the Radius and/or Ulna

Fractures of the radius and ulna may occur as a result of either indirect injury, such as twisting or pulling on the arm, or direct injury, such as that resulting from a fall. The usual treatment of radius fractures depends on the location. The proximal radial head may be fractured from a fall on an outstretched hand. Blood commonly collects in the elbow joint and must be aspirated. If the fracture is nondisplaced, a sling is applied. If the fracture is displaced, surgical intervention is required. After surgical repair of a displaced fracture, the arm is splinted with a posterior plaster splint. The client avoids movement for the first week, and then initiates movement gradually.

When both bones are broken, the fracture is usually displaced. The client complains of pain and inability to turn the palm of the hand up. A nondisplaced fracture is casted for about six weeks, and either a shorter cast or a brace is then applied for six more weeks. If the fracture is displaced, surgical intervention is performed. The physician reduces the fracture and may insert pins or screws to keep the bones in alignment. After the surgery, a cast is applied, and the client is encouraged to exercise the fingers.

Complications after a radius and/or ulnar fracture include compartment syndrome, delayed healing, and decreased wrist and finger movement. After surgery, the client also has an increased risk of infection. Nursing interventions focus on alleviating pain, maintaining immobilization, and educating clients in neurovascular assessments, the importance of elevation, and the need to inform the physician of changes in sensation or an increase in pain.

Fractures in the Wrist and Hand

Wrist fractures often result from a fall onto an outstretched hand or onto the back of the hand. A common type of wrist fracture is **Colles's fracture**, in which the distal radius fractures after a fall onto an outstretched hand. The client with a wrist fracture presents with a bony deformity, pain, numbness, weakness, and decreased ROM of the fingers. The capillary refill and sensation of the hand must be assessed.

The hand is composed of many bones. Most commonly, the metacarpals and phalanges are involved in a hand fracture. The injuring mechanism in a hand fracture varies greatly from striking an object with a closed fist to closing a hand in a door. The client presents with complaints of pain, edema, and decreased ROM. The cause of the injury usually focuses the assessment on circulation, sensation, and ROM.

Comparative X-rays may be obtained to compare left and right wrists and hands. Complications of wrist and hand fractures are compartment syndrome, nerve damage, ligament damage, and delayed union. A wrist fracture is commonly treated with closed reduction, cast application, and elevation of the injured extremity. A hand fracture is splinted and elevated.

Nursing interventions focus on alleviating pain and educating the client in neurovascular assessments, the importance of elevation, and how to exercise the fingers to prevent stiffness. If the dominant hand is injured, the client will require assistance in performing ADLs.

Fracture of the Ribs

Rib fractures commonly result from blunt chest trauma. The location of the fracture and involvement of underlying organs determine the severity of the injury. Fractures of the first through third ribs may result in injury to the subclavian artery or vein. Fractures of the lower ribs may result in spleen and liver injuries.

The client presents with a history of recent chest trauma. Typically, the client complains of pain along the lateral portion of the rib. Palpation of the rib reveals a bony deformity and increases pain. Deep inspiration also increases pain. The skin over the fracture site may be ecchymotic (bruised).

A complication of rib fractures is a **flail chest**, which results from the fracture of two or more adjacent ribs in two or more places and the formation of a free-floating segment that moves in the opposite direction of the rib cage. The bony instability impairs respirations (see Chapter 15). Treatment is aimed at stabilizing the flail segment and supporting respirations. Other complications of rib fractures include pneumothorax and/or hemothorax. The fractured rib may pierce the lung and injure it. The lower ribs may pierce the liver or spleen, resulting in intra-abdominal bleeding. Pneumonia may also develop from ineffective clearing of respiratory secretions.

A simple rib fracture is treated with pain medication and instructions for coughing, deep breathing, and splinting. The client is also instructed to return to the emergency room if shortness of breath develops. Nursing interventions focus on alleviating pain and teaching the client about splinting. Because deep inspiration increases pain, clients frequently avoid it. The client may be instructed to splint the injured rib with the hand or a pillow and take deep breaths and cough to decrease the chance of developing atelectasis. Incentive spirometry is encouraged.

Fracture of the Pelvis

The client with a pelvic fracture presents with pain in the back or hip area. A single fracture in the pelvis is treated conservatively with bed rest on a firm mattress. Log rolling increases client comfort. A pelvic fracture with two fracture sites is considered unstable and treated with surgery. An external fixator may be applied to stabilize the pelvis. In the client who is not stable for surgery, a pelvic sling may be used. The pelvic sling stabilizes the pelvis and allows the client to move in bed with less pain. Common complications include hypovolemia, spinal injury, bladder injury, urethral injury, kidney damage, and gastrointestinal trauma.

Nursing care focuses on alleviating discomfort, maintaining immobilization, and preparing the client for surgery if necessary. The nurse monitors the client for increased heart rate, decreased blood pressure, and decreasing hemoglobin levels. These findings may indicate impending hypovolemia due to bleeding into the pelvis. Any blood in the urine should be reported to the physician; this may indicate kidney, bladder, or urethral damage.

Fracture of the Shaft of the Femur

A large amount of force, such as from motor vehicle crashes, falls, or acts of violence, is required to fracture the shaft of the femur. Clients with femoral shaft fractures often have associated multiple trauma. A fracture of the femoral shaft is manifested by an edematous, deformed, painful thigh. The client is unable to move the hip or knee. Initial assessment focuses on the circulation and sensation present in the affected extremity. Pedal pulses and capillary refill in the affected extremity are compared to the unaffected extremity. Complications of a femoral shaft fracture include hypovolemia due to blood loss (which may be as great as 1.0 to 1.5 L), fat embolism, dislocation of the hip or knee, muscle atrophy, and ligament damage.

Treatment of fractures of the shaft of the femur initially includes skeletal traction to separate the bony fragments, and reduce and immobilize the fracture. Depending on the location and severity of the fracture, traction may be followed by either external or internal fixation. Strength in the affected extremity is maintained through gluteal and quadricep exercises. ROM exercises for unaffected extremities are critical in preparation for ambulation. Although full weight bearing is usually restricted until X-rays demonstrate bone union, the client may be allowed to carry out non-weight-bearing activities with an assistive device.

The nurse assesses pulses in the extremity and compares them bilaterally. Sensation is evaluated by asking whether the client can feel touch and discriminate sharp from dull objects. Nursing interventions include providing pain medication, providing reassurance and decreasing anxiety, and assisting with exercises of the lower legs, feet, and toes.

Fracture of the Hip

A hip fracture refers to a fracture of the femur at the head, neck, or trochanteric regions. Hip fractures are classified as intracapsular or extracapsular. **Intracapsular fractures** involve the head or neck of the femur; **extracapsular fractures** involve the trochanteric region. The majority of hip fractures involve the neck or trochanteric regions. The femoral head and neck lie within the joint capsule and are not covered in periosteum; thus, they do not have a large blood supply. Fractures here usually fragment and may further decrease blood supply, increasing the risk of nonunion and avascular necrosis. The trochanteric region is covered in periosteum and, therefore, has more blood supply than the head or neck.

Hip fractures are a significant problem, causing the greatest number of deaths and most serious health problems of all fractures. Most are the result of falls, which account for 87%

of all fractures for people 65 years or older (CDC, 2000). Statistics for hip fractures include the following:

- Approximately 75% to 80% of hip fractures are sustained by postmenopausal women, who have the highest incidence of osteoporosis.
- Most people with hip fractures are hospitalized for two weeks.
- Half of all older adults hospitalized for a hip fracture cannot return home or live independently after the fracture.
- By the year 2040, the number of hip fractures is expected to exceed 500,000, which reflects society's increasing older population. Factors contributing to falls include problems with gait and balance, neurological and musculoskeletal impairments, dementia, psychoactive medications, and visual impairments.

Hip fractures are common in older adults as a result of decreases in bone mass and the increased tendency to fall. Whether the femur breaks spontaneously and causes the fall or whether the fall causes the fracture is not always clear; regardless of the cause of the fracture, however, rapid interventions are required to prevent bone necrosis. Assessment findings commonly associated with a hip fracture are pain, shortening of the affected lower extremity, and external rotation. Rarely, the fracture dislocates posteriorly; if that occurs, the extremity may internally rotate.

A hip fracture may be treated with traction to decrease muscle spasms, followed by surgery; or surgery may be performed immediately or within the first 24 hours. The goal of surgery is to reduce and stabilize the fracture, thereby increasing mobility, decreasing pain, and preventing complications. Surgery usually consists of open reduction and internal fixation of the fracture. Fixation is accomplished by securing the femur in place with pins, screws, nails, or plates. An open reduction and internal fixation works well for fractures in the trochanteric area. Fractures of the femoral neck frequently disrupt blood supply to the femoral head. If blood supply is disrupted, the surgeon will replace the femoral head with a prosthesis. If the acetabulum has been damaged, the surgeon may insert a metal cup. Replacement of either the femoral head or the acetabulum with a prosthesis is called a hemiarthroplasty. Replacement of both the femoral head and the acetabulum is a total hip arthroplasty (THA), discussed in Chapter 30. Nursing care focuses on alleviating pain, maintaining circulation to the injured extremity, and increasing mobility.

Fracture of the Tibia and/or Fibula

Fractures of the lower extremities often result from a fall on a flexed foot, a direct blow, or a twisting motion. The client presents with edema, pain, bony deformity, and a hematoma at the level of injury.

Circulation and sensation are assessed to rule out common complications of the fracture, including damage to the peroneal nerve or tibial artery, compartment syndrome, hemarthroses, and ligament damage. Peroneal nerve damage may be indicated by the client's inability to point the toe on the affected side upward. Tibial artery damage may be the cause of an absent dorsalis pedis pulse on the affected side. Compartment syndrome may be present if the client develops pain on passive movement and paresthesias. An edematous knee may indicate a collection of blood in the knee joint. Ligament damage may be present if the client cannot move the knee and/or ankle.

If the fracture is closed, a closed reduction and casting are frequently performed. A long leg cast that allows for partial weight bearing is used. Partial weight bearing usually is prescribed by the physician within 10 days of the fracture. A short leg cast will be applied in three to four weeks. If the fracture is open, either external fixation or open reduction and internal fixation will be performed. After surgery, a cast may be applied, and weight bearing begins according to the physician's orders, usually in about six weeks.

Nursing care is designed to increase comfort, monitor neurovascular status, and prevent complications. The nurse instructs the client in cast care, the use of assistive devices, how to perform neurovascular assessment, and when to follow up with the physician.

Fracture in the Ankle and Foot

The client with an ankle fracture presents with pain, limited ROM, hematoma, edema, and difficulty ambulating. Most ankle fractures are treated by closed reduction and casting. Open fractures are treated by surgical intervention and splinting.

The client with a foot fracture presents with similar symptoms; however, range of motion of the ankle is not usually affected. Most foot fractures are nondisplaced and treated with closed reduction and casting. More severe displaced foot fractures may require surgery and the placement of wires to maintain reduction of the fracture.

Nursing care focuses on increasing comfort, increasing mobility, and educating the client. Analgesia is given for pain. The extremity should be elevated, and ice can be applied. The client is taught cast care, neurovascular assessment, and walking with crutches.

Nursing Care

In planning and implementing nursing care for the client with fractures, the nurse should consider the client's response to the traumatic experience. Although each client has individual needs, nursing care commonly focuses on client problems with pain, impaired physical mobility, impaired tissue perfusion, and neurovascular compromise.

Health Promotion

Trauma prevention can save lives. Many communities are educating people of all ages, from grade-schoolers to older adults, in trauma prevention. Young adults face a high risk of sustaining trauma. They need to be taught the importance of safety equipment, such as automobile seat belts, bicycle helmets, football pads, proper footwear, protective eyewear, and hard hats, in preventing or decreasing the severity of injury from trauma. Older adults should have regular screenings for osteoporosis, activity levels, cognitive and affective disorders, sensory impairments, and risk for falls. Educational programs about workplace and farm safety, including information about ergonomic principles, can also help prevent musculoskeletal injuries.

Having a regular exercise program and avoiding obesity are important factors in maintaining good bone health in all adults. An adequate intake of calcium is essential to ensure proper growth, development, and maintenance of strong bones throughout life. It is important that women ensure good bone health prior to menopause, as the loss of estrogen during and after menopause decreases calcium use. Strong bones are formed by calcium intake and weight-bearing exercise, both of which are equally important in the postmenopausal woman.

Older clients are at higher risk for musculoskeletal trauma due to falls. For these clients, home assessments must be performed and potential hazards removed.

Assessment

Collect the following data through the health history and physical examination (see Chapter 28).

- *Health history:* age, history of traumatic event, history of chronic illnesses, history of prior musculoskeletal injuries, medications. (Ask the older adult specifically about anticoagulants.)
- *Physical assessment:* pain with movement, pulses, edema, skin color and temperature, deformity, range of motion, touch. (These assessments include the five Ps of neurovascular assessment, as follows, included in both the initial assessment and ongoing focused assessments.)
  1. *Pain.* Assess pain in the injured extremity by asking the client to grade it on a scale of 0 to 10, with 10 as the most severe pain.
  2. *Pulses.* Assess distal pulses beginning with the unaffected extremity. Compare the quality of pulses in the affected extremity to those of the unaffected extremity.
  3. *Pallor.* Observe for pallor and skin color in the injured extremity. Paleness and coolness may indicate arterial compromise, whereas warmth and a bluish tinge may indicate venous blood pooling.
  4. *Paralysis/Paresis.* Assess ability to move body parts distal to the fracture site. Inability to move indicates paralysis. Loss of muscle strength (weakness) when moving is paresis. A finding of limited range of motion may lead to early recognition of problems, such as nerve damage and paralysis.
  5. *Paresthesia.* Ask the client if any change in sensation (paresthesia) has occurred.

Nursing Diagnoses and Interventions

Nursing care for clients with fractures ranges from teaching for home care treatments provided in the emergency or urgent care department, such as manual reduction and cast application, to providing interventions to maintain health and decrease the risk of complications in clients with complex or multiple fractures. Teaching is also necessary for caregivers of the older adult who is discharged home or to a long-term care or rehabilitation facility following a fractured hip.

Acute Pain

Pain is caused by soft tissue damage and is compounded by muscle spasms and swelling.

- Monitor vital signs. *Some analgesics decrease respiratory effort and blood pressure.*
- Ask the client to rate the pain on a scale of 0 to 10 (with 10 as the most severe pain) before and after any intervention. *This facilitates objective assessment of the effectiveness of the chosen pain relief strategy. Pain that increases in intensity or remains unrelieved with analgesics can indicate compartment syndrome.*
- For the client with a hip fracture, apply Buck's traction per physician's orders. *Buck's traction immobilizes the fracture and decreases pain and additional trauma.*
- Move the client gently and slowly. *Gentle moving helps to prevent the development of severe muscle spasms.*
- Elevate the injured extremity above the level of the heart. *Elevating the extremity promotes venous return and decreases edema, which decreases pain.*
- Encourage distraction or other noninvasive methods of pain relief, such as deep breathing and relaxation. *Distraction, deep breathing, and relaxation help decrease the focus on the pain and may lessen the intensity of pain.*

- Administer pain medications as prescribed. For home care, explain the importance of taking pain medications before the pain is severe. *Analgesics alleviate pain by stimulating opiate receptor sites.*

Risk for Peripheral Neurovascular Dysfunction

In the client with a fracture, compartment syndrome or deep vein thrombosis can impair circulation and, in turn, tissue perfusion.

- Assess the five Ps every one to two hours. Report abnormal findings immediately. *Unrelenting pain, pallor, diminished distal pulses, paresthesias, and paresis are strong indicators of compartment syndrome.*
- Assess nailbeds for capillary refill. *Delayed capillary refill may indicate decreased tissue perfusion.*
- Monitor the extremity for edema and swelling. *Excessive swelling and hematoma formation can compromise circulation.*
- Assess for deep, throbbing, unrelenting pain. *Pain that is not relieved by analgesics may indicate neurovascular compromise.*
- Assess the tightness of the cast. *Edema can cause the cast to become tight; a tight-fitting cast may lead to compartment syndrome or paralysis.*
- If cast is tight, be prepared to assist the physician with **bivalving.** *Bivalving, the process of splitting the cast down both sides, alleviates pressure on the injured extremity.*
- If compartment syndrome is suspected, assist the physician in measuring compartment pressure. Normal compartment pressure is 10 to 20 mmHg. *Compartment pressure greater than 30 mmHg indicates compartment syndrome.*
- Elevate the injured extremity above level of the heart. *Elevating the extremity increases venous return and decreases edema.*
- Administer anticoagulant per physician's order. *Prophylactic anticoagulation decreases the risk of clot formation.*

Risk for Infection

The client who undergoes surgical repair will have a postoperative wound. Any break in skin integrity must be monitored for infection.

- Monitor vital signs and lab reports of WBCs. *Increases in pulse rate, respiratory rate, temperature, and WBCs may indicate infection.*
- Use sterile technique for dressing changes. *The initial postoperative dressing will be changed by the surgeon. The nurse must change all subsequent dressings without introducing organisms into the operative site.*
- Assess the wound for size, color, and the presence of any drainage. *Redness, swelling, and purulent drainage indicate infection.*
- Administer antibiotics per physician's orders. *Short-term prophylactic antibiotic administration inhibits bacterial reproduction and thereby helps prevent skin flora from entering the wound. Antibiotics are usually only administered for 24 hours.*

Impaired Physical Mobility

The client who has experienced a fracture requires immobilization of the fractured bone(s). Immobilization alters normal gait and mobility. The client will need to use assistive devices, such as crutches, canes, slings, or walkers.

- Teach or assist client with ROM exercises of the unaffected limbs. *ROM exercises help prevent muscle atrophy and maintain strength and joint function. Flexion and extension exercises prevent the development of foot drop, wrist drop, or frozen joints.*

- Teach isometric exercises, and encourage the client to perform them every four hours. *Isometric exercises help prevent muscle atrophy and force synovial fluid and nutrients into the cartilage.*

- Encourage ambulation when able; provide assistance as necessary. *Ambulation maintains and improves circulation, helps prevent muscle atrophy, and helps maintain bowel function.*

- Teach and observe the client's use of assistive devices, such as canes, crutches, walkers, slings, in conjunction with the physical therapist. *Proper use of devices is necessary for safe ambulation and helps prevent the loss of joint function secondary to complications and falls.*

- Turn the client on bed rest every two hours. If the client is in traction, teach the client to shift his or her weight every hour. *Turning and shifting weight increase circulation and help prevent skin breakdown.*

Risk for Disturbed Sensory Perception: Tactile

The client who has sustained a fracture is at risk for nerve injury from the initial trauma, as well as from complications such as compartment syndrome.

- Assess the ability to differentiate between sharp and dull touch and the presence of paresthesias and paralysis every one to two hours. *Paresthesias develop as a result of pressure on nerves and may indicate compartment syndrome.*

- Elevate the injured extremity above the level of the heart. *Elevating the extremity decreases swelling and the risk of compartment syndrome and nerve entrapment. Check the cast for fit. A tightly fitting cast can decrease blood flow to distal tissues, compress nerves, and cause compartment syndrome.*

- Support the injured extremity above and below the fracture site when moving the client. *Supporting the injured extremity above and below the fracture site helps prevent displacement of bony fragments and decreases the risk of further nerve damage.*

Home Care

Client and family teaching focuses on individualized needs. The type of fracture and its location determine how much teaching the client and family will require. For example, a client who has a simple nondisplaced tibial fracture may need to be taught only cast care and walking with crutches. An older client who has sustained a hip fracture and requires surgical intervention, by contrast, has a wider array of teaching needs, including the use of an abduction pillow, proper bending, and proper sitting. Address the following topics for home care of the client who has fractured a hip:

- Encourage independence in ADLs.
- Explain that the client should sit only on high chairs to prevent excess flexion of the hip; a high toilet seat can be added to a regular toilet seat.
- Encourage the client and family to equip the shower with a rail to aid stability and prevent falls.
- If a walker is needed, teach the client its proper use: Do not carry the walker, but lift it, advance it, and then take two steps, or use a rolling walker.

- If a cane is needed, instruct the client to use it on the affected side.
- Stress the importance of well-balanced meals, and explain all prescribed medications.

Clients who have experienced a fracture or who have had orthopedic surgery often require an extended period of immobilization or limited activities. Address the following topics for home care:

- Do not try to scratch under a cast with a sharp object.
- Do not get a plaster cast wet.
- Follow the physician's order for weight bearing.
- Physical therapy departments or offices often can evaluate the home environment for safety and suggest modifications as needed. Physical therapists also teach walking with crutches, limited weight bearing, transferring, and other activities.
- Home care agencies can teach wound care and provide ongoing monitoring of wound healing.
- Local medical equipment and supply sources rent or sell durable equipment, such as crutches, walkers, wheelchairs, overhead trapeze units, shower chairs, elevated toilet seats, grab bars, and bedside commodes. Slings or braces may be purchased through medical equipment dealers.
- Local pharmacies are good resources for dressing supplies such as antiseptic solutions or ointments, dressings, and tape.
- Fitness equipment suppliers may be useful for rehabilitation needs, such as hand or ankle weights for strengthening exercises.

30 Nursing Care of Clients with Musculoskeletal Disorders

Various metabolic, autoimmune, inflammatory, degenerative, neoplastic, infectious, and structural disorders may affect the musculoskeletal system. Many of these diseases have significant physical, psychosocial, and financial consequences. When these problems occur, clients experience many different individualized responses to their altered health status. Nursing care is directed toward meeting physiologic needs, providing education, and ensuring psychologic support for the client and family.

Arthritis, meaning joint inflammation, and **arthralgia**, meaning joint pain, are terms used to describe many disease processes and manifestations involving the musculoskeletal system. These diseases affect not only the joints, but also the connective tissues of the body. The various types of arthritis are discussed in this chapter in different sections, depending on the primary etiology of the disorder. Arthritis and other rheumatic disorders (various conditions that affect the musculoskeletal system) are widespread, affecting more than 33 million people in the United States. Arthritic disorders are a leading cause of disability; however, their very prevalence may lead the public and health care professionals to treat them as normal aging processes, or discount the validity of the pain and disability experienced by the person with arthritis.

The etiology of most rheumatic disorders is not clear; in many cases, the pathophysiologic processes involved are often complex and poorly understood. Many are primary disorders; others occur as secondary processes associated with another disease. The wear and tear of aging, autoimmune processes, metabolic disorders, genetic factors, and infection are implicated as causative factors in some forms of rheumatic disease.

Metabolic Disorders

Metabolic bone disorders originate in the bone remodeling process, which normally involves a sequence of events of bone reabsorption and formation. In the adult, this process is primarily internal remodeling through replacement of trabecular bone. Adults replace about 25% of trabecular bone every four months through reabsorption of old bone by osteoclasts and formation of new bone by osetoblasts (Porth, 2002). Metabolic bone disorders may result from a variety of factors, including aging, calcium and phosphate imbalances, genetics, and changes in levels of hormones.

The Client with Osteoporosis

Osteoporosis, literally defined as "porous bones," is a metabolic bone disorder characterized by loss of bone mass, increased bone fragility, and an increased risk of fractures. The reduced bone mass is caused by an imbalance of the processes that influence bone growth and maintenance. Although osteoporosis may result from an endocrine disorder or malignancy, it is most often associated with aging.

Osteoporosis is a health threat for an estimated 28 million Americans; 10 million people have osteoporosis and 18 million have low bone mass, increasing their risk for the disease (National Institute of Health [NIH], 2002). Although osteoporosis can occur at any age and in both men and women, it is most common in aging women. Approximately 50% of all women and 13% of men over the age of 50 will experience an osteoporosis-related fracture in their lifetime, most frequently in the hip, wrist, and vertebrae.

Risk Factors

The risk of developing osteoporosis depends on how much bone mass is achieved between ages 25 and 35, and how much is lost later. Certain diseases, lifestyle habits, and ethnic backgrounds increase the risk of developing osteoporosis. Many different variables affect one's risk of osteoporosis—some can be modified and others cannot.

Unmodifiable Risk Factors

Both men and women are susceptible to osteoporosis as they age, because the osteoblasts and osteoclasts undergo alterations that diminish their activity. Women have a significantly higher risk for manifestations and complications of osteoporosis because their peak bone mass is 10% to 15% less than that of men. In addition, age-related bone loss begins earlier and proceeds more rapidly in women, beginning in the 30s and accelerating before menopause. Estrogen in women and testosterone in men appear to help prevent bone loss; decreasing levels of these hormones associated with aging contribute to bone loss. Age-related bone loss in men occurs 15 to 20 years later than in women and at a slower rate.

Caucasians and Asians are at a higher risk for osteoporosis than African-Americans, who have greater bone density (bone mass positively correlates with the amount of skin pigmentation). Premature osteoporosis is increasing in female athletes, who have a greater incidence of eating disorders and amenorrhea. Poor nutrition and intense physical training can result in a deficient production of estrogen. Decreased estrogen, combined with a lack of calcium and vitamin D, results in a loss of bone density (Porth, 2002).

Clients who have an endocrine disorder such as hyperthyroidism, hyperparathyroidism, Cushing's syndrome, or diabetes mellitus are at high risk for osteoporosis. These disorders affect the metabolism, in turn affecting nutritional status and bone mineralization.

Modifiable Risk Factors

Modifiable risk factors include behaviors that place a person at risk for developing osteoporosis, as well as physical changes, such as menopause, whose contribution to osteoporosis can be modified by preventive strategies. Calcium deficiency is an important modifiable risk factor contributing to osteoporosis. Calcium is an essential mineral in the process of bone formation and other significant body functions. When there is an insufficient intake of calcium in the diet, the body compensates by removing calcium from the skeleton, weakening bone tissue. Acidosis, which may result from a high-protein diet, contributes to osteoporosis in two ways. Calcium is withdrawn from the bone as the kidneys attempt to buffer the excess acid. Acidosis may also directly stimulate osteoclast function. A high intake of diet soda with a high phosphate content can also deplete calcium stores (McCance & Huether, 2002).

With menopause and decreasing estrogen levels, bone loss accelerates in women. Estrogen promotes the activity of osteoblasts, increasing new bone formation. In addition, estrogen enhances calcium absorption and stimulates the thyroid gland to secrete calcitonin, a hormone that suppresses osteoclast activity and increases osteoblast activity. Estrogen replacement therapy (ERT) in postmenopausal women can reverse the bone changes that occur as estrogen levels decline in earlymenopause.

Cigarette smoking has long been identified as a risk factor for osteoporosis. Smoking decreases the blood supply to bones. Nicotine slows the production of osteoblasts and impairs the absorption of calcium, contributing to decreased bone density.

Excess alcohol intake is another risk factor for osteoporosis. Alcohol has a direct toxic effect on osteoblast activity, suppressing bone formation during periods of alcohol intoxication. In addition, heavy alcohol use may be associated with nutritional deficiencies that contribute to osteoporosis. Interestingly, moderate alcohol consumption in postmenopausal women may actually increase bone mineral content, possibly by increasing levels of estrogen and calcitonin.

Sedentary lifestyle is another modifiable risk factor that can cause osteoporosis. Weight-bearing exercise, such as walking, influences bone metabolism in several ways. The stress of this type of exercise causes an increase in blood flow to bones, which brings growth-producing nutrients to the cells. Walking causes an increase in osteoblast growth and activity.

Prolonged use of medications that increase calcium excretion, such as aluminum-containing antacids, corticosteroids, and anticonvulsants, increase the risk of developing osteoporosis. Heparin therapy increases bone resorption, and its prolonged use is associated with osteoporosis. Antiretroviral therapy for people with AIDS or HIV infection may cause decreased bone density and osteoporosis (Porth, 2002).

Pathophysiology

While the exact pathophysiology of osteoporosis is unclear, it is known to involve an imbalance of the activity of osteoblasts that form new bone and osteoclasts that resorb bone. Until age 35, when peak bone mass occurs, formation occurs more rapidly than does reabsorption. After peak bone mass is achieved, slightly more is lost than is gained (about 0.3% to 0.5% per year); this loss is accelerated if the diet is deficient in vitamin D and calcium. In women, bone loss increases after menopause (with loss of estrogen), then slows, but does not stop, at about age 60. Older women may have lost between 35% and 50% of their bone mass, older men may have lost between 20% and 35% (Mayo Clinic, 2002).

Osteoporosis affects the diaphysis (shaft of the bone) and the metaphysis (portion of the bone between the diaphysis and the epiphysis). The diameter of the bone increases, thinning the outer supporting cortex. As osteoporosis progresses, trabeculae are lost from cancellous bone (the spongy tissue of bone) and the outer cortex thins to the point that even minimal stress will fracture the bone (Porth, 2002).

Manifestations and Complications

The most common manifestations of osteoporosis are loss of height, progressive curvature of the spine, low back pain, and fractures of the forearm, spine, or hip. Osteoporosis is often called the "silent disease," as bone loss occurs without symptoms.

The loss of height occurs as vertebral bodies collapse. Acute episodes generally are painful, with radiation of the pain around the flank into the abdomen. Vertebral collapse can occur with little or no stress; minimal movements such as bending, lifting, or jumping, may precipitate the pain. In some clients, vertebral collapse may occur slowly, accompanied by little discomfort. Along with loss of height, characteristic dorsal kyphosis and cervical lordosis develop, accounting for the "dowager's hump" often associated with aging. The abdomen tends to protrude and knees and hips flex as the body attempts to maintain its center of gravity.

Fractures are the most common complication of osteoporosis, with the disease being responsible for more than 1.5 million fractures each year. These include 700,000 vertebral compression fractures, 300,000 hip fractures, 250,000 wrist fractures, and 300,000 fractures at other sites (NIH, 2002). There may be no obvious manifestations of osteoporosis until fractures occur. Some fractures are spontaneous; others may result from everyday activities. While wrist and vertebral fractures have not been shown to increase disability or mortality, persistent pain and associated posture changes may restrict the client's activities or interfere with ADLs.

Collaborative Care

Care of the client with osteoporosis focuses on stopping or slowing the process, alleviating the symptoms, and preventing complications. Proper nutrition and exercise are important components of the treatment program.

Diagnostic Tests

The manifestations of osteoporosis can mimic those of other bone disorders, so diagnostic tests are needed to differentiate osteoporosis from other problems.

- *X-rays* provide a picture of skeletal structures; however, osteoporotic changes may not be seen until over 30% of the bone mass has been lost.
- *Quantitative computed tomography (QCT)* of the spine measures trabecular bone within vertebral bodies.
- *Dual-energy X-ray absorptiometry (DEXA)* measures bone density in the lumbar spine or hip and is considered to be highly accurate.
- *Ultrasound* transmits painless sound waves through the heel of the foot to measure bone density. This 1-minute test is not as sensitive as DEXA, but is accurate enough for screening purposes.
- *Alkaline phosphatase (AST)* may be elevated following a fracture.
- *Serum bone Gla-protein,* also called *osteocalcin,* can be used as a marker of osteoclastic activity and, therefore, is an indicator of the rate of bone turnover. This test is most useful to evaluate the effects of treatment, rather than as an indicator of the severity of the disease.

Medications

Estrogen replacement therapy reduces bone loss, increases bone density in the spine and hip, and reduces the risk of fractures in postmenopausal women. It is particularly recommended for women who have undergone surgical menopause before age 50, and often is prescribed for women with other osteoporosis risk factors. Estrogen therapy alone is associated with an increased risk of endometrial cancer, so it usually is prescribed in combination with progestin (hormone replacement therapy or HRT). The choice of using HRT to prevent osteoporosis is one that must be made between the woman and her health care provider.

Table 30-1. Medication Administration — The Client with Osteoporosis

Calcium

Postmenopausal women, regardless if they take replacement estrogens, are encouraged to take calcium to prevent osteoporosis.

Nursing Responsibilities
- Help clients maintain an adequate dietary intake of calcium. The best dietary source is milk and other dairy products, including yogurt.
- Postmenopausal women who take estrogens need 1000 mg of calcium daily. Those who do not take estrogens need about 1500 mg daily to minimize osteoporosis.
- Identify alternate sources, such as skim milk and low-fat yogurt, oysters, canned sardines or salmon, beans, cauliflower, and dark-green leafy vegetables.

Client and Family Teaching
- Take calcium carbonate in divided doses 30 to 60 minutes before meals to allow for absorption.
- Take calcium citrate with meals to minimize gastrointestinal distress.

Calcitonin

Calcitonin-salmon injection, synthetic
Calcimar
Miacalin (injection or nasal spray)

In postmenopausal osteoporosis, calcitonin prevents further bone loss and increases bone mass if the client consumes adequate amounts of calcium and vitamin D. Calcitonin may be used in postmenopausal women who cannot or will not take estrogen.

Nursing Responsibilities
- Calcitonin is protein in nature; both the parenteral and nasal spray forms may cause an anaphylactic-type allergic response. Observe the client for 20 minutes after administration; have appropriate emergency equipment and drugs available to treat anaphylaxis.
- Alternate nostrils daily when administering calcitonin nasal spray.
- Review medical history for conditions that contraindicate use of calcitonin products: hypersensitivity to salmon calcitonin and lactation (calcitonin is secreted in breast milk and may inhibit lactation).

Continued on the next page

Table 30-1. Continued

- Observe for side effects: nausea and vomiting, anorexia, mild transient flushing of the palms of the hands and the soles of the feet, and urinary frequency.
- Teach the client the proper technique for handling and injecting the drug at home.

Client and Family Teaching

- Take the medication in the evening to minimize side effects.
- Warm nasal spray to room temperature before using.
- Rhinitis (runny nose) is the most common side effect with calcitonin nasal spray. Other possible side effects include sores, itching, or other nasal symptoms. Report nosebleeds to your primary care provider.
- Nausea and vomiting may occur during initial stages of therapy; they disappear as treatment continues.
- While taking the medication, be sure to consume adequate amounts of calcium and vitamin D.

Fluoride

Fluoride is a mineral long recognized as essential for the normal formation of dentin and tooth enamel. Fluoride appears to decrease the solubility of bone mineral and, therefore, the rate of bone reabsorption. Its use in preventing and treating osteoporosis is relatively new but promising.

Nursing Responsibilities

- Monitor serum fluoride levels every three months.
- Have bone mineral density studies conducted at 6-month intervals to document progress of bone growth.

Client and Family Teaching

- Take sodium fluoride tablets after meals, and avoid milk or dairy products; these reduce gastrointestinal absorption of the medication.
- While taking fluoride, be sure to maintain an adequate calcium intake.
- Use fluoride mouth rinse immediately after brushing teeth and just before retiring at night. Do not swallow the rinse, and avoid eating or drinking for at least 30 minutes after use.
- Notify the physician if teeth become stained or mottled after repeated use of fluoride mouth rinse.

Raloxifene (Evista) is a selective estrogen receptor modulator (SERM) that appears to prevent bone loss by mimicking estrogen's beneficial effects on bone density in postmenopausal women. It does not have the risks of estrogen. Hot flashes are a common side effect, and this drug should not be taken by a woman with a history of blood clots.

Alendronate (Fosamax), risedronate (Actonel), and etidronate (Didronel) are from the class of drugs known as biphosphonates. Biphosphonates are potent inhibitors of bone resorption that may be used to prevent and treat osteoporosis. They inhibit bone breakdown, preserve bone mass, and increase bone density in the hip and vertebrae. These are especially useful for men, young adults, and to prevent or treat steroid-induced osteoporosis.

Calcitonin (Miacalcin) is a hormone that increases bone formation and decreases bone resorption. Calcitonin increases spinal bone density and reduces the risk of compression fractures; it may reduce the risk of hip fracture as well. Calcitonin usually is prescribed as a nasal spray, although it is also available in parenteral form. Because calcitonin is a protein, it can precipitate anaphylactic-type allergic responses.

Sodium fluoride stimulates osteoblast activity, increasing bone formation. When used to treat osteoporosis, bone mass of the spine increases and the risk of spinal fractures may be reduced. Fluoride therapy may, however, be associated with an increased risk of hip and other nonvertebral fractures (see Table 30-1).

Nursing Care

Osteoporosis is both preventable and treatable; therefore, nursing care focuses primarily on planning and implementing interventions to prevent the disease, its manifestations, and the resulting injuries. An important aspect of preventing osteoporosis is educating clients under age 35.

Health Promotion

Health promotion activities to prevent or slow osteoporosis focus on calcium intake, exercise, and health-related behaviors.

Diet

For clients of all ages, stress the importance of maintaining a daily calcium intake that meets NIH recommendations (see Chapter 39). This is particularly important for adolescent girls and young adult women who may avoid eating many high-calcium foods, such as dairy products, because of concerns about weight. Optimal calcium intake before age 30 to 35 probably increases peak bone mass. Emphasize that lowfat (or nonfat) dairy products also contain calcium, although some fat in the product may enhance calcium absorption.

Milk and milk products are the best sources of calcium. The lactose in milk facilitates calcium absorption as well. Other food sources of calcium include sardines, clams, oysters, and salmon, as well as dark green, leafy vegetables, such as broccoli, collard greens, bok choy, and spinach. For clients who avoid dairy products because of lactose intolerance or a vegetarian diet, suggest alternate sources.

Calcium supplements are available in many forms. Most supplements (including Tums) provide calcium carbonate in the range of 200 to 600 mg per tablet. Other forms of calcium, including citrate, gluconate, and lactate, generally provide a lower amount of elemental calcium per tablet. A combination of calcium with vitamin D is recommended, particularly for older adults who may have a vitamin D deficiency that impairs their ability to absorb and use calcium. (Calcium supplements are discussed in Chapter 39.)

Exercise

Teach clients the importance of physical activity and weight-bearing exercises in preventing and slowing bone loss. Suggest that clients participate in regular exercise, such as walking, for at least 20 minutes, four or more times a week. Inform clients that swimming and pool aerobic exercises are not as beneficial in maintaining bone density, because of the lack of weight-bearing activity.

Healthy Behaviors

Behaviors that help prevent osteoporosis include not smoking, avoiding excessive alcohol intake, and limiting caffeine intake to two or three cups of coffee each day.

Assessment

Collect the following data through the health history and physical examination (see Chapter 28):

- *Health history:* age, risk factors, history of fractures, smoking history, alcohol intake, medications, usual diet, menstrual history including menopause, usual exercise/activity level.
- *Physical examination:* height, spinal curves, low back pain.

Nursing Diagnoses and Interventions

Nursing care of clients who have osteoporosis focuses on teaching about the disease process, helping maintain physical mobility and nutrition, and solving problems associated with pain and injury.

Health-Seeking Behaviors

At multiple points in the client's lifetime, nurses can provide vital information that will help clients use self-care strategies to reduce their risk of developing osteoporosis.

- Assess the client's health habits, including diet, exercise, smoking, and alcohol use. *The risk of developing osteoporosis in later life is affected by such things as diet, regular participation in weight-bearing exercise, and personal habits, such as smoking and alcohol consumption.*
- Teach women and men of all ages about the importance of maintaining an adequate calcium intake. Provide a list of calcium-rich foods, and discuss the use of calcium supplements with clients who do not consume adequate dietary calcium. *Calcium needs vary during the course of a lifetime; however, many clients never consume adequate amounts of calcium. This affects their peak bone mass and the rate of bone loss with aging. Calcium in foods is more completely absorbed than that supplied by calcium supplements.*
- Discuss the importance of maintaining a regular schedule of weight-bearing exercise, either through an exercise program or regular physical activity. *Weight-bearing exercise promotes osteoblast activity, helping maintain bone strength and integrity.*
- Refer clients to smoking-cessation programs and alcohol treatment programs as appropriate. *Smoking interferes with estrogen's protective effects on bones, promoting bone loss. Excess alcohol intake affects the nutritional status of the client, increasing the risk of calcium and vitamin D deficiency.*
- Refer clients with significant risk factors for osteoporosis to primary care providers or clinics for bone-density evaluation as indicated. *Early identification and treatment of osteoporotic changes in bones can reduce the risk and possible long-term consequences of falls and fractures.*

Risk for Injury

Falls that would result in little or no injury in the healthy adult may cause fractures in the client with osteoporosis. Even normal movements such as twisting, bending, lifting, or rising from bed can precipitate a vertebral fracture.

- Implement safety precautions as necessary for the client who is hospitalized or in a long-term care facility. Maintain the client's bed in low position; use side rails if indicated to prevent the client from getting up alone; provide nighttime lighting to toilet facilities. *Most falls are preventable, particularly in hospitals and long-term care facilities.*

- Avoid using restraints (if hospitalized or a resident in a long-term care facility) if at all possible. *Restraints may actually increase the client's risk of falling and increase the risk of injury associated with a fall.*

- Teach clients who are able to participate in weight-bearing exercises to perform exercises at least three times a week for a sustained period of 30 to 40 minutes. The mechanical force of weight-bearing exercises promotes bone growth. *Bones weaken and demineralize without exercise. Walking is an easy, low-impact form of exercise. Swimming (including walking on the bottom of the pool) does not provide the needed weight-bearing activity.*

- Encourage older adults to use assistive devices to maintain independence in ADLs. *Walking sticks, canes, and other assistive devices encourage client independence and support activities that promote bone growth.*

- Teach older clients about safety and fall precautions. *A simple assessment of the client's home for safety and fall risks may reduce the risk of fractures and, in turn, the cost of hospitalization and potential disability and/or death.*

- Evaluate and closely monitor the client's medications. The reasons for, types of, and dosage of the client's medications should be evaluated, especially if the person has been falling frequently or has a change in mental status. *Falls may be related to the number of both prescribed and over-the-counter medications the client is taking.*

Imbalanced Nutrition: Less Than Body Requirements

Most Americans do not maintain their recommended daily intake of calcium. Clients must therefore be made aware of the relationship between an adequate calcium intake and maintaining strong bones.

- Teach adolescents, pregnant or lactating women, and adults through age 35 to eat foods high in calcium and to maintain a daily calcium intake of 1200 to 1500 mg. *The National Institutes of Health recommend a daily calcium intake of 1200 to 1500 mg per day for adolescents and young adults, as well as for pregnant and lactating women.*

- Encourage postmenopausal women to maintain a calcium intake of 1000 to 1500 mg daily, either through diet or a calcium supplement. *Calcium needs for postmenopausal women vary, depending on age and estrogen therapy.*

- Teach clients taking calcium supplements the importance of taking the medication at the proper time and the side effects that may occur. *Free hydrochloric acid is needed for calcium absorption. Calcium carbonate supplement (e.g., Tums) should be taken 30 to 60 minutes before meals to allow adequate absorption. Calcium citrate supplements should be taken with meals to prevent gastrointestinal distress.*

Acute Pain

Advanced stages of osteoporosis can result in pain and immobilization. Acute pain usually results from a complicating fracture, especially a compression fracture of the vertebrae.

- Review activity tolerance and suggest modifications in exercise schedules as indicated. *Clients with osteoporosis should remain active and participate in weight-bearing exercises;*

however, the client's abilities and severity of the disease may warrant a modification in the exercise regimen.

- Suggest anti-inflammatory pain medications for treatment of both acute and chronic phases of pain. Clients should be instructed in the amount and frequency as noted on the manufacturer's labels. *Continuous administration of ibuprofen or other NSAIDs can be useful to provide relief from pain.*

- Suggest the application of heat to relieve pain. *A heating pad may offer temporary pain relief. To avoid the "rebound effect," the heat should be removed every 20 to 30 minutes.*

Home Care

The client who has osteoporosis needs education on safety and preventing falls (see Chapter 38). In addition to home safety, outdoor safety is important, too. Clients should be taught to use assistive devices for added stability, to wear rubber-soled shoes for traction, to walk on the grass when sidewalks are slippery, and to sprinkle salt or kitty litter on icy sidewalks in the winter.

Address the following topics when discussing home care.

- Resources for medical supplies and assistive devices
- Diet, exercise, and medications
- Pain management
- Maintaining good posture to help prevent stress on the spine
- Helpful resources:
  1. National Osteoporosis Foundation
  2. Osteoporosis and Related Bone Diseases National Resource Center (National Institutes of Health)
  3. National Women's Health Resource Center
  4. Older Women's League.

Table 30-2. Differential Features of Osteoporosis, Osteomalacia, and Paget's Disease

Differentiating Features	Osteoporosis	Osteomalacia	Paget's Disease
Pathophysiology	Resorption greater than bone formation	Inadequate mineralization of bone matrix	Excessive osteoclastic activity and formation of poor-quality bone
Calcium level (serum)	Normal	Low or normal	Normal or elevated (especially in immobilized clients)
Phosphate level (serum)	Normal	Low or normal	Normal
Parathyroid hormone level (serum)	Normal	High or normal	Normal

Table 30-2. Continued

Alkaline phosphatase level (serum)	Normal	Elevated	Increased; not a reliable test for clients who have liver disease or are pregnant
Hydroxyproline (urine)	Not applicable	Not applicable	Increased
Radiographic findings	Osteopenia, fractures	Decreased bone density, radiolucent bands known as Looser's zones, or pseudofractures	"Punched-out" appearance of bone, increase in bone thickness, linear fractures, mosaic pattern of bone matrix

The Client with Gout

Gout is a syndrome that occurs from an inflammatory response to the production or excretion of uric acid resulting in high levels of uric acid in the blood (*hyperuricemia*) and in other body fluids, including synovial fluid (McCance & Huether, 2002). This metabolic disorder is characterized by deposits of urates (insoluble precipitates) in the connective tissues of the body. Gout has an acute onset, usually at night, and often involves the first metatarsophalangeal joint (great toe). The initial acute attack is usually followed by a period of months or years without manifestations. As the disease progresses, urates are deposited in various other connective tissues. Deposits in the synovial fluids cause acute inflammation of the joint (**gouty arthritis**). Over time, urate deposits in subcutaneous tissues cause the formation of small white nodules (called **tophi**). Deposits of crystals in the kidneys can form urate kidney stones and result in kidney failure.

Gout may occur as either a primary or secondary disorder. Primary gout is characterized by elevated serum uric acid levels resulting from either an inborn error of purine metabolism or a decrease in renal uric acid excretion due to an unknown cause. Purines are part of the structure of the nuclear compounds DNA and RNA; they may also be synthesized by the body. Impaired uric acid excretion leads to hyperuricemia in the majority of people with primary gout. In secondary gout, hyperuricemia occurs as a result of another disorder or treatment with certain medications. Disorders associated with rapid cell turnover, such as some malignancies (leukemia in particular), hemolytic anemia, and polycythemia, can increase purine metabolism. Chronic renal disease, hypertension, starvation, and diabetic ketoacidosis can interfere with uric acid excretion, as can certain drugs, including some diuretics, such as furosemide, ethacrynic acid, and chlorothiazide; pyrazinamide; cyclosporin; ethambutol; and low-dose salicylates. Ethanol ingestion appears to interfere with uric acid excretion and to accelerate its synthesis. In addition, hospitalized clients with gout are at risk for an acute attack from changes in their diet, abdominal surgery, or medications (Tierney, et al., 2001).

The peak age of onset of gout in men is between 40 and 50 years. It is rare in women before menopause. The disease is more common in Pacific Islanders.

Pathophysiology

Uric acid is the breakdown product of purine metabolism. Normally, a balance exists between its production and excretion, with approximately two-thirds of the amount produced each day excreted by the kidneys and the rest in the feces. The serum uric acid level is normally maintained between 3.4 and 7.0 mg/dL in men and 2.4 and 6.0 mg/dL in women. At levels greater than 7.0 mg/dL, the serum is saturated, and monosodium urate crystals may form. It is not known exactly how crystals of monosodium urate crystals are deposited in joints. Several mechanisms may be involved:

- Crystals tend to form in peripheral tissues of the body, where lower temperatures reduce the solubility of the uric acid.
- A decrease in extracellular fluid pH and reduced plasma protein binding of urate crystals are evident.
- Tissue trauma and a rapid change in uric acid levels may also lead to crystal deposition. A rapid increase in uric acid may occur with tissue trauma and release of cellular components.

The monosodium urate crystals may form in the synovial fluid or in the synovial membrane, cartilage, or other joint connective tissues. They may also form in the heart, earlobes, and kidneys. These crystals stimulate and continue the inflammatory process, during which neutrophils respond by ingesting the crystals. The neutrophils release their phagolysosomes, causing tissue damage, which perpetuates the inflammation.

Manifestations and Complications

The manifestations of gout are hyperuricemia, recurrent attacks of inflammation of a single joint, tophi in and around the joint, renal disease, and renal stones. Unless treated, the manifestations of gout appear in three stages: asymptomatic hyperuricemia, acute gouty arthritis, and tophaceous gout.

Asymptomatic Hyperuricemia

The first stage is asymptomatic hyperuricemia, with serum levels averaging 9 to 10 mg/dL. Most people with hyperuricemia do not progress to further stages of the disease.

Acute Gouty Arthritis

The second state is acute gouty arthritis. The acute attack, usually affecting a single joint, occurs unexpectedly, often beginning at night. It may be triggered by trauma, alcohol ingestion, dietary excess, or a stressor, such as surgery. It is often precipitated by an abrupt or sustained increase in uric acid levels. The affected joint becomes red, hot, swollen, and exquisitely painful and tender.

Approximately 50% of initial attacks of acute gouty arthritis occur in the metatarsophalangeal joint of the great toe. Other sites for acute attacks include the instep of the foot, ankles, heels, knees, wrists, fingers, and elbows. The pain, often intense, peaks within several hours and may be accompanied by fever and an elevated WBC and sedimentation rate. The affected joints are swollen, the skin over the joint is warm and dusky red.

Acute attacks of gouty arthritis last from several hours up to several weeks and typically subside spontaneously. There are no long-lasting sequelae, and the client enters an asymptomatic period called the intercritical period. The intercritical period may last up to 10 years; however, approximately 60% of people experience a recurrent attack within 1 year. Successive attacks tend to last longer, occur with increasing frequency, and resolve less completely than the initial attack.

Tophaceous (Chronic) Gout

Tophaceous or chronic gout occurs when hyperuricemia is not treated. The urate pool expands, and monosodium urate crystal deposits (tophi) develop in cartilage, synovial membranes, tendons, and soft tissues. They are seen most often in the helix of the ear; in tissues surrounding joints and bursae (especially around the elbows and knees); along tendons of the finger, toes, ankles, and wrists; on ulnar surfaces of the forearms; along the shins of the legs; and on other pressure points. The skin over tophi may ulcerate, exuding chalky material containing inflammatory cells and urate crystals. Tophi can also develop in the tissues of the heart and spinal epidura. Although tophi themselves are not painful, they may restrict joint movement and cause pain and deformities of the affected joints. Tophi may also compress nerves and erode and drain through the skin.

Kidney disease may occur in clients with untreated gout, particularly when hypertension is also present. Urate crystals are deposited in renal interstitial tissue. Uric acid crystals also form in the collecting tubules, renal pelvis, and ureter, forming stones. Renal stones are 1000 times more prevalent in people with primary gout (McCance & Huether, 2002). The stones can range in size from a grain of sand to a massive structure filling the spaces of the kidney. Uric acid stones can potentially obstruct urine flow and lead to acute renal failure.

Collaborative Care

The classic presentation of acute gouty arthritis is so distinctive that the diagnosis can often be based on the client's history and physical examination. Treatment is directed toward terminating an acute attack, preventing recurrent attacks, and reversing or preventing complications resulting from crystal deposition in tissues and formation of uric acid kidney stones.

Diagnostic Tests

Diagnostic testing is performed to establish an accurate diagnosis and direct long-term therapy.

- *Serum uric acid* is nearly always elevated (usually above 7.5 mg/dL) and is indicative of hyperuricemia.
- **WBC count** shows significant elevation, reaching levels as high as 20,000/mm³ during an acute attack.
- *Eosinophil sedimentation rate (ESR or sed rate)* is elevated during an acute attack from the acute inflammatory process that accompanies deposits of urate crystals in a joint.
- *A 24-hour urine specimen* is analyzed to determine uric acid production and excretion.
- *Analysis of fluid* aspirated from the acutely inflamed joint or material aspirated from a tophus shows typical needle-shaped urate crystals, providing the definitive diagnosis of gout.

Medications

Medications are used to terminate an acute attack, prevent further attacks, and reduce serum uric acid levels to prevent long-term sequelae of the disease. It is important to treat the acute attack of gouty arthritis before initiating treatment to reduce serum uric acid levels, because an abrupt decrease in serum uric acid may lead to further acute manifestations. Pharmacologic therapy is a mainstay of treatment in achieving these goals.

Acute Attack

NSAIDs are the treatment of choice for an acute attack of gout. Indomethacin (Indocin) is the most frequently used NSAID for gout, although others are equally effective. During an acute attack, indomethacin is usually prescribed at 50 mg every eight hours until the client's manifestations have resolved. Other NSAIDs which may be prescribed include ibuprofen (Motrin), naproxen (Naprosyn, Anaprox), tolmetin sodium (Tolectin), piroxicam (Feldene), and sulindac (Clinoril). While extremely effective, NSAIDs are contraindicated for clients with active peptic ulcer disease, impaired renal function, or a history of hypersensitivity reactions to the drugs. (NSAIDS are fully described in Chapter 41.)

Colchicine can dramatically affect the course of an acute attack. Joint pain begins to diminish within 12 hours of the initiation of treatment and disappears within 2 days. Colchicine apparently acts by interrupting the cycle of urate crystal deposition and inflammation in an acute attack of gout. It has no anti-inflammatory effect in other forms of arthritis, and its use is limited to gout. The use of colchicine is limited by significant side effects. When administered orally, the majority of clients develop significant abdominal cramping, diarrhea, nausea, or vomiting. Intravenous administration is limited by potential toxic effects including local pain, tissue damage if extravasation occurs during injection, bone marrow suppression, and disseminated intravascular coagulation (DIC). It is contraindicated for clients who have significant gastrointestinal, renal, hepatic, or cardiac disease.

Corticosteroids may also be prescribed for the client with acute gouty arthritis. If possible, the intra-articular route is preferred for monoarticular arthritis to avoid the multiple systemic effects of steroid therapy. When gout is polyarticular, corticosteroids may be administered either orally or intravenously.

Analgesics may also be prescribed during an acute episode of gouty arthritis. Either codeine or meperidine (Demerol) may be administered orally every four hours to manage the client's pain. Aspirin is avoided because it may interfere with uric acid excretion.

Prophylactic Therapy

In clients at high risk for future attacks of acute gout, prophylactic therapy with daily colchicine may be initiated. Prophylaxis is particularly useful during the first one to two years of treatment with antihyperuricemic agents. Although colchicine does not affect the serum uric acid directly, it reduces the frequency of attacks by preventing crystal deposition within the joint. The doses required to achieve this effect are small, and few side effects are associated with therapy.

Treatment to reduce serum uric acid levels is typically initiated for clients with recurring gout, tophi, or renal damage. Asymptomatic hyperuricemic clients require no treatment. Uricosuric agents are used for clients who do not eliminate uric acid adequately; allopurinol is prescribed for clients who produce excessive amounts of uric acid. Uricosuric drugs block the tubular reabsorption of uric acid, promoting its excretion and reducing serum levels. These drugs reduce the frequency of acute attacks, particularly when administered with colchicine. Probenecid (Benemid) and sulfinpyrazone (Aprazone, Anturane, Zynol) are the primary uricosuric drugs employed.

Allopurinol (Zyloprim) is a xanthine oxidase inhibitor that lowers plasma uric acid levels and facilitates the mobilization of tophi. Because of its effectiveness in lowering serum uric acid levels, it may trigger an attack of acute gout. The nursing implications for medications used to treat gout are included in Table 30-3.

Dietary Management

Dietary purines contribute only slightly to uric acid levels in the body, and no specific diets are recommended. If a low-purine diet is recommended, the client should be taught that high purine foods include all meats and seafood, yeast, beans, peas, lentils, oatmeal, spinach, asparagus, cauliflower, and mushrooms. The obese client is advised to lose weight, but fasting is contraindicated for clients with gout. Alcohol intake and specific foods that tend to precipitate attacks are to be avoided.

Other Treatments

During an acute attack of gouty arthritis, bed rest is prescribed. It is continued for approximately 24 hours after the attack has subsided, because early ambulation may bring about recurrence of acute manifestations (Tierney, et al., 2001). The affected joint may be elevated, and hot or cold compresses may be applied for comfort.

A liberal fluid intake to maintain a daily urinary output of 2000 mL or more is recommended to increase urate excretion and reduce the risk of urinary stone formation. Urinary alkalinizing agents, such as sodium bicarbonate or potassium citrate, may be prescribed as well to minimize the risk of uric acid stones. It is important to monitor clients receiving these preparations carefully for signs of fluid and electrolyte or acid-base imbalances.

Nursing Care

Clients with gout provide self-care at home. Teaching focuses on self-management of pain and altered mobility.

Nursing Diagnoses and Interventions

Pain is a primary focus for nursing interventions in the client experiencing an acute attack of gout. The client's mobility is also impaired during an acute attack, both because of discomfort and prescribed activity limitations.

Acute Pain

The pain associated with an attack of acute gouty arthritis is intense and accompanied by exquisite tenderness of the affected joint. Measures to alleviate the pain are vital in the initial period until anti-inflammatory medications become effective and the acute inflammatory response is relieved. The following are important in teaching about pain relief:

- Position the affected joint for comfort. Elevate the joint or extremity (usually the foot) on a pillow, maintaining alignment. *Elevation and normal body alignment facilitate blood return from the affected joint, alleviating some of the edema.*
- Protect the affected joint from pressure, placing a foot cradle on the bed to keep bed covers off the foot. *A foot cradle keeps bed linens from applying pressure on the affected joint.*
- Take anti-inflammatory and antigout medications as prescribed. In the initial period, colchicine may be given hourly. *These medications reduce the acute inflammatory response, gradually relieving discomfort.*
- Take analgesics as prescribed. *Supplemental analgesia may be necessary in the acute period until the inflammatory response is mediated.*
- Maintain bed rest. *It is important to immobilize the affected joint and promote rest to prevent exacerbation of joint inflammation.*

Table 30-3. Medication Administration – The Client with Gout

Colchicine

Colchicine is used to terminate an acute attack of gouty arthritis and to prevent recurrent episodes of the disease. Colchicine does not alter serum uric acid levels, but appears to interrupt the cycle of urate crystal deposition and inflammatory response. It may be administered either by mouth or intravenously. Colchicine is also available as a fixed-dose combination with a uricosuric agent, probenecid (Benemid). Only plain colchicine is used to treat an acute attack of gout; combination therapy is employed to prevent further attacks.

Nursing Responsibilities
- Assess for possible contraindications to colchicine therapy, including serious gastrointestinal, renal, hepatic, or cardiac disease.
- Administer the following as ordered:
  1. *Intravenous doses:* Give undiluted or diluted in up to 20 mL sterile normal saline for injection. Administer over a period of two to five minutes.
  2. *Oral doses:* Give on an empty stomach to facilitate absorption.
- Evaluate for adverse effects, including abdominal cramping, nausea, vomiting, and diarrhea, and report promptly, because these side effects may necessitate discontinuation of the drug.

Client and Family Teaching
- Drink three to four quarts of liquid per day.
- Report adverse responses, including gastrointestinal problems, fatigue, bleeding, easy bruising, or recurrent infections, to the physician.
- Do not drink alcohol.

Uricosuric Drugs

Probenecid (Benemid)
Sulfinpyrazone (Anturane)

Probenecid is a uricosuric drug that inhibits the tubular reabsorption of urate, promoting the excretion of uric acid and decreasing serum uric acid levels. Sulfinpyrazone is a uricosuric drug that potentiates the renal excretion of uric acid, reducing serum uric acid levels. It is used to prevent recurrent attacks of acute gouty arthritis and treat chronic gout.

Nursing Responsibilities
- Assess for prior hypersensitivity responses to this drug.
- Administer after meals or with milk to minimize gastric distress.
- Increase fluid intake to at least 3 L/day to prevent the formation of uric acid kidney calculi.
- Administer sodium bicarbonate or potassium citrate as ordered to maintain an alkaline urine.
- Do not administer aspirin to clients receiving probenecid because salicylates interfere with the action of the drug.
- Monitor clients receiving the following drugs concurrently with probenecid for increased or toxic effects: penicillin and related antibiotics, indomethacin, acetaminophen, naproxen, ketoprofen, meclofenamate, lorazepam, and rifampin.

Table 30-3. Continued

- Monitor for possible adverse effects of probenecid, including headache, dizziness, hepatic necrosis, nausea and vomiting, renal colic, bone marrow depression, anaphylaxis, fever, hives, and pruritus.
- Administer sulfinpyrazone with meals or antacid to minimize gastric distress.
- Monitor clients taking sulfinpyrazone with other sulfa drugs for increased or toxic effects; monitor for hypoglycemia in clients receiving insulin or oral hypoglycemics concurrently, and monitor for bleeding or increased anticoagulant effect in clients receiving warfarin concurrently.
- Assess for contraindications to therapy with sulfinpyrazone, including active peptic ulcer disease, a history of hypersensitivity to phenylbutazone or other pyrazoles, or blood dyscrasias.

Client and Family Teaching
- Do not take aspirin or products containing aspirin while taking probenecid. Use acetaminophen for relief of mild pain.
- Drink at least three quarts of fluids per day to minimize the risk of kidney stone formation.
- Take sulfinpyrazone with meals to minimize gastric distress, and report epigastric pain, nausea, or black stools to the physician promptly.

Allopurinol (Zyloprim)

Allopurinol acts on purine metabolism, reducing the production of uric acid and decreasing serum and urinary concentrations of uric acid. It is used for clients with manifestations of primary or secondary gout, including acute attacks, tophi, joint destruction, urinary stones, and nephropathy. It is not indicated for use in the treatment of asymptomatic hyperuricemia.

Nursing Responsibilities
- Monitor intake and output and increase fluid intake to approximately 3 L/day.
- Monitor for desired effect of decreased serum uric acid levels, and for adverse effects, such as nausea, diarrhea, and rash.
- Assess BUN and creatinine levels prior to the initiation of and during treatment with allopurinol. Report signs of impaired renal function, such as an elevated BUN and creatinine, decreased urine output, and dilute or frothy urine to the physician.
- Administer with meals to minimize gastric distress.
- Monitor CBC periodically because allopurinol therapy may cause bone marrow depression.
- In clients receiving warfarin concurrently, monitor prothrombin times and be alert to evidence of bleeding, because allopurinol prolongs the half-life of warfarin.
- Monitor clients receiving chlorpropamide, cyclophosphamide, hydantoin, theophylline, vidarabine, or ACE inhibitors concurrently for increased drug effects.
- Discontinue the drug and notify the physician immediately if the client develops a rash. Rash and hypersensitivity responses occur more frequently in clients receiving ampicillin, amoxicillin, or thiazide diuretics.

Client and Family Teaching
- Stop taking the drug and report any skin rash, painful urination, blood in the urine, eye irritation, or swelling of the lips or mouth to the physician immediately.

Continued on the next page

Table 30-3. Continued

- Take the medication after meals to minimize gastric distress.
- Drink three to four quarts of fluid daily to maintain a urinary output greater than 2 L/day.
- Acute gouty attacks may occur during the initial stages of allopurinol therapy; continue therapy prescribed for attacks, such as colchicine, to minimize acute episodes.
- Do not take a double dose of medication if you miss a dose.

Impaired Physical Mobility

Bed rest is prescribed to prevent further urate mobilization and joint inflammation as well as to protect the affected joint.

- Encourage active and passive ROM exercises of joints and muscle-tensing exercises on unaffected limbs. *These exercises help maintain joint mobility, muscle tone, and the client's sense of well-being.*
- When ambulation is allowed, suggest using a walker or cane as needed. *Weight bearing on the affected limb may be restricted until the inflammation is totally relieved.*
- Resume normal activities as allowed by the physician. *Initial acute attacks of gouty arthritis do not cause permanent damage to the affected joint, and the client can resume usual activities once the attack has subsided.*

Home Care

Discuss the following topics with the client:

- *The disease and its manifestations.* Tell the client that initial attacks cause no permanent damage, but that recurrent attacks can lead to permanent damage and joint destruction. Discuss other potential effects of continued hyperuricemia, including tophaceous deposits in subcutaneous and other connective tissues. Discuss the potential for kidney damage and kidney stones.
- *The rationale for and use of prescribed medication.* Stress the need to continue the medication until the physician discontinues it, even though the client is free of manifestations of gout.
- *The importance of a high intake of fluids each day and avoiding the use of alcohol.*

Degenerative Disorders

Degenerative disorders, especially degenerative joint disease, are the most common form of arthritis in the older adult. Both primary and secondary forms are seen in adults of all ages. Primary or idiopathic osteoarthritis, the most common type, occurs without a clear precipitating factor. Secondary osteoarthritis is associated with an identifiable cause. For instance, it may be related to trauma to a joint, inflammation, skeletal disorders, such as congenital hip dysplasia, or metabolic disorders. Regardless of cause, degenerative disorders of the joints and muscles can lead to impaired mobility and chronic pain. These problems may in turn cause disability, especially in the performance of ADLs by older adults.

The Client with Osteoarthritis

Osteoarthritis (OA) (also labeled *degenerative joint disease)* is the most commonly occurring of all forms of arthritis. This disease is characterized by loss of articular cartilage in articulating joints and hypertrophy of the bones at the articular margins. OA may be idiopathic (without known cause) or secondary (associated with known risk factors). Idiopathic OA affects more than 60 million people in the United States, affecting adult men more than women until after age 55, when the incidence becomes twice as high in women (McCance & Huether, 2002) The joints most affected are in the hand, wrist, neck, lower back, hip, knee, ankles, and feet. Men are more likely than women to have hip OA, while postmenopausal women more often have hand OA.

Localized OA affects only one or two joints. Generalized OA affects three or more joints. Generalized OA may also be classified as nodal (involving the hand) or nonnodal (no hand involvement). Nodal OA may also affect the knees, hips, cervical spine, and lumbar spine. Idiopathic OA most commonly affects the terminal interphalangeal joints (*Heberden's nodes*), and less often the proximal interphalangeal joints (*Bouchard's nodes*), the joints of the thumb, the hip, the knee, the metatarsophalangeal joint of the big toe, and the cervical and lumbar spine. Secondary OA may occur in any joint from an articular injury.

Risk Factors

Idiopathic OA is associated with increasing age, with more than 90% of individuals affected by age 40 but few experiencing manifestations until after 50 or 60 (Maher, Salmond, & Pellino, 2002). It has been suggested that OA may be inherited as an autosomal recessive trait, with genetic defects that cause premature destruction of the joint cartilage. The causes of secondary OA include trauma, mechanical stress, inflammation of joint structures, joint instability, neurologic disorders, endocrine disorders, and selected medications.

Excessive weight contributes to the development of OA, especially in the hip and knee. Inactivity is another risk factor. Moderate recreational exercise has been shown to both decrease the chance of developing OA and the progression of manifestations when OA is present. People involved in strenuous, repetitive exercise, such as participating in sports, have an increased risk of developing secondary OA.

Other risk factors that are linked to OA are hormonal factors, such as decreased estrogen in menopausal women, excessive growth hormone, and increased parathyroid hormone.

Pathophysiology

The cartilage that lines joints provides a smooth surface, so that the bones of the joint glide over one another without friction, and it distributes the load from one bone to the next, dissipating the mechanical stress that occurs with joint loading. This cartilage normally contains more than 70% water. More than 90% of its dry weight is collagen, which provides strength, and proteoglycans, which provide elasticity and stiffness to compression. Cartilage cells, the chondrocytes, nest in this meshwork of collagen and proteoglycans. Normal articular cartilage exudes some of its water with compression, providing lubrication for joint surfaces. This water is reabsorbed during relaxation of the joint.

In OA, proteoglycans and collagen are lost from the cartilage as a result of enzymatic degradation. The water content of the cartilage increases as the collagen matrix is destroyed.

With the loss of proteoglycans and collagen fibers, the cartilage becomes yellow or brownish gray and loses its tensile strength. Surface ulcerations occur, and fissures develop in deeper layers of the cartilage. Eventually, large areas of articular cartilage are lost, and underlying bone is exposed. The bone thickens in exposed areas, reducing its ability to absorb energy in joint loading. Cysts can also develop in the bone. Cartilage-coated **osteophytes** (bony outgrowths often called "joint mice") change the anatomy of the joint. As these spurs or projections enlarge, small pieces may break off, leading to mild synovitis (inflammation of the synovial membrane).

Manifestations and Complications

The onset of OA is usually gradual and insidious, and the course slowly progressive. Pain and stiffness in one or more joints (usually weight bearing) are the first manifestations of OA. The pain is localized to the affected joints and may be described as a deep ache. It is typically aggravated by use or motion of the joint and relieved by rest, although it may become persistent as the disease progresses. Pain at night may be accompanied by paresthesias (numbness, tingling). Pain may also be referred to other parts of the body; for example, OA of the lumbosacral spine may cause severe pain along the path of the sciatic nerve. Following periods of immobility, such as sleeping all night or after a long automobile ride, involved joints may stiffen. Usually only a few minutes of activity are necessary to relieve the stiffness. Range of motion of the joint decreases as the disease progresses, and grating or crepitus may be noted during movement. Bony overgrowth may cause joint enlargement, and flexion contractures may occur because of joint instability. In OA, enlarged joints are characteristically bony-hard and cool on palpation.

OA of the spine may involve the vertebral bodies and intervertebral disks, the diarthrodial joints, or both. Spondylosis is degenerative disk disease. As the intervertebral disks degenerate, disk space between the vertebrae is lost. Degenerative disk disease may be complicated by herniated disk, the protrusion of the nucleus pulposus of the disk. Herniation usually occurs in a lateral direction, potentially compressing nerve roots and causing radicular (distributed along the nerve) pain and muscle weakness. See Chapter 32 for further discussion of disk disorders.

Disk degeneration and joint space narrowing alter the mechanics of the spinal column, promoting osteoarthritic changes in the articular processes (the facet joints) of the vertebrae. The cartilage covering the inferior and superior articular processes degenerates, causing localized pain, stiffness, muscle spasm, and limited range of motion. Osteophytes may form on articular processes, further contributing to pain and muscle spasm.

The presentation of OA in older clients is similar to that in younger adults. However, in this population, the risk of debilitation because of OA is greater, and the disease may progress faster. In addition, pain, stiffness, and limited range of motion increase the risk of falls and fractures in the older adult.

Collaborative Care

At this time, no treatment is available to arrest the process of joint degeneration. Appropriate management, however, is important to relieve pain and maintain the client's function and mobility.

Diagnostic Tests
The diagnosis of OA is generally based on the client's history and physical examination, and X-rays of affected joints. Characteristic changes of OA are visible in X-ray studies of affected

joints. Initially, irregular joint space narrowing is seen. Progressive changes include increased density of subchondral (under cartilage) bone, osteophyte formation at the joint periphery, and the formation of cysts in the bone.

Medications

The pain of OA often can be managed through the use of analgesics, such as aspirin or acetaminophen. Acetaminophen is generally preferred for use in older clients because it has fewer toxic side effects. NSAIDs may also be prescribed. These medications are discussed in more detail in Chapter 41. Capsaicin cream can reduce joint pain and tenderness when applied topically to affected joints.

Medications that have proven effective in decreasing the pain and stiffness of OA are the NSAID COX-2 inhibitors meloxicam (Mobic), celecoxib (Celebrex), and rofecoxib (Vioxx). These medications provide analgesic/anti-inflammatory effects comparable to conventional NSAIDS, but have fewer adverse effects on the gastrointestinal and renal systems. Clients should be taught to report any signs of gastrointestinal bleeding to their health care providers. If meloxicam is prescribed, teach the client that it may decrease the effectiveness of ACE inhibitors and diuretics, may increase lithium levels and toxicity, and there is a risk of increased bleeding if taken at the same time as aspirin, warfarin, and the herbs feverfew, garlic, ginger, and ginko.

Potent anti-inflammatory medications, such as systemic corticosteroids, are seldom prescribed for clients with OA, although intra-articular corticosteroid injections may be used. With intra-articular injections, a long-acting corticosteroid medication, often mixed with a local anesthetic, such as lidocaine, is injected directly into the joint space of the affected joints. Although this procedure may provide marked pain relief, it can hasten the rate of cartilage breakdown if performed more frequently than every four to six months.

Conservative Treatment

Conservative treatment may include any or all of the following:

- Physical therapy for ROM exercises
- Resting the involved joint
- Using a cane, crutches, or a walker
- Weight loss, if indicated
- Analgesic and anti-inflammatory medications.

Surgery

Surgical procedures can provide dramatic results for clients with significant chronic pain and loss of joint function. Although elective surgical procedures are frequently avoided in the older adult, even aged clients can benefit significantly if they do not have a chronic medical condition that contraindicates surgery.

Arthroscopy

Although arthroscopic debridement and lavage of involved joints has been used, certain questions exist about its effectiveness and further research is ongoing (Reuters Health, 2002).

Osteotomy

An **osteotomy**, an incision into or transection of the bone, may be performed to realign an affected joint, particularly when significant bony overgrowth or osteophyte formation has occurred. This procedure may also be used to shift the joint load toward areas of less severely damaged cartilage. Although osteotomy does not halt the process of OA, it may have a beneficial effect on joint function and pain, delaying the need for a joint replacement by several years.

Joint Arthroplasty

A **joint arthroplasty** is the reconstruction or replacement of a joint. Arthroplasty is usually indicated when the client has severely restricted joint mobility and pain at rest. Pain is virtually eliminated, and the function of the joint is generally improved. Arthroplasty may involve partial joint replacement or reshaping of the bones of a joint. For most clients with OA, both surfaces of the affected joint are replaced with prosthetic parts in a procedure known as a **total joint replacement.** Joints that may be replaced include the hip, knee, shoulder, elbow, ankle, wrist, and joints of the fingers and toes.

In a total joint replacement, some or all of the synovium, cartilage, and bone on both sides of the joint are removed. A metallic prosthesis is inserted to replace one joint surface (generally the load-end or distal portion of a weight-bearing joint). The other joint surface is replaced by a silicone-lined ceramic or plastic prosthesis.

Most prosthetic joints are uncemented, that is, made of porous ceramic and metal components inserted so that they fit tightly into existing bone. The implant is secured by new bone growth into the prosthesis, a process that requires approximately six weeks. Although a longer non-weight-bearing period is necessary initially until the prosthesis is fixed in place by the bony growth, the implant appears to have a longer useful life span than cemented prostheses. In a cemented joint replacement, methyl methacrylate (a pliable polymer that hardens to hold the prosthesis in place) is used to secure the prosthesis to existing bone. Although the client is able to resume normal activities more rapidly following a cemented joint replacement, methyl methacrylate initiates an inflammatory response, and the joint eventually loosens.

- In a *total hip replacement,* the articular surfaces of the acetabulum and femoral head are replaced. The entire head of the femur and part of the femoral neck are removed and replaced with a prosthesis. The acetabulum is remodeled, and a prosthesis of high-molecular-weight polyethylene is inserted. The success rate for total hip replacement is reported to be greater than 90%. Approximately 250,000 total hip replacements are done each year in the United States; most are for treatment of OA (McCance & Huether, 2002). Potential problems associated with a total hip replacement include dislocation within the prosthesis, loosening of joint components from surrounding bone, and infection. If recurrent or ineffectively treated, these complications may necessitate removal of the prosthesis, resulting in severe shortening of the extremity and an unstable hip joint.

- *Total knee replacement* is performed if the client has intractable pain and X-ray films show evidence of arthritis of the knee. Several prosthetic devices involving removal of varying amounts of bone are available for knee joint replacement. The femoral side of the joint is replaced with a metallic surface, and the tibial side with polyethylene. More than 80% of clients obtain significant or total relief of pain with a total knee replacement. They must, however, engage in a vigorous program of rehabilitation to achieve the best results. Joint failure is more common with knee replacement than with a total hip replacement. Loosened joint components, often on the tibial side, are the most common cause of failure.

- *Total shoulder replacement* is indicated for unremitting pain and marked limitation of range of motion because of arthritic involvement of both the humeral and glenoid joint surfaces of the shoulder. The joint is immobilized in a sling or abduction splint for two to three weeks following arthroplasty. Dislocation, loosening of the prosthesis, and infection are potential problems associated with total shoulder replacement.

- *Total elbow replacement* involves replacement of the humeral and ulnar surfaces of the elbow joint with a metal and polyethylene prosthesis. Pain and disabling stiffness of the joint are indications for an elbow arthroplasty. Complications, including dislocation, fracture, tricep weakness, loosening, and infection, occur frequently.

Infection is the major complication associated with total joint replacement. Not only does infection interfere with healing and prolong recovery, but also it may necessitate removal of the prosthesis and may lead to loss of joint function. Other potential complications include circulatory impairment to the affected limb, thromboembolism, nerve damage, and dislocation of the joint.

Complementary Therapies

The following complementary therapies are examples of those that may be used by people with OA to relieve pain and stiffness (Springhouse, 1998).

- Bioelectromagnetic therapy
- Eliminating nightshade foods, such as potatoes, tomatoes, peppers, eggplant, tobacco
- Taking nutritional supplements, such as boron, zinc, copper, selenium, manganese, flavonoids, evening primrose oil
- Herbal therapy
- Osteopathic manipulation
- Vitamin therapy
- Yoga.

Nursing Care

OA is a chronic process for which there is no cure. The focus of nursing care for the client with OA is providing comfort, helping maintain mobility and ADLs, and assisting with adaptations to maintain life roles.

Health Promotion

Although OA cannot be prevented, maintaining a normal weight and having a program of regular, moderate exercise will reduce risk factors. Glucosamine and chrondroitin are popular nutritional supplements for OA that are increasingly popular and have been found to be of benefit in reducing manifestations. Clients should discuss these supplements with their health care provider before using them.

Assessment

Collect the following data through the health history and physical examination (see Chapter 28).

- *Health history:* family history of OA, occupation, recreational activities, joint pain and stiffness, ability to carry out ADLs and self-care activities.
- *Physical assessment:* height/weight; gait, joints: symmetry, size, shape, color, appearance, temperature, pain, crepitus, range of motion, Heberden's nodes, Bouchard's nodes.

Nursing Diagnoses and Interventions

Chronic Pain

Pain is a primary manifestation of OA. As joint tissues degenerate and changes in joint structure occur, the amount of discomfort generally increases. The pain associated with OA increases with activity, and tends to be relieved with rest. Nonpharmacologic comfort measures are appropriate, with mild analgesics used to supplement these as needed.

- Monitor the client's level of pain, including intensity, location, quality, and aggravating and relieving factors. *Accurate assessment of pain provides a basis for evaluation of the effect of interventions.*
- Teach clients to take prescribed analgesic or anti-inflammatory medication as needed. *Analgesics reduce the perception of pain and may decrease muscle spasm as well. Anti-inflammatory medication may be ordered to decrease local inflammatory response in affected joints.*
- Encourage rest of painful joints. *The pain of OA is often relieved by joint rest.*
- Suggest applying heat to painful joints using the shower, a tub or sitz bath, warm packs, hot wax baths, heated gloves, or diathermy, which uses high-frequency electrical currents to generate heat. *Heat application reduces accompanying muscle spasm, relieving pain. Moist heat penetrates deeper than dry heat; diathermy delivers heat directly to lesions in deeper body tissues.*
- Emphasize the importance of proper posture and good body mechanics for walking, sitting, lifting, and moving. *Good body mechanics and posture reduce stress on affected joints.*
- Encourage the overweight client to reduce. *Excess weight places abnormal stress on joints, particularly the knees.*
- Teach the client to use splints or other devices on affected joints as needed. *These assistive devices help maintain the correct anatomic position of the joint and relieve stress.*
- Encourage the client to use nonpharmacologic pain relief measures, such as progressive relaxation, meditation, visualization, and distraction. *These adjunctive pain relief measures can reduce the client's reliance on analgesics and increase comfort.*

Impaired Physical Mobility

As intra-articular cartilage degenerates and joint structures are altered, the client with OA experiences pain, stiffness, and decreased range of motion in affected joints. When the spine, large weight-bearing joints of the hips and knees, or the ankles and feet are affected, physical mobility can be significantly reduced.

- Assess the range of motion of affected joints. *Assessing joint mobility is important as a basis for planning appropriate interventions.*

- Perform a functional mobility assessment, evaluating the client's gait, ability to sit and rise from sitting, ability to step into and out of the tub or shower, and negotiation of stairs. *The functional assessment provides vital data about the client's ability to maintain ADLs.*
- Teach the client active and passive ROM exercises as well as isometric, progressive resistance, and low-impact aerobic exercises. *Active ROM exercises help maintain muscle tone and mobility of affected joints and prevent contractures. Isometric and progressive resistance exercises improve muscle tone and strength; aerobic exercise improves endurance and cardiovascular fitness.*
- Suggest the client take analgesics or other pain relief measures prior to exercise or ambulation. *With decreased pain, the client is able to perform exercises better and ambulate greater distances.*
- Encourage the client to plan periods of rest during the day. *Rest helps reduce fatigue, pain, and joint stress.*
- Teach the client how to use ambulatory aids such as a cane or walker, as prescribed. *These devices help relieve some weight bearing and stress on affected joints.*

Self-Care Deficit

Just as OA of the lower extremities can reduce the client's mobility, OA of the upper extremities (the wrist, hand, and finger joints in particular) can significantly interfere with performance of ADLs, such as cooking and brushing the hair. When the lower extremities are affected, bathing and toileting can be difficult.

- Perform a functional assessment of the upper and lower extremities. For upper extremities, assess the ability to touch the back of the head, and to hold and use small items, such as eating utensils. *The functional assessment provides important data about the client's ability to provide self-care.*
- Assess the client's home setting to determine the need for assistive devices, such as handrails, grab bars, walk-in shower stall, or shower chair and handheld showerhead. *Many assistive devices are relatively easy and inexpensive to obtain and can significantly improve the client's independence in performing ADLs.*
- Assist the client in obtaining other assistive devices such as long-handled shoehorns, zipper grabbers, long-handled tongs or grippers for retrieving items from the floor, jar openers, and special eating utensils. *These devices can prolong independence in performing ADLs.*

Home Care

Because of the chronicity of OA, clients and their families need appropriate teaching to manage the disease and its consequences effectively. Much of the teaching focus is on preservation of joint function and mobility. Discuss the following topics:

- Safeguard against hazards to safe mobility, such as scatter rugs. Encourage installation of safety devices, such as hand rails and grab bars.
- Understand the disease process and its chronic degenerative nature.
- Learn exercise techniques, including range of motion, isometric, postural, stretching, and strengthening, to maintain healthy cartilage, preserve range of motion, and develop supportive muscles and tendons. A walking program is beneficial for clients with OA of the knee.

- Do not overuse or stress affected joints with heavy lifting, excessive stair climbing or bending, or other repetitive actions.
- Balance exercise with rest of affected joints through the use of whole body rest, splints, or assistive devices. In addition, sit in a straight chair without slumping; avoid soft chairs or recliners, and sleep on a firm mattress or use a bed board.
- Use pain relief measures including prescribed or over-the-counter analgesic medications, and nonpharmacologic pain relief measures such as heat, rest, massage, relaxation, and meditation.
- For the client who has had a total joint replacement, discuss the following:
  1. Use and weight bearing of the affected limb
  2. Proper use of splints, braces, slings, or other devices to maintain the desired limb position during healing
  3. Appropriate environmental modifications, such as an overhead trapeze for getting out of bed, elevated toilet seats, and types of chairs to use and avoid when sitting
  4. Prescribed exercises
  5. Use of assistive devices for ambulation, such as crutches or a walker
  6. Possible complications, including signs of infection or dislocation, and the need to notify the physician promptly if these occur.
  7. Make referrals to home care, physical or occupational therapy, or other community agencies as indicated.

Autoimmune and Inflammatory Disorders

Autoimmune and inflammatory disorders of the musculoskeletal system are chronic systemic rheumatic disorders, characterized by diffuse inflammatory lesions and degenerative changes in connective tissues. The disorders have similar clinical features and may affect many of the same structures and organs.

The Client with Rheumatoid Arthritis

Rheumatoid arthritis (RA) is a chronic systemic autoimmune disease that causes inflammation of connective tissue, primarily in the joints. It is found worldwide, affecting 1% to 2% of the total population and all races. It affects three times as many women as men. The onset of RA occurs most frequently between the ages of 20 and 40 years. Its course and severity are variable, and the range of manifestations is broad. Manifestations of RA may be minimal, with mild inflammation of only a few joints and little structural damage, or relentlessly progressive, with multiple inflamed joints and marked deformity. Most clients exhibit a pattern of symmetric involvement of multiple peripheral joints and periods of remission and exacerbation.

The cause of RA is unknown. A combination of genetic, environmental, hormonal, and reproductive factors are thought to play a role in its development. It is speculated that infectious agents, such as bacteria, mycoplasmas, and viruses (especially Epstein-Barr virus). may play a role in initiating the autoimmune processes present in RA.

The course of RA is variable and fluctuating. Remissions are most likely to occur in the first year of the disease. The rate at which joint deformities develop is not constant. Disease progression is fastest during the first six years, slowing thereafter. RA contributes to disability and a tendency to shorten life expectancy.

The incidence of RA increases with age up to about 70 years. Although the onset and manifestations of RA are much the same in older and younger clients, differentiating between RA and OA in the older adult may be difficult at times. It is important to establish an accurate diagnosis, however, because the management of these disorders differs significantly. Clinical features distinguishing RA from OA are listed in Table 30-4.

For older clients, RA is managed much as it is for younger people. However, prolonged bed rest or inactivity is not prescribed for acute episodes, because it may result in irreversible immobility in the older adult. Also, pharmacologic therapy is used with greater caution, because of the increased risk of toxicity. In many cases, less emphasis is placed on preventing joint deformity and more emphasis on maintaining function for the older client with RA.

Table 30-4. A Comparison of the Manifestations of Rheumatoid Arthritis and Osteoarthritis

Feature	Rheumatoid Arthritis	Osteoarthritis
Onset	Usually insidious, may be abrupt	Insidious
Course	Generally progressive, characterized by remissions and exacerbations	Slowly progressive
Pain and stiffness	Predominant on arising, lasting .1 hour; also occurs after prolonged inactivity	Pain with activity; stiffness following periods of immobility generally relieved within minutes
Affected joints	• Appear red, hot, swollen; "boggy" and tender to palpation; decreased ROM, weakness	• Affected joints may appear swollen; cool and bony hard on palpation; decreased ROM
	• Multiple joints affected in symmetric pattern; PIP, MCP, wrists, knees, ankles, and toes often involved	• One or several joints affected including hips, knees, lumbar and cervical spine, PIP and DIP, wrist, and 1st MTP joint
Systemic manifestations	Fatigue, weakness, anorexia, weight loss, fever; rheumatoid nodules; anemia	Fatigue

Pathophysiology

It is believed that long-term exposure to an unidentified antigen causes an aberrant immune response in a genetically susceptible host. As a result, normal antibodies (immunoglobulins) become autoantibodies and attack host tissues. These transformed antibodies, usually found in people with RA, are called **rheumatoid factors (RFs).** The self-produced antibodies bind with their target antigens in blood and synovial membranes, forming immune complexes (see Chapter 42 for further information about autoimmune processes).

The damage to cartilage that occurs in RA is the result of at least three processes (McCance & Huether, 2002):

- Neutrophils, T cells, and other synovial fluid cells are activated and degrade the surface layer of the articular cartilage.
- Cytokines (especially interleukin-1 and tumor necrosis factor alpha) cause the chondrocytes to attack the cartilage.
- The synovium digests nearby cartilage, releasing inflammatory molecules containing interleukin-1 and tumor necrosis factor alpha.

Leukocytes are attracted to the synovial membrane from the circulation, where neutrophils and macrophages ingest the immune complexes and release enzymes that degrade synovial tissue and articular cartilage. Activation of B and T lymphocytes results in increased production of rheumatoid factors and enzymes that increase and continue the inflammatory process.

The synovial membrane is damaged by the inflammatory and immune processes. It swells from infiltration of the leukocytes and thickens as cells proliferate and abnormally enlarge. The inflammation spreads and involves synovial blood vessels. Small venules are occluded and vascular flow to the synovial tissue decreases. As blood flow decreases and metabolic needs increase (from the increased number and size of cells), hypoxia and metabolic acidosis occur. Acidosis stimulates synovial cells to release hydrolytic enzymes into surrounding tissues, starting erosion of the articular cartilage and inflammation of the supporting ligaments and tendons.

The inflammation also causes hemorrhage, coagulation, and deposits of fibrin on the synovial membrane, in the intracellular matrix, and in the synovial fluid. Fibrin develops into granulation tissue (**pannus**) over denuded areas of the synovial membrane. The formation of pannus leads to scar tissue formation that immobilizes the joint.

Joint Manifestations

The onset of RA is typically insidious, although it may be acute (precipitated by a stressor, such as infection, surgery, or trauma). Joint manifestations are often preceded by systemic manifestations of inflammation, including fatigue, anorexia, weight loss, and nonspecific aching and stiffness. Clients report joint swelling with associated stiffness, warmth, tenderness, and pain. The pattern of joint involvement is typically polyarticular (involving multiple joints) and symmetric. The proximal interphalangeal (PIP) and metacarpophalangeal (MCP) joints of the fingers, the wrists, the knees, the ankles, and the toes are most frequently involved, although RA can affect any joint. Stiffness is most pronounced in the morning, lasting more than one hour. It may also occur with prolonged rest during the day, and may be more severe following strenuous activity. Swollen, inflamed joints feel "boggy" or spongelike on palpation because of synovial edema. Range of motion is limited in affected joints, and weakness may be evident.

The persistent inflammation of RA causes deformities of the joint itself and supporting structures, such as ligaments, tendons, and muscles. As the joint is destroyed, ligaments, tendons, and the joint capsule are weakened or destroyed. Joint cartilage and bone are also destroyed. Weakening or destruction of these supporting structures results in lack of opposition to muscle pull, causing deformity.

Characteristic changes in the hands and fingers include ulnar deviation of the fingers and subluxation at the MCP joints. Swan-neck deformity is characterized by hyperextension of the PIP joint with compensatory flexion of the distal interphalangeal (DIP) joints. A flexion deformity of the PIP joints with extension of the DIP joint is called a boutonniere deformity. The ability to effect a pinch is limited by hyperextension of the interphalangeal joint and flexion of the MCP joint of the thumb.

Wrist involvement is nearly universal, leading to limited movement, deformity, and carpal tunnel syndrome. Inflammation of the elbows often causes flexion contracture.

The knees are frequently affected in RA, with visible swelling often obliterating normal contours. Instability of the knee joint along with quadriceps atrophy, contractures, and valgus (knock-knee) deformities can lead to significant disability. Ambulation may be limited by pain and deformities when the ankles and feet are involved. Typical deformities of the feet and toes include subluxation, hallux valgus (deviation of the great toe toward the other digits of the foot), lateral deviation of the toes, and cock-up toes (turned-up toes).

Spinal involvement is usually limited to the cervical vertebrae. Neck pain is common, and neurologic complications can occur.

Extra-Articular Manifestations

RA is a systemic disease with a variety of extra-articular manifestations. These are seen particularly in clients with high levels of circulating rheumatoid factor. Fatigue, weakness, anorexia, weight loss, and low-grade fever are common when the disease is active. Anemia resistant to iron therapy frequently affects clients with RA. Skeletal muscle atrophy is common, usually most apparent in the musculature around affected joints.

Rheumatoid nodules may develop, usually in subcutaneous tissue in areas subject to pressure: on the forearm, olecranon bursa, over the MCP joints, and on the toes. Rheumatoid nodules are granulomatous lesions that are firm and either movable or fixed. They may also be found in viscera, including the heart, lungs, intestinal tract, and dura.

Other possible extra-articular manifestations of RA include subcutaneous nodules, pleural effusion, vasculitis, pericarditis, and splenomegly (enlargement of the spleen).

Collaborative Care

The diagnosis of RA is based on the client's history, physical assessment, and diagnostic tests. Diagnostic criteria developed by the American Rheumatism Association are used as well. At least four of seven criteria must be present to establish the diagnosis.

Once the diagnosis of RA has been established, the goals of therapy are to:

*   Relieve pain.
*   Reduce inflammation.
*   Slow or stop joint damage.
*   Improve well-being and ability to function.

No cure currently exists for RA; the goal of treatment is to relieve its manifestations. A multidisciplinary approach is used, with a balance of rest, exercise, physical therapy, and suppression of the inflammatory processes.

Because a cure is not available and traditional therapies are not always fully effective, the client with RA is vulnerable to quackery. Many nontraditional treatments, including diets, topical preparations, vaccines, hormones, plant extracts, and copper bracelets, have been put forth. These treatments are often costly, and none has been shown to be effective.

Diagnostic Tests

Diagnostic tests are used to help establish the diagnosis of RA, although no test specific to the disease is available. Testing is also used to rule out other forms of arthritis and connective tissue disorders.

- Rheumatoid factors (RFs), autoantibodies to IgG, are present in approximately 75% of people with RA. High levels of RF are often associated with severe RA.
- *Erythrocyte sedimentation rate (ESR)* is typically elevated, and is often used as an indicator of disease and inflammatory activity when evaluating the effectiveness of treatment.
- *Synovial fluid examination* will demonstrate changes associated with inflammation, including increased turbidity (cloudiness), decreased viscosity, increased protein levels, and 3000 to 50,000 WBCs.
- *X-rays* of affected joints are taken, and are the most specific for diagnosis of RA. Early in the disease, few changes may be evident other than soft-tissue swelling and joint effusions. As the disease progresses, joint space narrowing and erosions are seen.
- CBC usually shows moderate anemia. The platelet count is often elevated.

Treatments

The primary objectives in treating RA are to reduce pain and inflammation, preserve function, and prevent deformity.

Medications

Four general approaches are used in the pharmacologic management of clients with RA.

- Aspirin and other NSAIDs and mild analgesics are used to reduce the inflammatory process and manage the signs and symptoms of the disease. Although these drugs may relieve manifestations of RA, they appear to have little effect on disease progression.
- The second approach uses low-dose oral corticosteroids to reduce pain and inflammation. Recent studies suggest that low-dose oral corticosteroids also may slow the development and progression of bone erosions associated with RA.
- A diverse group of drugs classified as disease-modifying or slow-acting antirheumatic drugs are employed in the third approach to treating RA. These drugs, which include gold compounds, D-penicillamine, antimalarial agents, and sulfasalazine, appear to alter the course of the disease, reducing its destruction of joints. Immunosuppressive and cytotoxic drugs are included in this category as well.
- Intra-articular corticosteroids may be used to provide temporary relief in clients for whom other therapies have failed to control inflammation.

Aspirin

Aspirin is often the first drug prescribed in the treatment of RA unless its use is contraindicated for the client. Aspirin is an inexpensive and effective anti-inflammatory and analgesic agent. The dose of aspirin required to achieve a therapeutic blood level of 15 to 30 mg/dL and its full anti-inflammatory effect is approximately 4 g per day in divided doses (three or four 5 g [325 mg] tablets qid). This effective dose is just under the toxic dose, which produces tinnitus and hearing loss. The client may be instructed to increase the dose of aspirin gradually until either maximal improvement or toxicity occurs. If tinnitus develops, the client reduces the dose by two to three tablets per day until the tinnitus stops.

Gastrointestinal side effects and interference with platelet function are the greatest hazards of aspirin therapy. Clients are instructed to take aspirin with meals, milk, or antacids to minimize gastrointestinal distress and reduce the risk of GI bleeding. Enteric-coated forms of aspirin and nonacetylated salicylate compounds produce less gastric distress than plain or buffered aspirin and reduce the risk of gastric ulceration, but they are more expensive. Salsalate (Disalcid, Mono-Gesic, Salflex) and choline magnesium trisalicylate (Trilisate, Tricosal) are examples of nonacetylated salicylate products. All salicylate products are contraindicated for clients with a history of aspirin allergy.

Other Nonsteroidal Anti-Inflammatory Drugs

A number of other nonsteroidal anti-inflammatory drugs (NSAIDs) are available for use in the management of RA if aspirin is not tolerated or effective. All NSAIDs act by inhibiting prostaglandin synthesis. Although the efficacy of all NSAIDs, including aspirin, is equivalent, client responses are individual. Several trials of different NSAIDs may be necessary to find the most effective drug.

Some NSAIDs are considerably more expensive than aspirin, but may cause less gastrointestinal distress and require fewer doses per day. Gastric irritation, ulceration, and bleeding remain the most common toxic effects of NSAIDs. They can also affect the lower intestinal tract, leading to perforation or aggravation of inflammatory bowel disorders. All NSAIDs can also be toxic to the kidneys.

NSAIDs commonly prescribed for clients with RA are listed in Table 30-5. Nursing implications of their administration are described in Chapter 41.

Corticosteroids

Systemic corticosteroids can dramatically relieve the symptoms of RA and appear to slow the progression of joint destruction. The long-term use of corticosteroids is associated with multiple side effects, such as poor wound healing, increased risk of infection, osteoporosis, and gastrointestinal bleeding. Severe rebound manifestations can occur when these medications are discontinued. For these reasons, the use of systemic corticosteroids is limited to low dosages daily. The nursing implications for corticosteroid therapy are discussed in Chapter 42.

Disease-Modifying Drugs

Disease-modifying drugs are a diverse group of medications including drugs that modify immune and inflammatory responses, gold salts, antimalarial agents, sulfasalazine, and D-penicillamine (Table 30-6). They share characteristics that make them useful in the treatment of RA. Although beneficial effects are not apparent for several weeks or months following the initiation of therapy, they can produce not only clinical improvement but also evidence of decreased disease activity. Because their anti-inflammatory effect is minimal, NSAIDs are continued during therapy. As many as two-thirds of clients taking disease-modifying drugs show improvement, although these drugs have not been shown to slow bone erosion or facilitate healing. All of these drugs are fairly toxic, and close monitoring is necessary during the course of therapy.

Table 30–5. *Examples of Nonsteroidal Anti-Inflammatory Drugs Used to Treat Rheumatoid Arthritis*

Drug	Average Dose	Comments and Precautions
Aspirin	600–900 mg 4 to 6 times daily	Least expensive NSAID; associated with risk of GI ulceration, bleeding, and possible hemorrhage; may cause hepatotoxicity
Diclofenac (Voltaren)	50 mg tid or qid; or 75 mg bid	Expensive; risk of hepatotoxicity
Etodolac (Lodine)	200–400 mg q6h	Expensive; may have less gastrointestinal toxicity
Fenoprofen (Nalfon)	300–600 mg tid or qid	Should not be administered to clients with impaired renal function; risk of GU effects, such as dysuria, cystitis, hematuria, acute interstitial nephritis, and nephrotic syndrome
Flurbiprofen (Ansaid)	50–100 mg tid or qid, not to exceed 300 mg/day	Expensive
Ibuprofen (Motrin, Advil, others)	300 mg qid; 400–800 mg tid or qid	Available in prescription and over-the-counter forms; less gastric distress reported than with aspirin or indomethacin; discontinue if visual disturbances develop
Indomethacin (Indocin)	25–50 mg bid or tid	A potent NSAID used for moderate to severe RA and acute episodes of chronic disease; higher incidence of adverse GI effects and CNS effects, such as headache, dizziness, and depression
Ketoprofen (Orudis)	50–75 mg tid or qid	Expensive; older adults and clients with renal insufficiency require lower doses
Meclofenamate sodium (Meclomen)	100 mg bid to qid	Increased risk of adverse effects in older adults; GI effects include diarrhea and abdominal pain; anemia may develop during therapy
Nabumetone (Relafen)	1000–2000 mg per day	Most common adverse effects include diarrhea, dyspepsia, and abdominal pain
Naproxen (Aleve, Anaprox, Naprosyn)	250–500 mg bid	Available in prescription and over-the-counter preparations
Oxaprozin (Daypro)	1200 mg daily	Expensive; risk of severe hepatotoxicity; rash may occur

Table 30-5. Continued

Piroxicam (Feldene)	20 mg daily in a single or divided dose	Expensive; GI side effects including stomatitis, anorexia, and gastric distress may occur more frequently than with other NSAIDs
Sulindac (Clinoril)	150–200 mg bid	May be safer for use than other NSAIDs in clients with chronic renal disease; rare fatal hypersensitivity reaction with fever, liver function abnormalities, and severe skin reaction
Tolmetin (Tolectin)	200–600 mg tid	Expensive; may have higher rate of side effects including GI distress, headache, dizziness, elevated blood pressure, edema, and weight gain

Drugs that modify the autoimmune and inflammatory responses in clients with RA include leflunomide (Arava) and etanercept (Enbrel). Leflunomide reversibly inhibits an enzyme involved in the autoimmune process and etanercept inhibits the binding of tumor necrosis factor to receptor sites.

Gold salts may be administered by mouth, but the intramuscular route is preferred because it is more effective. The mode of action of gold is unknown, but it may produce clinical remission in some clients and decrease new bony erosions. Weekly therapy is continued until significant improvement is noted unless toxic reactions occur. Clients experiencing benefit from gold therapy may be continued on monthly injections for several years. About 30% of clients on gold therapy experience toxic reactions, including dermatitis, stomatitis, bone marrow depression, and proteinuria. Mild skin reactions do not always necessitate discontinuation of therapy. CBC and urinalysis are monitored throughout treatment with gold to assess for more severe toxic responses.

Hydroxychloroquine (Plaquenil) is an antimalarial agent sometimes employed in the treatment of RA. Three to six months of therapy is required to achieve the desired response, and many clients do not experience significant benefit. Although hydroxychloroquine has a relatively low toxicity, it can cause pigmentary retinitis and vision loss. Clients receiving this drug require a thorough vision examination every six months.

Sulfasalazine, a drug regularly prescribed for chronic inflammatory bowel disease, may also be prescribed for RA. See Chapter 20 for further discussion of this drug and its nursing implications. For clients not responding to the above preparations, penicillamine may be prescribed. Although this agent may be effective in the management of RA, toxic reactions are common and can be severe, including bone marrow suppression, proteinuria, and nephrosis.

Table 30-6. Disease-Modifying Drugs Used to Treat Rheumatoid Arthritis

Class/Medications	Usual Dose	Adverse Effects	Comments/Nursing Responsibilities
Gold salts:			
Gold sodium thiomalate (Myochrysine)	Parenteral: 1st dose 10 mg; 2nd dose 25 mg, then 50 mg weekly IM	• Pruritus, dermatitis • Stomatitis, metallic taste • Renal toxicity • Blood dyscrasias • Gastrointestinal distress • CNS reactions including irritability, nightmares, psychoses • Retinopathy • Alopecia, pruritus • Blood dyscrasias • GI disturbances	• Frequent UA and CBC • Monitor client after injection for flushing, fainting, dizziness, sweating, possible anaphylactic reaction • Should not be used during pregnancy • Regular ophthalmologic examination required
Aurothioglucose (Solganal)	Oral: 6 mg daily		
Auranofin (Ridaura Capsules)	200–600 mg daily with meals		
Antimalarial:			
Hydroxychloroquine (Plaquenil)	2 g/day in divided doses with meals	• Anorexia, nausea, vomiting, gastric distress • Decreased sperm count • Headache • Rash • Blood dyscrasias • Hypersensitivity responses including Stevens-Johnson syndrome • CNS, liver, and renal toxicity • Skin rashes • Fever • Gastrointestinal distress • Oral ulcers, loss of taste • Fever • Bone marrow depression with thrombocytopenia, leukopenia, anemia • Renal toxicity • May induce immune complex disorders such as Goodpasture's syndrome and myasthenia gravis	• Administer in evenly divided doses • Maintain high fluid intake • May cause yellow-orange skin or urine discoloration • Regular CBCs necessary • Regular CBC and UA necessary • Administer on an empty stomach • Discontinue during pregnancy • May require 2 to 3 months of therapy before benefit is seen
Sulfasalazine (Azulfidine)			
Penicillamine (Cuprimine, Depen Titratable)	125–250 mg/day initially, slowly increased to a total of 1000–1500 mg/day		

Immunosuppressive Therapy

Immunosuppressive or cytotoxic drugs are increasingly employed in the management of RA. Indeed, many now consider methotrexate the treatment of choice for clients with aggressive RA. Methotrexate may be used along with NSAIDs in the initial treatment plan. A weekly dose can produce a beneficial effect in as few as two to four weeks. Gastric irritation and stomatitis are the most frequent side effects associated with methotrexate. Alcoholism, diabetes, obesity, advanced age, and renal disease increase the risk of toxic effects (hepatotoxicity, bone marrow suppression, interstitial pneumonitis).

Other immunosuppressive agents such as cyclosporine, azathioprine, and monoclonal antibodies, have also been employed in the treatment of clients with severe, progressive, crippling disease who have failed to respond to other measures.

Rest and Exercise

A balanced program of rest and exercise is an important component in the management of clients with RA. During an acute exacerbation of the disease, the client may be hospitalized, or a short period of complete bed rest may be prescribed. For most clients, regular rest periods during the day are beneficial to reduce manifestations of the disease. Additionally, splinting of inflamed joints reduces unwanted motion and provides local joint rest. A variety of orthotic devices are available to reduce joint strain and help maintain function.

Rest must be balanced with a program of physical therapy and exercise to maintain muscle strength and joint mobility. Range-of-motion exercises are prescribed to maintain joint function and prevent contractures. Isometric exercises are used to improve muscle strength without increasing joint stress. Isotonic exercises also help improve muscle strength and preserve function. Low-impact aerobic exercises, such as swimming and walking, have been shown to benefit clients with RA without adversely affecting joint inflammation or prompting acute episodes.

Physical and Occupational Therapy

Physical and occupational therapists can design and monitor individualized activity and rest programs.

Heat and Cold

Heat and cold are used for their analgesic and muscle-relaxing effects. Moist heat is generally the most effective, and can be provided by a tub bath. Joint pain is relieved in some clients through the application of cold.

Assistive Devices and Splints

Assistive devices, such as a cane, walker, or elevated toilet seat, are most useful for clients with significant hip or knee arthritis. Splints provide joint rest and prevent contractures. Night splints for the hands and/or wrists should maintain the extremity in a position of maximum function. The best "splint" for the hip is lying prone for several hours a day on a firm bed. In general, splints should be applied for the shortest period needed, should be made of lightweight materials, and should be easily removed to perform ROM exercises once or twice a day.

Diet

For most clients with RA, an ordinary, well-balanced diet is recommended. Some clients may benefit from substitution of usual dietary fat with omega-3 fatty acids found in certain fish oils.

Surgery

Surgical intervention may be employed for the client with RA at a variety of disease stages. Early in the course of the disease, synovectomy, excision of synovial membrane, can provide temporary relief of inflammation, relieve pain, and slow the destructive process, helping to preserve joint function. Arthrodesis, joint fusion, may be used to stabilize joints, such as cervical vertebrae, wrists, and ankles. Arthroplasty, or total joint replacement, may be necessary in cases of gross deformity and joint destruction. Total joint replacement and nursing care needs of clients undergoing this surgery are discussed in the preceding section on OA.

Other Therapies

Several newer treatments that are not yet in widespread use may be employed in clients with progressive RA. These experimental therapies are directed toward ameliorating the underlying immunologic process. Plasmapheresis has been used to remove circulating antibodies, moderating the autoimmune response. Total lymphoid irradiation decreases total lymphocyte levels, although serious adverse effects are associated with this treatment, and its continued efficacy has not been established.

Nursing Care

Clients with chronic, progressive, systemic disorders, such as RA, have multiple nursing care needs involving all functional health patterns. Physical manifestations of the disease often result in acute and chronic pain, fatigue, impaired mobility, and difficulty performing routine tasks. The disease also has many psychosocial effects. The client has an incurable chronic disease that may lead to severe crippling. Pain and fatigue can interfere with the client's ability to perform expected roles, such as home maintenance or job responsibilities. Even though the client's hands may appear swollen, other people may not understand the systemic nature of the disease or realize the difference between RA and OA.

Health Promotion

People with RA have control of their lives by becoming arthritis self-managers. They can help prevent deformities and the effects of arthritis by following prescriptions for exercise, rest, weight management, posture, and positioning. The following suggestions are outlined by the Moss Rehab Resource Net (2002):

- Never attempt an activity that cannot be stopped immediately if it proves to be beyond your power to complete it.
- Respect pain as a warning signal. When you experience pain, change your method of doing things, use equipment or tools if necessary, and take intermittent rest periods.
- Use the strongest joints available for an activity. For example, use the palm of your hand or the crook of your elbow instead of fingers for grasping while carrying.
- Avoid stress toward a position of deformity, such as when the fingers drift toward the little finger. For example, open a jar with your right hand and close a jar with your left hand.
- Avoid activities that need a tight grip, such as writing, wringing, and unscrewing.

Assessment

Collect the following data through the health history and physical examination (see Chapter 28).

- *Health history:* pain, stiffness, fatigue, joint problems: location, duration, onset, effect on function, fever, sleep patterns, past illnesses or surgery, ability to carry out ADLs and self-care activities.
- *Physical assessment:* height/weight; gait, joints: symmetry, size, shape, color, appearance, temperature, range of motion, pain; skin: nodules, purpura; respiratory: cough, crackles; cardiovascular: pericardial friction rub, apical bradycardia, S3.

Nursing Diagnoses and Interventions

Many nursing diagnoses may be appropriate for the client with RA. This section focuses on those related to its predominant manifestations and their effect on the client's life.

Chronic Pain

Pain is a constant feature of RA when the disease is active. Pain accompanies both acute inflammation and lower levels of chronic inflammation. Some clients say the pain in joints and surrounding tissue is like a deep, constant toothache. Pain can significantly affect the client's ability to provide self-care and maintain daily activities. It also contributes to the client's fatigue.

- Monitor the level of pain and duration of morning stiffness. *Pain and morning stiffness are indicators of disease activity. Increased pain may necessitate changes in the therapeutic treatment plan.*
- Encourage the client to relate pain to activity level and adjust activities accordingly. Teach the importance of joint and whole-body rest in relieving pain. *Pain is an indicator of excess stress on inflamed joints. Increasing pain indicates a need to decrease activity levels.*
- Teach the use of heat and cold applications to provide pain relief. The client may apply heat by showering or taking tub baths, or using warm compresses or other local applications, such as paraffin dips. For clients who find that heat increases pain and swelling during periods of acute inflammation, cold packs may be more effective. *Both heat and cold have analgesic effects and can help relieve associated muscle spasms.*
- Teach about the use of prescribed anti-inflammatory medications and the relationship of pain and inflammation. *Anti-inflammatory agents reduce chemical mediators of inflammation and swelling, relieving pain.*
- Encourage using other nonpharmacologic pain relief measures, such as visualization, distraction, meditation, and progressive relaxation techniques. *These techniques can reduce muscle tension and help the client focus away from the pain, decreasing the intensity of the pain experience.*

Fatigue

The pain and chronic inflammatory processes associated with RA lead to fatigue. Other factors contribute as well. Discomfort often disrupts the client's sleep patterns. Anemia, muscle atrophy, and poor nutrition also play a role in the development of fatigue. The client with RA may experience depression or hopelessness, with associated manifestations of fatigue.

- Encourage a balance of periods of activity with periods of rest. *Both joint and whole-body rest are important to reduce the inflammatory response.*

- Stress the importance of planned rest periods during the day. *Rest is vital during acute exacerbations of the disease, and is also important to maintain the client in remission.*

- Help in prioritizing activities, performing the most important ones early in the day. *Assigning priorities helps the client avoid performing relatively unimportant activities at the expense of more meaningful and important ones.*

- Encourage regular physical activity in addition to prescribed ROM exercises. *Aerobic exercise promotes a sense of well-being and restful sleep patterns.*

- Refer to counseling or support groups. *Counseling and support groups can help the client develop effective coping strategies and deal with depression and hopelessness.*

Ineffective Role Performance

Fatigue, pain, and the crippling effects of RA can interfere with the client's ability to pursue a career and fill other life roles, such as parent, spouse, or homemaker. As the client's role changes, so must the roles of other family members. This can contribute to changes in family processes, increased stress in the family, and further difficulty coping with the effects of the disease.

- Discuss the effects of the disease on the client's career and other life roles. Encourage the client to identify changes brought on by the disease. *Discussion helps the client to accept the changes and begin to identify strategies for coping with them.*

- Encourage the client and family to discuss their feelings about role changes and grieve lost roles or abilities. *Verbalization allows family members to validate and accept feelings about losses and changes, thus helping them to move into new roles.*

- Listen actively to concerns expressed by the client and family members; acknowledge the validity of concerns about the disease, prescribed treatment, and the prognosis. *Demonstrating acceptance of these feelings and concerns promotes trust and validates their reality.*

- Help the client and family identify strengths they can use to cope with role changes. *Identifying strengths helps the client and family to consider role changes that maintain self-esteem and dignity.*

- Encourage the client to make decisions and assume personal responsibility for disease management. *Clients who assume a personal and active role in managing their disease maintain a greater sense of self-control and self-esteem.*

- Encourage the client to maintain life roles as far as the disease allows. *Maintaining roles helps the client continue to feel useful and stay in contact with other people.*

Disturbed Body Image

The acute and long-term effects of RA can affect the client's body image, leading to feelings of hopelessness and powerlessness, social withdrawal, and difficulty adapting to changes. When inflammation and joint deformity occur despite compliance, the client may have difficulty accepting the need to continue therapeutic measures, particularly those that have side effects or are costly or time consuming. In addition, unproven alternative treatment strategies and quackery may become increasingly attractive to the client.

- Demonstrate a caring, accepting attitude toward the client. *This attitude helps the client accept the physical changes brought on by the disease.*

- Encourage the client to talk about the effects of the disease, both physical effects and effects on life roles. *Verbalization helps the client identify feelings and gives the nurse opportunity to validate these feelings.*

- Encourage the client to maintain self-care and usual roles to the extent possible. Discuss the use of clothing and adaptive devices that promote independence. *Independence enhances the client's self-esteem.*

- Provide positive feedback for self-care activities and adaptive strategies. *Positive reinforcement encourages the client to continue adaptive measures and maintain independence.*

- Refer to self-help groups, support groups, and other agencies that provide assistive devices and literature. *These groups and agencies can help the client develop adaptive strategies to cope with the effects of RA, enhancing the client's self-concept, body image, and independence.*

Home Care

RA is typically a chronic, progressive disease. As with most diseases of this nature, involvement of the client and family in its management is vital. Education is an important nursing role in caring for clients with RA and their families. Address the following topics for home care of the client and for family members:

- Disease process and treatments, including rest and exercise
- Medications
- Management of stiffness and pain
- Energy conservation
- Use of assistive devices to maintain independence, including self-care aids such as handheld showers, long-handled brushes and shoe horns, and eating utensils with oversized or special handles
- Clothing options such as elastic waist pants without zippers, Velcro closures, zippers with large pull-tabs, and slip-on shoes
- How to apply splints and take care of skin
- Home and equipment modifications, such as a raised toilet seat, grab bars in the bathroom, a bath chair, or adapted counter heights for clients in a wheelchair
- Physical therapy, occupational therapy, home health and homemaker services
- Helpful resources:
  1. National Institute of Arthritis and Musculoskeletal and Skin Diseases
  2. American College of Rheumatology
  3. Arthritis Foundation
  4. American Physical Therapy Foundation
  5. American Chronic Pain Association.

The Client with Systemic Lupus Erythematosus

Systemic lupus erythematosus (SLE) is a chronic inflammatory immune complex connective-tissue disease. It affects almost all body systems, including the musculoskeletal system. The manifestations of SLE are widely variable, thought to result from cell and tissue damage caused by deposition of antigen-antibody complexes in connective tissues. SLE affects multiple body systems, and it can range from a mild, episodic disorder to a rapidly fatal disease process.

Approximately 1 person in 2000 is affected by SLE, with women predominating by a ratio of 9:1 over men. The disease usually affects women of childbearing age (during which the incidence is 30 times greater than in men), but it can occur at any age. It is more common in African-Americans, Hispanics, and Asians than it is in Caucasians (Porth, 2002). The incidence is higher in some families.

Although the exact etiology of SLE is unknown, genetic, environmental, and hormonal factors play a role in its development. Twin studies and a familial pattern of the disease point to a genetic component, as does an increased incidence of other connective-tissue diseases in relatives of people with SLE. Certain human leukocyte antigen (HLA) genes are seen more frequently in people with SLE. Environmental factors, such as viruses, bacterial antigens, chemicals, drugs, or ultraviolet light, may play a role in activation of the pathologic mechanisms of the disease. In addition, it is felt that sex hormones may influence the development of SLE. Women with SLE have reduced levels of several active androgens that are known to inhibit antibody responses. Estrogens have been shown to enhance antibody responses and have an adverse effect in clients with SLE.

The course of SLE is mild and chronic in most clients, with periods of remission and exacerbation. The number and severity of exacerbations tend to decrease with time. In some clients, however, SLE is a virulent disease with significant organ system involvement.

Clients with active disease have an increased risk for infections, which are often opportunistic and severe. Infections such as pneumonia and septicemia are the leading cause of death in clients with SLE, followed by the effects of renal or central nervous system involvement.

Pathophysiology

The pathophysiology of SLE involves the production of a large variety of autoantibodies against normal body components, such as nucleic acids, erythrocytes, coagulation proteins, lymphocytes, and platelets. Autoantibody production results from hyperreactivity of B cells (humoral response) because of disordered T-cell function (cellular immune response). The most characteristic autoantibodies in SLE are produced in response to nucleic acids, including DNA, histones, ribonucleoproteins, and other components of the cell nucleus.

SLE autoantibodies react with their corresponding antigen to form immune complexes, which are then deposited in the connective tissue of blood vessels, lymphatic vessels, and other tissues. The deposits trigger an inflammatory response leading to local tissue damage. The kidneys are a frequent site of complex deposition and damage; other tissues affected include the musculoskeletal system, brain, heart, spleen, lung, GI tract, skin, and peritoneum. The autoantibodies produced and their target tissue determine the manifestations of SLE.

A number of drugs can cause a syndrome that mimics lupus in clients with no other risk factors for the disease. Procainamide (Procan-SR, Pronestyl, others) and hydralazine (Apresoline, Hydralyn) are the most common drugs implicated, along with isoniazid (INH).

Renal and CNS manifestations of SLE rarely occur with drug-induced lupus, but arthritic and other systemic symptoms are common. Manifestations of drug-induced lupus usually resolve when the medication is discontinued.

Manifestations and Complications

Typical early manifestations of SLE mimic those of rheumatoid arthritis, including systemic manifestations of fever, anorexia, malaise, and weight loss, and musculoskeletal manifestations of multiple arthralgias and symmetric polyarthritis. Joint symptoms affect more than 90% of clients with SLE. Although synovitis may be present, the arthritis associated with SLE is rarely deforming.

Most people affected by SLE have skin manifestations at some point during their disease. In fact, SLE was originally described as a skin disorder and named for the characteristic red butterfly rash across the cheeks and bridge of the nose. Many clients with SLE are photosensitive; a diffuse maculopapular rash on skin exposed to the sun is also common. Other cutaneous manifestations include discoid lesions (raised, scaly, circular lesions with an erythematous rim), hives, erythematous fingertip lesions, and splinter hemorrhages. Alopecia is common in clients with SLE, although the hair usually grows back. Painless mucous membrane ulcerations may occur on the lips or in the mouth or nose.

Approximately 50% of people with SLE experience renal manifestations of the disease, including proteinuria, cellular casts, and nephrotic syndrome. Up to 10% develop renal failure as a result of the disease.

Hematologic abnormalities, such as anemia, leukopenia, and thrombocytopenia, are common with SLE. Cardiovascular disorders. such as pericarditis, vasculitis, and Raynaud's phenomenon, often occur. Less frequently, myocarditis, endocarditis, and venous or arterial thrombosis may develop. Pleurisy, pleural effusions, and lupus pneumonitis are common pulmonary manifestations of SLE.

Many clients with SLE develop transient nervous system involvement, often within the first year of the disease. Organic brain syndrome manifestations include decline in intellect, memory loss, and disorientation. Other possible neurologic manifestations include psychosis, seizures, depression, and stroke. Ocular manifestations of SLE include conjunctivitis, photophobia, and transient blindness due to retinal vasculitis.

Gastrointestinal symptoms of SLE, such as anorexia, nausea, abdominal pain, and diarrhea, may affect up to 45% of clients with the disease. The liver may be enlarged, and liver function tests may yield abnormal results.

Clients with SLE who become pregnant may experience abrupt onset of hypertension, edema, and proteinuria (a syndrome similar to pregnancy-induced hypertension). Midtrimester fetal death may result.

Collaborative Care

Because of the diversity of organ system involvement and manifestations of SLE, diagnosis can be difficult. No one specific test is available to confirm the presence of this disease in all people suspected of having it. Instead, the diagnosis is based on the client's history and physical assessment, as well as laboratory studies.

As with rheumatoid arthritis, effective management of SLE requires teamwork, with active participation by both the client and the physician. Communication, trust, and emotional support are especially important. Although there is no cure for SLE, the 10-year survival rate is greater than 70% among clients with this disease, which was once considered fatal in most cases.

Diagnostic Tests

The multiple autoantibodies produced in SLE cause a number of abnormalities in laboratory studies.

*   *Anti-DNA antibody testing* is a more specific indicator of SLE, because these antibodies are rarely found in any other disorder.
*   *Eosinophil sedimentation rate (ESR)* is typically elevated, occasionally to >100 mm/hr.
*   *Serum complement levels* are usually decreased as complement is consumed or "used up" by the development of antigen-antibody complexes.
*   *CBC abnormalities* include moderate to severe anemia, leukopenia and lymphocytopenia, and possible thrombocytopenia.
*   *Urinalysis* shows mild proteinuria, hematuria, and blood cell casts during exacerbations of the disease when the kidneys are involved. *Renal function tests* including a serum creatinine and blood urea nitrogen (BUN) may also be ordered to evaluate the extent of renal disease.
*   *Kidney biopsy* may be performed to assess the severity of renal lesions and guide therapy.

Medications

The client with mild or remittent lupus erythematosus may need little or no therapy other than supportive care. Arthralgias, arthritis, fever, and fatigue can often be managed with aspirin or other NSAIDs. Aspirin is particularly beneficial for clients with SLE because its antiplatelet effects help prevent thrombosis. It may, however, cause liver toxicity and hepatitis.

Skin and arthritic manifestations of SLE may be treated with antimalarial drugs, such as hydroxychloroquine (Plaquenil). Hydroxychloroquine has also been shown to be effective in reducing the frequency of acute episodes of SLE in people with mild or inactive disease. Retinal toxicity and possibly irreversible blindness are the primary concerns with this drug. For this reason, the client taking hydroxychloroquine undergoes ophthalmologic exam every six months.

Clients with severe and life-threatening manifestations of SLE, such as nephritis, hemolytic anemia, myocarditis, pericarditis, or CNS lupus, require corticosteroid therapy in high doses. Such clients may require 40 to 60 mg of prednisone per day initially. The dosage is tapered as rapidly as the client's disease allows, although lowering the dosage may precipitate an acute episode. Some clients with SLE require long-term corticosteroid therapy to manage symptoms and prevent major organ damage. These clients are at increased risk for corticosteroid side effects, such as cushingoid effects, weight gain, hypertension, infection, accelerated osteoporosis, and hypokalemia.

Immunosuppressive agents, such as cyclophosphamide or azathioprine, may be used, alone or in combination with corticosteroids, to treat clients with active SLE or lupus nephritis. When these agents are used in combination, lower, less toxic doses of each drug can be used. The client receiving immunosuppressive agents is at increased risk for infection, malignancy, bone marrow depression, and toxic effects specific to the drug prescribed.

Other Treatments

Because of the photosensitivity associated with SLE, the client should be cautioned to avoid sun exposure. Clients should use sunscreens with a sun protection factor (SPF) rating of 15 or higher when out of doors. Topical corticosteroids may be used to treat skin lesions. Some physicians recommend avoiding the use of oral contraceptives, because estrogen can trigger an acute episode.

Clients with lupus nephritis who progress to develop end-stage renal disease are treated with dialysis (hemodialysis or peritoneal dialysis) and kidney transplantation. These treatment strategies are discussed in Chapter 24.

Nursing Care

Nursing care for the client with mild SLE may be limited to teaching. The client with severe disease, however, has many diverse nursing needs, which vary according to the organ systems involved. Because of the close link between rheumatoid arthritis and SLE, many of the nursing diagnoses and interventions identified for the client with arthritis may be appropriate for the client with lupus. The client with lupus nephritis or end-stage renal disease has the nursing care needs outlined in the sections of Chapter 27 related to glomerulonephritis and chronic renal failure. This section focuses on the unique needs of the client related to the dermatologic manifestations of lupus, an increased risk for infection, and health maintenance problems.

Nursing Diagnoses and Interventions

Impaired Skin Integrity

Skin lesions are a common manifestation of SLE. A rash or discoid lesion interrupts the integrity of the skin and the first line of protection against infection, increasing the client's already high risk of infection. These lesions, which usually appear on exposed parts of the skin, can also be disfiguring and cause the client emotional distress.

- Assess knowledge of SLE and its possible effects on the skin. *Assessment allows the nurse to base teaching and information on the client's existing knowledge, improving learning and retention.*
- Discuss the relationship between sun exposure and disease activity, both dermatologic and systemic. *It is important for the client to understand that sun exposure may not only cause dermatologic manifestations, but also trigger an acute episode.*
- Help the client identify strategies to limit sun exposure:
  1. Avoid being out of doors during hours of greatest sun intensity (10:00 a.m. to 3:00 p.m.).
  2. Use sunscreen with an SPF of 15 or higher when sun exposure cannot be avoided.
  3. Reapply sunscreen after swimming, exercising, or bathing.
  4. Wear loose clothing with long sleeves and wide-brimmed hats when out of doors.

These strategies can help the client maintain a normal lifestyle while helping to prevent acute episodes.

- Keep skin clean and dry; apply therapeutic creams or ointments to lesions as prescribed. *These measures promote healing and reduce the risk of infection.*

Ineffective Protection

Ineffective protection can be a problem for the client with SLE, who is at increased risk for infection and multiple organ system problems because of the disease. In addition, treatment with corticosteroids or immunosuppressive agents further impairs immune responses and the ability to fight infection. The following interventions are for the client who is hospitalized:

- Wash hands before and after providing direct care. *Handwashing removes transient organisms from the skin, reducing the risk of transmission to the client.*

- Use strict aseptic technique in caring for intravenous lines and indwelling urinary catheters or performing any wound care. *Aseptic technique offers protection against external and resident host microorganisms.*

- Assess frequently for signs and symptoms of infection. Monitor temperature and vital signs every four hours. Assess for signs of cellulitis, including tenderness, redness, swelling, and warmth. Report signs of infection to the physician promptly. *Therapy can suppress usual responses, such as elevated temperature and inflammation. The fever of infection may be mistaken for the fever commonly associated with lupus. The client receiving immunosuppressive therapy for the disease has an even higher risk for infection.*

- Monitor laboratory values, including CBC and tests of organ function; report changes to the physician. *An elevation in the WBC count with a shift to the left (increased numbers of immature leukocytes in the blood) may be an early indication of infection. Changes in liver function studies, renal function studies, myocardial enzymes, or other laboratory values may indicate organ system involvement.*

- Initiate reverse or protective isolation procedures as indicated by the client's immune status. *These procedures provide further protection from infection for the severely immunocompromised client.*

- Instruct family members and visitors to avoid contact with the client when they are ill. *A "minor" upper respiratory infection can be a significant illness for the client with SLE.*

- Help ensure an adequate nutrient intake, offering supplementary feedings as indicated or maintaining parenteral nutrition if necessary. *Adequate nutrition is important for healing and immune system function.*

- Teach the client the importance of good handwashing after using the bathroom and before eating. *Handwashing reduces the risk of infection with endogenous organisms.*

- Provide good mouth care. *Good oral hygiene reduces the population of microorganisms in the mouth and helps to keep oral mucous membranes intact.*

- Monitor for potential adverse effects of medications, including thrombocytopenia and possible bleeding, fluid retention with edema and possible hypertension, loss of bone density, osteoporosis, and possible pathologic fractures, renal or hepatic toxicity, and cardiac effects, particularly in the client with fluid retention and hypervolemia. *Medications used to treat SLE have many potential adverse effects that can impair normal protective and homeostatic mechanisms.*

Impaired Health Maintenance

As with other chronic diseases, much of the responsibility for maintaining optimal health rests with the client. Disease manifestations, such as fatigue, arthralgias, arthritis, and increased risk for infection, can interfere with the client's ability to maintain health. Psychosocial issues can also be a significant factor in health maintenance for the client with lupus. These issues may include denial of the significance of the disease, poor coping, lack of financial and other resources, and an inadequate support system.

- Assess the client's ability to maintain optimal health, identifying physical and psychosocial factors that may affect health maintenance. *Before intervening to improve the client's health maintenance, the nurse must identify and understand factors affecting it.*

- Provide care and teaching in a nonjudgmental manner. *To intervene effectively, the nurse must accept the client and family as they are.*
- Encourage the client and family members to discuss the effect of the disease on their lives. *Open discussion helps the client and the nurse identify barriers to health maintenance and begin exploring alternative strategies.*
- Initiate a multidisciplinary care conference with the client and family. *In this care conference, a number of perspectives can be expressed, improving the planning of strategies for health maintenance activities.*
- Refer the client and family to counseling as needed. *Counseling may help the client and family develop the necessary coping skills to accept and deal with the disease.*
- Refer the client and family to community and social service agencies, and local support groups. *These groups and agencies are valuable resources for the client and family.*

Home Care

Teaching is a critical factor in preparing clients with SLE to care for themselves at home. Address the following topics:

- The disease and its potential effects. Promote an optimistic outlook, stressing that the majority of clients do not require long-term corticosteroid therapy and that the disease may improve over time.
- The importance of skin care. Teach the client to avoid irritating soaps, shampoos, or chemicals (e.g., hair dyes and permanent wave solution) to prevent excessive drying of the skin. Encourage the client to use hypoallergenic products. Discuss the need to limit sun exposure, particularly between 10:00 a.m. and 3:00 p.m. Encourage the client to use sunscreen with an SPF of at least 15 and to wear long sleeves and wide-brimmed hats. For clients with hair loss, discuss the use of wigs, turbans, or other head coverings. Provide encouragement by reminding the client that the hair will grow back during periods of remission.
- The importance of avoiding exposure to infection. Encourage the client to avoid crowds and infectious individuals. Teach the client that getting adequate rest and nutrition and avoiding stress will increase resistance to infection.
- The need to follow the prescribed treatment plan, including rest and exercise, medications, and follow-up appointments. Discuss manifestations of an acute episode, including fever, chills; rash; increased fatigue and malaise; arthralgias; arthritis; urinary manifestations, such as oliguria or dysuria; chest pain; cough; or neurologic symptoms. Stress the importance of contacting the physician promptly if any of these symptoms occur.
- The significance of wearing a MedicAlert tag identifying their condition and therapy, such as corticosteroids or immunosuppressives.
- Family planning with the client and spouse. The use of oral contraceptives may be contraindicated for the client; if appropriate, provide information about alternative means of birth control. Pregnancy is not contraindicated for most women with lupus. However, the pregnant client requires close monitoring because acute episodes sometimes accompany pregnancy.
- Helpful resources:
  1. National Institute of Arthritis and Musculoskeletal and Skin Diseases
  2. Lupus Foundation of America.

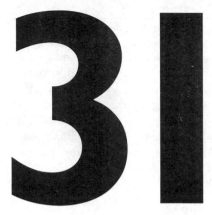

Assessing Clients with Neurologic Disorders

The nervous system regulates and integrates all body functions, mental abilities, and emotions. It collects information from the internal and external environments as sensory input, processes and interprets the input, and causes responses that are manifested as motor or sensory output.

Review of Anatomy and Physiology

The nervous system is divided into two regions: the central nervous system (CNS), which consists of the brain and spinal cord, and the peripheral nervous system (PNS), which consists of the cranial nerves, the spinal nerves, and the autonomic nervous system. These two highly integrated regions consist of just two types of cells: neurons, which receive impulses and send them on to other cells, and neuroglia, which protect and nourish the neurons.

Neurons

Each neuron consists of a dendrite, a cell body, and an axon. The dendrite is a short process (projection) from the cell body that conducts impulses toward (afferent) the cell body. Cell bodies, most of which are located within the CNS, are clustered in ganglia or nuclei. The cell bodies and dendrites comprise what is often called the gray matter of the CNS. The axon, a long process, conducts impulses away (efferent) from the cell body. Many axons are covered with a myelin sheath, a white lipid substance. It is interrupted at intervals in unmyelinated areas called nodes of Ranvier, which allow movement of ions between the axon and the extracellular fluid. The myelin sheath serves to increase the speed of nerve impulse conduction in axons and is essential for the survival of larger nerve processes. Myelinated nerve fibers comprise the white matter of the brain and spinal cord.

Action Potentials

Action potentials are impulses (movements of electrical charge along an axon membrane) that allow neurons to communicate with other neurons and body cells. They are initiated by stimuli and propagated by the rapid movement of charged ions through the cell membrane. When a neuron reaches a certain level of stimulation, an electrical impulse is generated and conducted along the length of its axon. The movement of impulses to and from the CNS is made possible by afferent and efferent neurons. Afferent, or sensory, neurons have receptors in skin, muscles, and other organs and relay impulses to the CNS. Efferent, or motor, neurons transmit impulses from the CNS to cause some type of action.

Nerve impulses occur when a stimulus reaches a point great enough to generate a change in electrical charge across the cell membrane of a neuron. A neuron that is not involved in impulse conduction is in a resting, or polarized, state, in which the number of positive ions in the fluid outside of the cell membrane is greater than in the fluid within the cell. The chief regulators of membrane potential are sodium and potassium: Sodium is the major positive ion in the extracellular fluid, and potassium is the major positive ion in the intracellular fluid. In response to an electrical stimulus, the cell membrane becomes permeable to sodium, which moves into the cell. This changes the polarity of the cell membrane, and the neuron is said to depolarize. This event stimulates an action potential, or a nerve impulse, to travel down the axon. When the charges and ions return to their original resting state, the neuron is repolarized. The events in an action potential are as follows:

- Initially, sodium permeability increases. As the membrane is depolarized, sodium channels open and sodium rushes into the cell to a point of depolarization (the inside of the cell becomes less negative in comparison to the outside of the cell).
- This is followed by a decrease in sodium permeability, lasting only about one millisecond. The sodium gates close and the sodium influx stops.
- The final event is an increase in potassium permeability. The potassium gates open, potassium rushes out of the cell, and the cell interior becomes progressively less positive. The membrane potential moves back to its resting state and is repolarized.

The action potential is generated only at the point of the stimulus; but once generated, it is propagated along the entire length of the axon regardless if the stimulus continues. Conduction of the impulse is rapid in myelinated fibers, with the action potential "jumping" from one node of Ranvier to the next. The conduction of the impulse is slower in unmyelinated fibers.

Neurotransmitters

Neurotransmitters are the chemical messengers of the nervous system. When the action potential reaches the end of the axon at the presynaptic terminal, a neurotransmitter is released and travels across the synaptic cleft to bind with receptors in the postsynaptic neuron dendrite or cell body. The neurotransmitter may either be inhibitory or excitatory. The excitatory neurotransmitter is almost always acetylcholine (ACh), which is rapidly degraded by the enzyme acetylcholinesterase. Norepinephrine (NE) is another major neurotransmitter. It may be either excitatory or inhibitory.

Nerves that transmit impulses through the release of ACh are called cholinergic. Receptors that bind ACh are found in the viscera, skeletal muscle cells, and the adrenal medulla (where they stimulate the release of epinephrine). The effect of ACh binding may be either to stimulate or to inhibit a response.

Nerves that transmit impulses through the release of NE are called adrenergic. Receptors that bind NE are found in the heart, lungs, kidneys, blood vessels, and all target organs stimulated by the sympathetic division except the heart. Adrenergic receptors are further divided into alpha and beta types. Alpha-adrenergic receptors help control such varied functions as arterial vasoconstriction and pupil dilation. Beta-adrenergic fibers may be either beta$_1$ or beta$_2$ receptors. Beta$_1$ receptors are found in the heart, where they regulate the rate and force of contraction. Beta$_2$ receptors are found in receptor cells of the lungs, arteries, liver, and uterus; they help regulate bronchial diameter, arterial diameter, and glycogenesis. Generally, binding of NE to alpha receptors stimulates a response, whereas binding to beta receptors inhibits a response.

Other neurotransmitters include gamma aminobutyric acid (GABA), which inhibits CNS function; dopamine, which may be inhibitory or excitatory and helps control fine movement and emotions; and serotonin, which is usually inhibitory and controls sleep, hunger, and behavior and also affects consciousness.

The Central Nervous System

The central nervous system (CNS) consists of the brain and spinal cord, highly evolved clusters of neurons which act to accept, interconnect, interpret, and generate a response to nerve impulses originating throughout the body.

The Brain The brain is the control center of the nervous system and also generates thoughts, emotions, and speech. Averaging 3 to 4 lb in weight, the brain is surrounded by the skull, a bony structure that provides support and protection. The brain has four major regions: the cerebrum, the diencephalon, the brainstem, and the cerebellum. The general functions of these regions are summarized in Table 31-1.

The two hemispheres of the cerebrum account for almost 60% of brain weight. The surface of the cerebrum is folded into elevated ridges of tissue called gyri, which are separated by shallow grooves called sulci. Deep grooves called fissures further divide the surface of the cerebrum. The longitudinal fissure separates the hemispheres, and the transverse fissure separates the cerebrum from the cerebellum. In addition, each cerebral hemisphere is divided into frontal, parietal, temporal, and occipital lobes.

The cerebral hemispheres are connected by a thick band of nerve fibers called the corpus callosum, which allows communication between the two hemispheres. Each hemisphere receives sensory and motor impulses from the opposite side of the body. One of the cerebral hemispheres tends to develop more than the other. Most people have a more highly developed left hemisphere, which is responsible for the control of language. The right hemisphere has greater control over nonverbal perceptual functions.

Table 31-1. General Functions of the Four Regions of the Brain

Region	Functions
Cerebrum	Interprets sensory input. Controls skeletal muscle activity. Processes intellect and emotions. Contains skills memory.
Diencephalon	Conducts sensory and motor impulses. Regulates autonomic nervous system. Regulates and produces hormones. Mediates emotional responses.
Brainstem	Serves as conduction pathway. Serves as site of decussation of tracts. Contains respiratory nuclei. Helps regulate skeletal muscles.
Cerebellum	Processes information. Provides information necessary for balance, posture, and coordinated muscle movement.

The cerebral cortex is the outer surface of the cerebrum. It consists of neuron cell bodies, unmyelinated fibers, neuroglia, and blood vessels. The functions of the different lobes of the cerebrum and the specific areas of the cerebral cortex are listed in Table 31-2.

The diencephalon is embedded in the cerebrum superior to the brainstem. It consists of the thalamus, hypothalamus, and epithalamus. The thalamus begins to process sensory impulses before they ascend to the cerebral cortex. It serves as a sorting, processing, and relay station for input into the cortical region. The hypothalamus, located inferior to the thalamus, regulates temperature, water metabolism, appetite, emotional expressions, part of the sleep-wake cycle, and thirst. The epithalamus forms the dorsal part of the diencephalon and includes the pineal body, which is part of the endocrine system that affects growth and development.

Table 31-2. Functions of Lobes of the Cerebrum and Areas of the Cerebral Cortex

Area	Functions
Parietal lobe (somatic sensory area of cerebral cortex)	Promotes recognition of pain, coldness, and light touch. The left side receives input from the right side of the body, and vice versa.
Occipital lobe	Receives and interprets visual stimuli.
Temporal lobe	Receives and interprets olfactory and auditory stimuli.
Frontal lobe	Controls movements of voluntary muscles.
Primary motor area	Facilitates voluntary movement of skeletal muscles.
Speech area	Promotes understanding of spoken and written words.
Motor speech area (Broca's area)	Promotes vocalization of words.

Brain Stem. The brainstem consists of the midbrain, pons, and medulla oblongata. The midbrain is a center for auditory and visual reflexes. In addition, it functions as a nerve pathway between the cerebral hemispheres and lower brain. The pons is located just below the midbrain. It consists mostly of fiber tracts, but it also contains nuclei that control respiration. The medulla oblongata, located at the base of the brainstem, is continuous with the superior portion of the spinal cord. Nuclei of the medulla oblongata play an important role in controlling cardiac rate, blood pressure, respiration, and swallowing.

The cerebellum is connected to the midbrain, pons, and medulla. Its functions include coordination of skeletal muscle activity, maintenance of balance, and control of fine movements.

Ventricles. The brain contains four ventricles, which are chambers filled with cerebrospinal fluid (CSF). They are linked by ducts that allow the CSF to circulate. One lateral ventricle is located within each hemisphere. These communicate with the third ventricle through the foramen of Monro. The third ventricle communicates with the fourth ventricle through the cerebral aqueduct that runs through the midbrain. The cerebral aqueduct is continuous with the central canal of the spinal cord.

Cerebrospinal Fluid. A clear and colorless liquid, cerebrospinal fluid (CSF) is formed by the choroid plexus, which are groups of capillaries located in the brain ventricles. It consists of 99% water and contains protein, sodium, chloride, potassium, bicarbonate, and glucose. The usual amount of CSF ranges from 80 to 200 mL, averaging about 150 mL, and is replaced several times each day. It is absorbed by arachnoid villi. CSF is normally produced and absorbed in equal amounts. CSF circulates from the lateral ventricles of the cerebral hemispheres into the third ventricle, through the midbrain, and into the fourth ventricle. Some CSF flows down the center of the spinal cord as the rest of it circulates into the subarachnoid space and returns to the blood through the arachnoid villi. CSF forms a cushion for the brain tissue, protects the brain and spinal cord from trauma, helps provide nourishment for the brain, and removes waste products of cerebrospinal cellular metabolism.

Meninges. The CNS is covered and protected by three connective tissue membranes called meninges. The meninges form divisions within the skull, enclose venous sinuses, and contain CSF. The meninges have three layers. The outermost layer is attached to the inner surface of the skull, and the innermost layer is the most external brain covering. The outermost, double layer is the dura mater. The middle layer is the arachnoid mater. It forms a space that contains CSF and is the site of all major cerebral blood vessels. The innermost layer, the pia mater, clings to the brain itself and is filled with small blood vessels.

Cerebral Circulation and the Blood-Brain Barrier

The cerebral hemispheres receive their blood supply from the anterior and middle internal cerebral arteries. These two arteries are branches of the common carotid arteries. The brainstem and cerebellum receive their blood supply from the basilar artery. The posterior cerebrum receives blood from the posterior cerebral arteries. These major arteries are connected by small anterior and posterior communicating arteries, which form a circle of connected blood vessels called the circle of Willis. This circle serves as a protective device, providing alternative routes for brain tissues to receive their blood supply. The brain receives about 750 mL of blood each minute and uses 20% of the body's total oxygen uptake. The large amount of oxygen is necessary for metabolism of glucose, which is the brain's sole source of energy.

The capillaries in the brain have low permeability because the cells that compose their walls join at very tight junctions and are surrounded by a basement membrane and by the processes of supporting cells in the brain (called astrocytes). As a result, the brain is protected from many harmful substances in the blood. This blood-brain barrier allows lipids, glucose, some amino acids, water, carbon dioxide, and oxygen to pass through it, thus maintaining a controlled environment. Substances, such as urea, creatinine, proteins, some toxins, and most antibiotics, cannot pass this barrier and enter brain tissue. However, injury to, or infection of, the brain may cause increased permeability of the blood-brain barrier, altering concentrations of proteins, water, and electrolytes.

The Limbic System and the Reticular Formation

The limbic system and the reticular formation are functional brain systems. These systems, made of networks of neurons, communicate across areas of the brain.

The limbic system consists of structures that form a ring of tissue in the medial side of each hemisphere, surrounding the upper portion of the brainstem and corpus callosum. The limbic system integrates and modulates input to make up the affective part of the brain, providing emotional and behavioral responses to environmental stimuli.

The reticular formation is located through the central core of the medulla oblongata, pons, and midbrain. This system has widespread connections throughout the brain and relays sensory input from all body systems to all levels of the brain. The reticular formation includes the reticular activating system (RAS). The RAS is a stimulating system for the cerebral cortex, keeping it alert and responsive to incoming sensory stimuli while filtering out repetitive or unwanted stimuli. The sleep center inhibits activity of the RAS and drugs and alcohol may depress it. Other parts of the reticular formation include motor nuclei that help maintain muscle tone and coordinated movements through interconnections with spinal nerves, and the vasomotor and cardiovascular regulatory centers, which are part of autonomic regulation of the cardiovascular system.

The Spinal Cord

The spinal cord is surrounded and protected by 33 vertebrae, including 7 cervical, 12 thoracic, 5 lumbar, 5 sacral, and 4 fused vertebrae, which form the coccyx. Each vertebra consists of a body and a vertebral arch formed by projections from the body. This arch encloses a space called the vertebral foramen. The vertebral foramina of all the vertebrae form the vertebral canal through which the spinal cord passes. Intervertebral foramina are spaces between the vertebrae through which spinal nerve roots pass as they exit the vertebral column.

Intervertebral discs are located between each of the movable vertebrae. Each disc is made of a thick capsule surrounding a gelatinous core called the nucleus pulposus. Ligaments that provide mobility and protection surround the vertebral column, which is discussed in greater detail in Chapter 33.

The spinal cord extends from the medulla to the level of the first lumbar vertebra. It serves as a center for conducting messages to and from the brain and as a reflex center. The spinal cord is about 17 inches (42 cm) long and 0.75 inch (1.8 cm) thick. The cord is protected by the vertebrae, the meninges, and cerebrospinal fluid. The gray matter of the cord is on the inside, and the white matter is on the outside (the reverse of the arrangement in the brain).

The roots of 31 pairs of spinal nerves, divided into the cervical, thoracic, and lumbar nerves, arise from the cord. Each separates into posterior (sensory) and anterior (motor) roots. Damage to the posterior roots results in loss of sensation, whereas damage to the anterior root results in flaccid paralysis.

Functions of the Spinal Cord and Spinal Roots

Messages to and from the brain are conducted via ascending (sensory) pathways and descending (motor) pathways. The major ascending tracts are the lateral and anterior spinothalamic tracts, which carry sensations for pain, temperature, and crude touch; and the posterior tracts, called the fasciculus gracilis and fasciculus cuneatus, which carry sensations for fine touch, position, and vibration. The lateral and anterior corticospinal (pyramidal) tracts are descending tracts consisting of fibers that originate in the motor cortex of the brain and travel to the brainstem and then down the spinal cord. They mediate voluntary purposeful movements and stimulate certain muscular actions while inhibiting others. They also carry fibers that inhibit muscle tone. The rubrospinal, anterior and lateral reticulospinal, and tectospinal (extrapyramidal) tracts include the pathways between the cerebral cortex, basal ganglia, brainstem, and spinal cord outside the pyramidal tract. They maintain muscle tone and gross body movements.

Upper and Lower Motor Neurons

Upper motor neurons, such as those of the corticospinal and extrapyramidal tract, carry impulses from the cerebral cortex to the anterior gray column of the spinal cord. Damage to upper motor neurons results in increased muscle tone, decreased muscle strength, decreased coordination, and hyperactive reflexes. Lower motor neurons, such as the peripheral and cranial nerves, begin in the anterior gray column of the spinal cord and end in the muscle. These are the "final common pathways." Damage to lower motor neurons results in decreased muscle tone and loss of reflexes.

The Peripheral Nervous System

The peripheral nervous system (PNS) links the CNS with the rest of the body. It is responsible for receiving and transmitting information from and about the external environment. The PNS consists of nerves, ganglia (groups of nerve cells), and sensory receptors located outside, or peripheral to, the brain and spinal cord. The PNS is divided into a sensory (afferent) division and a motor (efferent) division. Most nerves of the PNS contain fibers for both divisions, and all are classified regionally as either spinal nerves or cranial nerves.

Spinal Nerves

The 31 pairs of spinal nerves are named by their location:

- Cervical nerves: 8 pairs
- Thoracic nerves: 12 pairs
- Lumbar nerves: 5 pairs
- Sacral nerves: 5 pairs
- Coccygeal nerves: 1 pair.

Spinal nerves exit the vertebral column through intervertebral foramina to travel to the body regions they serve. The spinal cord does not reach the end of the vertebral column; as a result, the lumbar and sacral nerve roots travel inferiorly through the vertebral canal for some distance before exiting the vertebral column through their associated intervertebral foramina. This collection of descending nerve roots is called the cauda equina.

Each spinal nerve contains both sensory and motor fibers. The sensory fibers are located in the dorsal root, and their cell bodies are located within the dorsal root ganglion. The motor fibers are located in the ventral root, and their cell bodies are located within the spinal cord. The dorsal and ventral roots merge outside the vertebral canal just past the dorsal root ganglion, forming a spinal nerve. Each spinal nerve further divides into branches called rami.

The ventral rami of the cervical, brachial, lumbar, and sacral regions form complex clusters of nerves called plexuses. The main spinal nerve plexuses innervate the skin and the underlying muscles of the arms and legs. For example, the cervical plexus innervates the diaphragm through the phrenic nerve; the brachial plexus innervates the upper extremities through the median, ulnar, and radial nerves; and the lumbar plexus innervates the anterior thigh through the femoral nerve.

An area of skin innervated by cutaneous branches of a single spinal nerve is called a dermatome. The dorsal roots of the spinal nerves carry sensations from these specific dermatomes. Dermatomes provide anatomical landmarks that are useful for locating neurologic lesions.

Cranial Nerves

Twelve pairs of cranial nerves originate in the forebrain and brainstem. The vagus nerve extends into the ventral body cavity, but the 11 other pairs innervate only head and neck regions. Although most are mixed nerves, three pairs (olfactory, optic, and vestibulocochlear) are solely sensory. The cranial nerves and their related functions are listed in Table 31-3.

Reflexes

A reflex is a rapid, involuntary, predictable motor response to a stimulus. Reflexes are categorized as either somatic or autonomic. *Somatic reflexes* result in skeletal muscle contraction. *Autonomic reflexes* activate cardiac muscle, smooth muscle, and glands. A reflex occurs over a pathway called a reflex arc.

The essential components of a *reflex arc* are a receptor, a sensory neuron to carry afferent impulses to the CNS, an integration center in the spinal cord or brain, a motor neuron to carry efferent impulses, and an effector (the tissue that responds by contracting or secreting).

Somatic reflexes mediated by the spinal cord are called *spinal reflexes.* Many spinal reflexes occur without impulses traveling to and from the brain, with the cord serving as the integration center, while others require brain activity and modulation. *Deep-tendon reflexes (DTRs)* occur in response to muscle contraction and cause muscle relaxation and lengthening. DTRs depend on intact sensory and motor nerve roots, functional synapses in the spinal cord, a functional neuromuscular junction, and a competent muscle. Thus, an abnormal deep-tendon reflex could indicate a variety of health problems, including a lesion of a spinal nerve. Flexor, or withdrawal, reflexes are caused by actual or perceived painful stimuli and result in withdrawal of the part of the body that is threatened. Superficial responses result from gentle cutaneous stimulation. These responses depend on functional upper motor pathways and on an intact reflex arc.

Table 31-3.   Cranial Nerves

Name	Function
I Olfactory	Sense of smell
II Optic	Vision
III Oculomotor	Eyeball movement Raising of upper eyelid Constriction of pupil Proprioception
IV Trochlear	Eyeball movement
V Trigeminal	Sensation of the upper scalp, upper eyelid, nose, nasal cavity, cornea, and lacrimal gland Sensation of the palate, upper teeth, cheek, top lip, lower eyelid, and scalp Sensation of the tongue, lower teeth, chin, and temporal scalp Chewing
VI Abducens	Lateral movement of the eyeball
VII Facial	Movement of facial muscles Secretions of lacrimal, nasal, submandibular, and sublingual glands Sensation of taste

Table 31-3. Continued

VIII Vestibulocochlear	Sense of equilibrium
	Sense of hearing
IX Glossopharyngeal	Swallowing
	Gag reflex
	Secretions of parotid salivary gland
	Sense of taste
	Touch, pressure, and pain from pharynx and posterior tongue
	Pressure from carotid arteries
	Receptors to regulate blood pressure
X Vagus	Swallowing
	Regulation of cardiac rate
	Regulation of respirations
	Digestion
	Sensation from thoracic and abdominal organs
	Proprioception
	Sense of taste
XI Accessory	Movement of head and neck
	Proprioception
XII Hypoglossal	Movement of tongue for speech and swallowing

The Autonomic Nervous System

The autonomic nervous system (ANS) is a division of the PNS that regulates the internal environment of the body. It is also called the general visceral motor system, because it consists of motor neurons that innervate the body's viscera. Whereas skeletal muscle activity is regulated by a division of the PNS called the somatic nervous system, the ANS regulates the activity of cardiac muscle, smooth muscle, and glands.

The reticular formation in the brainstem is the primary controller of the ANS. Stimulation of centers in the medulla initiates reflexes that regulate cardiac rate, blood vessel diameter, and gastrointestinal function.

The ANS has sympathetic and parasympathetic divisions. Although fibers from both divisions affect the same structures, the actions of the two divisions are opposite in effect, and they serve to counterbalance each other. The major neurotransmitters for impulse transmission in the ANS are acetylcholine and norepinephrine. Acetylcholine is the primary neurotransmitter of the parasympathetic division. Norepinephrine is the primary neurotransmitter of the sympathetic division.

Sympathetic Division. The sympathetic division of the ANS prepares the body to handle situations that are perceived as harmful or stressful and to participate in strenuous activity. Cell bodies for this division arise in the lateral horns of the spinal cord in the area from T_1 through L_2. The fibers separate after leaving the cord, and form a chain of ganglia that extends from the neck to the pelvis. Long fibers then extend to the organs that are supplied by the sympathetic division. Stimulation of the sympathetic division can exert the following effects on target organs or tissues:

- Dilated pupils
- Inhibited secretions

- Copious production of sweat (**diaphoresis**)
- Increased rate and force of heartbeat
- Vasodilation of the coronary arteries
- Dilation of the bronchioles
- Decreased digestion
- Increased release of glucose by the liver
- Decreased urine output
- Vasoconstriction of arteries
- Vasoconstriction of abdominal and skin blood vessels
- Increased blood clotting
- Increased metabolic rate
- Increased mental alertness.

Parasympathetic Division. The parasympathetic division of the ANS operates during nonstressful situations. Cell bodies for this division are located in the brain stem (for the cranial nerves) and in the lateral gray matter of S_2 through S_4. The fibers, other than those supplying cranial nerves III, VII, IX, and X, are carried by the vagus nerve to body tissues, thoracic organs, and visceral organs. Stimulation of the parasympathetic division of the ANS produces the following effects:

- Constriction of pupils
- Stimulation of glandular secretions
- Decreased heart rate
- Vasoconstriction of coronary arteries
- Constriction of the bronchioles
- Increased peristalsis and secretion of gastrointestinal fluid.

Assessing Neurologic Function

The client's neurologic system is assessed by both a health assessment interview to collect subjective data and a physical assessment to collect objective data.

Health Assessment Interview

This section provides guidelines for collecting subjective data through a health assessment interview specific to the functions of the neurologic system. If the client's level of consciousness is altered, the nurse may need to rely on family members for information. The client's level of consciousness may be assessed by using the Glasgow Coma Scale, found in Table 31-4.

Table 31-4.   Glasgow Coma Scale

Assessment	Response	Score*
Eyes open (Record C if eyes are closed by swelling.)	Spontaneously	4
	To speech	3
	To pain	2
	No response	1
Best motor response (Record best upper arm response.)	Obeys commands	6
	Localizes pain	5
	Flexion-withdrawal	4
	Abnormal flexion	3
	Abnormal extension	2
	No response	1
Best verbal response (Record T if an endotracheal or tracheostomy tube is in place.)	Oriented	5
	Confused	4
	Inappropriate words	3
	Incomprehensible sounds	2
	No response	1
Total Score:		————

*A higher score indicates a higher level of functioning.

An interview to assess neurologic function may focus on a chief complaint or may be done as part of a total health assessment. If the client has a health problem involving any component of neurologic function, analyze its onset, characteristics and course, severity, precipitating and relieving factors, and any associated symptoms, noting the timing and circumstances. For example, ask the client the following:

- Describe the location and intensity of the pain you have experienced in your left leg. Is it made worse by coughing, sneezing, or walking?
- When did you first notice that you were having numbness in your fingers?
- Describe the difficulty you have when you try to walk.

Questions about present health status should include information about numbness, tingling sensations, tremors, problems with coordination or balance, or loss of movement in any part of the body. Ask the client about difficulty with speaking, seeing, hearing, tasting, or detecting odors. In addition, elicit information about memory; feeling state, such as anxiety or depression; recent changes in sleep patterns; ability to perform self-care and activities of daily living; sexual activity; and weight. If the client is taking prescribed or over-the-counter medications, ask about the type and purpose, as well as the frequency and duration of use.

Ask about any past history of seizures, fainting, dizziness, headaches, and any trauma, tumors, or surgery of the brain, spinal cord, or nerves. Discuss illnesses that may cause neurologic manifestations, including cardiac disease, strokes, pernicious anemia, sinus infections, liver disease, and/or renal failure. Also ask the client about family history of neurologic health problems, diabetes mellitus, hypertension, seizures, or mental health problems.

Question the client about occupational hazards, such as exposure to toxic chemicals or materials, use of protective headgear, and the amount of time spent performing repetitive motions (e.g., data entry and assembly). Ask questions about self-care to assess the client's diet and use of tobacco, drugs, or alcohol, and ask whether the client wears a helmet when riding a bike or motorcycle or participating in contact sports.

Physical Assessment

Physical assessment of the client begins when the nurse first meets the client and makes an overall evaluation of the client's mental and physical status. The mental status examination is conducted with both the nurse and the client seated. The rest of the neurologic examination may be performed with the client either sitting or standing.

The neurologic system is assessed through inspection, palpation, and percussion (with a reflex hammer). When conducting the mental status and cognitive portions of the examination, be aware that fatigue or illness may alter findings. Provide rest periods for the client as needed. When interpreting findings, consider the client's age, educational background, and cultural orientation.

Collect the equipment necessary for this assessment: a cotton ball and safety pin, tongue blade, tuning fork, ophthalmoscope, reflex hammer, pencil and paper, printed materials, and substances to test the senses of smell and taste. The assessment should take place in a private, comfortable setting. Ask the client to remove outer clothing, shoes, and stockings. Provide a gown for the client to wear. It is important to explain to the client that the neurologic examination is lengthy and may consist of questions and requests that seem strange to the client. Explain the rationale for each part of the examination.

A brief version of this physical assessment, often referred to as a *neuro check,* may be performed in a shorter time period when a client requires frequent ongoing assessments of neurologic status.

Table 31-5. Abbreviated Neurologic Assessment (Neuro Check)

---

1. Assess level of consciousness (response to auditory and/or tactile stimulus).
2. Obtain vital signs (BP, P, R).
3. Check pupillary response to light.
4. Assess strength of hand grip and movement of extremities bilaterally.
5. Determine ability to sense touch/pain in extremities.

Mental Status Assessment with Abnormal Findings (✓)

• Assess appearance.
• Observe dress, hygiene, and grooming.

- Observe gait and posture.
  - ✓ Unilateral neglect (inattention to one side of body) may occur with some strokes of the middle cerebral artery. Poor hygiene and grooming may be seen in clients with dementing disorders.
  - ✓ Abnormal gait and posture may be seen in transient ischemic attacks (TIAs), strokes, and Parkinson's disease.
- Assess behavior.
- Observe client's actions and affect.
- Note the content and quality of speech.
- Note level of consciousness. Use the Glasgow Coma Scale (see Table 31-4) to document findings. Scores may range from 3 (deeply comatose) to 15 (alert and oriented).
  - ✓ Emotional swings or changes in personality may be observed with strokes of the anterior cerebral artery.
  - ✓ The face appears masklike (very little expressive movement of facial muscles) in clients with Parkinson's disease.
  - ✓ Apathy is seen in dementing disorders.
  - ✓ **Aphasia** (defective or absent language function) may occur in TIAs. Receptive aphasia (inability to understand verbal or written language) is often noted in strokes of the posterior or anterior cerebral artery. Aphasias are seen with damage to the left cerebral cortex. Aphasias are more often seen with strokes of the right hemisphere than the left hemisphere.
  - ✓ **Dysphonia** (change in the tone of the voice) is common in strokes of the posterior inferior cerebral artery. Dysphonia is seen with paralysis of the vocal cords (cranial nerve X).
  - ✓ **Dysarthria** (difficulty speaking) is seen with lesions of upper and lower motor neurons, the cerebellum, and the extrapyramidal tract. It is also seen in strokes of the anterior inferior and superior cerebral arteries.
  - ✓ Damage to the brainstem and/or cerebral cortex may alter level of consciousness.
  - ✓ Drowsiness and decreased level of consciousness may be associated with brain trauma, infections, TIAs, stroke, and brain tumors.
  - ✓ Level of consciousness is usually altered and may progress to coma with stroke of the middle cerebral artery.
  - ✓ Confusion and coma may be seen in clients with strokes affecting the vertebralbasilar arteries.
- Assess cognitive function.
- Note orientation to time, place, and person.
- Note attention span and recent and remote memory. Ask the client to:
  1. Repeat five to seven numbers.
  2. Recall three items after five minutes.
  3. Recall his or her address, breakfast, or birthday.
- Assess thought processes (both content and perceptions) by noting responses to questions.

- Note ability to understand what is said and to express thoughts.
- Note ability to make logical and safe judgments.
  - ✓ Disorientation to time and place may occur in clients with stroke of the right cerebral hemisphere.
  - ✓ Memory deficits are often seen with strokes of the anterior cerebral artery and vertebralbasilar artery.
  - ✓ Perceptual deficits may be seen in strokes of the middle cerebral artery. These same deficits may occur following brain trauma and in dementing disorders.
  - ✓ Impaired cognition is often noted with strokes of the middle cerebral artery, cerebral trauma, and brain tumors.

Cranial Nerve Assessments with Possible Abnormal Findings (3)

- Test CN I (olfactory).
- Note client's ability to smell scents (e.g., soap, coffee) with each nostril. This test is usually done only if a problem with the ability to smell is reported.
  - ✓ **Anosmia** (an inability to smell) may be seen with lesions of the frontal lobe and may also occur with impaired blood flow to the middle cerebral artery.
- Test CN II (optic).
- Assess vision with Snellen chart.
  - ✓ Blindness in one eye may be seen with strokes of the internal carotid artery or with TIAs. Impaired vision or blindness in one side of both eyes (**homonymous hemianopia**) is associated with blockage of the posterior cerebral artery.
  - ✓ Impaired vision may also be seen with strokes of the anterior cerebral artery and brain tumors.
  - ✓ Blindness or double vision may be noted with involvement of the vertebralbasilar arteries. Double or blurred vision may also occur with TIAs.
  - ✓ **Papilledema** (swelling of the optic nerve) occurs with increased intracranial pressure.
- Test CN III, IV, and VI (oculomotor, trochlear, and abducens).
- Assess extraocular movements by asking the client to follow your finger as you write an *H* in the air.
- Assess PERRL ("pupils equally round and reactive to light") by covering one eye at a time and shining a bright light directly into the uncovered eye (use a penlight or the ophthalmoscope).
- Assess for **ptosis** (drooping eyelids).
  - ✓ **Nystagmus** (involuntary eye movement) may be seen with strokes of the anterior, inferior, and superior cerebellar arteries. Constricted pupils are associated with impaired blood flow to the vertebralbasilar arteries. Ptosis (also called Horner's syndrome) occurs with strokes of the posterior inferior cerebellar artery, myasthenia gravis, and palsy of CN III.
- Test CN V (trigeminal).
- Assess ability to feel light, dull, and sharp sensations on the face. With the client's eyes closed, check whether sensation is the same on both sides of the face. Stroke the cheek with a wisp of cotton for light touch, with a closed safety pin for dull touch, and with a tongue

blade for sharp touch. If the sharp point of a safety pin is used to assess sharp touch, be sure to avoid scratching the surface of the skin, and discard the pin after it is used.

- Assess the corneal reflex by touching the corneal surface with a wisp of cotton. This reflex is tested on unconscious clients. Normally the client blinks.

  ✓ Changes in facial sensations are noted with impaired blood flow to the carotid artery.

  ✓ Decreased sensations to the face and cornea on the same side of the body occur with strokes of the posterior inferior cerebral artery.

  ✓ Lip and mouth numbness occur with strokes of the vertebralbasilar artery.

  ✓ Loss of facial sensation or contraction of the masseter and temporal muscles is seen with lesions of CN V.

  ✓ Severe facial pain is seen with trigeminal neuralgia (tic douloureux).

  ✓ The corneal reflex may be impaired with lesions of CN V or VII.

- Test CN VII (facial).
- Assess ability to taste sweet, sour, and salt on the anterior two-thirds of the tongue by asking the client to stick out the tongue and applying a salty, sweet, or sour substance.
- Assess ability to frown, show teeth, blow out cheeks, raise eyebrows, smile, and close eyes tightly.

  ✓ Loss of ability to taste may occur with brain tumors or with nerve impairment.

  ✓ Asymmetry or decreased movement of facial muscles is noted with lesions of the upper and lower motor neurons.

  ✓ Paralysis of the lower motor neurons results in the inability to close eyes, a flat nasolabial fold, paralysis of lower face, and inability to wrinkle forehead.

  ✓ Paralysis of the upper motor neurons results in weakness of eyelids and paralysis of lower face.

  ✓ Pain, paralysis, and sagging of facial muscles is seen on the affected side in Bell's palsy.

- Test CN VIII (acoustic).
- Assess ability to hear the ticking of a watch and whispered and spoken words.

  ✓ Decreased hearing or deafness may occur with strokes of the vertebralbasilar arteries and/or tumors of CN VIII.

- Test CN IX and X (glossopharyngeal and vagus).
- Observe client swallowing a small drink of water.
- Observe for a symmetrical rise of the soft palate and uvula as the client says "ah."
- Assess gag reflex by touching back of client's throat with tongue blade.
- Assess ability to taste salty, sweet, and sour substances on the posterior third of the tongue (see previous description).

  ✓ **Dysphagia** (difficulty swallowing) is common with impaired blood flow to the vertebralbasilar arteries and to the posterior inferior, anterior inferior, or superior cerebellar arteries.

  ✓ Unilateral loss of the gag reflex occurs with lesions of CN IX and X.

- Test CN XI (spinal accessory).
- Assess the client's ability to shrug the shoulders and turn head against resistance: Ask

the client to turn the head to one side against the resistance of your hand; ask the client to shrug the shoulders while you exert downward pressure. Observe symmetry, strength, and size of muscles.

✓ Muscle weakness is noted with lower motor neuron disease. Contralateral hemiparesis is seen with strokes affecting the middle or internal carotid artery.

- Test CN XII (hypoglossal).
- Assess the client's ability to stick out the tongue and move the tongue from side to side against resistance of a tongue blade.

✓ Atrophy and **fasciculations** (twitches) of the tongue are seen in lower motor neuron disease. The tongue may deviate toward involved side of the body.

Sensory Function Assessments with Abnormal Findings (✓)

- Assess ability to perceive various sensations.

- Touch both sides of various parts of the body (the chest, abdomen, arms, and legs) with one or more of the following:
  1. Cotton wisp
  2. Sharp object
  3. Dull object
  4. Vibrating tuning fork placed on bony prominences

  ✓ Decreased sensation of pain occurs with injury to the spinothalamic tract.

  ✓ Decreased vibratory sensations are seen with injuries to the posterior column tract.

  ✓ Transient numbness of face, arm, or hand is seen with TIAs.

  ✓ Sensory loss on one side of the body is seen with lesions of higher pathways to the spinal cord.

  ✓ Bilateral sensory loss is seen in polyneuropathy. Sensations are impaired with strokes, brain tumors, and spinal cord trauma or compression.

- Assess sense of position (**kinesthesia**).
- Move the client's finger or big toe up or down. Ask the client to describe the movement.

  ✓ Lesions of the posterior column of the spinal cord may affect sense of position.

- Assess ability to discriminate fine touch.
- Ask the client to identify:
  1. Object in hand, such as a coin or key (tests stereognosis).
  2. Number written on hand (tests graphesthesia).
  3. Two points of simultaneous pinpricks on the hand (tests two-point discrimination).
  4. Where he/she is being touched (tests localization).
  5. How many sensations are felt when touched simultaneously on both sides of the body (tests extinction).

  ✓ Inability to discriminate fine touch (stereognosis, graphesthesia, two points, point localization and extinction) may occur with injury to the posterior columns or sensory cortex.

Motor Function Assessments with Abnormal Findings (✓)

- Assess bilateral symmetry and size of muscles.
  - ✓ Atrophy of muscles is seen with disease of the lower motor neurons.
- Assess for **tremors** (rhythmic movements) and fasciculations. Observe movements as client is at rest (not making a purposeful movement) and with activity (making a purposeful movement, such as reaching for a glass of water).
  - ✓ Tremors that occur with activity are seen in multiple sclerosis and disease of the cerebellar system.
  - ✓ Tremors that occur at rest and disappear with movement are common in Parkinson's disease.
  - ✓ Fasciculations occur in disease or trauma to the lower motor neurons, as a side effect of medications, in fever, in sodium deficiency, and in uremia.
- Assess muscle tone.
  - ✓ Muscle tone is decreased (**flaccidity**) in disease or trauma of the lower motor neurons and early stroke.
  - ✓ Muscle tone is increased (**spasticity**) in disease of the corticospinal motor tract.
  - ✓ Muscles are rigid in disease of the extrapyramidal motor tract.
  - ✓ Muscles move in small, regular jerky movements (cogwheel rigidity) in Parkinson's disease.
- Assess bilateral muscle strength and movement. The following criteria for recording the grading of muscle strength are often used.

  0 = no contraction

  1 = trace of contraction

  2 = active movement with gravity

  3 = active movement against gravity

  4 = active movement against gravity and resistance

  5 = normal power

  Ask the client to:

  1. Squeeze your hands.
  2. Push feet against the resistance of your hands.
  3. Raise both legs off the bed.
  - ✓ Weakness of the arms, legs, or hands is often seen with TIAs. **Hemiplegia** (paralysis of one-half of the body vertically) is noted with strokes of the internal carotid artery and posterior cerebral artery.
  - ✓ Weakness of extremities is often noted with strokes of the vertebralbasilar arteries.
  - ✓ Flaccid paralysis is noted with strokes of the anterior spinal artery.
  - ✓ Paralysis or decreased movement is seen in multiple sclerosis and myasthenia gravis.
  - ✓ There is total loss of motor function below the level of injury in complete spinal cord transection and in injuries to the anterior portion of the spinal cord.
  - ✓ Spasticity of muscles may occur as a result of incomplete spinal cord injuries.

Cerebellar Function Assessments with Abnormal Findings (✓)

- Assess the gait. Ask the client to walk normally, then in a heel-to-toe fashion, then on toes, and finally on heels.
- Perform Romberg's test: Ask the client to stand with the feet together and eyes closed. (Stand close to client to prevent falling). There should be minimal swaying for up to 20 seconds.

  ✓ **Ataxia** is a lack of coordination and a clumsiness of movements, with staggering, wide-based, and unbalanced gait. Ataxia is often seen with anterior strokes and cerebellar tumors. Swaying and falling is seen in cerebellar ataxia. Inability to walk on toes, then heels may indicate disease of the upper motor neurons.

  ✓ Spastic hemiparesis is often associated with strokes or upper motor neuron disease. The client walks with one leg stiffly dragging while the other leg circles out and forward. One arm is held flexed and close to the side.

  ✓ Steppage gait is noted with disease of the lower motor neurons. The client drags or lifts the foot high, then slaps the foot onto the floor. The client cannot walk on the heels.

  ✓ Sensory ataxia may be associated with polyneuropathy or damage to the posterior columns. The client walks on the heels before bringing down the toes and the feet are held wide apart. Gait worsens with the eyes closed.

  ✓ Parkinsonian gait is often seen in Parkinson's disease. The client stoops over while walking and shuffles the feet. The arms are held close to the side.

  ✓ A positive Romberg's test may be seen in cerebellar ataxia.

- Assess coordination.
- Observe ability to pat knees, alternating front and back of hands and increasing speed.
- Observe ability to touch each finger of one hand to the thumb.
- Observe ability to touch the nose, then one of your fingers, then the nose again.
- Observe ability to run each heel down each shin, while in a supine position.

  ✓ Ataxic movements are apparent in cerebellar disease.

Reflex Assessments with Abnormal Findings (✓)

A reflex hammer is used to strike the tendon of various reflex sites. To test deep-tendon reflexes, ask the client to lock the fingers of both hands together and then pull; this encourages relaxation and promotes reflexes of lower extremities. Superficial reflexes are assessed by lightly stroking the area with the end of a tongue blade. The following criteria for recording reflexes are often used. A score of 2 is considered normal.

  0 = absent or no response

  1 = hypoactive; weaker than normal (+)

  2 = normal (++)

  3 = stronger than normal (+++)

  4 = hyperactive (++++)

- Assess the patellar, biceps, brachioradialis, triceps, and achilles deep-tendon reflexes.

  ✓ Hyperactive reflexes are present with lesions of upper motor neurons.

  ✓ Decreased reflexes are present with lower motor neuron involvement.

- Assess for clonus by dorsiflexing the client's foot.
  - ✓ **Clonus,** a hyperactive, rhythmic dorsiflexion and plantar flexion of the foot, is noted with upper motor neuron disease.
- Assess the superficial abdominal and cremasteric reflexes.
- Abdominal reflex: Lightly stroke the abdomen with a tongue blade from the side to the midline. Normally the side of the abdomen being stroked will contract.
- Cremasteric reflex: Lightly stroke the inner thigh of the male client with a tongue blade. Normally, the testicle on the side being stroked will rise.
  - ✓ Superficial reflexes may be absent with disease of the lower and upper motor neurons.
- Assess the Babinski reflex.
  - ✓ Dorsiflexion of the big toe and fanning of the other toes is seen with upper motor neuron disease of the pyramidal tract.

Special Neurologic Assessments with Abnormal Findings (✓)

- Assess for Brudzinski's sign. With the client supine, flex the head to the chest.
  - ✓ Pain, resistance, and flexion of hips and knees occur with meningeal irritation.
- Assess for Kernig's sign. With the client supine, flex the knees and hips, then straighten the knee.
  - ✓ Excessive pain and/or resistance occurs with meningeal irritation.
- Assess for abnormal postures.
- Observe for **decorticate posturing,** in which the upper arms are close to the sides; the elbows, wrists, and fingers are flexed; the legs are extended with internal rotation; and the feet are plantar flexed.
- Observe for **decerebrate posturing,** in which the neck is extended, with the jaw clenched; the arms are pronated, extended, and close to the sides; the legs are extended straight out; and the feet are plantar flexed.
  - ✓ Decorticate posturing occurs with lesions of the corticospinal tracts.
  - ✓ Decerebrate posturing occurs with lesions of the midbrain, pons, or diencephalon.

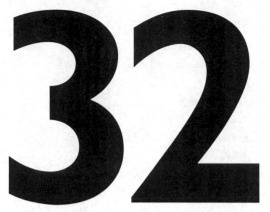

Nursing Care of Clients with Cerebrovascular and Spinal Cord Disorders

The health problems discussed in this chapter result from alterations in cerebral blood flow. Disorders of the spinal cord and brain affect an estimated 50 million Americans, costing the American public more than $400 billion a year in direct health care costs and indirect lifetime costs. Clients with disorders of cerebral blood flow and the spinal cord experience a wide variety of neurologic deficits that affect cognitive and perceptual health patterns.

Nursing care for clients with these disorders is tailored to meet the needs of the client and is individualized according to the client's responses to alterations in intracranial and spinal cord structure and function. This chapter's discussion of nursing care includes consideration of acute and long-term health care needs.

Cerebrovascular Disorders

The Client with a Stroke

A **stroke (cerebral vascular accident [CVA]),** also referred to as a *brain attack,* is a condition in which neurologic deficits result from decreased blood flow to a localized area of the brain. Strokes may be *ischemic* (when blood supply to a part of the brain is suddenly interrupted by a thrombus or embolus) or *hemorrhagic* (when a blood vessel breaks open, spilling blood into spaces surrounding neurons). The neurologic deficits caused by ischemia and the resultant necrosis of cells in the brain vary according to the area of the brain involved, the size of the affected area, and the length of time blood flow is decreased or stopped. A major loss of blood supply to the brain can cause severe disability or death. When the duration of decreased blood flow is short and the anatomical area involved is small, the person may not be aware that damage has been done.

Incidence and Prevalence

Strokes are the third leading cause of death in North America, where approximately 600,000 people suffer a stroke each year. Of those, 160,000 die, and many clients who survive are left with some type of functional impairment (Porth, 2002). The highest incidence occurs in people over 65 years of age. However, 28% of cerebral vascular accidents occur in people under the age of 65, and strokes occur in every age group. They occur more frequently in men than women.

Risk Factors

Certain diseases, lifestyle habits, and ethnic backgrounds increase the risk of a stroke including:

- *Hypertension.* Increased systolic and diastolic blood pressure is associated with damage to all blood vessels, including the cerebral vessels.

- *Diabetes mellitus.* Diabetes leads to vascular changes in both the systemic and cerebral circulation and increases the risk of hypertension.

- *Sickle cell disease.* Changes in the shape of the red blood cells increase blood viscosity and produce erythrocyte clumps that may occlude small cerebral vessels.

- *Substance abuse.* The injection of unpurified substances increases the risk for a stroke, and abuse of certain drugs can decrease cerebral blood flow and increase the risk for intracranial hemorrhage. Substances associated with strokes include alcohol, nicotine, heroin, amphetamines, and cocaine.

- *Atherosclerosis.* Occlusion of cerebral vessels by atherosclerotic plaque impairs or obstructs blood flow to specific areas of the brain.

Other risk factors include a family history of obesity, a sedentary lifestyle, hyperlipidemia, atrial fibrillation, cardiac disease, cigarette smoking, and previous transient ischemic attacks. Risk factors specific to women are oral contraceptive use, pregnancy, and menopause.

Overview of Normal Cerebral Blood Flow

The brain, which makes up only 2% of total body weight, receives approximately 20% of the cardiac output each minute (about 750 mL) and accounts for 20% of the body's oxygen consumption. Brain function depends on a consistent blood and oxygen supply. When cerebral blood flow is decreased or interrupted, the resulting ischemia may lead to death of brain cells and pathophysiologic alterations (Porth, 2002).

The brain is supplied with blood from the internal carotid arteries (anteriorly) and the vertebral arteries (posteriorly). Two sets of veins drain cerebral blood into venous plexuses and dural sinuses and then into the internal jugular veins at the base of the skull. The veins in the cerebral system do not have valves; therefore, the direction of flow depends on gravity or pressure differences between the venous sinuses and the extracranial veins.

Activities that increase intrathoracic pressure, such as sneezing, coughing, straining to have a bowel movement, or vomiting, also briefly increase intracranial pressure. This increased intracranial pressure occurs because the increased intrathoracic pressure is transmitted through the internal jugular veins and the dural sinuses.

Cerebral blood flow, especially in the deep cerebral vessels, is largely self-regulated by the brain to meet metabolic needs. This self-regulation (also called *autoregulation*) allows the brain to maintain a constant blood flow despite changes in systemic blood pressure. However, autoregulation is not effective when systemic blood pressure falls below 50 mmHg or rises above 160 mmHg. In the latter case, the increased systemic pressure (as in hypertension) causes an increase in cerebral blood flow with resultant overdistention of cerebral vessels. Cerebral blood flow is affected by concentrations of carbon dioxide, oxygen, and hydrogen ions. Cerebral blood flow increases in response to increased carbon dioxide concentrations, increased hydrogen ion concentrations, and decreased oxygen concentrations.

Pathophysiology

A stroke is characterized by a gradual or rapid onset of neurologic deficits due to compromised cerebral blood flow. Strokes may result from a variety of problems, including transient ischemic attack (TIA), cerebral thrombosis, cerebral embolism, and cerebral hemorrhage.

When blood flow to and oxygenation of cerebral neurons are decreased or interrupted, pathophysiologic changes at the cellular level take place in four to five minutes. Cellular metabolism ceases as glucose, glycogen, and adenosine triphosphate (ATP) are depleted and the sodium-potassium pump fails. Cells swell as sodium draws water into the cell. Cerebral blood vessel walls also swell, further decreasing blood flow. Even if circulation is restored, vasospasm and increased blood viscosity can continue to impede blood flow. Severe or prolonged ischemia leads to cellular death. A central core of dead or dying cells is surrounded by a band of minimally perfused cells, called the *penumbra*. Although cells in the penumbra have impaired metabolic activities, their structural integrity is maintained. The survival of these cells depends on a timely return of adequate circulation, the volume of toxic products released by adjacent dying cells, the degree of cerebral edema, and alterations in local blood flow. The potential survival of cells in the penumbra has led to the use of thrombolytic agents in the early treatment of ischemic stroke (Porth, 2002).

The neurologic deficits that occur as a result of a stroke can often be used to identify its location. Because the sensory-motor pathways cross at the junction of the medulla and spinal cord (decussation), strokes lead to loss or impairment of sensory-motor functions on the side of the body opposite the side of the brain that is damaged. This effect, known as a **contralateral deficit,** causes a stroke in the right hemisphere of the brain to be manifested by deficits in the left side of the body (and vice versa).

Ischemic Stroke

Ischemic strokes result from cerebrovascular obstruction by thrombosis or emboli. They include TIAs, thrombotic stroke, and embolic stroke.

Transient Ischemic Attack

A **transient ischemic attack (TIA)** is a brief period of localized cerebral ischemia that causes neurologic deficits lasting for less than 24 hours (usually less than 1 to 2 hours; Porth, 2002). The deficits may be present for only minutes or may last for hours. TIAs are often warning signals of an ischemic thrombotic stroke. One or many TIAs may precede a stroke, with the time between the TIA and a stroke ranging from hours to months.

The etiology of TIA includes inflammatory artery disorders, sickle cell anemia, atherosclerotic changes in cerebral vessels, thrombosis, and emboli. Transient cerebral ischemia may also occur as a result of subclavian steal syndrome, a relatively rare pathophysiologic process in which blood that normally flows from the vertebral arteries into the circulation of the brain changes direction and flows from the vertebral arteries into the arteries of the arm. This reverse flow occurs when the arm is exercised and the subclavian artery is occluded.

Neurologic manifestations of a TIA vary according to the location and size of the cerebral vessel involved. Manifestations have a sudden onset and often disappear within minutes or hours. Commonly occurring deficits include contralateral numbness or weakness of the hand, forearm, and corner of the mouth (due to middle cerebral artery involvement); aphasia (due to ischemia of the left hemisphere); and visual disturbances, such as blurring (due to involvement of the posterior cerebral artery; Porth, 2002).

Thrombotic Stroke

A **thrombotic stroke** is caused by occlusion of a large cerebral vessel by a thrombus (a blood clot). Thrombotic CVAs most often occur in older people who are resting or sleeping. The blood pressure is lower during sleep, so there is less pressure to push the blood through an already narrowed arterial lumen, and ischemia may result.

Thrombi tend to form in large arteries that bifurcate and have narrowed lumens as a result of deposits of atherosclerotic plaque. The plaque involves the intima of the arteries, causing the internal elastic lamina to become thin and frayed with exposure of underlying connective tissue. This structural change causes platelets to adhere to the rough surface and release the enzyme adenosine diphosphate. This enzyme initiates the clotting sequence, and the thrombus forms. A thrombus may remain in place and continue to enlarge, completely occluding the lumen of the vessel, or a part of it may break off and become an embolus.

The most common locations of thrombi are the internal carotid artery, the vertebral arteries, and the junction of the vertebral and basilar arteries. Thrombotic strokes affecting the smaller cerebral vessels are called **lacunar strokes,** because the infarcted areas slough off, leaving a small cavity or "lake" in the brain tissue. A thrombotic stroke usually affects only one region of the brain that is supplied by a single cerebral artery.

A thrombotic stroke occurs rapidly but progresses slowly. It often begins with a TIA, and continues to worsen over one to two days; the condition is called a stroke-in-evolution. When maximum neurologic deficit has been reached, usually in three days, the condition is called a completed stroke. At that time, the damaged area is edematous and necrotic.

Embolic Stroke

An **embolic stroke** occurs when a blood clot or clump of matter traveling through the cerebral blood vessels becomes lodged in a vessel too narrow to permit further movement. The area of the brain supplied by the blocked vessel becomes ischemic. The most frequent sites of cerebral emboli are at bifurcations of vessels, particularly those of the carotid and middle cerebral arteries. This type of stroke is typically seen in clients who are younger than those experiencing thrombotic strokes and occurs when the client is awake and active.

Many embolic strokes originate from a thrombus in the left chambers of the heart, formed during atrial fibrillation. These are referred to as *cardiogenic embolic strokes.* Emboli result when parts of the thrombus break off and are carried through the arterial system to the brain. Cerebral emboli may also be due to carotid artery atherosclerotic plaque, bacterial endocarditis, recent myocardial infarction, rheumatic heart disease, and ventricular aneurysm.

An embolic stroke has a sudden onset and causes immediate deficits. If the embolus breaks up into smaller fragments and is absorbed by the body, symptoms will disappear in a few hours to a few days. If the embolus is not absorbed, symptoms will persist. Even if the embolus is absorbed, the vessel wall where the embolus lodges may be weakened, increasing the potential for cerebral hemorrhage.

Hemorrhagic Stroke

A **hemorrhagic stroke,** or **intracranial hemorrhage,** occurs when a cerebral blood vessel ruptures. It occurs most often in people with sustained increase in systolic-diastolic pressure. Intracranial hemorrhage usually occurs suddenly, often when the affected person is engaged in some activity. Although hypertension is the most common cause, a variety of factors may contribute to a hemorrhagic stroke, including ruptured intracranial aneurysms, trauma, erosion of blood vessels by tumors, arteriovenous malformations, anticoagulant therapy, and blood disorders. Of all forms of stroke, this form is most often fatal.

As a result of the blood vessel rupture, blood enters the brain tissue, the cerebral ventricles, or the subarachnoid space, compressing adjacent tissues and causing blood vessel spasm and cerebral edema. Blood in the ventricles or subarachnoid space irritates the meninges and brain tissue, causing an inflammatory reaction and impairing absorption and circulation of cerebral spinal fluid.

The onset of manifestations from a hemorrhagic stroke is rapid. Manifestations depend on the location of the hemorrhage, but may include vomiting, headache, seizures, hemiplegia, and loss of consciousness. Pressure on the brain tissue from increased intracranial pressure (discussed in Chapter 33) may cause coma and death.

Manifestations and Complications

Manifestations and complications of a stroke vary according to the cerebral artery involved and the area of the brain affected. Manifestations are always sudden in onset, focal, and usually one sided. The most common manifestation is weakness involving the face and arm, and sometimes the leg. Other common manifestations are numbness on one side, loss of vision in one eye or to the side, speech difficulties, and difficulties with balance. The various deficits associated with involvement of a specific cerebral artery are collectively referred to as stroke syndromes, although the deficits often overlap.

Table 32-1. Manifestations of a Stroke by Involved Cerebral Vessel

---

Internal Carotid Artery

- Contralateral paralysis of the arm, leg, and face
- Contralateral sensory deficits of the arm, leg, and face
- If the dominant hemisphere is involved: aphasia
- If the nondominant hemisphere is involved: apraxia, agnosia, unilateral neglect
- Homonymous hemianopia

Middle Cerebral Artery

- Drowsiness, stupor, coma
- Contralateral hemiplegia of the arm and face
- Contralateral sensory deficits of the arm and face
- Global aphasia (if dominant hemisphere involved)
- Homonymous hemianopia

Continued on the next page

Table 32-1. Continued

Anterior Cerebral Artery

- Contralateral weakness or paralysis of the foot and leg
- Contralateral sensory loss of the toes, foot, and leg
- Loss of ability to make decisions or act voluntarily
- Urinary incontinence

Vertebral Artery

- Pain in face, nose, or eye
- Numbness and weakness of the face on involved side
- Problems with gait
- Dysphagia
- Dysarthria

Typical manifestations and complications include motor deficits, elimination disorders, sensory-perceptual deficits, language disorders, and behavioral changes. These may be transient or permanent, depending on the degree of ischemia and necrosis as well as time of treatment. As a result of the neurologic deficits, the client with a stroke has manifestations that involve many different body systems (see Table 32-2).

Motor Deficits

Body movement results from a complex interaction between the brain, spinal cord, and peripheral nerves. The motor areas of the cerebral cortex, the basal ganglia, and the cerebellum initiate voluntary movement by sending messages to the spinal cord, which then transmits the messages to the peripheral nerves. A stroke may interrupt the central nervous system component of this relay system and produce effects in the contralateral side ranging from mild weakness to severe limitation of any kind of movement.

Table 32-2. Manifestations and Complications of Stroke by Body System

Integument

- Decubitus (pressure) ulcers

Neurologic

- Hyperthermia
- Neglect syndrome
- Seizures
- Agnosias
- Communication deficits
    a. Expressive aphasia
    b. Receptive aphasia

Table 32-2. Continued

    c.   Global aphasia

    d.   Agraphia

- Visual deficits
  a. Homonymous hemianopia
  b. Diplopia
  c. Decreased acuity

- Cognitive changes
  a. Memory loss
  b. Short attention span
  c. Distractibility
  d. Poor judgment
  e. Poor problem-solving ability
  f. Disorientation

- Behavioral changes
  a. Emotional lability
  b. Loss of social inhibitions
  c. Fear
  d. Hostility
  e. Anger
  f. Depression

- Increased intracranial pressure
- Alterations in consciousness
- Sensory loss (touch, pain, heat, cold, pressure)

Respiratory

- Respiratory center damage
- Airway obstruction
- Decreased ability to cough

Gastrointestinal

- Dysphagia
- Constipation
- Stool impaction

Genitourinary

- Incontinence
- Frequency
- Urgency
- Urinary retention
- Renal calculi

Continued on the next page

Table 32-2. Continued

Musculoskeletal

- Hemiplegia
- Contractures
- Bony ankylosis
- Disuse atrophy
- Dysarthria

Depending on the area of the brain involved, strokes may cause weakness, paralysis, and/or spasticity. The deficits include:

- **Hemiplegia:** paralysis of the left or right half of the body.
- **Hemiparesis:** weakness of the left or right half of the body.
- **Flaccidity:** absence of muscle tone (hypotonia).
- **Spasticity:** increased muscle tone (hypertonia), usually with some degree of weakness. The flexor muscles are usually more strongly affected in the upper extremities and the extensor muscles are more strongly affected in the lower extremities.

When the corticospinal tract is involved, the affected arm and leg almost always are initially flaccid and then become spastic within six to eight weeks. Spasticity often causes characteristic body positioning: adduction of the shoulder, pronation of the forearm, flexion of the fingers, and extension of the hip and knee. There is often foot drop, outward rotation of the leg, and dependent edema in the involved extremities.

The motor deficits may result in altered mobility, further impairing body function. The complications of immobility involve multiple body systems and include orthostatic hypotension, increased thrombus formation, decreased cardiac output, impaired respiratory function, osteoporosis, formation of renal calculi, contractures, and decubitus ulcer formation.

Elimination Disorders

Disorders of bladder and bowel elimination are common. A stroke may cause partial loss of the sensations that trigger bladder elimination, resulting in urinary frequency, urgency, or incontinence. Control of urination may be altered as a result of cognitive deficits. Changes in bowel elimination are common; they result from changes in level of consciousness, immobility, and dehydration (Hickey, 2003).

Sensory-Perceptual Deficits

A stroke may involve pathologic changes in neurologic pathways that alter the ability to integrate, interpret, and attend to sensory data. The client may experience deficits in vision, hearing, equilibrium, taste, and sense of smell. The ability to perceive vibration, pain, warmth, cold, and pressure may be impaired, as may proprioception (the body's sense of its position). The loss of these sensory abilities increases the risk for injury. Deficits may include:

- **Hemianopia:** the loss of half of the visual field of one or both eyes; when the same half is missing in each eye, the condition is called homonymous hemianopia.

- **Agnosia:** the inability to recognize one or more subjects that were previously familiar; agnosia may be visual, tactile, or auditory.
- **Apraxia:** the inability to carry out some motor pattern (e.g., drawing a figure, getting dressed) even when strength and coordination are adequate.

Another form of sensory-perceptual deficit is the **neglect syndrome** (or unilateral neglect), in which the client has a disorder of attention. In this syndrome, the person cannot integrate and use perceptions from the affected side of the body or from the environment on the affected side, and ignores that part. In severe cases, the client may even deny the paralysis. This deficit is more common following a stroke of the right hemisphere where damage to the parietal lobe (a center for mediation of directed attention) results in perceptual deficits.

Communication Disorders

Communication is a complex process, involving motor functions, speech, language, memory, reasoning, and emotions. Communication problems are usually the result of a stroke affecting the dominant hemisphere. The left hemisphere is dominant in about 95% of right-handed people and 70% of left-handed people (Porth, 2002).

Many different impairments may occur, and most are partial. Disorders of communication affect both speech (the mechanical act of articulating language through the spoken word) and language (the vocal or written formulation of ideas to communicate thoughts and feelings). Language involves oral and written expression and auditory and reading comprehension. Among these disorders are:

- **Aphasia:** the inability to use or understand language; aphasia may be expressive, receptive, or mixed (global).
- **Expressive aphasia:** a motor speech problem in which one can understand what is being said but can respond verbally only in short phrases; also called *Broca's aphasia.*
- **Receptive aphasia:** a sensory speech problem in which one cannot understand the spoken (and often written) word. Speech may be fluent but with inappropriate content; also called *Wernicke's aphasia.*
- **Mixed or global aphasia:** language dysfunction in both understanding and expression.
- **Dysarthria:** any disturbance in muscular control of speech.

Cognitive and Behavioral Changes

A change in consciousness, ranging from mild confusion to coma, is a common manifestation of a stroke. It may result from tissue damage following ischemia or hemorrhage involving either the carotid or vertebral arteries. Altered consciousness may also be the result of cerebral edema or increased intracranial pressure.

Behavioral changes include emotional lability (in which the client may laugh or cry inappropriately), loss of self-control (manifested by such behavior as swearing or refusing to wear clothing), and decreased tolerance for stress (resulting in anger or depression). Intellectual changes may include memory loss, decreased attention span, poor judgment, and an inability to think abstractly.

Collaborative Care

The client with a stroke may receive medical and/or surgical treatment. The focus in the acute care phase is on diagnosing the type and cause of the stroke, supporting cerebral circulation, and controlling or preventing further deficits.

Diagnostic Tests

Diagnostic tests may be ordered to detect increased risk for a stroke or to identify pathophysiologic changes after a stroke has occurred.

- *Computed tomography (CT)* without contrast is the first imaging technique used to demonstrate the presence of hemorrhage, tumors, aneurysm, ischemia, edema, and tissue necrosis. A CT scan can also demonstrate a shift in intracranial contents, and is useful in distinguishing the type of stroke (e.g., a hemorrhagic stroke results in an increase in density).

- *Arteriography* of cerebral vessels is performed to demonstrate abnormal vessel structures, vasospasm, loss of vessel wall integrity, and stenosis of the carotid arteries.

- **Transcranial ultrasound Doppler (TCD)** studies are used to evaluate the velocity of the blood flow through the intracranial arteries and provide information about partial or complete occlusion.

- *Magnetic resonance imaging (MRI)* test may be conducted to detect shifting of brain tissues as a result of hemorrhage or edema. A *magnetic resonance angiography (MRA)* may be performed to detect occlusive disease of the large cerebral vessels.

- *Positron emission tomography (PET)* and *single-photon emission computed tomography (SPECT)* are used to examine cerebral blood flow distribution and metabolic activity of the brain. Both tests use very short-lived radionuclides that emit radioactive energy as they move through the circulation. PET allows the identification of the location and size of the stroke; SPECT provides information about the metabolism of and blood flow through the brain tissue affected by the stroke.

- *Lumbar puncture* may be performed to obtain cerebrospinal fluid for examination if there is no danger of increased intracranial pressure. (Removal of cerebrospinal fluid when intracranial pressure is increased can result in herniation of the brainstem.) A thrombotic stroke may elevate cerebrospinal fluid pressure; after a hemorrhagic stroke frank blood may be seen in the cerebrospinal fluid.

Medications

Medications are administered to prevent a stroke in clients with TIAs or a previous stroke, and to treat the client during the acute phase of a stroke.

Prevention   Antiplatelet agents are often used to treat clients with TIAs or who have had a previous stroke. Platelets are concentrated in high blood flow arteries, they adhere to endothelial tissue damaged by atherosclerosis and occlude the vessel. The drugs used to prevent clot formation and blood vessel occlusion include aspirin, clopidogrel (Plavix), dipyridamole (Persantine), pentoxifylline (Trental), and ticlopidine (Ticlid).

Daily low-dose aspirin reduces TIA occurrence and stroke risk by interfering with platelet aggregation. Ticlopidine (Ticlid) is a platelet-aggregation inhibitor that has shown reduction in thrombotic stroke risk.

Acute Stroke

Pharmacologic agents are used to treat the client during the acute phase of an ischemic stroke to prevent further thrombosis formation, increase cerebral blood flow, and protect cerebral neurons. The type of medication used varies according to the type of stroke.

Anticoagulant drug therapy (discussed in Chapter 12) is often ordered for thrombotic stroke during the stroke-in-evolution phase, but is contraindicated in completed stroke, because it may increase the risk of cerebral hemorrhage. Anticoagulants are never administered to a client with a hemorrhagic stroke. Anticoagulants do not dissolve an existing clot, but prevent further extension of the clot and formation of new clots. Sodium heparin may be given subcutaneously or by continuous IV drip, or warfarin sodium (Coumadin) may be given orally.

Thrombolytic therapy, using a tissue plasminogen activator, such as recombinant altephase (Activase rt-pa), sometimes given concurrently with an anticoagulant, is used to treat thrombotic stroke. The drug converts plasminogen to plasmin, resulting in fibrinolysis of the clot. To be effective, it must be given within three hours of the onset of manifestations (Tierney, et al., 2001).

Antithrombotic drugs, which inhibit the platelet phase of clot formation, have been used as a preventive measure for clients at risk for embolic and thrombotic CVA. Both aspirin and dipyridamole have been used for this purpose. These drugs are also sometimes used in combination with other drugs during acute treatment. Antiplatelet agents are contraindicated in clients with a hemorrhagic stroke.

Calcium channel blockers, such as nimodipine (Nimotop), are under investigation and have been used in clinical trials to reduce ischemic deficits and death from stroke. They block glutamate, an excitatory neurotransmitter, to reduce the sensitivity of neurons to ischemia.

Corticosteriods, such as prednisone or dexamethasone, have been used to treat cerebral edema, but the results are not always positive. If the client has increased intracranial pressure, hyperosmolar solutions, such as mannitol, or diuretics, such as furosemide, may be administered. Anticonvulsants, such as phenytoin (Dilantin), and barbiturates may be prescribed if increased intracranial pressure causes seizures.

Treatments

The treatments used in the medical management of a stroke include surgery, physical therapy, occupational therapy, and speech therapy.

Surgery   Surgery may be performed to prevent the occurrence of a stroke or to restore blood flow when a stroke has already occurred. In people who have had TIAs or are in danger of having another stroke, a carotid endarterectomy at the carotid artery bifurcation may be performed to remove atherosclerotic plaque.

When an occluded or stenotic vessel is not directly accessible, an extracranial-intracranial bypass may be performed. Bypass of the internal carotid, middle cerebral, or vertebral arteries may be required. The indications for the bypass are symptoms of ischemia caused by TIAs or a mild completed stroke. The procedure reestablishes blood flow to the affected area of the brain.

Physical/Occupational/Speech Therapy

Physical therapy may help prevent contractures and improve muscle strength and coordination. Occupational therapy provides assistive devices and a plan for regaining lost motor skills that greatly improve quality of life after a stroke. In addition, the client with a communication disorder requires speech therapy.

Nursing Care

Even though many people who have a stroke have full recovery, a substantial number are left with disabilities that affect their physical, emotional, interpersonal, and family status. The required nursing care is often complex and multidimensional, requiring consideration of continuity of care for clients in acute care settings, long-term care settings, rehabilitation centers, and the home.

Nurses caring for clients who have had a stroke require knowledge and skill to meet the client's needs during both the acute and the rehabilitative phases of care. The client often has multiple losses: loss of mobility, ability to provide self-care, communications, concept of self, and interpersonal or intimate relationships with others. Holistic, individualized nursing care is essential in all settings and focuses on promoting the achievement of maximum potential and quality of life.

The client's family is often faced with many changes. The young to middle-aged adult with a family member who has had a stroke may be faced with economic difficulties and social isolation. The middle-aged adult family member may become the caretaker for an older parent, in essence switching roles with the parent. An older adult may not be able to care for a spouse and may have to accept nursing home placement. In addition, the older adult who has no family may have to struggle alone to regain the ability to function independently. Although not all of these problems are amenable to nursing solutions, the nurse is most often the health care provider who assesses and identifies the needs of each individual and provides information and referrals to clients and families to help meet those needs.

Because a stroke has the potential to cause many different health problems, a wide variety of nursing diagnoses may be appropriate. It is important to remember that each person will be affected differently, depending on the degree of ischemia and the area of the brain involved. Nursing diagnoses discussed in this section focus on problems with cerebral tissue perfusion (specific to nursing care during the acute phase), physical mobility, self-care, communication, sensory-perceptual deficits, bowel and urine elimination, and swallowing (specific to prevention of complications and rehabilitation). See Table 32-2 for more information.

Health Promotion

Health promotion activities focus on stroke prevention, especially for those people with known risk factors. It is important to discuss the importance of stopping smoking and drug use with clients of all ages. Maintaining a normal weight through diet and exercise can help reduce obesity, which increases the risk of hypertension and Type 2 diabetes mellitus (both in turn increase the risk of a stroke). Cholesterol levels should be screened regularly to monitor for hyperlipidemia. Regular health care to monitor for and treat cardiovascular disorders and to detect and treat infections such as infective endocarditis are important. It is also important to increase public awareness of the signs of a TIA or stroke, and of the need to call 911 or to seek care immediately if the following warning signs or symptoms occur:

- Sudden weakness or numbness of the face, arm, or leg, especially on one side of the body.
- Sudden confusion, difficulty speaking, or difficulty understanding speech.
- Sudden trouble walking, dizziness, loss of coordination.

- Sudden difficulty with vision in one or both eyes.
- Sudden severe headache without a cause.

Assessment

The following data are collected through the health history and physical examination (see Chapter 31). Further focused assessments are described with the following nursing interventions:

- *Health history:* risk factors, drug use (medications and illegal), smoking history, when symptoms began, severity of symptoms, presence of incontinence, level of consciousness, family support system.
- *Physical assessment:* motor strength, coordination, communication, cranial nerves.

Nursing Diagnoses and Interventions

The acute phase of a stroke is most often the time from admission to the hospital until the client is stabilized: usually 24 to 72 hours after admission (Hickey, 2003). Depending on the severity of the stroke, the client may be admitted to the intensive care unit. Regardless of the hospital setting, the nurse provides interventions to maintain body functions and prevent complications.

Ineffective Tissue Perfusion (Cerebral)

The initial assessment and care of the client admitted for intensive care focuses on identifying changes that may indicate altered cerebral perfusion. The client's airway, breathing, circulation, and neurologic status are monitored and interventions are provided to maintain cerebral perfusion.

- Monitor respiratory status and airway patency. Auscultate pulmonary sounds and monitor respiratory rate and results of studies of arterial blood gases.
- Suction as necessary, using care to suction no longer than 10 to 15 seconds at any one time, and using sterile technique.
- Place in a side-lying position.
- Administer oxygen as prescribed.

The client is often unconscious and breathing may be impaired. Suctioning removes secretions that not only obstruct airflow but also pose the risk for aspiration and pneumonia. Suctioning for longer than 15 seconds at a time may increase intracranial pressure (Hickey, 2003). Respiratory complications develop rapidly, as manifested by crackles and wheezes, rapid respirations, and respiratory acidosis. The administration of oxygen decreases the risk for hypoxia and hypercapnia, which can increase cerebral ischemia and intracranial pressure.

- Monitor neurologic status.
- Assess mental status and level of consciousness: restlessness, drowsiness, lethargy, inability to follow commands, unresponsiveness.
- Monitor strength and reflexes, and assess for pain, headache, decreased muscle strength, sluggish pupillary reflexes, absent gag or swallowing reflexes, hemiplegia, Babinski's sign, and decerebrate or decorticate posturing.

Frequent monitoring of neurologic status is necessary to detect changes. Alterations in mental status, level of consciousness, movement, strength, and reflexes indicate increased intracranial pressure, the major cause of death in the acute phase of a stroke.

- Continuously monitor cardiac status, observing for dysrhythmias. *A stroke may cause cardiac dysrhythmias, including bradycardia, PVCs, tachycardia, and AV block. Characteristic ECG changes include a shortened PR interval, peaked T waves, and a depressed ST segment.*
- Monitor body temperature. *Hyperthermia may develop if the hypothalamus is affected.*
- Maintain accurate intake and output records; measure urinary output via a Foley catheter. *A stroke may damage the pituitary gland, resulting in diabetes insipidus and the possibility of dehydration from greatly increased urinary output.*
- Monitor seizures. Pad the side rails, and administer prescribed anticonvulsants. *Seizures may be the result of cerebral tissue damage or increased intracranial pressure. Padded side rails prevent injury if a seizure occurs. Anticonvulsants prevent or treat seizures.*

Impaired Physical Mobility

The broad goals of care for clients with impaired mobility are to maintain and improve functional abilities (by maintaining normal function and alignment, preventing edema of extremities, and reducing spasticity) and to prevent complications.

- Encourage active ROM exercises for unaffected extremities and perform passive ROM exercises for affected extremities every four hours during day and evening shifts and once during the night shift. Support the joint during passive ROM exercises. *Active ROM exercises maintain or improve muscle strength and endurance, and help to maintain cardiopulmonary function. Passive ROM exercises do not strengthen muscles, but do help maintain joint flexibility.*
- Turn body every two hours around the clock, following a posted schedule for side-to-side and supine-to-prone position changes (verify prone positioning with the physician). Maintain body alignment and support extremities in proper position with pillows. *Turning on a regular basis, accompanied by proper positioning, maintains joint function, alleviates pressure on bony prominences that can lead to skin breakdown, decreases dependent edema in hands and feet, and lessens the risk of complications resulting from immobility.*
- Monitor the lower extremities each shift for symptoms of thrombophlebitis. Assess for increased warmth and redness in calves; measure the circumference of the calves and thighs. *Clients on bed rest (especially those with loss of muscle strength and tone) are particularly prone to the development of deep vein thrombosis. Promptly report symptoms of thrombophlebitis.*
- Collaborate with the physical therapist as the client gains mobility, using consistent techniques to move the client from the bed to the wheelchair and to help the client ambulate. *The use of consistent techniques facilitates rehabilitation.*

Self-Care Deficit

The client who has had a stroke may have a self-care deficit as a result of impaired mobility or mental confusion. It is important for clients to perform as much of their own physical care and grooming as possible to promote functional ability, increase independence, decrease feelings of powerlessness, and improve self-esteem.

Before establishing a plan to increase self-care, determine which hand was dominant before the stroke. If the client's dominant side is affected, self-care will be more difficult.

- Encourage use of the unaffected arm to bathe, brush teeth, comb hair, dress, and eat. *Use of the unaffected arm promotes functional ability and independence.*

- Teach the client to put on clothing by first dressing the affected extremities and then dressing the unaffected extremities. *This technique facilitates self-dressing with minimal assistance.*

- Collaborate with the occupational therapist in scheduling times for training for upper extremity functioning necessary for activities of daily living. Encourage the use of assistive devices (if required) for eating, physical hygiene, and dressing. *Following a regular schedule in daily routines promotes learning. The use of assistive devices promotes independence and decreases feelings of powerlessness. Optimal grooming facilitates positive self-concept.*

Impaired Verbal Communication

The client who loses communication abilities requires intensive speech therapy and emotional support. It is important to determine the specific nature of the impairment when planning interventions and helping family members understand specific problem. Although the speech therapist is usually most involved with speech rehabilitation, nurses must plan interventions to meet communication needs during all phases of care.

Use the following guidelines:

- Approach and treat the client as an adult.

- Do not assume that the client who does not respond verbally cannot hear. Do not use a raised voice when addressing the client.

- Allow adequate time for the client to respond.

- Face the client and speak slowly.

- When you do not understand the client's speech, be honest and say so.

- Use short, simple statements and questions.

Providing the client with dignity and respect enhances the nurse-client relationship. Allowing adequate response time and using short verbal statements or questions while facing the client motivates the client to communicate and decreases frustration.

- Accept frustration and anger as a normal reaction to the loss of function. *Anger represents the client's frustration at the inability to control the loss of function.*

- Try alternate methods of communication, including writing tablets, flash cards, and computerized talking boards. *Clients unable to communicate verbally may use other methods effectively.*

Impaired Urinary Elimination and Risk for Constipation

Both urinary and bowel elimination may be altered because of neurologic deficits, impaired mobility, cognitive impairment, communication deficits, or preexisting problems (especially if the client is, as usual, an older adult). Other causes include changes in food and fluid intake and side effects of medications. Urinary incontinence or retention and constipation and fecal impaction are the usual manifestations.

- Assess for urinary frequency, urgency, incontinence, nocturia, and voiding in small amounts. In addition, assess the client's ability to respond to the need to void, the ability to use the call light, and the ability to use toileting equipment.

- Encourage bladder training by having client void on schedule, such as every two hours, rather than in response to the urge to void.

- Teach Kegel exercises. To perform Kegel exercises, the client contracts the perineal muscles as though stopping urination, holds the contraction for five seconds, and then releases.

- Use positive reinforcement (verbal praise) for successful management of urinary elimination.

Voiding every two hours or on schedule promotes bladder tone and urine storage. Kegel exercises increase pubococcygeal muscle tone and bladder control, decreasing incontinence. Positive reinforcement can be a useful part of the teaching program.

- Discuss prestroke bowel habits, as well as the pattern of bowel elimination since the stroke.

- If the client is able to swallow without difficulty, encourage fluids (up to 2000 mL per day) and a high-fiber diet.

- Increase physical activity as tolerated.

- Assist in using the toilet facilities at the same time each day (based on usual patterns of bowel elimination), ensuring privacy and having client sit in upright position if at all possible.

- Administer prescribed stool softeners if the client is following a bowel elimination routine or is not drinking sufficient fluids.

Increased fluids, fiber, and activity stimulate intestinal motility. Establishing a regular daily time for bowel movements in the upright position and in privacy promotes normal bowel elimination. Stool softeners help prevent the formation of hard stool that is more difficult to expel.

Impaired Swallowing

A stroke may impair the ability to swallow. Weakness or lack of coordination of the tongue, attention deficits, and deficits involving the swallowing reflex all play a role. Dysphagia (difficulty swallowing) may result in choking, drooling, aspiration, or regurgitation. Nursing care focuses on maintaining safety by preventing aspiration and on ensuring adequate nutrition.

- Ensure safety when eating.

- Position in upright sitting position with neck slightly flexed.

- Order puréed or soft food.

- Feed or teach client to eat by putting food behind the front teeth on the unaffected side of mouth and tilting the head slightly backward. Teach to swallow one bite at a time.

- Have suction equipment available at the bedside in case of choking or aspiration.

Sitting upright with the head and neck first slightly flexed and then tilted back helps the client swallow. The client can usually swallow puréed or soft foods more easily than liquid or solid foods. Using the unaffected side of the mouth helps prevent food from collecting in the mouth and makes swallowing safer; in addition, food is less likely to fall out of the mouth.

- Minimize distractions and, if necessary, give step-by-step instructions for eating. *Distractions increase the risk of aspiration. Complex activities are easier to perform when broken down into small steps.*

Home Care

Throughout the rehabilitation process, it is important to encourage self-care as much as possible but also to involve family members in the plan of care. Stress that ADLs may take twice as long as they did before the stroke. Emphasize that physical function may continue to improve for up to three months, and speech may continue to improve for even longer. Address the following topics in preparing the client and family for home care:

- Physical care, medications, physical therapy
- Realistic expectations
- Time off for the caregiver, respite care services
- Distributors for equipment and supplies
- Home environment conducive to using equipment (e.g., a wheel chair or walker)
- Home and equipment modifications (e.g., an elevated toilet seat, grab bars in the bathroom, a bath chair, a vise lid opener, a long-handled shoehorn)
- Home health services
- Community resources, such as Meals-on-Wheels, senior centers, eldercare, large-print telephone dials, stroke clubs, Life-line (emergency alerting systems through a local hospital or agency).
- Helpful organizational resources:
  1. American Heart Association
  2. National Stroke Association
  3. Stroke Clubs International
  4. The National Institute of Neurological Disorders and Stroke.

The Client with an Intracranial Aneurysm

An **intracranial aneurysm** is a saccular outpouching of a cerebral artery that occurs at the site of a weakness in the vessel wall. The weakness may be the result of atherosclerosis, a congenital defect, trauma to the head, aging, or hypertension. A ruptured cerebral aneurysm is the most common cause of a hemorrhagic stroke.

Incidence and Prevalence

Approximately 5 million North Americans have intracranial aneurysms; most go through life without any manifestations of bleeding. However, it is estimated that 30,000 people will have a rupture of an intracranial aneurysm each year, and two-thirds of the survivors will have serious disabilities. Intracranial aneurysms are most common in adults age 30 to 60 (Hickey, 2003; Porth, 2002).

The exact etiology is unknown, but theories of cause include (1) a developmental defect in the vessel wall and (2) degeneration or fragility of the vessel wall due to conditions, such as hypertension, atherosclerosis, connective tissue disease, or abnormal blood flow. Hypertension and cigarette smoking may be predisposing factors.

Pathophysiology

Intracranial aneurysms tend to occur at the bifurcations and branches of the carotid arteries and the vertebrobasilar arteries at the circle of Willis, with most aneurysms (85%) located anteriorly. They range in size from smaller than 15 mm to larger than 50 mm. Intracranial aneurysms tend to enlarge with time, making the vessel wall thin and increasing the probability of rupture.

There are several different types of intracranial aneurysms: A *berry aneurysm* is probably the result of a congenital abnormality of the tunica media of the artery. The aneurysm usually ruptures without warning. A *saccular aneurysm* is any aneurysm with a saccular outpouching, which distends only a small portion of the vessel wall. This type of aneurysm is often caused by trauma. In a *fusiform aneurysm,* the entire circumference of a blood vessel swells to form an elongated tube. Most aneurysms of this type occur as a result of the changes of arteriosclerosis. Fusiform aneurysms act as space-occupying lesions. In a *dissecting aneurysm,* the tunica intima pulls away from the tunica media of the artery, and blood is forced between the two layers. It may result from atherosclerosis, inflammation, or trauma.

Intracranial aneurysms typically rupture from the dome rather than the base, forcing blood into the subarachnoid space at the base of the brain. The aneurysm may also rupture and force blood into brain tissue, the ventricles, or the subdural space. This discussion focuses on intracranial hemorrhages due to rupture of a cerebral aneurysm.

Manifestations and Complications

An intracranial aneurysm is usually asymptomatic until it ruptures, although very large aneurysms may cause headache and/or neurologic deficits due to pressure on adjacent intracranial structures. Small leakages of blood may occur periodically, causing headache, nausea, vomiting, and pain in the neck and back. The client may also have prodromal manifestations before the rupture occurs, such as headache, eye pain, visual deficits, and a dilated pupil.

The manifestations of a ruptured intracranial aneurysm (and subsequent subarachnoid hemorrhage) include a sudden, explosive headache; loss of consciousness; nausea and vomiting; a stiff neck and photophobia (due to meningeal irritation); cranial nerve deficits; stroke syndrome manifestations; and pituitary malfunctions (that result primarily from changes in ADH secretion).

The severity of the rupture is often inferred from the manifestations of the subarachnoid hemorrhage. In one system, severity ranges from grade I, in which the client has no symptoms or a slight headache with some stiffness of the neck, to grade V, in which the client is in a deep coma with decerebrate posturing.

Fibrin and platelets seal off the bleeding point, but the escaped blood forms a clot that irritates the brain tissue. The resulting inflammatory response causes cerebral edema, and both the edema and the hemorrhage increase intracranial pressure (Hickey, 2003). Bleeding into the subarachnoid space causes meningeal irritation. Hypothalamic dysfunction and seizures are also potential complications. The major complications of a ruptured intracranial aneurysm are rebleeding, vasospasm, and hydrocephalus.

Rebleeding

The greatest risk for rebleeding is within the first day after the initial rupture, and again in 7 to 10 days (when the initial clot breaks down). Rebleeding is manifested by a sudden severe headache, nausea and vomiting, decreasing levels of consciousness, and new neurologic deficits (Hickey, 2003). The mortality from rebleeding is as high as from the initial rupture.

Vasospasm

Cerebral vasospasm is a common but dangerous complication that occurs between 3 and 10 days after a subarachnoid hemorrhage. It is associated with a large number of deaths and disability. A cerebral vasospasm narrows the lumen of one or more cerebral vessels, causing ischemia and infarction of tissue supplied by the affected vessels. The actual cause is unknown, but it occurs in blood vessels surrounded by thick blood clots, suggesting that some substance in the clot initiates the spasm. The manifestations vary according to the degree of spasm and the area of brain affected. Regional alterations may cause focal deficits, such as hemiplegia, whereas global alterations cause loss of consciousness.

Hydrocephalus

Hydrocephalus, an abnormal accumulation of cerebrospinal fluid (CSF) within the cranial vault and dilation of the ventricles, is a potential complication of a ruptured intracranial aneurysm. Hydrocephalus is thought to be the result of obstruction of reabsorption of CSF through the arachnoid villi. The obstruction is caused by an increased protein content of the CSF because of lysis of blood in the subarachnoid space (Porth, 2002). The accumulation of cerebrospinal fluid increases intracranial pressure. Initial manifestations of hydrocephalus are typically nonspecific, but commonly include decreasing levels of consciousness.

Collaborative Care

The care of the client with a ruptured intracranial aneurysm includes determining the location of the aneurysm, treating the manifestations of the hemorrhage, and preventing rebleeding and vasospasm. Surgery is the treatment of choice to repair the bleeding artery.

Diagnostic Tests

The following diagnostic tests may be conducted to identify the site and extent of a ruptured intracranial aneurysm, as well as rebleeding:

- *CT scan* of the brain demonstrates blood in the subarachnoid space in most clients within the first 24 to 48 hours after rupture.
- *Lumbar puncture* may be performed to withdraw cerebrospinal fluid for analysis. The presence of blood in the cerebrospinal fluid confirms a subarachnoid hemorrhage. However, this procedure poses a risk of rebleeding and brain herniation (Porth, 2002).
- *Bilateral carotid* and *vertebral cerebral angiography* may be conducted to determine the site and size of an aneurysm. A contrast medium (if used) is injected into an artery, and X-ray films are taken to visualize the cerebral vessels. This diagnostic test is not conducted unless the client's condition is stable enough for surgery.

Medications

If surgery is not possible because of the client's condition, medications may be used to reduce the risk of rebleeding and vasospasm until surgery is feasible.

Aminocaproic acid (Amicar, Epsikapron) is a fibrinolysis inhibitor used to treat excessive bleeding in acute, life-threatening situations. It prevents the lysis of any blood clot that has formed near the site of a rupture. This drug is used in the first two weeks after aneurysm rupture (or until the client has surgery) to reduce the risk of rebleeding. The drug is administered intravenously the first week and orally thereafter. Potential complications include pulmonary embolism, venous thrombosis, and focal ischemic neurologic deficits.

Calcium channel blockers, such as nimodipine (Nimotop), are used to improve neurologic deficits due to vasospasm following subarachnoid hemorrhage from ruptured intracranial aneurysms. The drug is administered orally for three weeks after the hemorrhage. It has been found to reduce the incidence of ischemic deficits from arterial spasm without side effects (Tierney, et al., 2001).

Other medications that may be prescribed include:

*   Anticonvulsants, such as phenytoin (Dilantin), to prevent seizures if the client has increased intracranial pressure.

*   Stool softeners, such as docusate, to prevent constipation and straining with a bowel movement (which increases intracranial pressure and blood pressure). These, in turn, may cause rebleeding.

*   Analgesics (e.g., acetaminophen or codeine) for headache.

Surgery

Surgery for the treatment of intracranial aneurysm is done either to prevent rupture or to isolate the vessel to prevent further bleeding. Clients with good neurologic status may have surgery soon after the rupture. In clients with significant neurologic deficits, surgery may be delayed until they are more stable and less at risk for vasospasm.

There are several different types of surgery to repair a ruptured intracranial aneurysm or to prevent the rupture of an existing large aneurysm. The skull is opened (craniotomy), and the aneurysm is located. The neck of the aneurysm may be clipped with a metal clip (preventing the entry of blood into the aneurysm), or the involved artery may be clipped both proximally and distally to the aneurysm to isolate the affected area. Endovascular Gudlielmi detachable coils (GDCs) are used to treat aneurysms with narrow necks. The coil is inserted into the dome of the aneurysm and an electric current is passed through the coil to cause coagulation. The procedure, performed by a neuroradiologist, may be conducted either under general or local anesthesia (Bucher & Melander, 1999).

Nursing Care

Nursing Diagnoses and Interventions

Nursing care is planned and implemented for the client with a ruptured intracranial aneurysm to prevent rebleeding as well as to meet needs resulting from neurologic deficits. Other appropriate nursing diagnoses and interventions are described earlier in the chapter in the discussion of nursing care for the client with a stroke.

Ineffective Tissue Perfusion (Cerebral)

This discussion focuses on the care of the client immediately after the intracranial aneurysm ruptures. The expected outcome of care is preventing rebleeding and improving cerebral tissue perfusion. Institute aneurysm precautions to prevent rebleeding, as follows:

- Keep the client in a private, quiet, darkened room. Disconnect or remove the telephone. Avoid using bright overhead lights. *A quiet environment helps prevent an increase in blood pressure, which could precipitate rebleeding. The client may experience photophobia (abnormal sensitivity to light) if hemorrhage has damaged the oculomotor nerve.*

- Elevate the head of the bed 30 to 45 degrees; follow prescribed activity orders (usually complete bed rest, but in some cases bathroom privileges may be approved). *Elevating the head of the bed promotes venous return from the brain and thus decreases intracranial pressure. Decreasing activity reduces the likelihood of increases in blood pressure.*

- Limit visitors to two family members at any one time, and limit the duration of visits. Monitor client response to visitors and decrease interactions if the client becomes agitated or upset. *Psychologic stress may increase blood pressure and the risk of rebleeding; however, social isolation may increase anxiety and stress. Each client (and family) must be individually evaluated.*

- Allow reading, watching television (if available), or listening to the radio (if available) to promote relaxation. *Although these passive activities were previously contraindicated for the client on aneurysm precautions, current therapy is based on the belief that these activities promote relaxation and help control blood pressure.*

- Prevent constipation and straining to have a bowel movement. Administer stool softeners as prescribed. Collaborate with the client and physician about use of a bedside commode or the bathroom. Do not administer enemas. *The client is at risk for constipation as a result of decreased mobility and the administration of narcotics, such as codeine, for headache. When straining to have a bowel movement, the client uses the Valsalva maneuver, which increases intracranial pressure and may precipitate rebleeding.*

- If the client is alert, and depending on physician preferences, allow to feed self and provide own personal care. *In many instances, self-care causes less anxiety and stress than care provided by the nurse. The extent of care provided varies according to client condition and physician preferences.*

- Monitor vital signs and neurologic status as indicated by client condition (frequency of assessments may range from every 15 minutes to every 4 hours). *Vital signs and neurologic assessments provide ongoing data for evaluation of changes indicative of increasing intracranial pressure and decreasing neurologic function. Report any change immediately to the physician.*

- Maintain seizure precautions: Have suction equipment and an oropharyngeal tube at the bedside, maintain the bed in the low position, and keep the side rails padded and raised. *Applying suction and inserting an oropharyngeal airway may be necessary to maintain an open airway in case of seizure. A lowered bed and padded, raised side rails prevent injury if a seizure occurs.*

- Avoid positioning and activities that increase intracranial pressure, such as coughing, sneezing, vomiting, sharply flexing the neck, blowing the nose, enemas, moving self up in bed, or cigarette smoking. *These measures help to prevent increasing intracranial pressure and rebleeding.*

33

Nursing Care
of Clients with
Intracranial Disorders

The client with an intracranial disorder presents a unique challenge to the nurse. Problems the client experiences in the acute stage of the disorder are often a prelude to long-term problems requiring ongoing management. These long-term problems range from alterations in the body's basic functioning to dysfunctions in the complex processes of the human mind. Systemic problems may accompany or develop secondary to an intracranial disorder. Intracranial disorders may affect the client's quality of life and that of the client's family. This chapter discusses altered level of consciousness and increased intracranial pressure.

Altered Cerebral Function

The manifestations of altered cerebral function occur as a result of illness or injury. Assessment of the patterns of those manifestations helps determine the extent of the cerebral dysfunction and improvement or deterioration of cerebral function. Except in the case of direct damage to the brainstem and **reticular activating system (RAS),** brain function deterioration usually follows a predictable rostral to caudal progression, that is, a pattern in which higher levels of function are impaired initially, progressing to impairment of more primitive functions. Altered level of consciousness and behavior changes are early manifestations of the deterioration of the function of the cerebral hemispheres. Structures in the midbrain and brainstem are affected sequentially, with characteristic changes in level of consciousness; patterns of respiration, pupillary and oculomotor responses; and motor function (Porth, 2002).

The Client with Altered Level of Consciousness

Consciousness is a condition in which the person is aware of self and environment and is able to respond appropriately to stimuli. Full consciousness requires both normal arousal and full cognition.

- *Arousal,* or alertness, depends on the RAS, a diffuse system of neurons in the thalamus and upper brainstem.
- *Cognition* is a complex process involving all mental activities controlled by the cerebral hemispheres, including thought processes, memory, perception, problem solving, and emotion.

These two components of consciousness depend on the normal physiologic function of and connection between the arousal mechanisms of the reticular formation and the cognitive functions of the cerebral hemispheres. Because arousal and cognition are independent components of consciousness, each can act separately on stimuli. For example, the RAS reacts to the discomfort caused by a full bladder by waking the person in the middle of the night. Once awake, however, the frontal cortex alerts the person that the bladder is full and prompts the person to go to the bathroom and empty it.

The physiologic seat of consciousness, the reticular formation, is a mass of nerve cells and fibers that make up the core of the brainstem, extending from the medulla to the midbrain. The axons of reticular neurons are exceptionally long and branch outward to cells in the hypothalamus, thalamus, cerebellum, and spinal cord. A system of reticular neurons within the RAS passes steady streams of impulses through thalamic relays in order to stimulate the cerebral cortex into wakefulness. The body's sensory tracts interact with RAS neurons; this interrelationship helps control the strength of the RAS's rousing effect on the cerebrum.

Conditions that affect either the RAS or the function of the cerebral hemispheres can interfere with the normal level of consciousness. Terms describing altered level of consciousness (LOC) are listed and defined in Table 33-1. Nurses should remember that consciousness is a dynamic state: A client may pass from full consciousness to coma within hours or experience a slow diminishment of consciousness that does not become evident for weeks or months. The nurse can help provide effective care for a client with an altered level of consciousness by looking beyond the diagnostic labels of consciousness and accurately assessing the client's behavior and response to stimuli.

Pathophysiology

Level of consciousness may be altered by processes that affect the arousal functions of the brainstem, the cognitive functions of the cerebral hemispheres, or both. The major causes are (1) lesions or injuries that affect the cerebral hemispheres directly and widely or that compress or destroy the neurons of the RAS and (2) metabolic disorders.

Table 33-1. Terms Used to Describe Level of Consciousness

Term	Characteristics of Client
Full consciousness	Alert; oriented to time, place, and person; comprehends spoken and written words.
Confusion	Unable to think rapidly and clearly; easily bewildered, with poor memory and short attention span; misinterprets stimuli; judgment is impaired.
Disorientation	Not aware of or not oriented to time, place, or person.
Obtundation	Lethargic, somnolent; responsive to verbal or tactile stimuli but quickly drifts back to sleep.
Stupor	Generally unresponsive; may be briefly aroused by vigorous, repeated, or painful stimuli; may shrink away from or grab at the source of stimuli.

Table 33-1. Continued

Semicomatose	Does not move spontaneously; unresponsive to stimuli, although vigorous or painful stimuli may result in stirring, moaning, or withdrawal from the stimuli, without actual arousal.
Coma	Unarousable; will not stir or moan in response to any stimulus; may exhibit nonpurposeful response (slight movement) of area stimulated but makes no attempt to withdraw.
Deep coma	Completely unarousable and unresponsive to any kind of stimulus, including pain; absence of brainstem reflexes, corneal, pupillary, and pharyngeal reflexes and tendon and plantar reflexes.

Arousal

Damage to the RAS impairs the person's ability to maintain wakefulness and arousal. Stroke is the most common cause of RAS destruction. Other causes include demyelinating diseases, such as multiple sclerosis, tumors, abscesses, and head injury. Function of the RAS may be suppressed by compression of the brainstem, which produces edema and ischemia. Pressure and compression of the brainstem may be due to tumors, increased intracranial pressure, hematomas or hemorrhage, or aneurysm (McCance & Huether, 2002). Although it is possible to assess level of consciousness or arousal in the client with RAS damage, the impairment in arousal may make it impossible to assess cognitive function.

The function of the brain, especially the cerebral hemispheres, depends on continuous blood flow with unimpeded supplies of oxygen and glucose. Processes that disrupt this flow of blood and nutrients may cause widespread damage to the cerebral hemispheres, impairing arousal and cognition. Bilateral hemispheric lesions, such as global ischemia, or metabolic disorders, such as hypoglycemia, are the most common causes of altered LOC related to cerebral dysfunction of the hemispheres. Localized masses, such as a hematoma or cerebral edema, that displace normal structures and cause direct or indirect pressure on the opposite hemisphere or brainstem can also affect LOC. The client who has widespread damage to the cerebral hemispheres but an intact RAS has sleep-wake cycles and may rouse in response to stimuli; the client cannot be said to be alert, however, because cognition is impaired.

Both localized neurologic processes and systemic disorders can alter LOC. Processes occurring within the brain, which may directly destroy or compress neurologic structures, include the following:

- Increased intracranial pressure
- Stroke
- Hematoma
- Intracranial hemorrhage
- Tumors
- Infections
- Demyelinating disorders.

Any systemic condition that affects the delivery of blood, oxygen, and glucose to the brain or alters cell membranes may also alter LOC. If cerebral blood flow is impaired or the client becomes hypoxic or hypoglycemic, cerebral metabolism is impaired and level of consciousness declines rapidly. Clients at particular risk include those with poorly controlled diabetes and those with cardiac or respiratory failure.

Other metabolic alterations that can affect LOC include fluid and electrolyte imbalances, such as hyponatremia or hyperosmolality, and acid-base alterations, such as hypercapnia (an elevated arterial carbon dioxide level). Accumulated waste products and toxins from liver or renal failure can affect neuronal and neurotransmitter function, altering LOC. Drugs that depress the central nervous system (e.g., alcohol, analgesics, anesthetics) suppress metabolic and membrane activities in the RAS and cerebral hemispheres, thereby affecting LOC.

Seizure activity, abnormal electrical discharges from a local area of the brain or from the entire brain, commonly affects LOC. It appears that the spontaneous, disordered discharge of activity that occurs during a seizure exhausts energy metabolites or produces locally toxic molecules, altering LOC for a time after the seizure. Consciousness returns when the metabolic balance of the neurons is restored.

As the impairment of brain function progresses, more stimuli are required to elicit a response from the client. Initially, the client may rouse to verbal stimuli and respond appropriately to questions, remaining oriented to time, place, and person. With deterioration of neurologic function, the client becomes more difficult to rouse and may become agitated and confused when awakened. Orientation to time is lost initially, followed by orientation to place and then to person. Continuous stimulation or vigorous shaking is required to maintain wakefulness as LOC decreases. Eventually, the client does not respond, even with deep painful stimuli.

Patterns of Breathing

Progressive impairment of neural function also causes predictable changes in breathing patterns as respiratory centers are affected. In normal respirations, a rhythmic pattern is maintained by neural centers in the pons and medulla that respond to changes in arterial levels of oxygen (PaO_2) and carbon dioxide ($PaCO_2$). When there is damage to the RAS or cerebral hemispheres, neural control of these centers is lost, and lower brainstem centers regulate breathing patterns by responding only to changes in $PaCO_2$, resulting in irregular respiratory patterns. Progressive deterioration in brain function is accompanied by decreasing LOC and changes in breathing patterns. The type of respirations, by area of cerebral damage, are as follows (Porth, 2002):

- *Diencephalon:* Cheyne-Stokes respirations
- *Midbrain:* neurogenic hyperventilation (may exceed 40 per minute), the result of uninhibited stimulation of the respiratory centers
- *Pons:* apneustic respirations, characterized by sighing on midinspiration or prolonged inhalation and exhalation; results from excessive stimulation of the respiratory centers
- *Medulla:* ataxic/apneic respirations (totally uncoordinated and irregular), probably as a result of the loss of responsiveness to CO_2.

Pupillary and Oculomotor Responses

The brainstem areas that control arousal are adjacent to areas that control the pupils. A predictable progression of pupillary and oculomotor responses occurs as level of consciousness deteriorates toward coma. If the lesion or process affecting neurologic function is localized, effects may initially be seen in the *ipsilateral pupil* (the pupil on the same side as the lesion). With generalized or systemic processes, pupils are affected equally. If the pupils are small and equally reactive, metabolic processes affecting LOC may be present. With compression of cranial nerve III at the midbrain, the pupils may become oval or eccentric (off center). As the level of functional impairment progresses, the pupils become fixed (unresponsive to light) and, eventually, dilated.

In deteriorating LOC and coma, spontaneous eye movement is lost and reflexive ocular movements are altered. Normally, both eyes move simultaneously in the same direction; injury to the cranial nerve nuclei in the midbrain and pons can impair normal movement. **Doll's eye movements** are reflexive movements of the eyes in the opposite direction of head rotation; they are an indicator of brainstem function. As a result of the oculocephalic reflex, the eyes move upward with passive flexion of the neck and downward with passive neck extension. As brainstem function deteriorates, this reflex is lost. The eyes fail to turn together and, eventually, remain fixed in the midposition as the head is turned.

Instilling cold water into the ear canal (cold caloric testing) tests the oculovestibular response. Normally, this stimulus causes **nystagmus** (lateral tonic deviation of the eyes) toward the stimulus. This reflex is also lost as brain function deteriorates.

Motor Responses

The level of brain dysfunction and the side of the brain affected may be assessed by motor responses. These responses are the most accurate identifier of changes in mental status. In altered LOC, motor responses to stimuli range from an appropriate response to a command (e.g., "squeeze my hand" or "push my hands away with your feet") to flaccidity. Initially, the client may be able to move purposefully away from a noxious stimulus, for example, to brush the examiner's hand away from the face. As function declines, movements become more generalized (withdrawal, grimacing) and less purposeful. Reflexive motor responses may occur, including *decorticate* posturing with flexion of the upper extremities accompanied by extension of the lower extremities. With further decline, *decerebrate* posturing is seen, with adduction and rigid extension of the upper and lower extremities. Without intervention, the client eventually becomes flaccid, with little or no motor response to stimuli.

Coma States and Brain Death

Possible outcomes of altered LOC and coma include full recovery with no long-term residual effects, recovery with residual damage, such as learning deficits, emotional difficulties, or impaired judgment, or more severe consequences, such as persistent vegetative state (cerebral death) or brain death.

Irreversible Coma

Irreversible coma (persistent vegetative state) is a permanent condition of complete unawareness of self and the environment, resulting from death of the cerebral hemispheres with continued function of the brainstem and cerebellum. While the homeostatic regulatory functions of the brain continue, the ability to respond meaningfully to the environment is lost.

The client in vegetative state has sleep-wake cycles and retains the ability to chew, swallow, and cough, but cannot interact with the environment. When awake, the client's eyes may wander back and forth across the room, but they cannot track an object or person. In a **minimally conscious state,** the client is aware of the environment and can follow simple commands, manipulate objects, gesture or verbalize to indicate "yes/no" responses, and make meaningful movements, such as blinking or smiling, in response to a stimulus (McCance & Huether, 2002). Vegetative state is usually the result of severe head injury or global anoxia. With appropriate supportive care, the client may remain in this state for two to five years.

Locked-In Syndrome

Locked-in syndrome is distinctly different from vegetative state, in that the client is alert and fully aware of the environment and has intact cognitive abilities, but is unable to communicate through speech or movement because of blocked efferent pathways from the brain. Motor paralysis affects all voluntary muscles, although the upper cranial nerves (I through IV) may remain intact, allowing the client to communicate through eye movements and blinking. In essence, the client is "locked" inside a paralyzed body in which he or she remains fully conscious of self and environment. Infarction or hemorrhage of the pons that disrupts outgoing nerve tracts, but spares the RAS, is the usual cause of locked-in syndrome. This condition may also result when the corticospinal tracts between the midbrain and pons are interrupted. Disorders of the lower motor neurons or muscles, such as acute polyneuritis, myasthenia gravis, or amyotrophic lateral sclerosis (ALS), may also paralyze motor responses, leading to locked-in syndrome.

Brain Death

Brain death is the cessation and irreversibility of all brain functions, including the brainstem. Although the exact criteria for establishing brain death may vary somewhat from state to state, it is generally agreed that brain death has occurred when there is no evidence of cerebral or brainstem function for an extended period (usually 6 to 24 hours) in a client who has a normal body temperature and is not affected by a depressant drug or alcohol poisoning. Generally recognized criteria are:

- Unresponsive coma with absent motor and reflex movements.
- No spontaneous respiration (apnea).
- Pupils fixed (unresponsive to light) and dilated.
- Absent ocular responses to head turning and caloric stimulation.
- Flat EEG and no cerebral blood circulation present on angiography (if performed).
- Persistence of these manifestations for 30 minutes to 1 hour and for 6 hours after onset of coma and apnea.

Apnea in the comatose client is determined by the apnea test. The ventilator is removed while maintaining oxygenation by tracheal cannula and allowing the Pco_2 to increase to 60 mmHg or higher. This level of carbon dioxide is high enough to stimulate respiration if the brainstem is functional. The electroencephalogram (EEG) may be used to establish the absence of brain activity when brain death is suspected. A flat (isoelectric) EEG over a period of 6 to 12 hours in a client who is not hypothermic or under the influence of drugs that depress the central nervous system is generally accepted as an indicator of brain death (McCance & Huether, 2002).

Prognosis

The prognosis for clients with altered levels of consciousness and coma varies according to the underlying cause and pathologic process. Age and general medical condition also play a role in determining outcome. Young adults may fully recover following deep coma from head injury, drug overdose, or other cause. Recovery of consciousness within two weeks is associated with a favorable outcome. In general, the prognosis is poor for clients who lack pupillary reaction or reflex eye movements six hours after the onset of coma.

Collaborative Care

Management of the client with an altered LOC or coma must begin immediately. The focus of management is to identify the underlying cause, preserve function, and prevent deterioration if possible. Airway and breathing must be maintained during the initial acute stage until the diagnosis and prognosis can be established. Intravenous fluids are used to support circulation and to correct fluid, electrolyte, and acid-base imbalances. Treatment protocols to reduce increased intracranial pressure or control seizure activity may be initiated. Changes in LOC associated with craniocerebral trauma, such as hematomas, often require immediate surgical intervention.

Diagnostic Tests

Although the client's history and physical examination findings often indicate the cause of alterations in LOC, several diagnostic tests may be useful in establishing the diagnosis. The following tests may be ordered to evaluate for possible metabolic, toxic, or drug-induced disorders.

- *Blood glucose* is measured immediately when coma is of unknown origin and hypoglycemia is suspected or possible. The brain contains minimal stores of glucose and is dependent on a continuous supply for metabolism. When the blood glucose falls to less than 40 to 50 mg/dL, cerebral function declines rapidly. The client with type 1 diabetes is at particular risk for hypoglycemia-induced coma.

- *Serum electrolytes*, sodium, potassium, bicarbonate, chloride, and calcium in particular, are measured to assess for metabolic disturbances and guide intravenous therapy. Hyponatremia, in which serum sodium levels are below 115 mEq/L (normal level: 135 to 145 mEq/L), is associated with coma and convulsions, especially if it develops rapidly.

- *Serum osmolality* is evaluated. Both hyperosmolar and hypoosmolar states may be associated with coma. Hyperosmolality (above 320 mOsm/kg H_2O) causes cellular dehydration of brain tissue as fluid is drawn into the vascular system by osmosis. Hypo-osmolality (less than 250 mOsm/kg H_2O), by contrast, leads to cerebral edema and swelling, impairing consciousness.

- *ABGs* are drawn to evaluate arterial oxygen and carbon dioxide levels as well as acid-base balance. Hypoxemia is a frequent cause of altered LOC; increased levels of carbon dioxide are also toxic to the brain and can induce coma, particularly when the onset of hypercapnia is acute.

- *Serum creatinine* and *BUN* are measured to evaluate renal function.

- *Liver function tests,* including bilirubin, AST, ALT, LDH, serum albumin, and serum ammonia levels, are determined to evaluate hepatic function. High ammonia levels seen in hepatic failure interfere with cerebral metabolism and neurotransmitters, affecting level of consciousness.

- *Toxicology screening* of blood and urine is done to determine if altered LOC is the result of acute drug or alcohol toxicity. Serum alcohol levels are measured and the blood is assessed for the presence of substances such as barbiturates, carbon monoxide, or lead.

- *CBC with differential* is done to assess for possible anemia or infectious causes of coma.
- *CT* and *MRI scanning* are done to detect neurologic damage due to hemorrhage, tumor, cyst, edema, myocardial infarction, or brain atrophy. These tests may also identify displacement of brain structures by large or expanding lesions. It is important to remember, however, that not all lesions or causes of altered LOC can be determined by CT scan or MRI.
- *EEG* is used to evaluate the electrical activity of the brain. The EEG is particularly valuable in identifying unrecognized seizure activity as a cause of altered LOC and is also useful in identifying certain infectious and metabolic causes of altered LOC. A normal EEG in an unresponsive client may identify locked-in syndrome. In addition to the baseline EEG, evoked responses may also be determined. The EEG is monitored as an auditory tone or other sensory stimulus is provided to assess the brain's responsiveness.
- *Radioisotope brain scan* is performed to identify abnormal lesions in the brain and evaluate cerebral blood flow.
- *Cerebral angiography* allows radiographic visualization of the cerebral vascular system. A radiopaque dye is injected into the carotid or vertebral arteries, followed by fluoroscopic and serial X-ray evaluation of the cerebral circulation. This exam can identify lesions, such as aneurysms, occluded vessels, or tumors, and may also be used to determine cessation of cerebral blood flow and brain death.
- *Transcranial Doppler studies* use an ultrasound velocity detector that records sound waves reflected from RBCs in blood vessels to assess cerebral blood flow.
- *Lumbar puncture with CSF analysis* is performed when infection and possible meningitis are suspected as a cause of altered LOC.

Medications

Medications are used to support homeostasis and normal function for the client with altered LOC, as well as to treat specific underlying disorders. An intravenous catheter is inserted, and fluid balance is maintained using isotonic or slightly hypertonic solutions, such as normal saline or lactated Ringer's solution. The client's response to fluid administration is monitored carefully for evidence of increased cerebral edema.

If hypoglycemia is present, 50% glucose is administered intravenously to restore cerebral metabolism rapidly. Conversely, insulin is administered to the client with hyperglycemia to reduce the blood glucose level and thus the serum osmolality. With narcotic overdose, naloxone is administered. Naloxone is a narcotic antagonist that competes for narcotic receptor sites, effectively blocking the depressant effect of the narcotic. Thiamine may be administered with glucose, particularly if the client is malnourished or known to abuse alcohol, to prevent exacerbation of Wernicke's encephalopathy, a hemorrhagic encephalopathy due to thiamine deficiency and associated with chronic alcoholism (Tierney, et al., 2001).

Any underlying fluid and electrolyte imbalance is corrected by administering medications or appropriate electrolytes. For the client who is hyponatremic and has a low serum osmolality, furosemide (Lasix) or an osmotic diuretic, such as mannitol, may be administered to promote water excretion. Appropriate antibiotics are administered intravenously to the client with suspected or confirmed meningitis.

Surgery

Although surgery is not indicated for most clients with altered LOC, it may be necessary if the cause of coma is a tumor, hemorrhage, or hematoma. When there is a risk of increased intracranial pressure, the client is monitored continuously. These measures are discussed in the section on increased intracranial pressure.

Other Therapeutic Measures

Support of the airway and respirations is vital in the client with an altered LOC. The client who is drowsy but rousable may need little more than an oral pharyngeal airway. With more severe alterations in consciousness, the client may need endotracheal intubation to maintain airway patency, particularly if the cough and gag reflexes are absent. Mechanical ventilation is indicated when hypoventilation or apnea is present. Unless a do-not-resuscitate (DNR) order is in effect, mechanical ventilation should be initiated, even if it has not been established that the disorder is reversible; without ventilatory support, cerebral anoxia develops rapidly, and brain death may ensue. ABGs are monitored frequently to determine the adequacy of ventilation. Hyperventilation may be used to reduce PCO_2 and promote cerebral vasoconstriction to reduce cerebral edema.

In clients with long-term alterations in consciousness, such as vegetative state or locked-in syndrome, measures to maintain nutritional status are initiated. Enteral feedings with a gastrostomy tube are preferred if the client is unable to take enough food by mouth without aspirating. In some cases, parenteral nutrition may be used.

Nursing Care

Nursing Diagnoses and Interventions

Nursing care of the client with an altered LOC is planned and implemented for a variety of responses. Nursing diagnoses and interventions discussed in this section are directed toward the unconscious client and focus on problems with airway maintenance, skin integrity, contractures, and nutrition.

Ineffective Airway Clearance

Ineffective airway clearance related to loss of the cough reflex and the inability to expectorate is a major problem for the unconscious client. The cough reflex may be absent or impaired when conditions that produce coma depress the function of the medullary centers.

- Assess ability to clear secretions. Monitor breath sounds, rate and depth of respirations, dyspnea, pulse oximeter, and the presence of cyanosis. *The client's ability to clear secretions serves as the initial assessment base for developing further interventions.*

- In unconscious clients, or those without an intact cough reflex, maintain an open airway by periodic suctioning, limiting the time of suctioning to 10 to 15 seconds or less. *Periodic suctioning may be necessary to clear the airway of mucus, blood, or other drainage. Suctioning for more than 15 seconds in the client with increased intracranial pressure may cause hypercapnia, which in turn vasodilates cerebral vessels, increases cerebral blood volume, and increases intracranial pressure.*

- Turn client from side to side every two hours, and maintain a side-lying position with the head of the bed elevated approximately 30 degrees. Do not position the unconscious client on the back. *Turning the client from side to side facilitates respirations, prevents the tongue from obstructing the airway, and helps prevent pooling of secretions in one area of the lungs, thus decreasing the risk of pneumonia.*

- If the client has a tracheostomy, provide tracheostomy care every four hours and suction when secretions are present, *to maintain an open airway.*

Risk for Aspiration

The unconscious client with a depressed or absent gag and swallowing reflex is at high risk for aspiration. Drainage, mucus, or blood may obstruct the airway and interfere with oxygenation. Pooling of aspiration secretions in the lungs also increases the risk of pneumonia.

- Assess swallowing and gag reflexes every shift as appropriate to the client's level of consciousness. *Deepening levels of unconsciousness may cause a loss in swallow and gag reflexes.*
- Monitor for and report manifestations of aspiration: crackles and wheezes, dullness to percussion over an area of the lungs, dyspnea, tachypnea, cyanosis. *Early recognition facilitates prompt intervention.*
- Provide interventions to prevent aspiration:
  1. Maintain NPO status.
  2. Place in the side-lying position.
  3. Provide oral hygiene and suctioning as needed.

The side-lying position allows secretions to drain from the mouth rather than into the pharynx. Oral hygiene and suctioning remove secretions that might otherwise be aspirated.

- Monitor the results of arterial blood gas analysis and pulse oximetry. Maintain records of trends. *Arterial blood gases and pulse oximetry directly measure the oxygen content of blood and are good indicators of the lungs' ability to oxygenate the blood.*

Risk for Impaired Skin Integrity

The unconscious client is at risk for impaired skin integrity as a result of immobility and the inability to provide self-care. On average, healthy people change positions during sleep every 11 minutes; the unconscious client often cannot maintain the movement needed to prevent pressure on the skin, especially over bony prominences. As a result, the skin and subcutaneous tissues may become ischemic and prone to develop pressure ulcers. Perspiration and incontinence of urine and stool may exacerbate the problem. Nursing interventions are directed to maintaining the integrity not only of the skin, but also of the lips and mucous membranes.

- Assess skin every shift, especially over bony prominences and around genitals and buttocks. The large surface area of the skin bears weight and is in constant contact with the surface of the bed. *The skin, subcutaneous tissue, and muscles, especially those tissues over bony prominences, undergo constant pressure. This impairs normal capillary blood flow, which interferes with the exchange of nutrients and waste products. Tissue ischemia and necrosis may result and lead to the development of pressure ulcers.*
- Provide proper positioning. Reposition bed-ridden clients at least every two hours if this is consistent with the overall treatment goals. Keep the head of the bed elevated no higher than 30 degrees. Provide special pads and mattresses that distribute weight more evenly (e.g., silicone-filled pads, egg-crate cushions, turning frames, flotation pads). Lift

the client instead of dragging the client across the sheet. *When the head of the bed is elevated above 30 degrees, the client's torso tends to slide down toward the foot of the bed. Friction and perspiration cause the skin and superficial fascia to remain fixed against the bed linens while the deep fascia and skeleton slide downward. When a person is pulled rather than lifted, the skin remains fixed to the sheet while the fascia and muscles are pulled upward. These sheering forces promote tissue breakdown.*

• Provide interventions to prevent breakdown of the skin and mucous membranes:

   1. Keep bed linens clean, dry, and wrinkle free.
   2. Provide daily bath with mild soap.
   3. Cleanse the skin after urine and fecal soiling with a mild cleansing agent.
   4. Provide oral care and lubricate the lips every two to four hours.
   5. Maintain accurate intake and output records.
   6. Keep the cornea moist by instilling methyl cellulose solution (0.5% to 1%) and apply protective eye shields or close the eyelids with adhesive strips if the corneal reflex is absent.

Keeping linens clean, dry, and wrinkle free decreases the risk of injury from the shearing force of bed rest and protects against environmental factors that cause drying. Adequate hydration of the stratum corneum appears to protect the skin against mechanical insult. Preventing dehydration maintains circulation and decreases the concentration of urine, thereby minimizing skin irritation in people who are incontinent. Proper eye care prevents corneal abrasion and irritation.

Impaired Physical Mobility

Clients who are unconscious are unable to maintain normal musculoskeletal movement and are at high risk for contractures related to decreased movement. Because the flexor and adductor muscles are stronger than the extensors and abductors, flexor and adductor contractures develop quickly without preventive measures. Passive ROM exercises must be performed routinely to maintain muscle tone and function, to prevent additional disability, and to help restore impaired motor function.

• Maintain extremities in functional positions by providing proper support devices. Remove support devices every four hours for skin care and passive ROM exercises. Provide pillows for the axillary region; rolled washcloths may be placed in elevated hands; use splints to prevent plantar flexion (footdrop). *Pillows in the axillary region help prevent adduction of the shoulder. Rolled washcloths help decrease edema and flexion contracture of the fingers. Splints are useful in preventing plantar flexion. Remove these support devices every four hours to increase circulation to the area.*

• Perform passive ROM exercises (unless contraindicated, as for the client with increased intracranial pressure) at least four times a day, keeping the following principles in mind:

   1. Place one hand above the joint being exercised. The other hand gently moves the joint through its normal range of motion.
   2. Move the body part to the point of resistance, and stop.

Placing one hand above the joint provides support against gravity and prevents unwanted movement. ROM exercises help prevent contractures by stretching muscles and tendons and maintaining joint mobility.

Risk for Imbalanced Nutrition: Less Than Body Requirements

The unconscious client is at risk for an alteration in nutrition related to a reduced or complete inability to eat. This is especially true for the client who is unconscious as the result of an infection or trauma, both of which increase metabolic requirements.

*   Monitor nutritional status through daily weights (on bed scales) and laboratory data. *For accuracy, weigh the client at the same time each day, using the same scales. Ensure that the client wears the same clothing. Changes in laboratory data with decreased nutrition include a decrease in the levels of serum albumin and serum transferrin.*

*   Assess the need for alternative methods of nutritional support (tube feeding or total parenteral nutrition) through collaboration with dietitian. *Clients unable to take oral food require parenteral nutrition or liquid feedings through a nasogastric, gastrostomy, or jejunostomy tube. Needs for protein, calories, zinc, and vitamin C increase during wound healing.*

Support of the Family

Family members of a client with an altered level of consciousness are often very anxious. It is difficult for the family to deal with the client's uncertain prognosis. They may experience various conflicting emotions, such as guilt and anger. Reinforce information provided by the physician, and encourage the family to talk to the client as though he or she were able to understand. Explain that this communication may initially seem awkward, but in time it will feel appropriate. Evaluate the family's readiness to receive explanations regarding the client's treatment and care. The presence of many tubes (e.g., intravenous line, catheter, ventilator) may be overwhelming to the family. They may misperceive the seriousness of the situation if a thorough explanation is not given. Include the family in the client's care as much as they wish to be involved.

Allow significant others to stay with the client when possible. Reinforce the need for family members to care for themselves by encouraging adequate meals and rest. Offer to contact support services, such as friends, neighbors, and social services that the hospital may provide. Ask family members to leave a telephone number where they can be reached, and assure them that they will be called if any significant changes occur. Encourage family members to call if they have questions or concerns.

The Client with a Seizure Disorder

Seizures are "paroxysmal motor, sensory, or cognitive manifestations of spontaneous, abnormally synchronous discharges of collections of neurons in the cerebral cortex" (Porth, 2002, p. 1189). This abnormal neuronal activity, which may involve all or part of the brain, disturbs skeletal motor function, sensation, autonomic function of the viscera, behavior, or consciousness. The term **epilepsy** is used to denote any disorder characterized by recurrent seizures. Epilepsy is categorized as a paroxysmal disorder because its manifestations are discontinuous; that is, minutes, days, weeks, or even years may elapse between seizures.

Incidence and Prevalence

Epilepsy and seizures affect approximately 2.3 million Americans, costing an estimated $12.5 billion in medical expenses and lost or reduced earnings. About 10% of Americans will experience a seizure. People of all ages are affected, but particularly children and the elderly.

The incidence of epilepsy is increasing. Researchers have suggested that the increase may be due to technologic advances in obstetric and pediatric care that allow extremely high-risk neonates to survive and to other technologic advances that have improved survival rates after craniocerebral trauma.

Isolated seizure episodes may occur in otherwise healthy people for a variety of reasons, including an acute febrile state, infection, metabolic or endocrine disorder, such as hypoglycemia, or exposure to toxins. Epilepsy may be idiopathic (i.e., it may have no identifiable cause), or it may be secondary to birth injury, infection, vascular abnormalities, trauma, or tumors. Older adults may experience seizures as a result of vascular diseases (the most common cause in adults over 60) and degenerative disorders, such as Alzheimer's disease.

Pathophysiology and Manifestations

Normally, when the mind is actively working, electrical activity in the brain is unsynchronized; when the mind is at rest, electrical activity is mildly synchronized. It is believed that most seizures arise from a few unstable, hypersensitive, and hyperreactive neurons in the brain. During a seizure, these neurons produce a rhythmic and repetitive hypersynchronous discharge. Although the exact initiating factor for seizure activity has not been identified, several theories have been proposed (Porth, 2002):

- Alterations in the permeability of, or ion distribution across, cell membranes
- Alterations in the excitability of neurons resulting from glial scarring or decreased inhibition of activity in the cerebral cortex or thalamic region
- Imbalances of excitatory and inhibitory neurotransmitters, such as acetylcholine (ACh) or gamma aminobutyric acid (GABA).

All people have a seizure threshold; when this threshold is exceeded, a seizure may result. In some people, the seizure threshold may be abnormally low, increasing their risk for seizure activity; in other people, pathologic processes may alter the seizure threshold (Porth, 2002). The neurons that initiate seizure activity are called the *epileptogenic focus*. Abnormal neuronal activity may remain localized, causing a partial or focal seizure, or it may spread to involve the entire brain, causing generalized seizure activity. Seizures may also be provoked or unprovoked. *Unprovoked (primary or idiopathic) seizures* have no identifiable cause, with multiple episodes diagnosed as a seizure disorder or epilepsy. *Provoked (secondary) seizure* etiologies include febrile seizures in children, toxemia of pregnancy, rapid withdrawal from alcohol or barbiturates, systemic metabolic conditions, such as hypoglycemia, hypoxia, uremia, and electrolyte imbalances, and pathologies of the brain, such as meningitis, cerebral bleeding, or cerebral edema.

Metabolic needs of the brain increase dramatically during seizure activity. The demand for adenosine triphosphate (ATP), the energy source of the brain, increases by approximately 250%. Consequently, the demand for glucose and oxygen (which are needed to produce ATP) increases, and oxygen consumption increases by about 60%. To supply this increased oxygen need and remove carbon dioxide and other metabolic by-products, cerebral blood flow increases to about 2.5 times that of the normal rate. As long as oxygenation, blood glucose levels, and cardiac function remain normal, cerebral blood flow can respond to this increased metabolic demand of the brain. If cerebral blood flow cannot meet these needs, however, cellular exhaustion and cellular destruction may result.

Although seizures may be categorized in several different ways, the classification developed by the International League Against Epilepsy is the most useful clinically (Tierney, et al., 2001). Seizures are divided into those that affect only part of the brain (partial seizures) and those that are generalized.

Partial Seizures

Partial seizures involve the activation of only a restricted part of one cerebral hemisphere. A partial seizure accompanied by no alteration in consciousness is called a *simple partial seizure;* one in which consciousness is impaired is called a *complex partial seizure.*

The manifestations of simple partial seizures depend on the involved area of the brain. Manifestations may include alterations in motor function, sensory signs, or autonomic or psychic symptoms. Typically, the motor portion of the cortex is affected, causing recurrent muscle contractions of a contralateral part of the body, such as a finger or hand, or the face. This motor activity may stay confined to one area or spread sequentially to adjacent parts, a phenomenon known as a *Jacksonian march* or *Jacksonian seizure.* Manifestations of a simple partial seizure involving the sensory portion of the brain may include abnormal sensations or hallucinations. Disruptions in the function of the autonomic nervous system, with resulting tachycardia, flushing, hypotension, and hypertension, or psychic manifestations, such as a sense of déjà vu or inappropriate fear or anger, may also be experienced during a simple partial seizure.

During a complex partial seizure, consciousness is impaired and the client may engage in repetitive, nonpurposeful activity, such as lip smacking, aimless walking, or picking at clothing. These behaviors are known as *automatisms.* During the seizure, the client loses conscious contact with the environment; amnesia is common after the seizure, and several hours may elapse before the client regains full consciousness. Complex partial seizures usually originate in the temporal lobe and may be preceded by an aura, such as an unusual smell, a sense of déjà vu, or a sudden intense emotion.

Generalized Seizures

Generalized seizures involve both hemispheres of the brain as well as deeper brain structures, such as the thalamus, basal ganglia, and upper brainstem. Consciousness is always impaired with generalized seizures. Absence and tonic-clonic seizures are the common forms of generalized seizure activity; they occur more frequently (especially in children) than partial seizures.

Absence Seizures

Absence (petit mal) seizures are characterized by a sudden brief cessation of all motor activity accompanied by a blank stare and unresponsiveness. Absence seizures are more common in children than in adults. The seizure typically lasts only 5 to 10 seconds, although some may last for 30 seconds or more. Movements such as eyelid fluttering or automatisms such as lip smacking may occur during an absence seizure. Seizure activity may vary from occasional episodes to several hundred per day.

Tonic-Clonic Seizures

Tonic-clonic seizures are the most common type of seizure activity in adults. This type of seizure activity follows a typical pattern. An aura may precede generalized seizure activity. The aura may be a vague sense of uneasiness or an abnormal sensation, such as a smell of burning rubber or seeing bright light. Often, however, the seizure occurs without warning.

The seizure begins with a sudden loss of consciousness and sharp tonic muscle contractions (the *tonic phase* of the seizure). With the muscle contraction, air is forced out of the lungs, and the client may cry out. Postural control is lost, and the client falls to the floor in the opisthotonic posture. Muscles are rigid, with the arms and legs extended and the jaw clenched. Urinary incontinence is common; bowel incontinence may also occur. Breathing ceases and cyanosis develops during the tonic phase of a seizure. The pupils are fixed and dilated. The tonic phase lasts an average of 15 seconds, although it may persist for up to a minute.

The *clonic phase,* which follows the tonic phase, is characterized by alternating contraction and relaxation of the muscles in all the extremities along with hyperventilation. The eyes roll back, and the client froths at the mouth. The clonic phase varies in duration and subsides gradually. The entire tonic-clonic portion of the seizure generally lasts no more than 60 to 90 seconds.

Following the clonic phase of seizure activity, the client remains unconscious and unresponsive to stimuli. This period is known as the *postictal period* or *phase.* The client is relaxed and breathes quietly. The client regains consciousness gradually, and may be confused and disoriented on waking. Headache, muscle aches, and fatigue often follow the seizure, and the client may sleep for several hours. Amnesia of the seizure is usual; also, the client might be unable to recall events just prior to the seizure activity.

Because of the lack of warning with tonic-clonic seizures, the client may experience injury. Head injury, fractures, burns, or motor vehicle crashes may occur as a result of seizure activity.

Status Epilepticus

Status epilepticus can develop during seizure activity. In this case, the seizure activity becomes continuous, with only very short periods of calm between intense and persistent seizures. The repetitive seizures may be of any type, although they are usually generalized tonic-clonic (Porth, 2002). Repeated seizures have a cumulative effect, producing muscular contractions that can interfere with respirations. The client is in great danger of developing hypoxia, acidosis, hypoglycemia, hyperthermia, and exhaustion if the convulsive activity is not halted. Status epilepticus is considered a life-threatening medical emergency that requires immediate treatment.

Collaborative Care

Initial treatment focuses on controlling the seizure; the long-term goal is to determine the cause and prevent future seizures. Collaborative care includes diagnostic testing, medications, and, in some cases, surgery.

Diagnostic Tests

Diagnostic testing is performed to confirm the seizure diagnosis and to determine any treatable causes and precipitating factors. The tests include:

* *Complete neurologic exam* to determine the focal neurologic deficit or the focus or origin of seizure activity.
* *Electroencephalogram (EEG)* to help confirm the seizure diagnosis and localize any lesion(s).

- *Skull X-rays* to identify possible fractures, deformities in bony structures, or calcification.
- *MRI* or *CT scan* to determine the presence of a tumor, congenital lesions, edema, infarct, hemorrhage, arteriovenous malformation, or a structural deviation, such as ventricular enlargement.
- *Lumbar puncture* to determine the presence of infection (meningitis) or elevated protein levels in the CSF.
- *Blood studies* to assess blood count, electrolytes, blood urea, and blood glucose.
- *Electrocardiogram (ECG)* to rule out underlying cardiac dysrhythmias.

Medications

Anticonvulsant medications can reduce or control most seizure activity. These medications do not cure the disorder; they only manage its manifestations. Anticonvulsant medications generally act in one of two ways: by raising the seizure threshold or by limiting the spread of abnormal activity within the brain.

The goals of medications for epilepsy are to protect the client from harm and to reduce or prevent seizure activity without impairing cognitive function or producing undesirable side effects. Ideally, the lowest possible dose of a single medication that will control the client's seizures is prescribed; often, however, several medications must be tried before the most effective is identified, and a combination of drugs may be needed to manage the client's seizures. Therapy is individualized, based on the type of seizure activity and the client's response to the medication. Nursing implications for these drugs are described in Table 33-2. The success rate is higher in clients with partial and secondary tonic-clonic seizures when carbamazepine (Tegretol), phenytoin (Dilantin), or valproic acid (Depakote) is used. Another medication approved for partial seizures is tiagabine (Gabitril), a GABA inhibitor. If the client has been seizure free for at least three years, withdrawal of medications may be considered, with the dose of one drug at a time reduced over weeks or months. There is no way of predicting which clients can remain seizure free without medication, but if seizures reoccur, the same medications usually provide good control.

Status epilepticus requires immediate intervention to preserve life. Establishing and maintaining the airway is a priority. A solution of 50% dextrose is administered intravenously to prevent hypoglycemia. Diazepam (Valium) or lorazepam (Ativan) is given intravenously, and the dose is repeated after ten minutes if necessary to stop seizure activity. Phenytoin (Dilantin) is also administered intravenously for longer-term control of seizures. Phenobarbital may also be administered to clients in status epilepticus.

Table 33-2. Medication Administration — Seizures

Anticonvulsants

Examples of anticonvulsants are:

Phenytoin (Dilantin)	Ethosuximide (Zarontin)
Phenobarbital	Clonazepam (Klonopin)
Primidone (Mysoline)	Gabapentin (Neurontin)
Carbamazepine (Tegretol)	Lamotrigine (Lamictal)
Valproic acid (Depakene)	Tiagabine HCL (Gabitril)

Table 33-2. Continued

Anticonvulsant agents are used to control chronic seizures and involuntary muscle spasms or movements characteristic of certain neurologic diseases. These drugs act in the motor cortex of the brain to reduce the spread of electrical discharges from the rapidly firing epileptic foci in this area. These agents control seizures without impairing the normal functions of the CNS. Drugs effective against one type of seizure may not be effective against another; anticonvulsant therapy must be individualized.

Nursing Responsibilities
- Monitor blood pressure, pulse, and respirations.
- Note evidence of CNS side effects, such as blurred vision, dimmed vision, slurred speech, nystagmus, or confusion. Gingival hyperplasia may be noted in clients taking phenytoin.
- Recognize that if clients are to be on prolonged therapy, they may need a diet rich in vitamin D.
- Monitor the serum calcium level as ordered; phenytoin can contribute to demineralization of bone.
- When administering anticonvulsants intravenously, monitor closely for respiratory depression and cardiovascular collapse.
- Administer gabapentin two hours after antacids.
- Administer tiagabine HCL with food.

Client and Family Teaching
- Take the exact dosage prescribed. Do not increase, decrease, or discontinue the dosage without obtaining the primary care provider's approval; doing so may lead to convulsions.
- Avoid hazardous tasks until the drug has been regulated. Anticonvulsant drugs may at first decrease mental alertness and cause drowsiness, headache, dizziness, and incoordination of muscles. These effects are usually dose related and may disappear with a change of dosage or continued therapy.
- If you are taking phenytoin (Dilantin), maintain good oral hygiene: Use a soft toothbrush, massage the gums, and floss daily.
- It is very important to obtain liver function studies regularly as ordered by the primary care provider. This will help detect early signs of hepatitis and other liver problems. Report for all scheduled laboratory studies, including complete blood count, kidney and liver function studies, and drug levels.
- Carry identification indicating the type of seizures for which you are being treated.
- Do not take gabapentin one hour before or less than two hours after an antacid.
- If you are taking lamotrigine and develop a rash, tell your health care provider.
- Take Tiagabine HCL (Gabitril) with food.

Treatments

Surgery
When all attempts to control the client's seizures fail, excision of the tissue involved in the seizure activity may be an effective and safe treatment alternative. An estimated 5% of clients

with epilepsy may be candidates for surgery. The goal of surgery is to reduce the client's uncontrollable seizures.

To be selected as a candidate for surgery, the client must be highly motivated and psychologically prepared. A psychologic screening is required because the preoperative preparation is extensive and time-consuming, and because the surgery is long and requires that the client remain awake during surgery, so that he or she can cooperate and respond to commands. The EEG is monitored during surgery to identify the epileptogenic focus and evaluate the effect of surgical intervention.

Resective surgery, with removal of the epileptogenic focus, is an option that is still in its early stages. Candidates for this type of surgery include those who are unresponsive to medical management, who have a unilateral focus, and who have impaired quality of life from seizures. Resections of the temporal lobe are most commonly performed and are most effective for partial complex seizures.

Vagal Nerve Stimulation

Vagal nerve stimulation is approved as a treatment for clients with partial-onset seizures who do not respond to drugs and are not candidates for surgery. The mechanism of action is unknown.

Nursing Care

Health Promotion

Health promotion activities for the client with seizures focus on teaching to reduce the incidence of seizure activity and to promote safety. Stress the following:

- Know the importance of follow-up care, of keeping medical appointments, and of continuing to take anticonvulsant medications as prescribed even when no seizures are experienced.
- Review any state and local laws that apply to people with seizure disorders. Driving a motor vehicle is usually prohibited for six months to two years after a seizure episode. Usually, a driver's license can be reinstated or obtained after a seizure-free period and a letter from the nurse practitioner or physician.
- Teach client and family members measures to prevent injury at home:
  1. Avoid smoking when alone or in bed.
  2. Avoid alcohol.
  3. Avoid becoming excessively tired.
  4. Install grab bars in the shower and tub area.
  5. Do not lock doors of the bedroom or bathroom.
  6. Avoid an excessive intake of caffeine.

Assessment

Collect the following data through the health history and physical examination:

- Health history: past seizures: age when the client's first seizure occurred, most recent seizure, factors precipitating a seizure, any warning signs (aura), prophylactic anticonvulsant therapy, and specific concerns the client may have about the seizures
- Physical assessment: important data used in determining an accurate diagnosis that describe manifestations obtained from nursing assessments before, during, and after a seizure. (Table 33-3 lists nursing assessments with rationale.)

Nursing Diagnoses and Interventions

Nursing care of clients with a seizure disorder focuses on providing care during and immediately after the seizure and on client teaching. The client with seizures has a wide variety of responses to actual or potential changes in health status; interventions discussed in this section focus on facilitating physical and psychologic comfort and safety.

Risk for Ineffective Airway Clearance

During a seizure, the tongue may fall back and obstruct the airway, the gag reflex may be depressed, and secretions may pool at the back of the throat. These may put the client at risk for an obstructed airway. Most seizures occur in the home or community; teach these interventions also to the client's family.

- Provide interventions to maintain a patent airway:
    1. Loosen clothing around the neck.
    2. Turn on the side.
    3. Do not force anything into the mouth.
- If prescribed and available, administer oxygen by mask.

Although it was at one time believed that it was necessary to place a padded tongue blade in the client's mouth during a seizure, this is no longer recommended; an improperly placed tongue blade can obstruct the airway. Turning the client on the side allows secretions to drain from the mouth.

- Teach family members how to care for the client during a seizure to prevent airway obstruction. *Family members are often the only people present to provide this emergency intervention.*

Table 33-3. Nursing Assessments Before, During, and After a Seizure

Assessment	Rationale
What was the client's level of consciousness? If consciousness was lost, at what point?	Indicates area of brain involved and type of seizure.
What was the client doing just before the attack?	May suggest precipitating factors.
In what part of the body did the seizure start?	May indicate the site of seizure activity in the brain tissue; for example, if jerking movements were first observed in right hand, the seizure focus may be in left motor cortex in the area of the hand.
Was there an epileptic cry?	Usually indicates the tonic stage of a generalized tonic-clonic seizure.
Were any automatisms such as eyelid fluttering, chewing, lip smacking, or swallowing observed?	Often seen in complex, partial, and absence seizures.

Continued on the next page

Table 33-3. Continued

Assessment	Rationale
How long did movements last? Did the location or character change (tonic to clonic)? Did movements involve both sides of the body or just one?	Indicates areas in which focal activity originated.
Did the head and/or eyes turn to one side and, if so, which side?	Helps localize the focus of the seizure. During the seizure, the head and eyes typically will turn away from the side of the epileptogenic focus.
Were there changes in pupillary reactions?	Indicates involvement of the autonomic nervous system.
If the client fell, was the head hit?	Skull X-ray studies may be needed to rule out subdural hematoma or fracture.
Was there foaming or frothing from the mouth?	Usually indicates a tonic-clonic seizure.

Anxiety

The client with a seizure disorder is understandably anxious about the future, with questions about ability to go to school, work, have a family, and drive a car. Feelings of embarrassment about having a seizure in public and rejection by others are common and also increase the client's anxiety.

- Provide support by explaining that concerns are normal. *It is important to be sensitive to the effect of seizures on the client's self-concept and body image; alterations in these areas not only increase anxiety, but also cause withdrawal from socialization with others. Demonstrating acceptance of the client's concerns allows further discussion.*
- Help identify safe leisure activities. *Worrying about being hurt if a seizure occurs may cause withdrawal from social activities that are pleasurable.*
- Provide information about sources and support groups. *Sharing information with other people with similar health problems allows for a more realistic viewpoint; accurate information can clear up misconceptions that cause anxiety.*
- Provide accurate information about hiring practices and legal limitations on driving or operating heavy or dangerous machinery. *Accurate information decreases anxiety about the unknown. The American Disabilities Act prohibits discrimination; however, there are legal limitations on driving until the person is proved free of seizures.*

Home Care

Teaching follows a systematic assessment of the needs of both the client and family. Include family members so that they can learn seizure management, including the care and observations necessary before and during a seizure. Stress the importance of safety and keeping the airway patent.

Help both the client and family adjust to a diagnosis of epilepsy. Address the following topics:

- Misconceptions, common fears, and myths about epilepsy.
- The importance of wearing a MedicAlert band or carrying a medical alert card at all times.
- Avoiding alcoholic beverages and limiting coffee intake.
- Taking showers versus tub baths, because of safety issues during a generalized seizure.
- Factors that may trigger a seizure, such as abrupt withdrawal from medication, constipation, fatigue, excessive stress, fever, menstruation, sights and sounds, such as television, flashing video, and computer screens.
- Helpful resources:
  - American Epilepsy Society
  - Epilepsy Foundation.

34

Nursing Care of Clients with Neurologic Disorders

This chapter discusses a variety of neurologic disorders. For many of the disorders, nursing care is based on similar nursing diagnoses. To avoid repeating those diagnoses and interventions for each disorder, they have been divided among the nursing care discussions as appropriate.

Degenerative Neurologic Disorders

Degenerative neurologic disorders can affect the central nervous system and the peripheral nerves. By progressively disrupting cognitive processes or motor functions, disorders such as multiple sclerosis, Alzheimer's disease, and Parkinson's disease strike at the core of an individual's sense of personal autonomy and well-being and can be psychologically and emotionally devastating to family members and caregivers.

Ongoing medical research into degenerative neurologic disorders offers an increasing measure of hope to clients and their families. The discovery of genetic or biochemical markers associated with some of these disorders is leading to the development of effective screening and diagnostic methods. In addition, new drugs may make it possible to halt the progression of the disorders in some clients, transforming the disorders into manageable conditions.

The Client with Alzheimer's Disease

Alzheimer's disease (AD) (also called *dementia of Alzheimer type [DAT]* or *senile disease complex*) is a form of dementia characterized by progressive, irreversible deterioration of general intellectual functioning. **Dementia** is defined by the World Health Organization as a chronic or progressive disease of the brain in which multiple cortical functions, calculation, learning capacity, language, and judgment are disturbed. Impairments of cognitive function are usually accompanied by deterioration in emotional control, social behavior, and motivation.

Memory loss is usually the first sign of Alzheimer's disease. Memory deficits are initially subtle, and family members and friends may not suspect a problem until the disease progresses and symptoms become more noticeable. Family members may also deny the symptoms and ignore deficits until the person exhibits unsafe or extremely unusual behavior.

Progression of the disease varies, but the course is one of deteriorating cognition and judgment with eventual physical decline and total inability to perform ADLs. With the loss of the ability to perform even the most basic ADLs, the burden of meeting the client's needs shifts to the caregiver.

Incidence and Prevalence

Alzheimer's disease is the most common degenerative neurologic illness and the most common cause of cognitive impairment (Porth, 2002). It accounts for about two-thirds of cases of dementia in America, affecting adults in middle to late life. Scientists estimate that more than 4 million people have AD, and the number of people with AD doubles every 5 years beyond age 65.

Risk Factors and Warning Signs

As one ages, the risk of developing AD increases. With numbers of older people increasing, this type of dementia is predicted to also increase. The risk factors for AD are older age, family history, and female gender. Warning signs are:

- Memory loss that affects job skills
- Difficulty performing familiar tasks
- Problems with language
- Disorientation to time and place
- Poor or decreased judgment
- Problems with abstract thinking
- Misplacing things
- Changes in mood or behavior
- Changes in personality
- Loss of initiative.

Recognizing early symptoms is important, because the cause of dementia, such as from depression or hypothyroidism, may be reversible. Dementia from AD is not reversible. Treatment, however, can maximize quality of life and allow the affected person to plan for the future.

Pathophysiology

The exact cause of AD is unknown. Theories include loss of neurotransmitter stimulation by choline acetyltransferase, mutation for encoding amyloid precursor protein, and alteration in apolipoprotein E. Other possible causes are gene defects on chromosomes 14, 19, or 21, which may lead to clumping and precipitation of insoluble amyloid as plaques. The role of protein kinase C, the link between AD and aluminum, a viral cause, an autoimmune cause, and mitochondrial defects that alter cell metabolism and protein processing are being studied (McCance & Huether, 2002).

Two types of AD exist: *Familial AD* follows an inheritance pattern and *sporadic AD* has no obvious inheritance pattern. AD is further described as early onset (occurring in people younger than 65) and late onset (occurring in people age 65 and older). Early-onset AD usually affects people ages 30 to 60, is relatively rare, and often progresses more rapidly than late-onset AD.

Several structural and chemical changes in the brain occur with AD, especially in the hippocampus and the frontal and temporal lobes of the cerebral cortex. As AD destroys neurons in the hippocampus and related structures, short-term memory fails and the ability to perform easy and familiar tasks declines. The effect of AD on neurons in the cerebral cortex is loss of language skills and judgment. Emotional outbursts and behavior changes, such as wandering and agitation, begin to occur and become more frequent as the disease progresses. Eventually, other areas of the brain are affected; all affected areas begin to atrophy, and the person becomes totally helpless and unresponsive.

Characteristic findings in the brains of AD clients are loss of nerve cells and the presence of *neurofibrillary tangles* and *amyloid plaques*. Neurofibrillary tangles result when a tau, a kind of protein in the neurons, becomes distorted and twisted. Tau normally holds together the microtubles, which guide nutrients and molecules to the end of the axon. In AD, tau changes and twists into pairs of filaments, which then join to form tangles. As tau no longer maintains the transport system, communication is lost between neurons. Death of neurons may follow, contributing to the development of dementia.

Groups of nerve cells (especially the terminal axons) degenerate and clump around an amyloid core as plaque. They are found in the spaces between the neurons of the brain. These plaques, which develop first in areas used for memory and cognition, disrupt transmission of nerve impulses. The plaques consist primarily of insoluble deposits of beta-amyloid, a protein fragment from a larger protein called amyloid precursor protein (APP), mixed with other neurons and nonnerve cells. It is not yet known if plaque formation causes AD or if plaques are a by-product of the AD process.

Blood flow to the affected areas of the brain is decreased. The brain atrophies, and corresponding enlargement of ventricles and sulci is evident. As AD progresses, more areas of the brain are affected, with symptoms correlating to those affected areas of the brain. For example, neuronal and neurotransmitter losses in the parietal lobe result in problems with perception and interpretation of environmental stimuli; deficits in the frontal lobe cause changes in personality and emotional lability.

Manifestations

Alzheimer's disease is classified into three stages based on the client's manifestations and abilities, as outlined in Table 34-1. It is important to note that the progression of AD varies for each individual and may not precisely follow the model.

Stage I AD

In stage I, a client typically appears physically healthy and alert, and cognitive deficits can go undetected unless thorough and periodic evaluations are performed. Usually, family members are the first to notice lapses in memory, subtle changes in personality, or problems in doing simple calculations. AD clients and families may consciously or unconsciously compensate for cognitive deficits by adjusting schedules and routines. Clients may seem restless, forgetful, or uncoordinated.

Table 34-1. Manifestations of Alzheimer's Disease

Stage I: Approximately 2 to 4 Years

- Short-term memory loss: Forgets location and names of objects and has difficulty learning new information; long-term memory is unaffected.
- Decreased attention span.
- Subtle personality changes: Lacks spontaneity; denial, irritability, and depression are possible.
- Mild cognitive deficits: Attempts to adjust to and cover up memory loss.
- Visuospatial deficits: Some problems with depth perception.

Stage II: Approximately 2 to 12 Years

- Impaired cognition: Obvious memory deficits and confusion; loss of abstract thinking; astereognosis and agraphia; inability to do math calculations; loss of ability to tell time and time disorientation, manifested as "sundowning"; wandering behavior.
- Personality changes: Becomes easily agitated and irritable; may have delusions or hallucinations.
- Visuospatial deficits: Is unable to dress self; has poor spatial orientation.
- Impaired motor skills: Paces and is restless at times; motor apraxia is evident when using familiar objects.
- Impaired judgment: Diminished social skills; inability to drive a car; inability to make decisions (e.g., choose clothing).

Stage III: Approximately 2 to 4 Years or Longer

- Cognitive abilities grossly decreased or absent: Is usually disoriented to time, place, and person.
- Communication skills usually absent: Is frequently mute.
- Motor skills grossly impaired or absent: Limb rigidity and posture flexion; bowel and bladder incontinence.

Stage II AD

In stage II, memory deficits are more apparent, and the client is less able to behave spontaneously. Clients may wander and get lost, even in their own homes. Although progression of manifestations continues and orientation to place and time deteriorates, AD clients may still have periods of mental lucidity and engage in time-oriented conversations. Generally, however, clients become more confused and lose their sense of time, leading to changes in sleeping patterns, agitation, and stress. AD clients are less able to make even simple decisions and to adapt to environmental changes. Some AD clients develop severe attacks related to seemingly minor events; this reaction may result from a progressively lowered stress threshold. **Sundowning** is another behavioral change, characterized by increased agitation, time disorientation, and wandering behaviors during afternoon and evening hours; it is accelerated on overcast days.

Language deficits are common in stage II. They include *paraphasia* (using the wrong word), *echolalia* (repetition of words or phrases), and *scanning speech,* in which the client appears to search for words. Eventually, total *aphasia* (absence of speech) may occur. Frustration and depression are common among AD clients as the full extent and implications of the deficits become obvious.

The AD client slowly loses the ability to perform simple tasks required for hygiene or eating because sequencing of tasks is lost. For example, the client may open a can of soup but not remember to pour it into a pan to heat it. Instead, the client might place the can directly on the burner and leave the heat on high even after a smoke alarm sounds. The AD client may falsely interpret the smoke alarm as a telephone ringing, a tornado warning siren, or an ambulance siren. Thus, safety is a high priority for the client in stage II.

Sensorimotor deficits in stage II include *apraxia,* the inability to perform purposeful movements and use objects correctly; *astereognosis,* the inability to identify objects by touch; and *agraphia,* the inability to write. Problems related to malnutrition and decreased fluid intake, such as anemia and constipation, may be evident. Sleep pattern disturbances are also common and are related to the loss of time orientation, sundowning phenomenon, and depression.

Stage III AD

Stage III brings increasing dependence, with inability to communicate, loss of continence, and progressive loss of cognitive abilities. Common complications include pneumonia, dehydration, malnutrition, falls, depression, delusions, and paranoid reactions. The prognosis of a client with AD is poor, with an average life expectancy of 7 years from time of diagnosis. Death frequently occurs from pneumonia secondary to aspiration.

Collaborative Care

There is no cure for AD, and the main objective of care is to provide an environment that matches the client's functional abilities. Nurses, physicians, physical therapists, and social workers collaborate with the client's family to provide the least restrictive environment in which the client can safely function.

Diagnostic Tests

Alzheimer's disease is diagnosed by ruling out causes for the client's manifestations. The only definitive method of diagnosis is postmortem examination of brain tissue. An extensive workup is especially important, because the dementia may be due to a reversible or treatable condition. For example, an older client's misuse of medications can lead to overdosing and resulting confusion. Other categories of conditions that may be considered and ruled out include depression, infection, hypothyroidism, dehydration, heart disease, stroke, and chronic obstructive respiratory disease.

The following diagnostic tests may be done:

- *EEG* may reveal a slowed pattern in the later stages of the disorder.
- *MRI* and *CT scan of the brain* demonstrates shrinkage of the hippocampus as well as changes in other parts of the brain.

- *Positron emission tomography (PET) scan* allows visualizing the activity and interactions of various parts of the brain as they are used during cognitive operations involving information processing.
- *Psychometric evaluation* using the Folstein Mini Mental Status Examination form or a similar instrument reflects the loss of memory and other cognitive skills over time.

Other tests may be performed, depending on the client's manifestations. For example, if the client has hypertension and memory changes, cerebral vascular studies are indicated to exclude multi-infarct dementia or other problems. Ruling out reversible dementia disorders requires evaluation of specific laboratory studies, such as thyroid function studies and measurement of electrolyte and vitamin levels.

Guidelines for the early recognition and assessment of AD have been established by the Agency for Healthcare Research and Quality. A diagnosis of Alzheimer's disease requires the presence of dementia, onset between age 40 and 90 years (most often after age 65), and absence of systemic or brain disorders that could cause mental changes.

Medications

Cholinesterase inhibitors are used to treat mild to moderate dementia in AD. Tacrine hydrochloride (Cognex) was the first medication specifically approved for the treatment of AD. Donepezil hydrochloride (Aricept) is used to treat mild to moderate AD dementia with some success. Rivastigmine tartrate (Exelon) is also used to treat mild to moderate AD symptoms. It improves the ability to carry out ADLs, decreases agitation and delusions, and improves cognitive function. See Table 34-2 for information about medications used to treat AD.

Table 34-2. Medication Administration

The Client with Alzheimer's Disease (AD)

Cholinergic (Parasympathomimetics); Cholinesterase Inhibitors

Tacrine hydrochloride (Cognex)
Donepezil hydrochloride (Aricept)
Rivastigmine tartrate (Exelon)

In the early stages of AD, the pathologic changes in neurons result in a deficiency of acetylcholine (a key neurotransmitter involved in cognitive functioning). Cholinesterase inhibitors slow the breakdown of acetylcholine release by the remaining intact neurons. In addition, rivastigmine tartrate inhibits the G_1 form of acetylcholinesterase (found in higher levels in the brain of clients with AD), so less acetylcholine is degraded. The drugs are used to improve memory in mild to moderate AD dementia.

Nursing Responsibilities
- Administer tacrine hydrochloride one hour before meals, if possible.
- Administer donepezil hydrochloride at bedtime.
- Administer rivastigmine tartrate (both capsules and liquid) with food. Liquid form may be administered undiluted or mixed with water, juice, or soda. Stir to completely dissolve.

Table 34-2. Continued

- Monitor for jaundice, increased bilirubin levels, and other signs of liver involvement, such as rising serum aminotransferase (AST, ALT) levels. Therapy is usually decreased when the enzyme level exceeds four times normal limits and discontinued when the level reaches five times normal.
- Observe for gastrointestinal bleeding and gastric ulcer pain.
- Monitor for cholinergic-related problems: bladder outlet obstruction, seizures, and slowed cardiac rate.
- Assist with ambulation as dizziness is a common side effect.
- Monitor glycemic control in clients with diabetes.
- Assess for improvement in AD symptoms, especially in reasoning, memory, and ADLs.

Client and Family Teaching
- Notify the physician promptly if jaundice, seizures, slowed heart rate, GI bleeding, or difficulty urinating occurs.
- Follow directions for times and instructions about administration of specific medication.
- Follow your health care provider's recommendation for periodic EEG, blood tests, and urine tests.
- These medications do not cure AD, and will at some point become ineffective as the disease progresses.

Depression often accompanies AD and is treated with the appropriate medication. Antihistamines and tricyclic antidepressants that have high anticholinergic activity are usually avoided because they can increase AD symptoms. Occasionally clients with AD require tranquilizers such as thioridazine (Mellaril) or haloperidol (Haldol), to manage severe agitation. Other therapies under study to prevent or delay the onset of AD include antioxidants, such as vitamin E, anti-inflammatory agents, and estrogen replacement therapy in women.

Complementary Therapy

The following types of complementary therapy may be used in treating the manifestations of AD.

- Massage, which decreases agitation
- Herbs
- Ginko biloba, which is thought (among other actions) to improve cognition
- Huperzine A, a traditional Chinese medicine, which acts as an acetylcholinesterase inhibitor
- Coenzyme Q10, an antioxidant that naturally occurs in the body
- Supplements, such as zinc, selenium, and evening primrose oil
- Therapies involving art, music, sound, and dance.

Nursing Care

Clients with AD often require intensive, supportive nursing interventions directed at the physical and psychosocial responses to illness. Equally important, the nurse can facilitate the long-term support of these clients by providing teaching and referrals to follow-up care in the community.

Health Promotion

Health promotion for the client with AD focuses on maintaining functional abilities and safety. If the client will be cared for at home, address safety considerations as well as the caregivers' abilities to meet the client's basic needs, such as maintaining hygiene and other ADLs. Adapt nursing interventions and teaching to the client's stage of Alzheimer's disease.

Assessment

Collect the following data through the health history and physical examination (see Chapter 40). Further focused assessments are described with nursing interventions below.

- *Health history:* family member/caregiver support, living arrangements, ability to carry out ADLs, drug use, work history (e.g., exposure to metals), previous history of multiple strokes, brain injury or brain infection, family history of dementia, sleep pattern, changes in cognition and memory, ability to communicate, changes in behavior.
- *Physical assessment:* height/weight, orientation, abstract reasoning, mental status.

Nursing Diagnoses and Interventions

During the early stage of AD, nursing care focuses on helping the client make minor adaptations to his or her environment. As the client becomes progressively unable to manage self-care tasks, more adaptations are required. Equally important, the caregiver needs more support—both physical and psychosocial—as the client becomes increasingly dependent.

Impaired Memory

Impaired memory is an appropriate nursing diagnosis in stage I AD. At this stage, techniques to help with the memory loss should be included in teaching for both the client and the caregiver.

- Suggest complementary therapies, such as meditation, massage, or exercise. *These activities can help reduce stress, which can aggravate memory loss.*
- Suggest using a calendar, keeping lists of reminders, or asking someone else to remind of appointments and events. *Written or verbal reminders are helpful if memory is impaired.*
- Recommend using a medication box labeled with days and times. *A medication box is a good way to remember to take medications.*
- If safety is a concern, such as turning on the stove and forgetting it, suggest using alternatives, such as a microwave. Program emergency numbers into the telephone. Ask client to consider a Life-line telephone program. *These measures can increase safety.*
- Suggest using cues, such as an alarm on a watch or a pocket computer, to trigger actions at designated times. *Cues are often helpful when memory loss is a problem.*

Chronic Confusion

Clients with AD often have memory deficits that make functioning in a nonstructured environment difficult. Many of the nursing interventions for this diagnosis need to be modified over time as the client continues to lose cognitive function.

- Label rooms, drawers, and other items as needed. *Visual cues promote the highest possible degree of independence for the client.*
- Remove potential hazards, such as sharp knives or potentially harmful liquids or chemicals, from the environment. *Ensuring safety is a critical factor in providing care.*

- Keep environmental stimuli to a minimum: Decrease noise levels; speak in a calm, low voice; and take an unhurried approach. *Minimizing sensory input and maintaining a calm manner may decrease anxiety.*

- Begin each interaction by identifying self and calling client by name. *These techniques provide information for the client with memory loss.*

- Limit questions to those that require a simple yes or no response. *Questions need to be appropriate to the client's ability as decision making and verbal skills decline.*

- Orient to the environment, person, and time as able; place large, easy-to-read calendars and clocks in the client's line of vision. Make references to the season or day of the week when conversing with the client. *Orient the client according to his or her level of ability; orienting to precise time may not be possible in the later stages of AD.*

- Provide boundaries by placing red or yellow tape on the floor. *Boundaries help the client stay within safe areas.*

- Provide continuity in nursing staff. *This not only promotes consistency of care for the client but also allows the nurse to determine more accurately changes in the client's condition.*

- Repeat explanations simply and as needed to decrease anxiety. *Loss of short-term memory leads to loss of a point of reference; eventually, AD clients think they are experiencing everything for the first time.*

Table 34-3. Communication Techniques for the Client with AD

< Face the client and talk directly to him or her; call the client by name.

< When first approaching the client, identify yourself.

< Use simple sentences and words with few syllables.

< Speak in a calm, low voice.

< Ask one question at a time. Use questions that require only a yes or no response.

< Keep nonverbal communication relaxed and parallel to the verbal communication.

< Avoid giving the impression of being in a hurry; try to have a relaxed approach.

< Observe for anxiety—wringing hands, pacing, darting eye movements—and alter your approach to decrease anxiety.

< Avoid arguing with clients; do not insist on orienting client to reality; the client's point of reference may not be based in reality.

< Give plenty of time for the client with AD to process what you are trying to say; do not expect clients to perform skills beyond their abilities.

< Repeat explanations in simple terms.

Anxiety

Managing the AD client's behaviors associated with anxiety, restlessness, and confusion is a major challenge confronting nurses and caregivers. Frequently, clients are relatively calm in the morning hours, only to experience increasing periods of agitation in the afternoon and evening hours. The AD client may even waken from the night's sleep with confusion, fearfulness, or panic attacks.

- Monitor for early behaviors of fatigue and agitation. *Early assessment of problems results in prompt intervention to promote rest or to remove the client from the situation causing anxiety.*

- Remove client from situations that are causing increased anxiety, such as noisy activities involving large groups. *High-stimulus situations may increase anxious feelings and agitation.*

- Keep daily routine as consistent as possible. *Providing a structured day enhances feelings of familiarity and decreases stress.*

- Schedule rest periods or quiet times throughout the day. *Fatigue contributes to anxiety and lowers the stress threshold.*

- Provide quiet activities, such as listening to favorite music, in the afternoon or early evening. *Quiet activities may help decrease sundowning.*

- If confusion and agitation persist or escalate, assess for physical causes, such as decreased oxygenation, infections, fatigue, constipation, and electrolyte imbalance. *Physical factors can increase agitation in clients with AD.*

- Use therapeutic touch or gentle hand massage. *These activities induce relaxation and have a calming effect.*

Hopelessness

As the client and family recognize the impact of AD on their lives, they may feel a sense of hopelessness and powerlessness. They may not have the coping skills to deal effectively with the diagnosis and anticipated problems. The increasingly degenerative, irreversible nature of the disorder tends to diminish hope; only the ability to adapt to the many problems can restore it.

- Assess the client's and family's response to the diagnosis and understanding of AD; encourage expression of feelings. *Understanding the client/family's perspective enables the nurse to dispel myths about AD.*

- Provide realistic information about the disorder; provide information at the client/family's level of understanding. *Client and family may need to have separate sessions. Factual information provides a foundation for decision making.*

- Avoid criticizing or judging expressed feelings. *An environment accepting of the expression of real feelings promotes both further expression of feelings and willingness to discuss other issues.*

- Support positive family bonds and enhance communication among family members; promote mutual positive regard. *Strong family relationships can provide direction for living and convey a willingness to share the burden.*

- Encourage the client to make as many decisions as possible. *Self-determination enhances a feeling of control over a situation and may give a sense of hope.*

- Encourage the client and family to seek spiritual guidance that previously inspired hope. *The client's church is a legitimate support system. Belief in God can inspire hope beyond present circumstances.*

Caregiver Role Strain

Most caregivers of clients with AD are spouses or other family members. Because AD is a chronic and eventually debilitating disorder, caregivers may feel overwhelmed by their responsibilities. The caregiving spouse faces not only the responsibility for the client's multiple physical demands, but also economic and psychosocial stressors. An area that must be discussed is the ability and safety of the client in driving an automobile. Although is may be necessary, the loss of independence represented by the loss of the ability to drive may further trigger anxiety and anger. Fear of the future, loss of income, loss of companionship and a mate—combined with fatigue—make the caregiver vulnerable. Caregivers may become physically and mentally exhausted and socially isolated because of the overwhelming responsibilities of providing total care to the incapacitated family member.

- Teach the caregivers self-care techniques, such as taking rest periods and avoiding fatigue. *Fatigue adds to stress and potentially leads to poor decision making.*
- Have the caregivers list and regularly take part in physical activities they enjoy, such as walking or swimming. *Regular physical exercise decreases stress.*
- Refer the caregivers to local AD support groups. Suggest books pertinent to the subject. *Explicit suggestions in locating support systems and providing specific information promotes coping.*
- Refer the caregivers to Meals-on-Wheels, home health, respite care, and other community services. *Community agencies can relieve some of the daily care burdens, thus providing time for other activities. Programs that support caregivers have been shown to delay nursing home placement.*
- Ensure the family knows that hospice care is available during the end stages of AD. *Hospice services can support the family during this difficult time.*

Home Care

Teaching for clients and families centers initially on explaining the disorder and exploring available support systems. Anticipate the need to reexplain the disorder and its consequences, as clients and families may be in shock or denial during the initial period of the disease.

In addition to explaining the anticipated changes with AD, suggest practical solutions to identified problems. It is important to evaluate both the client and caregivers; interventions must be appropriate for the family's situation and resources. Maintaining the least restrictive environment that promotes safety for the client is a major goal of teaching. Using memory cues, such as labeling drawers to indicate the specific types of clothing and labeling rooms, can help orient the client and foster independence. Consistency in the environment and daily routine is an essential part of care. Emphasizing realistic expectations means adjusting care and communication techniques to the client's level of ability.

Address the following topics for home care of the client and for the caregiver:

- Support groups and peer counseling are helpful in handling caregiver stress.
- A person with AD who is confused or agitated is not comfortable and is usually frightened.
- Plan care that matches the person's level of coping, using a consistent routine.
- Provide regular rest periods to decrease the client's stress and fatigue (these do not increase nighttime wandering).
- Plan care for the caregiver. Periodic respite care during the initial stages, with plans for increasing assistance to meet the client's daily needs as the disease progresses, may be sufficient. Referrals to the appropriate agency for long-term care, including skilled nursing facilities, may be indicated. Family members may need help adjusting to the idea of extended care but may be relieved to relinquish the physical care needs.

- Suggest the following resources:
    1. Alzheimer's Association
    2. Alzheimer's Disease and Related Disorders Association
    3. Alzheimer's Disease Education and Referral Center
    4. National Institute of Neurological and Communicative Disorders and Stroke

The Client with Multiple Sclerosis

Multiple sclerosis (MS) is a chronic demyelinating disease of the central nervous system, associated with an abnormal immune response to an environmental factor. The symptoms of MS vary according to the area of the nervous system affected. The initial onset may be followed by a total remission, making diagnosis difficult. In about 60% of clients, MS is characterized by periods of exacerbation, when symptoms are highly pronounced, followed by periods of remission. The end result, however, is progression of the disease with increasing loss of function.

Incidence and Prevalence

Approximately 500,000 people in the United States have MS. Females are affected 2 times more often than males, and the incidence is highest in young adults (age 20 to 40). The disease occurs more commonly in temperate climates, including the northern United States. This association is established by approximately age 15, and moving to or from a temperate climate after that age does not change it.

The onset of MS is usually between 20 and 50 years of age, with a peak at age 30. MS is the most prevalent CNS demyelinating disorder, and is a leading cause of neurologic disability in young adults. Although all races are affected, MS is primarily a disease of Caucasians. Although a definite genetic factor has not been established, 15% of those with MS have a relative with the disease (McCance & Huether, 2002).

Pathophysiology

MS is believed to occur as a result of an autoimmune response to a prior viral infection in a genetically susceptible person. The infection, which is thought to occur early in life, activates T cells. T cells usually move in and out of the CNS across the blood-brain barrier, but for an unknown reason, they remain in the CNS in people with MS. The T cells facilitate infiltration by other leukocytes, and an inflammatory process follows. Inflammation destroys myelin and oligodendrocytes (myelin-producing cells), leading to axon dysfunction. The myelin sheaths are fatty, segmented wrappings that normally protect and insulate nerve fibers and increase the speed of transmission of nerve impulses. In multiple sclerosis, these myelin sheaths of the white matter of the spinal cord, brain, and optic nerve are destroyed in patches, called plaques, along the axon. The **demyelination** of nerve fibers slows and distorts the conduction of nerve impulses and sometimes results in the total absence of impulse transmission. The neurons usually affected by MS are located in the spinal cord, brainstem, cerebral and cerebellar areas, and the optic nerve.

Table 34-4. Classifications of Multiple Sclerosis

Relapsing-remitting: The most common clinical course of MS, characterized by exacerbations (acute attacks) with either full recovery or partial recovery with disability.

Primary progressive: Steady worsening of disease from the onset with occasional minor recovery.

Secondary progressive: Begins as with relapsing-remitting, but the disease steadily becomes worse between exacerbations.

Progressive-relapsing: This rare form continues to progress from the onset but also has exacerbations.

Both plaques and diffuse lesions form as demyelinating lesions. Plaques typically are scattered through the white matter of the CNS, although they may extend into adjacent gray matter. Early manifestations are the result of inflammatory edema in and around the plaque and partial demyelination. These manifestations typically disappear within weeks after the initial episode. With progression of the disease, the demyelination and plaque formation result in scarring of glia (*gliosis*) and degeneration of axons. Continued loss of function leads to permanent disability, usually over about 20 years.

There are four classifications of MS: relapsing-remitting, primary progressive, secondary progressive, and progressive-relapsing. Most individuals with MS present with the relapsing-remitting type.

Various stressors have been suggested as triggers for MS. These stressors include febrile states, pregnancy, extreme physical exertion, and fatigue. These precipitating factors can also cause a relapse of the manifestations during the course of the disease.

Manifestations

The manifestations of MS vary according to the areas destroyed by demyelination and the affected body system. Fatigue is one of the most disabling manifestations, and affects almost all clients with MS. The manifestations, categorized by the established syndromes of MS, include:

Mixed or Generalized Type (50% of cases)

- Manifestations include optic nerve involvement, with visual blurring, fogginess, or haziness; and impaired color perception. There is also decreased central visual acuity, area of diminished vision in the visual fields, acquired color vision deficit (especially to red and green), and an altered pupillary reaction to light.
- Brainstem lesions (cranial nerves III to XII) are noted, with nystagmus, dysarthria, deafness, vertigo, vomiting, tinnitus, facial weakness, and decreased sensation. Other manifestations include diplopia and eye pain, and cognitive dysfunctions involving concentration, short-term memory, word finding, and planning.
- Mood alterations are manifested as depression more often than euphoria.

Spinal Type (25% of cases)

- Weakness and/or numbness is noted in one or both extremities (most often the legs).
- Upper motor neuron involvement is manifested by stiffness, slowness, weakness (spastic paresis).
- Bladder dyfunctions include urgency, hesitancy, and incontinence.
- Bowel dysfunction is most often seen as constipation.
- Neurogenic impotence is noted.

Cerebellar Type (5% of cases)

- Client shows manifestations of nystagmus, ataxia, and hyptonia.

Amaurotic Form (5% of cases)

- Client develops blindness.

Short-lived attacks of neurologic deficits indicate the temporary appearance or worsening of manifestations. Conditions that cause short-lived attacks include (1) minor increases in body temperature or serum calcium concentrations (both increase the leakage of current through demyelinated neurons) and (2) functional demands that exceed conduction capacity. Paroxysmal attacks are sensory or motor manifestations that occur abruptly and last for only seconds or minutes; the manifestations are paresthesias, dysarthria and ataxia, and tonic head turning. Paroxysmal attacks, which may occur many times a day, result from the direct transmission of nerve impulses between adjacent demyelinated axons (McCance & Huether, 2002).

Collaborative Care

Management of the client with MS varies according to the severity of the manifestations. The focus is on retaining the optimal level of functioning possible, given the degree of disability. Rehabilitation—physical, occupational/vocational, and psychosocial—is a cornerstone of a team approach to treatment. During exacerbations, the focus of interventions shifts to controlling manifestations and quickly returning to remission.

Diagnostic Tests

Diagnosis of MS is challenging because the disease does not manifest uniformly. Initially, a thorough history and physical examination are completed, and their importance in establishing a diagnosis cannot be overemphasized. Diagnostic tests vary with the presenting complaints. MRI is the most definitive test available; however, it is one of several laboratory and diagnostic tests that may be performed when establishing the diagnosis.

- *Cerebral spinal fluid (CSF) analysis* reveals an increased number of T lymphocytes that are reactive with antigens, indicating the presence of an immune response in the client. Of MS patients, 80% have elevated levels of immunoglobulin G (IgG) in the CSF. IgG may not be increased during the initial period of the disease.
- *MRI studies* are performed. Cerebral MRI detects multifocal lesions in the white matter. Serial MRIs may be performed to chart the course of the disease. MRI of the spinal cord or optic nerves can detect lesions in these areas.
- *CT scan* of the brain shows atrophy and white matter lesions. In about 25% of clients with MS, enlarged ventricles are visible on CT.

- *Positron emission tomography (PET) scan* measures brain activity. In MS clients, the scan reveals areas with changes in glucose metabolism.

- *Evoked response testing* of visual, auditory, or somatosensory impulses may show delayed conduction.

Medications

Medications slow the progression of MS and decrease the number of attacks. See Table 34-5 for information about these medications.

The medications used during an exacerbation are aimed at decreasing inflammation to inhibit manifestations and induce remission. Frequently, a combination of adrenocorticotrophic hormone (ACTH) and glucocorticoids is used to decrease inflammation and suppress the immune system. Immunosuppressive agents, including azathioprine (Imuran) and cyclophosphamide (Cytoxan), are also used. Some centers administer cyclophosphamide monthly to prevent exacerbations.

Other medications treat the manifestations of MS, such as muscle spasms. Anticholinergics are sometimes administered for bladder spasticity; cholinergics are given if the client has a problem with urinary retention related to flaccid bladder.

Treatments

Although medications are the primary method of controlling manifestations, other treatments include surgery, dietary management, and rehabilitative therapies.

Table 34-5. Medication Administration – The Client with Multiple Sclerosis

Immunomodulators

Interferon beta-1a (Avonex)
Interferon beta-1b (Betaseron)
Glatiramer acetate (Copaxone, Copolymer-1)

Interferon beta-1a, interferon beta-1b, and glatiramer acetate are administered to clients with relapsing-remitting MS to prolong the time of onset to disability. Their use is based on the assumption that MS is an immunologically mediated disease. Interferon beta-1b produces a decrease in the MS lesions in some clients. Some clients, however, develop a decrease in the absolute neutrophil count and increases in the levels of liver enzymes. Anxiety, confusion, and depression with suicidal tendencies also have been reported. Other adverse reactions include pain, inflammation, hypersensitivity at the injection site, and generalized flulike manifestations. Some women experience menstrual disorders. Pregnant women should not take these medications.

Nursing Responsibilities
- Assess baseline parameters to evaluate drug side effects: psychologic profile, liver function tests, and CBC with differential. Monitor CBC and liver function tests every three months or as prescribed.

- Assess injection site and report ulceration promptly (pain and redness are common reactions).

Continued on the next page

Table 34-5. Continued

- Evaluate client's baseline neurologic, sensory, and motor function. Monitor changes in condition and function.
- Report if client is pregnant or breast-feeding.

Client and Family Teaching

- This drug may cause depression and thoughts of suicide; report these feelings immediately to the physician.
- The medication is reconstituted and should be discarded if it becomes discolored or precipitates out. Administer the medication within three hours of reconstitution. Rotate injection sites, and avoid any areas that are red or show other skin reactions.
- Seek follow-up care to monitor neurologic changes, CBC, and liver function.
- Avoid prolonged exposure to sunlight.

Adrenocorticosteroid Therapy

Adrenocorticotropic hormone (ACTH) (Acthar)
Prednisone (Deltasone, Meticorten, Orasone)
Methylprednisolone (Medrol, Solu-Medrol)

Adrenocorticosteroids are used both to sustain a remission and to treat exacerbations of MS. ACTH is usually given to induce a remission; it is administered intravenously for one week and may be followed by oral prednisone therapy. Another protocol involves administering ACTH intravenously for 3 days followed by intramuscular injections every 12 hours for 1 week (Hickey, 2002). The drugs are given to suppress the immune system, implicated in the etiology of MS. If the drug is used long term, the usual steroid precautions are indicated, such as monitoring for glucose intolerance, osteoporosis, and cataract formation. The drugs are used with caution in pregnant and lactating women.

Muscle Relaxants

Baclofen (Lioresal)
Dantrolene (Dantrium)
Diazepam (Valium)

Muscle relaxants are given to clients with MS to relieve muscle spasms. Baclofen and diazepam act by suppressing CNS reflexes that regulate muscle activity; neither drug affects muscle strength. Baclofen therapy should be discontinued over one to two weeks; sudden withdrawal may cause seizures and paranoid ideation. In contrast to diazepam and baclofen, dantrolene acts directly on skeletal muscles, and it may affect muscle strength. Dantrolene may cause hepatotoxicity and should not be administered when hepatitis or cirrhosis is present.

Nursing Responsibilities

- Evaluate baseline muscle strength and spasticity, ROM, and dexterity.
- Maintain safety or fall precautions; dizziness and drowsiness are common side effects.
- For the client taking dantrolene, monitor liver function tests (enzymes and bilirubin) for signs of hepatotoxicity.

Client and Family Teaching

- These drugs may cause sedative effects. Take appropriate safety measures (e.g., avoid driving).

Table 34-5. Continued

- Avoid CNS depressants (antihistamines, alcohol); they can increase the sedative effects of the medication.
- Continue follow-up care; if you are taking dantrolene, for example, liver function will need to be monitored.
- If you are taking baclofen, do not suddenly stop the medication.
- Increase fiber and fluids in the diet to prevent constipation.
- Change positions slowly to minimize dizziness and other effects of orthostatic hypotension.

Immunosuppressants

Azathioprine (Imuran)
Cyclophosphamide (Cytoxan)

Immunosuppressants are given to clients with MS because of the autoimmune component of the disease. Both medications can cause bone marrow suppression and increase the risk of cancer. Azathioprine may produce hepatitis. Toxic effects of cyclophosphamide include hemorrhagic cystitis, sterility, and stomatitis.

Nursing Responsibilities
- Monitor baseline parameters: CBC with platelet count and differential, urinalysis, liver function tests, hepatitis profile.
- Assess for anemia: fatigue, lethargy, pallor.
- Watch for signs of bleeding.
- Protect against and observe for subtle signs of infection.

Client and Family Teaching
- Report signs of infection, bleeding, and anemia immediately.
- Drink at least 2 L (2 quarts) of fluid a day, and observe urine for blood.
- Report jaundice immediately.
- Check oral cavity daily for changes or ulcers.
- Avoid becoming pregnant while taking these drugs.
- Obtain follow-up care, including frequent blood tests.

Surgery

Surgery may be indicated for clients who experience severe spasticity and deformity. However, physical therapy can prevent most severe problems. Foot drop from severe plantar flexion can be relieved with an Achilles tenotomy, a surgical procedure in which the Achilles tendon is transected.

Dietary Management

Several diets involving manipulation of fats are currently under investigation. Clients with MS may be overweight because of their inability to ambulate; depression may contribute to the problem because people who are depressed tend to eat more and burn fewer calories. Ideally, the client should maintain a weight as close as possible to that recommended for the client's height and body type.

As MS progresses, the client's ability to prepare food and eat is compromised. Changes in muscle tone, tremor, weakness, and ataxia all contribute to nutritional problems. Dysphagia is also a common problem. The diet must be adapted to accommodate changes in the client's ability to chew and swallow.

Rehabilitation

Physical and rehabilitative therapies are tailored to the client's level of functioning. The long-term goal is to enable the client to retain as much independence as possible. One major intervention is to maintain and increase existing muscle strength.

Spasticity is managed with stretching exercises, gait training, and braces, splints, or other assistive devices. To maintain balance, the client is encouraged to widen the base of support by standing with the feet slightly further apart. Walkers and canes may be weighted to provide support and balance for the ataxic client.

A team approach to rehabilitation will provide supportive services: speech therapy for problems with phonation, occupational therapy to maintain strength in the upper extremities and carry out ADLs, and occupational counseling. Consultations with a urologist are indicated for problems with urinary incontinence, urinary tract infections, retention, and impotence. Consultation with a respiratory therapist may be needed if the client develops chronic respiratory infections from inability to cough, move secretions, or breathe deeply, especially with increased debilitation.

Nursing Care

Because the disease most often affects young adults in the prime of life, the psychosocial and economic impact can be devastating. People with MS have to make adjustments to the body image changes while simultaneously adapting to the altered relationships and decreased earnings usually encountered with the disease. A once-healthy spouse becomes wheelchair-bound; a person once independent may eventually become dependent for even the most basic ADLs. The unpredictable course of MS is a challenge for long-term planning.

Health Promotion

Following an overview of the disorder, the client needs to understand how to prevent fatigue and exacerbations. Teach the client to avoid stress, extremes of cold and heat, high humidity, physical overexertion, and infections. Because pregnancy can exacerbate symptoms, counseling about this risk is indicated. Also, address preventive measures to avoid risk of respiratory and urinary tract infections.

Assessment

Collect the following data through the health history and physical examination (see Chapter 31):

- *Health history:* history of childhood viral illnesses, geographical residence when a child, exposure to physical or emotional stressors (pregnancy/delivery, extremes of heat), medications, symptom onset, severity of symptoms.
- *Physical assessment:* affect, mood, speech, eye movements, gait, tremors, vision and hearing, reflexes, muscle strength and movement, sensation.

Nursing Diagnoses and Interventions

Interventions for the client with MS vary with the acuity of exacerbations and the presenting problems. Many nursing diagnoses relate to the inability to perform ADLs, for example, *self-care deficit, impaired home maintenance management,* and *powerlessness.* Others reflect problems with musculoskeletal changes or altered nerve conduction, for example, *impaired physical mobility, ineffective breathing pattern, social isolation, constipation,* and *urinary incontinence.* The nursing diagnoses discussed in this section are *fatigue* and *self-care deficit.*

Fatigue

Fatigue is defined by NANDA (2001) as an overwhelming sustained sense of exhaustion and decreased capacity for physical and mental work at the usual level. Fatigue affects every aspect of the MS client's life—the ability to remain independent and perform self-care, sexual function, mobility, airway clearance, and ultimately self-concept and coping. A great deal of teaching is needed to help the client and family understand fatigue and how to adapt. Clients and families need assistance managing fatigue in a society in which energy is highly valued.

- Assess degree of fatigue and identify contributing factors. *Fatigue is a subjective experience that needs to be evaluated thoroughly before planning can begin.*

- Arrange daily activities to include rest periods. *Rest is essential to manage feelings of fatigue; periods of relaxation may help replenish energy reserves.*

- Ask the client to consider which activities are really necessary and to set priorities. *Prioritizing activities promotes independence and self-control.*

- Suggest performing tasks in the morning hours. *Biorhythm studies indicate that people usually have greater energy reserves in the morning hours and diminished reserves in the afternoon.*

- Advise to avoid temperature extremes, such as hot showers or exposure to cold. *Maintaining a relatively constant body temperature may avoid exacerbation of the disorder. Heat can delay impulse transmission across demyelinated nerves, which contributes to fatigue.*

- Refer to the appropriate professionals to manage fatigue: stress management groups, support groups, occupational or physical therapist, as indicated. *Support groups and therapy can facilitate self-management and improving coping.*

Self-Care Deficits

Clients with MS may need assistance with bathing, toileting, dressing, grooming, and feeding. The help needed can range from minimal guidance to total dependence. The client's ability to perform self-care activities is the gauge by which family members and caregivers need to adjust assistance. Self-care encompasses both the decisions about care and the provision of care; most clients are capable of making decisions even after physical limitations prevent physical self-care. The need to maintain self-determination cannot be overemphasized and must be incorporated into each intervention.

- Assess the extent of the client's self-care deficit; refer to other health team members for assessment as appropriate. For example, refer to a speech pathologist to assess swallowing and gag reflex, if indicated. *An accurate assessment is crucial to individualizing interventions.*

- Suggest adaptive devices, such as arm or wrist braces, as needed. *Meeting hygiene needs and feeding self are essential for positive self-concept, self-esteem, and socialization.*

- Teach to use assistive devices, such as plate guards; to modify consistency of foods; and to eat when energy level is better. If unable to buy and prepare meals, provide referral to Meals-on-Wheels. *Proper nutrition is basic to health; adapting utensils and foods can ensure that nutritional needs are met.*

- Teach interventions related to altered bowel and bladder function: fluid intake of at least 2000 mL daily, bowel routine as indicated to prevent constipation, self-catheterization skills as necessary. *Maintaining optimal bowel and bladder function decreases the risk of urinary tract infection and bowel impaction.*

Home Care

The nurse adapts teaching approaches based on the MS client's needs. The inconsistent and erratic nature of the disease can make teaching difficult. Initial teaching focuses on a realistic explanation of MS. Referral to a support group early in the course of the disease is also recommended. Social support can make a positive difference in a client's ability to cope with MS. Address the following topics in preparing the client for home care:

- Various treatment options and their side effects
- Information about medications, particularly steroid use, and about possible interactions with prescription or over-the-counter medications
- Ongoing care from nurses, counselors, and physical, occupational, and speech therapists, as well as the physician and community health nurse.
- Helpful resources:
  1. National Multiple Sclerosis Society
  2. National Institute of Neurological and Communicative Disorders and Stroke.

The Client with Parkinson's Disease

Parkinson's disease (PD) is a progressive, degenerative neurologic disease characterized by *tremor at rest* (resting or **nonintention tremor**), muscle rigidity, and *akinesia* (poverty of movement). People with PD are faced with multiple problems involving independence in ADLs, emotional well-being, financial security, and relationships with caregivers.

Incidence and Prevalence

Parkinson's disease is one of the most common neurologic disorders affecting older adults, affecting up to 1 million people in the United States. Although it may occur in younger people, the onset of PD is most often after age 40, with the mean age being 60. Men are affected more than women.

Parkinson's-like manifestations, called *secondary parkinsonism,* may result from other disorders, such as trauma, encephalitis, tumors, toxins, and drugs. Drug-induced parkinsonism, which is usually reversible, may occur in people taking neuroleptics, antiemetics, antihypertensives, and illegal designer drugs containing the chemical MPTP (McCance & Huether, 2002). Carbon monoxide or cyanide poisoning can also cause secondary parkinsonism. This discussion focuses on primary Parkinson's disease, the cause of which is unknown.

Pathophysiology

Coordinated, voluntary body movement is achieved through the actions of neurotransmitters in the basal ganglia of the brain. Some neurotransmitters facilitate the transmission of excitatory nerve impulses, while other neurotransmitters inhibit their transmission. Together, this system allows control of movement. A disturbed balance between excitatory and inhibitory neurotransmitters causes disorders of voluntary motor function.

In PD, neurons in the cerebral cortex atrophy and are lost, and the dopaminergic nigrostriatal (pigmented) pathway degenerates. Also, the number of specific dopamine receptors in the basal ganglia decreases. These pathologic processes cause a decrease in dopamine (a neurotransmitter that helps regulate nerve impulses involved in motor function). The usual balance of dopamine (an inhibitory neurotransmitter) and acetylcholine (an excitatory neurotransmitter) in the brain is disrupted, and dopamine no longer inhibits acetylcholine. The failure to inhibit acetylcholine is the underlying basis for the manifestations of the disorder. Parkinson's disease has five stages, outlined in Table 34-6.

Manifestations

Parkinson's disease begins with subtle symptoms. Clients complain of feeling tired and seem to move more slowly; a slight tremor may accompany the fatigue. In a small percentage of clients, dementia is the initial presenting symptom.

Table 34-6. Stages of Parkinson's Disease

I   Unilateral involvement only, usually with minimal or no functional impairment.

II Bilateral or midline involvement, without impairment of balance.

III First sign of impaired righting reflexes, evidenced as unsteadiness as the client turns or demonstrated when the client is pushed from standing equilibrium with the feet together and eyes closed. Functionally, the client is somewhat restricted in activities but may have some employment potential, depending on the type of employment. Clients are physically capable of leading independent lives, and their disability is mild to moderate.

IV Fully developed, severely disabling disease; the client is still able to walk and stand unassisted but is markedly incapacitated.

V   Client is confined to bed or wheelchair unless aided.

Tremor at Rest

Tremor at rest is usually the first manifestation experienced, with upper extremities more often affected. Resting tremors of the hand show a "pill rolling" motion of the thumb and fingers (given this name as this is the way in which medicinal pills were formed in the early days of medicine). The tremor may be controlled with purposeful, voluntary movement, and is worsened by stress and anxiety. Clients have progressive impairment in performing skills that require dexterity and fine muscle control, such as writing and eating.

Rigidity and Akinesia

Manifestations related to motor and postural effects include rigidity, akinesia, and uncoordinated movements. *Rigidity* (resulting from involuntary contraction of all skeletal muscles) makes both active and passive movement difficult. It is manifested as increased resistance to passive range of motions. Although the extremity moves, it does so in a jerky motion, called *cogwheel rigidity.* The first manifestation of rigidity may be muscle cramps in the toes or hands, but most often the client describes stiffness, heaviness, or aching in muscles.

Akinesia is the most common and crippling manifestation. All striated muscles are affected, including those that involve chewing, swallowing, and speaking. Slowed or delayed movements affect the eyes, mouth, and voice, causing a masklike face and softened or muffled voice. Disorders of swallowing result in problems with eating and with drooling. Clients have a staring gaze with minimal change in expression. Akinetic movements include both hypokinesia and bradykinesia. *Hypokinesia* (decreased frequency or absence of associated movements) is one of the earliest manifestations. Clients describe being "frozen" in place as voluntary movement is lost, and they sit or lie in one position without movement for long periods of time. *Bradykinesia* (slow movement) is experienced as difficulty in starting, continuing, or coordinating movements. Both of these disorders of movement are interspersed with freezing, which is brought about by turning, increasing the effort to move, or making visual or touch contacts.

Table 34-7. Manifestations of Parkinson's Disease

Manifestations Related to Motor Dysfunction

- Nonintention tremor
- Bradykinesia or akinesia
  a. Slowed movements; inability to initiate voluntary movements
  b. Slowed speech, low amplitude
  c. Poor articulation
  d. Decreased eye movements (i.e., blinking)
  e. Masklike, expressionless face
- Rigidity
- Posture and gait disturbances
  a. Trunk tilted forward
  b. Shuffling gait, propulsive at times
  c. Retropulsion
- Complications: falls, fractures, impaired communication, social isolation

Manifestations Related to Autonomic System Dysfunction

- Skin problems
  a. Seborrhea
  b. Excess sweating on face and neck, absence of sweating of trunk and extremities
  c. Mottled skin

Table 34-7. Continued

- Heat intolerance
- Postural hypotension
- Constipation
- Complications: skin breakdown, dizziness, falls, constipation

Manifestations Related to Cognitive and Psychologic Dysfunction

- Dementia
    a. Memory loss
    b. Lack of insight and problem-solving ability
    c. Declining intellectual abilities
- Anxiety
- Depression
- Complications: loss of ability to function, social isolation

Abnormal Posture

The loss of normal postural reflexes results in postural abnormalities, including disorders of postural fixation, equilibrium, and righting. Involuntary flexion of the head and shoulders means the person with PD cannot maintain an upright position of the trunk when sitting or standing. This problem of postural fixation results in the characteristic stooped, leaning forward position. Disorders of equilibrium follow loss of postural fixation with an inability to make adjustments when leaning or falling. The client takes short, accelerated steps, also characteristic of PD, to try to maintain an upright position when walking.

Autonomic and Neuroendocrine Effects

Many manifestations result from the loss of functions controlled by the autonomic nervous system. Elimination problems include constipation and urinary hesitation or frequency. Clients may experience problems related to orthostatic hypotension, including dizziness with position change. Eczematous skin changes and seborrhea are related to the increase in sweat gland activity secondary to increased sebotropic hormone production.

Mood and Cognition

Both depression and dementia are pathologies associated with PD. Depression occurs in half of all clients and a third have dementia. Dementia, resulting from loss of cholinergic cells, loss of neurons, senile plaques, neurofibrillary tangles, and amyloid changes in small blood vessels, is seen more often in clients over the age of 70. The client manifests confusion, disorientation, memory loss, distractibility, and changes in abstraction and judgment. *Bradyphrenia* may also occur, resulting in slow thinking and a decreased ability to form thoughts, plan, and decide.

Sleep Disturbances

Clients with PD also have sleep disturbances, although they may experience decreased manifestations during sleep in the early stages. The ability to fall and stay sleep is affected by acetylcholine. Muscle rigidity may compromise sleep because of the inability to change position. This lack of muscle movement causes the client to awaken and consciously shift position.

Interrelated Effects

Some of the manifestations that clients with PD experience have multiple contributing factors. For example, constipation is common because of decreased peristalsis. However, decreased peristalsis is not the only cause: Immobility, tremors (resulting in being unable to drink from a glass easily), and dietary changes from dysphagia all contribute to the problem of constipation.

The following complications are associated with Parkinson's disease.

*   Oculogyric crisis, in which the eyes become fixed with a lateral and upward gaze
*   Paranoia and hallucinations, which may accompany dementia
*   Impaired communication due to changes in speech, handwriting, and expressiveness
*   Falls from balance, posture, and motor changes
*   Infections, such as pneumonia, related to immobility
*   Malnutrition related to dysphagia and inability to prepare meals
*   Altered sleep patterns due to loss of dopamine, l-dopa side effects (nightmares, dreams), or side effects of anticholinergics (hyperreflexia, muscle twitching), and depression
*   Skin breakdown and pressure ulcers associated with urinary incontinence, malnutrition, and sweat reflex changes
*   Depression and social isolation.

Prognosis

Prognosis is poor, owing to the progressive degeneration that ultimately affects multiple physiologic systems and their function. Psychosocial effects are equally devastating, and the family needs more support as the client's debilitation increases. Total disability is usually seen 10 to 20 years after diagnosis. The leading cause of death is pneumonia.

Collaborative Care

Diagnosis is based primarily on a thorough history and physical examination, and is made based on two of the following manifestations: tremor at rest, bradykinesia, rigidity, and postural instability. Interventions vary with the clinical stage of the disorder and include medication, surgery, and rehabilitation to retain the optimal level of functioning possible. A team approach is essential for these clients.

Diagnostic Tests

Diagnostic studies may support a potential diagnosis of Parkinson's disease; however, no test clearly differentiates Parkinson's disease from other neurologic disorders. However, PET scan will show decreased uptake of 6-[18F]-fluoro-dopa. Tests are usually performed to rule out disorders that produce secondary parkinsonism. The following tests may be ordered:

*   *Drug screens* determine the presence of medications or toxins that cause secondary parkinsonism, such as methyldopa, reserpine, or carbon monoxide.
*   *EEG* may indicate slowed pattern and disorganization.
*   *Upper GI X-ray series* with small bowel follow-through shows delayed emptying, distention, and possibly megacolon with severe constipation.
*   *CBC* may show low hemoglobin and hematocrit levels due to anemia.

- *Chemistry profile* may reflect low protein and albumin levels related to the client's inability to buy and prepare meals.

Medications

The goal of drug therapy is to control symptoms to the extent possible. Generally, medications vary with the stage of the disease; however, response is individualized and guides the selection of medications. Types of drugs used include monoamine oxidase (MAO) inhibitors, dopaminergics, dopamine agonists, and anticholinergics. Information about these drugs is presented in Table 34-8.

Initially clients are treated with selegiline (Carbex, Eldepryl), amantadine (Symmetrel), or anticholinergics. As the disease progresses, levodopa (Dopar, Larodopa) in combination with carbidopa (Lodosyn) is used in a medication named carbidopa-levodopa (Sinemet). Because levodopa eventually loses its effectiveness, dopamine agonists are added to increase the effectiveness of levodopa. Eventually, pharmacotherapeutic agents lose their efficacy, and the disease continues to progress despite treatment. Response to the drugs fluctuate; this phenomenon is called the "on-off" response.

Bromocriptine (Parlodel) and pergolide (Permax), agents that inhibit the breakdown of dopamine, are used to delay progression of the disease. COMT inhibitors (tolcapone [Tasmar] and entacapone [Comtan]) are used in conjunction with carbidopa-levodopa therapy to reduce the metabolism of levodopa, leading to more sustained dopaminergic stimulation of the brain.

Other medications may be used to treat problems related to Parkinson's disease. Antidepressants may be prescribed. Propranolol (Inderal) may be used to treat tremors; it should be used cautiously when clients have orthostatic hypotension.

Treatments

Treatments to control manifestations and to improve function include electrical stimulation, surgery, and physical therapy, occupational therapy, and speech therapy.

Electrical Stimulation

Activa TM tremor control therapy uses an implanted pacemaker-like device to deliver mild electrical stimulation to block the brain impulses that cause tremor. In this procedure, an insulated wire is surgically placed in the thalamus and connected to an implanted pulse generator (similar to an advanced cardiac pacemaker) near the clavicle. Clients can increase or decrease the stimulation depending on their tremor suppression needs (National Parkinson Foundation, 2001).

Surgery

Pallidotomy is a surgical technique for Parkinson's disease, and its results have been helpful for many clients. In this procedure, the neurosurgeon locates the affected areas of the globus pallidus and destroys the involved tissue. As a result, clients who could not previously ambulate are able to walk, and tremors cease. The long-term effects are still being evaluated.

Table 34 -8. Medication Administration — The Client with Parkinson's Disease

Dopaminergics

Levodopa (Larodopa, Dopar)
Carbidopa-levodopa (Sinemet)
Amantadine (Symmetrel)

These drugs have their major effect on the akinesia of Parkinson's disease, improving mobility while decreasing muscle rigidity and tremor. Levodopa is a metabolic precursor of dopamine, but unlike dopamine, it can cross the blood–brain barrier. Levodopa is converted to dopamine in the brain by decarboxylase, a catalytic enzyme, and stimulates dopamine receptors to balance the dopamine/acetylcholine concentrations. Carbidopa prevents decarboxylase from converting levodopa to dopamine in the peripheral tissues; therefore, carbidopa is frequently given in combination with levodopa. Amantadine is used to treat dyskinesia and also elevates mood.

Levodopa is avoided in clients with narrow-angle glaucoma, severe angina pectoris, transient ischemic attacks, or melanoma. The "on-off" phenomenon occurs after the client takes levodopa for several years; this phenomenon is characterized by unexpected dyskinesias and lack of symptom control.

Common side effects are nausea and vomiting; darkening of urine and sweat; dyskinesias, especially in the first few months of therapy; dysrhythmias; orthostatic hypotension; and psychologic reactions, such as hallucinations and vivid dreams. Older adults are particularly susceptible to psychologic disturbances.

Nursing Responsibilities

- Establish the client's baseline functional abilities in performing ADLs and administering the medication; assess motor control and coordination.
- To avoid adverse reactions, assess the client's overall health status before initiating therapy.
- Monitor medications known to cause adverse drug interactions: anticholinergics, pyridoxine, and antipsychotic agents alter the effectiveness of levodopa; MAO-B inhibitors can cause severe hypertension because of their vasoconstrictive effects.
- Withhold levodopa for eight hours prior to administering Sinemet to avoid potentiating the effects of the circulating levodopa.

Client and Family Teaching

- Levodopa may not take effect for several weeks to months.
- Do not alter dosages of medications; taking more of a medication may not result in better symptom control and can cause severe side effects.
- Your protein intake should be divided into equal amounts for the day's meals. Avoid foods high in pyridoxine, such as pork, beef, ham, avocado, beans, and oatmeal.
- Levodopa may cause a change in color of urine; this is harmless, however.
- To prevent side effects:
  1. Prevent nausea by taking medication with food.
  2. Change position slowly to avoid a drop in blood pressure and risk of falling.
  3. Prevent constipation by increasing fluid intake and exercising regularly.

Table 34-8. Continued

4. Notify practitioner if you begin to have difficulty making voluntary movements or cardiac or psychologic symptoms develop.

5. Watch for the "on-off" phenomenon, in which periods of symptom control alternate with periods when the drug fails to control symptoms.

Monoamine Oxidase (MAO) Inhibitors

Selegiline (Eldepryl, Deprenyl)

Selegiline works by selectively inhibiting the enzyme that inactivates dopamine in the brain. It may be administered alone or as an adjunct therapy with levodopa: Selegiline inhibits the enzyme system that would otherwise break down and destroy dopamine. This synergistic effect lasts approximately one to two years. The combination of selegiline and levodopa increases the adverse reactions of dopamine; nurses must be alert for orthostatic hypotension, changes in movement, hallucinations, and confusion. These responses can be modified by lowering the dose of levodopa. Because it is highly selective for the MAO-A enzyme, selegiline does not have antidepressant effects like the MAO-B inhibitors. The risk of severe hypertension is low.

Nursing Responsibilities
- Establish baseline functional abilities: motor control and movements, position changes, mental status.
- Monitor problems with insomnia.
- Assess for orthostatic hypotension; look for unsteadiness with position change and complaints of dizziness.
- Assess for hypertension, which can occur with higher than usual doses.

Client and Family Teaching
- It is very important to take the medication as directed, especially dose and time of administration.
- Notify the practitioner if insomnia occurs.
- Report signs of dizziness when changing positions or standing, changes in ability to move, or psychologic changes.
- Change positions slowly, especially when moving from a sitting to standing position.
- Keep follow-up appointments for evaluation of the medication's effectiveness.

Dopamine Agonists

Bromocriptine (Parlodel)   Pramipexole (Mirapex)
Pergolide (Permax)   Ropinirole (Requip)

Dopamine agonists act by directly activating dopamine receptors in the brain. They are frequently used in combination with levodopa therapy: When dopamine agonists are given with levodopa, they increase the therapeutic effects of levodopa and reduce fluctuations in motor symptoms. Adverse reactions are similar to those of levodopa: nausea, orthostatic hypotension, and psychologic disturbances are common. Nursing responsibilities and client and family teaching information are similar to those that apply to the dopaminergics.

Continued on the next page

Table 34-8. Continued

COMT Inhibitors

Tolcapone (Tasmar)
Entacapone (Comtess)

COMT inhibitors inhibit catechol-O-methyltransferase (COMT), which is responsible for metabolizing dopamine. The concurrent administration of a COMT inhibitor with levodopa increases the amount of levodopa available to the brain to control Parkinson's disease.

Nursing Responsibilities

- Monitor liver function test results and manifestations of liver impairment (dark urine, jaundice).
- Administer with food.
- If given concurrently with warfarin, monitor PT and INR.

Client and Family Teaching
- Avoid using alcohol and sedatives.
- Rise slowly from a sitting or lying position to avoid falling.
- Nausea is common at the beginning of therapy.
- Do not abruptly stop taking the medication.
- Report increased loss of muscle control, yellow skin or eyes, dark urine, hallucinations, severe diarrhea.

Anticholinergics

Trihexyphenidyl (Artane)   Procyclidine (Kemadrin)
Benztropine (Cogentin)   Chlorphenoxamine
Biperiden (Akineton)   (Phenoxene)
Cycrimine (Pagitane)

Anticholinergics are effective in Parkinson's disease because they block the excitatory action of the neurotransmitter acetylcholine. They are frequently used during the early stages of the disease or when the client can no longer take levodopa. They may be given in combination with carbidopa-levodopa therapy. These medications ease drooling, tremors, and rigidity; however, side effects are common and may include blurred vision, dry mouth, constipation, delayed gastric emptying, urinary retention, photophobia, and tachycardia. Older adults are especially susceptible to heat stroke and psychologic side effects, including confusion, depression, delusions, and hallucinations. Anticholinergics should be tapered slowly when discontinued to avoid enhancing parkinsonian symptoms.

Nursing Responsibilities
- Perform baseline assessment for presence of glaucoma, cardiac dysfunction, and prostatic hypertrophy.
- Note other medications, including over-the-counter medications that have anticholinergic effects, such as antihistamines and tricyclic antidepressants.
- Monitor for side effects, especially changes in vision, elimination, gastric emptying, and mentation.

Table 34-8. Continued

Client and Family Teaching

- Inform your practitioner if you begin taking any new medications or notice any new symptoms.
- Avoid overexposure to heat, and take precautions to avoid heat stroke: Drink fluids, keep cool, and avoid strenuous activity on hot days.
- Drink adequate amounts of fluid to minimize constipation.
- Practice home safety to prevent falls associated with blurred vision.
- Avoid taking over-the-counter antihistamines or sleeping aids; these have anticholinergic activity.
- Have the eyes examined annually to check for glaucoma; wear dark glasses if photophobia develops.
- Do not suddenly stop taking anticholinergics.

Stereotaxic thalamotomy (an X-ray is taken during neurosurgery to guide the insertion of a needle into a specific area of the brain) has been used only for clients who do not respond to medications—generally, younger people with extreme unilateral tremor. The surgeon destroys a small amount of tissue by creating a lesion in the ventrolateral nucleus of the thalamus. This surgery decreases tremors and rigidity in the contralateral extremity.

Autologous adrenal medullary transplant is another procedure that has been used when medications do not adequately control a client's symptoms. The client must be a good surgical risk and free of dementia and end-stage cardiac, pulmonary, or renal disease. First an adrenalectomy and then a craniotomy are performed. Use of this procedure remains controversial.

Fetal tissue transplantation is another controversial surgical procedure limited to select medical centers. In this procedure, tissue of the substantia nigra is transplanted into the client's caudate nucleus.

Rehabilitation

Depending on their individual needs, clients frequently benefit from rehabilitation therapy with a physical therapist, social worker, psychologist, and/or speech therapist.

Physical therapists (PT) can implement an individual exercise program to improve coordination, balance, gait, and transfers. Preventing contractures is an important goal of exercise therapy. It is crucial that family and health care personnel permit the client adequate time to perform not only exercise regimens but also ADLs. Activities should not be rushed.

An occupational therapist (OT) helps the client adapt to changing abilities pertinent to work, self-care, and recreational activities. Some rehabilitation centers assign OT personnel the responsibility of addressing the client's upper extremity functions while assigning PT personnel to manage lower extremity problems. For example, skills related to cooking and grooming would be supervised by the OT, whereas mobility and posture skills would be supervised by the PT.

Speech therapists frequently address not only the client's speech but also chewing and swallowing. These therapists evaluate clients and plan treatment regimens. The challenge with clients who have PD is that they not only have vocalization problems, but also dexterity deficits; speech therapists therefore must evaluate the potential benefits of assistive devices, such as a magic slate, voice synthesizer, or computer, for each client.

Nursing Care

The chronic and eventually debilitating nature of PD poses many challenges to clients, families, and health care professionals. Dependence due to declining physical and mental abilities is of major concern. In the early stages, most clients are able to remain at home, with the family assisting with or providing many of the client's ADL needs. As the disease progresses and the burden of care increases, the client and family may prefer placement in a long-term care facility.

Health Promotion

Teaching preventive measures is extremely important when caring for clients who have Parkinson's disease. Preventing malnutrition, falls and other environmental accidents, constipation, skin breakdown from incontinence or immobility, and joint contracture requires teaching and reinforcement.

In addition to incorporating information about safety needs, teach ways to prevent orthostatic hypotension when the client changes positions; some clients may also benefit from wearing elastic hose. In addition, address safety considerations about proper administration of medications.

Assessment

Collect the following data through the health history and physical examination (see Chapter 31). Further focused assessments are described with nursing interventions below.

- *Health history:* brain trauma, stroke, infection, exposure to heavy metals or carbon monoxide, medication and drug use, incontinence, constipation, weight loss, sweating, sleep problems, muscle pain, mood.
- *Physical assessment:* affect; appearance; speech, scalp, eyelashes, and skin; drooling; tremor; coordination; posture; gait; muscle rigidity; mental status.

Nursing Diagnoses and Interventions

Clients with PD have complex and, ultimately, multisystem needs. Deficits in mobility and self-care are common. Psychosocial needs may include problems related to ineffective coping, powerlessness, and disturbed body image. Refer to the nursing care sections throughout this chapter for discussions of fatigue, self-care deficit, ineffective airway clearance, and other pertinent diagnoses. This section focuses on the nursing diagnoses related to impaired physical mobility, impaired verbal communication, imbalanced nutrition: less than body requirements, and disturbed sleep pattern.

Impaired Physical Mobility

Clients with PD have impaired mobility for several reasons, including tremors, gait pattern disturbances, and alterations in body positioning, such as forward bending of the trunk. Poor self-esteem may contribute to the client's lack of motivation and willingness to be mobile.

- Request the physical therapist teach caregivers how to do ROM exercises at least twice a day, emphasizing the trunk, neck, arms, hips, and legs. *Maintaining joint mobility promotes better function and strength, improving gait pattern. Consistent ROM exercises can prevent contractures.*

- Consult with a physical therapist to develop an individualized exercise program. *A program specific to the client supplies motivation as well as helping the client maintain muscle tone, flexibility, and mobility.*
- Ask caregivers to ambulate the client at least four times a day if possible. *Exercise fosters independence and self-esteem.*
- Recommend assistive devices, such as canes, splints, or braces, as indicated. *Adaptive equipment improves balance, protects joints, and promotes proper anatomic positioning.*
- To promote mobility and safety:
    1. Slightly elevate the back legs of chairs and raise the toilet seat to help rise from a sitting position to a standing position.
    2. Wear shoes with Velcro closures.
    3. Remove potential hazards, such as unanchored throw rugs.
    4. Install hand rails and nonskid surfaces in bath tubs and showers.
    5. Ensure adequate lighting throughout the home and in outside areas, especially in areas where transfers are common.

Safety measures prevent potential complications that may result from falls or other accidents and promote self-esteem through self-care.

Impaired Verbal Communication

Diminished vocal amplitude and loss of muscular control can impair the client's ability to speak. Both caregivers and family members must remember to give clients enough time for self-expression; an unhurried approach is recommended. Seek input from family members when determining alternative methods of communicating with the client.

- Assess current communication abilities in speech, hearing, and writing. *Communication involves both sending and receiving messages.*
- Develop methods of communication appropriate to coordination abilities, such as a magic slate; flash cards with common phrases; pointing to objects. *Individualizing a method of communication decreases anxiety and isolation.*
- Consult with a speech pathologist to develop oral exercises and interventions that will facilitate speaking. *The muscles of speech and swallowing are affected by the Parkinson's disease process.*
- Remind to speak more loudly, if possible. *A low, monotonous voice is characteristic of the client with Parkinson's disease.*

Imbalanced Nutrition: Less Than Body Requirements

Tremors, altered gait, and impaired chewing and swallowing can cause nutritional problems in the client with PD. As the disorder progresses, interventions for ensuring optimal nutrition need to be adapted to the client's functional abilities. Assess the client's swallow reflex before starting any feeding program. During the initial stages of the disorder, some clients may have the nursing diagnosis, *Imbalanced nutrition: More than body requirements,* if kcal intake exceeds energy expenditure.

- Assess nutritional status and self-feeding abilities; consult with occupational or speech therapist, if needed. *An initial assessment of abilities ensures that interventions are personalized to the client's current functional abilities.*

- Teach caregivers how to prepare foods of proper consistency as determined by swallowing function. *The client may aspirate food that is too liquid.*
- Weigh weekly. *Early recognition of weight loss allows for intervention.*
- Teach eating methods to decrease tremors, such as holding a piece of bread in the hand that is not holding an eating utensil. *Nonintention tremor may be reduced through purposeful activity.*
- Encourage diet that is high in bulk and fluids. *Several anti-Parkinson's medications can cause constipation.*

Disturbed Sleep Pattern

Rigidity and weakness can cause clients with Parkinson's disease to lose the ability to move and change positions during sleep. The resulting discomfort causes periods of wakefulness. Medications to treat Parkinson's disease contribute to sleep pattern disturbance; for example, levodopa can cause vivid dreams. Nurses can help accurately assess the sleep pattern disturbance and in planning interventions to improve or increase sleep time.

- Assess sleep pattern and existing conditions that may affect sleep, such as depression or pain. *Clients experiencing anxiety, depression, and dementia have a difficult time falling asleep and may wake up more at night.*
- Explain the disease process and the effects of decreased dopamine on the sleep-wake cycle. *Depending on the dosage, levodopa causes less REM sleep and deep sleep.*
- Review the client's medication. *Bromocriptine and levodopa, especially if used with an anticholinergic, can cause vivid dreams. Other medications (diuretics, theophylline, hypnotics) also may interfere with sleep.*
- Teach how to modify lifestyle activities that affect sleep:
    1. Institute a routine of activities with limited rest periods during the day; avoid napping close to bedtime. Avoid strenuous exercise in the evening. *Daytime sleeping may contribute to decreased nighttime sleeping. Vigorous exercise just before bedtime may act as a stimulant.*
    2. Incorporate diet modifications, such as limiting caffeine and alcohol intake. *Caffeine is a stimulant, and alcohol may cause early-morning awakenings, increased daytime sleepiness, and nightmares.*
    3. Drink a glass of milk before bedtime. *Milk contains L-tryptophan, which produces sedative effects by shortening the time taken to fall asleep (sleep latency).*
    4. Adapt the environment to aid in sleep (e.g., darken the room and decrease noises). *Reducing environmental stimuli decreases external sleep disturbances.*

Home Care

It is important for both the client and the family to maintain independence and self care as long as possible. To maintain function and quality of life, the following topics should be addressed:

- Realistic expectations.
- Equipment suppliers.
- Home environment conducive to using equipment.
- Referrals to speech therapist, occupational therapist, physical therapist, dietitian.

- Gait training and exercises for improving ambulation, speech, swallowing, and self-care.
- Increased fluid intake of 3000 mL/day and increased fiber in every meal.
- Stool softeners or laxatives as needed for bowel elimination.
- Swallowing during eating and taking medications. (Have suction equipment available and know the Heimlich maneuver if choking occurs.)
- Foods that can be easily swallowed, such as pureed or soft, and feed six small meals a day if possible.
- Helpful resources:
  1. American Parkinson's Disease Association
  2. National Parkinson Foundation, Inc.
  3. Parkinson's Disease Foundation
  4. The National Institute of Neurological Disorders and Stroke.

35

Assessing Clients with Integumentary Disorders

The skin, the hair, and the nails make up the integumentary system. The skin provides an external covering for the body, separating the body's organs and tissues from the external environment. It is the largest organ of the body and has many functions. The integumentary system:

- Protects the body from injury from the external environment.
- Provides a barrier to the loss of body fluids and electrolytes.
- Maintains the integrity of the body surface through wound repair.
- Serves as a sense organ for touch, pressure, pain, and temperature.
- Provides a film over the body through the action of glandular secretions, which protects the body from bacterial and fungal invasion.
- Dissipates body heat through the evaporation of sweat.
- Participates in the production of vitamin D.
- Serves as an indicator of emotions and health or illness through color changes.

Review of Anatomy and Physiology

The Skin
The **skin** has a total surface area of 15 to 20 square feet and weighs about 9 pounds. It has been estimated that each square inch of skin contains 15 feet of blood vessels, 4 yards of nerves, 650 sweat glands, 100 oil glands, 1500 sensory receptors, and over 3 million cells that are constantly dying and being replaced. The skin is composed of two regions: the epidermis and the dermis.

The Epidermis
The **epidermis,** which is the surface or outermost part of the skin, consists of epithelial cells. The epidermis has either four or five layers, depending on its location; there are five layers over the palms of the hands and the soles of the feet, and four layers over the rest of the body.

The stratum basale is the deepest layer of the epidermis. It contains melanocytes, cells that produce the pigment melanin, and keratinocytes, which produce keratin. **Melanin** forms a protective shield to protect the keratinocytes and the nerve endings in the dermis from the damaging effects of ultraviolet light. Melanocyte activity probably accounts for the difference in skin color in humans. **Keratin** is a fibrous, water-repellent protein that gives the epidermis its tough, protective quality. As keratinocytes mature, they move upward through the epidermal layers, eventually becoming dead cells at the surface of the skin. Millions of these cells are worn off by abrasion each day, but millions are simultaneously produced in the stratum basale. The next layer of the epidermis is the stratum spinosum. Several cells thick, this layer contains abundant Langerhans cells that arise from the bone marrow and migrate to the epidermis. Mitosis occurs at this layer, although not as abundantly as in the stratum basale.

The stratum granulosum is only two to three cells thick, and also contains Langerhans cells. The cells of the stratum granulosum contain a glycolipid that slows water loss across the epidermis. *Keratinization,* a thickening of the cells' plasma membranes, begins in the stratum granulosum. The stratum lucidum is present only in areas of thick skin. It is made up of flattened, dead keratinocytes.

The outermost layer of the epidermis, the stratum corneum, is also the thickest, making up about 75% of the epidermis's total thickness. It consists of about 20 to 30 sheets of dead cells filled with keratin fragments arranged in "shingles" that flake off as dry skin.

The Dermis

The **dermis** is the second, deeper layer of skin. Made of a flexible connective tissue, this layer is richly supplied with blood cells, nerve fibers, and lymphatic vessels. Most of the hair follicles, sebaceous glands, and sweat glands are located in the dermis. The dermis consists of a papillary and a reticular layer. The papillary layer contains ridges that indent the overlying epidermis. It also contains capillaries and receptors for pain and touch. The deeper, reticular layer contains blood vessels, sweat and sebaceous glands, deep pressure receptors, and dense bundles of collagen fibers. The regions between these bundles form lines of cleavage in the skin. Surgical incisions parallel to these lines of cleavage heal more easily and with less scarring than incisions or traumatic wounds across cleavage lines.

Superficial Fascia

Underlying the skin is a layer of subcutaneous tissue called the **superficial fascia.** It consists primarily of adipose (fat) tissue, and helps the skin adhere to underlying structures.

Skin Color

The color of the skin is the result of varying levels of pigmentation. Melanin, a yellow-to-brown pigment, is darker and is produced in greater amounts in persons with dark skin color than in those with light skin. Exposure to the sun causes a buildup of melanin and a darkening or tanning of the skin in people with light skin. Carotene, a yellow-to-orange pigment, is found most in areas of the body where the stratum corneum is thickest, such as the palms of the hands. Carotene is more abundant in the skins of persons of Asian ancestry and, together with melanin, accounts for their golden skin tone. The epidermis in Caucasian skin has very little melanin and is almost transparent. Thus, the color of the hemoglobin found in red blood cells circulating through the dermis shows through, lending Caucasians a pinkish skin tone.

Skin color is influenced also by emotions and illnesses. **Erythema,** a reddening of the skin, may occur with embarrassment (blushing), fever, hypertension, or inflammation. It may also result from a drug reaction, sunburn, acne rosacea, or other factors. A bluish discoloration of the skin and mucous membranes, called **cyanosis,** results from poor oxygenation of hemoglobin. **Pallor,** or paleness of skin, may occur with shock, fear, or anger or in anemia and hypoxia. **Jaundice** is a yellow-to-orange color visible in the skin and mucous membranes; it is most often the result of a hepatic disorder.

Glands of the Skin

The skin contains sebaceous (oil) glands, sweat (sudoriferous) glands, and ceruminous glands. Each of these glands has a different function.

Sebaceous glands are found all over the body except on the palms and soles. These glands secrete an oily substance called sebum, which usually is ducted into a hair follicle. Sebum softens and lubricates the skin and hair and also decreases water loss from the skin in low humidity. Sebum also protects the body from infection by killing bacteria. The secretion of sebum is stimulated by hormones, especially androgens. If a sebaceous gland becomes blocked, a pimple or whitehead appears on the surface of the skin; as the material oxidizes and dries, it forms a blackhead. Acne vulgaris is an inflammation of the sebaceous glands.

There are two types of sweat glands: eccrine and apocrine. **Eccrine sweat glands** are more numerous on the forehead, palms, and soles. The gland itself is located in the dermis; the duct to the skin rises through the epidermis to open in a pore at the surface. **Sweat,** the secretion of the eccrine glands, is composed mostly of water, but also contains sodium, antibodies, small amounts of metabolic wastes, lactic acid, and vitamin C. The production of sweat is regulated by the sympathetic nervous system and serves to maintain normal body temperature. Sweating also occurs in response to emotions. Most **apocrine sweat glands** are located in the axillary, anal, and genital areas. The secretions from apocrine glands are similar to those of sweat glands, but they also contain fatty acids and proteins. Their function is unknown.

Ceruminous glands are modified apocrine sweat glands. Located in the skin of the external ear canal, they secrete yellow-brown waxy cerumen. This substance provides a sticky trap for foreign materials.

The Hair

Hair is distributed all over the body, except the lips, nipples, parts of the external genitals, the palms of the hands, and the soles of the feet. Hair is produced by a hair bulb, and its root is enclosed in a hair follicle. The exposed part, called the shaft, consists mainly of dead cells. Hair follicles extend into the dermis and in some places, such as the scalp, below the dermis. Many factors, including nutrition and hormones, influence hair growth.

Hair in various parts of the body has protective functions: The eyebrows and eyelashes protect the eyes; hair in the nose helps keep foreign materials out of the upper respiratory tract; and hair on the head protects the scalp from heat loss and sunlight.

The Nails

A **nail** is a modified scalelike epidermal structure. Like hair, nails consist mainly of dead cells. They arise from the stratum germinativum of the epidermis. The body of the nail rests on the nail bed. The nail matrix is the active, growing part of the nail. The proximal visible end of the nail has a white crescent, called a lunula. The sides of the nail are overlapped by skin, called nail folds. The proximal nail fold is thickened and is called the eponychium or cuticle. Nails form a protective coating over the dorsum of each digit on the fingers and toes.

Assessing the Integumentary System

The function of the integumentary system (skin, glands, hair, and nails) is assessed by both a health assessment interview to collect subjective data and a physical assessment to collect objective data.

The Health Assessment Interview

This section provides guidelines for collecting subjective data through a health assessment interview specific to the skin and its appendages. A health assessment interview to determine problems with the integumentary system may be conducted as part of a health screening or total health assessment, or it may focus on a chief complaint, such as itching or a rash. If the client has a skin problem, analyze its onset, characteristics and course, severity, precipitating and relieving factors, and any associated symptoms, noting the timing and circumstances. For example, ask the client:

- What type of itching have you experienced?
- When did you first notice a change in this mole?
- Did you change to any different kinds of shampoo or other hair products just before you started to lose your hair?

Ask about any change in health, rashes, itching, color changes, dryness or oiliness, growth of or changes in warts or moles, and the presence of lesions. Precipitating causes, such as medications, the use of new soaps, skin-care agents, cosmetics, pets, travel, stress, or dietary changes, must also be explored. In assessing hair problems, ask about any thinning or baldness, excessive hair loss, change in distribution of hair, use of hair-care products, diet, and dieting. When assessing nail problems, ask about nail splitting or breakage, discoloration, infection, diet, and exposure to chemicals.

The client's medical history is important. Questions focus on previous problems, allergies, and lesions. Skin problems may be manifestations of other disorders, such as cardiovascular disease, endocrine disorders, hepatic disease, and hematologic disorders. Occupational and social history may provide cues to skin problems; ask the client about travel, exposure to toxic substances at work, use of alcohol, and responses to stress.

Assess the presence of risk factors for skin cancer carefully. These include male gender; age over 50; family history of skin cancer; extended exposure to sunlight; tendency to sunburn; history of sunburn or other skin trauma; light-colored hair or eyes; residence in high altitudes or near the equator; and exposure to radiation, X-rays, coal, tar, or petroleum products.

Also explore the risk factors for malignant melanoma. These include a large number of moles, the presence of atypical moles, a family history of melanoma, prior melanoma, repeated severe sunburns, ease of freckling and sunburning, or inability to tan.

Physical Assessment

Physical assessment of the skin, hair, and nails may be performed either as part of a total assessment or alone for clients with known or suspected problems. Conduct the physical examination of the skin, hair, and nails by inspection and palpation. Assess the skin for color, presence of lesions (observable changes from normal skin structure), temperature, texture, moisture, turgor, and presence of edema. Characteristics of lesions to note include location and distribution, color, pattern, edges, size, elevation, and type of exudate (if present). Examine the hair for color, texture, quality, and scalp lesions. Determine the shape, color, contour, and condition of the nails.

The equipment necessary for assessment of the skin includes a ruler (to measure lesions), a flashlight (to illuminate lesions), and disposable rubber gloves to protect the examiner. Prior to the examination, collect all necessary equipment and explain techniques to the client to decrease anxiety.

The examination should be conducted in a warm, private room. The client removes all clothing and puts on a gown or drape. The areas to be examined should be fully exposed, but protect the client's modesty by keeping other areas covered. The client may be standing, sitting, or lying down at various times of the examination.

Integumentary Assessments with Abnormal Findings (✓)

- **Inspect skin color.**
  - ✓ Pallor and/or cyanosis are seen with exposure to cold and with decreased perfusion and oxygenation. In cyanotic dark-skinned clients, skin loses glow and appears ashen. Cyanosis may be more visible in the mucous membranes and nail beds of these clients.
  - ✓ In dark-skinned clients, jaundice may be most apparent in the sclera of the eyes.
  - ✓ Redness, swelling, and pain are seen with various rashes, inflammations, infections, and burns. First-degree burns cause areas of painful erythema and swelling. Red, painful blisters appear in second-degree burns, whereas white or blackened areas are common in third-degree burns.
  - ✓ **Vitiligo,** an abnormal loss of melanin in patches, typically occurs over the face, hands, or groin. Vitiligo is thought to be an autoimmune disorder.

- **Inspect the skin for lesions.** Primary and secondary lesions are described Table 35–1.
  - ✓ Pearly edged nodules with a central ulcer are seen in basal cell carcinoma.
  - ✓ Scaly, red, fast-growing papules are seen in squamous cell carcinoma.
  - ✓ Dark, asymmetric, multicolored patches (sometimes moles) with irregular edges appear in malignant melanoma.
  - ✓ Circular lesions are usually present in ringworm and in tinea versicolor.
  - ✓ Grouped vesicles may be seen in contact dermatitis.
  - ✓ Linear lesions appear in poison ivy and herpes zoster.
  - ✓ **Urticaria** (hives) appears as patches of pale, itchy wheals in an erythematous area.
  - ✓ In psoriasis, scaly red patches appear on the scalp, knees, back, and genitals.
  - ✓ In herpes zoster, vesicles appear along sensory nerve paths, turn into pustules, and then crust over.
  - ✓ Bruises are raised bluish or yellowish vascular lesions. Multiple bruises in various stages of healing suggest abuse.

- **Palpate skin temperature.**
  - ✓ Skin is warm and red in inflammation and is generally warm with elevated body temperature.
  - ✓ Decreased blood flow decreases the skin temperature; this may be generalized, as in shock, or localized, as in arteriosclerosis.

- **Palpate skin texture.**
  - ✓ Changes in the texture of the skin may indicate irritation or trauma.
  - ✓ The skin is soft and smooth in hyperthyroidism and coarse in hypothyroidism.

- **Palpate skin moisture.**
  - ✓ Dry skin often is present in the elderly and clients with hypothyroidism.
  - ✓ Oily skin is common in adolescents and young adults. Oily skin may be a normal finding, or it may accompany a skin disorder such as acne vulgaris.
  - ✓ Excessive perspiration may be associated with shock, fever, increased activity, or anxiety.
- **Palpate skin turgor.**
  - ✓ Pinch the client's skin gently over the collarbone. Tenting, in which the skin remains pinched for a few moments before resuming its normal position, is common in elderly clients who are thin.
  - ✓ Skin turgor is decreased in dehydration. It is increased in edema and scleroderma.
- **Assess for edema.**

  Assess **edema** (accumulation of fluid in the body's tissues) by depressing the client's skin over the ankle. Record findings as follows:

  1+ Slight pitting, no obvious distortion.

  2+ Deeper pit, no obvious distortion.

  3+ Pit is obvious; extremities are swollen.

  4+ Pit remains with obvious distortion.

  - ✓ Edema is common in cardiovascular disorders, renal failure, and cirrhosis of the liver. It also may be a side effect of certain drugs.

Table 35-1. Characteristics of Skin Lesions

Primary Skin Lesions

Macule, Patch	Flat, nonpalpable change in skin color. Macules are smaller than 1 cm, with a circumscribed border, and patches are larger than 1 cm and may have an irregular border. **Examples** Macules: freckles, measles, and petechiae. Patches: Mongolian spots, port-wine stains, vitiligo, and chloasma.
Papule, Plaque	Elevated, solid, palpable mass with circumscribed border. Papules are smaller than 0.5 cm; plaques are groups of papules that form lesions larger than 0.5 cm. **Examples** Papules: elevated moles, warts, and lichen planus. Plaques: psoriasis, actinic keratosis, and also lichen planus.
Nodule, Tumor	Elevated, solid, hard or soft palpable mass extending deeper into the dermis than a papule. Nodules have circumscribed borders and are 0.5 to 2 cm; tumors may have irregular borders and are larger than 2 cm. **Examples** Nodules: small lipoma, squamous cell carcinoma, fibroma, and intradermal nevi. Tumors: large lipoma, carcinoma, and hemangioma.
Vesicle, Bulla	Elevated, fluid-filled, round or oval shaped, palpable mass with thin, translucent walls and circumscribed borders. Vesicles are smaller than 0.5 cm; bullae are larger than 0.5 cm. **Examples** Vesicles: herpes simplex/zoster, early chickenpox, poison ivy, and small burn blisters. Bullae: contact dermatitis, friction blisters, and large burn blisters.

Table 35-1. Continued

Wheal	Elevated, often reddish area with irregular border caused by diffuse fluid in tissues rather than free fluid in a cavity, as in vesicles. Size varies. **Examples** Insect bites and hives (extensive wheals).
Pustule	Elevated, pus-filled vesicle or bulla with circumscribed border. Size varies. **Examples** Acne, impetigo, and carbuncles (large boils).
Cyst	Elevated, encapsulated, fluid-filled or semisolid mass originating in the subcutaneous tissue or dermis, usually 1 cm or larger. **Examples** Varieties include sebaceous cysts and epidermoid cysts.

Secondary Skin Lesions

Atrophy	A translucent, dry, paperlike, sometimes wrinkled skin surface resulting from thinning or wasting of the skin due to loss of collagen and elastin. **Examples** Striae, aged skin.
Erosion	Wearing away of the superficial epidermis causing a moist, shallow depression. Because erosions do not extend into the dermis, they heal without scarring. **Examples** Scratch marks, ruptured vesicles.
Lichen-ification	Rough, thickened, hardened area of epidermis resulting from chronic irritation such as scratching or rubbing. **Example** Chronic dermatitis.
Scales	Shedding flakes of greasy, keratinized skin tissue. Color may be white, gray, or silver. Texture may vary from fine to thick. **Examples** Dry skin, dandruff, psoriasis, and eczema.
Crust	Dry blood, serum, or pus left on the skin surface when vesicles or pustules burst. Can be red-brown, orange, or yellow. Large crusts that adhere to the skin surface are called scabs. **Examples** Eczema, impetigo, herpes, or scabs following abrasion.
Ulcer	Deep, irregularly shaped area of skin loss extending into the dermis or subcutaneous tissue. May bleed. May leave scar. **Examples** Decubitus ulcers (pressure sores), stasis ulcers, chancres.
Fissure	Linear crack with sharp edges, extending into the dermis. **Examples** Cracks at the corners of the mouth or in the hands, athlete's foot.
Scar	Flat, irregular area of connective tissue left after a lesion or wound has healed. New scars may be red or purple; older scars may be silvery or white. **Examples** Healed surgical wound or injury, healed acne.
Keloid	Elevated, irregular, darkened area of excess scar tissue caused by excessive collagen formation during healing. Extends beyond the site of the original injury. Higher incidence in people of African descent. **Examples** Keloid from ear piercing or surgery.

- **Inspect distribution and quality of hair.**

  A deviation in the normal hair distribution in the male or female genital area may indicate an endocrine disorder. **Hirsutism** (increased growth of coarse hair, usually on the face and trunk) is seen in Cushing's syndrome, acromegaly, and ovarian dysfunction. **Alopecia** (hair loss) may be related to changes in hormones, chemical or drug treatment, or radiation. In adult males whose hair loss follows the normal male pattern, the cause is usually genetic.

- **Palpate hair texture.**

  ✓ Some systemic diseases change the texture of the hair. For instance, hypothyroidism causes the hair to coarsen, whereas hyperthyroidism causes the hair to become fine.

- **Inspect the scalp for lesions.**

  ✓ Mild dandruff is normal, but excessive, greasy flakes indicate seborrhea requiring treatment.

  ✓ Hair loss, pustules, and scales appear on the scalp in tinea capitis (scalp ringworm).

  ✓ Red, swollen pustules appear around infected hair follicles and are called furuncles.

  ✓ Head lice may be seen as oval nits (eggs) adhering to the base of the hair shaft. Head lice are usually accompanied by itching.

- **Inspect nail curvature.**

  ✓ Clubbing, in which the angle of the nail base is greater than 180 degrees, is seen in respiratory disorders, cardiovascular disorders, cirrhosis of the liver, colitis, and thyroid disease. The nail becomes thick, hard, shiny, and curved at the free end.

- **Inspect the surface of the nails.**

  ✓ The nail folds become inflamed and swollen and the nail loosens in paronychia, an infection of the nails.

  ✓ Inflammation and transverse rippling of the nail is associated with chronic paronychia and/or eczema.

  ✓ The nail plate may separate from the nail bed in trauma, psoriasis, and Pseudomonas and Candida infections. This separation is called oncolysis.

  ✓ Nail grooves may be caused by inflammation, by planus, or by nail biting.

  ✓ Nail pitting may be seen with psoriasis.

  ✓ A transverse groove (Beau's line) may be seen in trachoma and/or acute diseases.

  ✓ Thin spoon-shaped nails may be seen in anemia.

- **Inspect nail color.**

  ✓ The sudden appearance of a pigmented band may indicate melanoma. However, pigmented bands are normally found in over 90% of African Americans.

  ✓ Yellowish nails are seen in psoriasis and fungal infections.

  ✓ Dark nails occur with trauma, Candida infections, and hyperbilirubinemia.

  ✓ Blackish-green nails are apparent in injury and in Pseudomonas infection.

  ✓ Red splinter longitudinal hemorrhages may be seen in injury and/or psoriasis.

- **Inspect nail thickness.**

  ✓ Trauma to the nails usually causes thickening. Other causes of thick nails include psoriasis, fungal infections, and decreased peripheral vascular blood supply.

  ✓ Thinning of the nails is seen in nutritional deficiencies.

36

Nursing Care of Clients with Integumentary Disorders

The skin and its accessory structures (the integumentary system) enclose the body, providing protection by serving as a barrier between the internal and external environments. The skin contains receptors for touch and sensation, helps regulate body temperature, and maintains fluid and electrolyte balance. The skin also provides cues to racial and ethnic background, and plays a major role in determining self-concept, roles, and relationships.

There are many disorders of the integument. The client with minor or benign disorders is usually treated in a health care provider's office or outpatient setting; but the client with disorders that involve large areas of the body, are chronic, or are malignant may require inpatient care. This chapter discusses disorders of the skin, hair, and nails; Chapter 37 discusses the client with burns.

Common Skin Problems and Lesions

The disorders discussed in this section of the chapter are those experienced by a large number of people. Although they are considered minor health problems in terms of health care, they may cause major problems for the person experiencing a high level of discomfort and/or chronicity.

The Client with Psoriasis

Psoriasis is a chronic skin disorder characterized by raised, reddened, round circumscribed plaques covered by silvery white scales. The size of these lesions varies. The lesions may appear anywhere on the body; but they are most commonly found on the scalp, extensor surfaces of the arms and legs, elbows, knees, sacrum, and around the nails. The characteristic lesions in psoriasis are well-demarcated regions of erythematous plaques that shed thick gray flakes. As with any chronic illness, the skin manifestations may occur and disappear throughout life, with no discernible pattern to the recurrence.

Pathophysiology

Psoriasis affects about 1% of the U.S. population. The incidence is lower in warm, sunny climates. Onset usually occurs in the 20s, but it may occur at any age. Psoriasis occurs more often in Caucasians, but men and women are affected equally.

Sunlight, stress, seasonal changes, hormone fluctuations, steroid withdrawal, and certain drugs, such as alcohol, corticosteroids, lithium, and chloroquine, appear to exacerbate the disorder. About one-third of clients have a family history of psoriasis. Trauma to the skin from such events as surgery, sunburn, or excoriation is also a common precipitating factor; lesions that result from trauma are called Koebner's reaction (Porth, 2002).

Normally, the keratinocyte (an epidermal cell making up 95% of the epidermis) migrates from the basal cell to the stratum corneum (the outer skin layer) in about 14 days and is sloughed off 14 days later. Psoriatic skin cells, by contrast, have a shorter cycle of growth, completing the journey to the stratum corneum in only four to seven days, a condition called *hyperkeratosis*. These immature cells produce an abnormal keratin that forms thick, flaky scales at the surface of the skin. The increased cell metabolism stimulates increased vascularity, which contributes to the erythema of the lesions.

Psoriasis vulgaris is the most common form of psoriasis. The lesions can be found anywhere on the skin but most commonly involve the skin over the elbows, knees, and scalp. Initially, the lesions are papules that form into well-defined erythematous plaques with thick, silvery scales. The plaques in darker-skinned persons may appear purple.

Permanent remission of psoriasis is rare. The prognosis depends on the type, extent, and severity of the initial attack. The age of onset is also a factor; early-onset disease is usually more severe.

Manifestations and Complications

Pruritus is common over the psoriatic lesions. If the lesions are located in an intertriginous zone, such as between the toes, under the breasts, or in the perianal region, the psoriatic scales may soften, allowing painful fissures to form. When psoriasis affects the nails, pitting and a yellow or brown discoloration results. The nail may separate from the nail bed, thicken, and crumble. The involved nails, which are more often fingernails than toenails, are at high risk for infection.

Collaborative Care

Treatment is based on the type of psoriasis, the extent and location of the lesions, the age of the client, and the degree of disfigurement or disability.

Diagnostic Tests
- *Skin biopsy* may be done if the client presents with atypical manifestations, or to differentiate psoriasis from other inflammatory or infectious skin disorders.
- *Ultrasonography* may be performed to measure skin thickness; results reveal typical psoriatic changes in the stratum corneum and dermal inflammation.

Medications
A variety of medications and treatments may be prescribed, including topical medications and photochemotherapy. Although there is no cure, treatment decreases the severity and pain of the lesions.

Topical medications are administered to decrease inflammation, prolong the maturity time of keratinocytes, and increase remission time. Corticosteroids, tar preparations, anthralin, and the retinoids are typically used.

Topical corticosteroids decrease inflammation, suppress mitotic activity of psoriatic cells, and delay the movement of keratinocytes to the surface of the skin (thus giving them time to mature and decreasing hyperkeratinosis). Tazarotene gel, a topical retinoid, is useful in treating clients with mild to moderate cases. The most effective topical corticosteroids are potent preparations that are well absorbed through the skin and are used under an occlusive dressing. Corticosteroids may also be taken systemically or injected directly into the lesions.

Tar preparations, such as Estar, Psorigel, and Fototar, suppress mitotic activity and are also anti-inflammatory. Their exact mechanism of action is unknown, but they are effective in removing scales and increasing remission time. Preparations made of coal tar are messy, cause staining, and have an unpleasant odor, but they are an effective form of treatment.

Topical anthralin (dithranol) inhibits the mitotic activity of epidermal cells and is effective in some cases of chronic, localized psoriasis that do not respond to other topical agents. The medication is applied to the plaque patches at bedtime and left in place for 8 to 12 hours. Clients should be tested for sensitivity to the drug before use, and it should not be applied to inflamed or open areas of skin.

Calcipotriene (Dovonex) has been shown to be effective and safe in both the short-term and long-term treatment of psoriasis. It inhibits cell proliferation in the epidermis and facilitates cell differentiation. Although a derivative of topical vitamin D, calcipotriene does not seem to affect bone or calcium metabolism.

Treatments

Photochemotherapy
Photochemotherapy is the preferred treatment modality for severe psoriasis (Porth, 2002). A light-activated form of the drug methoxsalen is used. This drug is an antimetabolite that inhibits DNA synthesis and, thereby, prevents cell mitosis, decreasing hyperkeratosis. Exposure to ultraviolet-A (UVA) rays activates methoxsalen; it is administered orally, and the client is exposed to UVA 2 hours later. Treatments are administered 2 to 3 times a week; usually 10 to 20 total treatments are given over 1 to 2 months. The eyes are covered by dark glasses during the treatment. Treatment causes tanning, and direct sunlight must be avoided for 8 to 12 hours thereafter. If the client exhibits erythema, the treatments are stopped until the redness and swelling resolve.

Photochemotherapy has had a high success rate in achieving remission of psoriasis, but it can accelerate aging of exposed skin, induce cataract development, alter immune function, and increase the risk of melanoma.

Ultraviolet Light Therapy
Ultraviolet-B (UVB) light is often used to treat psoriasis. UVB light decreases the growth rate of epidermal cells, thereby decreasing hyperkeratosis. Mercury vapor lights or fluorescent UV tubes provide the UVB light; the latter are often arranged in a cabinet so the client can stand and expose psoriatic lesions more easily. These units may be purchased or constructed to be used in the client's home.

The light therapy is administered in gradually increasing exposure times, until the client experiences a mild erythema, like a mild sunburn. Treatments are given daily and are measured in seconds of exposure. The eyes are shielded during the treatment. The erythema response occurs in about eight hours. Careful assessment is necessary to prevent more severe burning, which could exacerbate the psoriasis. In clients with extensive psoriasis, UVB treatments may be combined with tar preparations, which increase the photosensitivity of the skin.

Nursing Care

The client with psoriasis requires nursing care to meet physical and psychologic responses to the illness. The nursing interventions discussed in this section focus on common problems of the client with psoriasis: risk for impaired skin integrity and body image disturbance.

Nursing Diagnoses and Interventions

Impaired Skin Integrity

Psoriatic lesions range from several scales to large, open areas. Typical psoriatic skin lesions increase the risk of infection, which can further compromise healing. In addition, certain treatments (e.g., the use of UVA or retinoids) may cause erythema or peeling of the skin, further altering skin integrity.

- Demonstrate methods to reduce injury to the skin when taking therapeutic baths or treatments:
  1. Use warm, not hot, water.
  2. Gently rub lesions with a soft washcloth, using a circular motion.
  3. Dry the skin with a soft towel, using a blotting or patting motion.
  4. Keep the skin lubricated at all times.

Hot water and dry skin increase pruritus, further stimulating the itch-scratch-itch cycle. Dry skin also worsens psoriasis. Washing or drying the skin with rough linens or pressure may excoriate the skin over the psoriatic lesions.

- Demonstrate application of topical medications:
  1. Apply the medication as prescribed in a thin layer, using hands (gloved, if appropriate), wooden tongue depressors, or a gauze pad.
  2. Avoid getting medications in the eyes, on mucous membranes, or in skinfolds.
  3. Apply a covering (occlusive dressing) over the medicated areas as prescribed, especially when using corticosteroids. Usually, the covering is applied for only 12 hours, often during the evening and night hours. Choose some type of plastic wrap that covers the area well.

Applying a thin layer of medication more frequently is often more effective than applying a single thick layer of medication. The medications used to treat psoriasis may irritate the eyes and mucous membranes; when applied in skinfolds, they may also cause maceration (skin breakdown due to prolonged exposure to moisture). Topical corticosteroids are often covered with occlusive dressing to increase absorption and thus facilitate treatment. However, constant occlusion may increase the effects of the medications to undesired levels and also increases the risk for infections.

- Teach manifestations of infection and how to contact the health care provider if these occur: elevated temperature, increased swelling, redness, pain, increase in drainage, and any change in the color of the drainage. *The client with skin lesions is at high risk for infection, as the skin is the body's first line of defense.*

- Teach manifestations of the complications of treatment: excoriation, increased erythema, increased peeling, and blister formation. *The medications or treatments may damage cells through chemical burns or excessive exposure to ultraviolet light. Times and methods of treatment need to be adjusted if these manifestations occur.*

Disturbed Body Image

The obvious skin lesions that accompany psoriasis often cause clients to isolate themselves from social contacts, withdraw from normal roles and responsibilities, and feel helpless or powerless.

- Establish a trusting relationship by expressing acceptance of the client, both verbally and nonverbally. For example, touch the client during social communications, demonstrating that the lesions are not contagious or offensive. *One's body image is affected not only by self-perception, but also by the responses of others. Nonjudgmental acceptance helps the client adapt to the change in body image. By touching the client during interactions, the nurse demonstrates that acceptance.*

- Encourage to verbalize feelings about self-perception in view of the chronic nature of psoriasis and to ask questions about the disease and treatment. *The client adapts to a changed body image through a process of recognition, acceptance, and resolution. Each person responds individually to disfigurement and loss.*

- Promote social interaction through family involvement in care, and referral to support groups of people with psoriasis or other chronic skin conditions. Acceptance by others is critical to acceptance of self. *Psoriasis treatment is lifelong, time consuming, and often unappealing. By becoming involved in care, the family communicates acceptance. Sharing experiences with others who have the same health problem is a source of strength in adjusting to a visible, chronic illness.*

Home Care

Client and family teaching focuses on treatments and skin care needs. The following topics should be addressed:

- The chronic nature of the disease, factors that may precipitate an exacerbation, and methods to reduce stress

- Interventions for pruritus and dry skin, and specific care for psoriasis:
  1. Expose the skin to sunlight, but avoid sunburn.
  2. Avoid trauma to the skin (e.g., do not scrub off scales, and use only an electric razor).
  3. Avoid exposure to contagious illnesses such as influenza and colds.
  4. Discuss current medications with the health care provider. Certain drugs, such as indomethacin (Indocin), lithium, and beta-adrenergic blocking agents, are known to precipitate exacerbations of psoriasis.
  5. In addition, suggest the National Psoriasis Foundation as a resource.

Infections and Infestations of the Skin

The skin's resistance to infections and infestations is provided by protective mechanisms, including skin flora, sebum, and the immune response. Although the skin is normally resistant to infections and infestations, these disorders may occur as a result of a break in the skin surface, a virulent agent, and/or decreased resistance due to a compromised immune system. This section discusses skin disorders resulting from bacterial infections, fungal infections, parasitic infestations, and viral infections.

The Client with a Bacterial Infection of the Skin

A number of bacteria normally inhabit the skin and do not cause an infection. However, when a break in the skin allows invasion by pathogenic bacteria, an infection, called a **pyoderma,** may occur. The most common bacterial infections are caused by gram-positive *Staphylococcus aureus* and beta-hemolytic streptococci.

Bacterial infections of the skin may be primary or secondary. Primary infections are caused by a single pathogen and arise from normal skin; secondary infections develop in traumatized or diseased skin.

Most bacterial infections are treated by a primary care provider, and the client remains at home for care. If the infection becomes more serious, however, inpatient care is required. In addition, nosocomial infections of wounds or open lesions in hospitalized clients are often the result of bacterial infections, especially by methicillin-resistant *Staphylococcus aureus (MRSA)*.

Pathophysiology

Bacterial infections of the skin arise from the hair follicle, where bacteria can accumulate and grow and cause a localized infection. However, the bacteria also can invade deeper tissues and cause a systemic infection, a potentially life-threatening disorder. Various types of bacterial infections involve the skin, including folliculitis, furuncles, carbuncles, cellulitis, erysipelas, and impetigo.

Folliculitis

Folliculitis is a bacterial infection of the hair follicle, most commonly caused by *Staphylococcus aureus.* The infection begins at the follicle opening and extends down into the follicle. The bacteria release enzymes and chemical agents that cause an inflammation. The lesions appear as pustules surrounded by an area of erythema on the surface of the skin. Folliculitis is found most often on the scalp and extremities. It is also often seen on the face of bearded men (called sycosis barbae), on the legs of women who shave, and on the eyelids (called a *stye*). Although folliculitis may appear without any apparent cause, contributing factors include poor hygiene, poor nutrition, prolonged skin moisture, and trauma to the skin.

Furuncles

Furuncles, often called boils, are also inflammations of the hair follicle. They often begin as folliculitis, but the infection spreads down the hair shaft, through the wall of the follicle, and into the dermis. The causative organism is commonly *Staphylococcus aureus.* A furuncle is initially a deep, firm, red, painful nodule from 1 to 5 cm in diameter. After a few days, the nodule changes into a large, tender cystic nodule. The cysts may drain substantial amounts of purulent drainage.

One or more furuncles may occur on any part of the body that has hair. Contributing factors include poor hygiene, trauma to the skin, areas of excessive moisture (including perspiration), and systemic diseases, such as diabetes mellitus and hematologic malignancies.

Carbuncles

A **carbuncle** is a group of infected hair follicles. The lesion begins as a firm mass located in the subcutaneous tissue and the lower dermis. This mass becomes swollen and painful and has multiple openings to the skin surface. Carbuncles are most frequently found on the back of the neck, the upper back, and the lateral thighs. In addition to the local manifestations, the client may experience chills, fever, and malaise. The contributing factors for carbuncles are the same as for furuncles. Both infections are more common in hot, humid climates.

Cellulitis

Cellulitis is a localized infection of the dermis and subcutaneous tissue. Cellulitis can occur following a wound or skin ulcer or as an extension of furuncles or carbuncles. The infection spreads as a result of a substance produced by the causative organism, called spreading factor (hyaluronidase). This factor breaks down the fibrin network and other barriers that normally localize the infection. The area of cellulitis is red, swollen, and painful. In some cases, vesicles may form over the area of cellulitis. The client may also experience fever, chills, malaise, headache, and swollen lymph glands.

Erysipelas

Erysipelas is an infection of the skin most often caused by group A streptococci. Chills, fever, and malaise are prodromal symptoms, occurring from 4 hours to 20 days before the skin lesion appears. The initial infection appears as firm red spots that enlarge and join to form a circumscribed, bright red, raised, hot lesion. Vesicles may form over the surface of the erysipelas lesion. The area usually is painful, itches, and burns. Erysipelas most commonly appears on the face, ears, and lower legs.

Impetigo

Impetigo is an infection of the skin caused by either *Staphylococcus aureus* or beta-hemolytic streptococci. Impetigo typically begins with a vesicle or pustule. This lesion ruptures, leaving an open area that discharges a honey-colored serous liquid that hardens into a crust. Within hours, more vesicles form. The pruritus that accompanies the eruptions causes scratching and excoriation, which spreads the infection. This disease occasionally occurs in adults, but is much more common in children.

Collaborative Care

The diagnosis of a bacterial infection of the skin is made by assessing the appearance of the lesion and by identifying the causative organism. Antibiotics specific to the organism are used in treatment.

Diagnostic Tests

- Culture and sensitivity of the drainage from the lesion may be ordered to identify the organism and to target the most effective antibiotics.
- If the infection is systemic, a blood culture may be ordered to identify a causative organism.
- People who experience repeated bacterial skin infections, or who provide care for others who exhibit infections, may have a culture taken from the external nares to determine whether they are carriers of bacteria (e.g., MSRA) and are reinfecting themselves or others.

Medications

The primary treatment for bacterial infections of the skin is an antibiotic specific to the organism. The antibiotic is usually taken orally, and may also be applied topically. Multiple furuncles and carbuncles may be treated with cloxacillin (a penicillinaseresistant penicillin); the cephalosporins are also often effective.

Nursing Care

Nursing care focuses on preventing the spread of infection and restoring normal skin integrity. Most clients provide self-care at home, but the incidence of secondary bacterial infections in the inpatient population is great enough to warrant their inclusion in planning and implementing care. Nursing interventions for inpatient and long-term care clients include the following:

- Practice good handwashing and teach its importance. Careful handwashing is one of the most effective methods to reduce the spread of infection both in and out of the hospital setting. Health care providers must wash their hands with soap and water before and after client care and between each client contact. All clients, family members, and visitors (both in the home and hospital setting) should be taught the importance of handwashing, but it is even more important for the client with a bacterial infection.
- Assess the client for any increase in infection, which may be manifested systemically by fever, tachycardia, chills, and malaise. Local manifestations of the spread of the infection include an increase in erythema, the size of the lesion, and drainage. This assessment is especially important for older, debilitated, or immunosuppressed clients, and for those who have large or dirty wounds.
- Place the client on isolation precautions to limit the spread of the organisms to other patients. All health care providers and visitors follow the procedures and protocols of the institution exactly to prevent cross-contamination.
- Cover draining lesions with a sterile dressing, and handle soiled dressings or linens according to standard precautions. When changing dressings, always wear disposable rubber gloves and masks.

Home Care

Client and family teaching focuses on facilitating tissue healing and eliminating the infection. Address the following topics:

- The importance of maintaining good nutrition.
- The importance of maintaining cleanliness through careful handwashing and proper handling and disposal of dressings.
- Preventing the spread of infection in the home by not sharing linens and towels and washing clothing and linens in hot water.
- The importance of not squeezing or trying to open a bacterial lesion.
- Avoiding the plucking of nasal hair or picking the nose.
- The importance of taking the full course of prescribed antibiotics on a regular schedule until the prescribed supply is finished.
- Bathing daily with an antibacterial soap. (The client can gently wash off crusts during the bath. Warm compresses may be applied to the lesions two to three times a day to increase comfort and decrease swelling.)

Inflammatory Disorders of the Skin

Inflammatory skin disorders are rarely associated with systemic manifestations. The inflammatory skin disorders discussed in this section include dermatitis, acne, pemphigus, lichen planus, and toxic epidermal necrolysis.

The Client with Dermatitis

Dermatitis is an inflammation of the skin characterized by erythema and pain or pruritus. Dermatitis may be acute or chronic.

Pathophysiology

In dermatitis, various exogenous and endogenous agents cause an inflammatory response of the skin. Different types of skin eruptions occur, often specific to the causative allergen, infection, or disease. The initial skin responses to these agents or illnesses include erythema, formation of vesicles and scales, and pruritus. Subsequently, irritation from scratching promotes edema, a serous discharge, and crusting. Long-term irritation in chronic dermatitis causes the skin to become thickened and leathery (a condition called *lichenification*) and darker in color.

Contact Dermatitis

Contact dermatitis is a type of dermatitis caused by a hypersensitivity response or chemical irritation. The major sources known to cause contact dermatitis are dyes, perfumes, poison plants (ivy, oak, sumac), chemicals, and metals. A contact dermatitis common in the health care field is latex (glove) dermatitis.

Allergic contact dermatitis is a cell-mediated or delayed hypersensitivity to a wide variety of allergens. Sensitizing antigens include microorganisms, plants, chemicals, drugs, metals, or foreign proteins. On initial contact with the skin, the allergen binds to a carrier protein, forming a sensitizing antigen. The antigen is processed and carried to the T cells, which in turn become sensitized to the antigen. The first exposure is the sensitizing contact; skin manifestations occur with subsequent exposures. These manifestations include erythema, swelling, and pruritic vesicles in the area of allergen contact. For example, a person hypersensitive to metal may have lesions under a ring or watch.

Irritant contact dermatitis is an inflammation of the skin from irritants; it is not a hypersensitivity response. Common sources of irritant contact dermatitis include chemicals, such as acids; soaps; and detergents. The skin lesions are similar to those seen in allergic contact dermatitis.

Atopic Dermatitis

Atopic dermatitis is an inflammatory skin disorder that is also called **eczema.** The exact cause is unknown, but related factors include depressed cell-mediated immunity, elevated IgE levels, and increased histamine sensitivity. The disorder is seen more often in children, but chronic forms persist throughout life.

Clients with atopic dermatitis have a family history of hypersensitivity reactions, such as dry skin, eczema, asthma, and allergic rhinitis. Although up to one-third of clients with atopic dermatitis also have food allergies, a positive correlation has not been found.

The dermatitis results when mast cells, T lymphocytes, monocytes, and other inflammatory cells are activated and release histamine, lymphokines, and other inflammatory mediators. The immune response interacts with the allergen to create a chronic inflammatory condition. In the adult form of atopic dermatitis, characteristic lesions include chronic lichenification, erythema, and scaling, the result of pruritus and scratching. The lesions are usually found on the hands, feet, or flexor surfaces of the arms and legs. Scratching and excoriation increase the risk of secondary infections, as well as invasion of the skin by viruses such as herpes simplex.

Seborrheic Dermatitis

Seborrheic dermatitis is a chronic inflammatory disorder of the skin that involves the scalp, eyebrows, eyelids, ear canals, nasolabial folds, axillae, and trunk. The cause is unknown. This disorder is seen in all ages, from the very young (called "cradle cap") to the very old. Clients taking methyldopa (Aldomet) for hypertension occasionally develop this disorder, and it is a component of Parkinson's disease. Seborrheic dermatitis is also frequently seen in clients with AIDS.

The lesions are yellow or white plaques with scales and crusts. The scales are often yellow or orange and have a greasy appearance. Mild pruritus is also present. Diffuse dandruff with erythema of the scalp often accompanies the skin lesions.

Exfoliative Dermatitis

Exfoliative dermatitis is an inflammatory skin disorder characterized by excessive peeling or shedding of skin. The cause is unknown in about half of all cases, but a preexisting skin disorder, such as psoriasis, atopic dermatitis, contact dermatitis, or seborrheic dermatitis, is found in about 40% of the cases (Tierney, et al., 2001). Exfoliative dermatitis is also associated with leukemia and lymphoma.

Both systemic and localized manifestations may appear. Systemic manifestations include weakness, malaise, fever, chills, and weight loss. Scaling, erythema, and pruritus may be localized or involve the entire body. In addition to peeling of skin, the client may lose the hair and nails.

Generalized exfoliative dermatitis may cause debility and dehydration. The impairment of skin integrity increases the risk for local and systemic infections.

Collaborative Care

The client with dermatitis is treated primarily with topical medications and therapeutic baths. If the dermatitis is due to hypersensitivity to an allergen, the client avoids exposure to environmental irritants and suspected foods. The client also discontinues as many medications as possible to determine whether the dermatitis is the result of a drug allergy.

Diagnostic Tests
The diagnosis is often based on the manifestations of the disorder. Diagnostic tests may include the following:

- Scratch tests and intradermal tests are conducted to identify a specific allergen.
- Serum studies may find elevated eosinophil and IgE levels in atopic dermatitis.
- Skin biopsy may reveal specific changes in inflammatory dermatitis.

Medications
The medications used depend on the cause of the dermatitis and the severity of the manifestations. Minor cases are treated with antipruritic medications, whereas more severe cases are treated with oral antihistamines, oral and/or topical corticosteroids, and wet dressings. Topical anti-infectives may be prescribed if necessary.

Nursing Care

Nursing care of the client with dermatitis focuses primarily on providing information for self-care at home. The client is responsible for managing skin problems and requires education and support. Address the following topics:

- Medications and treatments do not cure the disease; they only relieve the symptoms.
- Dry skin increases pruritus, which stimulates scratching. Scratching may in turn cause excoriation, and excoriation increases the risk of infection.
- It may be necessary to change the diet or environment to avoid contact with allergens.
- When using steroid preparations, apply only a thin layer to slightly damp skin (e.g., after taking a bath).
- If occlusive dressings are necessary, a plastic suit may be used.
- When using oral corticosteroids, never abruptly stop taking the medication. Rather, follow instructions to taper the dosage gradually.
- Antihistamines cause drowsiness. When using these medications, avoid alcohol and use caution when driving or working around machinery.

The Client with Acne

Acne is a disorder of the pilosebaceous (hair and sebaceous gland) structure, which opens to the skin surface through a pore. The sebaceous glands, which empty directly into the hair follicle, produce sebum, a lipid substance. Sebaceous glands are present over the entire skin surface except the soles of the feet and the palms of the hands, but the largest glands are on the face, scalp, and scrotum. Sebum production is a response to direct hormonal stimulation by testicular androgens in men and adrenal and ovarian androgens in women.

Pathophysiology

Acne may be noninflammatory or inflammatory. Noninflammatory acne lesions are primarily *comedones,* more commonly called pimples, whiteheads, and blackheads. Whiteheads are pale, slightly elevated papules categorized as closed comedones. Blackheads are plugs of material that accumulate in the sebaceous glands. They are categorized as open comedones. The color is the result of the movement of melanin into the plug from surrounding epidermal cells. Inflammatory acne lesions include comedones, erythematous pustules, and cysts. Inflammation close to the skin surface results in pustules; deeper inflammation results in cysts. The inflammation is believed to result from irritation from fatty acid constituents of the sebum and from substances produced by *Propionibacterium acnes* bacteria, both of which escape into the dermis when the follicular wall of closed comedones ruptures.

Several forms of acne occur at different periods of the life span. The most common are acne vulgaris, acne rosacea, and acne conglobata.

Acne Vulgaris

Acne vulgaris is the form of acne common in adolescents and young to middle adults. Although the lesions may persist longer in women, the incidence is greater in men. The actual cause of acne vulgaris is unknown. Possible causes include androgenic influence on the sebaceous glands, increased sebum production, and proliferation of the organism *Propionibacterium acnes.* Many factors once thought to cause acne vulgaris, including high-fat diets, chocolate, infections, and cosmetics, have been disproved (Porth, 2002).

Mild cases may involve only a few scattered comedones, but severe cases are manifested by multiple lesions of all types. Most acne vulgaris lesions form on the face and neck, but they also occur on the back, chest, and shoulders. The lesions are usually mildly painful and may itch. The complications of acne vulgaris, especially in severe cases, are formation of cysts, pigment changes in persons with dark skin, severe scarring, and lowered self-concept from the obvious skin eruptions.

Acne Rosacea

Acne rosacea is a chronic type of facial acne that occurs more often in middle and older adults. The cause is unknown. The lesions of acne rosacea begin with erythema over the cheeks and nose. Other skin lesions may or may not appear. Over years of time, the skin color changes to dark red, and the pores over the area become enlarged. The soft tissue of the nose may exhibit *rhinophyma,* an irregular bullous thickening that can be treated with plastic surgery.

Acne Conglobata

Acne conglobata is also a chronic type of acne of unknown cause that begins in middle adulthood. This type causes serious skin lesions: Comedones, papules, pustules, nodules, cysts, and scars occur primarily on the back, buttocks, and chest, but may occur on other body surfaces. The comedones have multiple openings and a discharge that ranges from serous to purulent with a foul odor.

Collaborative Care

The management of acne is similar, regardless of type. Because acne vulgaris is most common, the discussions of collaborative and nursing care focus on that type.

Treatment is primarily by medications and continues for several weeks. Treatment is based on the type and severity of the lesions.

Diagnostic Tests

The disease is diagnosed by the typical location and appearance of lesions. If the client has pustules, a culture of the drainage is performed to differentiate viral or bacterial dermatitis from acne.

Medications

The treatment of acne is tailored to the individual and is based on the severity of the lesions. For acne with comedones, tretinoin (retinoic acid, Retin-A) or benzoyl peroxide preparations are prescribed. Azelaic acid (Azelex) may also be used. Benzoyl peroxide preparations are found in over-the-counter medications, such as Fostex, Acne-Dome, Desquam-X, Benzagel, Clear By Design, and Xerac BP. These products are keratolytic and loosen the comedones.

Mild forms of papular inflammatory acne are treated with topical clindamycin (Cleocin T), a bacteriostatic agent that decreases the amount of fatty acids on the skin surface. This medication may be combined with tretinoin therapy.

Moderate forms of papular inflammatory acne are treated with oral or topical antibiotics, such as tetracycline, erythromycin, and minocycline. These antiacne antibiotics are administered for three to four months; if the client's skin is clear, the dose is lowered gradually to a maintenance dose that will maintain clear skin.

Severe forms of papular inflammatory acne are treated with isotretinoin (Accutane). This drug is effective, but has serious side effects. Isotretinoin, with nursing responsibilities, is discussed below.

Table 36-1. Medication Administration — Acne Medications

Antiacne Retinoids

Tretinoin (Retin-A)   Isotretinoin (Accutane)

Tretinoin is a vitamin A derivative classified as an acne agent. This topical agent acts as an irritant to decrease cohesiveness of follicular epithelial cells, thereby decreasing comedone formation while increasing the extrusion of comedones from the skin surface.

Isotretinoin is a vitamin A analogue classified as an acne product. It reduces the size of sebaceous glands, inhibits sebaceous gland differentiation to decrease sebum production, and alters sebum lipid composition.

Nursing Responsibilities
* Administer tretinoin with caution to pregnant women, the effects of absorption on the developing fetus are not clearly defined.

Continued on the next page

Table 36-1. Continued

- Isotretinoin is absolutely contraindicated for pregnant women or for women who want to become pregnant. The medication poses a high risk of major deformities in the infant if pregnancy occurs during use, even use that continues only for short periods.
- Do not administer to clients with eczema or to those who are hypersensitive to the sun.

Client and Family Teaching

Tretinoin

- Use the cream in a test area twice at night to test for sensitivity; if no reaction occurs, increase applications gradually to the prescribed frequency.
- A pea-sized amount of the cream is enough to cover the entire face.
- Apply the cream to clean, dry skin.
- Do not apply the cream to the eyes, mouth, angles of the nose, or mucous membranes.
- Wash your face no more than two to three times a day, using a mild soap. Do not use skin preparations, such as after-shave lotion or perfumes, that contain alcohol, menthol, spice, or lime, they may irritate your skin.
- The medication may cause a temporary stinging or warm sensation, but should not cause pain.
- The skin where you apply the cream will be mildly red and may peel; if you experience a more severe reaction, consult your health care provider.
- The medication may cause increased sensitivity to sunlight, use sunscreens and wear protective clothing when outdoors.
- Your acne may become worse during the first two weeks of treatment; this is an expected response.

Isotretinoin

- Take the pills with food.
- Your acne may become worse during the initial period of treatment; this is an expected response.
- The medication causes dryness of the eyes, so you may have trouble wearing contact lenses during and after treatment.
- Do not take vitamin A supplements; they will increase the effects of the medication.
- Avoid prolonged exposure to sunlight; use sunscreen and protective clothing when in the sun.
- Notify the physician at once if you have abdominal pain, severe diarrhea, rectal bleeding, headache, nausea or vomiting, or visual disturbances.
- Do not drink alcohol while taking this medication (it causes an increase in triglycerides).
- Night vision may become worse; use caution when driving at night.
- Do not donate blood while or for one month after taking this medication.
- (*For female clients*) You must use two reliable forms of contraception simultaneously for at least one month before, during, and at least one month after therapy with this medication. The medication may cause deformities in a baby conceived at this time.

Treatments

Dermabrasion and Laser

Dermabrasion of inactive acne lesions can improve the client's appearance, especially if the scars are flat. Laser excision of deep scars may also be used.

Nursing Care

Nursing care is individualized to the client's developmental needs and is conducted primarily through teaching in clinics or the home setting. Regardless of the client's age or gender, it is important to remember that almost all clients with acne are embarrassed by and self-conscious of their appearance. Prior to teaching, establish rapport with the client and clarify beliefs; for example, the client may believe the lesions result from poor hygiene, masturbation, use of cosmetics, eating the wrong types of foods, or lack of sexual activity. It is critical to teach the client about the causes of and factors involved in acne prior to teaching self-care.

Home Care

The teaching plan for the client with acne includes general guidelines for skin care and health as well as specific guidelines for care of the acne lesions. The following topics should be addressed:

- Wash the skin with a mild soap and water at least twice a day to remove accumulated oils.
- Shampoo the hair often enough to prevent oiliness.
- Eat a regular, well-balanced diet. Foods do not cause or increase acne.
- Expose the skin to sunlight, but avoid sunburn.
- Get regular exercise and sleep.
- Try to avoid putting your hands on your face.
- Do not squeeze a pimple. Squeezing forces the material of the pimple deeper into the skin and usually causes the pimple to become larger and infected.
- The treatment for acne lasts months, in some cases for the rest of one's life. It is very important to take the medications each day for the prescribed length of time.

Skin Trauma

Trauma to the skin can be unintentional or intentional (as in the case of surgery). Chemicals, radiation, pressure, or thermal changes cause skin trauma. This section discusses pressure ulcers and frostbite, as well as intentional trauma from cutaneous and plastic surgery or treatment. Thermal injury, or burns, is discussed in Chapter 37.

The Client with a Pressure Ulcer

Pressure ulcers are ischemic lesions of the skin and underlying tissue caused by external pressure that impairs the flow of blood and lymph (Porth, 2002). The ischemia causes tissue necrosis and eventual ulceration. These ulcers, also called bed sores or decubitus ulcers, tend to develop over a bony prominence, such as the heels, greater trochanter, sacrum, and ischia, but they may appear on the skin of any part of the body subjected to external pressure, friction, or shearing forces.

Incidence

The incidence of pressure ulcers in hospitals, long-term care facilities, and home settings is high enough to warrant concern for health care providers. The incidence in hospitals has been reported as ranging from 3.5% to 29%, whereas the incidence in long-term care facilities is reported to be around 23%. Little research has been done to determine the extent of the problem in the home setting. However, with increasing numbers of clients (and especially older adult clients) being cared for in the home, it is probable that the incidence is great enough to warrant plans of care to prevent their occurrence.

Pathophysiology

Pressure ulcers develop from external pressure that compresses blood vessels or from friction and shearing forces that tear and injure vessels. Both types of pressure cause traumatic injury and initiate the process of pressure ulcer development.

External pressure that is greater than capillary pressure and arteriolar pressure interrupts blood flow in capillary beds. When pressure is applied to skin over a bony prominence for two hours, tissue ischemia and hypoxia from external pressure cause irreversible tissue damage. For example, when the body is in the supine position, the body's weight applies pressure to the sacrum. The same amount of pressure causes more damage when it is applied to a small area than when it is distributed over a large surface.

Shearing forces result when one tissue layer slides over another. The stretching and bending of blood vessels cause injury and thrombosis. Clients in hospital beds are subject to shearing forces when the head of the bed is elevated and the torso slides down toward the foot of the bed. Pulling the client up in bed also subjects the client to shearing forces. (For this reason, always lift clients up in bed). In both cases, friction and moisture cause the skin and superficial fascia to remain fixed to the bed sheet, while the deep fascia and bony skeleton slides in the direction of body movement.

When a person lies or sits in one position for an extended length of time without moving, pressure on the tissue between a bony prominence and the external surface of the body distorts capillaries and interferes with normal blood flow. If the pressure is relieved, blood flow to the area increases, and a brief period of reactive hyperemia occurs without permanent damage. However, if the pressure continues, platelets aggregate in the endothelial cells surrounding the capillaries and form microthrombi. These microthrombi impede blood flow, resulting in ischemia and hypoxia of tissues. Eventually, the cells and tissues of the immediate area of pressure and of the surrounding area die and become necrotic.

Alterations in the involved tissue depend on the depth of the injury. Injury to superficial layers of skin results in blister formation, whereas injury to deeper structures causes the pressure ulcer area to appear dark reddish-blue. As the tissues die, the ulcer becomes an open wound that may be deep enough to expose the bone. The necrotic tissue elicits an inflammatory response, and the client experiences increases in temperature, pain, and white blood cell count. Secondary bacterial invasion is common. Enzymes from bacteria and macrophages dissolve necrotic tissue, resulting in a foul-smelling drainage.

Pressure ulcers are graded or staged to classify the degree of damage. The stages are listed in Table 36-2.

Table 36-2. Pressure Ulcer Staging

Stage I Nonblanchable erythema of intact skin; the heralding lesion of skin ulceration. Identification of stage I pressure ulcers may be difficult in clients with darkly pigmented skin. *Note:* Reactive hyperemia can normally be expected to be present for one-half to three-fourths as long as the pressure occluded blood flow to the area. This should not be confused with stage I pressure ulcer.

Stage II Partial-thickness skin loss involving epidermis and/or dermis. The ulcer is superficial and presents clinically as an abrasion, blister, or shallow crater.

Stage III Full-thickness skin loss involving damage or necrosis of subcutaneous tissue that may extend down to, but not through, underlying fascia. The ulcer presents clinically as a deep crater with or without undermining of adjacent tissue.

Stage IV Full-thickness skin loss with extensive destruction, tissue necrosis, or damage to muscle, bone, or supporting structures (e.g., tendon or joint capsule). Sinus tracts may also be associated with stage IV ulcers.

Note: When eschar is present, accurate staging of the pressure ulcer is not possible until the eschar has sloughed or the wound has been debrided.

Note: Text is from *Pressure Ulcers in Adults: Prediction and Prevention* by the Agency for Health Care Policy and Research, 1992, Rockville, MD: U.S. Department of Health and Human Services.

Risk Factors

Although a pressure ulcer may develop in an adult of any age who has an impairment in mobility, those most at risk are older adults with limited mobility, people with quadriplegia, and clients in the critical care setting (Porth, 2002). Other clients prone to develop pressure ulcers are those with fractures of large bones (e.g., hip or femur) or who have undergone orthopedic surgery or sustained spinal cord injury. In addition to deficits in mobility and activity, incontinence and nutritional deficit also increase the risk of pressure ulcer development. Clients with chronic illnesses, such as renal failure and anemia, and those with edema or infection are also at increased risk.

Because of age-related skin changes, the older adult is at increased risk for the development of pressure ulcers. The skin of the older adult has a thicker epidermis, a thinner dermis with decreased vascularity, decreased sebaceous gland activity, and decreased strength and elasticity. As a result, the more fragile and less nourished dermal layer is more prone to shear and friction problems. In addition, the skin of the older adult responds more slowly to inflammation, and wounds heal more slowly; when pressure ulcers occur, they are more difficult to reverse.

Collaborative Care

For the client at risk for pressure ulcers, the goal is prevention. Existing ulcers require collaborative treatment to promote healing and restore skin integrity.

Diagnostic tests are conducted to determine the presence of a secondary infection and to differentiate the cause of the ulcer. If the ulcer is deep or appears infected, drainage or biopsied tissue is cultured to determine the causative organism.

Topical and systemic antibiotics specific to the infectious organism eradicate any infection present. Additionally, a variety of topical products promote healing. Examples are listed in Table 36–3.

Surgical debridement may be necessary if the pressure ulcer is deep; if subcutaneous tissues are involved; or if an eschar (a scab or dry crust that forms over skin damaged by burns, infections, or excoriations) has formed over the ulcer, preventing healing by granulation. Large wounds may require skin grafting for complete closure.

Table 36-3. Products Used to Treat Pressure Ulcers

Stage	Product	Purpose
I	Skin Prep	Toughens intact skin and preserves skin integrity.
	Granulex	Prevents skin breakdown, increases blood supply, adds moisture, contains trypsin to aid in removal of necrotic tissue.
	Hydrocolloid dressing (e.g., DuoDerm)	Prevents skin breakdown and promotes healing without the formation of a crust over the ulcer. Is permeable to air and water vapor; prevents the growth of anaerobic organisms.
	Transparent dressing (e.g., Tegaderm)	Prevents skin breakdown; prevents entrance of moisture and bacteria, but allows oxygen and moisture vapor permeability.
II	Transparent dressing	Enhances healing (see above).
	Hydrocolloid dressing	Enhances healing (see above). *Note:* If infection is present, these types of dressings are contraindicated. A sterile dressing should be applied instead.
III	Wet-to-dry gauze dressing with sterile normal saline	Allows necrotic material to soften and adhere to the gauze, so that the wound is debrided.
	Hydrocolloid dressing	Enhances healing (see above).
	Proteolytic enzymes (such as Elase)	Proteolytic enzymes serve as a debriding agent in inflamed and infected lesions.
IV	Wet-to-dry gauze dressing with sterile normal saline	Enhances healing (see above). *Note:* Transparent or hydrocolloid dressings or skin barriers are contraindicated.
	Vacuum-assisted closure (V.A.C.)	Creates a negative pressure to help reduce edema, increase blood supply and oxygenation, and decrease bacterial colonization. Also helps promote moist wound healing and the formation of granulation tissue.

Nursing Care

The client with one or more pressure ulcers not only has impaired skin integrity, but also is at increased risk for infection, pain, and decreased mobility. Pressure ulcers also prolong treatment for other conditions, increase health care costs, and diminish the client's quality of life.

Nursing Diagnoses and Interventions

The following interventions and rationales are adapted from the clinical guidelines developed by the Agency for Health Care Policy and Research (1992, 1994) in identifying adults at risk and treating those with stage I pressure ulcers.

Risk for Impaired Skin Integrity

- Identify at-risk individuals needing prevention and the specific factors placing them at risk.
- Assess bed- and chair-bound clients, as well as those who are unable to reposition themselves, for additional risk factors: immobility, incontinence, nutritional factors, such as inadequate dietary intake and impaired nutritional status, and altered level of consciousness.
- Assess clients on admission to acute care and rehabilitation hospitals, nursing homes, home care programs, and other health care facilities.
- Use a systematic risk assessment by using a validated risk assessment tool, such as the Braden scale.
- Document all assessments of risk.

Individuals at risk for pressure ulcers must be identified so that risk factors can be reduced through intervention. The primary risk factors for pressure ulcers are immobility and limited activity; therefore, assess clients who cannot reposition themselves or whose activity is limited to bed or chair. Validated tools ensure systematic evaluation of individual risk factors. The client requires periodic reassessment for pressure ulcers. Accurate and complete documentation of all risk assessments ensures continuity of care and may be used as a foundation for the skin care plan.

- Conduct a systematic skin inspection at least once a day, paying particular attention to the bony prominences. Systematic, comprehensive, and routine skin care may decrease pressure ulcer incidence (although the exact role is unknown. Inspect the following to assess a pressure ulcer:
  - Location of any lesion or ulcer.
  - Estimation of the stage.
  - Dimensions of the ulcer: length, width, depth.
  - Presence of any abnormal pathways in the wound:
    1. Sinus tract: a cavity or channel underneath the wound.
    2. Tunneling: a passageway or opening that may be visible at skin level, but with most of the tunnel under the surface of the skin.
    3. Undermining: areas of tissue destruction underneath intact skin along wound margins.
    4. Visible necrotic tissue. (Slough is necrotic tissue that is in the process of separating from viable tissue.)

5. Presence of an exudate

6. Presence or absence of granulation tissue

Skin inspection provides data the nurse uses in designing interventions to reduce risk and in evaluating outcomes of those interventions.

- Clean the skin at the time of soiling and at routine intervals, as frequently as the client's need or preference dictates. Avoid hot water, use a mild cleansing agent, and clean the skin gently, applying as little force and friction as possible. *Metabolic wastes and environmental contaminants accumulate on the skin; these potentially irritating substances should be removed frequently. Feces and urine cause chemical irritation and should be removed as soon as possible. Hot water may cause skin injury. Mild cleansing agents are less likely to remove the skin's natural barrier.*

- Minimize environmental factors leading to skin drying, such as low humidity and exposure to cold. Treat dry skin with moisturizers. *Well-hydrated skin resists mechanical trauma. Hydration decreases as the ambient air temperature decreases, especially when the air humidity is low. Poorly hydrated skin is less pliable, and severe dryness is associated with fissuring and cracking of the stratum corneum. Moisturizers reduce dry skin.*

- Avoid massage over bony prominences. *Although massage has been practiced for years, evidence now suggests that massage over bony prominences may lead to deep tissue trauma in clients at risk for or with beginning skin manifestations of a pressure ulcer.*

- Minimize skin exposure to moisture due to incontinence, perspiration, or wound drainage. When these sources of moisture cannot be controlled, use underpads or briefs made of materials that absorb moisture and present a quick-drying surface to the skin. Change underpads and briefs frequently. Do not place plastic directly against the skin. *Moisture from incontinence, perspiration, or wound drainage may contain factors that irritate the skin; moisture alone can increase the susceptibility of the skin to injury.*

- To minimize skin injury due to friction and shearing forces, use proper positioning, transferring, and turning techniques. Lubricants, such as cornstarch or creams, protective films, such as transparent dressings and skin sealants, protective dressings, such as hydrocolloids, and protective padding may also reduce friction injuries. *Shear injury occurs when skin remains stationary and the underlying tissue shifts. This shift diminishes the blood supply to the skin and results in ischemia and tissue damage. Proper positioning, however, can eliminate most shear injuries. Friction injuries to the skin occur when it moves across a coarse surface, such as bed linens. Most friction injuries can be avoided by using appropriate techniques to move clients so that their skin is never dragged across the linens. Any agent that eliminates contact or decreases the friction between the skin and the linens reduces the potential for injury.*

- Assess factors involved in inadequate dietary intake of protein or kilocalories. Offer nutritional supplements, and support the client during mealtimes. If dietary intake remains inadequate, consult with a dietitian about other dietary interventions. *The role nutrition plays in the development of (and to a lesser degree, the healing of) pressure ulcers is not understood, but poor dietary intake of kilocalories, protein, and iron has been associated with the development of pressure ulcers.*

- Maintain the client's current level of activity, mobility, and range of motion. *Frequent turning, repositioning, and movement are essential in reducing the risk of pressure ulcers.*
- For the client on bed rest or who is immobile, provide interventions against the adverse effects of external mechanical forces of pressure, friction, and shear:
  1. Reposition all at-risk clients at least every two hours, using a written schedule for systematic turning and repositioning.
  2. For clients on bed rest, use positioning devices, such as pillows or foam wedges, to protect bony prominences.
- For completely immobile clients, use devices to totally relieve pressure on the heels (the most common method is to raise the heels off the bed). Do not use donut-type devices.
- Avoid placing clients in the side-lying position directly on the trochanter.
- Maintain the head of the bed at the lowest degree of elevation consistent with the client's medical condition and other restrictions. Limit the amount of time the head of the bed is elevated.
- Use assistive devices, such as a trapeze or bed linen, to move clients in bed who cannot assist during transfers and position changes.
- Place any at-risk client on a pressure-reducing device, such as foam, static air, alternating air, gel, or water mattress.

Data indicate that the more spontaneous movements that bedridden, older adult clients make, the lower the incidence of pressure ulcers. Studies reveal that fewer pressure ulcers develop in at-risk clients who are turned every two to three hours. Proper positioning can reduce pressure on bony prominences. It is difficult to redistribute pressure under heels; suspending the heels is the best method. Donut cushions are more likely to cause than to prevent pressure ulcers. Shearing forces are exerted on the body when the head of the bed is elevated. Lifting (rather than dragging) is less likely to cause injury from friction. Pressure-reducing devices and beds can decrease the incidence of pressure ulcers.

- For chair-bound clients, use pressure-reducing devices. Consider postural alignment, distribution of weight, balance and stability, and pressure relief when positioning these clients. Avoid uninterrupted sitting in a chair or wheelchair. Reposition the client every hour. Teach clients who can do so to shift their weight every 15 minutes. Use a written plan for positioning, movement, and the use of positioning devices. Do not use donut devices. *Prolonged, uninterrupted mechanical pressure results in tissue breakdown. The client's weight should be shifted at least every hour.*

Home Care

Client and family teaching for care of a pressure ulcer also focuses on prevention and includes much of the same information presented in the preceding section. Because many clients with pressure ulcers are older or have other serious illnesses, a caregiver may require teaching on such topics as the following:

- Definition and description of pressure ulcers
- Common locations of pressure ulcers
- Risk factors for the development of pressure ulcers

- Skin care
- Ways to avoid injury
- Diet.

Depending on the stage of the pressure ulcer, the nurse teaches the client or caregiver how to care for ulcers that are already present: how to change wet-to-dry dressings, apply skin barriers, and avoid injury and infection. Referrals to a home health agency or community health department can help the family through the lengthy healing process.

37

Nursing Care of Clients with Burns

A **burn** is an injury resulting from exposure to heat, chemicals, radiation, or electric current. A transfer of energy from a source of heat to the human body initiates a sequence of physiologic events that in the most severe cases leads to irreversible tissue destruction. Burns range in severity from a minor loss of small segments of the outermost layer of the skin to a complex injury involving all body systems. Treatments vary from simple application of a topical antiseptic agent in an outpatient clinic to an invasive, multisystem, interdisciplinary health team approach in the aseptic environment of a burn center.

It is estimated that more than 2 million burn injuries occur each year in the United States, and, of those, about 70,000 require hospitalization (Braunwald & Fauci, 2001). The home is the most common site for fire-related burns. Home fires cause 73% of all fire-related deaths, with about 12 people dying in home fires each day. Factors associated with deaths from burns are age (especially children and older adults), careless smoking, alcohol or drug intoxication, and physical and mental disabilities. Occupation is also a factor, with electricians and chemical workers among those at greatest risk (Rutan, 1998).

Types of Burn Injury

The four types of burn injury are thermal, chemical, electrical, and radiation. Although all four types can lead to generalized tissue damage and multisystem involvement, the causative agents and priority treatment measures are unique to each.

Thermal Burns

Thermal burns result from exposure to dry heat (flames) or moist heat (steam and hot liquids). They are the most common burn injuries and occur most often in children and older adults. Direct exposure to the source of heat causes cellular destruction that can result in charring of vascular, bony, muscle, and nervous tissue.

Chemical Burns

Chemical burns are caused by direct skin contact with either acid or alkaline agents. More than 25,000 products found in the home or workplace can cause chemical burns. The chemical destroys tissue protein, leading to necrosis. Burns caused by alkalis, such as lye, are more difficult to neutralize than are burns caused by acids. They also tend to have deeper penetration with a correspondingly more severe burn than from acid. Organic compound burns, such as by petroleum distillates, cause cutaneous damage through fat solvent action and may also cause renal and liver failure if absorbed.

Chemical agents are further classified according to the manner by which they structurally alter proteins. Oxidizing agents, such as household bleach, alter protein configuration through the chemical process of reduction. Corrosives, such as lye, cause extensive protein denaturation. Protoplasmic poisons, such as organic compounds, form salts with proteins, inhibiting calcium and other ions needed for cell viability. The severity of the chemical burn is related to the type of agent, the concentration of the agent, the mechanism of action, the duration of contact, and the amount of body surface area exposed.

Electrical Burns

The severity of electrical burns depends on the type and duration of current, and amount of voltage. It is particularly difficult to assess the extent of the electrical burn injury, because the destructive processes initiated by the electrical insult are concealed and may persist for weeks beyond the time of the incident. It is difficult to assess the depth and extent of the burn, as electricity follows the path of least resistance, which in the human body tends to lie along muscles, bone, blood vessels, and nerves. Necrosis of the tissue results from impaired blood flow, secondary to blood coagulation at the site of the electrical injury. More than 90% of electrical burn wounds of the extremities that develop gangrene result in amputation.

Alternating current, as is found in conventional households, produces repeated electrical surges that lead to tetanic muscle contractions. Such sustained muscle contractions inhibit respiratory efforts for the duration of contact and result in respiratory arrest. The contractions also cause the person to clamp down on the power source, such as an electrical cord, and thus may increase the duration of contact with the source. Direct current, as in injury from a lightning bolt, exposes the body to very high voltage for an instantaneous period of time. High voltage (lightning) injury usually results in entry and exit wounds. The flash-over effect, a phenomenon unique to lightning injury, actually saves the client from death. It is seen in those instances in which the current travels over the moist surface of the skin rather than through deeper structures.

Radiation Burns

Radiation burns are usually associated with sunburn or radiation treatment for cancer. These kinds of burns tend to be superficial, involving only the outermost layers of the epidermis. All functions of the skin remain intact. Symptoms are limited to mild systemic reactions: headache, chills, local discomfort, nausea, and vomiting. More extensive exposure to radiation or radioactive substances, as in nuclear power accidents, leads to the same degree of tissue damage and multisystem involvement associated with other types of burns.

Factors Affecting Burn Classification

Tissue damage following a burn is determined primarily by two factors: depth of the burn (the layers of underlying tissue affected) and the extent of the burn (the percentage of body surface area involved).

Depth of the Burn

The depth of burn of injury is determined by the elements of the skin that have been damaged or destroyed. Burn depth results from a combination of the temperature of the burning agent and the length of contact. Burns are classified as either superficial, partial thickness, or full thickness.

Superficial Burns

A **superficial burn** (often called a first-degree burn) involves only the epidermal layer of the skin. This type of burn most often results from damage from sunburn, ultraviolet light, minor flash injury (from a sudden ignition or explosion), or mild radiation burn associated with cancer treatment. Because the skin remains intact, this degree of burn is not calculated into the estimates of burn injury. The skin color ranges from pink to bright red, and there may be slight edema over the burned area. Superficial burns involving large body surface areas may be manifested by chills, headache, nausea, and vomiting. The injury usually heals in three to six days, with dryness and peeling of the outer layer of skin. There is no scar formation. Superficial burns are treated with mild analgesics and the application of water-soluble lotions. Extensive superficial burns, especially in older adults, may require intravenous fluid treatment.

Partial-Thickness Burns

Partial-thickness burns (often called second-degree burns) may be subdivided into superficial partial-thickness and deep dermal partial-thickness burns. The classification depends on the depth of the burn.

A *superficial partial-thickness burn* involves the entire dermis and the papillae of the dermis. Causes may include such injuries as a brief exposure to flash flame or dilute chemical agents, or contact with a hot surface. This burn is often bright red, but has a moist, glistening appearance with blister formation. The burned area will blanch on pressure, and touch and pain sensation remain intact. Pain in response to temperature and air is usually severe. These injuries heal within 21 days with minimal or no scarring, but pigment changes are common. Analgesics are administered, and if large blistered areas are disrupted, skin substitutes may be used.

A *deep partial-thickness burn* also involves the entire dermis, but extends further into the dermis than a superficial partial-thickness burn. Hair follicles, sebaceous glands, and epidermal sweat glands remain intact (Porth, 2002). Hot liquids or solids, flash flame, direct flame, intense radiant energy, or chemical agents may cause this level of burn wound. The surface of the burn wound appears pale and waxy and may be moist or dry. Large, easily ruptured blisters may be present, or the blisters may look like flat, dry tissue paper. Capillary refill is decreased, and sensation to deep pressure is present. The burn wound is less painful than a superficial partial-thickness burn, but areas of pain and areas of decreased sensation may be present. Deep partial-thickness burn wounds often require more than 21 days for healing and may convert to a full-thickness injury as necrosis extends the depth of the wound. Contractures are possible, as are hypertrophic scarring and functional impairment. Excision and grafting may be necessary to decrease scarring and loss of function.

Full-Thickness Burns

A **full-thickness burn** (often called a third-degree burn) involves all layers of the skin, including the epidermis, the dermis, and the epidermal appendages. The burn wound may extend into the subcutaneous fat, connective tissue, muscle, and bone. Full-thickness burns are caused by prolonged contact with flames, steam, chemicals, or high-voltage electric current.

Depending on the cause of injury, the burn wound may appear pale, waxy, yellow, brown, mottled, charred, or nonblanching red. The wound surface is dry, leathery, and firm to the touch. Thrombosed blood vessels may be visible under the surface of the wound. There is no sensation of pain or light touch, as pain and touch receptors have been destroyed. Full-thickness burns require skin grafting to heal.

Extent of the Burn

The extent of the burn injury is expressed as a percentage of the total body surface area (TBSA). There are several methods used for determining the extent of injury. The "rule of nines" is a rapid method of estimation used during the prehospital and emergency care phases. In this method, the body is divided into five surface areas—head, trunk, arms, legs, and perineum—and percentages that equal or total a sum of nines are assigned to each body area. For example, a client with burns of the face, anterior right arm, and anterior trunk has burn injury involving 27% of the total body surface area (in this example, face = 4.5%, arm = 4.5%, and trunk = 18% to total 27%). Only partial- and full-thickness burns are included in the estimation.

On the client's admission to the hospital, critical care area, or burn center, more accurate methods for estimating the extent of injury are employed. For example, the Lund and Browder method determines surface area measurements for each body part according to the age of the client.

A recognized system for describing a burn injury, developed by the American Burn Association, uses both the extent and depth of burn to classify burns as minor, moderate, or major.

Burn Wound Healing

Burns heal in the same processes as do other wounds, but the wound healing phases occur more slowly and last longer. The healing process involves four phases: hemostasis, inflammation, proliferation, and remodeling. The following physiologic events occur (Carrougher, 1998):

* *Hemostasis.* Immediately following the injury, platelets coming in contact with the damaged tissue aggregate and degranulate (releasing growth factors). Fibrin is deposited, trapping further platelets, and a thrombus is formed. The thrombus, combined with local vasoconstriction, leads to hemostasis which walls off the wound from the systemic circulation.

* *Inflammation.* Local vasodilation and an increase in capillary permeability follows hemostasis. Neutrophils infiltrate the wound and peak in about 24 hours, and then monocytes predominate. The monocytes are converted into macrophages, which consume pathogens and dead tissue, and also secrete various growth factors. These growth factors stimulate the proliferation of fibroblasts and a deposit of a provisional wound matrix.

* *Proliferation.* Within three to four days postburn, fibroblasts are the major cell within the wound. Their number peaks at about 14 days after the injury. Granulation tissue

begins to form, with complete reepithelialization occurring during this stage. Epithelial cells cover the wound as each cell stretches across the wound surface to join with other epithelial cell sheets or the other side of the wound. The proliferation phase lasts until complete reepithelialization occurs, by epithelial cell migration, surgical intervention, or a combination of the two.

- *Remodeling.* This phase may last for years. Collagen fibers, laid down during the proliferative phase, are reorganized into more compact areas. Scars contract and fade in color. In normal healing following a minor burn injury, the newly formed skin closely resembles its neighboring tissue. However, when a burn injury extends into the dermal layer of skin, two types of excessive scar may develop. A **hypertrophic scar** is an overgrowth of dermal tissue that remains within the boundaries of the wound. A **keloid** is a scar that extends beyond the boundaries of the original wound. People with dark skin are at greater risk for hypertrophic scars and keloids.

The Client with a Minor Burn

Minor burn injuries consist of superficial burns that are not extensive, superficial split-thickness burns that involve less than 15% of TBSA, and full-thickness burns that involve less than 2% of TBSA, excluding the special care areas (eyes, ears, face, hands, feet, perineum, and joints). Minor burn injuries are not associated with immunosuppression, hypermetabolism, or increased susceptibility to infection.

A minor burn injury is usually treated in an outpatient facility. The goal of therapy is to promote wound healing, eliminate discomfort, maintain mobility, and prevent infection.

Pathophysiology

Sunburn

Sunburns result from exposure to ultraviolet light. Such injuries, which tend to be superficial, are more commonly seen in clients with lighter skin. Because the skin remains intact, the manifestations in most cases are mild and are limited to pain, nausea, vomiting, skin redness, chills, and headache. Treatment is performed on an outpatient basis and generally consists of applying mild lotions, increasing liquid intake, administering mild analgesics, and maintaining warmth. Older adults should be monitored for evidence of dehydration. Proper use of sunscreen and limiting sun exposure to the less hazardous hours of the day (before 10 A.M. and after 3 P.M.) can prevent sunburn.

Scald Burn

Minor scald burns result from exposure to moist heat and involve superficial and superficial split-thickness burns of less than 15% of TBSA. The goals of therapy are to prevent wound contamination and to promote healing. The nurse teaches the client to apply antibiotic solutions and light dressings and to maintain adequate nutritional intake. Mild analgesics may be ordered to help the client carry out activities of daily living. Tetanus toxoid is administered as appropriate.

Collaborative Care

In the outpatient facility, the wound may be washed with mild soap and water. Tar and asphalt can be removed with mineral oil, petroleum ointments, or Medisol (a citrus and petroleum distillate with hydrocarbon structure). Tetanus toxoid booster is recommended for all clients whose immunization histories are in doubt. Although controversy regarding the care of blisters remains, blisters may be managed in one of three ways: left intact, evacuated, or debrided. Follow-up care for the minor burn injury includes twice daily wound cleansing with application of bland ointment, range-of-motion exercises to affected joints, and weekly clinic appointments until the wound heals completely.

Nursing Care

Although the nurse seldom treats the minor burn in the acute care environment, the burn treatment methods used in the outpatient setting follow the same standard approaches to care. General nursing measures include taking the history, estimating the extent and depth of the injury, cleansing the wound, applying topical agents, dressing the wound, controlling pain, and establishing follow-up care.

Home Care

The nurse should address the following topics to facilitate self-care at home of minor burns.

- How to identify and report manifestations of impaired wound healing:
  1. Change in healthy appearance of the wound (altered skin integrity, swelling, blister formation, erythema).
  2. Signs of infection (fever, purulent drainage, foul odor).
- Wound care:
  1. Daily cleansing with mild soap and water.
  2. Using sterile technique to change dressings.
  3. Correct application of ordered topical agents.
- Pain management:
  1. Use mild analgesics as ordered.
  2. Use alternative pain management therapies.

The Client with a Major Burn

A major burn involves serious injury to the underlying layers of skin and covers a large body surface area. The American Burn Association defines a major burn as one that involves:

- >25% TBSA in adults less than 40 years of age.
- >20% TBSA in adults more than 40 years of age.
- >10% TBSA full-thickness burn.
- Injuries to the face, eyes, ears, hands, feet, or perineum.
- High-voltage electrical injuries.
- All burn injuries with inhalation injury or major trauma.

Pathophysiology

The pathophysiologic changes that result from major burn injuries involve all body systems. Extensive loss of skin (the body's protective barrier) can result in massive infection, fluid and electrolyte imbalances, and hypothermia. Often the person inhales the products of combustion, thus compromising respiratory function. Cardiac dysrhythmias and circulatory failure are common manifestations of serious burn injuries. A profound catabolic state dramatically increases caloric expenditure and nutritional deficiencies. An alteration in gastrointestinal motility predisposes the client to developing paralytic ileus, and hyperacidity leads to gastric and duodenal ulcerations. Dehydration slows glomerular filtration rates and renal clearance of toxic wastes and may lead to acute tubular necrosis and renal failure. Overall body metabolism may be profoundly altered.

Integumentary System

Heat transfer to skin is a complex phenomenon. If the microcirculation of the skin remains intact during burning, it cools and protects the deeper portions of the skin and cools the outer surface once the heat source is removed. With extensive burn injury, the integrity of the microcirculation is lost, and the burning process continues even after the heat source is removed.

Burns have a characteristic skin surface appearance that resembles a bull's-eye, with the most severe burn located centrally and the lesser burns located along the peripheral wound edges. Depending on their intensity, burns consist of one, two, or three concentric three-dimensional zones closely corresponding on the skin surface to the depth of the burn.

- The outer zone of hyperemia blanches on pressure and heals in two to seven days postburn.
- The medial zone of stasis is initially moist, red, and blistered and blanches on pressure. It becomes pale and necrotic on days three to seven postburn.
- The inner zone of coagulation immediately appears leathery and coagulated. It merges with the necrotic zone of stasis in three to seven days postburn.

The overall thickness of the dermis and epidermis varies considerably from one area of the body to another. Similar temperatures produce different depths of injury to different body parts. For example, in the adult, skin covering the medial aspect of the forearm is thinner and more easily damaged than the skin covering the back of the same person. Skin dissipates heat maximally in areas of greatest vascularization. When heat absorption exceeds the rate of dissipation, cellular temperatures rise, and skin tissue is destroyed.

The burn injury results in the formation of necrotic skin and subcutaneous tissue. During the acute stage of the injury, a hard crust (**eschar**) forms, which covers the wound and harbors necrotic tissue. The eschar is characteristically leathery and rigid. Removal of the eschar facilitates healing.

Cardiovascular System

The effects of a major burn are manifested in all components of the vascular system, and include hypovolemic shock (burn shock); cardiac dysrhythmias, such as ventricular fibrillation); cardiac arrest; and vascular compromise.

Hypovolemic Shock (Burn Shock)

Within minutes of the burn injury, a cascade of cellular events is initiated, and a massive amount of fluid shifts from the intracellular and intravascular compartments into the interstitium. This shift is a type of hypovolemic shock called **burn shock,** and it continues until capillary integrity is restored, usually within 24 to 36 hours of the injury. Although the pathophysiologic mechanisms of postburn vascular changes and fluid volume shifts are not clearly understood, three processes occur early in the postburn phase in clients with ≥ 40% TBSA:

- Increase in microvascular permeability at the burn wound site.
- Generalized impairment of cell wall function, resulting in intracellular edema.
- Increase in osmotic pressure of the burned tissue, leading to extensive fluid accumulation.

During burn shock, the shifting of fluid is the direct result of a loss of cell wall integrity at the site of injury and in the capillary bed. Fluid leaks from the capillaries into interstitial compartments located at the burn wound site and throughout the body, resulting in a decrease in fluid volume within the intravascular space. Plasma proteins and sodium escape into the interstitium, enhancing edema formation. Blood pressure falls as cardiac output diminishes.

Vasoconstriction results as the vascular system attempts to compensate for fluid loss. Abnormal platelet aggregation and white blood cell (WBC) accumulation result in ischemia in the deeper tissue below the burn, leading to eventual thrombosis. Red blood cells (RBCs) and WBCs remain in the circulation, producing an elevation in erythrocyte and leukocyte counts secondary to hemoconcentration.

The leakage of fluid into the interstitium compromises the lymphatic system, resulting in intravascular hypovolemia and edema at the burn wound site. Edematous body surfaces impair peripheral circulation and result in necrosis of the underlying tissue. During burn shock, potassium ions leave the intracellular compartment, predisposing the client to developing cardiac dysrhythmias. The process of burn shock continues until capillary integrity is restored, usually within 24 hours of the injury.

Burn shock reverses when fluid is reabsorbed from the interstitium into the intravascular compartment. The blood pressure rises as cardiac output increases, and urinary output improves. Diuresis continues from several days to two weeks postburn. During this phase, the extra cardiac workload may predispose the older client, or the client with cardiovascular disease, to fluid volume overload.

Cardiac Rhythm Alterations

Burns of more than 40% TBSA cause significant myocardial dysfunction, with a decrease in myocardial contractibility and cardiac output. These changes, which occur prior to a decrease in plasma volume, are believed to be due to the release of substances and oxygen-free radicals from the burn wound and from ischemic myocardial cells. Electrical burns often result in cardiac dysrrhythmias or cardiac arrest caused by heat damage to the myocardium or electrical interference with cardiac electrical activity.

Peripheral Vascular Compromise

Direct heat damage to extremities, especially if circumferential burns are present, results in damage to blood vessels. Circulation to extremities may be further impaired by edema and by peripheral vasoconstriction that occurs during burn shock. In addition, **compartment syndrome** (in which the tissue pressure within a muscle compartment exceeds microvascular pressure, interrupting cellular perfusion) may result from circumferential burns and edema.

Respiratory System

Pulmonary damage may result from either direct inhalation injury or as part of the systemic response to the injury. Inhalation injury is a frequent and often lethal complication of burns. The injury may range from mild respiratory inflammation to massive pulmonary failure. Exposure to heat, asphyxiants, and smoke initiates the pathophysiologic process associated with inhalation injury.

Inflammation occurs at localized sites within the airway and is manifested as hyperemia. As a result, cells are destroyed and the bronchial cilia are rendered inactive. Because the mucociliary transport mechanism no longer functions, the client may develop bronchial congestion and infection.

Interstitial pulmonary edema develops secondary to the escape of fluid from the pulmonary vasculature into the interstitial compartment of the lung tissue. Surfactant is inactivated, resulting in atelectasis and alveolar collapse. Sloughing of the damaged and dead lung tissue occasionally produces debris that may lead to complete airway obstruction.

Upper airway (above the level of the glottis) thermal injury results from the inhalation of heated air or chemicals dissolved in water. Physical findings include the presence of soot, charring, edema, blisters, and ulcerations along the mucosal lining of the oropharynx and larynx. The resulting edema in the airway peaks within the first 24 to 48 hours of injury. Lower airway thermal injury is a rare occurrence. Because the lower airway is protected by laryngeal reflexes, thermal injury below the vocal cords is seldom seen. However, when it does occur, it is typically associated with the inhalation of steam or explosive gases or the aspiration of hot liquids.

Smoke poisoning results when toxic gases and particulate matter, the products of incomplete combustion, deposit directly onto the pulmonary mucosa. The composition of the products of combustion depends on the combustible material, the rate at which the temperature increases, and the amount of ambient oxygen present. Irritant gases and particulate matter have a direct cytotoxic effect. The degree of injury is determined by their solubility in water, duration of exposure, and the size of the particulate or aerosol droplet.

Carbon monoxide, a common asphyxiant, is a colorless, tasteless, odorless gas that has a 200 times greater affinity for hemoglobin than does oxygen. It displaces oxygen to bind with hemoglobin, forming carboxyhemoglobin. As a result, the decrease in arterial oxyhemoglobin produces tissue hypoxia. Carbon monoxide impairs both oxygen delivery and cellular oxygen use.

Gastrointestinal System

Dysfunction of the gastrointestinal system is directly related to the size of the burn wound. Clients with ≥ 20% TBSA experience decreased peristalsis with resultant gastric distention and increased risk of aspiration. A decrease in or absence of bowel sounds is a manifestation of paralytic ileus (adynamic bowel) secondary to burn trauma. The resulting cessation of intestinal motility leads to gastric distention, nausea, vomiting, and hematemesis.

Stress ulcers (**Curling's ulcers**) are acute ulcerations of the stomach or duodenum that form following the burn injury. Abdominal pain, acidic gastric pH levels, hematemesis, and melana in the stool may indicate a gastric ulcer.

In addition, ischemia of the intestine from splanchnic vasoconstriction increases the intestinal mucosal permeability. As a result, normal intestinal bacteria move from the lumen of the bowel to extraluminal sites, a process called *bacterial translocation*. This process is believed to be one of the mechanisms causing systemic sepsis and multiple organ dysfunction syndrome.

Urinary System

During the early stages of the burn injury, renal blood flow and glomerular filtration rates are greatly reduced from the decreased intravascular blood volume and the release of antidiuretic hormone (ADH) by the posterior pituitary. Urine output decreases, and serum creatinine and blood urea nitrogen increase.

Dark brown concentrated urine may indicate myoglobinuria, the result of the release of large amounts of dead or damaged erythrocytes after a major burn injury. When large amounts of these pigments are released, the liver cannot keep pace with conjugation and the pigments pass through the glomeruli. The pigments can occlude the renal tubules and cause renal failure, especially when dehydration, acidosis, or shock is also present.

Immune System

The function of the immune system is to protect the human body from invasion by foreign microorganisms. The capillary leak that occurs in the early stages of the burn injury continues throughout the burn shock phase and impairs the active components of both the cell-mediated and humoral immune systems.

The humoral immune system relies on B cells to produce antibodies or immunoglobulins (see Chapter 42). In the burn client, the serum levels of all immunoglobulins are significantly diminished. Serum protein levels remain persistently low throughout the clinical course until wound closure is effected. A marked decrease in T-cell counts results in a reduction of cytotoxic activity and suppression of the cell-mediated immune system.

The compromise in the humoral and cell-mediated immune systems constitutes a state of acquired immunodeficiency, which places the burn client at risk for infection. The period of vulnerability is transient and may last from one to four weeks following the onset of the burn injury. During this time frame, opportunistic infections can be fatal despite aggressive antimicrobial therapy.

Metabolism

Two distinct phases characterize the body's metabolic response to the burn injury. The ebb phase, occurring during the first three days of the injury, is manifested by decreased oxygen consumption, fluid imbalance, shock, and inadequate circulating volume. These responses protect the body from the initial impact of the injury.

A second phase, the flow phase, occurs when adequate burn resuscitation has been accomplished. This phase is characterized by increases in cellular activity and protein catabolism, lipolysis, and gluconeogenesis. The basal metabolic rate (BMR) significantly increases, reaching twice the normal rate. Body weight and heat drop dramatically. Total energy expenditure may exceed 100% of normal BMR. Hypermetabolism persists until after wound closure has been accomplished and may reappear if complications occur.

Collaborative Care

The burn team is composed of an interdisciplinary group of health care professionals, who together plan the care and treatment of the burn-injured client during the acute and rehabilitative stages. The burn team consists of the nurse, physician, physical therapist, dietitian, social worker, and burn technician. The team members meet regularly to discuss client progress and to determine collaboratively the most effective regimen of care and psychosocial support.

Stages of Collaborative Care

The clinical course of treatment for the burn client is divided into three stages: the emergent/resuscitative stage, the acute stage, and the rehabilitative stage. Although these stages are useful predictors of the clinical needs of the burn client, it is important to recognize that the process of burn injury is dynamic and that, in many cases, the clinical stage may not be clearly delineated. Assessment and management of the burn-injured client are ongoing processes determined by the clinical picture; they last throughout the course of treatment. During each stage, different groups of nurses, physicians, and allied health care specialists collaborate to manage the client's recovery.

The Emergent/Resuscitative Stage

The emergent/resuscitative stage lasts from the onset of injury through successful fluid resuscitation. During this stage, health care workers estimate the extent of burn injury, institute first-aid measures, and implement fluid resuscitation therapies. The client is assessed for shock and evidence of respiratory distress. If indicated, intravenous lines are inserted, and the client may be prophylactically intubated. During this stage, health care workers determine whether the client is to be transported to a burn center for the complex intervention strategies of the professional, interdisciplinary burn team.

Although many burn injuries are treated in local tertiary care facilities, the American Burn Association has developed guidelines for determining whether the client should be transported to a burn center for interdisciplinary approaches to treatment and rehabilitation. Adult clients who should be treated at burn centers include those with:

- Second- or third-degree burns >10% TBSA and older than 50 years of age.
- Second- or third-degree burns >20% TBSA in adults to the age of 50.
- Third-degree burns >5% TBSA in adults of any age.
- Burns involving the hands, feet, face, eyes, ears, or perineum.
- Electrical (including lightning), chemical, and inhalation injuries.
- Circumferential burns of the extremities and/or chest.
- Any burn associated with extenuating problems, preexisting illness, fractures, or other trauma.

Acute Stage

The acute stage begins with the start of diuresis and ends with closure of the burn wound (either by natural healing or by using skin grafts). During this stage, wound care management, nutritional therapies, and measures to control infectious processes are initiated. Hydrotherapy and excision and grafting of full-thickness wounds are performed as soon as possible after injury. Enteral and parenteral nutritional interventions are started early in the treatment plan to address caloric needs resulting from extensive energy expenditure. Measures to combat infection are implemented during this stage, including the administration of topical and systemic antimicrobial agents. Pain management constitutes a significant segment of the nursing care plan throughout the clinical course of the burn-injured client. The administration of narcotic pharmaceutical agents must precede all invasive procedures to maximize client comfort and to reduce the anxieties associated with wound debridement and intensive physical therapy.

Rehabilitative Stage

The rehabilitative stage begins with wound closure and ends when the client returns to the highest level of health restoration, which may take years. During this stage, the primary focus is the biopsychosocial adjustment of the client, specifically the prevention of contractures and scars and the client's successful resumption of work, family, and social roles through physical, vocational, occupational, and psychosocial rehabilitation. The client is taught to perform range-of-motion exercises to enhance mobility and to support injured joints.

Prehospital Client Management

Treatment at the injury scene includes measures to limit the severity of the burn and support vital functions. Before attempting to remove the client from the source of burn injury, rescuers must ensure their own safety. Depending on the causative agent, rescuers may need to consult with experts to determine the best way to eliminate the source of the injury. Once the safety of the rescuers has been established, all prehospital interventions are aimed at eliminating the heat source, stabilizing the client's condition, identifying the type of burn, preventing heat loss, reducing wound contamination, and preparing for emergency transport. Restrictive jewelry and clothing is removed at the scene to prevent circumferential constriction of the torso and extremities.

Stop the Burning Process

Emergency measures, by type of injury, include:

Thermal Burns. If the thermal injury has been caused by dry heat, smother inflamed clothing or lavage with water. Help the person "stop, drop, and roll" to extinguish the flame and limit the extent of burn. Once the flame has been extinguished, cover the body to prevent hypothermia. If the thermal injury has been caused by moist heat, lavage the area with cool water. Ice is not used for cooling as it causes vasoconstriction and may result in further injury.

Chemical Burns. For chemical burns, immediately remove the clothing and use a hose or shower to lavage the involved area thoroughly for a minimum of 20 minutes. Many chemicals are in powder form and as much dry chemical needs to be removed as possible before flushing the surface with water. Unusual chemicals may require consultation with the poison control center about appropriate treatment. Protective clothing should be worn during this process to protect the rescuer from chemical exposure.

Electrical Burns. Electrical injuries pose serious potential harm to both rescuer and burn victim. Ensure that the source of electrical current has been disconnected, or move the person to safety and away from the energy source using a nonconductive device, such as a broomstick. If the person is unresponsive, assess for the presence of cardiac and respiratory function. If indicated, begin cardiopulmonary resuscitation (CPR). A spinal cord injury may be present secondary to the forceful contraction of the muscles of the neck and back during exposure to the current. If possible, place the person in a cervical collar and transport on a spinal board.

Radiation Burns. Radiation injuries are usually minor and involve only the epidermal layer of skin. Treatment focuses on helping normal body mechanisms promote wound healing. For severe radiation burns, such as those that result from industrial radiation accidents, trained personnel may need to render the area safe for entry prior to rescue. All interventions are aimed at shielding, establishing distance, and limiting the time of exposure to the radioactive source.

Support Vital Function

The initial assessment of the client's respiratory and hemodynamic status begins with an evaluation of the client's airway, breathing, and circulation (the ABCs of care).

*   If the client has no pulse and is not breathing, begin CPR. Establish an airway, and start mouth-to-mouth breathing and chest compressions. Continue CPR until spontaneous cardiopulmonary function returns or until the emergency management team takes over.

*   Position the client with the head elevated at greater than 30 degrees, and administer 100% humidified oxygen by face mask. Use nasotracheal suction as necessary to maintain a patent airway. Endotracheal intubation may be necessary if the client has facial edema and inhalation injury. Auscultate the lungs often onsite to monitor respiratory status. Continuous pulse oximetry provides ongoing assessment of the client's oxygen saturation levels.

*   Monitor for cardiac dysrrhythmias or arrest. When available, connect the client to a cardiac monitor and observe for dysrhythmias. Elevate burned extremities above the level of the heart to facilitate circulation.

*   Initiate fluid replacement therapy for burn wounds that involve more than 20% of the total body surface area. Continuously assess heart and lung sounds and observe level of consciousness, cardiac rate and rhythm, blood pressure, and urine output.

*   Cover the client to maintain body temperature and to prevent further wound contamination and tissue damage.

Emergency and Acute Care

Prehospital personnel report to the emergency department staff all findings and medical interventions that occurred at the scene of the injury. The nurse obtains a history of the injury, estimates the depth and extent of the burn, begins fluid resuscitation, and maintains ventilation according to protocol.

Fluid Resuscitation

Fluid resuscitation is the administration of intravenous fluids to restore the circulating blood volume during the acute period of increasing capillary permeability. To counteract the effects of burn shock, fluid resuscitation guidelines are used to replace the extensive fluid and electrolyte losses associated with major burn injuries. Fluid replacement is necessary in all burn wounds that involve ≥ 20% TBSA.

Crystalloid fluids are administered through two large-bore (14 to 16 gauge) catheters, preferably inserted through unburned skin. Warmed Ringer's lactate solution is the intravenous fluid most widely used during the first 24 hours after burn injury, as it most closely approximates the body's extracellular fluid composition. Several formulas may be used to replace fluid loss. Two commonly used formulas are as follows:

- Parkland formula, in which lactated Ringer's solution is administered 4 mL X kg X % TBSA burn.

- Modified Brooke formula, in which lactated Ringer's solution is administered 2 mL X kg X % TBSA burn.

These formulas specify the volume of fluid to be infused in the first 24 hours after the injury, with 50% of the fluid to be infused during the first 8 hours, followed by the remaining 50% over the next 16 hours (25% per 8 hours). Over the second 24 hours, fluids for clients with larger burns, such as more than 30% TBSA, are changed to a crystalloid solution of 5% dextrose in water titrated to maintain urine output (Bucher & Melander, 1999).

Hourly urine output is often used as the indicator of effective fluid resuscitation, with 30 to 50 cc for an adult considered adequate. (With electrical burns, a urine output of 75 to 100 cc should be maintained). Another valuable indicator is heart rate; if fluid resuscitation is adequate, the rate should be less than 120 beats per minute or in the upper limits of normal for age. A higher rate may indicate a need for additional fluid (Bucher & Melander, 1999).

During the fluid resuscitation stage, the client may require invasive hemodynamic monitoring. A pulmonary artery catheter can be used to monitor cardiac output, cardiac index, and pulmonary artery wedge pressures. All measurements must be maintained within normal limits to effect adequate fluid resuscitation.

Respiratory Management

Upon the client's admission to the emergency department, several baseline assessments of respiratory status must be obtained: chest X-ray study, ABGs, vital signs, and carboxyhemoglobin levels. Intubation is indicated for all clients with burns of the chest, face, or neck. The primary treatment plan is oriented toward preventing atelectasis and maintaining alveolar oxygen exchange. The following interventions should be initiated:

- Maintain the head of the bed at 30 degrees or greater to maximize the client's ventilatory efforts. Turn the client side to side every two hours to prevent hypostatic pneumonia.

- To keep airway passages clear, suction the client frequently, encourage the client to use incentive spirometry hourly, and help the client perform coughing and deep-breathing exercises every two hours.

- In the face of impending airway obstruction, the client will require intubation. Nasotracheal tube placement is the preferred route because it seems to be better tolerated and can be more effectively secured. If the client has suffered nasolabial burns, however, the orotracheal route is preferred. Nasotracheal and orotracheal intubation is reserved for short-term ventilatory management. For long-term ventilatory management (i.e., greater than three weeks), a tracheostomy is performed.

- Humidification of either room air or oxygen helps prevent the drying of tracheal secretions. Ambient air or oxygen flow is based on ABG results. The client may be placed on a face mask, steam collar, T-piece, mechanical ventilation with PEEP, pressure support ventilation, or high-frequency jet ventilation. The goal of all therapies is to maintain adequate tissue oxygenation with the least amount of inspired oxygen flow necessary.

- Medications to dilate constricted bronchial passages are administered intravenously and as inhalants to control bronchospasms and wheezing. Mucolytic agents liquefy tenacious sputum and aid in expectoration.
- An arterial line is placed in the client with major burn injury for continuous assessment of ABGs. Pulmonary artery pressure catheters may be inserted to measure pulmonary vascular resistance (PVR), pulmonary artery pressure (PAP), pulmonary capillary wedge pressure (PCWP), and mixed venous oxygen saturation (SVO2). The PVR and PAP rise in the presence of hypoxia. The SVO2 is the average percentage of hemoglobin bound with oxygen in the venous blood and reflects overall tissue utilization of oxygen. Pulse oximetry monitors arterial oxygen saturation levels.
- Pain medications are administered if the client is not in shock.

After stabilization in the emergency department, the client is transferred to the critical care unit or a specialized burn center (a facility that has a burn physician as director of a specialized nursing unit with dedicated burn beds). In both settings, continuous monitoring of diagnostic tests, administration of medications, pain control, wound management, and nutrition support therapies constitute the initial plan of care.

Diagnostic Tests

The following diagnostic tests are used to evaluate the client's progress and to modify intervention strategies:

- *Urinalysis* indicates the adequacy of renal perfusion and the client's nutritional status. In catabolic states, nitrogen is excreted in large amounts into the urine. Nitrogen loss is measured through 24-hour urine collections for total nitrogen, urea nitrogen, and amino acid nitrogen. *Myoglobinuria,* which manifests as a dark brown, wine-colored urine, signals the development of acute tubular necrosis. Loss of plasma protein and dehydration lead to proteinuria and elevated urine specific gravity. Glycosuria is a transient development following major burn injury; it indicates a need to adjust the nutritional program.
- The *complete blood count* is monitored regularly. Hematocrit is elevated secondary to hemoconcentration and fluid shifts from the intravascular compartment. Hemoglobin is decreased secondary to hemolysis. White blood cells are elevated if infection is present.
- *Serum electrolytes* are monitored regularly. Sodium levels are decreased secondary to massive fluid shifts into the interstitium. Potassium levels initially are elevated during burn shock, as a result of cell lysis and fluid shifts into the extracellular space. Potassium levels decrease after burn shock resolves, as fluid shifts back to intracellular and intravascular compartments.
- *Renal function* test results are closely monitored. Blood urea nitrogen (BUN) is elevated secondary to dehydration. Creatinine is elevated in the presence of renal insufficiency.
- *Total protein, albumin, transferrin, prealbumin, retinol binding protein, alpha 1-acid glycoprotein, and C-reactive protein* indicate protein synthesis and nutritional status. Because of the fluid shifts that occur during the early stages of the burn injury, they are more useful markers during the rehabilitative phase of care.
- *Creatine phosphokinase (CPK)* is elevated following an electrical burn, secondary to extensive muscle damage.

- *Blood glucose* is transiently elevated after major burn injury.

- *Serial ABGs* indicate the presence of hypoxia and acid-base disturbances, and indicate client responses to changes in oxygen therapies. The burn-injured client may demonstrate elevated or lowered pH, decreased Pco_2, decreased Po_2, and low-normal bicarbonate levels.

- *Pulse oximetry* allows continuous assessment of oxygen saturation levels. The burn-injured client may have saturation levels below 95%.

- *Serial chest X-ray* studies document changes within the first 24 to 48 hours that may reflect the presence of atelectasis, pulmonary edema, or acute respiratory disease (ARD).

- *Serial electrocardiograms (EKGs)* are necessary to monitor the development of dysrhythmias, especially those associated with hypokalemic and hyperkalemic states.

Medications

Pain Control

Burns often cause excruciating pain. In the early stages of care, intravenously administered narcotics, such as morphine, meperidine, or fentanyl, are the best means of managing pain. Morphine is the drug of choice. Once the client has been stabilized, it is appropriate to administer narcotics prior to initiating hydrotherapy or intensive exercising routines. The oral, subcutaneous, or intramuscular route of administration should be avoided until hemodynamic stability and unimpaired tissue perfusion returns.

As the client enters the rehabilitative stage of care, alternative therapies for pain control may be added to the plan of care. Distraction, self-hypnosis, guided imagery, and relaxation techniques are helpful adjuncts in managing pain and coping with loss. Patient-controlled analgesia (PCA) enhances the client's ability to cope with pain. See Chapter 38 for a discussion of strategies for managing pain.

Antimicrobial Agents

Systemic infection is a leading cause of death in major burn patients. Gram-positive organisms, such as Staphylococcus and Streptococcus colonize the burn surface during the first week postburn; gram-negative enteric organisms become more common with longer periods of hospitalization. To eliminate infection on the surface of the burn wound, topical antimicrobial therapy is used, depending on protocol. Of the many antimicrobial agents available, the three most widely used are mafenide acetate (Sulfamylon) cream, sulfadiazine (Silvadene) cream, and silver nitrate 0.5% soaks. All three are broad-spectrum antibiotics. The choice of topical antibiotic is based on the extent of the burn wound, the presence of identified bacterial organisms, whether an open (exposing the wound to the air) or closed (using bulky dressings) method of treatment is used, and client response.

The increasing trend is toward prophylactic antibiotic administration in burn clients (Tierney, McPhee, & Papadakis, 2001). Systemic antimicrobial therapy is indicated in the immediate preoperative and postoperative period associated with excision and autografting. Postoperatively, the therapy is discontinued as soon as the client's hemodynamic status returns to normal, usually within the first 24 hours. In the long-term treatment of identified infectious processes, drug administration is limited to the least amount of time required to eradicate the infection.

Tetanus Prophylaxis

If the client's immunization status is in doubt, tetanus toxoid is administered intramuscularly early in the acute phase of care to prevent *Clostridium tetani* infection.

Preventing Gastric Hyperacidity

Hyperacidity must be controlled to prevent Curling's ulcer. A nasogastric tube is placed during the emergent phase of care, and gastric aspirant is obtained hourly. The gastric pH should be assessed and maintained at levels above 5. To control gastric acid secretion during the acute phase of care, histamine H_2 blockers (e.g., famotidine [Pepcid] and ranitidine [Zantac]) can be administered intravenously, either intermittently or as continuous infusions. As soon as bowel sounds become audible, the client is placed on an antacid regimen.

Treatments

Surgery

Three surgical interventions are commonly employed to manage the burn wound: surgical debridement, escharotomy, and autografting.

Escharotomy. When the burn eschar forms circumferentially around the torso or extremities, it acts as a tourniquet, impairing circulation. Left unchecked, the affected body part becomes gangrenous.

To prevent circumferential constriction of the torso or extremity, an **escharotomy** is performed by the physician with a scalpel or by electrocautery. A sterile surgical incision is made longitudinally along the extremity or the trunk to release taut skin and allow for expansion caused by edema formation. In the first 24 hours following the procedure, the incision should be gently packed with fine mesh gauze. After 24 hours, the site may be treated with a direct application of a topical antimicrobial agent.

Surgical Debridement. **Surgical debridement** refers to the process of excising the wound to the level of fascia (fascial excision) or sequentially removing thin slices of the burn wound to the level of viable tissue (sequential excision). Because **fascial excision,** or **fasciectomy,** sacrifices potentially viable fat and lymphatic tissue, its use is reserved for clients with extensive or full-thickness burns. The most common technique is electrocautery with cutting and coagulating current capabilities. Sequential excision is performed with the use of a dermatome. Shallow burns and some of moderate depth bleed briskly after one slice. If bleeding does not occur, the procedure is repeated until a viable bed of dermis or subcutaneous fat is reached. Following surgical debridement, the client is returned to the burn unit.

Autografting. A procedure performed in the surgical suite, **autografting** is used to effect permanent skin coverage. Early burn wound excision and skin grafting decreases the hospital stay and enhances rehabilitation. Skin is removed from healthy tissue (donor site) of the burn-injured client and applied to the burn wound. After the autograft is applied, the grafted area is immobilized. The site is assessed daily for evidence of adherence. The client resumes range-of-motion exercises five days postgraft. As the wound heals, the client may complain of itching, which can be treated with mild lotions.

Cultured epithelial autografting is a technique in which skin cells are removed from unburned sites on the client's body, then minced and placed in a culture medium for growth. Over a 5- to 7-day period, the cells expand 50 to 70 times the size of the initial biopsies. The cells are again separated out and placed in a new culture medium for continued growth. With this technique, enough skin can be grown over a period of three to four weeks to cover an entire human body. The cells are prepared in sheets and attached to petroleum jelly gauze backing, which is applied to the burn wound site. Problems with infection and lack of attachment have occurred.

Biologic and Biosynthetic Dressings

The terms *biologic dressing* and *biosynthetic dressing* refer to any temporary material that rapidly adheres to the wound bed, promotes healing, and/or prepares the burn wound for permanent autograft coverage. Ideally, these kinds of dressings should be easy to apply and remove, inexpensive, nonantigenic, elastic, able to reduce pain, able to serve as a bacterial barrier, and able to enhance the natural healing process. The dressings are applied to the burn wound as soon as possible. Covering the wound eliminates the loss of water through evaporation, reduces infection, and promotes wound healing. Biologic and biosynthetic dressings that are currently in use include homograft (allograft), heterograft (xenograft), amnionic membranes, and synthetic materials.

Homograft, or **allograft,** is human skin that has been harvested from cadavers. It is stored in skin banks located throughout the nation. The development of methods to achieve prolonged storage of frozen, viable skin has increased the use of this dressing; however, its short supply and expense still pose problems. It is manufactured as strips cut to the pattern of the burn and applied using sterile technique. Under normal circumstances, a homograft is rejected within 14 to 21 days following application.

Heterograft, or **xenograft,** is skin obtained from an animal, usually a pig. Although fresh porcine heterograft is available to some centers, frozen heterograft is much more commonly used. Once applied, heterograft appears to undergo early softening and lysis from enzymatic action from the wound. As a result, frequent changes of the heterograft dressing are necessary. Because of the high infection rates associated with this dressing, silver-nitrate-treated porcine heterograft has been developed to retard microbial growth.

The multiple problems associated with the use of biologic dressings have driven the development of synthetic materials. One such material is Biobrane, a composite material consisting of nylon mesh bonded to silicone that has proved successful in the temporary coverage of second- and third-degree burns. Whereas Biobrane adheres well to moderately clean wounds, it cannot adhere to or lower bacterial counts in grossly contaminated wounds. Biobrane dressing is supplied in various sizes, cut to fit the wound site, and secured with tape or Steri-Strips. It spontaneously separates from the wound when the underlying tissue heals. Hydrocolloid dressings are another type of biosynthetic material. They are occlusive wafers of gumlike materials that provide a water-resistant outer layer for coverage of the donor site. They protect healing tissue from excessive drying, liquefy necrotic tissue, and absorb wound drainage.

If dermal thickness is lost in deep partial-thickness or full-thickness burns, several products can serve as a dermal replacement. Integra is a synthetic dermal substitute and Alloderm is human cadaver allograft dermis that is nonimmunogenic. These products are placed in the wound, and split-thickness autografts are then placed over the dermal replacement. These products are used to provide temporary wound coverage, reduce pain, and facilitate healing.

The most recent temporary skin substitute is TransCyte. This bioengineered substance is derived from human fibroblast cells grown within mesh. As the cells grow, they secrete human dermal collagen, matrix proteins, and growth factors. The product is produced, extensively tested for any infectious agents, and then frozen. It is used for temporary covering for surgically debrided full-thickness and deep partial-thickness burn wounds, and is an alternative to silver sulfadiazine and cadaver skin. TransCyte forms a transparent, protective barrier over the wound surface and is typically applied only once. The best results have been obtained when it was applied within 24 hours of injury.

Wound Management

The outcomes of care for the client with a major burn depends on the prevention and treatment of infection through daily topical wound care, wound monitoring, and wound excision and closure. The goals of wound management are as follows (Bucher & Melander, 1999):

- Remove nonviable tissue.
- Control microbial colonization.
- Promote reepithelialization.
- Achieve wound coverage as early as possible.

Debriding the Wound. Burned tissue releases chemical mediators that stimulate phagocytosis in an attempt to digest debris left by decaying necrotic tissue. Necrotic tissue that remains despite phagocytic action retards healing and prolongs inflammation. **Debridement** is the process of removing all loose tissue, wound debris, and eschar (dead tissue) from the wound. Three methods of debridement are employed: mechanical, enzymatic, and surgical (surgical debridement was previously discussed).

A nurse may perform mechanical debridement by applying and removing gauze dressings (wet-to-dry or wet-to-moist), hydrotherapy, irrigation, or scissors and tweezers. During hydrotherapy (in an immersion tank, a shower, or on a spray table) the burn injury may be gently washed with a mild soap or wound cleaner solution to remove dead skin and separate eschar. The solution is then rinsed off with warm saline or tap water. Body hair (except for eyebrows) should be shaved within the burn and to within 2.5 cm of the wound edges. Blistered skin is grasped with a dry gauze and gently removed. The edges of blisters or eschar are trimmed with blunt scissors. The wound is then covered with a topical antimicrobial agent.

Enzymatic debridement involves the use of a topical agent to dissolve and remove necrotic tissue. An enzyme, such as sutilains, collagenase (Santyl), or fibrinolysis-deoxyribonuclease (Elase) is applied in a thin layer directly to the wound and covered with one layer of fine mesh gauze. A topical antimicrobial agent is then applied and covered with a bulky wet dressing; the wound is immobilized with expandable mesh gauze.

Dressing the Wound. Once the wound has been cleaned and debrided, it may be dressed using one of two methods. In the open method, the burn wound remains open to air, covered only by a topical antimicrobial agent. This method allows the wound to be easily assessed. Topical agents must be frequently reapplied because they tend to rub off onto the bedding.

In the closed method, a topical antimicrobial agent is applied to the wound site, which is covered with gauze or a nonadherent dressing and then gently wrapped with a gauze roll bandage. With the closed method, burn wounds are usually dressed twice daily and as needed. Dressings are applied circumferentially in a distal-to-proximal manner. All fingers and toes are wrapped separately.

Positioning, Splints, and Exercise. During therapy, the client must be maintained in positions that prevent **contractures** from forming. Because flexion is the natural resting position of joints and extremities, early physical therapy may include maintaining antideformity positions. Splints immobilize body parts and prevent contractures of the joints. They are applied and removed according to schedules established by the physical therapist.

Early in the acute phase of care, the physical therapist prescribes active and passive ROM exercises, which are performed every two hours at the bedside, most often by physical therapy. Early ambulation is also part of the plan of care once the client's condition becomes stable.

Support Garments. Applying uniform pressure can prevent or reduce hypertrophic scarring. Tubular support bandages are applied five to seven days postgraft to maintain a tension ranging from 10 to 20 mmHg to control scarring. The client wears custom-made elastic pressure garments for six months to a year postgraft.

Nutritional Support

The client with a major burn is in a hypermetabolic and catabolic state. The resting energy expenditure after severe burn injury can increase by as much as 100% above normal levels, depending on the extent of catabolism and the client's physical activity, size, age, and gender. This increase is believed due to heat loss from the burn wound, an increase in beta-adrenergic activity, pain, and infection. As a result, total caloric needs may be as great as 4000 to 6000 kcal per day.

Traditional dietary management based on oral intake seldom meets the kcal requirements necessary to reverse negative nitrogen balance and begin the healing process. Enteral feedings with a nasointestinal feeding tube are therefore instituted within 24 to 48 hours of the burn injury to offset hypermetabolism, improve nitrogen balance, and decrease length of hospital stay. A nasointestinal feeding tube is placed under fluoroscopy, with the tip extending past the pylorus to prevent reflux and aspiration.

Although enteral feeding is the preferred nutritional therapy, it is contraindicated in Curling's ulcer, bowel obstruction, feeding intolerance, pancreatitis, or septic ileus. When the enteral route cannot be used, a central venous catheter is inserted via the subclavian or jugular vein for the administration of total parenteral nutrition (TPN).

Nursing Care

The client with a major burn has complex, multisystem needs.

Health Promotion

Although treatments have improved significantly over the last several decades, there is no cure for burns. Prevention remains the primary goal. With the public's increasing attention to health promotion and disease prevention, the nursing profession currently is well positioned to collaborate with other disciplines to develop initiatives to reduce the number of burn injuries. For example, as client advocates, nurses can alert political leaders to the need to pass legislation aimed at reducing the incidence of burns. Appropriate legislative themes might center on safety in the workplace (e.g., requirements for smoke alarms and sprinkler systems), on the highways (e.g., regulations regarding the transportation of flammable liquids), and in the home (e.g., requirements for safety devices for water heaters and wood-burning stoves, and for self-extinguishing cigarettes). As educators, nurses can develop teaching plans for families and communities to heighten awareness of the problem. As researchers, nurses can investigate conditions leading to burn injury and suggest methods to reduce its prevalence. Working together with health care policymakers and community leaders, nurses can join the effort to lower the number of annual burn cases.

Assessment

Nursing assessment is continuous from the initial contact with the client with a burn injury. This section describes the secondary survey, conducted when the client arrives at the emergency department. Once there, the staff must act quickly to obtain the client's history of the burn injury, including the time of injury, causative agents, early treatment, medical history, and client's age and body weight. In most cases, the client is awake and oriented and able to relate the information during the emergent phase of care. Because changes in sensorium will become evident within the first few hours following a major burn injury, the nurse obtains as much information as is possible immediately on the client's arrival.

- *Time of injury.* In many cases, the client is admitted to the emergency department an hour or more after the injury occurred. The time of the burn injury must be documented as precisely as possible at the scene, because all fluid resuscitation calculations are based on the time of the burn injury, not on the client's time of arrival at the ER.

- *Cause of the injury.* Because the type of burn injury determines which nursing measures take priority, identify the specific causative agent to establish the appropriate plan of care.

- *First-aid treatment.* Prior to the arrival of medical personnel, the client or family may have applied home remedies to treat the burn wound. It is important for the nurse to ascertain and document the nature of all home treatment interventions, including the application of neutralizing agents, liquids, and immobilizing devices used to splint associated injuries.

- *Past medical history.* Clients with histories of respiratory, cardiac, renal, metabolic, neurologic, gastrointestinal, or skin diseases; alcohol abuse; or altered immune states require more intense observation. Known allergies are obtained.

- *Age.* Older adults tend to require more supportive care.

- *Medications.* Drugs, either prescribed or recreational, taken by the client prior to the burn injury may further complicate the treatment regimen. Drugs that affect any of the major body systems or cause mood alterations will need to be factored into the treatment plan. As part of the early assessment, obtain and document blood levels of therapeutic pharmaceutical agents and mood-altering substances.

- *Body weight.* During the acute and rehabilitative phases of the burn injury, the client will lose as much as 20% of preburn weight. This fact will have significant implications for all clients, especially for those who are underweight or cachectic at the time of the injury.

Nursing Diagnoses and Interventions

A major burn affects virtually every body system, as well as social, cultural, economic, psychological, and spiritual well-being. Immediate treatment in an intensive care setting is followed by years of rehabilitation and a lifetime of change in what was possible for an individual before the injury. Many nursing diagnoses are appropriate for the client with a major burn injury; those described here are *Impaired Skin Integrity, Deficient Fluid Volume, Acute Pain, Risk For Infection, Impaired Physical Mobility, Imbalanced Nutrition: Less Than Body Requirements, Powerlessness,* and *Home Care.*

Impaired Skin Integrity

The burn injury significantly impairs skin integrity. The severity of wounds varies according to the depth and extent of the burn. General treatment measures are designed to restore normal skin function as quickly as possible. Nursing care focuses on assessing and cleansing the wound and controlling infection.

*   Estimate the extent and depth of the burn wound and recalculate extent of unhealed burns weekly. *The severity of the burn injury is the basis for determining which type of interventions are appropriate. Reassessment on a regular basis is necessary to monitor the healing process.*

*   Provide daily wound care (including debridement method, dressing method, and medication administration) as prescribed, *to remove dead tissue, control infection, and promote reepithelialization as soon as possible.*

*   Provide special skin care to sensitive body areas:

    1. Clean burns involving the eyes with normal saline or sterile water, *to prevent corneal and conjunctival drying and adherence.* If contracture of the eyelid develops, apply drops or ointment to the eye, *to prevent corneal abrasion.*

    2. Gently wipe burns of the lips with saline-soaked pads. Apply an antibiotic ointment as prescribed. Assess the mouth frequently, and perform mouth care routinely. If an oral endotracheal tube is in place, reposition it often, *to prevent pressure ulcer formation.*

    3. Gently debride burns of the nose, and apply mafenide acetate (Sulfamylon) cream. Position nasogastric and nasotracheal tubes, *to prevent excessive pressure.*

    4. Apply mafenide acetate (Sulfamylon) cream to burns of the ear. Gently debride and thoroughly clean the wound with a water spray. Do not cover ears with dressings. Do not use pillows; to reduce pressure to the area, use a foam doughnut instead. *Burns of the ears are prone to infection; special positioning devices are necessary to decrease pressure ulcer formation.*

Deficient Fluid Volume

Fluid resuscitation rates are adjusted periodically throughout the emergent stage of care. The nurse should be particularly aware of several situations that may warrant the administration of fluids at rates in excess of the calculations needed to maintain adequate urine output: initial underestimation of the burn size, sequestration of fluid into the lung tissue in inhalation injury, electrical injury (which tends to cause more extensive damage than is immediately visible), full-thickness burns, and inordinately delayed starts of fluid resuscitation.

*   Assess blood pressure and heart rate frequently. *Vital signs rapidly deteriorate when fluid resuscitation is inadequate.*

*   Monitor hemodynamic status, including CVP and PCWP. *Inadequate fluid resuscitation is manifested by a drop in the central venous pressure and pulmonary capillary wedge pressure.*

- Follow prescribed protocols for intravenous fluid resuscitation. *Therapy for burn shock is aimed at supporting the client through the period of hypovolemic instability.*

- Monitor intake and output hourly. *Report urine outputs of less than 50 mL/h. Intake and output measurements indicate the adequacy of fluid resuscitation, and should range from 30 to 50 mL per hour in an adult.*

- Weigh daily. *Body weight is used to calculate fluid requirements.*

- Test all stools and emesis for the presence of blood. *Occult blood in emesis or stool indicates gastrointestinal bleeding.*

- Maintain a warm environment. *Hypothermia leads to shivering and further loss of body fluid through increased energy expenditure and catabolism.*

- Monitor for fluid volume overload. *Older clients and those with underlying cardiac disease may demonstrate symptoms of congestive heart failure during the fluid resuscitation stage.*

Acute Pain

The client experiences excruciating pain with extensive superficial and all partial-thickness burns. Intense pain is also experienced during wound care and physical therapy. In addition, increased levels of anxiety about treatments and outcomes may further increase the perception of pain.

- Measure the client's level of pain, using a consistent measurement tool. *Pain tolerance is the duration and intensity of pain that the client is able to endure. Pain tolerance differs from one client to the next and may vary in the same client in different situations.*

- Medicate before painful procedures and determine when PCA is appropriate. *The inability to manage pain results in feelings of despair and frustration.*

- Administer intravenous narcotic analgesics as prescribed. *Nurses' fear of precipitating addiction often makes them reluctant to administer narcotics. During the acute stage of burn injury, however, invasive procedures and exposed neurosensory nerve endings dictate the need for narcotic pharmaceutical agents.*

- Explain all procedures and expected levels of discomfort. *Clients who are prepared for painful procedures and know beforehand the actual sensations they will feel experience less stress.*

- Use methods of nonnarcotic pain control in combination with medications for pain. *Noninvasive pain relief measures (e.g., relaxation, massage, distraction) can enhance the therapeutic effects of pain relief medications.*

- Allow the client to verbalize the pain experience. *Each person experiences and expresses pain in his or her own manner, using various sociocultural adaptation techniques.*

Risk for Infection

From the onset of the burn injury, loss of the body's natural barrier to the external environment increases the risk of infection. Nursing interventions focus on controlling infectious processes. Monitor the results of diagnostic tests, maintain nutritional therapies, and apply antimicrobial agents to monitor and prevent the spread of infection, a major complication of the burn injury.

- Monitor daily for manifestations of wound infection. Remove topical medications and wound exudate and examine the entire wound. *Early manifestations of wound infection include swelling and inflammation in intact skin surrounding the wound; a change in the color, odor, or amount of exudate; increased pain; and loss of previously healed skin grafts.*

- Monitor for positive blood cultures, *which indicate bacteremia.*
- Monitor for hyperermia, cough, chest pain, wheezing, rhonchi, decreased oxygen saturation, and purulent sputum, *which are manifestations of pneumonia.*
- Monitor for the presence of bacteria in the urine, fever, urgency, frequency, dysuria and superpubic pain, *which are manifestations of urinary tract infections.*
- Obtain daily WBC counts. *Leukocyte counts are indicators of immune system function, and increase in the presence of infection.*
- Determine tetanus immunization status. *Burn clients are at risk for anaerobic infection caused by* Clostridium tetani.
- Maintain high kcal intake. *Nutritional support provides the nutrients needed to maintain the body's defense mechanisms.*
- Maintain an aseptic environment, using standard precautions, including gloving, gowning, and sterile procedures. *Strict isolation technique deters the development of nosocomial infection.*
- Culture all wounds and body secretions per protocol. *Culture and sensitivity reports identify the presence of infectious microbes and indicate appropriate antimicrobial therapies.*
- Administer prescribed antimicrobial medications, *to decrease invasive wound infections.*

Impaired Physical Mobility

As the burn wound heals and new skin tissue forms, the involved area tends to shrink. Contractures form at the site and significantly limit mobility, especially when a joint is involved. Physical therapy is important, beginning in the early stages of treatment. The nurse institutes ambulation and planned exercise regimens as soon as the client's condition stabilizes.

- Perform active or passive ROM exercises to all joints every two hours. Ambulate when stable. *Regular exercise prevents further loss of motion, restores movement, and improves functional status.*
- Apply splints as prescribed. Maintain antideformity positions, and reposition the client hourly. *Splinting and positioning retard the formation of contractures.*
- Maintain limbs in functional alignment, *to preserve joint mobility.*
- Anticipate the need for analgesia. *Administering analgesics promotes the client's comfort during exercising sessions.*

Imbalanced Nutrition: Less Than Body Requirements

The burn injury initiates a complex series of events that have a profound effect on the body's use of nutrients and expenditure of energy. Daily kcal requirements are determined by the nutritionist, and as soon as possible, enteral feedings are initiated. Duodenal tubes are placed to enhance intestinal absorption and retard gastric reflux. Parenteral nutrition is reserved for instances in which enteral feedings are contraindicated. Nursing measures focus on assessing feeding tolerance and use of nutrients.

- Maintain nasogastric/nasointestinal tube placement. *Correct tube placement ensures appropriate absorption of nutrients and prevents aspiration.*
- Maintain enteral/parenteral nutritional support as prescribed. Observe and report any evidence of feeding intolerance: diarrhea, vomiting, excessive gastric residue, abdominal distention, absent bowel sounds, and constipation. *The dietitian, in collaboration with the physician, selects and individualizes the feeding formula according to the client's daily*

energy expenditure requirements and feeding tolerance. Failure to maintain rates of infusion predisposes the client to continued catabolism and negative nitrogen balance.

- Weigh the client daily. *Anthropometric measurements indicate the adequacy of nutritional support therapies.*
- Obtain daily laboratory values for protein, iron, CBC, glucose, and albumin. *Decreased serum values indicate inadequate nutritional intake.*

Powerlessness

Usually, the client with a major burn injury endures a lengthy hospital stay involving many treatments and care protocols that are beyond his or her control. During the early stages, much of the care regimen involves excruciating pain. Further, the foreign environment of the burn unit makes it difficult for the client to relate to the immediate surroundings. For example, the need to control infection in the burn unit requires hospital personnel and family members to don sterile clothing prior to coming to the client's bedside. Family members and nursing personnel appear radically different when they are masked and gowned, and their odd appearance can add to the burn-injured client's sense of alienation.

- Allow the client as much control over the surroundings and daily routine as possible. For example, allow the client to choose times of dressing changes. *Powerlessness derives from the belief that one is unable to influence the outcome of a situation.*
- Keep needed items within reach, such as call bell, urinal, water pitcher, and tissues, *to reinforce the client's feelings of control.*
- Allow the client to express feelings. *The nurse can help the client cope by therapeutically listening, displaying a caring presence, clarifying misconceptions, and providing positive feedback.*
- Set short-term, realistic goals (e.g., set a goal for the client to ambulate from bedside to chair twice daily). *Small incremental gains are easier to achieve and allow for frequent positive reinforcement.*

Home Care

Client and family teaching is an important component of all phases of burn care. As treatment progresses, the nurse encourages family members to assume more responsibility in providing care. From admission to discharge, the nurse teaches the client and family to assess all findings, implement therapies, and evaluate progress. The following topics should be addressed in preparing the client and family for home care:

- The long-term goals of rehabilitation care: to prevent soft tissue deformity, protect skin grafts, maintain physiologic function, manage scars, and return the client to an optimal level of independence.
- Avoiding exposure to people with colds or infections and following aseptic technique meticulously when caring for the wound.
- The need for progressive physical activity.
- How to apply splints, pressure support garments, and other assistive devices.
- Dietary requirements with required kcal.
- Alternative pain control therapies, such as guided imagery, relaxation techniques, and diversional activities.
- Care of the graft and donor sites.

- Referral for occupational therapy, social service, clergy, and/or psychiatric services as appropriate.
- Helpful resources:
    1. American Burn Association
    2. International Society for Burn Injuries
    3. American Academy of Facial Plastic and Reconstructive Surgery
    4. The Phoenix Society for Burn Survivors, Inc.

section three

Special Considerations

38 Nursing Care of Clients in Pain

Pain is a subjective response to both physical and psychologic stressors. All people experience pain at some point during their lives. Although pain usually is experienced as uncomfortable and unwelcome, it also serves a protective role, warning of potentially health-threatening conditions. For this reason, pain is increasingly referred to as the *fifth* vital sign, with recommendations to assess pain with each vital sign assessment. The JCAHO (2000) has established pain standards that identify the relief of pain as a client right and requires health care facilities to implement specific procedures for, and provider education on, pain assessment and management.

Each individual pain event is a distinct and personal experience influenced by physiologic, psychologic, cognitive, sociocultural, and spiritual factors. Pain is the symptom most associated with describing oneself as ill, and it is the most common reason for seeking health care. Among the many definitions and descriptors of pain is the one most relevant: Pain is "whatever the person experiencing it says it is, and existing whenever the person says it does" (McCaffery, 1979, p. 11). This definition acknowledges the client as the only person who can accurately define and describe his or her own pain and serves as the basis for nursing assessment and care of clients in pain. It also supports the values and beliefs about pain necessary for holistic nursing care, including the following:

- Only the person affected can experience pain; that is, pain has a personal meaning.
- If the client says he or she has pain, the client is in pain. All pain is real.
- Pain has physical, emotional, cognitive, sociocultural, and spiritual dimensions.
- Pain affects the whole body, usually negatively.
- Pain may serve as both a response to and a warning of actual or potential trauma.

Theories and Neurophysiology of Pain

One well-known theory, gate control, suggests that the interaction of two systems determines pain and its perception (Melzack & Wall, 1965, 1968). The first of these interrelated systems is the substantia gelatinosa in the dorsal horns of the spinal cord. The substantia gelatinosa regulates impulses entering or leaving the spinal cord. The second system is an inhibitory system within the brainstem.

Small-diameter A-delta and C fibers in the spinal cord carry fast and slow pain impulses. In addition, large-diameter A-beta fibers carry impulses for tactile stimulation from the skin. In the substantia gelatinosa, these impulses encounter a "gate" that is thought to be opened and closed by the domination of either the large-diameter touch fibers or the small-diameter pain fibers. If impulses along the small-diameter pain fibers outnumber impulses along the large-diameter touch fibers, then the gate is open and pain impulses travel unimpeded to the brain. If impulses from the touch fibers predominate, then they will close the gate and the pain impulses will be turned away there. This explains why massaging a stubbed toe can reduce the intensity and duration of the pain.

The second system described by the gate control theory, the inhibitory system, is thought to be located in the brainstem. It is believed that cells in the midbrain, activated by a variety of stimuli such as opiates, psychologic factors, or even simply the presence of pain itself, signal receptors in the medulla. These receptors in turn stimulate nerve fibers in the spinal cord to block the transmission of impulses from pain fibers.

Ongoing research has demonstrated that the control and modulation of pain is much more complex than the description in the gate control theory, which served as a base for further research about pain-modulating systems. Tactile information is now known to be transmitted by both large-diameter and small-diameter fibers, and interactions between sensory neurons is known to occur at multiple levels of the central nervous system (Porth, 2002).

Stimuli

Nerve receptors for pain are called *nociceptors*. They are located at the ends of small afferent neurons and are woven throughout all the tissues of the body except the brain. Nociceptors are especially numerous in the skin and muscles. Pain occurs when biologic, mechanical, thermal, electrical, or chemical factors stimulate nociceptors (Table 38–1). The intensity and duration of the stimuli determine the sensation. Long-lasting, intense stimulation produces greater pain than brief, mild stimulation.

Nociceptors are stimulated either by direct damage to the cell or by the local release of biochemicals secondary to cell injury. *Bradykinin,* an amino acid, appears to be the most abundant and potent pain-producing chemical; other biochemical sources of pain include prostaglandins, histamine, hydrogen ions, and potassium ions. These biochemicals are thought to bind to nociceptors in response to noxious stimuli, causing the nociceptors to initiate pain impulses.

Table 38–1. Pain Stimuli

Causative Factor	Example
Microorganisms (e.g., bacteria, viruses)	Meningitis
Inflammation	Sore throat
Impaired blood flow	Angina
Invasive tumor	Colon cancer
Radiation	Radiation for cancer
Heat	Sunburn
Obstruction	Kidney stone
Spasm	Colon cramping
Compression	Carpal tunnel syndrome
Decreased movement	Pain after cast removal

Table 38-1. Continued

Stretching or straining	Sprained ankle
Fractures	Fractured hip
Swelling	Arthritis
Deposits of foreign tissue	Endometriosis
Chemicals	Skin rash
Electricity	Electrical burn
Conflict, difficulty in life	Psychogenic pain

Pain Pathway

The neural pathway of pain is summarized as follows:

1. Pain is perceived by the nociceptors in the periphery of the body (e.g., in the skin or viscera). Cutaneous pain is transmitted through small afferent A-delta and even smaller C nerve fibers to the spinal cord. A-delta fibers are myelinated and transmit impulses rapidly. They produce sharp, well-defined pain sensations, such as those that result from cuts, electric shocks, or the impact of a blow. A-delta fibers are associated with acute pain. C fibers are not myelinated and thus transmit pain impulses more slowly. The pain from deep body structures, such as muscles and viscera, is primarily transmitted by C fibers, producing diffuse burning or aching sensations. C fibers are associated with chronic pain. Both A-delta and C fibers are involved in most injuries. For example, if a person bangs the elbow, A-delta fibers transmit this pain stimulus within 0.1 second. The person feels this pain as a sharp, localized, smarting sensation. One or more seconds after the blow, the person experiences a duller, aching, diffuse sensation of pain impulses carried by the C fibers.

2. Secondary neurons transmit the impulses from the afferent neurons through the dorsal horn of the spinal cord, where they synapse in the substantia gelatinosa. The impulses then cross over to the anterior and lateral spinothalamic tracts.

3. The impulses ascend the anterior and lateral spinothalamic tracts and pass through the medulla and midbrain to the thalamus.

4. In the thalamus and cerebral cortex, the pain impulses are perceived, described, localized, and interpreted, and a response is formulated. A noxious impulse becomes pain when the sensation reaches conscious levels and is perceived and evaluated by the person experiencing the sensation.

Some pain impulses ascend along the paleospinothalamic tract in the medial section of the spinal cord. These impulses enter the reticular formation and the limbic systems, which integrate emotional and cognitive responses to pain. Interconnections in the autonomic nervous system may also cause an autonomic response to the pain. In addition, deep nociceptors often converge on the same spinal neuron, resulting in pain that is experienced in a part of the body other than its origin.

Inhibitory Mechanisms

Efferent fibers run from the reticular formation and midbrain to the substantia gelatinosa in the dorsal horns of the spinal cord. Along these fibers, pain may be inhibited or modulated. The analgesia system is a group of midbrain neurons that transmits impulses to the pons and medulla, which in turn stimulate a pain inhibitory center in the dorsal horns of the spinal cord. The exact nature of this inhibitory mechanism is unknown.

The most clearly defined chemical inhibitory mechanism is fueled by *endorphins* (endogenous morphines), which are naturally occurring opioid peptides present in neurons in the brain, spinal cord, and gastrointestinal tract. Endorphins in the brain are released in response to afferent noxious stimuli, whereas endorphins in the spinal cord are released in response to efferent impulses. Endorphins work by binding with opiate receptors on the neurons to inhibit pain impulse transmission.

Types and Characteristics of Pain

Acute Pain

Acute pain has a sudden onset, is usually temporary, and is localized. Pain that lasts for less than six months and has an identified cause is classified as acute pain. The sudden onset usually results from tissue injury from trauma, surgery, or inflammation. The pain is usually sharp and localized, although it may radiate. The three major types of acute pain are:

*   *Somatic pain,* which arises from nerve receptors originating in the skin or close to the surface of the body. Somatic pain may be either sharp and well localized or dull and diffuse. It is often accompanied by nausea and vomiting.

*   *Visceral pain,* which arises from body organs. Visceral pain is dull and poorly localized because of the low number of nociceptors. The viscera are sensitive to stretching, inflammation, and ischemia but relatively insensitive to cutting and temperature extremes. Visceral pain is associated with nausea and vomiting, hypotension, and restlessness. It often radiates or is referred.

*   *Referred pain,* which is perceived in an area distant from the site of the stimuli. It commonly occurs with visceral pain, as visceral fibers synapse at the level of the spinal cord, close to fibers innervating other subcutaneous tissue areas of the body. Pain in a spinal nerve may be felt over the skin in any body area innervated by sensory neurons that share that same spinal nerve route. Body areas defined by spinal nerve routes are called dermatomes (see Chapter 31).

Acute pain warns of actual or potential injury to tissues. As a stressor, it initiates the fight-or-flight autonomic stress response. Characteristic physical responses include tachycardia, rapid and shallow respirations, increased blood pressure, dilated pupils, sweating, and pallor. The person experiencing the pain responds to this threat with anxiety and fear. This psychologic response may further increase the physical responses to acute pain.

Chronic Pain

Chronic pain is prolonged pain, usually lasting longer than six months. It is not always associated with an identifiable cause and is often unresponsive to conventional medical treatment. Chronic pain is often described as dull, aching, and diffuse. Unlike acute pain, chronic pain has a much more complex and poorly understood purpose.

Chronic pain can be subdivided into four categories:

*   *Recurrent acute pain* is characterized by relatively well-defined episodes of pain interspersed with pain-free episodes. Examples of recurrent acute pain include migraine headaches and sickle cell crises.

- *Ongoing time-limited pain* is identified by a defined time period. Some examples are cancer pain, which ends with control of the disease or death, and burn pain, which ends with rehabilitation or death.
- *Chronic nonmalignant pain* is non-life-threatening pain that nevertheless persists beyond the expected time for healing. Chronic lower back pain falls into this category.
- *Chronic intractable nonmalignant pain syndrome* is similar to simple chronic nonmalignant pain, but is characterized by the person's inability to cope well with the pain and sometimes by physical, social, and/or psychologic disability resulting from the pain.

The client with chronic pain often is depressed, withdrawn, immobile, irritable, and/or controlling. Although chronic pain may range from mild to severe and may be continuous or intermittent, the unrelenting presence of the pain often results in the pain itself becoming the pathologic process requiring intervention. The most common chronic pain condition is lower back pain. Other common chronic pain conditions include the following (McCance & Huether, 2002):

- *Neuralgias* are painful conditions that result from damage to a peripheral nerve caused by infection or disease. Postherpetic neuralgia (following shingles) is an example.
- Reflex sympathetic *dystrophies* are characterized by continuous severe, burning pain. These conditions follow peripheral nerve damage and present the symptoms of pain, vasospasm, muscle wasting, and vasomotor changes (vasodilation followed by vasoconstriction).
- *Hyperesthesias* are conditions of oversensitivity to tactile and painful stimuli. Hyperesthesias result in diffuse pain that is usually increased by fatigue and emotional lability.
- Myofascial pain syndrome is a common condition marked by injury to or disease of muscle and fascial tissue. Pain results from muscle spasm, stiffness, and collection of lactic acid in the muscle. Fibromyalgia is an example.
- Cancer often produces chronic pain, usually due to factors associated with the advancing disease. These factors include a growing tumor that presses on nerves or other structures, stretching of viscera, obstruction of ducts, or metastasis to bones. The malignant tumor may also mechanically stimulate pain or the production of biochemicals that cause pain. Pain may also be associated with chemotherapy and radiation therapy.
- Chronic postoperative pain is rare but may occur following incisions in the chest wall, radical mastectomy, radical neck dissection, and surgical amputation.

Central Pain

Central pain is related to a lesion in the brain that may spontaneously produce high-frequency bursts of impulses that are perceived as pain. A vascular lesion, tumor, trauma, or inflammation may cause central pain. Thalamic pain, one of the most common types, is severe, spontaneous, and often continuous. Hyperesthesia (an abnormal sensitivity to touch, pain, or other sensory stimuli) may occur on the side of the body opposite to the lesion in the thalamus. The perception of body position and movement may also be lost.

Phantom Pain

Phantom pain is a syndrome that occurs following amputation of a body part. The client experiences pain in the missing body part even though he or she is completely mentally aware that it is gone. This pain may include itching, tingling, or pressure sensations, or it may be more severe, including burning or stabbing sensations. In some cases, the client may describe a sensation that an amputated limb is twisted or cramped. It is thought that this type of pain may be due to stimulation of the severed nerves at the site of the amputation. Treatment is complex and often unsuccessful.

Psychogenic Pain

Psychogenic pain is experienced in the absence of any diagnosed physiologic cause or event. Typically psychogenic pain involves a long history of severe pain. It is thought that the client's emotional needs prompt the pain sensations. Psychogenic pain is real, and may in turn lead to physiologic changes, such as muscle tension, which may produce further pain. This condition may result from interpersonal conflicts, a need for support from others, or a desire to avoid a stressful or traumatic situation. Depression is often present.

Factors Affecting Responses to Pain

Physical response to pain involves specific and often predictable neurologic changes. In fact, everyone has the same pain threshold and perceives pain stimuli at the same stimulus intensity. For example, heat is perceived as painful at 44∞ to 46∞ C, the range at which it begins to damage tissue. What varies is the person's perception of and reaction to pain. The individualized response to pain is shaped by multiple and interacting factors including age, sociocultural influences, emotional state, past experiences with pain, source and meaning of the pain, and knowledge base.

When describing a person as being highly sensitive to pain, one is referring to the person's **pain tolerance,** which is the amount of pain a person can endure before outwardly responding to it. The ability to tolerate pain may be decreased by repeated episodes of pain, fatigue, anger, anxiety, and sleep deprivation. Medications, alcohol, hypnosis, warmth, distraction, and spiritual practices may increase pain tolerance.

Age

Age influences a person's perception and expression of pain. The older adult with normal age-related changes in neurophysiology may have decreased perception of sensory stimuli and a higher pain tolerance. In addition, chronic disease processes more common in the older adult, such as peripheral vascular disease or diabetes, may interfere with normal nerve impulse transmission. Individuals in this age group may have atypical responses to pain: decreased perception of acute pain, heightened perceptions of chronic pain, and/or increased incidence of referred pain.

Often believing that pain is a part of growing older, the client may ignore pain or self-medicate with over-the-counter medications. As a result of these behaviors, the older adult is at increased risk of injury or serious illness. Table 38-2 lists age-related changes and their effects on pain.

Table 38-2. Nursing Care of the Older Adult: Age-Related Changes and Their Effects on Pain

Factors Related to Aging	Effects	Outcomes
Decreased blood flow	Ischemia, decreases in brain function	Client forgets to take medication
Changes in neurotransmitters related to sleep and mood	Decreased sleep resulting in vulnerability to pain	Greater risk of chronic pain, fatigue, increased withdrawal
Reduced levels of norepinephrine	Lowered transmission of pain	Less likely to notice an injury
Changes in sensory interpretation	Lowered pain sensation	Client may not take appropriate protective action
Decreased peripheral nerve conduction	Lowered response to pain	Not seeking appropriate care
Slowed reaction time	Slower avoidance response	Client receives more serious injury
Reduced movement	Increased risk for muscle wasting	May cause immobility

Sociocultural Influences

Each person's response to pain is strongly influenced by the family, community, and culture. Sociocultural influences affect the way in which a person tolerates pain, interprets the meaning of pain, and reacts verbally and nonverbally to the pain. For example, if the client's family believes that males should not cry and must tolerate pain stoically, then the male client often will appear withdrawn and refuse pain medication. If a family encourages open and intense emotional expression, then the client may cry freely and appear comfortable requesting pain medication.

Cultural standards also teach an individual how much pain to tolerate, what types of pain to report, to whom to report the pain, and what kind of treatment to seek. Note, however, that behaviors vary greatly within a culture and from generation to generation. The nurse should approach each client as an individual, observing the client carefully, taking the time to ask questions, and avoiding assumptions.

The nurse also has a set of sociocultural values and beliefs about pain. If these values and beliefs differ from those of the client, the assessment and management of pain may be based on the values of the nurse rather than on the needs of the client. The nurse must be familiar with ethnic and cultural diversity in pain expression and management and respect cultural differences. It is particularly important to remember that pain behaviors are not an objective indicator of the amount of pain present for any individual client. Finally, most experts agree that cultural differences in the expression of, response to, and interpretation of the meaning of pain need further research.

Emotional Status

Emotional status influences the pain perception. The sensation of pain may be blocked by intense concentration (e.g., during sports activities) or may be increased by anxiety or fear. Pain often is increased when it occurs in conjunction with other illnesses or physical discomforts, such as nausea or vomiting. The presence or absence of support people or caregivers that genuinely care about pain management may also alter emotional status and the perception of pain.

Anxiety may increase the perception of pain, and pain in turn may cause anxiety. In addition, the muscle tension common with anxiety can create its own source of pain. This association explains why nonpharmacologic interventions, such as relaxation or guided imagery, are helpful in relieving or decreasing pain.

Fatigue, lack of sleep, and depression are also related to pain experiences. Pain interferes with a person's ability to fall asleep and stay asleep, and thus induces fatigue. In turn, fatigue can lower pain tolerance. Depression is clearly linked to pain: Serotonin, a neurotransmitter, is involved in the modulation of pain in the central nervous system (CNS). In clinically depressed people, serotonin is decreased, leading to an increase in pain sensations. The reverse is also true: In the presence of pain, depression is common.

Past Experiences with Pain

Previous experiences with pain are likely to influence the person's response to a current pain episode. If supportive adults responded to childhood experiences with pain appropriately, the adult usually will have a healthy attitude to pain. If, however, the person's pain was responded to with exaggerated emotions or neglectful indifference, that person's future responses to pain may be exaggerated or denied.

The responses of health care providers to the person in pain can influence the person's response during the next pain episode. If providers respond to pain with effective strategies and a caring attitude, the client will remain more comfortable during any subsequent pain episode, and anxiety will be avoided. If, however, the pain is not adequately relieved, or if the client feels that empathetic care was not given, anxiety about the next pain episode sets up the client for a more complex and, therefore, more painful event.

Source and Meaning

The meaning associated with the pain influences the experience of pain. For example, the pain of labor to deliver a baby is experienced differently from the pain following removal of a major organ for cancer. Because pain is the major signal for health problems, it is strongly linked to all associated meanings of health problems, such as disability, loss of role, and death. For this reason, it is important to explain to clients the etiology and prognosis for the pain assessed.

If the client perceives the pain as deserved (e.g., "just punishment for sins"), then the client may actually feel relief that the "punishment" has commenced. If the client believes that the pain will relieve him or her from an unrewarding job, dangerous military service, or even stressful social obligations, there may similarly be a feeling of relief. In contrast, pain that is perceived as meaningless (e.g., chronic low back pain or the unrelieved pain of arthritis) can cause anxiety and depression.

Knowledge

A lack of understanding of the source, outcome, and meaning of the pain can contribute negatively to the pain experience. It is important to assess the client's readiness to learn, use methods of teaching that are effective for the client and family, and evaluate learning carefully. Teaching must include the process of the pain, its predictable course (if possible), and the proposed plan of care. In addition, encourage clients to communicate preferences for pain relief. Learning how to let significant others know of the presence of pain and how to use their help can also promote effective pain management.

Myths and Misconceptions About Pain

Myths and misconceptions about pain and its management are common in both health care providers and clients. Following are some of the most common of these myths:

Myth 1: *Pain is a result, not a cause.* According to the traditional view, pain is only a symptom of a condition. However, it is now recognized that unrelieved or poorly relieved pain itself sets up further responses, such as immobility, anger, and anxiety; pain may also delay healing and rehabilitation.

Myth 2: *Chronic pain is really a masked form of depression.* Serotonin plays a chemical role in pain transmission, and is also the major modulator of depression. Therefore, pain and depression are chemically related, not mutually exclusive. It is common to find them coexisting.

Myth 3: *Narcotic medication is too risky to be used in chronic pain.* This common misconception often deprives clients of the most effective source of pain relief. It is true that other methods should be tried first; if, however, they prove ineffective, narcotics should be considered as an appropriate alternative.

Myth 4: *It is best to wait until a client has pain before giving medication.* It is now widely accepted that anticipating pain has a noticeable effect on the amount of pain a client experiences. Offering pain relief before a pain event is well on its way can lessen the pain.

Myth 5: *Many clients lie about the existence or severity of their pain.* Very few clients lie about their pain.

Myth 6: *Postoperative pain is best treated with intramuscular injections.* The most commonly used postoperative pain relief for many years was meperidine (Demerol) given intramuscularly. However, meperidine has many adverse effects, such as irritating tissues and producing the CNS stimulant normeperidine. In addition, meperidine is short acting. Most contemporary experts do not recommend its use to manage postoperative pain.

Collaborative Care

Effective pain relief results from collaboration among health care providers. Pain clinics are centers staffed by a team of health care professionals who use a multidisciplinary approach to managing chronic pain. Therapies may include traditional pharmacologic agents, as well as herbs, vitamins, and other dietary supplements; nutritional counseling; psychotherapy; biofeedback; hypnosis; acupuncture; massage; and other treatments. Hospices for dying clients also provide a multifaceted approach to pain management. Chapter 43 provides information about pain management during end-of-life care.

Medications

Medication is the most common approach to pain management. Various drugs with many kinds of delivery systems are available. These drugs include nonnarcotic analgesics, nonsteroidal anti-inflammatory drugs (NSAIDs), narcotics, synthetic narcotics, antidepressants, and local anesthetic agents. In addition to administering prescribed medications, the nurse may act independently in choosing the dosage and timing. The nurse is also responsible for assessing the side effects of medications, evaluating a medication's effectiveness, and providing client teaching. The nurse's role in pain relief is client advocate and direct caregiver.

The World Health Organization "ladder of analgesia" effectively guides the use of medications (WHO, 1986/1990). NSAIDs and narcotic pain medications are used progressively until pain is relieved, reflecting the interactive nature of these two types of analgesics. Table 38-3 describes terms associated with pain medication.

Nonnarcotic Analgesics

Nonnarcotic analgesics, such as acetaminophen (Tylenol) produce analgesia and reduce fever. The exact mechanism of action is unknown. They are used to treat mild to moderate pain.

NSAIDs

NSAIDs act on peripheral nerve endings and minimize pain by interfering with prostaglandin synthesis. Examples are aspirin, ibuprofen, and celecoxib (Celebrex). The NSAIDs have anti-inflammatory, analgesic, and antipyretic actions. NSAIDs are the treatment of choice for mild to moderate pain and continue to be effective when combined with narcotics for moderate to severe pain.

Table 38-3. Terms Associated with Pain Medication

< *Addiction:* The compulsive use of a substance despite negative consequences, such as health threats or legal problems.

< *Drug abuse:* The use of any chemical substance for other than a medical purpose.

< *Physical drug dependence:* A biologic need for a substance. If the substance is not supplied, physical withdrawal symptoms occur.

< *Psychologic drug dependence:* A psychologic need for a substance. If the substance is not supplied, psychologic withdrawal symptoms occur.

< *Drug tolerance:* The process by which the body requires a progressively greater amount of a drug to achieve the same results.

< *Equianalgesic:* Having the same pain-killing effect when administered to the same individual. Drug dosages are equianalgesic if they have the same effect as morphine sulfate 10 mg administered intramuscularly.

< *Pseudoaddiction:* Behavior involving drug seeking; a result of receiving inadequate pain relief.

Narcotics (Opioids)

Narcotics, or opioids, are derivatives of the opium plant. These drugs (and their synthetic forms) are the pharmacologic treatment of choice for moderate to severe pain. Examples are morphine, codeine, and fentanyl (Durgesic, Actiq). Narcotic analgesics produce analgesia by binding to opioid receptors both within and outside the CNS.

A common myth among health care professionals is that using narcotics for pain treatment poses a real threat of addiction. Actually, when the medications are used as recommended, there is little to no risk of addiction. Rather, if pain is not adequately treated, the client may seek more and more narcotic relief, thus increasing the risk of tolerance. Nursing implications for narcotics are found in Table 38-4.

Antidepressants

Antidepressants within the tricyclic and related chemical groups act on the production and retention of serotonin in the CNS, thus inhibiting pain sensation. They also promote normal sleeping patterns, further alleviating the suffering of the client in pain.

Local Anesthetics

Drugs, such as benzocaine and zylocaine are part of a large group of substances that block the initiation and transmission of nerve impulses in a local area, thus blocking pain as well. Local anesthetics can be delivered by a variety of methods. They are sometimes used to enable a client to begin moving and using a painful area to diminish long-term pain.

Duration of Action

Each of the pharmacologic agents has a unique absorption and duration of action. The nurse caring for the client in pain must understand that no drug will have a totally predictable course of action, because each person absorbs, metabolizes, and excretes medications at different dosage levels. The only way to obtain reliable data about the effectiveness of the medication for the individual client is to assess how that client responds. Therefore, the best choice is to individualize the dosing schedule.

The two major descriptors of dosing schedules are *around the clock* (ATC) or *as necessary* (PRN). (The abbreviation PRN stands for *pro re nata,* Latin for "as circumstances may require.") An ATC administration is appropriate if the client experiences pain constantly and predictably during a 24-hour period. A PRN administration is appropriate for pain that is not predictable or constant. The PRN medication should be administered as soon as the pain begins.

Giving analgesics before the pain occurs or increases gives the client confidence in the certainty of pain relief and thereby avoids some of the untoward effects of pain. The benefits of a preventive approach can be summarized as follows:

- The client may spend less time in pain.
- Frequent analgesic administration may allow for smaller doses and less analgesic administration.
- Smaller doses will in turn mean fewer side effects.
- The client's fear and anxiety about the return of pain will decrease.
- The client will probably be more physically active and avoid the difficulties caused by immobility.

The side effects of a drug can become difficult to manage if the dosage is too high. The best formula for adequate dosage is a balance between effective pain relief and minimal side effects. Within prescribed limits, the nurse can choose the correct dose according to the client's response. It is also the role of the nurse to inform the physician if the prescribed dosage does not meet the client's needs.

Routes of Administration

The route of administration significantly affects how much of the medication is needed to relieve pain. For example, oral doses of some narcotics must be up to five times greater than parenteral doses to achieve the same degree of pain relief. Different narcotics have different recommended dosages. Consulting an equianalgesic dosage chart helps ensure that dosages of different narcotics administered by different routes will have the same analgesic effect when administered to the same client. These charts are based on a comparison of an analgesic to 10 mg (IM) of morphine.

Oral. The simplest route for both client and nurse is the oral (PO) route. Special nursing care is still required, because some medications must be given with food, some are irritating to the gastrointestinal system, and some clients have trouble swallowing pills. Liquid and timed-release forms are available for special applications.

Rectal. The rectal route is helpful for clients who are unable to swallow. Several of the opioid narcotics are available in this form. The rectal route is effective and simple, but the client and family may not accept it. To be effective, any rectal medication must be placed above the rectal sphincter.

Transdermal. The transdermal, or patch, form of medication is increasingly being used because it is simple, painless, and delivers a continuous level of medication. Although expensive, transdermal medications are easy to store and apply. Additional short-acting medication is often needed for breakthrough pain.

To apply a medication transdermally, the nurse or client must clip any hair from the area, clean the site (which should be on the upper torso) with clear water, dry the cleansed area, apply the patch immediately upon opening the package, and ensure that the contact is complete, especially around the edges. The effectiveness of a patch lasts for a variable amount of time, and the next patch should be applied on a different site.

Intramuscular. Once the most popular route for pain medication administration, the intramuscular (IM) route is being reconsidered. Its disadvantages include uneven absorption from the muscle, discomfort on administration, and time consumed to prepare and administer the medication.

Intravenous. The intravenous (IV) route provides the most rapid onset, usually ranging from 1 to 15 minutes. Medication can be given by drip, bolus, or **patient-controlled analgesia (PCA),** a pump with a control mechanism that affords the client self-management of pain. Studies of PCA use for postoperative pain have shown that clients require less overall medication because of the even blood level of medication maintained, the feeling of control maintained by the client, and the absence of anxiety. Several drugs are available for this route. The disadvantages are the nursing care needed for any intravenous line, the potential for infection, and the cost of disposable supplies. The PCA method of administration requires careful client teaching.

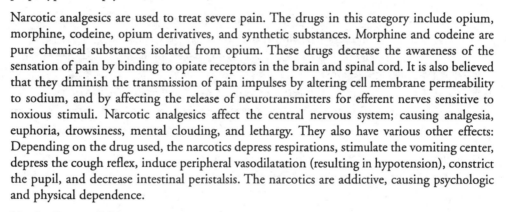

Table 38-4. Medication Administration – Narcotic Analgesics

Examples of narcotic analgesics are:

buprenorphine HCl (Buprenex)
codeine
hydromorphone HCl (Dilaudid)
meperidine HCl (Demerol)
morphine sulfate
nalbuphine HCl (Nubain)
oxymorphone HCl (Numorphan)
pentazocine (Talwin)
propoxyphene napsylate (Darvocet-N)

Narcotic analgesics are used to treat severe pain. The drugs in this category include opium, morphine, codeine, opium derivatives, and synthetic substances. Morphine and codeine are pure chemical substances isolated from opium. These drugs decrease the awareness of the sensation of pain by binding to opiate receptors in the brain and spinal cord. It is also believed that they diminish the transmission of pain impulses by altering cell membrane permeability to sodium, and by affecting the release of neurotransmitters for efferent nerves sensitive to noxious stimuli. Narcotic analgesics affect the central nervous system; causing analgesia, euphoria, drowsiness, mental clouding, and lethargy. They also have various other effects: Depending on the drug used, the narcotics depress respirations, stimulate the vomiting center, depress the cough reflex, induce peripheral vasodilatation (resulting in hypotension), constrict the pupil, and decrease intestinal peristalsis. The narcotics are addictive, causing psychologic and physical dependence.

Nursing Responsibilities

- Narcotics are regulated by federal law; the nurse must record the date, time, client name, type and amount of the drug used, and sign the entry in a narcotic inventory sheet. If the drug must be wasted after it is signed out, the act must be witnessed and the narcotic sheet signed by the nurse and the witness. Computerized narcotic documentation methods are also available.

- Keep a narcotic antagonist, such as naloxone, immediately available to treat respiratory depression.

- Assess allergies or adverse effects from narcotics previously experienced by the client.

- Meperidine (Demerol) is associated with CNS toxicity, and thus involves significant patient risk. For any client who is receiving more than one dose, monitor for nervousness, restlessness, tremors, twitching, shakiness, myoclonic jerks, diaphoresis, changes in level of awareness, agitation, disorientation, confusion, delirium, hallucinations, violent shivering, and/or seizures. This toxicity can occur with any route of administration or any dosing regimen. This risk is increased with oral administration and in clients with decreased renal function (including normal changes with aging). Report these manifestations to the physician.

- Assess for any respiratory disease, such as asthma, that might increase the risk of respiratory depression.

- Assess the characteristics of the pain and the effectiveness of drugs that have been previously used to treat the pain.

Continued on the next page

Table 38-4. Continued

- Take and record baseline vital signs before administering the drug.
- Administer the drugs, following established guidelines.
- Monitor vital signs, level of consciousness, pupillary response, nausea, bowel function, urinary function, and effectiveness of pain management.
- Teach noninvasive methods of pain management for use in conjunction with narcotic analgesics.
- Provide for client safety.

Client and Family Teaching

- The use of narcotics to treat severe pain is unlikely to cause addiction.
- Do not drink alcohol.
- Do not take over-the-counter medications unless approved by the health care provider.
- Increase intake of fluids and fiber in the diet to prevent constipation.
- The drugs often cause dizziness, drowsiness, and impaired thinking; use caution when driving or making decisions.
- Report decreasing effectiveness or the appearance of side effects to the physician.

Subcutaneous. The subcutaneous (SC) route is accepted, but it is less commonly used than other methods. Its advantages and disadvantages are similar to those of the intravenous route.

Intraspinal. The intraspinal route is invasive and requires more extensive nursing care.

Nerve Blocks. In a nerve block, anesthetics, sometimes in combination with steroidal anti-inflammatory drugs, are injected by a physician or nurse anesthetist into or near a nerve, usually in an area between the nociceptor and the dorsal root. The procedure may be performed to determine the precise location of the pain source: Pain relief indicates that the injection site is the site of the source of the pain.

Temporary (local) nerve blocks may give the client enough relief to (1) develop a more hopeful attitude that pain relief is possible, (2) allow local procedures to be performed without causing discomfort, or (3) exercise and move the affected part. Nerve blocks may also be performed to predict the results of neurosurgery. For long-term pain relief, a permanent neurolytic agent is used. Neurolytic blocks usually are reserved for terminally ill clients because of the risks of weakness, paralysis, and bowel and bladder dysfunction.

Nursing Care

Nursing care of the client with pain presents perhaps more of a challenge than almost any other type of illness or injury. Regardless of the type of pain, the goal of nursing care is to assist the client to achieve optimal control of the pain.

Assessment

A comprehensive approach to pain assessment is essential to ensure adequate and appropriate interventions. The assessment areas are client perceptions, physiologic responses, behavioral responses, and self-management of pain and the effectiveness of pain management strategies.

Client Perceptions

The most reliable indicator of the presence and degree of pain is the client's own statement about the pain. The McGill Pain Questionnaire is a useful tool in assessing the client's subjective experience of the pain. It asks the client to locate the pain, to describe the quality of the pain, to indicate how the pain changes with time, and to rate the intensity of the pain.

The client's perception of the pain can also be assessed by using the following PQRST technique:

- P = What precipitated (triggered, stimulated) the pain? Has anything relieved the pain? What is the pattern of the pain?
- Q = What are the quality and quantity of the pain? Is the pain sharp, stabbing, aching, burning, stinging, deep, crushing, viselike, gnawing?
- R = What is the region (location) of the pain? Does the pain radiate to other areas of the body?
- S = What is the severity of the pain?
- T = What is the timing of the pain? When does it begin, how long does it last, and how is it related to other events in the client's life?

The most common method to assess the severity of pain is a pain rating scale. For clients who do not understand English or numerals, a scale using colors (e.g., light blue for no pain through bright red for worst possible pain) or pictures may be helpful. The following nursing interventions will help the nurse use a pain rating scale to achieve optimal results.

- To ensure consistent communication, explain the specific pain rating scale being used. If a word descriptor scale is used, verify that the client can read the language being used. If a numerical scale is used, be sure the client can count to 10. If the client is not able to report pain because of communication difficulties, intubation, emotional disturbances, or cognitive impairments, follow these guidelines (Pasero & McCaffrey, 2000):
    1. Be sure the client is unable to report pain. Researchers have found that even residents in a nursing home who are cognitively impaired can validly self-report pain.
    2. Consider pathologic conditions and procedures that might cause pain and treat the client for pain.
    3. Look for indicators of pain, such as grimacing, restlessness, stillness, verbal or nonverbal vocalizations, and grasping an object.
    4. Ask a family member or caretaker about the client's pain to serve as a proxy pain rating.
- Discuss the definition of the word pain to ensure that the client and the provider are communicating on the same level. It is often helpful to use the client's own words when describing the pain.
- Explain that the report of pain is important for promoting recovery, not just for achieving temporary comfort.

Physiologic Responses

Predictable physiologic changes occur in the presence of acute pain. These may include muscle tension; tachycardia; rapid, shallow respirations; increased blood pressure; dilated pupils; sweating; and pallor. Over time, however, the body adapts to the pain stimulus, and these physiologic changes may be extinguished in clients with chronic pain.

Behavioral Responses

Some behaviors are so typical of people in pain that the behaviors are referred to as *pain behaviors*. They include bracing or guarding the painful part, taking medication, crying, moaning, grimacing, withdrawing from activity and socialization, becoming immobile, talking about pain, holding the painful area, breathing with increased effort, exhibiting a sad facial expression, and being restless.

Behavioral responses to pain may or may not coincide with the client's report of pain and are not reliable cues to the pain experience. For example, one client may rate pain at an 8 on a 1 to 10 scale while laughing or walking down the hall; another may deny pain completely while tachycardic, hypertensive, and grimacing. Discrepancies between the client's report of pain and behavioral responses may be the result of cultural factors, coping skills, fear, denial, or the utilization of relaxation or distraction techniques.

Clients may deny pain for a variety of reasons, including fear of injections, fear of drug/narcotic addiction, misinterpretation of terms (the client may not think that aching, soreness, or discomfort qualify as pain), or the misconception that health care providers know when clients experience pain. Some clients may deny pain as part of an attempt to deny that there is something wrong with them. Other clients, by contrast, may think that "as needed" medications will be given only if their pain rating is high. Clients may also use pain as a mechanism to gain attention from family and health care providers.

Self-Management of Pain

The client's attempts to manage pain are useful additions to the assessment database. This information is individualized and client specific, including many factors such as culture, age, and client knowledge. Collect detailed descriptions of actions the client or significant others took, when and how these measures were applied, and how well they worked.

Nursing Diagnoses and Interventions

The primary nursing diagnoses for clients in pain are acute pain and chronic pain. The interventions for these diagnoses are combined in this discussion.

Acute Pain or Chronic Pain

- Assess the characteristics of the pain by asking the client to:
  1. Point to the pain location or to mark the pain location on a figure drawing. *Pain location provides information about the etiology of the pain and the type of pain being experienced.*
  2. Rate the intensity of the pain by using a pain scale (1 to 10, with 10 being the worst pain ever experienced), a visual analog scale (a scale on which pain is marked on a continuum from no pain to severe pain), or with word descriptors, such as the McGill Pain Questionnaire. Use the same scale with each assessment. *The intensity of pain is a subjective experience. The perception of the intensity of pain is affected by the client's degree of concentration or distraction, state of consciousness, and expectations. Some body tissues are more sensitive than others.*
  3. Describe the quality of the pain, saying, for example, "Describe what your pain feels like." If necessary, provide word descriptors for the client to select. *Descriptive terms provide insight into the nature and perception of the pain. In addition, the location and type of pain (e.g., acute versus chronic) affect the quality.*

4. Describe the pattern of the pain, including time of onset, duration, persistence, and times without pain. It is also important to ask if the pain is worse at regular times of the day and if it has any relationship to activity. *The pattern of pain provides clues about cause and location.*

5. Describe any precipitating or relieving factors, such as *sleep deficits, anxiety, temperature extremes, excessive noise, anxiety, fear, depression, and activity.*

6. Describe the meaning of the pain, including its effects on lifestyle, self-concept, roles, and relationships. *Clients with acute pain may believe the pain is a normal response to injury or that it signals serious illness and death. Pain is a stressor that may affect the ability of the client to cope effectively. The client with chronic pain often has concerns about addiction to pain medication, costs, social interactions, sexual activities, and relationships with significant others.*

7. Monitor manifestations of pain by taking vital signs; assessing skin temperature and moisture; observing pupils; observing facial expressions, position in bed, guarding of body parts; and noting restlessness. *Autonomic responses to pain may result in an increased blood pressure, tachycardia, rapid respirations, perspiration, and dilated pupils. Other responses to pain include grimacing, clenching the hands, muscle rigidity, guarding, restlessness, and nausea. The client with chronic pain may have an unexpressive, tired facial appearance.*

- Communicate belief in the client's pain by verbally acknowledging the presence of the pain, listening carefully to the description of pain, and acting to help the client manage the pain. *Because pain is a personal, subjective experience, the nurse must convey belief in the client's pain. By doing so, the nurse reduces anxiety and thereby lessens pain.*

- Provide optimal pain relief with prescribed analgesics, determining the preferred route of administration. Provide pain-relieving measures for severe pain on a regular around-the-clock basis or by self-administration, such as with a PCA pump. *The client is a part of the decision-making process and can exert some control over the situation by choosing the administration route. Analgesics are usually most effective when they are administered before pain occurs or becomes severe. Around-the-clock administration has been proven to provide better pain management for both acute and chronic pain.*

- Teach the client and family nonpharmacologic methods of pain management, such as relaxation, distraction, and cutaneous stimulation. *These techniques are especially useful when used in conjunction with pain medications and may also be useful in managing chronic pain.*

- Provide comfort measures, such as changing positions, back massage, oral care, skin care, and changing bed linens. *Basic comfort measures for personal cleanliness, skin care, and mobility promote physical and psychosocial well-being, lessening the perception of pain.*

- Provide client and family teaching and make referrals if necessary to assist with coping, financial resources, and home care. *The client (and family) with pain requires information about medications, noninvasive techniques for pain management, and sources of assistance with home-based care. The client with acute pain requires information about the expected course of pain resolution.*

Home Care

Teaching the client and family includes:

- Specific drugs to be taken, including the frequency, potential side effects, possible drug interactions, and any special precautions to be taken, such as taking with food or avoiding alcohol.
- How to take or administer the drugs.
- The importance of taking pain medications before the pain becomes severe.
- An explanation that the risk of addiction to pain medications is small when they are used for pain relief and management.
- The importance of scheduling periods of rest and sleep.

Suggest the following resources:

- Pain clinics
- Community support groups
- American Cancer Society
- American Pain Society.

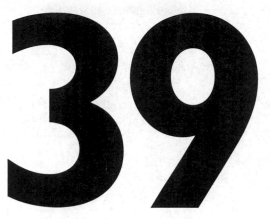

Nursing Care of
Clients with Altered
Fluid, Electrolyte or
Acid-Base Balance

Changes in the normal distribution and composition of body fluids often occur in response to illness and trauma. These changes affect fluid balance of the intracellular and extracellular compartments of the body, the concentration of electrolytes within fluid compartments, and the body's hydrogen ion concentration (pH). Normal physiologic processes depend on a relatively stable state in the internal environment of the body. The fluid volume, electrolyte composition, and pH of both intracellular and extracellular spaces must remain constant within a relatively narrow range to maintain health and life.

Homeostasis is the body's tendency to maintain a state of physiologic balance in the presence of constantly changing conditions. Homeostasis is necessary if the body is to function optimally at a cellular level and as a total organism. Homeostasis depends on multiple factors in both the external and internal environments, such as available oxygen in the air and nutrients in food, as well as normal body temperature, respiration, and digestive processes. The normal volume, composition, distribution, and pH of body fluids reflect a state of homeostasis.

The goal in managing fluid, electrolyte, and acid-base imbalances is to reestablish and maintain a normal balance. Nursing care includes assessing clients who are likely to develop imbalances, monitoring clients for early manifestations, and implementing collaborative and nursing interventions to prevent or correct imbalances. Effective nursing interventions require an understanding of the multiple processes that maintain fluid, electrolyte, and acid-base balance and an understanding of the causes and treatment of imbalances that occur.

Overview of Normal Fluid and Electrolyte Balance

Fluid and electrolyte balance in the body involves regulatory mechanisms that maintain the composition, distribution, and movement of fluids and electrolytes. This section provides an overview of fluid and electrolyte balance in the body. It is followed by discussion of fluid volume and electrolyte balance disorders.

Body Fluid Composition
Body fluid is composed of water and various dissolved substances (solutes).

Water

Water is the primary component of body fluids. It functions in several ways to maintain normal cellular function. Water:

- Provides a medium for the transport and exchange of nutrients and other substances, such as oxygen, carbon dioxide, and metabolic wastes, to and from cells.
- Provides a medium for metabolic reactions within cells.
- Assists in regulating body temperature through the evaporation of perspiration.
- Provides form for body structure and acts as a shock absorber.
- Provides insulation.
- Acts as a lubricant.

Total body water constitutes about 60% of the total body weight, but this amount varies with age, gender, and the amount of body fat. Total body water decreases with aging; in people over age 65, body water may decrease to 45% to 50% of total body weight. Fat cells contain comparatively little water: In the person who is obese, the proportion of water to total body weight is less than in the person of average weight; in a person who is very thin, the proportion of water to total body weight is greater than in the person of average weight. Adult females have a greater ratio of fat to lean tissue mass than adult males; therefore, they have a lower percentage of body water content.

To maintain normal fluid balance, body water intake and output should be approximately equal. The average fluid intake and output usually is about 2500 mL over a 24-hour period.

Electrolytes

Body fluids contain both water molecules and chemical compounds. These chemical compounds can either remain intact in solution or separate (dissociate) into discrete particles. **Electrolytes** are substances that dissociate in solution to form charged particles called ions. *Cations* are positively charged electrolytes; *anions* are negatively charged electrolytes. For example, sodium chloride (NaCl) in solution dissociates into a sodium ion, a cation carrying a positive charge (Na^+); and a chloride ion, an anion carrying a negative charge (Cl^-). Electrolytes may be *univalent,* with only one unit of electrical charge, such as sodium (Na^+) and chloride (Cl^-); or they may be *divalent,* carrying two units of electrical charge, such as magnesium (Mg^{2+}) and phosphate (HPO_4^{2-}).

Electrolytes have many functions. They:

- Assist in regulating water balance.
- Help regulate and maintain acid-base balance.
- Contribute to enzyme reactions.
- Are essential for neuromuscular activity.

The concentration of electrolytes in body fluids generally is measured in milliequivalents per liter of water (mEq/L). A milliequivalent is a measure of the chemical combining power of the ion. For example, 100 mEq of sodium (Na^+) can combine with 100 mEq of chloride (Cl^-) to form sodium chloride (NaCl). Sodium, potassium, and chloride usually are measured in milliequivalents. In some cases, the amount of an electrolyte in body fluid may be measured by weight in milligrams per 100 mL (1 deciliter [dL]) of water (mg/dL). Calcium, magnesium, and phosphorus often are measured by weight in milligrams per deciliter.

Body Fluid Distribution

Body fluid is classified by its location inside or outside of cells. *Intracellular fluid (ICF)* is found within cells. It accounts for approximately 40% of total body weight. ICF is essential for normal cell function, providing a medium for metabolic processes. *Extracellular fluid (ECF)* is located outside of cells. It accounts for approximately 20% of the total body weight. ECF is classified by location.

- Interstitial fluid is located in the spaces between most of the cells of the body. It accounts for approximately 15% of total body weight.

- Intravascular fluid, called plasma, is contained within the arteries, veins, and capillaries. It accounts for approximately 5% of total body weight.

- Transcellular fluid includes urine; digestive secretions; perspiration; and cerebrospinal, pleural, synovial, intraocular, gonadal, and pericardial fluids.

A trace amount of water is found in bone, cartilage, and other dense connective tissues; this water is not exchangeable with other body fluids.

ECF is the transport medium that carries oxygen and nutrients to and waste products from the cells. For example, plasma transports oxygen from the lungs and glucose from the digestive system to the tissues. These solutes diffuse through the capillary wall into the interstitial space, and from there across the cell membrane into the cells. Waste products of metabolism (e.g., carbon dioxide and hydrogen ion) diffuse from the intracellular space into the interstitial space, and from there into plasma via the capillary walls. Plasma then transports these waste products to the lungs and kidneys for elimination.

The concentration of various electrolytes in ICF and ECF differs significantly. ICF contains high concentrations of potassium (K^+), magnesium (Mg^{2+}), and phosphate (PO_4^{2-}), as well as other solutes, such as glucose and oxygen. Sodium (Na^+), chloride (Cl^-), and bicarbonate (HCO_3^-) are the principal extracellular electrolytes. The high sodium concentration in ECF is essential to regulating body fluid volume. The concentration of potassium in ECF is low. There is a minimal difference in electrolyte concentration between plasma and interstitial fluid. Normal values for electrolytes in plasma are shown in Table 39–1.

The body fluid compartments are separated by several types of membranes.

- Cell membranes separate interstitial fluid from intracellular fluid.

- Capillary membranes separate plasma from interstitial fluid.

- Epithelial membranes separate transcellular fluid from interstitial fluid and plasma. These membranes include the mucosa of the stomach, intestines, and gallbladder; the pleural, peritoneal, and synovial membranes; and the tubules of the kidney.

A cell membrane consists of layers of lipid and protein molecules. The layering of these molecules controls the passage of fluid and solutes between the cell and interstitial fluid. The cell membrane is selectively permeable; that is, it allows the passage of water, oxygen, carbon dioxide, and small water-soluble molecules, but bars proteins and other intracellular colloids.

The capillary membrane separating the plasma from the interstitial space is made of squamous epithelial cells. Pores in the membrane allow solute molecules, such as glucose and sodium, dissolved gases, and water to cross the membrane. Minute amounts of albumin and other proteins can also pass through the pores of a capillary membrane, but normally plasma proteins stay in the intravascular compartment.

Body Fluid Movement

Four chemical and physiologic processes control the movement of fluid, electrolytes, and other molecules across membranes between the intracellular and interstitial space and the interstitial space and plasma. These processes are osmosis, diffusion, filtration, and active transport.

Osmosis. The process by which water moves across a selectively permeable membrane from an area of lower solute concentration to an area of higher solute concentration is **osmosis**. A *selectively permeable membrane* allows water molecules to cross, but is relatively impermeable to dissolved substances (*solutes*). Osmosis continues until the solute concentration on both sides of the membrane is equal. For example, if pure water and a sodium chloride solution are separated by a selectively permeable membrane, then water molecules will move across the membrane to the sodium chloride solution. Osmosis is the primary process that controls body fluid movement between the ICF and ECF compartments.

Table 39-1. Normal Values for Electrolytes and Serum Osmolality

Serum Component	Values
Electrolytes	
Sodium (Na^+)	135–145 mEq/L
Chloride (Cl^-)	98–106 mEq/L
Bicarbonate (HCO_3)	22–26 mEq/L
Calcium (Ca^{2+}) (total)	8.5–10 mg/dL
Potassium (K^+)	3.5–5.0 mEq/L
Phosphate/inorganic phosphorus (PO_4^{-2})	1.7–2.6 mEq/L (2.5–4.5 mg/dL)
Magnesium (Mg^{2+})	1.6–2.6 mg/dL (1.3–2.1 mEq/L)
Serum osmolality	275–295 mOsm/kg

Osmolarity and Osmolality. The concentration of a solution may be expressed as the osmolarity or osmolality of the solution. *Osmolarity* refers to the amount of solutes per liter of solution (by volume); it is reported in milliosmoles per liter (mOsm/L) in a solution. *Osmolality* refers to the number of solutes per kilogram of water (by weight); it is reported in milliosmoles per kilogram (mOsm/kg). Because osmotic activity in the body is regulated by the number of active particles (solutes) per kilogram of water, osmolality is used to describe the concentration of body fluids. The normal osmolality of both ICF and ECF ranges between 275 and 295 mOsm/kg. The osmolality of the extracellular fluid depends chiefly on sodium concentration. Serum osmolality may be estimated by doubling the serum sodium concentration (approximately 142 mEq/L).

Osmotic Pressure and Tonicity. The power of a solution to draw water across a membrane is known as the *osmotic pressure* of the solution. The composition of interstitial fluid and intravascular plasma is essentially the same except for a higher concentration of proteins in the plasma. These proteins (especially albumin) exert osmotic pressure, pulling fluid from the interstitial space into the intravascular compartment. This osmotic activity is important in maintaining fluid balance between the interstitial and intravascular spaces, helping hold water within the vascular system.

Tonicity refers to the effect a solution's osmotic pressure has on water movement across the cell membrane of cells within that solution. *Isotonic* solutions have the same concentration of solutes as plasma. Cells placed in an isotonic solution will neither shrink nor swell as there is no net gain or loss of water within the cell, and no change in cell volume. Normal saline (0.9% sodium chloride solution) is an example of an isotonic solution.

Hypertonic solutions have a greater concentration of solutes than plasma. In their presence, water is drawn out of a cell, causing it to shrink. A 3% sodium chloride solution is hypertonic. *Hypotonic* solutions (such as 0.45% sodium chloride) have a lower solute concentration than plasma. When red blood cells are placed in a hypotonic solution, water moves into the cells, causing them to swell and rupture (*hemolyze*).

The concepts of osmotic draw and tonicity are important in understanding the pathophysiologic changes that occur with fluid and electrolyte imbalances, as well as treatment measures. For example, an increased sodium concentration of extracellular fluid causes water to shift from the ICF compartment to the ECF compartment. In this case, administering a hypotonic intravenous solution will facilitate water movement back into the intracellular space.

Diffusion. The process by which solute molecules move from an area of high solute concentration to an area of low solute concentration to become evenly distributed is **diffusion**. The two types of diffusion are simple and facilitated diffusion. *Simple diffusion* occurs by the random movement of particles through a solution. Water, carbon dioxide, oxygen, and solutes move between plasma and the interstitial space by simple diffusion through the capillary membrane. Water and solutes move into the cell by passing through protein channels or by dissolving in the lipid cell membrane. *Facilitated diffusion*, also called carrier-mediated diffusion, allows large water-soluble molecules, such as glucose and amino acids, to diffuse across cell membranes. Proteins embedded in the cell membrane function as *carriers*, helping large molecules cross the membrane.

The rate of diffusion is influenced by a number of factors, such as the concentration of solute and the availability of carrier proteins in the cell membrane. The effect of both simple and facilitated diffusion is to establish equal concentrations of the molecules on both sides of a membrane.

Filtration. The process by which water and dissolved substances (solutes) move from an area of high hydrostatic pressure to an area of low hydrostatic pressure is **filtration**. This usually occurs across capillary membranes. *Hydrostatic pressure* is created by the pumping action of the heart and gravity against the capillary wall. Filtration occurs in the glomerulus of the kidneys, as well as at the arterial end of capillaries.

A balance of hydrostatic (filtration) pressure and osmotic pressure regulates the movement of water between the intravascular and interstitial spaces in the capillary beds of the body. Hydrostatic pressure within the arterial end of the capillary pushes water into the interstitial space. Hydrostatic pressure within the interstitial space opposes this movement to some degree. At the venous end of the capillary, the osmotic force of plasma proteins draws fluid back into the capillary.

Active Transport. **Active transport** allows molecules to move across cell membranes and epithelial membranes against a concentration gradient. This movement requires energy (adenosine triphosphate, or ATP) and a carrier mechanism to maintain a higher concentration of a substance on one side of the membrane than on the other. The sodium-potassium pump is an important example of active transport. High concentrations of potassium in intracellular fluids and of sodium in extracellular fluids are maintained because cells actively transport potassium from interstitial fluid (where the concentration of potassium is about 5 mEq/L) into intracellular fluid (where the potassium concentration is about 150 mEq/L).

Body Fluid Regulation

Homeostasis requires several regulatory mechanisms and processes to maintain the balance between fluid intake and excretion. These include thirst, the kidneys, renin-angiotensin-aldosterone mechanism, antidiuretic hormone, and atrial natriuretic factor. These mechanisms affect the volume, distribution, and composition of body fluids.

Thirst

Thirst is the primary regulator of water intake. Thirst plays an important role in maintaining fluid balance and preventing dehydration. The thirst center, located in the brain, is stimulated when the blood volume drops because of water losses or when serum osmolality (solute concentration) increases.

The thirst mechanism is highly effective in regulating extracellular sodium levels. Increased sodium in ECF causes the serum osmolality to increase, stimulating the thirst center. Fluid intake in turn reduces the sodium concentration of ECF and lowers serum osmolality. Conversely, a drop in serum sodium and low serum osmolality inhibit the thirst center.

Kidneys

The kidneys are primarily responsible for regulating fluid volume and electrolyte balance in the body. They regulate the volume and osmolality of body fluids by controlling the excretion of water and electrolytes. In adults, about 170 L of plasma are filtered through the glomeruli every day. By selectively reabsorbing water and electrolytes, the kidneys maintain the volume and osmolality of body fluids. About 99% of the glomerular filtrate is reabsorbed, and only about 1500 mL of urine is produced over a 24-hour period.

Renin-Angiotensin-Aldosterone System

The renin-angiotensin-aldosterone system works to maintain intravascular fluid balance and blood pressure. A fall in blood flow or blood pressure to the kidneys stimulates specialized receptors in the juxtaglomerular cells of the nephrons to produce *renin*, an enzyme. Renin converts angiotensinogen (a plasma protein) in the circulating blood into angiotensin I. Angiotensin I travels through the bloodstream to the lungs, where it is converted to angiotensin II by angiotensin-converting enzyme (ACE). Angiotensin II is a potent vasoconstrictor; it raises the blood pressure. It also stimulates the thirst mechanism to promote fluid intake and acts directly on the kidneys, causing them to retain sodium and water. Angiotensin II stimulates the adrenal cortex to release aldosterone. Aldosterone promotes sodium and water retention in the distal nephron of the kidney, restoring blood volume.

Antidiuretic Hormone

Antidiuretic hormone (ADH) regulates water excretion from the kidneys. Osmoreceptors in the hypothalamus respond to increases in serum osmolality and decreases in blood volume, stimulating ADH production and release. ADH acts on the distal tubules of the kidney, making them more permeable to water and thus increasing water reabsorption. With increased water reabsorption, urine output falls, blood volume is restored, and serum osmolality drops as the water dilutes body fluids.

Two disorders of ADH production illustrate this effect. First, diabetes insipidus is a condition characterized by a deficiency in ADH production. The lack of ADH causes the distal tubules and collecting ducts of the kidney to be impermeable to water, resulting in copious, very dilute urine output. ADH is not released in response to resulting serum hyperosmolality, but the thirst mechanism is stimulated and the client drinks additional fluids, maintaining high urine output. Second, in the syndrome of inappropriate ADH secretion (SIADH), excess ADH is released. Increased water reabsorption causes increased fluid volume and scant, concentrated urine output.

Atrial Natriuretic Factor

Atrial natriuretic factor (ANF) is a hormone released by atrial muscle cells in response to distension from fluid overload. ANF affects several body systems, including the cardiovascular, renal, neural, gastrointestinal, and endocrine systems, but it primarily affects the renin-angiotensin-aldosterone system. ANF opposes this system by inhibiting renin secretion and blocking the secretion and sodium-retaining effects of aldosterone. As a result, ANF promotes sodium wasting and diuresis (increased urine output) and causes vasodilation.

Fluid and Electrolyte Imbalances

The Client with Fluid Volume Deficit

Fluid volume deficit (FVD) is a decrease in intravascular, interstitial, and/or intracellular fluid in the body. Fluid volume deficits may be due to excessive fluid losses, insufficient fluid intake, or failure of regulatory mechanisms and fluid shifts within the body. Fluid volume deficit is a relatively common problem that may exist alone or in combination with other electrolyte or acid-base imbalances. The term **dehydration** refers to loss of water alone, even though it often is used interchangeably with fluid volume deficit.

Pathophysiology

The most common cause of fluid volume deficit is excessive loss of gastrointestinal fluids from vomiting, diarrhea, gastrointestinal suctioning, intestinal fistulas, and intestinal drainage. Other causes of fluid losses include:

- Excessive renal losses of water and sodium from diuretic therapy, renal disorders, or endocrine disorders.
- Water and sodium losses during sweating from excessive exercise or increased environmental temperature.
- Hemorrhage.
- Chronic abuse of laxatives and/or enemas.

Inadequate fluid intake may result from lack of access to fluids, inability to request or to swallow fluids, oral trauma, or altered thirst mechanisms. Older adults are at particular risk for fluid volume deficit.

Fluid volume deficit can develop slowly or rapidly, depending on the type of fluid loss. Loss of extracellular fluid volume can lead to **hypovolemia**, decreased circulating blood volume. Electrolytes often are lost along with fluid, resulting in an **isotonic fluid volume deficit**. When both water and electrolytes are lost, the serum sodium level remains normal, although levels of other electrolytes, such as potassium, may fall. Fluid is drawn into the vascular compartment from the interstitial spaces as the body attempts to maintain tissue perfusion. This eventually depletes fluid in the intracellular compartment as well.

Hypovolemia stimulates regulatory mechanisms to maintain circulation. The sympathetic nervous system is stimulated, as is the thirst mechanism. ADH and aldosterone are released, prompting sodium and water retention by the kidneys.

Third Spacing

Third spacing is a shift of fluid from the vascular space into an area where it is not available to support normal physiologic processes. The trapped fluid represents a volume loss and is unavailable for normal physiologic processes. Fluid may be sequestered in the abdomen or bowel, or in such other actual or potential body spaces as the pleural or peritoneal space. Fluid may also become trapped within soft tissues following trauma or burns. Assessing the extent of fluid volume deficit resulting from third spacing is difficult. It may not be reflected by changes in weight or intake-and-output records, and it may not become apparent until after organ malfunction occurs (Metheny, 2000).

Manifestations

With a rapid fluid loss, such as hemorrhage or uncontrolled vomiting, manifestations of hypovolemia develop rapidly. When the loss of fluid occurs more gradually, the client's fluid volume may be very low before symptoms develop.

Rapid weight loss is a good indicator of fluid volume deficit. Each liter of body fluid weighs about 1 kg (2.2 lb). Loss of interstitial fluid causes skin turgor to diminish. When pinched, the skin of a client with FVD remains elevated. Loss of skin elasticity with aging makes this assessment finding less accurate in older adults. Tongue turgor is not generally affected by age; therefore, assessing the size, dryness, and longitudinal furrows of the tongue may be a more accurate indicator of fluid volume deficit.

Postural or orthostatic hypotension is a sign of hypovolemia. A drop of more than 15 mmHg in systolic blood pressure when changing from a lying to standing position often indicates loss of intravascular volume. Venous pressure falls as well, causing flat neck veins, even when the client is recumbent. Loss of intravascular fluid causes the hematocrit to increase.

Compensatory mechanisms to conserve water and sodium and maintain circulation account for many of the manifestations of fluid volume deficit, such as tachycardia; pale, cool skin (vasoconstriction); and decreased urine output. The specific gravity of urine increases as water is reabsorbed in the tubules. Table 39–2 compares assessment findings for fluid deficit and fluid excess.

Collaborative Care

The primary goals of care related to fluid volume deficit are to prevent deficits in clients at risk and to correct deficits and their underlying causes. Depending on the acuity of the imbalance, treatment may include replacement of fluids and electrolytes by the intravenous, oral, or enteral route. When possible, the oral or enteral route is preferred for administering fluids. In acute situations, however, intravenous fluid administration is necessary.

Diagnostic Tests

Laboratory and diagnostic tests may be ordered when fluid volume deficit is suspected. Such tests measure:

- *Serum electrolytes.* In an isotonic fluid deficit, sodium levels are within normal limits; when the loss is water only, sodium levels are high. Decreases in potassium are common.
- *Serum osmolality.* To help differentiate isotonic fluid loss from water loss. With water loss, osmolality is high; it may be within normal limits with an isotonic fluid loss.
- *Serum hemoglobin and hematocrit.* The hematocrit often is elevated due to loss of intravascular volume and hemoconcentration.
- *Urine specific gravity and osmolality.* As the kidneys conserve water, both the specific gravity and osmolality of urine increase.
- *Central venous pressure (CVP).* The CVP measures the mean pressure in the superior vena cava or right atrium, providing an accurate assessment of fluid volume status.

Fluid Management

A fluid challenge may be done to evaluate fluid volume when urine output is low and cardiac or renal function is questionable. A fluid challenge helps prevent fluid volume overload resulting from intravenous fluid therapy when cardiac or renal function is compromised. Nursing responsibilities for a fluid challenge are as follows:

1. Obtain and document baseline vital signs, breath sounds, urine output, and mental status.
2. Administer (by IV infusion) an initial fluid volume of 200 to 300 mL over 5 to 10 minutes.
3. Reevaluate baseline data at the end of the 10-minute infusion period.
4. Administer additional fluid until a specified volume is infused or the desired hemodynamic parameters are achieved.

Table 39-2. *Comparison of Assessment Findings in Clients with Fluid Imbalance*

Assessment	Fluid Deficit	Fluid Excess
Blood pressure	Decreased systolic Postural hypotension	Increased
Heart rate	Increased	Increased
Pulse amplitude	Decreased	Increased

Continued on the next page

Table 39–2. Continued

Respirations	Normal	Moist crackles Wheezes
Jugular vein	Flat	Distended
Edema	Rare	Dependent
Skin turgor	Loose, poor turgor	Taut
Output	Low, concentrated	May be low or normal
Urine specific gravity	High	Low
Weight	Loss	Gain

Intravenous fluids are often prescribed to correct FVD. Table 39–3 describes the types, tonicity, and uses of commonly administered intravenous fluids. Isotonic electrolyte solutions (0.9% NaCl or Ringer's solution) are used to expand plasma volume in hypotensive clients or to replace abnormal losses, which are usually isotonic in nature. Five percent dextrose in water (D5W) is given to provide water to treat total body water deficits. D5W is isotonic (similar in tonicity to the plasma), and thus does not provoke hemolysis of red blood cells. The dextrose is metabolized to carbon dioxide and water, leaving free water available for tissue needs.

Hypotonic saline solution (0.45% NaCl with or without added electrolytes) or hypotonic mixed electrolyte solutions are used as maintenance solutions. These solutions provide additional electrolytes, such as potassium; a buffer (lactate or acetate) as needed; and water.

Nursing Care

Nurses are responsible for identifying clients at risk for fluid volume deficit, initiating and carrying out measures to prevent and treat fluid volume deficit, and monitoring the effects of therapy.

Health Promotion

Health promotion activities focus on teaching clients to prevent fluid volume deficit. Discuss the importance of maintaining adequate fluid intake, particularly when exercising and during hot weather. Advise clients to use commercial sports drinks to replace both water and electrolytes when exercising during warm weather. Instruct clients to maintain fluid intake when ill, particularly during periods of fever or when diarrhea is a problem.

Table 39-3.   Commonly Administered Intravenous Fluids

	Fluid and Tonicity	**Uses**
Dextrose in Water Solutions	5% dextrose in water (D5W) Isotonic	Replaces water losses
		Provides free water necessary for cellular rehydration
		Lowers serum sodium in hypernatremia
	10% dextrose in water (D10W)	Provides free water

Table 39-3. Continued

	Hypertonic	Provides nutrition (supplies 340 kcal/L)
	20% dextrose in water (D20W) Hypertonic	Supplies 680 kcal/L May cause diuresis
	50% dextrose in water (D50W) Hypertonic	Supplies 1700 kcal/L Used to correct hypoglycemia
Saline Solutions	0.45% sodium chloride Hypotonic	Provides free water to replace hypotonic fluid losses Maintains levels of plasma sodium and chloride
	0.9% sodium chloride Isotonic	Expands intravascular volume Replaces water lost from extracellular fluid Used with blood transfusions Replaces large sodium losses (as from burns)
	3% sodium chloride Hypertonic	Corrects serious sodium depletion
Combined Dextrose and Saline Solution	5% dextrose & 0.45% sodium chloride Isotonic	Provides free water Provides sodium chloride Maintenance fluid of choice if there are noelectrolyte imbalances
Multiple Electrolyte Solutions	Ringer's solution Isotonic (electrolyte concentrations of sodium, potassium, chloride, and calcium are similar to plasma levels)	Expands the intracellularfluid Replaces extracellular fluid losses
	Lactated Ringer's solution Isotonic (similar in composition of electrolytes to plasma but does not contain magnesium)	Replaces fluid losses from burns and the lower gastrointestinal tract Fluid of choice for acute blood loss

Discuss the increased risk for fluid volume deficit with older adults and provide information about prevention. Teach older adults (and their caretakers) that thirst decreases with aging and urge them to maintain a regular fluid intake of about 1500 mL per day, regardless of perception of thirst.

Carefully monitor clients at risk for abnormal fluid losses through routes, such as vomiting, diarrhea, nasogastric suction, increased urine output, fever, or wounds. Monitor fluid intake in clients with decreased level of consciousness, disorientation, nausea and anorexia, and physical limitations.

Assessment

Collect assessment data through the health history interview and physical examination.

- *Health history:* Risk factors, such as medications, acute or chronic renal or endocrine disease; precipitating factors, such as hot weather, extensive exercise, lack of access to fluids, recent illness (especially if accompanied by fever, vomiting, and/or diarrhea); onset and duration of symptoms.

- *Physical assessment:* Weight; vital signs including orthostatic blood pressure and pulse; peripheral pulses and capillary refill; jugular neck vein distention; skin color, temperature, turgor; level of consciousness and mentation; urine output.

Nursing Diagnoses and Interventions

The focus for nursing diagnoses and interventions for the client with fluid volume deficit is on managing the effects of the deficit and preventing complications.

Deficient Fluid Volume

Clients with fluid volume deficit due to abnormal losses, inadequate intake, or impaired fluid regulation require close monitoring as well as immediate and ongoing fluid replacement.

- Assess intake and output accurately, monitoring fluid balance. In acute situations, hourly intake and output may be indicated. *Urine output should be 30 to 60 mL per hour (unless renal failure is present). Urine output of less than 30 mL per hour indicates inadequate renal perfusion and an increased risk for acute renal failure and inadequate tissue perfusion.*

- Assess vital signs, CVP, and peripheral pulse volume at least every four hours. *Hypotension, tachycardia, low CVP, and weak, easily obliterated peripheral pulses indicate hypovolemia.*

- Weigh daily under standard conditions (time of day, clothing, and scale). *In most instances (except third spacing), changes in weight accurately reflect fluid balance.*

- Administer and monitor the intake of oral fluids as prescribed. Identify beverage preferences and provide these on a schedule. *Oral fluid replacement is preferred when the client is able to drink and retain fluids.*

- Administer intravenous fluids as prescribed using an electronic infusion pump. Monitor for indicators of fluid overload if rapid fluid replacement is ordered: dyspnea, tachypnea, tachycardia, increased CVP, jugular vein distension, and edema. *Rapid fluid replacement may lead to hypervolemia, resulting in pulmonary edema and cardiac failure, particularly in clients with compromised cardiac and renal function.*

- Monitor laboratory values: electrolytes, serum osmolality, BUN, and hematocrit. *Rehydration may lead to changes in serum electrolytes, osmolality, BUN, and hematocrit. In some cases, electrolyte replacement may be necessary during rehydration.*

Ineffective Tissue Perfusion

A fluid volume deficit can lead to decreased perfusion of renal, cerebral, and peripheral tissues. Inadequate renal perfusion can lead to acute renal failure. Decreased cerebral perfusion leads to changes in mental status and cognitive function, causing restlessness, anxiety, agitation, excitability, confusion, vertigo, fainting, and weakness.

- Monitor for changes in level of consciousness and mental status. *Restlessness, anxiety, confusion, and agitation may indicate inadequate cerebral blood flow and circulatory collapse.*

- Monitor serum creatinine, BUN, and cardiac enzymes, reporting elevated levels to the physician. *Elevated levels may indicate impaired renal function or cardiac perfusion related to circulatory failure.*
- Turn client at least every two hours. Provide good skin care and monitor for evidence of skin or tissue breakdown. *Impaired circulation to peripheral tissues increases the risk of skin breakdown. Turn frequently to relieve pressure over bony prominences. Keep skin clean, dry, and moisturized to help maintain integrity.*

Risk for Injury

The client with fluid volume deficit is at risk for injury because of dizziness and loss of balance resulting from decreased cerebral perfusion secondary to hypovolemia.

- Institute safety precautions, including keeping the bed in a low position, using side rails as needed, and slowly raising the client from supine to sitting or sitting to standing position. *Using safety precautions and allowing time for the blood pressure to adjust to position changes reduce the risk of injury.*
- Teach client and family members how to reduce orthostatic hypotension:
  a. Move from one position to another in stages; for example, raise the head of the bed before sitting up, and sit for a few minutes before standing.
  b. Avoid prolonged standing.
  c. Rest in a recliner rather than in bed during the day.
  d. Use assistive devices to pick up objects from the floor rather than stooping.

Teaching measures to reduce orthostatic hypotension reduces the client's risk for injury. Prolonged bed rest increases skeletal muscle weakness and decreases venous tone, contributing to postural hypotension. Prolonged standing allows blood to pool in the legs, reducing venous return and cardiac output.

Home Care

Depending on the severity of the fluid volume deficit, the client may be managed in the home or residential facility, or may be admitted to an acute care facility. Assess the client's understanding of the cause of the deficit and the fluids necessary for providing replacement. Address the following topics when preparing the client and family for home care:

- The importance of maintaining adequate fluid intake (at least 1500 mL per day; more if extra fluid is being lost through perspiration, fever, or diarrhea).
- Manifestations of fluid imbalance, and how to monitor fluid balance.
- How to prevent fluid deficit:
  Avoid exercising during extreme heat.
  1. Increase fluid intake during hot weather.
  2. If vomiting, take small frequent amounts of ice chips or clear liquids, such as weak tea, flat cola, or ginger ale.
  3. Reduce intake of coffee, tea, and alcohol, which increase urine output and can cause fluid loss.
- Replacement of fluids lost through diarrhea with fruit juices or bouillon, rather than large amounts of tap water
- Alternate sources of fluid, such as gelatin, frozen juices, or ice cream, for effective replacement of lost fluids

The Client with Fluid Volume Excess

Fluid volume excess results when both water and sodium are retained in the body. Fluid volume excess may be caused by fluid overload (excess water and sodium intake) or by impairment of the mechanisms that maintain homeostasis. The excess fluid can lead to excess intravascular fluid (**hypervolemia**) and excess interstitial fluid (**edema**).

Pathophysiology

Fluid volume excess usually results from conditions that cause retention of both sodium and water. These conditions include heart failure, cirrhosis of the liver, renal failure, adrenal gland disorders, corticosteroid administration, and stress conditions causing the release of ADH and aldosterone. Other causes include an excessive intake of sodium-containing foods, drugs that cause sodium retention, and the administration of excess amounts of sodium-containing intravenous fluids, such as 0.9% NaCl or Ringer's solution. This iatrogenic cause of fluid volume excess primarily affects clients with impaired regulatory mechanisms.

In fluid volume excess, both water and sodium are gained together in about the same proportions as normally exists in extracellular fluid. The total body sodium content is increased, which in turn causes an increase in total body water. Because the increase in sodium and water is isotonic, the serum sodium and osmolality remain normal, and the excess fluid remains in the extracellular space.

Manifestations and Complications

Excess extracellular fluid leads to hypervolemia and circulatory overload. Excess fluid in the interstitial space causes peripheral or generalized edema. The following manifestations of fluid volume excess relate to both the excess fluid and its effects on circulation.

- The increase in total body water causes weight gain (more than 5% of body weight) over a short period.
- Circulatory overload causes manifestations such as:
  1. A full, bounding pulse.
  2. Distended neck and peripheral veins.
  3. Increased central venous pressure (>11–12 cm of water).
  4. Cough, **dyspnea** (labored or difficult breathing), **orthopnea** (difficulty breathing when supine).
  5. Moist crackles (rales) in the lungs; pulmonary edema (excess fluid in pulmonary interstitial spaces and alveoli) if severe.
  6. Increased urine output (**polyuria**).
  7. **Ascites** (excess fluid in the peritoneal cavity).
  8. Peripheral edema, or if severe, *anasarca* (severe, gener alized edema).
- Dilution of plasma by excess fluid causes a decreased hematocrit and BUN.
- Possible cerebral edema (excess water in brain tissues) can lead to altered mental status and anxiety.

Heart failure is not only a potential cause of fluid volume excess, but it is also a potential complication of the condition if the heart is unable to increase its workload to handle the excess blood volume. Severe fluid overload and heart failure can lead to pulmonary edema, a medical emergency.

Collaborative Care

Managing fluid volume excess focuses on prevention in clients at risk, treating its manifestations, and correcting the underlying cause. Management includes limiting sodium and water intake and administering diuretics.

Diagnostic Tests

The following laboratory tests may be ordered:

* *Serum electrolytes* and *serum osmolality* are measured. Serum sodium and osmolality usually remain within normal limits.
* *Serum hematocrit* and *hemoglobin* often are decreased due to plasma dilution from excess extracellular fluid.

Additional tests of *renal* and *liver function*, such as serum creatinine, BUN, and liver enzymes, may be ordered to help determine the cause of fluid volume excess if it is unclear.

Medications

Diuretics are commonly used to treat fluid volume excess. They inhibit sodium and water reabsorption, increasing urine output. The three major classes of diuretics, each of which acts on a different part of the kidney tubule, are as follows:

* Loop diuretics act in the ascending loop of Henle.
* Thiazide-type diuretics act on the distal convoluted tubule.
* Potassium-sparing diuretics affect the distal nephron.

Treatments

Fluid Management

Fluid intake may be restricted in clients who have fluid volume excess. The amount of fluid allowed per day is prescribed by the primary care provider. All fluid intake must be calculated, including meals and that used to administer medications orally or intravenously.

Table 39-4. Medication Administration – Diuretics for Fluid Volume Excess

Diuretics increase urinary excretion of water and sodium. They are categorized into three major groups: loop diuretics, thiazide and thiazide-like diuretics, and potassium-sparing diuretics. Diuretics are used to enhance renal function and to treat vascular fluid overload and edema. Common side effects include orthostatic hypotension, dehydration, electrolyte imbalance, and possible hyperglycemia. Diuretics should be used with caution in the older adult. Examples of each major type follow.

Continued on the next page

Table 39-4. Continued

Loop Diuretics

Furosemide (Lasix)   Ethacrynic Acid (Edecrin)
Bumetanide (Bumex)   Torsemide (Demadex)

Loop diuretics inhibit sodium and chloride reabsorption in the ascending loop of Henle (see Chapter 22 for the anatomy of the kidneys). As a result, loop diuretics promote the excretion of sodium, chloride, potassium, and water.

Thiazide and Thiazidelike Diuretics

Bendroflumethiazide (Naturetin)   Polythiazide (Renese)
Chlorothiazide (Diuril)   Chlorthalidone (Hygroton)
Hydrochlorothiazide   Trichlormethiazide
(HydroDIURIL, Oretic)   (Naqua)
Metolazone (Zaroxolyn)   Indapamide (Lozol)

Thiazide and thiazidelike diuretics promote the excretion of sodium, chloride, potassium, and water by decreasing absorption in the distal tubule.

Potassium-Sparing Diuretics

Spironolactone (Aldactone)
Amiloride HCl (Midamor)
Triamterene (Dyrenium)

Potassium-sparing diuretics promote excretion of sodium and water by inhibiting sodium-potassium exchange in the distal tubule.

Client and Family Teaching

* The drug will increase the amount and frequency of urination.
* The drugs must be taken even when you feel well.
* Take the drugs in the morning and afternoon to avoid having to get up at night to urinate.
* Change position slowly to avoid dizziness.
* Report the following to your primary health care provider: dizziness; trouble breathing; or swelling of face, hands, or feet.
* Weigh yourself every day, and report sudden gains or losses.
* Avoid using the salt shaker when eating.
* If the drug increases potassium loss, eat foods high in potassium, such as orange juice and bananas.
* Do not use salt substitute if you are taking a potassium-sparing diuretic.

Dietary Management

Because sodium retention is a primary cause of fluid volume excess, a sodium-restricted diet often is prescribed. Americans typically consume about 4 to 5 grams (g) of sodium every day; recommended sodium intake is 500 to 2400 mg per day. The primary dietary sources of sodium are the salt shaker, processed foods, and foods themselves.

A mild sodium restriction can be achieved by instructing the client and primary food preparer in the household to reduce the amount of salt in recipes by half, avoid using the salt shaker during meals, and avoid foods that contain high levels of sodium (either naturally or because of processing). In moderate and severely sodium-restricted diets, salt is avoided altogether, as are all foods containing significant amounts of sodium.

Nursing Care

Nursing care focuses on preventing fluid volume excess in clients at risk and on managing problems resulting from its effects.

Health Promotion

Health promotion related to fluid volume excess focuses on teaching preventive measures to clients who are at risk (e.g., clients who have heart or kidney failure). Discuss the relationship between sodium intake and water retention. Provide guidelines for a low-sodium diet, and teach clients to carefully read food labels to identify "hidden" sodium, particularly in processed foods. Instruct clients at risk to weigh themselves on a regular basis, using the same scale, and to notify their primary care provider if they gain more than 5 lb in a week or less.

Carefully monitor clients receiving intravenous fluids for signs of hypervolemia. Reduce the flow rate and promptly report manifestations of fluid overload to the physician.

Assessment

Collect assessment data through the health history interview and physical examination.

- Health history: Risk factors such as medications, heart failure, acute or chronic renal or endocrine disease; precipitating factors such as a recent illness, change in diet, or change in medications. Recent weight gain; complaints of persistent cough, shortness of breath, swelling of feet and ankles, or difficulty sleeping when lying down.
- Physical assessment: Weight; vital signs; peripheral pulses and capillary refill; jugular neck vein distention; edema; lung sounds (crackles or wheezes), dyspnea, cough, and sputum; urine output; mental status.

Nursing Diagnoses and Interventions

Nursing diagnoses and interventions for the client with fluid volume excess focus on the multisystem effects of the fluid overload.

Excess Fluid Volume

Nursing care for the client with fluid volume excess includes collaborative interventions, such as administering diuretics and maintaining a fluid restriction, as well as monitoring the status and effects of the fluid volume excess. This is particularly critical in older clients because of the age-related decline in cardiac and renal compensatory responses.

- Assess vital signs, heart sounds, CVP, and volume of peripheral arteries. *Hypervolemia can cause hypertension, bounding peripheral pulses, a third heart sound (S_3) due to the volume of blood flow through the heart, and high CVP readings.*

- Assess for the presence and extent of edema, particularly in the lower extremities, the back, sacral, and periorbital areas. *Initially, edema affects the dependent portions of the body—the lower extremities of ambulatory clients and the sacrum in bedridden clients. Periorbital edema indicates more generalized edema.*

- Obtain daily weights at the same time of day, using approximately the same clothing and a balanced scale. *Daily weights are one of the most important gauges of fluid balance. Acute weight gain or loss represents fluid gain or loss. Weight gain of 2 kg is equivalent to 2 L of fluid gain.*

- Administer oral fluids cautiously, adhering to any prescribed fluid restriction. Discuss the restriction with the client and significant others, including the total volume allowed, the rationale, and the importance of reporting all fluid taken. *All sources of fluid intake, including ice chips, are recorded to avoid excess fluid intake.*

- Provide oral hygiene at least every two hours. *Oral hygiene contributes to client comfort and keeps mucous membranes intact; it also helps relieve thirst if fluids are restricted.*

- Teach client and significant others about the sodium-restricted diet, and emphasize the importance of checking before bringing foods to the client. *Excess sodium promotes water retention; a sodium-restricted diet is ordered to reduce water gain.*

- Administer prescribed diuretics as ordered, monitoring the client's response to therapy. *Loop or high-ceiling diuretics such as furosemide can lead to rapid fluid loss and signs of hypovolemia and electrolyte imbalance.*

Risk for Impaired Skin Integrity

Tissue edema decreases oxygen and nutrient delivery to the skin and subcutaneous tissues, increasing the risk of injury.

- Frequently assess skin, particularly in pressure areas and over bony prominences. *Skin breakdown can progress rapidly when circulation is impaired.*

- Reposition the client at least every two hours. Provide skin care with each position change. *Frequent position changes minimize tissue pressure and promote blood flow to tissues.*

- Provide an eggcrate mattress or alternating pressure mattress, foot cradle, heel protectors, and other devices to reduce pressure on tissues. *These devices, which distribute pressure away from bony prominences, reduce the risk of skin breakdown.*

Risk for Impaired Gas Exchange

With fluid volume excess, gas exchange may be impaired by edema of pulmonary interstitial tissues. Acute pulmonary edema is a serious and potentially life-threatening complication of pulmonary congestion.

- Auscultate lungs for presence or worsening of crackles and wheezes; auscultate heart for extra heart sounds. *Crackles and wheezes indicate pulmonary congestion and edema. A gallop rhythm (S_3) may indicate diastolic overloading of the ventricles secondary to fluid volume excess.*

- Place in Fowler's position if dyspnea or orthopnea is present. *Fowler's position improves lung expansion by decreasing the pressure of abdominal contents on the diaphragm.*

- Monitor oxygen saturation levels and **arterial blood gases (ABGs)** for evidence of impaired gas exchange (Sao_2 < 92%–95%; Pao_2 < 80 mmHg). Administer oxygen as indicated. *Edema of interstitial lung tissues can interfere with gas exchange and delivery to* *body tissues. Supplemental oxygen promotes gas exchange across the alveolar-capillary membrane, improving tissue oxygenation.*

Home Care

Teaching for home care focuses on managing the underlying cause of fluid volume excess and preventing future episodes of excess fluid volume. Address the following topics when preparing the client and family for home care:

- Signs and symptoms of excess fluid and when to contact the care provider.
- Prescribed medications: when and how to take, intended and adverse effects, what to report to care provider.
- Recommended or prescribed diet; ways to reduce sodium intake; how to read food labels for salt and sodium content; use of salt substitutes, if allowed.
- If restricted, the amount and type of fluids to take each day; how to balance intake over 24 hours.
- Monitoring weight; changes reported to care provider.
- Ways to decrease dependent edema:
  a. Change position frequently.
  b. Avoid restrictive clothing.
  c. Avoid crossing the legs when sitting.
  d. Wear support stockings or hose.
  e. Elevate feet and legs when sitting.
- How to protect edematous skin from injury:
  a. Do not walk barefoot.
  b. Buy well-fitting shoes; shop in the afternoon when feet are more likely to be swollen.
- Using additional pillows or a recliner to sleep, to relieve orthopnea.

Potassium Imbalance

Potassium, the primary intercellular cation, plays a vital role in cell metabolism, cardiac, and neuromuscular function. The normal serum (ECF) potassium level is 3.5 to 5.0 mEq/L.

Overview of Normal Potassium Balance

Most potassium in the body is found within the cells (ICF), which have a concentration of 140 to 150 mEq/L. This significant difference in the potassium concentrations of ICF and ECF helps maintain the resting membrane potential of nerve and muscle cells; either a deficit or an excess of potassium can adversely affect neuromuscular and cardiac function. The higher intracellular potassium concentration is maintained by the sodium-potassium pump.

To maintain its balance, potassium must be replaced daily. Normally, potassium is supplied in food. Virtually all foods contain potassium, although some foods and fluids are richer sources of this element than others.

The kidneys eliminate potassium very efficiently; even when potassium intake is stopped, the kidneys continue to excrete it. Because the kidneys do not conserve potassium well, significant amounts may be lost through this route. However, because the kidneys are the principal organs involved in the elimination of potassium, renal failure can lead to potentially serious elevations of serum potassium.

Aldosterone helps regulate potassium elimination by the kidneys. An increased potassium concentration in ECF stimulates aldosterone production by the adrenal gland. The kidneys respond to aldosterone by increasing potassium excretion. Changes in aldosterone secretion can profoundly affect the serum potassium level.

Normally only small amounts of potassium are lost in the feces, but substantial amounts may be lost from the gastrointestinal tract with diarrhea or through drainage from an ileostomy (a permanent opening into the small bowel).

Potassium constantly shifts into and out of the cells. This movement between ICF and ECF can significantly affect the serum potassium level. For example, potassium shifts into or out of the cells in response to changes in hydrogen ion concentration (pH) as the body strives to maintain a stable acid-base balance. Table 39-5 summarizes potassium imbalances, their causes, and manifestations.

Table 39-5. Causes and Manifestations of Potassium Imbalances

Imbalance	Causes	Manifestations
Hypokalemia Serum potassium <3.5 mEq/L	• Excess GI losses: vomiting, diarrhea, ileostomy drainage • Renal losses: diuretics, hyperaldosteronism • Inadequate intake • Shift into cells: Alkalosis, rapid tissue repair	**Cardiovascular** • Dysrhythmias • ECG changes **Gastrointestinal** • Nausea and vomiting • Anorexia • Decreased bowel sounds • Ileus **Musculoskeletal** • Muscle weakness • Leg cramps
Hyperkalemia Serum potassium >5.0 mEq/L	• Renal failure • Potassium-sparing diuretics • Adrenal insufficiency • Excess potassium intake (e.g., excess potassium replacement) • Aged blood • Shift out of cells: Cell and tissue damage, acidosis	**Cardiovascular** • Tall, peaked T waves, widened QRS • Dysrhythmias • Cardiac arrest **Gastrointestinal** • Nausea and vomiting • Abdominal cramping • Diarrhea **Neuromuscular** • Muscle weakness • Paresthesias • Flaccid paralysis

The Client with Hypokalemia

Hypokalemia is an abnormally low serum potassium (less than 3.5 mEq/L). It usually results from excess potassium loss, although hospitalized clients may be at risk for hypokalemia because of inadequate potassium intake.

Pathophysiology and Manifestations

Excess potassium may be lost through the kidneys or the gastrointestinal tract. These losses cause depletion of total potassium stores in the body.

- Excess potassium loss through the kidneys often is secondary to drugs, such as potassium-wasting diuretics, corticosteroids, amphotericin B, and large doses of some antibiotics. Hyperaldosteronism, a condition in which the adrenal glands secrete excess aldosterone, also causes excess elimination of potassium through the kidneys. Glucosuria and osmotic diuresis (e.g., associated with diabetes mellitus) also cause potassium wasting through the kidneys (Metheny, 2000).

- Gastrointestinal losses of potassium result from severe vomiting, gastric suction, or loss of intestinal fluids through diarrhea or ileostomy drainage.

Potassium intake may be inadequate in clients who are unable or unwilling to eat for prolonged periods. Hospitalized clients are at risk, especially those on extended parenteral fluid therapy with solutions that do not contain potassium. Clients with anorexia nervosa or alcoholism may develop hypokalemia due to both inadequate intake and loss of potassium through vomiting, diarrhea, or laxative or diuretic use.

A *relative* loss of potassium occurs when potassium shifts from ECF into the cells. This usually is due to loss of hydrogen ion and alkalosis, although it also may occur during periods of rapid tissue repair (e.g., following a burn or trauma), in the presence of excess insulin (insulin promotes potassium entry into skeletal muscle and liver cells), during acute stress, or because of hypothermia. In these instances, the total body stores of potassium remain adequate.

Hypokalemia affects the transmission of nerve impulses, interfering with the contractility of smooth, skeletal, and cardiac muscle, as well as the regulation and transmission of cardiac impulses.

- Characteristic electrocardiogram (ECG) changes of hypokalemia include flattened or inverted T waves, the development of U waves, and a depressed ST segment. The most serious cardiac effect is an increased risk of atrial and ventricular **dysrhythmias** (abnormal rhythms). Hypokalemia increases the risk for digitalis toxicity in clients receiving this drug used to treat heart failure.

- Hypokalemia affects both the resting membrane potential and intracellular enzymes in skeletal and smooth muscle cells. This causes skeletal muscle weakness and slowed peristalsis of the gastrointestinal tract. Muscles of the lower extremities are affected first, then the trunk and upper extremities.

Hypokalemia can also affect kidney function, particularly the ability to concentrate urine. Severe hypokalemia can lead to **rhabdomyolysis**, a condition in which muscle fibers disintegrate, releasing myoglobin to be excreted in the urine.

Collaborative Care

The management of hypokalemia focuses on prevention and treatment of a deficiency.

Diagnostic Tests

The following laboratory and diagnostic tests may be ordered:

- *Serum potassium (K+)* is used to monitor potassium levels in clients who are at risk for or who are being treated for hypokalemia. A serum K+ of 3.0 to 3.5 mEq/L is considered mild hypokalemia. Moderate hypokalemia is defined as a serum K+ of 2.5 to 3.0 mEq/L, and severe hypokalemia as a serum K+ of less than 2.5 mEq/L (Metheny, 2000).

- *Arterial blood gases (ABGs)* are measured to determine acid-base status. An increased pH (alkalosis) often is associated with hypokalemia.

- *ECG recordings* are obtained to evaluate the effects of hypokalemia on the cardiac conduction system.

Medications

Oral and/or parenteral potassium supplements are given to prevent and, as needed, treat hypokalemia. To prevent hypokalemia in the client taking nothing by mouth, 40 mEq of potassium chloride per day is added to intravenous fluids. The dose used to treat hypokalemia includes the daily maintenance requirement, replacement of ongoing losses (e.g., gastric suction), and additional potassium to correct the existing deficit. Several days of therapy may be required.

Table 39-6. Medication Administration – Hypokalemia

Potassium Sources

Potassium acetate (Tri-K)
Potassium bicarbonate (K + Care ET)
Potassium citrate (K-Lyte)
Potassium chloride (K-Lease, Micro-K 10, Apo-K)
Potassium gluconate (Kaon Elixir, Royonate)

Potassium is rapidly absorbed from the gastrointestinal tract; potassium chloride is the agent of choice, because low chloride often accompanies low potassium. Potassium is used to prevent and/or treat hypokalemia (e.g., with parenteral nutrition and potassium-wasting diuretics, and prophylactically after major surgery).

Nursing Responsibilities
- When giving oral forms of potassium:
    a. Dilute or dissolve effervescent, soluable, or liquid potassium in fruit or vegetable juice or cold water.
    b. Chill to increase palatability.
    c. Give with food to minimize GI effects.

- When giving parenteral forms of potassium:
    a. Administer slowly.

Table 39-6. Continued

    b.   *Do not* administer undiluted.

    c.   Assess injection site frequently for signs of pain and inflammation.

    d.   Use an infusion control device.

- Assess for abdominal pain, distention, gastrointestinal bleeding; if present, do not administer medication. Notify health care provider.
- Monitor fluid intake and output.
- Assess for manifestations of hyperkalemia: weakness, feeling of heaviness in legs, mental confusion, hypotension, cardiac arrhythmias, changes in ECG, increased serum potassium levels.

Client and Family Teaching

- Do not take potassium supplements if you are also taking a potassium-sparing diuretic.
- When parenteral potassium is discontinued, eat potassium-rich foods.
- Do not chew enteric-coated tablets or allow them to dissolve in the mouth; this may affect the potency and action of the medications.
- Take potassium supplements with meals.
- Do not use salt substitutes when taking potassium (most salt substitutes are potassium based).

Dietary Management

A diet high in potassium-rich foods is recommended for clients at risk for developing hypokalemia or to supplement drug therapy.

Nursing Care

Health Promotion

When providing general health education, discuss using balanced electrolyte solutions (e.g., Pedialyte or sports drinks) to replace abnormal fluid losses (excess perspiration, vomiting, or severe diarrhea). Discuss the necessity of preventing hypokalemia with clients at risk. Provide diet teaching and refer clients with anorexia nervosa for counseling. Stress the potassium-losing effects of taking diuretics and using laxatives to enhance weight loss. Discuss the potassium-wasting effects of most diuretics with clients taking these drugs, and encourage a diet rich in high-potassium foods, as well as regular monitoring of serum potassium levels.

Assessment

Assessment data related to hypokalemia include the following:

- *Health history:* Current manifestations, including anorexia, nausea and vomiting, abdominal discomfort, muscle weakness or cramping, other symptoms; duration of symptoms and any precipitating factors, such as diuretic use, prolonged vomiting or diarrhea; chronic diseases, such as diabetes, hyperaldosteronism, or Cushing's syndrome; current medications.
- *Physical assessment:* Mental status; vital signs including orthostatic vitals, apical and peripheral pulses; bowel sounds, abdominal distension; muscle strength and tone.

Nursing Diagnoses and Interventions

Activity Intolerance

Muscle cramping and weakness are common early manifestations of hypokalemia. The lower extremities are usually affected initially. This muscle weakness can cause the client to fatigue easily, particularly with activity.

* Monitor skeletal muscle strength and tone, which are affected by moderate hypokalemia. *Increasing weakness, paresthesias, or paralysis of muscles or progression of affected muscles to include the upper extremities or trunk can indicate a further drop in serum potassium levels.*

* Monitor respiratory rate, depth, and effort; heart rate and rhythm; and blood pressure at rest and following activity. *Tachypnea, dyspnea, tachycardia, and/or a change in blood pressure may indicate decreasing ability to tolerate activities. Report changes to the care provider.*

* Assist with self-care activities as needed. *Increasing muscle weakness can lead to fatigue and affect the ability to meet self-care needs.*

Decreased Cardiac Output

Hypokalemia affects the strength of cardiac contractions and can lead to dysrhythmias that further impair cardiac output. Hypokalemia also alters the response to cardiac drugs, such as digitalis and the antidysrhythmics.

* Monitor serum potassium levels, particularly in clients at risk for hypokalemia (those with excess losses due to drug therapy, gastrointestinal losses, or who are unable to consume a normal diet). Report abnormal levels to the care provider. *Potassium must be replaced daily, as the body is unable to conserve it. Either lack of intake or abnormal losses of potassium in the urine or gastric fluids can lead to hypokalemia.*

* Monitor vital signs, including orthostatic vitals and peripheral pulses. *As cardiac output falls, the pulse becomes weak and thready. Orthostatic hypotension may be noted with decreased cardiac output.*

* Monitor clients taking digitalis for toxicity. Monitor response to antidysrhythmic drugs. *Hypokalemia potentiates digitalis effects and increases resistance to certain antidysrhythmics.*

* Dilute intravenous potassium and administer using an electronic infusion device. In general, potassium is given no faster than 10 to 20 mEq/hour. Closely monitor intravenous flow rate and response to potassium replacement. *Rapid potassium administration is dangerous and can lead to hyperkalemia and cardiac arrest.*

Risk for Imbalanced Fluid Volume

* Maintain accurate intake and output records. *Gastrointestinal fluid losses can lead to significant potassium losses.*

* Monitor bowel sounds and abdominal distention. *Hypokalemia affects smooth muscle function and can lead to slowed peristalsis and paralytic ileus.*

Acute Pain

Discomfort is common when intravenous potassium chloride at a concentration of more than 40 mEq/L is given into a peripheral vein.

- When possible, administer intravenous KCl through a central line. *The rapid blood flow through central veins dilutes the KCl solution, decreasing discomfort.*

- Spread the total daily dose of KCl over 24 hours to minimize the concentration of intravenous solutions. *High concentrations of KCl are irritating to vein walls, particularly if inflammation is present.*

- Discuss with the physician using a small amount of lidocaine prior to or with the infusion. *Both a lidocaine bolus given at the infusion site and a small amount of lidocaine in the intravenous infusion have been shown to at least partially relieve discomfort associated with concentrated potassium solutions (Metheny, 2000).*

Home Care

The focus in preparing the client with or at risk for hypokalemia is prevention. Discharge planning focuses on teaching self-care practices. Include the following topics when preparing the client and family for home care:

- Recommended diet, including a list of potassium-rich foods.

- Prescribed medications and potassium supplements, their use, and desired and unintended effects.

- Using salt substitutes (if recommended) to increase potassium intake; avoiding substitutes if taking a potassium supplement or potassium-sparing diuretic.

- Manifestations of potassium imbalance (hypokalemia or hyperkalemia) to report to health care provider.

- Recommendations for monitoring serum potassium levels.

- If taking digitalis, manifestations of digitalis toxicity to report to health care provider.

- Managing gastrointestinal disorders that cause potassium loss (vomiting, diarrhea, ileostomy drainage) to prevent hypokalemia.

The Client with Hyperkalemia

Hyperkalemia is an abnormally high serum potassium (greater than 5 mEq/L). Hyperkalemia can result from inadequate excretion of potassium, excessively high intake of potassium, or a shift of potassium from the intracellular to the extracellular space. *Pseudohyperkalemia* (an erroneously high serum potassium reading) can occur if the blood sample hemolyzes, releasing potassium from blood cells, before it is analyzed. Hyperkalemia affects neuromuscular and cardiac function.

Pathophysiology and Manifestations

Impaired renal excretion of potassium is a primary cause of hyperkalemia. Untreated renal failure, adrenal insufficiency (e.g., Addison's disease or inadequate aldosterone production), and medications, such as potassium-sparing diuretics, the antimicrobial drug trimethoprim, and some NSAIDs, impair potassium excretion by the kidneys.

In clients with normal renal excretion of potassium, excess oral potassium (e.g., by supplement or use of salt substitutes) rarely leads to hyperkalemia. Rapid intravenous administration of potassium or transfusion of aged blood can lead to hyperkalemia.

A shift of potassium ions from the intracellular space can occur in acidosis, with severe tissue trauma, during chemotherapy, and due to starvation. In acidosis, excess hydrogen ions enter the cells, causing potassium to shift into the extracellular space. The extent of this shift is greater with metabolic acidosis than with respiratory acidosis.

Hyperkalemia alters the cell membrane potential, affecting the heart, skeletal muscle function, and the gastrointestinal tract. The most harmful consequence of hyperkalemia is its effect on cardiac function. The cardiac conduction system is affected first, with slowing of the heart rate, possible heart blocks, and prolonged depolarization. ECG changes include peaked T waves, a prolonged PR interval, and widening of the QRS complex. Ventricular dysrhythmias develop, and cardiac arrest may occur. Severe hyperkalemia decreases the strength of myocardial contractions.

Skeletal muscles become weak and paralysis may occur with very high serum potassium levels. Hyperkalemia causes smooth muscle hyperactivity, leading to gastrointestinal disturbances.

The seriousness of hyperkalemia is based on the serum potassium (K^+) level and ECG changes.

- Mild hyperkalemia: serum K^+ between 5 and 6.5 mEq/L; ECG changes limited to peaked T wave.
- Moderate hyperkalemia: serum K^+ between 6.5 and 8 mEq/L; ECG changes limited to peaked T wave.
- Severe hyperkalemia: serum K^+ greater than 8 mEq/L; ECG shows absent P waves and widened QRS pattern.

The manifestations of hyperkalemia result from its effects on the heart, skeletal, and smooth muscles. Early manifestations include diarrhea, colic (abdominal cramping), anxiety, paresthesias, irritability, and muscle tremors and twitching. As serum potassium levels increase, muscle weakness develops, progressing to flaccid paralysis. The lower extremities are affected first, progressing to the trunk and upper extremities.

Collaborative Care

The management of hyperkalemia focuses on returning the serum potassium level to normal by treating the underlying cause and avoiding additional potassium intake. The choice of therapy for existing hyperkalemia is based on the severity of the hyperkalemia.

Diagnostic Tests
The following laboratory and diagnostic tests may be ordered:

- *Serum electrolytes* show a serum potassium level greater than 5.0 mEq/L. Low calcium and sodium levels may increase the effects of hyperkalemia; therefore, these electrolytes are usually measured as well.
- *ABGs* are measured to determine if acidosis is present.
- An *ECG* is obtained and *continuous ECG monitoring* is instituted to evaluate the effects of hyperkalemia on cardiac conduction and rhythm.

Medications
Medications are administered to lower the serum potassium and to stabilize the conduction system of the heart. For moderate to severe hyperkalemia, calcium gluconate is given

intravenously to counter the effects of hyperkalemia on the cardiac conduction system. While the effect of calcium gluconate lasts only for one hour, it allows time to initiate measures to lower serum potassium levels. To rapidly lower these levels, regular insulin and 50 g of glucose are administered. Insulin and glucose promote potassium uptake by the cells, shifting potassium out of ECF. In some cases, a 2-agonist, such as albuterol, may be given by nebulizer to temporarily push potassium into the cells. Sodium bicarbonate may be given to treat acidosis. As the pH returns toward normal, hydrogen ions are released from the cells and potassium returns into the cells.

To remove potassium from the body, sodium polystyrene sulfonate (Kayexalate), a resin that binds potassium in the gastrointestinal tract, may be administered orally or rectally. If renal function is normal, diuretics, such as furosemide, are given to promote potassium excretion.

Dialysis

When renal function is severely limited, either peritoneal dialysis or hemodialysis may be implemented to remove excess potassium. These measures are invasive and typically used only when other measures are ineffective.

Nursing Care

Nursing care focuses related to hyperkalemia include identifying clients at risk, preventing hyperkalemia, and addressing problems resulting from the systemic effects of hyperkalemia.

Health Promotion

Clients at the greatest risk for developing hyperkalemia include those taking potassium supplements (prescribed or over-the-counter), using potassium-sparing diuretics or salt substitutes, and experiencing renal failure. Athletes participating in competition sports, such as body building, and using anabolic steroids, muscle-building compounds, or "energy drinks" may also be at risk for hyperkalemia.

Teach all clients to carefully read food and dietary supplement labels. Discuss the importance of taking prescribed potassium supplements as ordered, and not increasing the dose unless prescribed by the care provider. Advise clients taking a potassium supplement or potassium-sparing diuretic to avoid salt substitutes, which usually contain potassium. Discuss the importance of maintaining an adequate fluid intake (unless a fluid restriction has been prescribed) to maintain renal function to eliminate potassium from the body.

Assessment

Assessment data related to hyperkalemia include the following:

- *Health history:* Current manifestations, including numbness and tingling, nausea and vomiting, abdominal cramping, muscle weakness, palpitations; duration of symptoms and any precipitating factors, such as use of salt substitutes, potassium supplements, or reduced urine output; chronic diseases, such as renal failure or endocrine disorders; current medications.
- *Physical assessment:* Apical and peripheral pulses; bowel sounds; muscle strength in upper and lower extremities; ECG pattern.

Nursing Diagnoses and Interventions

Risk for Activity Intolerance

Both hypokalemia (low serum potassium levels) and hyperkalemia (high serum potassium levels) affect neuromuscular activity and the function of cardiac, smooth, and skeletal muscles. Hyperkalemia can cause muscle weakness and even paralysis.

- Monitor skeletal muscle strength and tone. *Increasing weakness, muscle paralysis, or progression of affected muscles to affect the upper extremities or trunk can indicate increasing serum potassium levels.*

- Monitor respiratory rate and depth. Regularly assess lung sounds. *Muscle weakness due to hyperkalemia can impair ventilation. In addition, medications, such as sodium bicarbonate or sodium polystyrene sulfonate, can cause fluid retention and pulmonary edema in clients with preexisting cardiovascular disease.*

- Assist with self-care activities as needed. *Increasing muscle weakness can lead to fatigue and affect the ability to meet self-care needs.*

Risk for Decreased Cardiac Output

Hyperkalemia affects depolarization of the atria and ventricles of the heart. Severe hyperkalemia can cause dysrhythmias with ventricular fibrillation and cardiac arrest. The cardiac effects of hyperkalemia are more pronounced when the serum potassium level rises rapidly. Low serum sodium and calcium levels, high serum magnesium levels, and acidosis contribute to the adverse effects of hyperkalemia on the heart muscle.

Table 39-7. Medication Administration – Hyperkalemia

Diuretics

Potassium-wasting diuretics, such as furosemide (Lasix), may be used to enhance renal excretion of potassium.

Nursing Responsibilities
- Monitor serum electrolytes.
- Monitor and record weight at regular intervals under standard conditions (same time of day, balanced scale, same clothing).
- Monitor intake and output.

Insulin, Hypertonic Dextrose, and Sodium Bicarbonate

Insulin, hypertonic dextrose (10% to 50%), and sodium bicarbonate are used in the emergency treatment of moderate to severe hyperkalemia. Insulin promotes the movement of potassium into the cell, and glucose prevents hypoglycemia. The onset of action of insulin and hypertonic dextrose occurs within 30 minutes and is effective for approximately 4 to 6 hours.

Sodium bicarbonate elevates the serum pH; potassium is moved into the cell in exchange for hydrogen ion. Sodium bicarbonate is particularly useful in the client with metabolic acidosis. Onset of effects occurs within 15 to 30 minutes and is effective for approximately 2 hours.

Table 39-7. Continued

Nursing Responsibilities
- Administer intravenous insulin and dextrose over prescribed interval of time using an infusion pump.
- Administer sodium bicarbonate as prescribed. It may be administered as an intravenous bolus or added to a dextrose-in-water solution and given by infusion.
- In clients receiving sodium bicarbonate, monitor for sodium overload, particularly in clients with hypernatremia, heart failure, and renal failure.
- Monitor the ECG pattern closely.
- Monitor serum electrolytes (K^+, Na^+, Ca^{2+}, Mg^{2+}) frequently during treatment.

Calcium Gluconate and Calcium Chloride

Intravenous calcium gluconate or calcium chloride is used as a temporary emergency measure to counteract the toxic effects of potassium on myocardial conduction and function.

Nursing Responsibilities
- Closely monitor the ECG of the client receiving intravenous calcium, particularly for bradycardia.
- Calcium should be used cautiously in clients receiving digitalis, because calcium increases the cardiotonic effects of digitalis and may precipitate digitalis toxicity, leading to dysrhythmias.

Sodium Polystyrene Sulfonate (Kayexalate) and Sorbitol

Sodium polystyrene sulfonate (Kayexalate) is used to treat moderate or severe hyperkalemia. Categorized as a cation exchange resin, Kayexalate exchanges sodium or calcium for potassium in the large intestine. Sorbitol is given with Kayexalate to promote bowel elimination. Kayexalate and sorbitol may be administered orally, through a nasogastric tube, or rectally as a retention enema. The usual dosage is 20 g three or four times a day with 20 mL of 70% sorbitol solution.

Nursing Responsibilities
- Because Kayexalate contains sodium, monitor clients with heart failure and edema closely for water retention.
- Monitor serum electrolytes (K^+, Na^+, Ca^{2+}, Mg^{2+}) frequently during therapy.
- Restrict sodium intake in clients who are unable to tolerate increased sodium load (e.g., those with CHF or hypertension).
- Closely monitor the response to intravenous calcium gluconate, particularly in clients taking digitalis. *Calcium increases the risk of digitalis toxicity.*

Risk for Imbalanced Fluid Volume

Renal failure is a major cause of hyperkalemia. Clients with renal failure are also at risk for fluid retention and other electrolyte imbalances.

- Closely monitor serum potassium, BUN, and serum creatinine. Notify the physician if serum potassium level is greater than 5 mEq/L, or if serum creatinine and BUN levels are increasing. *Serum creatinine and BUN are the primary indicators of renal function. Levels of these substances rise rapidly in acute renal failure, more slowly in chronic renal failure.*

- Maintain accurate intake and output records. Report an imbalance of 24-hour totals and/or urine output less than 30 mL/hour. *Oliguria (scant urine) or anuria (no urine output) may indicate renal failure and an increased risk for hyperkalemia and fluid volume excess.*

- Monitor clients receiving sodium bicarbonate for fluid volume excess. *Increased sodium from injection of a hypertonic sodium bicarbonate solution can cause a shift of water into the extracellular space.*

- Monitor clients receiving cation exchange resins and sorbitol for fluid volume excess. *The resin exchanges potassium for sodium or calcium in the bowel. Excessive sodium and water retention may occur.*

Home Care

Preventing future episodes of hyperkalemia is the focus when preparing the client for home care. Include the family, a significant other, or a caregiver when teaching the following topics.

- Recommended diet and any restrictions including salt substitutes and foods high in potassium.

- Medications to be avoided, including over-the-counter and fitness supplements.

- Follow-up appointments for lab work and evaluation.

Acid-Base Disorders

Homeostasis and optimal cellular function require maintenance of the hydrogen ion (H^+) concentration of body fluids within a relatively narrow range. Hydrogen ions determine the relative acidity of body fluids. **Acids** release hydrogen ions in solution; **bases** (or **alkalis**) accept hydrogen ions in solution. The hydrogen ion concentration of a solution is measured as its pH. The relationship between hydrogen ion concentration and pH is inverse; that is, as hydrogen ion concentration increases, the pH falls, and the solution becomes more acidic. As hydrogen ion concentration falls, the pH rises, and the solution becomes more alkaline or basic. The pH of body fluids is slightly basic, with the normal pH ranging from 7.35 to 7.45 (a pH of 7 is neutral).

Regulation of Acid-Base Balance

A number of mechanisms work together to maintain the pH of the body within this normal range. Metabolic processes in the body continuously produce acids, which fall into two categories: volatile acids and nonvolatile acids. **Volatile acids** can be eliminated from the body as a gas. Carbonic acid (H_2CO_3) is the only volatile acid produced in the body. It dissociates (separates) into carbon dioxide (CO_2) and water (H_2O); the carbon dioxide is then eliminated from the body through the lungs. All other acids produced in the body are *nonvolatile acids* that must be metabolized or excreted from the body in fluid. Lactic acid, hydrochloric acid, phosphoric acid, and sulfuric acid are examples of nonvolatile acids. Most acids and bases in the body are weak; that is, they neither release nor accept a significant amount of hydrogen ion.

Three systems work together in the body to maintain the pH despite continuous acid production: buffers, the respiratory system, and the renal system.

Buffer Systems

Buffers are substances that prevent major changes in pH by removing or releasing hydrogen ions. When excess acid is present in body fluid, buffers bind with hydrogen ions to minimize the change in pH. If body fluids become too basic or alkaline, buffers release hydrogen ions, restoring the pH. Although buffers act within a fraction of a second, their capacity to maintain pH is limited. The major buffer systems of the body are the bicarbonate-carbonic acid buffer system, phosphate buffer system, and protein buffers.

The bicarbonate-carbonic acid buffer system can be illustrated by the following equation:

$$CO_2 + H_2O \leftrightarrow H_2CO_3 \leftrightarrow H^+ + HCO_3^-$$

Bicarbonate (HCO_3^-) is a weak base; when an acid is added to the system, it combines with bicarbonate, and the pH changes only slightly. Carbonic acid (H_2CO_3) is a weak acid produced when carbon dioxide dissolves in water. If a base is added to the system, it combines with carbonic acid, and the pH remains within the normal range. Although the amounts of bicarbonate and carbonic acid in the body vary to a certain extent, as long as a ratio of 20 parts bicarbonate (HCO_3^-) to 1 part carbonic acid (H_2CO_3) is maintained, the pH remains within the 7.35 to 7.45 range. The normal serum bicarbonate level is 24 mEq/L, and that of carbonic acid is 1.2 mEq/L. Thus, the ratio of bicarbonate to carbonic acid is 20:1. It is this ratio that maintains the pH within the normal range. Adding a strong acid to extracellular fluid depletes bicarbonate, changing the 20:1 ratio and causing the pH to drop below 7.35. This is known as **acidosis**. Addition of a strong base depletes carbonic acid as it combines with the base. The 20:1 ratio again is disrupted and the pH rises above 7.45, a condition known as **alkalosis**.

Intracellular and plasma proteins also serve as buffers. Plasma proteins contribute to buffering of extracellular fluids. Proteins in intracellular fluid provide extensive buffering for organic acids produced by cellular metabolism. In red blood cells, hemoglobin acts as a buffer for hydrogen ion when carbonic acid dissociates. Inorganic phosphates also serve as extracellular buffers, although their roles are not as important as the bicarbonate-carbonic acid buffer system. Phosphates are, however, important intracellular buffers, helping to maintain a stable pH.

Respiratory System

The respiratory system (and the respiratory center of the brain) regulates carbonic acid in the body by eliminating or retaining carbon dioxide. Carbon dioxide is a potential acid; when combined with water, it forms carbonic acid (see previous equation). Acute increases in either carbon dioxide or hydrogen ions in the blood stimulate the respiratory center in the brain. As a result, both the rate and depth of respiration increase. The increased rate and depth of lung ventilation eliminates carbon dioxide from the body, and carbonic acid levels fall, bringing the pH to a more normal range. Although this compensation for increased hydrogen ion concentration occurs within minutes, it becomes less effective over time. Clients with chronic lung disease may have consistently high carbon dioxide levels in their blood.

Alkalosis, by contrast, depresses the respiratory center. Both the rate and depth of respiration decrease, and carbon dioxide is retained. The retained carbon dioxide then combines with water to restore carbonic acid levels and bring the pH back within the normal range.

Renal System

The renal system is responsible for the long-term regulation of acid-base balance in the body. Excess nonvolatile acids produced during metabolism normally are eliminated by the kidneys. The kidneys also regulate bicarbonate levels in extracellular fluid by regenerating bicarbonate ions as well as reabsorbing them in the renal tubules. Although the kidneys respond more slowly to changes in pH (over hours to days), they can generate bicarbonate and selectively excrete or retain hydrogen ions as needed. In acidosis, when excess hydrogen ion is present and the pH falls, the kidneys excrete hydrogen ions and retain bicarbonate. In alkalosis, the kidneys retain hydrogen ions and excrete bicarbonate to restore acid-base balance.

Assessment of Acid-Base Balance

Acid-base balance is evaluated primarily by measuring arterial blood gases.

Arterial blood is used because it reflects acid-base balance throughout the entire body better than venous blood. Arterial blood also provides information about the effectiveness of the lungs in oxygenating blood. The elements measured are pH, the $PaCO_2$, the PaO_2, and bicarbonate level.

Table 39-8. Normal Arterial Blood Gas Values

Value	Normal Range	Significance
pH	7.35 to 7.45	Reflects hydrogen ion (H^+) concentration • <7.35 = acidosis • >7.45 = alkalosis
$PaCO_2$	35 to 45 mmHg	Partial pressure of carbon dioxide (CO_2) in arterial blood • <35 mmHg = hypocapnia • >45 mmHg = hypercapnia
PaO_2	80 to 100 mmHg	Partial pressure of oxygen (O_2) in arterial blood • <80 mmHg = hypoxemia
HCO_3^-	22 to 26 mEq/L	Bicarbonate concentration in plasma
BE	−3 to +3	Base excess; a measure of buffering capacity

The $PaCO_2$ measures the pressure exerted by dissolved carbon dioxide in the blood. The $PaCO_2$ reflects the respiratory component of acid-base regulation and balance. The $PaCO_2$ is regulated by the lungs. The normal value is 35 to 45 mmHg. A $PaCO_2$ of less than 35 mmHg is known as *hypocapnia;* a $PaCO_2$ greater than 45 mmHg is *hypercapnia.*

The PaO_2 is a measure of the pressure exerted by oxygen that is dissolved in the plasma. Only about 3% of oxygen in the blood is transported in solution; most is combined with hemoglobin. However, it is the dissolved oxygen that is available to the cells for metabolism. As dissolved oxygen diffuses out of plasma into the tissues, more is released from hemoglobin. The normal value for PaO_2 is 80 to 100 mmHg. A PaO_2 less than 80 mmHg is indicative of *hypoxemia*. The PaO$_2$ is valuable for evaluating respiratory function, but is not used as a primary measurement in determining acid-base status.

The **serum bicarbonate** (HCO$_3^-$) reflects the renal regulation of acid-base balance. It is often called the metabolic component of arterial blood gases. The normal HCO$_3^-$ value is 22 to 26 mEq/L.

The **base excess (BE)** is a calculated value also known as buffer base capacity. The measurement of base excess reflects the degree of acid-base imbalance by indicating the status of the body's total buffering capacity. It represents the amount of acid or base that must be added to a blood sample to achieve a pH of 7.4. This is essentially a measure of increased or decreased bicarbonate. The normal value for base excess for arterial blood is − 3.0 to + 3.0. Normal ABG values are summarized in Table 39-8.

ABGs are analyzed to identify acid-base disorders and their probable cause, to determine the extent of the imbalance, and to monitor treatment. When analyzing ABG results, it is important to use a systematic approach. First evaluate each individual measurement, then look at the interrelationships to determine the client's acid-base status (see Table 39-9).

Acid-Base Imbalance

Acid-base disorders fall into two major categories: acidosis and alkalosis. Acidosis occurs when the hydrogen ion concentration increases above normal (pH below 7.35). Alkalosis occurs when the hydrogen ion concentration falls below normal (pH above 7.45).

Acid-base imbalances are further classified as *metabolic* or *respiratory* disorders. In metabolic disorders, the primary change is in the concentration of bicarbonate. In **metabolic acidosis**, the amount of bicarbonate is decreased in relation to the amount of acid in the body. It can develop as a result of abnormal bicarbonate losses or because of excess nonvolatile acids in the body. The pH falls below 7.35 and the bicarbonate concentration is less than 22 mEq/L. **Metabolic alkalosis**, by contrast, occurs when there is an excess of bicarbonate in relation to the amount of hydrogen ion. The pH is above 7.45 and the bicarbonate concentration is greater than 26 mEq/L.

In respiratory disorders, the primary change is in the concentration of carbonic acid. **Respiratory acidosis** occurs when carbon dioxide is retained, increasing the amount of carbonic acid in the body. As a result, the pH falls to less than 7.35, and the PaCO$_2$ is greater than 45 mmHg. When too much carbon dioxide is "blown off," carbonic acid levels fall and **respiratory alkalosis** develops. The pH rises to above 7.45 and the PaCO$_2$ is less than 35 mmHg.

Acid-base disorders are further defined as *primary* (simple) and *mixed*. Primary disorders usually are due to one cause. For example, respiratory failure often causes respiratory acidosis due to retained carbon dioxide; renal failure usually causes metabolic acidosis due to retained hydrogen ion and impaired bicarbonate production. Table 39-10 summarizes primary acid-base imbalances with common causes of each. Mixed disorders occur from combinations of respiratory and metabolic disturbances. For example, a client in cardiac arrest develops a mixed respiratory and metabolic acidosis due to lack of ventilation (and retained CO$_2$) and hypoxia of body tissues that leads to anaerobic metabolism and acid by-products (excess nonvolatile acids).

Table 39-9. Interpreting Arterial Blood Gases

1. Look at the pH.
   - pH <7.35 = acidosis
   - pH >7.45 = alkalosis

2. Look at the $Paco_2$.
   - $Paco_2$ <35 mmHg = hypocapnia; more carbon dioxide is being exhaled than normal
   - $Paco_2$ >45 mmHg = hypercapnia; carbon dioxide is being retained

3. Evaluate the pH–$Paco_2$ relationship for a possible respiratory problem.
   - If the pH is <7.35 (acidosis) and the $Paco_2$ is >45 mmHg (hypercapnia), retained carbon dioxide is causing increased H^+ concentration and respiratory acidosis.
   - If the pH is >7.45 (alkalosis) and the $Paco_2$ is <35 mmHg (hypocapnia), low carbon dioxide levels and decreased H^+ concentration are causing respiratory alkalosis.

4. Look at the bicarbonate.
   - If the HCO_3^- is <22 mEq/L, bicarbonate levels are lower than normal.
   - If the HCO_3^- is >26 mEq/L, bicarbonate levels are higher than normal.

5. Evaluate the pH, HCO_3^-, and BE for a possible metabolic problem.
   - If the pH is <7.35 (acidosis), the HCO_3^- is <22 mEq/L, and the BE is <–3 mEq/L, then low bicarbonate levels and high H^+ concentrations are causing *metabolic acidosis.*
   - If the pH is >7.45 (alkalosis), the HCO_3^- is >26 mEq/L, and the BE is > + 3 mEq/L, then high bicarbonate levels are causing *metabolic alkalosis.*

6. Look for compensation.
   - *Renal compensation:*
     - In respiratory acidosis (pH < 7.35, $Paco_2$ > 45 mmHg), the kidneys retain HCO_3^- to buffer the excess acid, so the HCO_3^- is > 26 mEq/L.
     - In respiratory alkalosis (pH >7.45, $Paco_2$ <35 mmHg), the kidneys excrete HO_3^- to minimize the alkalosis, so the HCO_3^- is <22 mEq/L.
   - *Respiratory compensation:*
     - In metabolic acidosis (pH <7.35, HCO_3^- <22 mEq/L), the rate and depth of respirations increase, increasing carbon dioxide elimination, so the $Paco_2$ is <35 mmHg.
     - In metabolic alkalosis (pH >7.45, HCO_3^- >26 mEq/L), respirations slow, carbon dioxide is retained, so the $Paco_2$ is >45 mmHg.

7. Evaluate oxygenation.
   - Pao_2 <80 mmHg = hypoxemia; possible hypoventilation
   - Pao_2 >mmHg = hyperventilation

Compensation

With primary acid-base disorders, compensatory changes in the other part of the regulatory system occur to restore a normal pH and homeostasis. In metabolic acid-base disorders, the change in pH affects the rate and depth of respirations. This, in turn, affects carbon dioxide elimination and the $PaCO_2$, helping restore the carbonic acid to bicarbonate ratio. The kidneys compensate for simple respiratory imbalances. The change in pH affects both bicarbonate conservation and hydrogen ion elimination (see Table 39-11).

Table 39-10. Common Causes of Primary Acid-Base Imbalances

Imbalance	Common Causes
Metabolic acidosis pH < 7.35 HCO_3^- <22 mEq/L	↑ Acid production • Lactic acidosis • Ketoacidosis related to diabetes, starvation, or alcoholism • Salicylate toxicity ↓ Acid excretion • Renal failure ↑ Bicarbonate loss • Diarrhea, ileostomy drainage, intestinal fistula • Biliary or pancreatic fistulas ↑ Chloride • Sodium chloride IV solutions • Renal tubular acidosis • Carbonic anhydrase inhibitors
Metabolic alkalosis pH >7.45 HCO_3^- >26 mEq/L	↑ Acid loss or excretion • Vomiting, gastric suction • Hypokalemia ↑ Bicarbonate • Alkali ingestion (bicarbonate of soda) • Excess bicarbonate administration
Respiratory acidosis pH <7.35 $PaCO_2$ >45 mmHg	Acute respiratory acidosis • Acute respiratory conditions (pulmonary edema, pneumonia, acute asthma) • Opiate overdose • Foreign body aspiration • Chest trauma Chronic respiratory acidosis • Chronic respiratory conditions (COPD, cystic fibrosis) • Multiple sclerosis, other neuromuscular diseases • Stroke
Respiratory alkalosis pH >7.45 $PaCO_2$ <35 mmHg	• Anxiety-induced hyperventilation (e.g., anxiety) • Fever • Early salicylate intoxication • Hyperventilation with mechanical ventilator

Table 39-11. Compensation for Simple Acid-Base Imbalances

Primary Disorder	Cause	Compensation	Effect on ABGs
Metabolic acidosis	Excess nonvolatile acids; bicarbonate deficiency	Rate and depth of respirations increase, eliminating additional CO_2	↓ pH ↓ HCO_3^- ↓ $Paco_2$
Metabolic alkalosis	Bicarbonate excess	Rate and depth of respirations decrease, retaining CO_2	↑ pH ↑ HCO_3^- ↑ $Paco_2$
Respiratory acidosis	Retained CO_2 and excess carbonic acid	Kidneys conserve bicarbonate to restore carbonic acid:bicarbonate ratio of 1:20	↓ pH ↑ $Paco_2$ ↑ HCO_3^-
Respiratory alkalosis	Loss of CO_2 and deficient carbonic acid	Kidneys excrete bicarbonate and conserve H^+ to restore carbonic acid: bicarbonate ratio	↑ pH ↓ $Paco_2$ ↓ HCO_3^-

Compensatory changes in respirations occur within minutes of a change in pH. These changes, however, become less effective over time. The renal response takes longer to restore the pH, but is a more effective long-term mechanism. If the pH is restored to within normal limits, the disorder is said to be *fully compensated*. When these changes are reflected in ABG values, but the pH remains outside normal limits, the disorder is said to be *partially compensated*.

40

Nursing Care
of Clients
Experiencing
Shock

The Client Experiencing Shock

Shock is a clinical syndrome characterized by a systemic imbalance between oxygen supply and demand. This imbalance results in a state of inadequate blood flow to body organs and tissues, causing life-threatening cellular dysfunction.

Overview of Cellular Homeostasis and Hemodynamics

To maintain cellular metabolism, cells of all body organs and tissues require a regular and consistent supply of oxygen and the removal of metabolic wastes. This homeostatic regulation is maintained primarily by the cardiovascular system and depends on four physiologic components.

1. A cardiac output sufficient to meet bodily requirements.
2. An uncompromised vascular system, in which the vessels have a diameter sufficient to allow unimpeded blood flow and have good tone (the ability to constrict or dilate to maintain normal pressure).
3. A volume of blood sufficient to fill the circulatory system, and a blood pressure adequate to maintain blood flow.
4. Tissues that are able to extract and use the oxygen delivered through the capillaries.

In a healthy person, these components function as a system to maintain tissue perfusion. During shock, however, one or more of these components are disrupted. An understanding of basic hemodynamics is necessary to understand the pathophysiology of shock.

- **Stroke volume (SV)** is the amount of blood pumped into the aorta with each contraction of the left ventricle.
- **Cardiac output (CO)** is the amount of blood pumped per minute into the aorta by the left ventricle. CO is determined by multiplying the stroke volume (SV) by the heart rate (HR): CO = SV X HR.
- **Mean arterial pressure (MAP)** is the product of cardiac output and systemic vascular resistance (SVR): MAP = CO X SVR. When CO, SVR, or total blood volume rises, MAP and tissue perfusion increase. Conversely, when CO, SVR, or total blood volume falls, MAP and tissue perfusion decrease.

- The sympathetic nervous system maintains the smooth muscle surrounding the arteries and arterioles in a state of partial contraction called sympathetic tone. Increased sympathetic stimulation increases vasoconstriction and SVR; decreased sympathetic stimulation allows vasodilatation, which decreases SVR.

Pathophysiology

When one or more cardiovascular components do not function properly, the body's hemodynamic properties are altered. Consequently, tissue perfusion may be inadequate to sustain normal cellular metabolism. The result is the clinical syndrome known as shock. The manifestations of shock result from the body's attempts to maintain vital organs (heart and brain) and to preserve life following a drop in cellular perfusion. However, if the injury or condition triggering shock is severe enough or of long enough duration, then cellular hypoxia and cellular death occur.

Shock is triggered by a sustained drop in mean arterial pressure. This drop can occur after a decrease in cardiac output, a decrease in the circulating blood volume, or an increase in the size of the vascular bed due to peripheral vasodilatation. If intervention is timely and effective, the physiologic events that characterize shock may be stopped; if not, shock may lead to death.

Stage I: Early, Reversible, and Compensatory Shock

The initial stage of shock begins when baroreceptors in the aortic arch and the carotid sinus detect a sustained drop in MAP of less than 10 mmHg from normal levels. The circulating blood volume may decrease (usually to less then 500 mL), but not enough to cause serious effects.

The body reacts to the decrease in arterial pressure as it would to any physical stressor. The cerebral integration center initiates the body's response systems, causing the sympathetic nervous system to increase the heart rate and the force of cardiac contraction, thus increasing cardiac output. Sympathetic stimulation also causes peripheral vasoconstriction, resulting in increased systemic vascular resistance and a rise in arterial pressure. The net result is that the perfusion of cells, tissues, and organs is maintained.

Symptoms are almost imperceptible during the early stage of shock. The pulse rate may be slightly elevated. If the injury is minor or of short duration, arterial pressure is usually maintained, and no further symptoms occur.

Compensatory shock begins after the MAP falls 10 to 15 mmHg below normal levels. The circulating blood volume is reduced by 25% to 35% (1000 mL or more), but compensatory mechanisms are able to maintain blood pressure and tissue perfusion to vital organs, thereby preventing cell damage.

- Stimulation of the sympathetic nervous system results in the release of epinephrine from the adrenal medulla and the release of norepinephrine from the adrenal medulla and the sympathetic fibers. Both hormones rapidly stimulate the alpha- and beta-adrenergic fibers. Stimulated alpha-adrenergic fibers cause vasoconstriction in the blood vessels supplying the skin and most of the abdominal viscera. Perfusion of these areas decreases. Stimulated beta-adrenergic fibers cause vasodilatation in vessels supplying the heart and skeletal muscles (beta one response), and increase the heart rate and force of cardiac contraction (beta two response). Further, blood vessels in the respiratory system dilate, and the respiratory rate increases (beta two response). Thus, stimulation of the sympathetic nervous system results in increased cardiac output and oxygenation of these tissues.

• The renin-angiotensin response occurs as the blood flow to the kidneys decreases. Renin released from the kidneys converts a plasma protein to angiotensin II, which causes vasoconstriction and stimulates the adrenal cortex to release aldosterone. Aldosterone causes the kidneys to reabsorb water and sodium and to lose potassium. The absorption of water maintains circulating blood volume while increased vasoconstriction increases SVR, maintaining central vascular volume and raising blood pressure.

• The hypothalamus releases adrenocorticotropic hormone (ACTH), causing the adrenal glands to secrete aldosterone. Aldosterone promotes the reabsorption of water and sodium by the kidneys, preserving blood volume and pressure.

• The posterior pituitary gland releases antidiuretic hormone (ADH), which increases renal reabsorption of water to increase intravascular volume. The combined effects of hormones released by the hypothalamus and posterior pituitary glands work to conserve central vascular volume.

• As MAP falls in the compensatory stage of shock, decreased capillary hydrostatic pressure causes a fluid shift from the interstitial space into the capillaries. The net gain of fluid raises the blood volume.

Working together, these compensatory mechanisms can maintain MAP for only a short period of time. During this period, the perfusion and oxygenation of the heart and brain are adequate. If effective treatment is provided, the process is arrested, and no permanent damage occurs. However, unless the underlying cause of shock is reversed, these compensatory mechanisms soon become harmful, and shock perpetuates shock.

Stage II: Intermediate or Progressive Shock

The progressive stage of shock occurs after a sustained decrease in MAP of 20 mmHg or more below normal levels and a fluid loss of 35% to 50% (1800 to 2500 mL of fluid). Although the compensatory mechanisms in the previous state remain activated, they are no longer able to maintain MAP at a level sufficient to ensure perfusion of vital organs.

The vasoconstriction response that first helped sustain MAP eventually limits blood flow to the point that cells become oxygen deficient. To remain alive, the affected cells switch from aerobic to anaerobic metabolism. The lactic acid formed as a by-product of anaerobic metabolism contributes to an acidotic state at the cellular level. As a result, adenosine triphosphate (ATP), the source of cellular energy, is produced inefficiently. Lacking energy, the sodium-potassium pump fails. Potassium moves out of the cell, while sodium and water move inward. As this process continues, the cell swells, cell membrane integrity is lost, and cell organelles are damaged. Lysosomes within the cell spill out their digestive enzymes, which disintegrate any remaining organelles. Some enzymes spread to adjacent cells, where they erode and rupture cell membranes.

The acid by-products of anaerobic metabolism dilate the precapillary arterioles and constrict the postcapillary venules. This causes increased hydrostatic pressure within the capillary, and fluid shifts back into the interstitial space. The capillaries also become increasingly permeable, allowing serum proteins to shift from the vascular space into the interstitium. The buildup of plasma proteins increases the osmotic pressure in the interstitium, further accelerating the fluid shift out of the capillaries.

Throughout this period, the heart rate and vasoconstriction increase; however, perfusion of the skin, skeletal muscles, kidneys, and gastrointestinal organs is greatly diminished. Cells in the heart and brain become hypoxic, while other body cells and tissues become ischemic and anoxic. A generalized state of acidosis and hyperkalemia ensues. Unless this stage of shock is treated rapidly, the client's chances of survival are poor.

Stage III: Refractory or Irreversible Shock

If shock progresses to the irreversible stage, tissue anoxia becomes so generalized and cellular death so widespread that no treatment can reverse the damage. Even if MAP is temporarily restored, too much cellular damage has occurred to maintain life. Death of cells is followed by death of tissues, which results in death of organs. Death of vital organs contributes to subsequent death of the body.

Effects of Shock on Body Systems

Whatever its causes, shock produces predictable effects on the body's organ systems.

Cardiovascular System

The perfusion and oxygenation of the heart are adequate in the early stages of shock. As shock progresses, myocardial cells become hypoxic, and myocardial muscle function diminishes. Initially, the blood pressure may be normal or even slightly elevated (as a result of compensatory mechanisms) and the heart rate only slightly increased. Sympathetic stimulation increases the heart rate (a sinus tachycardia of 120 beats per minute is common) in an effort to increase cardiac output. As a result of vasoconstriction and decreased blood volume, the palpated pulse is rapid, weak, and thready; as shock progresses, peripheral pulses are usually nonpalpable.

Tachycardia reduces the time available for left ventricular filling and coronary artery perfusion, further reducing cardiac output. With progressive shock, altered acid-base balance, hypoxia, and hyperkalemia damage the heart's electrical systems and contractility. Consequently, cardiac dysrhythmias may develop. Decreased blood volume with decreased venous return also decreases cardiac output, and blood pressure falls.

The blood pressure changes produced by shock are characterized by a progressive decrease in both systolic and diastolic pressures and a narrowing pulse pressure. Auscultation of blood pressure is often difficult or impossible and is an inaccurate reflection of blood pressure status. For this reason, hemodynamic monitoring is usually instituted to follow the client's cardiovascular status accurately.

Respiratory System

During shock, oxygen delivery to cells may be impaired by a drop in circulating blood volume or, in the case of blood loss, by an insufficient number of red blood cells that carry oxygen. Although the respiratory rate increases because of compensatory mechanisms that promote oxygenation, the number of alveoli that are perfused decreases, and gas exchange is impaired. As a result, oxygen levels in the blood decrease, and carbon dioxide levels increase. As perfusion of the lungs diminishes, carbon dioxide is retained, and respiratory acidosis occurs.

A complication of decreased perfusion of the lungs is acute respiratory distress syndrome (ARDS), or "shock lung." The exact mechanism that produces ARDS is unknown, but some contributing factors have been identified. The pulmonary capillaries become increasingly permeable to proteins and water, resulting in noncardiogenic pulmonary edema. Production of surfactant (which controls surface tension within alveoli) is impaired, and the alveoli collapse or fill with fluid. This potentially lethal form of respiratory failure may result from any condition that causes hypoperfusion of the lungs, but it is more common in shock caused by hemorrhage, severe allergic responses, trauma, and infection.

Gastrointestinal and Hepatic Systems

The gastrointestinal organs normally receive 25% of the cardiac output through the splanchnic circulation. Shock constricts the splanchnic arterioles and redirects arterial blood flow to the heart and brain. Consequently, gastrointestinal organs become ischemic and may be irreversibly damaged.

Gastric mucosa tends to ulcerate when it becomes ischemic. Lesions of the gastric and duodenal mucosa (called *stress ulcers*) can develop within hours of severe trauma, sepsis, or burns (Porth, 2002). Gastrointestinal ulcers may hemorrhage within two to ten days following the original cause of shock. In addition, the permeability of damaged mucosa increases, allowing enteric bacteria or their toxins to enter the abdominal cavity and then progress to the circulation, resulting in sepsis.

Gastric and intestinal motility is impaired during shock, and paralytic ileus may result. If the episode of shock is prolonged, necrosis of the bowel may occur. In many cases, alterations in the structure and function of the gastrointestinal tract impair absorption of nutrients, such as protein and glucose.

Shock also alters the metabolic functions of the liver. Initially, *gluconeogenesis* (the process of forming glucose from noncarbohydrate sources) and *glycogenolysis* (the breakdown of glycogen into glucose) increase. This process allows blood glucose levels to increase as the body attempts to respond to the stressor; however, as shock progresses, liver functions are impaired, and hypoglycemia develops. Metabolism of fats and protein is impaired, and the liver can no longer effectively remove lactic acid, contributing to the development of metabolic acidosis.

The destruction of the liver's reticuloendothelial Kupffer cells (phagocytes that destroy bacteria) causes a further problem. Bacteria may proliferate within the circulatory system, causing overwhelming bacterial infection and toxicity.

Neurologic System

The primary effects of shock on the neurologic system involve changes in mental status and orientation. Cerebral hypoxia produces altered levels of consciousness, beginning with apathy and lethargy and progressing to coma. A common early symptom of cerebral hypoxia is restlessness. Continued ischemia of brain cells eventually causes swelling, resulting in cerebral edema, neurotransmitter failure, and irreversible brain cell damage.

As cerebral ischemia worsens, the sympathetic activity and vasomotor centers are depressed. This leads to a loss of sympathetic tone, causing systemic vasodilatation and pooling of blood in the periphery. As a result, venous return and cardiac output further decrease.

Renal System

Blood that normally perfuses the kidneys is shunted to the heart and brain during the progressive stage of shock, resulting in renal hypoperfusion. The drop in renal perfusion is reflected in a corresponding decrease in the glomerular filtration rate. Urine output is reduced, and the urine that is produced is highly concentrated. Oliguria of less than 20 mL per hour indicates progressive shock.

Healthy kidneys can tolerate a drop in perfusion for only about 20 minutes; thereafter, acute tubular necrosis develops (Porth, 2002). As tubular necrosis occurs, epithelial cells slough off and block the tubules, disrupting nephron function. The accumulating loss of functional nephrons eventually causes renal failure. Without normal renal function, metabolic waste products are retained in the plasma.

If treatment restores renal perfusion, the kidneys can regenerate the lost epithelial cells in the tubules, and renal function usually returns to normal. However, in the older or chronically ill client or in the client with sustained shock, loss of renal function may become permanent.

Effects on Skin, Temperature, and Thirst

In most types of shock, blood vessels supplying the skin are vasoconstricted, and the sweat glands are activated. As a result, changes in skin color occur. The skin of Caucasian clients becomes pale. In people with darker skin, such as those of African, Hispanic, or Mediterranean descent, shock-related skin color changes may be assessed as paleness of the lips, oral mucous membranes, nail beds, and conjunctiva. The skin is usually cool and moist and, in the later stages of shock, often edematous.

The body temperature decreases as shock progresses, the result of a decrease in overall body metabolism. Some people in shock become thirsty, probably a response to decreased blood volume and increased serum osmolality (Porth, 2002).

Types of Shock

Shock is identified according to its underlying cause. All types of shock progress through the same stages and exert similar effects on body systems. Any differences are noted in the following discussion.

Hypovolemic Shock

Hypovolemic shock is caused by a decrease in intravascular volume of 15% or more (Porth, 2002). In hypovolemic shock, the venous blood returning to the heart decreases, and ventricular filling drops. As a result, stroke volume, cardiac output, and blood pressure decrease. Hypovolemic shock is the most common type of shock, and it often occurs simultaneously with other types.

The decrease in circulating blood volume that triggers hypovolemic shock may result from:

- Loss of blood volume from hemorrhage (from surgery, trauma, gastrointestinal bleeding, blood coagulation disorders, ruptured esophageal varices).
- Loss of intravascular fluid from the skin due to injuries, such as burns.
- Loss of blood volume from severe dehydration.
- Loss of body fluid from the gastrointestinal system due to persistent and severe vomiting or diarrhea, or continuous nasogastric suctioning.
- Renal losses of fluid due to the use of diuretics or to endocrine disorders, such as diabetes insipidus.
- Conditions causing fluid shifts from the intravascular compartment to the interstitial space.

• Third spacing due to such disorders as liver diseases with ascites, pleural effusion, or intestinal obstruction.

Hypovolemic shock affects all body systems. Its effects vary depending on the client's age, general state of health, extent of injury or severity of illness, length of time before treatment is provided, and the rate of volume loss.

The manifestations of hypovolemic shock result directly from the decrease in circulating blood volume and the initiation of compensatory mechanisms. The loss of circulating blood volume reduces cardiac output by decreasing venous return to the heart. As a result, blood pressure drops. The carotid and cardiac baroreceptors sense the decrease in blood pressure and communicate it to the vasomotor centers in the brainstem. The vasomotor centers then induce the sympathetic compensatory responses. If the fluid loss is less than 500 mL, activation of the sympathetic response is generally adequate to restore cardiac output and blood pressure to near normal, although the heart rate may remain elevated.

With a sustained loss of blood volume (1000 mL or more), the shock stage progresses. Heart rate and vasoconstriction increase, and blood flow to the skin, skeletal muscles, kidneys, and abdominal organs decreases. Several renal mechanisms and a decline in capillary pressure help conserve blood volume. Eventually, the amount of blood flowing to cells is too low to oxygenate them and sustain production of cellular energy. Anaerobic metabolism begins, producing an acidotic environment for cells. As a result, cells lose their physical integrity. If untreated, shock causes multiple organ failure, and death results.

Cardiogenic Shock

Cardiogenic shock occurs when the heart's pumping ability is compromised to the point that it cannot maintain cardiac output and adequate tissue perfusion.

Table 40-1. Assessment Findings in Clients in Hypovolemic Shock

Initial Stage

< Blood pressure: normal to slightly decreased
< Pulse: slightly increased from baseline
< Respirations: normal (baseline)
< Skin: cool, pale (in periphery), moist
< Mental status: alert and oriented
< Urine output: slight decrease
< Other: thirst, decreased capillary refill time

Compensatory and Progressive Stages

< Blood pressure: hypotension
< Pulse: rapid, thready
< Respirations: increased
< Skin: cool, pale (includes trunk); poor turgor with fluid loss, edematous with fluid shift
< Mental status: restless, anxious, confused, or agitated

Continued on the next page

Table 40-1. Continued

< Urine output: oliguria (less than 30 mL/hour)
< Other: marked thirst, acidosis, hyperkalemia, decreased capillary refill time, decreased or absent peripheral pulses

Irreversible Stage

< Blood pressure: severe hypotension (often, systolic pressure is below 80 mmHg)
< Pulse: very rapid, weak
< Respirations: rapid, shallow; crackles and wheezes
< Skin: cool, pale, mottled with cyanosis
< Mental status: disoriented, lethargic, comatose
< Urine output: anuria
< Other: loss of reflexes, decreased or absent peripheral pulses

The loss of the pumping action of the heart may be caused by the following conditions:

• Myocardial infarction
• Cardiac tamponade
• Restrictive pericarditis
• Cardiac arrest
• Dysrhythmias, such as fibrillation or ventricular tachycardia
• Pathologic changes in the valves
• Cardiomyopathies from hypertension, alcohol, bacterial or viral infections, or ischemia
• Complications of cardiac surgery
• Electrolyte imbalances (especially changes in normal potassium and calcium levels)
• Drugs affecting cardiac muscle contractility
• Head injuries causing damage to the cardioregulatory center.

Myocardial infarction is the most common cause of cardiogenic shock. Clients admitted to the hospital for treatment of myocardial infarction or cardiac surgery are at risk for cardiogenic shock. The severity and progression of shock are related to the amount of myocardial damage.

Whatever the cardiogenic cause, the decrease in cardiac output causes a decrease in MAP. Heart rate may increase in response to compensatory mechanisms. However, tachycardia increases myocardial oxygen consumption and decreases coronary perfusion. The myocardium becomes progressively depleted of oxygen, causing further myocardial ischemia and necrosis. The typical sequence of shock is essentially unchanged in cardiogenic shock.

Table 40-2. Assessment Findings in Clients in Cardiogenic Shock

< Blood pressure: hypotension
< Pulse: rapid, thready; distention of veins of hands and neck

Table 40-2. Continued

< Respirations: increased, labored; crackles and wheezes; pulmonary edema

< Skin: pale, cyanotic, cold, moist

< Mental status: restless, anxious, lethargic progressing to comatose

< Urine output: oliguria to anuria

< Other: dependent edema; elevated CVP; elevated pulmonary capillary wedge pressure; arrhythmias

Cyanosis, however, is more common in cardiogenic shock, because stagnating blood increases extraction of oxygen from the hemoglobin at the capillary beds. As a result, the skin, lips, and nail beds may appear cyanotic. As cardiac failure (and cardiogenic shock) progresses, left ventricular end-diastolic pressure increases. The increase is transmitted to the pulmonary capillary bed, and pulmonary edema may occur. Retention of blood in the right side of the heart increases right atrial pressure, which leads to jugular venous distention as a result of backflow through the vena cava. Manifestations of cardiogenic shock are listed in Table 40–2.

Obstructive Shock

Obstructive shock is caused by an obstruction in the heart or great vessels that either impedes venous return or prevents effective cardiac pumping action. The causes of obstructive shock are impaired diastolic filling (e.g., pericardial tamponade or pneumothorax), increased right ventricular afterload (e.g., pulmonary emboli), and increased left ventricular afterload (e.g., aortic stenosis, abdominal distention). The manifestations are the result of decreased cardiac output and blood pressure, with reduced tissue perfusion and cellular metabolism.

Distributive Shock

Distributive shock (also called **vasogenic shock**) includes several types of shock that result from widespread vasodilatation and decreased peripheral resistance. As the blood volume does not change, relative hypovolemia results.

Septic Shock

Septic shock, the leading cause of death for clients in intensive care units, is one part of a progressive syndrome called systemic inflammatory response syndrome (SIRS). This condition is most often the result of gram-negative bacterial infections (i.e., *Pseudomonas, E. coli, Klebsiella*), but may also follow gram-positive infections from *Staphyloccus* and *Streptococcus* bacteria. Gram-negative sepsis has greatly increased in the past 10 years, with a 60% mortality rate despite treatment. The pathophysiology of septic shock is complex and not completely understood.

Clients at risk for developing infections leading to septic shock include those who are hospitalized, have debilitating chronic illnesses, or have poor nutritional status. The risk is heightened after invasive procedures or surgery. Other clients at risk of septic shock include older adults and those who are immunocompromised. Portals of entry for infection that may lead to septic shock are as follows:

• Urinary system: catheterizations, suprapubic tubes, cystoscopy.

• Respiratory system: suctioning, aspiration, tracheostomy, endotracheal tubes, respiratory therapy, mechanical ventilators.

- Gastrointestinal system: peptic ulcers, ruptured appendix, peritonitis.
- Integumentary system: surgical wounds, intravenous catheters, intra-arterial catheters, invasive monitoring, decubitus ulcers, burns, trauma.
- Female reproductive system: elective surgical abortion, ascending infections from transmission of bacteria during the intrapartal and postpartal periods, tampon use, sexually transmitted diseases.

Septic shock begins with *septicemia* (the presence of pathogens and their toxins in the blood). As pathogens are destroyed, their ruptured cell membranes allow endotoxins to leak into the plasma. The endotoxins disrupt the vascular system, coagulation mechanism, and immune system, and trigger an immune and inflammatory response. For this reason, the initial effects of septic shock differ from those of hypovolemic and cardiogenic shock; cardiac output is high and systemic vascular resistance is low.

Endotoxins directly damage the endothelial lining of small blood vessels first; the small blood vessels of the kidneys and lungs are most susceptible. Cellular damage stimulates the release of vasoactive proteins and activates coagulation factor XII. The vasoactive proteins stimulate peripheral vasodilatation and increase capillary permeability; the activation of coagulation factors results in the production of multiple intravascular blood clots.

As a result of the increased capillary permeability and vasodilatation, fluid shifts from the intravascular space to the interstitial space. Hypovolemia results as fluid volume is lost from the circulating blood. Hypovolemia and intravascular coagulation alter oxygenation and cellular metabolism, leading to anaerobic metabolism, lactic acidosis, and cellular death.

Septic shock has an early phase and a late phase. In early septic shock (sometimes called the *warm* phase), vasodilatation results in weakness and warm, flushed skin, and the septicemia often causes high fever and chills. In late septic shock (sometimes called the *cold* phase), hypovolemia and activity of the compensatory mechanisms result in typical shock manifestations, including cold, moist skin; oliguria; and changes in mental status. Death may result from respiratory failure, cardiac failure, or renal failure.

Toxic shock syndrome is an especially virulent form of septic shock, occurring most frequently in menstruating women who use tampons. It is thought that bacterial toxins diffuse from the site of infection in the vagina into the circulation. The toxins then trigger a widespread inflammatory response and septic shock. The manifestations of toxic shock syndrome include extreme hypotension, hyperpyrexia, headache, myalgia, confusion, skin rash, vomiting, and diarrhea (Porth, 2002).

Table 40-3. Assessment Findings in Clients in Septic Shock

Early (Warm) Septic Shock

- Blood pressure: normal to hypotension
- Pulse: increased, thready
- Respirations: rapid and deep
- Skin: warm, flushed
- Mental status: alert, oriented, anxious
- Urine output: normal

Table 40-3. Continued

< Other: increased body temperature; chills; weakness; nausea, vomiting, diarrhea; decreased CVP

Late (Cold) Septic Shock

< Blood pressure: hypotension

< Pulse: tachycardia, arrhythmias

< Respirations: rapid, shallow, dyspneic

< Skin: cool, pale, edematous

< Mental status: lethargic to comatose

< Urine output: oliguria to anuria

< Other: normal to decreased body temperature; decreased CVP

Disseminated intravascular coagulation (DIC), a generalized response to injury, is a potential risk in septic shock. This condition is characterized by simultaneous bleeding and clotting throughout the vasculature. Sepsis injures blood cells, causing platelet aggregation and decreased blood flow. As a result, blood clots form throughout the microcirculation. The clotting slows circulation further while stimulating excess fibrinolysis. As the body's stores of clotting factors are depleted, generalized bleeding begins.

Neurogenic Shock

Neurogenic shock is the result of an imbalance between parasympathetic and sympathetic stimulation of vascular smooth muscle. If parasympathetic overstimulation or sympathetic understimulation persists, sustained vasodilatation occurs, and blood pools in the venous and capillary beds.

Neurogenic shock causes dramatic reduction in systemic vascular resistance as the size of the vascular compartment increases. As systemic vascular resistance decreases, pressure in the blood vessels becomes too low to drive nutrients across capillary membranes, and cellular metabolism is impaired.

The following conditions can cause neurogenic shock by increasing parasympathetic stimulation or inhibiting sympathetic stimulation of the smooth muscle of blood vessels.

• Head injury
• Trauma to the spinal cord
• Insulin reactions (which cause hypoglycemia, decreasing glucose to the medulla)
• Central nervous system depressant drugs (such as sedatives, barbiturates, or narcotics)
• Anesthesia (spinal and general)
• Severe pain
• Prolonged exposure to heat.

Bradycardia occurs early, but tachycardia begins as compensatory mechanisms are initiated. Central venous pressure drops as veins dilate, venous return to the heart decreases, stroke volume decreases, and MAP falls. In early stages, the extremities are warm and pink (from the pooling of blood), but as shock progresses, the skin becomes pale and cool.

Anaphylactic Shock

Anaphylactic shock is the result of a widespread hypersensitivity reaction (called *anaphylaxis*). The pathophysiology in this type of shock includes vasodilatation, pooling of blood in the periphery, and hypovolemia with altered cellular metabolism. These physiologic alterations occur when a sensitized person has contact with an *allergen* (a foreign substance to which an individual is hypersensitive). Many different allergens can cause anaphylactic shock, including medications, blood administration, latex, foods, snake venom, and insect stings.

Anaphylactic shock does not occur with the first exposure to an allergen. With the first exposure to a foreign substance (the *antigen*), the body produces specific immunoglobulin E (IgE) antibodies against this antigen. The person is thus sensitized to that specific antigen. With subsequent exposure, the antigen reacts with the already formed IgE antibodies, disrupting cellular integrity. In addition, large amounts of histamine and other vasoactive amines are released and distributed through the circulatory system. These substances cause increased capillary permeability and massive vasodilatation, resulting in profound hypotension and eventual vascular collapse.

Histamine also causes constriction of smooth muscles in the bladder, uterus, intestines, and bronchioles. Respiratory distress, bronchospasm, laryngospasm, and severe abdominal cramping result. Serotonin (a neurotransmitter with vasoconstrictive properties) is released, further affecting respiratory status by increasing capillary permeability in the lungs. As a result, plasma leaks into the alveoli, gas exchange is impaired, and pulmonary edema may occur.

Anaphylactic shock begins and progresses rapidly. Manifestations may begin within 20 minutes of contact with an antigen. Unless appropriate intervention is provided, death can occur within a matter of minutes. Because anaphylaxis is rapid and potentially lethal, people with known allergies should carry some form of warning, such as a MedicAlert bracelet, informing others of their susceptibility. Health care providers should be extremely careful to assess and document allergies or previous drug reactions.

Collaborative Care

Medical care for the client in shock focuses on treating the underlying cause, increasing arterial oxygenation, and improving tissue perfusion. Depending on the cause and type of shock, interventions include emergency care measures, oxygen therapy, fluid replacement, and medications. Emergency care is often the first course of collaborative action taken to arrest shock.

Diagnostic Tests

The following diagnostic tests can help identify the type of shock and assess the client's physical status. Measurements include:

- *Blood hemoglobin and hematocrit.* Changes in hemoglobin and hematocrit concentrations usually occur in hypovolemic shock. These changes reflect the underlying etiology. In hypovolemic shock resulting from hemorrhage, the hemoglobin and hematocrit concentrations are lower than normal; in hypovolemic shock resulting from intravascular fluid loss, by contrast, the hemoglobin and hematocrit concentrations are higher than normal.

- *Arterial blood gases (ABGs),* to determine oxygen and carbon dioxide levels and pH. The effects of shock and of the body's compensatory mechanisms cause a decrease in pH (indicating acidosis), a decrease in the partial pressure of oxygen (Pao_2) and in total oxygen saturation, and an increase in the partial pressure of carbon dioxide ($Paco_2$).

- *Serum electrolytes,* to monitor the severity and progression of shock. As shock progresses, glucose levels decrease, sodium levels decrease, and potassium levels increase.

- *Blood urea nitrogen (BUN), serum creatinine levels, urine specific gravity,* and *osmolality,* to check renal function. As perfusion of the kidneys is decreased and renal function is reduced, the BUN and creatinine levels increase as does urine specific gravity and osmolality.

- *Blood cultures,* to identify the causative organism in septic shock.

- *White blood cell count and differential,* in the client with septic or anaphylactic shock. The total WBC count is increased in septic shock. Elevated neutrophils indicate acute infection, increased monocytes indicate a bacterial infection, and increased eosinophils indicate an allergic response.

- *Serum cardiac enzymes,* which are elevated in cardiogenic shock: lactate dehydrogenase (LDH), creatine phosphokinase (CPK), and serum glutamic-oxaloacetic transaminase (SGOT).

- *Central venous catheter,* to aid in the differential diagnosis of shock and to provide information about the preload of the heart. A pulmonary artery catheter may be inserted to monitor cardiac dynamics, fluid balance, and the effects of vasoactive medications.

Other diagnostic tests may be ordered to determine the extent of injury or damage or to locate the site of internal hemorrhage. These tests might include X-ray studies, computerized tomography (CT) scans, magnetic resonance imaging (MRI), endoscopic examinations, and echocardiograms. Newer diagnostic methods for hypoperfusion include gastric tonometry and sublingual Pco_2. Gastric tonometry measures the partial pressure of carbon dioxide in the gastric lumen. The measurement of sublingual carbon dioxide correlates well with decreased MAP (Sole, Lamborn, & Hartshorn, 2001).

Medications

When fluid replacement alone is not sufficient to reverse shock, vasoactive drugs (drugs causing vasoconstriction or vasodilatation) and inotropic drugs (drugs improving cardiac contractility) may be administered. When used to treat shock, these drugs increase venous return through vasoconstriction of peripheral vessels; they also improve the pumping ability of the heart by facilitating myocardial contractility and by dilating coronary arteries to increase perfusion of the myocardium.

Drugs that may be administered to the client in shock include:

- Diuretics to increase urine output after fluid replacement has been initiated.
- Sodium bicarbonate to treat acidosis.
- Calcium to replace calcium lost as a result of blood transfusions.
- Antiarrhythmic agents to stabilize heart rhythm.
- Antibiotics to suppress organisms responsible for septic shock.
- A cardiotonic glycoside, such as digitalis, to treat cardiac failure.
- Steroids to treat anaphylactic shock.

Oxygen Therapy

Establishing and maintaining a patent airway and ensuring adequate oxygenation are critical interventions in reversing shock. All clients in shock (even those with adequate respirations) should receive oxygen therapy (usually by mask or nasal cannula) to maintain the PaO_2 at greater than 80 mmHg during the first four to six hours of care. If the client's unassisted respiration cannot maintain PaO_2 at this level, ventilatory assistance may be necessary.

Fluid Replacement

The most effective treatment for the client in hypovolemic shock is the administration of intravenous fluids or blood. Fluids also treat septic and neurogenic shock. However, the client with cardiogenic shock may require either fluid replacement or restriction, depending on pulmonary artery pressure.

Various fluids may be administered alone or in combination as part of fluid replacement therapy in treating shock. Whole blood or blood products increase the oxygen-carrying capacity of the blood, and thus increase oxygenation of cells. Fluid replacements, such as crystalloid and colloid solutions, increase circulating blood volume and tissue perfusion. Fluid replacements are administered in massive amounts through two large-bore peripheral lines or through a central line.

Crystalloid Solutions

Crystalloid solutions contain dextrose or electrolytes dissolved in water; they are either isotonic or hypotonic. Isotonic solutions include normal saline (0.9%), lactated Ringer's solution, and Ringer's solution. Hypotonic solutions include one-half normal saline (0.45%) and 5% dextrose in water (D5W).

All crystalloid solutions increase fluid volume in both the intravascular and the interstitial space. Of the total amount infused, only about 25% remains in the intravascular system; the remaining 75% moves into the interstitial space. Consequently, fluid volume is only minimally expanded and the potential for peripheral edema is increased when crystalloid solutions are used. However, Ringer's lactate (an electrolyte solution) and 0.9% saline are the fluids of choice in treating hypovolemic shock, especially in the emergency phase of care while blood is being typed and crossmatched. Large amounts of these solutions may be infused rapidly, increasing blood volume and tissue perfusion.

Colloid Solutions

Colloid solutions contain substances (colloids) that should not diffuse through capillary walls. Hence, colloids tend to remain in the vascular system and increase the osmotic pressure of the serum, causing fluid to move into the vascular compartment from the interstitial space. As a result, plasma volume expands. Colloid solutions used to treat shock include 5% albumin, 25% albumin, hetastarch, plasma protein fraction, and dextran.

Colloid products reduce platelet adhesiveness and have been associated with reductions in blood coagulation. Consequently, the client's prothrombin time (PT), INR, platelet count, and activated partial thromboplastin time (PTT) should be monitored when these solutions are administered. Normal values are as follows:

PT	10–15 seconds
INR	1–1.2 seconds
Platelets	150,000–400,000
APTT	< 35 seconds

Blood and Blood Products

If hypovolemic shock is due to hemorrhage, the infusion of blood and blood products may be indicated. The goal of blood administration is to keep the hematocrit at 30% to 35% and the hemoglobin level between 12.5 and 14.5 g/100 mL. Available blood and blood products include fresh whole blood, stored whole blood, packed red blood cells, platelet concentrate, fresh-frozen plasma, and cryoprecipitate. Often, packed red blood cells are given to provide hemoglobin concentration and are supplemented with crystalloids to maintain an adequate circulatory volume.

Table 40-4. Types of Blood Components Used in Transfusion Therapy

Type	Use	Limitations
Whole blood	Replaces blood volume and oxygen-carrying capacity in hemorrhage and shock. Contains RBCs, plasma proteins, clotting factors, and plasma.	Contains few platelets or granulocytes; deficient in clotting factors V and VII. Greatest risks are for incompatibility or circulatory overload.
Red cells	Increase oxygen-carrying capacity in slow bleeding or in clients with anemia, with leukemia, or having surgery.	Has no viable platelets or granulocytes. Incompatibility may cause hemolytic reactions.
Platelets	Used to control or prevent bleeding in clients with platelet deficiencies.	If given for an extended period of time, antibodies may develop. Hypersensitivity reactions may occur.
Plasma	Expands blood volume; can be administered to any blood group or type. Contains all clotting factors and is used to restore those deficient in bleeding disorders.	May cause vascular overload, hypersensitivity reactions, or hemolytic reactions.
Albumin	Expands blood volume in shock and trauma. Used to treat clients in shock from trauma or infection and in surgery to replace blood volume and proteins.	Is not a substitute for whole blood. May cause hypersensitivity reactions.
Clotting factors	Factor VIII concentrate is used to treat clients with hemophilia A and von Willebrand's disease. Factor IX concentrate is used to treat clients with hemophilia B and other clotting factor deficiencies.	
Prothrombin complex	Contains prothrombin, clotting factors VII, IX, X, and part of XI. Used to treat clients with deficiencies of these factors.	
Cryoprecipitate	Contains factor VIII, factor XIII, von Willebrand's factor, and fibrinogen. Used to treat clients with clotting factor deficiencies.	May cause ABO incompatibilities.

Table 40-5. Blood Group Types and Compatibilities

Blood Group	RBC Agglutinogens	Serum Agglutinogens	Compatible Donor Blood Groups	Incompatible Donor Blood Groups
A	A	Anti-B	A, O	B, AB
B	B	Anti-A	B, O	A, AB
AB	A, B	None	A, B, AB, O	None
O	None	Anti-A, Anti-B	O	A, B, AB

Nursing Care

Nursing assessments and interventions to prevent shock are an essential part of the nursing care of every client. The primary nursing interventions to prevent shock are assessment and monitoring.

Health Promotion and Assessment

Nursing assessments are critical in preventing shock. Identifying clients at risk and making focused assessments are essential. Although shock may occur at any age, physiologic changes with aging make the older adult a high-risk population.

- *Hypovolemic shock:* Clients who have undergone surgery, have sustained multiple traumatic injuries, or have been seriously burned are most likely to develop hypovolemic shock. Monitoring fluid status is essential in preventing shock and includes daily assessments of weight, fluid intake by all routes, measurable fluid loss (e.g., urine, vomitus, wound drainage, gastric drainage, and chest tube drainage), and fluid loss that must be estimated, such as profuse perspiration and wound drainage. Assessments for the critically ill client are ongoing and include fluid balance, hemodynamic values, and vital signs.

- *Cardiogenic shock:* Clients with left anterior wall myocardial infarctions are at risk for developing cardiogenic shock. Nursing care to prevent the development of cardiogenic shock focuses on maintaining or improving myocardial oxygen supply by providing immediate pain relief, maintaining rest, and administering supplemental oxygen.

- *Neurogenic shock:* The risk of neurogenic shock is increased in clients who have spinal cord injuries and those who have received spinal anesthesia. Preventive nursing care includes maintaining immobility of clients with spinal cord trauma and elevating the head of the bed 15 to 20 degrees following spinal anesthesia. Elevations of more than 20 degrees, however, can potentiate headaches following spinal anesthesia and should be avoided.

- *Anaphylactic shock:* Prevent anaphylactic shock by collecting information about allergies and drug reactions during the health history. Note these allergies clearly on all documents and place a special armband on the client. Careful and frequent assessments during blood administration may prevent serious reactions to blood or blood products.

- *Septic shock:* Clients who are hospitalized, are debilitated, are chronically ill, or have undergone invasive procedures or tube insertions are at high risk for septic shock. Nursing care to prevent septic shock includes careful and consistent handwashing, the use of aseptic techniques for procedures (e.g., catheterizations, suctioning, changing dressings, starting and maintaining intravenous fluids or medications), and monitoring for local and systemic manifestations (e.g., white blood cell and differential counts) of infection.

Nursing Diagnoses and Interventions

Nursing care for the client in shock focuses on assessing and monitoring overall tissue perfusion and on meeting psychosocial needs of the client and the family. This section discusses nursing diagnoses that are appropriate for the client with hypovolemic shock.

Decreased Cardiac Output

Decreased cardiac output is the primary problem for the client in shock. Although much of the care related to this diagnosis is collaborative, many independent nursing interventions are critical to the care of the client in shock.

- *Assess and monitor cardiovascular function via the following:*
  1. Blood pressure.
  2. Heart rate and rhythm.
  3. Pulse oximetry.
  4. Peripheral pulses.
  5. Hemodynamic monitoring of arterial pressures, pulmonary artery pressures, and central venous pressures (CVPs).

A baseline assessment is necessary to establish the stage of shock. If palpable peripheral pulses and audible (to auscultation) blood pressure are lost, inserting central arterial, venous, and pulmonary artery catheters is essential to establish progression of shock accurately and to evaluate the client's response to therapy.

- Measure and record intake and output (total output and urinary output) hourly. *A decrease in circulating blood volume with hypotension and the effect of the compensatory mechanisms associated with shock can cause renal failure. Urinary output of less than 30 mL per hour in an acutely ill adult indicates reduced renal blood flow.*
- Monitor bowel sounds, abdominal distention, and abdominal pain. *Decreased splanchnic blood flow reduces bowel motility and peristalsis; paralytic ileus may result.*
- Monitor for sudden sharp chest pain, dyspnea, cyanosis, anxiety, and restlessness. *Hemoconcentration and increased platelet aggregation may result in pulmonary emboli.*
- Maintain bed rest and provide (to the extent possible) a calm, quiet environment. Place in a supine position with the legs elevated to about 20 degrees, trunk flat, and head and shoulders elevated higher than the chest. *Limiting activity and ensuring rest decreases the workload of the heart. The supine position with legs elevated increases venous return; however, this position should not be used for clients in cardiogenic shock. The Trendelenburg position is no longer recommended, because it causes the abdominal organs to press against the diaphragm (limiting respirations), decreases filling of the coronary arteries, and initiates aortic and carotid sinus reflexes.*

Altered Tissue Perfusion

As shock progresses, diminished tissue perfusion causes ischemia and hypoxia of major organ systems. As shock worsens, blood flow and oxygenation of the lungs, heart, and brain are also impaired. Hypoxia and ischemia result from decreased tissue perfusion in the kidneys, brain, heart, lungs, gastrointestinal tract, and the periphery.

- Monitor skin color, temperature, turgor, and moisture. *Decreased tissue perfusion is evidenced by the skin's becoming pale, cool, and moist; as hemoglobin concentrations decrease, cyanosis occurs.*

- Monitor cardiopulmonary function by assessing/monitoring the following:
  1. Blood pressure (by auscultation or by hemodynamic monitoring).
  2. Rate and depth of respirations.
  3. Lung sounds.
  4. Pulse oximetry.
  5. Peripheral pulses (brachial, radial, dorsalis pedis, and posterior tibial); include presence, equality, rate, rhythm, and quality. (If unable to palpate pulses, use a device, such as a Doppler ultrasound flowmeter to assess peripheral arterial blood flow.)
  6. Jugular vein distention.
  7. CVP measurements.

Baseline vital signs are necessary to determine trends in subsequent findings. As shock progresses, the blood pressure decreases, and the pulse becomes rapid, weak, and thready. As perfusion of the lungs decreases, crackles, wheezes, and dyspnea are commonly assessed. Capillary refill is prolonged, and peripheral pulses are weak or nonpalpable. Neck veins that cannot be seen when the client is in the supine position indicate decreased intravascular volume. CVP is an accurate means of determining fluid status in the client in shock; the findings will be low (5 to 15 cm of water is normal) in hypovolemic shock because of the decreased blood volume.

- Monitor body temperature. *An elevated body temperature increases metabolic demands, depleting reserves of bodily energy. It also increases myocardial oxygen demand and may place the client with previous cardiac problems at even greater risk for hypoperfusion.*

- Monitor urinary output per Foley catheter hourly, using a urimeter. *Urine output is a reliable indicator of renal perfusion.*

- Assess mental status and level of consciousness. *The appropriateness of the client's behavior and responses reflects the adequacy of cerebral circulation. Restlessness and anxiety are common early in shock; in later stages, the client may become lethargic and progress to a comatose state. Altered levels of consciousness are the result of both cerebral hypoxia and the effects of acidosis on brain cells.*

Anxiety

Many clients in hypovolemic shock have experienced some form of major trauma and may have life-threatening, multiple injuries. Following on-the-scene treatment, the client is usually admitted to the health care setting through the emergency department. Surgery may be required to treat injuries, followed by care in a critical care unit. Throughout this sequence of crisis events, treatment is invasive, and contact with family is minimal. Client and family responses to these situations of uncertainty, instability, and change include anxiety, fear, and powerlessness. These responses are affected by age, developmental level, cultural and ethnic group, experience with illness and the health care system, and support systems.

- Assess the cause(s) of the anxiety, and manipulate the environment to provide periods of rest. *Reducing stimuli that cause anxiety is calming and facilitates rest, which is necessary in the client at risk for bleeding.*
- Administer prescribed pain medications on a regular basis. *Pain precipitates and/or aggravates anxiety.*
- Provide interventions to increase comfort and reduce restlessness:
  1. Maintain a clean environment.
  2. Provide skin and oral care.
  3. Monitor the effectiveness of ventilation or oxygen therapy.
  4. Eliminate all nonessential activities.
  5. Remain with the client during procedures.
  6. Speak slowly and calmly, using short sentences.
  7. Use touch to provide support.

Unfamiliar sounds, sights, and odors can increase anxiety. Damp skin or a dry mouth increases discomfort. Inadequate gas exchange with a decrease in oxygen or an increase in carbon dioxide in the blood may cause the client to experience a "feeling of doom." Activity increases the body's need for oxygen. Listening and touch provide support in an environment in which the client often feels alone and abandoned. Severe anxiety interferes with the ability to understand others and to respond appropriately.

- Provide support for the client and family:
  1. Provide time, space, and privacy for family members.
  2. Allow family members access to the client when feasible.
  3. Encourage the expression of feelings and concerns. Provide anticipatory guidance to prepare for recovery or death and to support realistic hope.
  4. Acknowledge the beliefs, values, and expectations of the client and family.

Allowing the family access to the client reduces anxiety and gives both the client and the family some feeling of control. If prognosis is poor, access and involvement allow the family to begin the grieving process. If recovery is expected, contact provides the client and family with a feeling of hope. Supporting the client and family facilitates concrete problem solving, promotes acceptance of the illness and its implications, and helps them begin to establish ways of managing the illness experience.

- Provide information about the current setting to both the client and family; give the family information about available resources, such as pastoral care, social services, temporary housing, meals. *Knowing what to expect and how to control the environment to meet basic needs reduces anxiety.*

Home Care

Home care for the client who has experienced shock is highly individualized, depending on the cause and the illness or injury that caused shock. Therefore, topics for consideration are not included in this section.

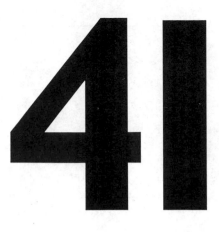

Nursing Care of Clients with Infection

The human body is continually threatened by foreign substances, infectious agents, and abnormal cells. The immune system is the body's major defense mechanism against infectious organisms and abnormal or damaged cells. Recent years have seen the emergence of resistant microorganisms, such as methicillin-resistant *Staphylococcus aureus,* and altered strains of familiar diseases, such as multiple-drug-resistant tuberculosis. New diseases have also emerged, such as Lyme disease and human immunodeficiency virus (HIV).

A thorough knowledge of the immune system increases understanding of the local and systemic inflammatory response, resistance to infectious disease, and the importance of immunization. This foundation can help the nurse teach clients and families to follow recommended treatment regimens, to promote and maintain health, and to prevent disease. In addition, the nurse can prescribe appropriate rehabilitative measures, such as increased rest and attention to optimal nutrition.

Overview of the Immune System

The immune system is a complex and intricate network of specialized cells, tissues, and organs. Cells of the immune system seek out and destroy damaged cells and foreign tissue, yet recognize and preserve host cells (Porth, 2002). The immune system performs the following functions:

- Defending and protecting the body from infection by bacteria, viruses, fungi, and parasites.
- Removing and destroying damaged or dead cells.
- Identifying and destroying malignant cells, thereby preventing their further development into tumors.

The immune system is activated by minor injuries, such as small lacerations or bruises, or by major injuries, such as burns, surgeries, and systemic diseases (e.g., pneumonia). The response of the immune system may be nonspecific or specific. Nonspecific responses prevent or limit the entry of invaders into the body, thereby limiting the extent of tissue damage and reducing the workload of the immune system. **Inflammation** is a nonspecific response activated by both minor and major injuries. When the inflammatory process is unable to destroy invading organisms or toxins, a more specific response, called the immune response, is activated.

Immune System Components

The immune system consists of molecules, cells, and organs that produce the immune response (Table 41-1). These components may be involved in the nonspecific inflammatory response, the specific immunologic response, or both.

Leukocytes

Leukocytes, or white blood cells (WBCs), are the primary cells involved in both nonspecific and specific immune system responses. Like all blood cells, leukocytes derive from stem cells, the hemocytoblasts, in the bone marrow. Unlike red blood cells (RBCs), which are confined to the circulation, leukocytes use the circulation to transport themselves to the site of an inflammatory or immune response. As the mobile units of the immune system, leukocytes detect, attack, and destroy anything that is recognized as "foreign." They are able to move through tissue spaces, locating damaged tissue and infection by responding to chemicals released by other leukocytes and damaged tissue.

Table 41-1. Cells and Tissues of the Immune System

Component	Location	Function
Leukocytes		
Granulocytes		
Neutrophils	Circulation	Phagocytosis and chemotaxis
Eosinophils	Circulation, respiratory tract, and gastroin testinal tract	Phagocytosis Protection against parasites Involved in allergic response
Basophils	Circulation	Release of chemotactic substances
Monocytes and macrophages	Circulation (monocytes) and body tissue, such as skin (histocytes), liver (Kupffer's cells), alveoli, spleen, tonsils, lymph nodes, bone marrow, brain	Trapping and phagocytizing of foreign sub stances and cellular debris Secretion of interleukin-1 to stimulate lymphocyte growth
Lymphocytes		
T cells	Circulation, lymph system, tissues	Activation of T and B cells
(mature in thymus gland)		Control of viral infections and destruction of cancer cells
		Involved in hypersensitivity reactions and graft tissue rejection
B cells (mature in bone marrow)	Circulation, spleen	Production of antibodies (immunoglobulins) to specific antigens
NK (natural killer) cells	Circulation	Cytotoxic; killing of tumor cells, fungi, viral infected cells, and foreign tissue

Table 41-1. Continued

Lymphoid Tissues

Primary or central lymphoid structures	Bone marrow and thymus gland	Production of immune cells; sites for cell maturation
Secondary or peripheral lymphoid structures	Circulation	
	Lymph nodes, spleen, tonsils, intestinal lym phoid tissue, lymphoid tissue in other organs	Sites for activation of immune cells by antigens

The normal number of circulating leukocytes is 4,500 to 10,000 cells per cubic millimeter (mm³) of blood (Kee, 2001). Many more leukocytes are marginated; that is, they adhere to vascular epithelial cells along the vessel walls, in other tissue spaces, or in the lymph system. In the presence of an attack, such as an infection, additional WBCs are released from the bone marrow, leading to **leukocytosis,** a WBC count of greater than 10,000/mm³. As WBCs move out of the bone marrow into the blood, the bone marrow increases its production of additional leukocytes. A decrease in the number of circulating leukocytes, known as **leukopenia,** occurs when bone marrow activity is suppressed or when leukocyte destruction increases.

Leukocytes are divided into three major groups: granulocytes, monocytes, and lymphocytes. The granulocytes and monocytes derive from the myeloid stem cells of the bone marrow and are instrumental in the inflammatory response. Lymphocytes derive from the lymphoid stem cells of the bone marrow and are the primary cells involved in the specific immune response. In laboratory tests, the WBC count indicates the total number of circulating leukocytes. The WBC differential identifies the portion of the total represented by each type of leukocyte.

Granulocytes. Granulocytes constitute 60% to 80% of the total number of normal blood leukocytes. Their cytoplasm has a granular appearance, and their nuclei are distinctively multilobular. Granulocytes have a short life span, measured in hours to days, compared to the life span of monocytes, which is measured in months to years. Granulocytes play a key role in protecting the body from harmful microorganisms during acute inflammation and infection. There are three types of granulocytes: neutrophils, eosinophils, and basophils.

Neutrophils, also called polymorphonuclear leukocytes (PMNs or polys), are the most plentiful of the granulocytes, constituting 55% to 70% of the total number of circulating leukocytes. Neutrophils are *phagocytic* cells, responsible for engulfing and destroying foreign agents, particularly bacteria and small particles. Neutrophils are the first phagocytic cells to arrive at the site of invasion, drawn by chemicals released by damaged tissue and invading organisms.

Neutrophils are produced in the bone marrow and released into the circulation when they mature. Segmented neutrophils (or segs) are mature forms, and usually account for about 55% of total leukocytes. *Bands* are immature neutrophils and usually comprise 5% of leukocytes. It takes about ten days for a neutrophil to mature and be released into the circulation. Once released, neutrophils have a circulating half-life of six to ten hours. They cannot replicate and must be replaced constantly to maintain adequate numbers in the circulation. They do not return to the bone marrow.

Eosinophils account for 1% to 4% of the total number of circulating leukocytes. They mature in the bone marrow in three to six days before being released into the circulation. Eosinophils have a circulating half-life of 30 minutes and a tissue half-life of 12 days. They too are phagocytic cells, but are less efficient at this process than neutrophils. Eosinophils are found in large numbers in the respiratory and gastrointestinal tracts, where they are thought to be responsible for protecting the body from parasitic worms, including tapeworms, flukes, pinworms, and hookworms. Eosinophils surround the parasite and release toxic enzymes from their cytoplasmic granules. The parasite, although too large to be phagocytized, is destroyed. Eosinophils are also involved in a hypersensitivity response, inactivating some of the inflammatory chemicals released during the inflammatory response.

Basophils constitute about 0.5% to 1% of the circulating leukocytes. These cells are not phagocytic. Granules within basophils contain proteins and chemicals, such as heparin, histamine, bradykinin, serotonin, and a slow-reacting substance of anaphylaxis (leukotrienes). These substances are released into the bloodstream during an acute hypersensitivity reaction or stress response.

Monocytes and Macrophages. *Monocytes* are the largest of the leukocytes and constitute 2% to 3% of circulating leukocytes. After their release from the bone marrow, monocytes are mobile for one to two days. They then migrate to various tissues throughout the body, attaching themselves to the tissues, where they remain for months or even years until they are activated. Monocytes mature into **macrophages** after settling into the tissues. Once they have migrated and matured, macrophages are differentiated by the tissues in which they reside. *Histiocytes* are tissue macrophages in loose connective tissue, *Kupffer cells* are found in the liver, *alveolar macrophages* in the lungs, and *microglia* in the brain. Tissue macrophages are also found in the spleen, tonsils, lymph nodes, and bone marrow.

Monocytes and macrophages are actively phagocytic, with the capacity to phagocytize large foreign particles and cell debris. Once they are in the tissue, macrophages can multiply to encapsulate and trap foreign matter that cannot be phagocytized. Like neutrophils, macrophages are drawn to an inflamed area by chemicals released from damaged tissue, a process known as chemotaxis. Monocytes and macrophages are particularly important in the body's defense against chronic infections, such as tuberculosis, viral infections, and certain intracellular parasitic infections.

Lymphocytes. Small and nondescript cells, the **lymphocytes** account for 20% to 40% of circulating leukocytes. Lymphocytes are the principal effector and regulator cells of specific immune responses. Along with monocytes and macrophages, lymphocytes protect the body from microorganisms, foreign tissue, and cell mutations or alterations. Through a process known as immune surveillance, lymphocytes monitor the body for cancerous cells and eliminate or destroy them.

Like other leukocytes, lymphocytes derive from the stem cells in the bone marrow. Lymphocytes have "homing" patterns: They constantly circulate, then return to concentrate in lymphoid tissues (the lymph nodes, spleen, thymus, tonsils, Peyer's patches in the submucosa of the distal ileum, and the appendix). On contact with an **antigen,** lymphocytes are activated and mature into either effector cells (e.g., plasma cells or cytotoxic cells), which are instrumental in destruction of the antigen, or memory cells. Memory cells stay inactive, sometimes for years, but activate immediately with subsequent exposure to the same antigen. They then proliferate rapidly, producing an intense immune response. Memory cells are responsible for providing acquired immunity.

Lymphocyte types are difficult to distinguish by appearance. They have distinct differences in how and where they mature, and in life cycle, surface characteristics, and function.

The three types of lymphocytes are **T lymphocytes (T cells)**, **B lymphocytes (B cells)**, and **natural killer cells (NK cells** or **null cells).** None of these cells acts independently. Their functions are closely interrelated.

T cells mature in the thymus gland, whereas B cells complete their maturation in the bone marrow. T cells and B cells are integral to the specific immune response.

NK cells are large, granular cells found in the spleen, lymph nodes, bone marrow, and blood. They constitute 15% of circulating lymphocytes. NK cells provide immune surveillance and resistance to infection, and they play an important role in the destruction of early malignant cells. Like B cells and T cells, NK cells are cytotoxic, but whereas T cells and B cells can attack only specific infected cells or malignant cells, NK cells can attack any target.

Antigens. Substances that are recognized as foreign or "non-self" are called antigens; they provoke a specific immune response when introduced into the body. Typically, antigens are large protein molecules, although polysaccharides, polypeptides, and nucleic acids may also be antigenic. Many antigens are proteins found on the cell membrane or cell wall of microorganisms or tissues, such as transplanted tissue or organs, incompatible blood cells, vaccines, pollen, egg white, and insect or snake venom.

Complete antigens, known as immunogens, have two characteristics:

- *Immunogenicity* is the ability to stimulate a specific immune response.
- *Specific reactivity* is the stimulation of specific immune system components.

The portion of an antigen that incites a specific immune response is called its antigenic determinant site (epitope). Complete antigens typically are large molecules with multiple antigenic sites; examples include proteins and certain polysaccharides. Small molecules (e.g., chemical toxins, drugs, and dust) that cannot evoke an antigenic response alone may link to proteins to function as complete antigens. These substances are known as haptans.

When an antigen is encountered in the body, a specific receptor on a lymphocyte "recognizes" it, and an immune response is generated. Two separate but overlapping immune responses may occur, depending on the antigen itself and the type of immune cell activated by contact with the antigen. Antigens, such as bacteria, bacterial toxins, and free viruses, usually activate B cells to produce **antibodies,** molecules that bind with the antigen and inactivate it. This is the **antibody-mediated (humoral) immune response.** Other antigens, such as viral-infected cells, cancer cells, and foreign tissue, activate T cells, which are the primary agents of the **cell-mediated (cellular) immune response.** In this immune response, the lymphocytes themselves inactivate the antigen, either directly or indirectly.

Lymphoid System

The *lymphoid system* consists of the lymph nodes, spleen, thymus, tonsils, lymphoid tissue scattered in connective tissues and mucosa, and the bone marrow. The thymus and bone marrow, in which T cells and B cells mature, are considered central lymphoid organs. The spleen, lymph nodes, tonsils, and other peripheral lymphoid tissue are peripheral lymphoid organs.

Lymph nodes, the most numerous elements of the lymphoid system, are small, round or bean-shaped encapsulated bodies that vary in size from 1 mm to 2 cm. Distributed throughout the body, lymph nodes generally occur in groups at the junction of the lymphatic vessels. They can be found in the neck, axillae, abdomen, and groin.

Lymph nodes have two functions: (1) to filter foreign products or antigens from the lymph, and (2) to house and support proliferation of lymphocytes and macrophages. Lymph, a clear, protein-containing fluid transported by lymph vessels, enters the node through afferent lymphatic vessels. Inside the node, the lymph flows through sinuses in the cortex of the lymph node where T and B lymphocytes and macrophages are abundant, then through sinuses of the medulla of the lymph node, which contains macrophages and plasma cells. The presence of a foreign antigen stimulates lymphocytes and macrophages to proliferate in the lymph nodes. Macrophages destroy the antigen by phagocytosis. Immune cells and lymph then leave the lymph node through efferent vessels. An abundant blood supply to the node also facilitates lymphocyte movement.

The *spleen* is the largest lymphoid organ in the body and the only lymphoid organ that can filter blood. The spleen is located in the upper left quadrant of the abdomen. The spleen has two kinds of tissue, white pulp and red pulp. White pulp is lymphoid tissue that serves as a site for lymphocyte proliferation and immune surveillance. B cells predominate in the white pulp. Blood filtration occurs in the red pulp. In blood-filled venous sinuses, phagocytic cells dispose of damaged or aged RBCs and platelets. Other debris and foreign matter, such as bacteria, viruses, and toxins, are also removed from the blood. The spleen also stores blood and the breakdown products of RBCs for future use. The spleen is not essential for life. If it is removed because of disease or trauma, the liver and the bone marrow assume its functions.

The *thymus gland* is located in the superior anterior mediastinal cavity beneath the sternum. It reaches its maximum size at puberty, then begins to atrophy slowly. By adulthood, it is difficult to differentiate from surrounding adipose tissue even though it remains active. In the elderly, the vast majority of thymus tissue has been replaced by adipose and fibrous connective tissue. During fetal life and childhood, the thymus serves as a site for the maturation and differentiation of thymic lymphoid cells, the T cells. Thymosin, an immunoregulatory hormone of the thymus, stimulates lymphopoiesis, the formation of lymphocytes or lymphoid tissue.

Bone marrow is soft organic tissue found in the hollow cavity of the long bones, particularly the femur and humerus, as well as the flat bones of the skull, sternum, ribs, and vertebrae. Bone marrow produces and stores hematopoietic stem cells, from which all cellular components of the blood are derived.

Lymphoid tissues are also located at key sites of potential invasion by microorganisms: the submucosa of the genitourinary, respiratory, and gastrointestinal tracts and the skin. Plasma cells in these lymphoid tissues defend the body against bacterial invasion at areas exposed to the external environment. In general, these tissues are known as *mucosa-associated lymphoid tissue* (MALT). Diffuse collections of lymphocytes, plasma cells, and phagocytes are scattered throughout the respiratory tract, concentrating at bifurcations of the bronchi and bronchioles. Gastrointestinal lymphoid tissue occurs as both diffusely scattered MALT and in more clearly defined tissues, such as the appendix and Peyer's patches, which are lymph nodules located on the distal ileum near its junction with the colon. Tonsils and adenoids protect the body from inhaled or ingested foreign agents. Skin-associated lymphoid tissue contains lymphocytes and Langerhans cells in the epidermis, which transport antigens to regional lymph nodes for phagocytosis.

Nonspecific Inflammatory Response

Barrier protection is the body's first line of defense against infection. The skin is the primary barrier. When intact, it prevents invasion by external organisms. When the skin is damaged or lost (e.g., as a result of injury, surgery, or burns), infection is much more likely. The membranes lining inner surfaces of the body are protected by a barrier of mucus, which traps microorganisms and other foreign substances. These can then be removed by other protective mechanisms, such as ciliary movement or the washing action of tears or urine. In addition, many body fluids contain bactericidal substances that provide barrier protection. These include acid in gastric fluid, zinc in prostatic fluid, and lysozyme in tears, nasal secretions, saliva, and sweat (Copstead & Banasik, 2000).

When these first-line defenses are breached, resulting tissue damage or foreign material entering the body induces a nonspecific immune response known as inflammation. Inflammation is an adaptive response to injury that brings fluid, dissolved substances, and blood cells into the interstitial tissues where the invasion or damage has occurred. The response is called nonspecific because the same events occur regardless of cause of the inflammatory process. Through the inflammatory reaction, the invader is neutralized and eliminated, destroyed tissue removed, and the process of healing and repair initiated.

There are three stages in the inflammatory response: (1) a vascular response characterized by vasodilation and increased permeability of blood vessels, (2) a cellular response and phagocytosis, and (3) tissue repair.

Vascular Response

After tissue cells are damaged, local blood vessels briefly constrict. Vasodilation follows almost immediately as inflammatory mediators such as histamine and kinins are released from damaged tissue. Increased blood flow causes vasocongestion at the injury site with resultant redness and heat. The congestion also increases local hydrostatic pressure. This, along with increased vessel permeability that results from chemical mediators, moves fluid out of the capillaries and into the interstitial spaces of the tissue. The escaping fluid, called fluid exudate, contains large amounts of protein and causes local edema. Fluid exudate has three functions: (1) It provides protection to the injured tissue by bringing certain nutrients needed for tissue healing; (2) it dilutes bacterial toxins; and (3) it transports cells needed for phagocytosis. Mild tissue damage, such as a blister, produces a *serous* exudate of primarily plasma fluid and a few proteins. With moderate to severe tissue damage, fluid exudate is *sanguineous* or *hemorrhagic*, containing large amounts of RBCs. A mixture of RBCs and serum is referred to as *serosanguineous* exudate. *Fibrinous* exudate forms a thick, sticky meshwork of fibrinogen, in effect "walling off" inflamed tissues and preventing the spread of infection (Porth, 2002). In more severe or acute inflammation, the fluid contains fibrin, RBCs, and dead and live bacteria. This type of exudate, called *purulent* exudate, has an odor and color characteristic of the bacteria present.

The vascular response localizes invading bacteria and keeps them from spreading. Increased capillary permeability enhances the release of clotting factors, such as fibrinogen, which converts to fibrin threads, entrapping the bacteria and walling them off from contact with the rest of the body.

Cellular Response

The cellular stage of the inflammatory process begins within less than an hour after the injury. This stage is marked by the margination and emigration of leukocytes into the damaged tissue, chemotaxis, and phagocytosis (Porth, 2002).

As serous fluid escapes the capillaries, the viscosity of blood in the area increases and its flow becomes more sluggish. Leukocytes marginate, moving to the edges of the blood vessels, and begin to adhere to the capillary endothelium. This process is known as pavementing. After margination and pavementing, leukocytes emigrate from the blood vessel into the tissue spaces. Within hours, millions of leukocytes emigrate into the area of inflammation (Price & Wilson, 1997).

Once leukocytes have emigrated, they are drawn to the damaged or inflamed tissues by chemotactic signals. Infectious agents, damaged tissues, and activated plasma substances, such as complement fractions, provide chemotaxic signals that attract an army of neutrophils, monocytes, and macrophages to the injury site.

The number of neutrophils around the site increases to about 15,000/mm^3 to 25,000/mm^3, and they begin their role in phagocytosis within a few hours. Monocytes become transient macrophages to augment the activity of the fixed macrophages; together they engulf dead cells, damaged tissue, nonfunctioning neutrophils, and invading bacteria.

Phagocytosis

Phagocytosis is a process by which a foreign agent or target cell is engulfed, destroyed, and digested. Neutrophils and macrophages, known as *phagocytes,* are the primary cells involved in phagocytosis. Once attracted to the inflammatory site, phagocytes select and engulf foreign material.

The following factors or processes help phagocytes differentiate foreign tissue from normal cells.

- *Smooth surface.* Normal tissue has a smooth surface that is resistant to phagocytosis, whereas the rough surface of a foreign agent or target cell promotes phagocytosis.

- *Surface charge.* Healthy body cells present an electronegative surface charge that repels phagocytes. Cellular debris and foreign agents, by contrast, have an electropositive charge that attracts them.

- *Opsonization.* This immune system process coats the surface of bacteria or target cells with a substance (an opsonin) as in the complement system. Opsonization enables the phagocyte to bind tightly with the foreign tissue, facilitating phagocytosis.

Phagocytes engulf the foreign agent or target cell by projecting pseudopodia ("false feet") in all directions around it. This produces a chamber called a *phagosome* containing the antigen, which is ingested into the cytoplasm. Once the phagosome has been engulfed, lysosomes fuse with the phagosome, killing any live organism and releasing digestive enzymes which destroy the antigen.

Phagocytes—in particular, neutrophils and macrophages—contain bactericidal agents that kill most of the bacteria they ingest before the bacteria can multiply and destroy the phagocyte itself. The phagocyte kills bacteria in a number of ways; for example, it alters the intracellular pH and produces bactericidal agents. Oxidizing agents, such as superoxide, hydrogen peroxide, and hydroxyl ions, are bactericidal. Two lysosomal substances that kill bacteria are lysozyme and phagocytin.

Some antigens, such as the tubercle bacterium, have coats or secrete substances that are resistant to lysosomal and bactericidal agents. To destroy such antigens, lysosomes release digestive enzymes into the phagosome. The lysosomes of neutrophils and macrophages contain an abundance of proteolytic (protein-destroying) enzymes that digest bacteria and other foreign protein components. The macrophage's lysosomes also contain lipases (fat-splitting enzymes) capable of digesting the thick lipid membranes of such bacteria as *Mycobacterium tuberculosis* and *Mycobacterium leprae*.

Once neutrophils have ingested toxic substances to their capacity, they in turn are killed. Neutrophils have the capacity to phagocytize 5 to 20 bacteria before they become inactive. Macrophages then digest the dead neutrophils. Monocytes or macrophages are capable of phagocytizing up to 100 bacteria. Because of their size, they can ingest larger particles than neutrophils can ingest, such as whole RBCs, necrotic tissue, cell fragments, malarial parasites, and dead neutrophils. Macrophages have the ability to extrude (release) the toxic substances and lysosomal enzymes within their phagosomes. As a result, they can continue to function for months and even years.

Healing

Inflammation is the first phase of the healing process. During the inflammatory process, particulate matter, bacteria, damaged cells, and inflammatory exudate are removed by phagocytosis. This process, called debridement, prepares the wound for healing.

The second phase of the healing process, known *as reconstruction,* may overlap the inflammatory phase. The ideal result of the healing process is *resolution,* the restoration of the original structure and function of the damaged tissue. Simple resolution occurs when there is no destruction of the normal tissue and the body is able to neutralize and remove the offending agent through the inflammatory process.

Resolution may also occur when the damaged tissue is capable of regeneration. The ability to regenerate, or replace lost parenchyma (functional tissue) with new, functional cells varies by tissue and cell type. *Labile cells* continue to regenerate throughout life. These cells are found in tissues where there is a daily turnover of cells—namely, bone marrow and the epithelial cells of the skin, mucous membranes, cervix, gastrointestinal tract, and genitourinary tract. *Stable cells* normally stop replicating when growth ceases, but are capable of regeneration when stimulated by an injury. Osteocytes (which are found in bone) and parenchymal cells of the kidneys, liver, and pancreas are stable cells. *Permanent* or *fixed cells* are unable to regenerate. When these cells are destroyed, they are replaced by fibrous scar tissue. Nerve cells, skeletal muscle cells, and cardiac muscle cells are fixed cells (Porth, 1998).

When regeneration and complete resolution is not possible, healing occurs by replacement of the destroyed tissue with collagen scar tissue. This process is known as *repair.* Although tissue that has undergone repair lacks the physiologic function of the destroyed tissue, the scar fills the lesion and provides tensile tissue strength.

Specific Immune Response

The introduction of antigens into the body causes a more specific reaction than the nonspecific inflammatory response. On the first exposure to an antigen, a change occurs in the host, resulting in a specific and rapid response following subsequent exposures. This specific response is known as the *immune response.*

The immune response to an antigen has the following distinctive properties:

- The immune response typically is directed against materials recognized as foreign (i.e., from outside the body) and is not usually directed against the self (i.e., cells or structures produced by the body). This property is known as self-recognition.

- The immune response is *specific*. It is initiated by and directed against particular antigens, such as a specific virus, bacterium, or transplanted tissue.
- Unlike a localized inflammatory response, the immune response is systemic. Immunity is generalized; it is not restricted to the initial site of infection or entry of foreign tissue.
- The immune response has memory. Repeated exposures to an antigen produce a more rapid response.

A client whose immune system is able to identify antigens and effectively destroy or remove them is said to be **immunocompetent.** Health problems may occur when the immune response is altered.

Antibody-Mediated Immune Response

The antibody-mediated (humoral) immune response is produced by B lymphocytes (B cells). B cells are constantly replaced through cell division and proliferation in the bone marrow. It is believed that B cells mature in the bone marrow, and then migrate to the spleen to await activation. They normally constitute 10% to 15% of circulating lymphocytes.

B cells are activated by contact with an antigen and by T cells (discussed in the next section). Each B cell has receptor sites for a specific antigen or antigens. When the antigen is encountered, the activated B cell proliferates and differentiates into antibody-producing plasma cells and memory cells. Plasma cells are short-lived, lasting only about one day. While alive, however, they can produce thousands of antibody molecules per second. Memory cells retain antibody-producing information, allowing a rapid response if the antigen is again encountered.

An antibody is an **immunoglobulin (Ig)** molecule with the ability to bind to and inactivate a specific antigen. Immunoglobulins comprise the gamma globulin portion of the blood proteins. The immune system produces numerous antibodies, each active against a specific antigen. Antibodies fall into five classes of immunoglobulins: IgG, IgA, IgM, IgD, and IgE. Each has a slightly different structure and function.

Table 41-2. Immunoglobulin Characteristics and Functions

Class	Percentage of Total	Characteristics and Function
IgG	75%	Most abundant Ig; also known as gamma globulin; found in blood, lymph, and intestines
		Active against bacteria, bacterial toxins, and viruses
		Activates complement
		The only Ig to cross the placenta, providing immune protection to neonate
IgA	10% to 15%	Found in saliva, tears, and bronchial, gastrointestinal, prostatic, and vaginal secretions, as well as blood and lymph
		Provides local protection on exposed mucous membrane surfaces and potent antiviral activity by preventing binding of the virus to cells of the respiratory and gastrointestinal tracts
		Levels decrease during stress

Table 41-2. Continued

IgM	5% to 10%	Found in blood and lymph
		First antibody produced with primary immune response
		High concentrations early in infection, decreases within about a week
		Mediates cytotoxic response and activates complement
IgD	<1%	Found in blood, lymph, and surfaces of B cells
		Exact function unknown; may be receptor-binding antigens to B-cell surface
IgE	<0.1%	Found on mast cells and basophils
		Involved in release of chemical mediators responsible for immediate hypersensitivity (allergic and anaphylactic) response

Antibodies are Y-shaped molecules of two light and two heavy polypeptide chains. The top portion of the Y, called the *Fab* or *antigen-binding fragment,* is chemically variable and specific to the antigen. The lower portion, the F_c or *crystallized fragment,* is constant for its class of immunoglobulin and directs the biologic activity of the immunoglobulin (the manner in which it functions). For example, the lower portion of immunoglobulin molecules produced against hepatitis A and hepatitis B are the same (IgG), but the upper portion is different and specific to the virus.

The antibodies produced by B cells link with the antigen and inactivate it through one of the following processes:

- Promoting phagocytosis of the antigen by neutrophils.
- Precipitation: combining with soluble antigens to form an insoluble complex or precipitate.
- Neutralization: combining with a toxin to neutralize its effects; the antigen-antibody complex is then destroyed by the process of phagocytosis.
- Lysis of the antigen cell membrane caused by combination with antibodies and complement.
- Agglutination (clumping) of antigens to form a noninvasive aggregate.
- Opsonization: coating of the antigen with antibodies and complement, making them more susceptible to phagocytosis.

The complete antibody-mediated response occurs in two phases. With initial exposure to an antigen, the primary response develops. B cells are activated to proliferate and begin producing antibodies. There is a latency period of three to six days before antibodies become detectable in the blood. Levels then continue to rise, peaking at 10 to 14 days after the initial exposure. With many illnesses (e.g., chickenpox), this peak correlates with recovery.

Subsequent exposure to the same antigen elicits a secondary response. Memory cells formed during the primary response stimulate the production of plasma cells, and an almost immediate rise in antibody levels occurs. This rapid secondary response is the basis of acquired immunity and is instrumental in preventing disease. It is also the mechanism through which vaccines provide protection from disease.

Cell-Mediated Immune Response

Many antigens cannot stimulate the antibody-mediated response, or are "hidden" from it because they live inside the body's cells (viruses and mycobacteria are examples of such antigens). The immune response providing protection against these antigens is the cell-mediated immune response, also called *cellular immunity.* T lymphocytes (T cells) initiate this type of immune response.

Approximately 70% to 80% of circulating lymphocytes are T cells. T cells migrate to the thymus during fetal and early life, establishing the lifetime pool of cells. T cells have a life span measured in years, maintaining their numbers through proliferation, primarily in the lymph nodes.

T cells are much more complex than B cells. There are two major classes of T cells, *effector cells* and *regulator cells.* The main effector T cell is the *cytotoxic cell,* also called the *killer T cell.* Regulator T cells are further classified into two groups: *helper T cells* and *suppressor T cells.*

T cells are antigen specific; that is, each subset is activated by a particular antigen. The antigens that activate T cells must be presented on another cell surface, such as pieces of virus presented on the surface of an infected cell, or the histocompatibility locus antigen (HLA) on a cell of transplanted tissue. When activated, T cells divide and proliferate, forming antigen-specific clones. (A clone is an exact copy of another cell.)

Cytotoxic T cells bind with cell surface antigens on virus-infected or foreign cells. Killer T cells destroy the antigen by combining with it and then either destroying its cell membrane or releasing cytotoxic substances into the cell. They are vital in the control of viral and bacterial infections.

Regulator T cells play a key role in controlling the immune response. The majority of regulator T cells are helper T cells. They stimulate the proliferation of other T cells, amplify the cytotoxic activity of killer T cells, and activate B cells to proliferate and differentiate. They interact directly with B cells to promote their multiplication and conversion into plasma cells capable of producing antibodies. The other regulatory T-cell group, suppressor T cells, provide negative feedback, making the immune response a self-limiting process.

On activation, both effector and regulator T cells synthesize and release lymphokines, a type of soluble protein. Lymphokines are a subgroup of nonspecific defense mechanisms known as **cytokines**. Lymphokines secreted by cytotoxic and helper T cells are important in amplifying the immune response and the nonspecific inflammatory response. They stimulate the following:

- B cells to become plasma cells and produce antibodies.
- Macrophages to become activated macrophages (the most aggressive phagocyte).
- Proliferation of killer T cells.

Suppressor T cells release lymphokines, which inhibit the activity of other T cells and B cells.

Although T cells can be activated only by specific antigens, much of the resulting effect is nonspecific—in other words, an enhanced inflammatory response. Like the antibody-mediated response, the cell-mediated response has memory. Subsequent exposures to an antigen result in a more rapid and effective inflammatory response and more effective phagocytosis by macrophages. This memory provides the basis for skin testing. A client previously exposed to tuberculosis, for example, develops a more pronounced inflammatory response when minute amounts are injected under the skin.

Normal Immune Responses

The Client with Tissue Inflammation and Healing

As noted, inflammation is a nonspecific response to injury that serves to destroy, dilute, or contain the injurious agent or damaged tissue. Inflammation may be either acute or chronic. Acute inflammation is a short-term reaction of the body to all types of tissue damage. It is immediate and aimed at protecting the body and preventing further invasion or injury. Acute inflammation usually lasts less than one to two weeks. Once the injurious agent is removed, the inflammation subsides. Healing with tissue repair or scar formation occurs, and the body functions in normal or near-normal capacity.

Chronic inflammation is slower in onset and may not have an acute phase. Its clinical manifestations occur over months or years. It involves cell proliferation and is debilitating, with long-term adverse effects. There is increased cellular exudate, necrosis, fibrosis, and sometimes tissue scarring, resulting in severe tissue damage.

Pathophysiology of Tissue Inflammation

The tissue damage that evokes an inflammatory response may be caused by specific or nonspecific agents. These agents may be *exogenous,* from outside the body, or *endogenous,* from within the body. Causes of inflammation include the following:

* Mechanical injuries, such as cuts or surgical incisions
* Physical damage, such as burns
* Chemical injury from toxins or poisons
* Microorganisms, such as bacteria, viruses, or fungi
* Extremes of heat or cold
* Immunologic responses, such as hypersensitivity reactions
* Ischemic damage or trauma, such as a stroke or myocardial infarction

Acute Inflammation

Regardless of the cause, location, or extent of the injury, the acute inflammatory response follows the previously outlined sequence of vascular response, cellular and phagocytic response, and healing.

Many of the manifestations of inflammation are produced by inflammatory mediators, such as histamine and prostaglandins, released when tissue is damaged.

The cardinal signs of inflammation include the following:

* Erythema (redness)
* Local heat caused by the increased blood flow to the injured area (hyperemia)

- Swelling due to accumulated fluid at the site
- Pain from tissue swelling and chemical irritation of nerve endings
- Loss of function caused by the swelling and pain.

The degree of functional loss depends on the location and extent of the injury. With increased tissue damage, more fluid exudate is formed, resulting in more swelling, pain, and functional impairment. Pain may be immediate or delayed. Prostaglandins intensify and prolong the pain. Kinins cause irritation to the nerve endings and contribute to the pain sensation.

Dead neutrophils, necrotic tissue, and digested bacteria accumulate as a result of inflammation and phagocytosis, forming *pus*. It usually forms and remains until after the infection subsides. Pus may push itself to the surface of the body or become internalized. In the latter case, pus is gradually autolyzed (self-digested) by enzymes over a period of days. The end product is then absorbed by the body. On occasion, pus may remain after the infection is resolved. Pockets of pus, called abscesses, may need to be artificially drained with a procedure called *incision and drainage (I&D)*. Ectopic calcifications are another possible result of residual collections of pus.

Systemic responses to inflammation include an increase in the size of lymph nodes due to the accumulation of bacteria, phagocytes, and destroyed lymph tissue. Enlarged lymph nodes are usually noted in the groin, axillae, and neck. Fever, often precipitated by inflammatory mediators or bacterial toxins, inhibits the growth of many microorganisms and increases tissue repair functions. Loss of appetite and fatigue may occur in the effort to conserve energy during the inflammatory process. Leukocytosis occurs with increased WBC production to support inflammation and phagocytosis.

Chronic Inflammation

Whereas acute inflammation is a self-limiting process lasting less than two weeks, chronic inflammation tends to be selfperpetuating, lasting weeks to months or years. Chronic inflammation may develop when the acute inflammatory process has been ineffective in removing the offending agent. For example, mycobacteria have cell walls with high lipid and wax content, making them resistant to phagocytosis. Chronic inflammation and granuloma formation is common with *Mycobacterium tuberculosis* infection. Persistent irritation by chemicals, particulate matter, or physical irritants such as talc, asbestos, or silica may also result in chronic inflammation.

The chronic inflammatory process is characterized by a dense infiltration of the site by lymphocytes and macrophages. The macrophages mass or coalesce to form a multinucleated giant cell surrounded by lymphocytes, in a lesion called a *granuloma*. The granuloma is effective in walling off the offending agent, isolating it from the rest of the body; however, the infectious agent or offending irritant may not be destroyed and can survive within the granuloma for a long period of time. The granuloma formed in tuberculosis is called a tubercle. *Mycobacterium tuberculosis* may survive for many years within the tubercle, emerging when the client's immune system is no longer able to contain it.

Complications

Inflammation and wound healing are highly metabolic processes that may be affected by a number of factors. Without adequate nutrition, blood supply, and oxygenation, tissues cannot effectively complete the process. Impaired inflammatory and immune processes can interfere with phagocytosis and preparation of the wound for healing. Infection prolongs the inflammatory process and delays healing.

Chronic diseases may also impair healing. Diabetes mellitus is a prominent example. With high blood glucose levels associated with poorly controlled diabetes, chemotaxic and phagocytic function is decreased. Collagen formation and tensile strength of the wound are also impaired. Small blood vessel disease is common in people with diabetes, a factor that further impairs the healing process.

Drug therapy, particularly corticosteroid medications, may suppress the immune and inflammatory responses, delaying healing (Porth, 2002). Other external factors, such as exposure to ionizing radiation and wound cleansing agents, can also affect healing.

Collaborative Care

Management of the client with inflamed tissue focuses on promoting healing. Care is generally supportive, allowing the client's own physiologic processes to remove foreign matter and damaged cells. Wound care may be minimal, involving only simple cleaning, or extensive, involving irrigations and debridement. The client is encouraged to rest, to increase fluid intake, and to eat a well-balanced, nutritious diet. Anti-inflammatory medications are administered only when the inflammatory process has become problematic. Antibiotics may also be prescribed to help eliminate infectious causes of inflammation.

Diagnostic Tests

The following diagnostic tests may be ordered to identify the source and extent of inflammation.

- *WBC with differential* provides information about the type and extent of inflammatory response. The differential count (the percentage of the total WBC made up by each type of leukocyte) provides further clues about inflammatory processes (Table 41-3).

Table 41-3. The White Blood Cell Count and Differential

Cell Type and Normal Value	Increased	Decreased
Total WBCs: 4000 to 10,000 per mm^3	*Leukocytosis:* Infection or inflammation, leukemia, trauma or stress, tissue necrosis	*Leukopenia:* Bone marrow depression, overwhelming infection, viral infections, immunosuppression, autoimmune disease, dietary deficiency
Neutrophils (segs, PMNs, or polys): 55% to 70%	*Neutrophilia:* Acute infection or stress response, myelocytic leukemia, inflammatory or metabolic disorders	*Neutropenia:* Bone marrow depression, overwhelming bacterial infection, viral infection, Addison's disease
Eosinophils (eos): 1% to 4%	*Eosinophilia:* Parasitic infections, hyper sensitivity reactions, autoimmune disorders	*Eosinopenia:* Cushing's syndrome, autoimmune disorders, stress, certain drugs

Continued on the next page

Table 41-3. Continued

Basophils (basos): 0.5% to 1%	*Basophilia:* Hypersensitivity responses, chronic myelogenous leukemia, chickenpox or smallpox, splenectomy, hypothyroidism	*Basopenia:* Acute stress or hypersensitivity reactions, hyperthyroidism
Monocytes (monos): 2% to 8%	*Monocytosis:* Chronic inflammatory disorders, tuberculosis, viral infections, leukemia, Hodgkin's disease, multiple myeloma	*Monocytopenia:* Bone marrow depression, corticosteroid therapy
Lymphocytes (lymphs): 20% to 40%	*Lymphocytosis:* Chronic bacterial infection, viral infections, lymphocytic leukemia	*Lymphocytopenia:* Bone marrow depression, immunodeficiency, leukemia, Cushing's syndrome, Hodgkin's disease, renal failure

Note: Data are from *Laboratory Tests and Diagnostic Procedures* (2nd ed.) by R. Chernecky and B. J. Berger, 1997, Philadelphia: W. B. Saunders; and *Mosby's Diagnostic and Laboratory Test Reference* (3rd ed.) by K. D. Pagana and T. J. Pagana, 1997, St. Louis: Mosby-Year Book.

- *Erythrocyte sedimentation rate (ESR or sed rate)* is a nonspecific test to detect inflammation. The rate at which RBCs fall to the bottom of a vertical tube is an indicator of inflammation. An increased ESR may indicate acute or chronic inflammation, tuberculosis, autoimmune disorders, some malignancies, and nephritis. Decreased ESR is found in congestive heart failure, sickle cell anemia, and polycythemia vera.

- *C-reactive protein (CRP) test* is used to detect CRP. This abnormal glycoprotein is produced by the liver and is excreted into the bloodstream during the acute phase of an inflammatory process. The expected result of this test is negative for CRP. A positive result indicates an acute or chronic inflammatory process. It may also indicate the client's response to therapy, because it decreases when inflammation subsides (Kee, 2001).

In addition to the above diagnostic tests, cultures of the blood and other body fluids may be ordered to determine if infection is the cause of inflammation.

Medications

Medications may be prescribed for the client with an inflammatory response to help alleviate distressing symptoms or destroy infectious agents.

Acetaminophen (Tylenol) may be administered to reduce the fever and pain associated with inflammation. Acetaminophen has no anti-inflammatory effect; it will not reduce the inflammatory process, but will relieve associated symptoms. Acetaminophen decreases fever by acting directly on the hypothalamus heat-regulating center. It also works on the central nervous system to relieve pain sensations.

Antibiotics may be used either prophylactically to prevent infection from interfering with the healing process of damaged tissue, or therapeutically to treat the infection. If infection is present, the organism and its response or sensitivity to various antibiotics are used to guide therapy.

Although inflammation is a beneficial process to prepare acutely injured tissue for healing, it can have damaging effects as well. When these effects are a concern or the manifestations of inflammation are deleterious to the client, anti-inflammatory medications may be prescribed. Anti-inflammatory medications fall into three broad groups: salicylates, such as aspirin; other nonsteroidal anti-inflammatory drugs (NSAIDs); and corticosteroids.

Aspirin (also called acetylsalicylic acid, or ASA) is an NSAID that has antipyretic, analgesic, and antiplatelet effects. Its beneficial effects are largely dose related. Low doses (as little as 81 mg per day) inhibit platelet aggregation and normal blood clotting. Higher doses (650 to 1000 mg 4 to 5 times per day) are required to accomplish its anti-inflammatory effects. However, 650 mg of aspirin is an effective analgesic and antipyretic dosage. To relieve pain, aspirin acts primarily on peripheral sensory nerves by inhibiting the synthesis of prostaglandins and kinins, which are chemical stimuli of sensory nerves. As an antipyretic, aspirin acts both centrally and peripherally. It inhibits the formation of pyrogenic substances that raise the hypothalamic thermostat. It also dilates peripheral blood vessels and promotes diaphoresis, increasing the dissipation of heat (Shannon, Wilson, & Stang, 2001).

In therapeutic doses, aspirin mediates the inflammatory process by inhibiting the synthesis of prostaglandins and acting on the mobility and activation of leukocytes. Inflammation is reduced, along with the swelling, redness, and impaired function that accompanies it.

The other NSAIDs have activity similar to that of aspirin. They inhibit prostaglandin synthesis, reducing the inflammatory and pain response. NSAIDs fall into the following classifications:

- *Salicylates,* which include aspirin and related compounds
- *Acetic acids,* including indomethacin (Indocin), ketorolac (Toradol), sulindac (Clinoril), and tolmetin (Tolectin)
- *Propionic acids,* including ibuprofen (Motrin and numerous nonprescription preparations), fenoprofen (Nalfon), and naproxen (Naprosyn)
- *Fenamates,* including meclofenamate (Meclomen)
- *Pyrazoles,* including phenylbutazone (Butazolidin)
- *Oxicams,* including piroxicam (Feldene).

Each group has a slightly different mode of action for prostaglandin inhibition. Clients may have varying degrees of relief with different NSAIDs; sometimes, several different agents must be tried before the most effective is identified. Side effects also differ to a certain extent; however, all have a potential cross-sensitivity with aspirin, all irritate the gastrointestinal tract, and all cause some degree of sodium and water retention. They also are more costly than aspirin, but they have a longer duration of action; therefore, fewer daily doses are required to achieve the desired effect. Indomethacin and phenylbutazone are the most toxic of the NSAIDs. Their use is limited to short-term therapy.

For acute hypersensitivity reactions, such as reactions to poison oak, or for inflammation that cannot be managed by aspirin or NSAID therapy, corticosteroid therapy may be prescribed. The glucocorticoids are hormones produced by the adrenal cortex that have widespread effects on body metabolism and the immune response. Glucocorticoids inhibit inflammation and may be lifesaving in acute fulminating or chronic progressive inflammation. They do not cure disease; they are palliative to manage the inflammatory process.

When glucocorticoids are prescribed to manage inflammation, the following principles are used to guide therapy:

- The smallest possible effective dose is used.
- If a local-acting preparation, such as a topical agent or intra-articular injection, proves effective, it can be prescribed.
- To minimize suppression of adrenal gland activity, an alternate-day dose schedule is used when possible.
- High-dose corticosteroid therapy is never stopped abruptly, but tapered, allowing the client's adrenal glands to resume normal function.

The incidence of potentially harmful side effects increases with higher doses and prolonged therapy.

Nutrition

Healing depends on cell replication, protein synthesis, and the function of specific organs—the liver, heart, and lungs in particular. Weight loss and protein depletion are risk factors for poor healing and wound complications. Even a few days of severely impaired nutritional intake can noticeably affect healing.

The client with an inflammatory process or healing wound requires a well-balanced diet of sufficient kilocalories to meet the metabolic needs of the body. Inflammation often produces *catabolism,* a state in which body tissues are broken down. Healing, by contrast, is a process of *anabolism,* or building up. Without sufficient kilocalories and nutrients, catabolism may predominate, impairing healing.

Carbohydrates are important to meet energy demands, as well as to support leukocyte function. Adequate protein is necessary for tissue healing and the production of antibodies and WBCs. Lack of adequate protein increases the risk of infection. Complete protein sources, those that provide the essential amino acids, are preferred. Dietary fats are used in the synthesis of cell membranes.

Vitamins A, B-complex, C, and K are also important to the healing process. Vitamin A is necessary for capillary formation and epithelialization. B-complex vitamins promote wound healing, and vitamin C is necessary for collagen synthesis. Vitamin K provides a vital component for the synthesis of clotting factors in the liver.

Although it has been established that minerals contribute to the inflammatory and healing processes, less is known about required amounts. Zinc appears to be important for tissue growth, skin integrity, cell-mediated immunity, and other general immune mechanisms (Lutz & Przytulski, 2001).

Nursing Care

Acute inflammation may be self-limiting or extensive and require hospitalization. Nursing care includes teaching clients with acute and chronic inflammatory conditions self-management at home.

Health Promotion

Health promotion activities to prevent inflammation focus on reducing the risk for accidents and exposure to harmful agents that can result in subsequent injury. It is important to educate the public about potential hazards in both the work and home environments. In addition, safety education guidelines, such as not drinking and driving, wearing a protective helmet when riding a bicycle, and using a safety belt in the car are important areas for discussion. Because most injuries occur at home, it is also important to discuss ways to make the home safer.

Assessment

The following data are collected through the health history and physical examination. Further focused assessments are described with nursing interventions in the next section.

*   *Health history:* risk factors, nutrition, medication use (anti-inflammatory and corticosteroids), location, duration, and type (redness, heat, pain, swelling, and impaired function) of symptoms.
*   *Physical assessment:* movement of injured area, circulation, wounds, lymph nodes.

Nursing Diagnoses and Interventions

The nursing care needs of the client with an inflammatory process are related to the manifestations of inflammation (pain in particular) and altered tissue integrity. Priority nursing diagnoses include *pain, impaired tissue integrity,* and *risk for infection.*

Pain

Along with redness, warmth, swelling, and impaired function, pain is one of the cardinal manifestations of inflammation. Depending on the cause, affected area, and degree of inflammation, pain may be acute and immobilizing or chronic and demoralizing. It is important to remember that pain is a subjective experience and that client responses to pain vary.

*   Assess pain using a scale of 0 to 10, with 0 being no pain and 10 being the worst pain; note the character and location of the pain. *Because pain is subjective, the client provides the most accurate information regarding his or her pain experience.*
*   Use physical and nonverbal cues to further assess the level of pain. *This intervention is especially important if the client is nonverbal or tends to underreport pain.*
*   Administer anti-inflammatory medications as prescribed. *These medications help reduce the pain resulting from acute inflammation.*
*   Administer analgesic medications as prescribed. *Although most analgesics do little to reduce inflammation, they provide additional pain relief by reducing the perception of pain.*
*   Monitor effectiveness of interventions. *Results may call for modifications in the regimen.*
*   Provide comfort measures, such as back rubs, position changes, or relaxation techniques. *These measures reduce muscle tension, relieve areas of pressure, and provide distraction.*
*   Encourage activities, such as reading, watching television, and taking part in social interactions. *Such activities provide distraction from the pain experience.*
*   Encourage rest. *Strenuous activity or exercising an inflamed body part may increase discomfort and tissue damage.*

- Provide cold or heat as pain-relief measures, as ordered. *For an acute injury, cold reduces swelling and relieves pain; after the initial stage, heat increases blood flow to the affected tissue and relieves pain and swelling by promoting absorption of edema. Either heat or cold may be contraindicated with some inflammatory processes; for example, if the appendix is acutely inflamed, applying heat to the abdomen may prompt the appendix to rupture, increasing the risk of peritonitis. If unsure, check with the client's primary care provider.*
- Elevate the inflamed area if possible. *Elevation promotes venous return and reduces swelling.*
- Teach about the appropriate use and expected effects of anti-inflammatory medications. *If the client's pain continues after the initial doses of anti-inflammatory medication, he or she may become discouraged and stop taking the medication before it becomes fully effective.*

Impaired Tissue Integrity

The inflammatory response can either precipitate or result from an impairment in the integrity of skin, support, or other tissues. Whatever the cause of the tissue alteration, it is vital that the nurse consider this alteration in delivering care.

- Assess general health and nutritional status. *Poor general health or chronic diseases, such as diabetes mellitus or renal failure, interfere with the healing processes and increase the risk of infection.*
- Assess circulation to the affected area. *Adequate tissue perfusion and oxygenation are necessary for healing.*
- Monitor the skin and surrounding tissue for increased signs of inflammation. *Inflammation can spread to adjacent tissues leading to conditions, such as cellulitis.*
- Provide protection and support for inflamed tissue. *This reduces discomfort and decreases the risk of further tissue damage.*
- Clean inflamed tissue gently; if possible, use water, normal saline, or nontoxic wound cleansers, such as Comfeel (Coloplast Corporation) only. *Soap and harsh cleansers, such as povidone-iodine (Betadine) and hydrogen peroxide, can cause further drying and tissue damage. Granulation tissue in a healing wound is fragile and easily damaged.*
- Keep the inflamed area dry, and expose it to air as much as possible. *This promotes healing and helps prevent infection.*
- Balance rest with the tolerable degree of mobility. *Rest decreases metabolic demands and allows for cell regeneration while mobility helps to promote oxygenation and perfusion of the tissues.*
- Provide supplemental oxygen as ordered. *Supplemental oxygen improves tissue oxygenation and reduces hypoxia.*
- Provide a well-balanced diet with adequate kilocalories to meet the body's metabolic and healing needs. If the client is allowed nothing by mouth (NPO), suggest parenteral or enteral nutrition. For the client who is unable to consume an adequate diet, consult with a dietitian for between-meal supplements, and/or multivitamin supplements. *Careful attention to diet and nutrient intake is important to provide the nutrients necessary for immune function and healing, and to prevent catabolism.*

Risk for Infection

The inflammatory response often indicates that body defense mechanisms have been set in motion to protect against invading microorganisms. Wounds, whether traumatic or surgical in nature, are typically contaminated, as attested to by subsequent wound infections. The client with a healing wound is at particular risk for infection.

- Assess the wound for specific signs of infection, including purulent drainage, odor, and poor healing. *The normal inflammatory response can indicate infection and, on occasion, mask its presence.*

- Monitor temperature, pulse, and respirations at least every four hours. *In response to the inflammatory process the temperature rises, usually in the range of 99°F (37.2°C) to 100.9°F (38.2°C). A temperature of 101.0°F (38.3°C) or above indicates infection. Fever is usually accompanied by increased heart and respiratory rates.*

- Culture purulent or odorous wound drainage. *Wound culture is used to determine the infectious organism and to direct antibiotic therapy.*

- Apply dry or moist heat to the affected area for no longer than 20 minutes several times a day. *Heat increases the circulation of blood to and from the inflamed tissue. Time is limited to prevent burns.*

- Provide fluid intake of 2500 mL per day. *Adequate hydration promotes blood flow and nutrient supply to the tissues, as well as dilutes and removes waste products from the body.*

- Assure adequate nutrition. *Adequate nutrition enhances the function and production of T cells and B cells, which are important in the immune response.*

- Use good handwashing techniques. *Handwashing removes transient microorganisms and is the best mechanism to prevent the spread of infection to a susceptible person.*

- Wear sterile gloves when providing wound care. *Using sterile gloves helps prevent further contamination of the wound and the spread of infection to other clients.*

Home Care

Client and family teaching enhances understanding of the inflammatory process, its cause, and its management. Teaching is also important to prevent further compromise that could result in infection.

Instructions, verbal and written, should include the following:

- Increase fluid intake to 2500 mL (approximately 2.5 quarts) per day.

- Eat a well-balanced diet high in vitamins and minerals and with adequate protein and kilocalories for healing.

- Use good handwashing techniques, particularly when caring for wounds or inflamed tissue and after using the bathroom.

- Elevate the inflamed area to reduce swelling and pain.

- Apply heat or cold for no longer than 20 minutes at a time to reduce the risk of tissue damage from burns or frostbite.

- Take all medications as prescribed, notifying the physician if adverse effects or hypersensitivity responses are noted.

- Rest acutely inflamed tissue; do not engage in strenuous activity until the inflammation has subsided.

42 Impaired Immune Responses

Recent years have seen the emergence of new diseases affecting the immune system. These diseases include human immunodeficiency virus (HIV) infection and altered strains of familiar diseases such as multidrug-resistant tuberculosis.

Disorders of impaired immune system responses may be either congenital or acquired. Often the function of either T or B cells is impaired, reducing the body's ability to defend against foreign antigens or abnormal host tissue.

No matter what the cause, clients with immunodeficiency disorders demonstrate an unusual susceptibility to infection. When the antibody-mediated response is primarily affected, the client is at particular risk for severe and chronic bacterial infections. These clients also do not develop long-lasting immunity to such diseases as chickenpox and are prone to recurrent cases. Clients with a defect of cell-mediated immunity tend to develop disseminated viral infections, such as herpes simplex and CMV. Candidiasis and other fungal infections are also common. Because T cells are involved with activating antibody-mediated immune responses as well, overwhelming bacterial infections may occur. Immunodeficiency in its most severe form occurs when both antibody-mediated and cell-mediated responses are impaired. Clients with combined immunodeficiency are susceptible to all varieties of infectious organisms, including those not normally considered to be pathogens.

Most immunodeficiency diseases are genetically determined and rare. They affect children more than adults. The noted exception is AIDS, an infectious disease caused by a virus.

The Client with HIV Infection

In 1981, five cases of *Pneumocystis carinii* pneumonia (PCP) and 26 cases of a rare cancer, Kaposi's sarcoma, were diagnosed in young, previously healthy homosexual males in Los Angeles and New York City. The term **acquired immunodeficiency syndrome (AIDS)** was ascribed to this new phenomenon to describe the immune system deficits associated with these opportunistic disorders. Prior to this time, both PCP and Kaposi's had been seen only in elderly, debilitated, or severely immunodeficient people. Other groups at risk for AIDS were soon identified: injection drug users, persons with hemophilia, recipients of blood transfusions, and immigrants from Haiti.

Research to identify the cause of this apparently new disease progressed feverishly, and in 1983, a common antibody was identified in clients with AIDS. The **human immunodeficiency virus (HIV)** was isolated in 1984. It then became apparent that AIDS was the final, fatal stage of HIV infection.

> It began, like so many epidemics, with a few isolated cases, a whisper that caught the ear of only a few in medical research. Today, that whisper has become a roar heard around the world. AIDS—acquired immunodeficiency syndrome—is now the epidemic of our generation, invading our lives in ways we never imagined—testing our scientific knowledge, probing our private values, and sapping our strength. AIDS no longer attracts our attention—it commands it. (Novello, 1993)

Incidence and Prevalence

As of December 2000, the CDC estimated that 800,000 to 900,000 persons in the United States were infected with HIV, with AIDS as the fifth leading cause of death among adults age 25 to 44. As many as one-third of those infected are unaware of their HIV infection. By the end of June 2000, a cumulative total of 753,907 cases of AIDS had been reported. By 1999, death rates among people with AIDS had decreased (Bihari, Levin, Malebranche, & Valdez, 2000), the result of a slowing of the epidemic and improved treatments.

Among men with new HIV infection, 60% were men who have sex with men, 25% were those injecting drugs, and 15% were people having heterosexual contact (primarily with injecting drug users). The majority (75%) of women were infected through heterosexual contact, with the remaining 25% through injection drug use. Among risk groups, the most rapid increases are noted in young gay and bisexual men, women, and inner-city intravenous drug users, especially African-Americans and Hispanics (Bihari et al., 2000). In the United States, the reported rate of adult/adolescent AIDS cases (per 100,000 population) reported was 84.2 among African Americans, 34.6 among Hispanics, 11.3 among American Indians/Alaska Natives, 9.0 among Caucasians, and 4.3 among Asians/Pacific Islanders (National Institute of Allergy and Infectious Diseases [NIAID], 2001). The rapid increase of AIDS cases among women is of special concern; those numbers increased from 7% of cases in 1985 to 23% of newly reported cases in 2000 (NIAID, 2000).

In addition, AIDS in the adult over age 50 accounts for 10% of all reported cases in the United States. Declining immune system function in older adults significantly increases their risk for contracting HIV/AIDS, along with the belief that they cannot be affected by it. Just as younger persons with HIV/AIDS contract the diseases primarily through sexual intercourse, so does the elderly population. Because older adults are beyond childbearing years, they often fail to use condoms when engaging in sexual activity. Manifestations may be overlooked by health care professionals, leading to a delayed diagnosis and increased severity of the disease.

There are an estimated 36.2 million people infected with AIDS worldwide, with virtually every country in the world reporting cases of AIDS (Joint United Nations Programme on HIV/AIDS [UNAIDS], 2000). The highest incidence is found in sub-Saharan Africa, South and Southeast Asia, the United States, western Europe, South America, and Canada. Approximately 70% of all people infected with HIV or who have AIDS live in sub-Saharan Africa, and another 16% live in South and Southeast Asia, especially in Thailand and India. The most common mode of transmission is heterosexual intercourse. The cofactors of general health status, the presence of genital ulcers, and the number of sexual partners correlate with incidence (Tierney, et al., 2001).

HIV is a retrovirus transmitted by direct contact with infected blood and body fluids. Significant concentrations of the virus are present in blood, semen, vaginal and cervical secretions, and cerebrospinal fluid (CSF) of infected individuals. It is also found in breast milk and saliva. Sexual contact is the primary mode of transmission. HIV is also transmitted through contact with infected blood via needle sharing during injection drug use or by transfusion. Approximately 15% to 30% of infants born to HIV-positive mothers are infected perinatally.

The risk factors for HIV infection are behavioral. Among adults in the United States, 60% of reported cases are in men who have sex with other men, including homosexuals, bisexuals, and such groups as prison populations. Unprotected anal intercourse is the major route of transmission in this group. Injection drug use is the second leading risk factor, accounting for approximately 25% of cases. Sharing of needles and other drug paraphernalia is the primary route of transmission in this group. Heterosexual intercourse with an infected drug user and exchanging sex for drugs are major risk factors for women. Hemophiliacs who require large amounts of intravenous clotting factors and people infected through blood transfusion account for a small number of cases, approximately 2% to 3%.

Among the general population of the United States, the prevalence of HIV infection is very low. Less than 0.04% of people voluntarily donating blood (a process that generally excludes people with high-risk behavior) are found to be HIV positive. HIV is not transmitted by casual contact, nor is there any evidence of its transmission by vectors, such as mosquitoes. Blood donation also poses no risk of contracting HIV to the donor, because only new sterile equipment is used. A small but real occupational risk exists for health care workers. Percutaneous exposure to infected blood or body fluids through a needle-stick injury or nonintact skin is the primary route of transmission. Documented evidence indicates that parenteral exposure poses a 0.3% risk of becoming HIV positive (Carrico, 2001). Mucosal exposures, such as splashing in the eyes or mouth, pose a much smaller risk.

Pathophysiology and Manifestations

HIV is a retrovirus, meaning it carries its genetic information in RNA. On entry into the body, the virus infects cells which have the CD4 antigen. Once inside the cell, the virus sheds its protein coat and uses an enzyme called *reverse transcriptase* to convert the RNA to DNA. This viral DNA is then integrated into host cell DNA and duplicated during normal processes of cell division. Within the cell, the virus may remain latent or become activated to produce new RNA and to form virions. The virus then buds from the cell surface, disrupting its cell membrane and leading to destruction of the host cell.

Although the virus may remain inactive in infected cells for years, antibodies are produced to its proteins, a process known as **seroconversion.** These antibodies are usually detectable six weeks to six months after the initial infection. Helper T or CD4 cells are the primary cells infected by HIV. It also infects macrophages and certain cells of the CNS. Helper T cells play a vital role in normal immune system function, recognizing foreign antigens and infected cells and activating antibody-producing B cells. They also direct cell-mediated immune activity and influence the phagocytic activity of monocytes and macrophages. The loss of these helper T cells leads to the immunodeficiencies seen with HIV infection (Porth, 2002).

Pathologic changes are also noted in the CNS of many infected individuals. Although the mechanism of neurologic dysfunction is unclear, neurologic manifestations of HIV infection may be seen in clients who have no apparent immune deficiency (Porth, 2002; Tierney et al., 2001). The clinical manifestations of HIV infection range from no symptoms to severe immunodeficiency with multiple opportunistic infections and cancers. It appears that the majority of clients develop an acute mononucleosis-type illness within days to weeks after contracting the virus. Typical manifestations include fever, sore throat, arthralgias and myalgias, headache, rash, and lymphadenopathy. The client may also experience nausea, vomiting, and abdominal cramping. The client often attributes this initial manifestation of HIV infection to a common viral illness such as influenza, upper respiratory infection, or stomach virus.

Following this acute illness, clients enter a long-lasting asymptomatic period. Although the virus is present and can be transmitted to others, the infected host has few or no symptoms. Clearly, the majority of HIV-infected persons are in this stage of the disease. The length of the asymptomatic period varies widely, but its mean length is estimated to be eight to ten years.

Some clients with few other symptoms develop persistent generalized lymphadenopathy. This is defined as enlargement of two or more lymph nodes outside the inguinal chain with no other illness or condition to account for the lymphadenopathy.

The move from asymptomatic disease or persistent lymphadenopathy to AIDS is often not clearly defined. The client may complain of general malaise, fever, fatigue, night sweats, and involuntary weight loss. Persistent skin dryness and rash may be a problem. Diarrhea is common, as are oral lesions, such as hairy leukoplakia, candidiasis, and gingival inflammation and ulceration.

With the development of significant constitutional disease, neurologic manifestations, or opportunistic infections or cancers, the client has manifestations that are characteristic of AIDS and a very poor prognosis. HIV infection and AIDS may be classified by using the CDC's matrix classification system. Under this system, HIV disease is determined by the presence of clinical symptoms (clinical categories A, B, and C) and by T4 cell counts (categories 1, 2, and 3).

When clinical manifestations develop, the outcome varies. With improvements in therapy, many clients are living longer after being diagnosed with AIDS. For example, in San Francisco, mean survival after a first bout with PCP is 18 to 24 months. The time of survival has increased from about 12 months at the start of the epidemic; however, survival after diagnosis of HIV-related lymphomas still averages less than eight months.

AIDS Dementia Complex and Neurologic Effects

Neurologic manifestations of HIV are common, affecting 40% to 60% of clients with AIDS. They result from both the direct effects of the virus on the nervous system and opportunistic infections.

AIDS dementia complex is the most common cause of mental status changes for clients with HIV infection. This dementia results from a direct effect of the virus on the brain and affects cognitive, motor, and behavioral functioning. Fluctuating memory loss, confusion, difficulty concentrating, lethargy, and diminished motor speed are typical manifestations of AIDS dementia complex. Clients become apathetic, losing interest in work and social and recreational activities. As the complex progresses, the client develops severe dementia with motor disturbances, such as ataxia, tremor, spasticity, incontinence, and paraplegia (Braunwald, et al., 2001; Porth, 2002).

Infections and lesions common with AIDS may also affect the CNS. Toxoplasmosis and non-Hodgkin's lymphoma are space-occupying lesions that may cause headache, altered mental status, and neurologic deficits. Cryptococcal meningitis and CMV infection are also common in people with AIDS.

Peripheral nervous system manifestations are also common in HIV-infected clients. Sensory neuropathies with manifestations of numbness, tingling, and pain in the lower extremities affect about 30% of clients with AIDS. A Guillain-Barré type of inflammatory demyelinating polyneuropathy can also occur, resulting in progressive weakness and paralysis.

Opportunistic Infections

Opportunistic infections are the most common manifestations of AIDS, often occurring simultaneously. The risk of opportunistic infections is predictable by the T4 or CD4 cell count. The normal CD4 cell count is greater than $1000/mm^3$. When the CD4 count falls to less than $500/mm^3$, manifestations of immunodeficiency are seen. With a count of less than $200/mm^3$, opportunistic infections and cancers are likely.

Pneumocystis Carinii Pneumonia

Pneumocystis carinii pneumonia (PCP) is the most common opportunistic infection affecting clients with AIDS. Approximately 75% to 80% of clients develop PCP at some point in their disease (Tierney, et al., 2001). It tends to be recurrent, and is the cause of death in about 20% of clients with AIDS. PCP is caused by a common environmental fungus that is not pathogenic in clients with intact immune systems.

Unlike many pneumonias, the manifestations of PCP are nonspecific and may progress insidiously. Clients often present with fever, cough, shortness of breath, tachypnea, and tachycardia. Complaints of mild chest pain and sputum may also be present. Breath sounds may initially be normal. With severe disease, the client may present with cyanosis and significant respiratory distress.

Tuberculosis

An estimated 4% of clients with AIDS develop tuberculosis, contributing significantly to the rise in incidence of this disease in the United States. In some clients, active tuberculosis results from reactivation of a prior infection. In other clients, it is a new, primary disease facilitated by impaired immune function. Rapid progression, diffuse pulmonary infiltrates, and disseminated disease occur more commonly in clients with AIDS. Multidrug-resistant strains of tuberculosis present a significant problem (Tierney, et al., 2001).

Clients with pulmonary tuberculosis present with a cough productive of purulent sputum, fever, fatigue, weight loss, and lymphadenopathy. Disseminated disease affects the bone marrow, bone, joints, liver, spleen, CSF, skin, kidneys, gastrointestinal tract, lymph nodes, brain, and other sites.

Candidiasis

Candida albicans infection is a common opportunistic infection in clients with AIDS. It is usually manifested as oral thrush or esophagitis. In women, vaginal candidiasis is frequent and often recurrent. Oral thrush presents as white, friable plaques on the buccal mucosa or tongue and, in the HIV-infected client, is often the first indication of progression to AIDS. Clients with esophagitis have difficulty swallowing and substernal pain or burning which increases with swallowing.

Mycobacterium Avium Complex

Mycobacterium avium complex (MAC) affects up to 25% of clients with AIDS, typically occurring late in the course of the disease when CD4 cell counts are less than $50/mm^3$. MAC is more common in women than men. MAC is caused by organisms commonly found in food, water, and soil. It is a major cause of "wasting syndrome" in persons with AIDS. Manifestations of MAC include chills and fever, weakness, night sweats, abdominal pain and diarrhea, and weight loss. Nearly every organ can be infected, and most people with MAC develop disseminated disease.

Other Infections

Herpes virus infections are common in clients with AIDS and may be severe. CMV can affect the retina, the gastrointestinal tract, or lungs. Disseminated herpes simplex or herpes zoster may occur, although severe mucocutaneous manifestations are more common.

Parasitic infections with *Toxoplasma gondii* and *Cryptococcus neoformans* commonly affect the CNS. Toxoplasmosis occurs as encephalitis or an intracerebral mass lesion. Changes in mental status, focal neurologic signs, and seizures may result. *Cryptococcus* infection may present as either meningitis or disseminated disease, primarily affecting the lungs. *Cryptosporidium,* a protozoon affecting the gastrointestinal tract, is an important cause of prolonged diarrhea in AIDS clients. Bacterial salmonella infections are also a relatively common cause of diarrhea.

Women with AIDS have a high incidence of pelvic inflammatory disease (PID). Although the pathogens appear to be the same as those in PID affecting non-HIV-infected women, the disease is more severe. Inpatient treatment with intravenous antibiotics is often necessary.

Secondary Cancers

As cell-mediated immune function declines, the risk of malignancy increases. The CDC classification of AIDS currently includes four cancers: Kaposi's sarcoma, non-Hodgkin's lymphoma, primary lymphoma of the brain, and invasive cervical carcinoma.

Kaposi's Sarcoma

Kaposi's sarcoma (KS) is often the presenting symptom of AIDS. It remains the most common cancer associated with the disease. KS predominantly affects homosexual males with AIDS, occurring much less commonly in injection drug users and heterosexuals. At this time, the reason for the discrepancy is unknown.

A tumor of the endothelial cells lining small blood vessels, KS presents as vascular macules, papules, or violet lesions affecting the skin and viscera. The face is a common site for skin lesions, especially the tip of the nose and pinnae of the ears. Common sites for visceral disease include the gastrointestinal tract, lungs, and lymphatic system.

The lesions of KS are usually painless initially, but may become painful as the disease progresses. Internally, the tumors may obstruct organ function or cause bleeding. When the lungs are involved, gas exchange may be severely impaired, resulting in pulmonary hemorrhage. This disease may progress slowly or rapidly. KS is an indicator of late-stage HIV disease, with an average survival time of 18 months after diagnosis.

Lymphomas

Lymphomas are malignancies of the lymphoid tissue, including lymphocytes, lymph nodes, and the lymphoid organs, such as the spleen and bone marrow. In AIDS, two lymphomas are common, non-Hodgkin's lymphoma and primary lymphoma of the brain. Hodgkin's disease also occurs five times more frequently in clients with HIV infection. The CNS is the usual site for these lymphomas, although they may be found in the bone marrow, gastrointestinal tract, liver, skin, and mucous membranes. They are aggressive tumors, growing and spreading rapidly. Headache and changes in mental status are common early symptoms of lymphomas affecting the CNS.

Cervical Cancer

Of women with HIV infection, 40% have cervical dysplasia. Cervical cancer develops frequently and tends to be aggressive. Women with concurrent HIV infection and cervical cancer usually die of the cervical cancer, not AIDS. Because of this, it is recommended that women with HIV infection have Papanicolaou (Pap) smears every six months and aggressive treatment of cervical dysplasia with colposcopic examination and cone biopsy.

Collaborative Care

Although multiple research studies to identify a cure for HIV infection and AIDS are underway, no cure is currently available. This fact, plus the apparent universally fatal nature of the disease, make prevention a vital strategy in HIV care. New treatments are under investigation.

The goals of care for the client with HIV disease are as follows:

- Early identification of the infection
- Promoting health-maintenance activities to prolong the asymptomatic period as long as possible
- Prevention of opportunistic infections
- Treatment of disease complications, such as cancers
- Providing emotional and psychosocial support.

Diagnostic Tests

Diagnostic testing is used to screen and identify the infection, as well as to monitor the client's disease and immune status. The following diagnostic tests may be ordered:

- *Enzyme-linked immunosorbent assay (ELISA)* is the most widely used screening test for HIV infection. The ELISA test was developed in 1985 to screen blood donors. ELISA tests for HIV antibodies; it does not detect the virus. Therefore, a client may have a negative ELISA test early in the course of infection, before detectable antibodies have developed. The test has a 99.5% or higher sensitivity when performed at least 12 weeks after infection. This means that more than 99.5% of tests performed on blood containing HIV antibodies will show a positive result. False positives can occur; therefore, an initial positive result is always tested repeatedly and confirmed using a different method of antibody detection, usually the Western blot.
- *Western blot antibody testing* is more reliable but more time consuming and more expensive than ELISA. When combined with ELISA, however, a specificity of greater

than 99.9% is achieved. Specificity is a measure of the probability that a negative test result indicates that no antibodies are present. In this test, the client's serum is mixed with HIV proteins to detect reaction. If antibodies to HIV are present, a detectable antigen-antibody response will occur.

- *HIV viral load tests* measure the amount of actively replicating HIV. Levels correlate with disease progression and response to antiretroviral medications. Levels greater than 5000 to 10,000 copies/mL indicate the need for treatment.

- *CBC* is performed to detect anemia, leukopenia, and thrombocytopenia, which are often present in HIV infection. Lymphopenia (or low levels of lymphocytes) is especially common in this disease.

- *CD4 cell count* is the most widely used test to monitor the progress of the disease and guide therapy. The CD4 cell count correlates so closely with the immunodeficiency disorders seen in AIDS. AIDS is now defined not only by the presence of opportunistic infections and other diseases indicative of immunodeficiency, but also by HIV-seropositive status and a CD4 count of less than $200/mm^3$ or a percentage of CD4 lymphocytes of less than 14%. CD4 counts are recommended every three to six months for all people with HIV disease.

In addition to these widely used tests, several other diagnostic, tests may be performed:

- *Blood culture for HIV* provides the most specific diagnosis but is an expensive and cumbersome test that is not widely available in the United States.

- *Immune-complex-dissociated p24 assay* is a test for p24 (HIV) antigen in the blood. This antigen indicates active reproduction of HIV and tends to be positive prior to seroconversion and with advanced disease. It is most useful in monitoring disease progress and the antiviral activity of medications (Tierney, et al., 2001).

Other diagnostic tests are used primarily to detect secondary cancers and opportunistic infections in the client with HIV. Tests ordered are both general and specific to the client's manifestations and may include the following:

- *Tuberculin skin testing* to detect possible tuberculosis infection.
- *Magnetic resonance imaging (MRI)* of the brain to identify lymphomas.
- *Specific cultures and serology examinations for opportunistic infections,* such as PCP, toxoplasmosis, and others.
- *Pap smears* every six months for early detection of cervical cancer in women.

Medications

Pharmacologic management of the client with HIV disease has two primary foci: (1) *to suppress the infection itself,* decreasing symptoms and prolonging life, and (2) *to treat opportunistic infections and malignancies.* Effectiveness of treatment is monitored by viral load and CD4 cell counts; positive results are indicated by a reduction in viral load along with preserving the CD4 count above $500 mm^3$.

Three classes of drugs used in antiretroviral treatment include nucleoside reverse transcriptase inhibitors (NRTIs), nonnucleoside reverse transcriptase inhibitors (NNRTIs), and protease inhibitors. The new treatment protocol, highly active antiretroviral therapy (HAART), combines three or four antiretroviral drugs to reduce the incidence of drug resistance. However, when clients with AIDS at earlier stages or at lower risk of rapid progression are treated, combination therapies may burden them with complicated and expensive medication schedules and increase the potential of developing drug toxicities and drug resistance (Tierney, et al., 2001). Clients beginning the HAART protocol must understand the benefits, risks, costs, and affects on daily life. HAART medications are expensive, costing more than $15,000 per year, and this does not include medications to prevent or treat opportunistic infections or cancer. Medications are scheduled for specific times throughout the day; therefore, leading a normal life becomes a challenge. In addition, all HAART medications cause major adverse reactions. Adherence to the treatment regimen is less than perfect, as with most chronic diseases, but in this case, the outcome could be fatal.

Table 42-1. Medication Administration – Antiretroviral Nucleoside Analogs

Zidovudine (AZT, Retrovir, ZDT)

Zidovudine is the first antiretroviral agent developed to treat HIV infection. It interferes with reverse transcriptase, thus inhibiting replication of the virus. Zidovudine is used for clients with CD4 cell counts of less than 500/μL. The usual dose is 500 to 600 mg per day in divided doses. It is administered orally.

Nursing Responsibilities
- Assess for possible contraindications to therapy including allergic response or a CD4 count of greater than 500/mm³.
- Administer by mouth, instructing the client to swallow capsules whole.
- Assess for adverse effects. Nausea and headache are common. They may be self-limiting, decreasing with time, or significant and continuing, necessitating a change of therapy. Other adverse effects include insomnia, malaise, and confusion.
- Assess CBC and differential. Notify the physician of significant changes.

Client and Family Teaching
- Zidovudine will not cure HIV infection but slows its progress and reduces significant symptoms.
- Take the drug as prescribed every four to six hours to maintain an effective blood level.
- Take the drug at least 1/2 hour before or one hour after meals if tolerated.
- With this and all antiretroviral drugs, it is important to emphasize that the client is still infective and can pass the infection to others. Use safer sex practices and other measures to prevent transmission to partners. Do not donate blood.
- Notify the physician if signs of an infection or adverse response to zidovudine develop: sore throat, swollen lymph glands, fever; unusual fatigue or weakness; easy bruising, bleeding gums, or an injury that will not heal; persistent or intractable nausea; muscle pain or wasting.
- Continue all scheduled follow-up visits and laboratory studies to monitor for drug toxicity.
- Check with the physician before taking any prescription or over-the-counter drug containing aspirin or other NSAID.

Continued on the next page

Table 42-1. Continued

Didanosine (DDI, Videx)

As with zidovudine, didanosine does not kill HIV but inhibits its replication within the cells. Its activity is similar to that of zidovudine. Didanosine has been shown to increase CD4 cell counts and lower p24 antigen levels (Tierney, et al., 2001). Didanosine is used alone for clients who are intolerant or resistant to zidovudine. It is also being used with zidovudine in combination therapy regimens. Didanosine does not cause the anemia associated with zidovudine, but it may cause granulocytopenia. Didanosine is also associated with an increased risk of pancreatitis, peripheral neuritis, and dry mouth.

Nursing Responsibilities

- Assess for possible contraindications to didanosine therapy, including previous episodes of pancreatitis and impaired renal or liver function.

- Administer as directed. Tablets are to be chewed thoroughly or dissolved in one ounce of water at room temperature. The powder form is dissolved in water prior to administration.

- Administer with caution to clients taking vincristine, rifampin, pentamidine, ethambutol, or metronidazole; the action of both drugs may be affected by concurrent administration. Intravenous pentamidine and trimethoprim-sulfamethoxazole taken concurrently may increase the risk of acute and fatal pancreatitis.

- Didanosine interferes with the absorption of ketoconazole and dapsone. Doses of these drugs should be scheduled at least two hours apart from didanosine doses.

- Evaluate for therapeutic response and possible adverse effects. Notify the physician if manifestations of peripheral neuropathy, diarrhea, depression, or other adverse effects develop.

- Stop the drug and notify the physician immediately if the client develops manifestations of pancreatitis or hepatic failure, including nausea and vomiting, severe abdominal pain, elevated bilirubin, or elevated serum enzymes (e.g., amylase, AST, ALT).

Client and Family Teaching

- Take the drug as directed. The prescribed two-tablet dose must always be taken to get the required amount of antacid to prevent the drug from being destroyed by stomach acid.

- Take on an empty stomach, at least one hour before or two hours after meals.

- Do not use alcohol while taking didanosine; alcohol may increase the risk of pancreatitis.

- Stop the drug and call the doctor immediately if nausea, vomiting, abdominal pain, or diarrhea develops. These may indicate pancreatitis.

- Call the doctor if extremity pain, weakness, numbness, or tingling occurs. These side effects usually disappear when didanosine is discontinued.

- Other side effects to report to the physician include unusual bleeding or bruising, fatigue, weakness, fever, or persistent sore throat.

Table 42-1. Continued

Zalcitabine (DDC, HIVID)

Another inhibitor of retroviral replication, zalcitabine is generally used in combination therapy regimens with zidovudine. It may also be used alone in clients who have become resistant to zidovudine. Unlike zidovudine and didanosine, zalcitabine is not toxic to the bone marrow, is inexpensive, and easy to administer (Tierney, et al., 2001). It is, however, associated with severe peripheral neuropathy and an increased risk of pancreatitis. Other adverse effects include stomatitis, rash, fever, and arthritis.

Nursing Responsibilities

- Assess for possible contraindications to zalcitabine: history of pancreatitis or evidence of impaired hepatic function.
- Check with the physician prior to administering the drug concurrently with vincristine, rifampin, intravenous pentamidine, ethambutol, pyrimethamine, dapsone, acyclovir, or metronidazole.
- Administer as prescribed, generally every eight hours.
- Evaluate for desired effect of increased CD4 counts and lower blood levels of p24 antigen.
- Notify the physician if the client develops evidence of pancreatitis, impaired hepatic function, or painful peripheral neuropathy.

Client and Family Teaching

- Take the medication on an empty stomach, one hour before or two hours after meals.
- Check with the physican before taking any other prescription or over-the-counter medication.
- Do not consume alcohol while taking this medication; alcohol increases the risk of pancreatitis.
- Notify the physician immediately if symptoms of peripheral neuropathy (see above section on didanosine) or pancreatitis develops.
- Report to the physician signs of infection or changes in condition.

Nucleoside Reverse Transcriptase Inhibitors

The NRTIs (also called nucleoside analogs) inhibit the action of viral reverse transcriptase, a retroviral enzyme that catalyzes the substrates for conversion and copying of viral RNA to DNA sequences. This enzyme is necessary for viral integration into cellular DNA and replication. The nucleoside analogs act as a chemical decoy for building blocks of the formation of the DNA copy, preventing the RNA from being copied into DNA. Each drug substitutes for a particular nucleoside base at different points on the chain.

- Zidovudine (Retrovir, AZT) was the first antiretroviral agent approved for use with HIV infection. It remains in widespread use and has been shown to decrease symptoms and prolong the lives of clients with AIDS. Zidovudine is often given to clients with a CD4 cell count of less than 500 because of evidence that it slows the progression to severe disease (Tierney, et al., 2001). Zidovudine may also be used prophylactically following a documented parenteral exposure to HIV. AZT is used in combination with ddI, ddC, or 3TC.

- Didanosine (ddI, Videx) also inhibits reverse transcriptase and viral replication. It is used in combination therapy with AZT.
- Zalcitabine (ddC, Hivid) is also a retroviral inhibitor that interferes with the reproduction of HIV. It provides a valuable combination agent with AZT.
- Stavudine (d4T, Zerit) is a retroviral inhibitor that has been shown to increase CD4 cell counts and decrease serum p24 antigen levels. Current use is for clients who are intolerant of AZT.
- Lamivudine (3-TC, Epivir) is used for low CD4 cell counts or symptomatic disease as a first-line treatment in combination with AZT.
- Abacavir (Ziagen) is a potent inhibitor of reverse transcriptase; however, it may cause serious hypersensitivity reactions.
- Zidovudine plus lamivudine (Combivir) is the first combination drug and currently decreases HIV zidovudine-resistant strains.

Protease Inhibitors

Protease is a viral enzyme necessary for the formation of specific viral protein needs for viral assembly and maturation. Protease inhibitors bond chemically with protease to block the function of the enzyme and result in the production of immature, noninfectious viral particles. When combined with other antiviral drugs, these chemicals increase the chance of eliminating the virus by interfering with different stages of its life cycle. However, viral resistance occurs rather quickly.

- Saquinavir (Invirase) is used in combination with nucleoside analogs to treat progression of the disease.
- Ritonavir (Norvir) is used in combination with nucleoside analogs to treat progression of the disease.
- Indinavir (Crixivan) is used in combination with nucleoside analogs to treat progression of the disease.
- Nelfinavir (Viracept) is used in cases of failure of or intolerance to other protease inhibitors.
- Amprenavir (Agenerase) is the newest protease inhibitor.
- Lopinavir/Ritonavir (Kaletra) is the first combination of protease inhibitors active against some HIV strains resistant to other protease inhibitors.

Nonnucleoside Reverse Transcriptase Inhibitors

Nevirapine (Viramune), Delavirdine (Rescriptor), and Efavirenz (Sustiva) are NNRTIs that may be used in combination with nucleoside analogs and protease inhibitors. However, one limitation to NNRTIs is the high incidence of cross-resistance to NRTIs. Some studies have shown that Nevirapine and Efavirenz may significantly reduce serum levels of the protease inhibitors. Optimal combinations of these agents have not been established.

Other agents may also be administered in combination with antiretroviral therapy. Interferons, which are naturally occurring lymphokines, have been used alone and in combination. Alpha-interferon may be used to treat KS and in combination with zidovudine to slow disease progression. Gamma-interferon is also used.

A number of pharmacologic agents are used to prevent and treat opportunistic infections and malignancies in the client with HIV. These agents are outlined in Table 42-2.

Many clients at some point require an implanted venous access device, such as a Groshong catheter, to facilitate blood sampling, intravenous medication administration, transfusions, and parenteral nutrition.

It is recommended that all HIV-infected clients receive pneumococcal, influenza, hepatitis B, and *Haemophilus influenzae b* vaccines. Persons with a positive PPD and negative chest X-ray are given prophylactic isoniazid (INH). When the client's CD4 cell count falls to less than 200, prophylactic treatment for PCP is begun, usually with trimethoprimsulfamethoxazole. Clients with a CD4 count of less than 100 are started on prophylactic treatment for MAC.

Table 42-2. Pharmacologic Treatment of Common Opportunistic Infections and Malignancies in HIV Disease

Condition	Treatment	Potential Adverse Effects
Infections		
Pneumocystis carinii pneumonia	Trimethoprim/ sulfamethoxazole	Rash, neutropenia, anemia, thrombocytopenia, Stevens-Johnson syndrome
	Pentamidine	Hypotension, altered blood glucose levels, hypocalcemia, anemia and leukopenia, liver and renal toxicity, pancreatitis
Tuberculosis	Combination drug therapy using isoniazid, rifampin, ethambutol, pyrazinamide, or streptomycin	Multiple
Candidiasis Oral thrush	Clotrimazole troches Nystatin suspension	Few toxic responses noted for either medication
Esophagitis or recurrent vaginitis	Ketoconazole Fluconazole	Hepatitis, adrenal insufficiency Hepatitis
	Amphotericin B	Bone marrow toxicity, acute renal or hepatic failure; nausea, vomiting; chills, fever, headache
Mycobacterium avium complex	Combination therapy using • Clarithromycin, plus • Clofazimine • Ethambutol • Rifampin • Ciprofloxacin • Amikacin	• Hepatitis, nausea, diarrhea • Diarrhea, nausea, vomiting; skin discoloration, pruritus, rash • Thrombocytopenia, hepatitis, optic neuritis • Bone marrow depression, renal failure, hepatitis • Nausea, rash • Bone marrow depression, renal failure, ototoxicity, hepatitis

Continued on the next page

Table 42-2. Continued

Cytomegalovirus	Ganciclovir	Bone marrow depression, fever
	Foscarnet	Renal failure, electrolyte imbalances, seizures
Herpes simplex or herpes zoster	Acyclovir	Nausea, vomiting, diarrhea; CNS effects; renal failure
Toxoplasmosis	Pyrimethamine, plus	Bone marrow depression, rash; respiratory failure; nausea, vomiting, abdominal pain; hematuria
	Sulfadiazine or clindamycin and folinic acid	Bone marrow depression, rash; respiratory failure; nausea, vomiting, abdominal pain; hematuria

Malignancies

Kaposi's sarcoma	Intralesional vinblastine	Inflammation and pain at injection site
Lymphoma	Combination chemotherapy	Nausea, vomiting; bone marrow toxicity; alopecia

Nursing Care

The client with HIV and AIDS has many care needs, including both physical and psychosocial support. Because there is as yet no cure or effective treatment for HIV disease, many of these needs fall within the realm of nursing to promote knowledge and understanding, self-care, comfort, and quality of life. As with many diseases that have an ultimately fatal outcome, the course of HIV infection may well be affected by the client's social support systems, control, perceived self-efficacy in management, and coping mechanisms.

As the epidemic spreads, nurses are providing care for increasing numbers of clients with HIV infection. These clients are not only in special care settings, but also on general units, maternal-child units, hospice, and home settings. As clients with HIV disease live longer, nurses will increasingly encounter clients in whom HIV disease is a secondary diagnosis, with another primary diagnosis, for example, heart disease, diabetes mellitus, or an operative procedure.

Prevention

To date, no safe immunization to protect against HIV infection has been developed. Education, counseling, and behavior modification are the primary tools for AIDS prevention. The benefit of education and behavior modification is evident in the homosexual male population. The incidence of new HIV infections in this population has declined dramatically in high-prevalence cities such as San Francisco. Nurses play a vital role in providing education about this epidemic and infection prevention for individuals and communities.

All sexually active individuals need to know how HIV is spread. Following are the only *totally* safe sex practices:

- No sex.
- Long-term mutually monogamous sexual relations between two uninfected people.
- Mutual masturbation without direct contact.

Clients who do engage in sexual activity need to know and practice safer sex. Reducing the number of sexual partners—for example, by entering into and remaining in a long-term mutually monogamous relationship with an uninfected partner—reduces the risk. Clients should not engage in unprotected sex, especially if the HIV status of the partner is unknown. Latex condoms have been shown to reduce the risk of transmitting HIV. Their effectiveness is improved when nonoxynol-9, a spermicide, is used for lubrication; however, it may cause genital ulcers which can facilitate HIV transmission. To be effective, condoms must be used with every sexual encounter involving vaginal, oral, or anal intercourse. They also need to be applied and removed properly. A female condom is also available for use.

The most difficult group of high-risk people to reach and educate has been injection drug users. People in this group should never share needles, syringes, or other drug paraphernalia. Many cities have initiated needle-exchange programs, providing a sterile needle and syringe in exchange for a used one. A fresh solution of household bleach and water in a 1:10 ratio is effective to clean "works" when sterile supplies are not available. It is important to also teach people in this population about safer sex practices, because most heterosexual HIV transmission occurs between injection drug users and their partners.

Screening of voluntary blood donors and donated blood supplies has reduced the risk of transmission by transfusion to 1 in 100,000. Because current blood-screening methods use antibody testing, receiving donated blood continues to carry a small risk. Clients in the *window period* between contraction of the virus and the development of detectable antibodies are able to transmit the virus to others, even though they do not yet test positive for HIV. This window period usually lasts from six weeks to six months; rarely, it lasts up to one year. When possible, encourage clients to use autologous transfusion, donating their own blood prior to an anticipated surgery. Seeking donations from family members is not encouraged for several reasons. Family members may have engaged in high-risk behaviors, but lie about their risk because of embarrassment or fear of discovery. Furthermore, the family member may have a different blood type or have other contraindications to donating.

Encourage HIV-positive clients to abstain from donating blood, organs, or sperm. They should understand tactics to avoid exchange of body fluids by not sharing needles or other drug paraphernalia, not sharing razors, and not obtaining a tattoo. Stress the importance of informing all medical personnel providing direct care (especially anyone performing a dental, surgical, or obstetric procedure) about the diagnosis.

Health care workers can prevent most exposures to HIV by using standard precautions. Testing to determine HIV status remains voluntary and relies on the use of antibody-screening methods. It is therefore impossible to identify every client who is HIV positive. With standard precautions, all clients are treated alike, eliminating the need to know the client's HIV status. All high-risk body fluids are treated as if they are infectious, and barrier precautions are used to prevent skin, mucous membrane, or percutaneous exposure to them. Counseling and testing are provided to health care workers with a documented needle-stick exposure. Some clinicians and facilities recommend prophylactic AZT therapy after needle-stick or splash exposure; however, it must be initiated immediately, and its effectiveness has yet to be established.

Assessment

Collect the following data through health history and physical examination. Further focused assessments are described with nursing interventions below.

- *Health history:* risk factors (transfusion, unprotected sex, needle exposure), infections (sexually transmitted diseases, hepatitis, TB), medications, recreational drug use, foreign travel, pets.
- *Physical assessment:* height, weight, nutrition, skin and mucous membranes, vision, lymph nodes, breath sounds, abdominal tenderness, motor strength, coordination, cranial nerves, gait, deep tendon reflexes, genitourinary examination, mental status.

Nursing Diagnoses and Interventions

Nursing care needs for the client with HIV infection change over the course of the disease. Preventive health care measures, health maintenance activities, education, and support of coping mechanisms are important in the early stages of the disease. Counseling the client with a new diagnosis of HIV infection is vital. HIV infection and AIDS continue to carry a social stigma that may interfere with the client's usual support systems and coping mechanisms. As the disease progresses and the client experiences more physical symptoms, direct care needs become more important while the need for psychosocial support continues. Acute exacerbation of opportunistic infections may necessitate hospitalization, but typically the client is managed at home.

Ineffective Coping

On receiving the test results indicating HIV seropositive status, the person with HIV infection is faced with multiple issues rarely affecting other clients. First and foremost, HIV is a disease for which there is no known cure and which is, at this time, thought to be almost universally fatal. Social support systems, family relationships, and the ability to obtain and retain useful work and health insurance may be disrupted by the disease. The client may experience guilt about his or her lifestyle and how the disease was contracted. As the disease progresses, social isolation, fatigue, body image changes, medication side effects, and multiple other issues affect the client's abilities to cope.

- Assess social support network and usual methods of coping. *This will help both the nurse and the client identify people and mechanisms that can help the client cope more effectively with the disease.*
- If possible, assign a primary nurse, whether the setting is home health, hospice, or acute care. *This helps promote the development of a therapeutic and trusting relationship and provides for continuity of care.*
- Plan for consistent, uninterrupted time with the client. *Time and a consistent presence encourage the client to express feelings and work through issues related to HIV infection.*
- Interact at every opportunity outside of providing specific nursing care treatments. *This purposeful interaction communicates caring and acceptance without fear of HIV disease.*
- Support the client's social network. *Nontraditional families may offer more support than the traditional family. This in turn may necessitate a liberal interpretation of the term family if unit policy is* immediate family only.

- Promote interaction between the client, significant others, and family. *Hospitalization and manifestations of HIV disease may bring about isolation from others and decrease the client's ability to cope.*

- Encourage involvement in making care decisions. *This gives the client a greater sense of self-worth and control over the situation, increasing coping abilities.*

- Set and maintain limits on manipulative and other destructive behaviors. *The client who is unable to limit inappropriate behaviors needs the external control established by setting limits.*

- Assist to accept responsibility for actions without blaming others. *Effective coping cannot occur without accepting responsibility for one's actions.*

- Support positive coping behaviors, decisions, actions, and achievements. *As self-esteem is enhanced, coping improves.*

Impaired Skin Integrity

Dryness, malnutrition, immobility from fatigue, and skin lesions on pressure sites contribute to impaired integrity of the skin for the client with HIV disease. Maintaining skin integrity is important because of the progressive and debilitating nature of the disease. It is also a consideration both as the first line of defense against infection in an immunosuppressed client and as a site for secondary manifestations, such as KS and herpes.

- Monitor the skin frequently for lesions and areas of breakdown. *Early identification of impaired skin integrity allows prompt intervention.*

- Monitor lesions for signs of infection or impaired healing. *Infection or poor tissue perfusion not only impairs healing but may lead to further skin breakdown.*

- Turn at least every two hours, more frequently if necessary. *Turning decreases unrelieved pressure on bony prominences and improves circulation to the tissues.*

- Use pressure-relieving devices, such as pressure and egg crate mattresses, or sheep skin pads for elbows and heels. *These devices provide prophylactic relief of pressure.*

- Keep skin clean and dry using mild, nondrying soaps or oils for cleansing. *Night sweats and diarrhea, if present, can cause breakdown and damage to the skin. Frequent cleansing with nondrying products discourages bacterial growth, thus reducing the risk of infection.*

- Massage around but not over affected pressure sites to increase circulation to the surrounding tissue. *Massaging over the affected area can cause skin breakdown.*

- If blisters are noted, leave intact, and dress with a hydrocolloid (Duoderm) dressing. *Blisters provide natural sterile coverings for damaged tissue, improving healing and preventing bacterial invasion.*

- Caution against scratching. If confused, trim fingernails and use mitts or soft restraints to prevent scratching. Check for circulation of hands and fingers frequently if mitts or restraints are used. *Scratching and skin damage allow bacteria to be introduced into lesions, increasing the risk of infection. Tight or restrictive restraints or mitts may compromise circulation.*

- Avoid the use of heat or occlusive dressings. *Heat can further dry and damage the skin; occlusive dressings may impair circulation and lead to ulceration.*

- Prevent skin shearing by using a turnsheet and adequate personnel when repositioning. *Shearing causes tissue trauma that can lead to decubitus ulcers.*

- Encourage ambulation if possible; if the client is confined to bed, encourage active or passive range-of-motion exercises. *Activity increases circulation, decreases pressure and skin breakdown, and helps maintain muscle tone.*
- Monitor nutritional intake and albumin levels. *Maintenance of optimal nutrition decreases the risk of tissue breakdown and improves resistance to infection.*

Imbalanced Nutrition: Less Than Body Requirements

Many factors associated with HIV disease, including manifestations of the disease itself, put the client at risk for altered nutrition and weight loss. Nausea and anorexia may be manifestations of the disease or the result of antiretroviral therapy. Chronic diarrhea is a common manifestation of constitutional HIV disease. Wasting syndrome is also common. It is manifested by involuntary weight loss of greater than 10% to 15% of baseline weight, severe diarrhea, fever, and chronic fatigue and weakness. The exact cause of wasting syndrome is unclear, but the diarrhea and fatigue contribute, as does the increased metabolic rate associated with fever. Oral and esophageal candidiasis and KS of the gastrointestinal tract may cause painful swallowing, making eating difficult and thereby contributing to anorexia. Poor nutritional status in the client with HIV can ultimately result in altered comfort, a change in body image, muscle wasting, increased risk of infection, and higher mortality and morbidity.

- Assess nutritional status, including weight; body mass; caloric intake; and laboratory studies, such as total protein and albumin levels, hemoglobin, and hematocrit. *These factors provide a baseline to determine the effectiveness of interventions.*
- Identify possible causes of altered nutrition. *Identification of causes provides direction for planned interventions.*
- Administer prescribed medications for candidiasis and other manifestations as ordered. *Eliminating this opportunistic infection improves comfort and facilitates food intake. Topical viscous anesthetic can help reduce pain and improve oral intake.*
- Administer antidiarrheal medications after stools and antiemetics prior to meals. Provide antipyretics as needed to control fever. *Reducing diarrhea will improve nutrient absorption; preprandial medication with an antiemetic reduces nausea and improves food intake. Reduction of fever lowers the body's metabolic demands.*
- Provide a diet high in protein and kilocalories. *A high-protein, high-kilocalorie diet provides the necessary nutrients to meet metabolic and tissue healing needs.*
- Offer soft foods and serve small portions. *Soft foods are easily digested. Small portions are more appealing to the anorectic or nauseated client.*
- Involve in meal planning and encourage significant others to bring favorite foods from home. *The client is more likely to consume adequate amounts of preferred foods. Allowing food choices enhances the client's sense of control.*
- Assist with eating as needed. *Fatigue and weakness can prevent the client from eating an adequate amount of food.*
- Provide supplementary vitamins and enteral feedings, such as Ensure. *This improves nutritional status and caloric intake.*
- Provide or assist with frequent oral hygiene. *Oral hygiene improves comfort and appetite, and reduces the risk of mucosal lesions.*
- Administer appetite stimulants, such as megestrol (Megace) and dronabinol (Marinol) as ordered. *Both drugs may increase appetite and promote weight gain.*

Ineffective Sexuality Patterns

The diagnosis of HIV infection can significantly alter the client's expressions of sexuality. Guilt over the diagnosis may interfere with libido. The client may be angry with a partner if that person was the probable source of infection. The client may fear spreading the disease to others via sexual relations. As the disease progresses, its manifestations can affect body image and self-esteem, impairing sexuality. Other symptoms, such as nausea, fatigue, and weakness, may also interfere with libido and sexual satisfaction.

- Examine your feelings about sexuality, your role in dealing with a client's sexuality, the client's lifestyle, and sexual preferences. *To deal effectively with the client's concerns, it is vital that the nurse be comfortable with his or her own feelings of sexuality and be able to accept the client's lifestyle. Referring the client to another nurse or counselor may be necessary.*

- Establish a trusting, therapeutic relationship through the use of time, active listening, caring, and self-disclosure. Maintain a nonthreatening, nonjudgmental attitude toward the client. *Sexuality is a private issue that will be uncomfortable or impossible for the nurse and client to discuss without a mutually trusting relationship.*

- Provide factual information about HIV infection and its effects. *This helps the client separate fears and myths from reality.*

- Discuss safer sex practices, including hugging, cuddling, nonsexual contact, the use of latex condoms and spermicidal lubricant, and mutual masturbation. *Alternative forms of sexual activity and expressing affection can allow the client and significant other to remain close throughout the course of the disease.*

- Encourage discussion of fears and concerns with significant other. *Open communication helps them to deal with issues related to sexuality.*

- For the client without a significant other, stress the need to continue to meet people and develop social relationships while practicing safer sex. *The risk of isolation is high in the client with HIV infection, and relationships with others help the client to cope with the disease.*

- Refer the client and significant other to local support groups for people and partners of people with HIV. *Support groups provide a social and support network of people facing the same issues.*

Home Care

Teaching needs for both the client and significant other are extensive. The primary need is information about the disease, its spread, and its expected course. The client and family need current factual information to plan realistically and to combat myths, misperceptions, and prejudices. At the same time, it is important to include information about current research and progress in treating the disease to maintain a sense of hopefulness.

The following topics should be discussed with the client and family to prepare for home care:

- Guidelines for safer sex practices
- Nutrition, rest and exercise, stress reduction, lifestyle changes, and maintaining a positive outlook
- Infection prevention and transmission, including handwashing and wearing gloves when handling client's secretions or excretions
- Importance of regular medical follow-up and monitoring of immune status

- Signs and symptoms of opportunistic infections and malignancies, as well as other symptoms that should be reported
- Medications and adverse effects
- Use and care of implanted venous access devices, total parenteral nutrition, intravenous pumps and continuous medication delivery systems, and intravenous or aerosolized medications
- Cessation of smoking, alcohol, and recreational or illicit drug use
- Home health services
- Hospice and respite care services
- Community resources, such as support groups, social agencies, and counselors
- Helpful resources:
    1. CDC National AIDS Hotline
    2. Gay Men's Health Crisis Network
    3. National Association of People with AIDS
    4. National Organization for HIV over Fifty.

43

Nursing Care of Clients Experiencing Loss, Grief, and Death

Loss may be defined as an actual or potential situation in which a valued object, person, body part, or emotion that was formerly present is lost or changed and can no longer be seen, felt, heard, known, or experienced. A loss may be temporary or permanent, complete or partial, objectively verifiable or perceived, physical or symbolic. Only the person who experiences the loss can determine the meaning of the loss.

Loss always results in change. The stress associated with the loss may be the precipitating factor leading to physiologic or psychologic change in the person or family. The effective or ineffective resolution of feelings surrounding the loss determines the person's ability to deal with the resulting changes.

Grief is the emotional response to loss and its accompanying changes. Grief as a response to loss is an inevitable dimension of the human experience. The loss of a job, a role (e.g., the loss of the role of spouse, as occurs in divorce), a goal, body integrity, a loved one, or the impending loss of one's own life may trigger grief. Loss is also integral to death. Although death is the ultimate loss, losses that occur in any phase of the life cycle may produce grief responses as intensely painful as those observed in the death experience.

Grieving may be thought of as the internal process the person uses to work through the response to loss. *Bereavement,* a form of depression accompanied by anxiety, is a common reaction to the loss of a loved one. *Mourning* describes the actions or expressions of the bereaved, including the symbols, clothing, and ceremonies that make up the outward manifestations of grief. Both grieving and mourning are healthy responses to loss because they ultimately lead the person to invest energy in new relationships and to develop positive self-regard.

Death is defined in many ways. One commonly used definition of death is an irreversible cessation of circulatory and respiratory functions or irreversible cessation of all functions of the entire brain, including the brainstem. With the current life-support systems available, the most often used criterion for determining death is whole-brain death (permanent irreversible cessation of the functioning of all areas of the brain).

Although death is an inevitable part of life, it is often an immensely difficult loss for the person who is dying and for his or her loved ones. Death may be accidental, such as from trauma, or the end of a long and painful struggle with a terminal illness, such as cancer or AIDS. It may also be purposeful, if a person commits suicide.

Theories of Loss, Grief, and Dying

Medical-surgical nurses often care for clients exhibiting responses typical of various stages of the grieving process. Highly individual in quality and duration, the grief process may range from discomforting to debilitating, and it may last a day or a lifetime, depending on what the loss means to the person experiencing it. Although each person experiences loss in a different manner, knowledge of some of the major theories of loss, grief, and dying can give the nurse a framework for holistic care of the client and family anticipating or experiencing a loss. Table 43–1 summarizes these theories.

Freud: Psychoanalytic Theory

Freud (1917, 1957) wrote about grief and mourning as reactions to loss. Freud described the process of mourning as one in which the person gradually withdraws attachment from the lost object or person. He observed that with normal grieving, this withdrawal of attachment is followed by a readiness to make new attachments. In comparing melancholia (prolonged gloominess, depression) with the "normal" emotions of grief, and its expression in mourning, Freud observed that the "work of mourning" is a nonpathologic condition that reaches a state of completion after a period of inner labor.

Table 43-1. Summary of Theories of Loss

Theorist	Dynamics
Freud	Grief and mourning are reactions to loss. Grieving is the inner labor of mourning a loss. Inability to grieve a loss results in depression.
Bowlby	The successful grieving process initiated by a loss or separation during childhood ends with feelings of emancipation from the lost person or object.
Engel	After the person perceives and evaluates the loss, the person adapts to it. Shock and disbelief, developing awareness, and restitution occur during the first year following the loss; in the months following, the person puts the lost relationship into perspective.
Lindemann	A sequence of responses is experienced following a catastrophic event; defined concepts of anticipatory grieving and morbid grief reactions.
Caplan	Periods of psychologic crisis are precipitated by hazardous circumstances; successful resolution of grief involves feelings of hope and engaging in activities of ordinary living.
Kübler-Ross	There are five stages defining the response to loss: denial, anger, bargaining, depression, and acceptance. Stages are not necessarily sequential.
Carter	Identified the quality of grief's changing character, the need to hold on to that which was good in the loved one's lost existence, expectations of how to react to the experience, and the ways in which personal history affects the quality and meaning of the loss.

Bowlby: Protest, Despair, and Detachment

Bowlby (1973, 1980) believed that the grieving process initiated by a loss or separation from a loved object or person successfully ends when the grieving person experiences feelings of emancipation from the lost object or person. He divided the grieving process into three phases and identified behaviors characteristic of each phase.

- *Protest.* The protest phase is marked by a lack of acceptance of the loss. All energy is directed toward protesting the loss. The person experiences feelings of anger toward self and others, and feelings of ambivalence toward the lost object or person. Crying and angry behaviors characterize this phase.

- *Despair.* The person's behavior becomes disorganized. Despair mounts as efforts to deny the loss compete with acceptance of permanent loss. Crying and sadness, coupled with a desire for the lost object or person to return, result in disorganized thoughts as the client recognizes the reality of the loss.

- *Detachment.* As the person realizes the permanence of the loss and gradually relinquishes attachment to the lost object, a reinvestment of energy occurs. Both the positive and negative aspects of the relationship are remembered. Expressions of hopefulness and readiness to move forward are characteristic of this phase.

Engel: Acute Grief, Restitution, and Long-Term Grief

Engel (1964) related the grief process to other methods of coping with stress: After the person perceives and evaluates the loss (the stressful event), the person adapts to it. Engel's recognition of the impact of cognitive factors on the grieving process was an important contribution to our understanding of grieving.

Engel described three main stages in the grief process: an acute stage, a restitution stage, and a long-term stage. The acute stage occurs in two phases. The first phase, shock and disbelief, begins immediately after the person receives the news of the loss. The initial response may be denial, which may help the person to cope with the overwhelming pain. Alternatively, the grieving person in this phase may appear to accept the loss, making statements such as, "It was for the best," while repressing his or her feelings. This phase of shock and disbelief normally lasts only a few hours; however, it may continue for one or two days.

As the shock and disbelief begin to fade, the second phase, developing awareness, follows. The finality of the loss becomes a reality, and pain, anguish, anger, guilt, and blame surface. The person feels a need to make someone responsible for the loss. "If only" and "why" frequently punctuate the expressed or inner dialogue of the bereaved. Crying is common. "It is during this time that the greatest degree of anguish or despair, within the limits imposed by cultural patterns, is experienced or expressed" (Engel, 1964, p. 93). Culturally patterned behaviors, such as maintaining a stoic pose in public or weeping openly, characterize this phase.

The acute stage is followed by a stage of restitution, in which the mourning is institutionalized. Friends and family gather to support the grieving person through rituals dictated by the culture. As time passes, the mourner continues to feel a painful void and is preoccupied with thoughts of the loss. The mourner may join a support group or seek other social support for coping with the loss.

After the restitution stage, which lasts at least a year, the mourner begins to come to terms with the loss. In this long-term stage, interest in people and activities is renewed. The person puts the lost relationship in perspective as he or she begins to form new relationships. Engel observed that this period might last another one to two years.

Lindemann: Categories of Symptoms

Lindemann (1944) interviewed people who had lost a loved one during the course of medical treatment, disaster victims, and relatives of members of the armed forces who had died. Lindemann's research led him to describe normal grief, anticipatory grieving, and morbid grief reactions. He described symptoms characteristic of normal grief into categories of somatic (physical symptoms without an organic cause) distress, preoccupation with the image of the deceased, feelings of guilt, hostile reactions, and loss of patterns of conduct

Anticipatory grieving was defined as a cluster of predictable responses to an anticipated loss. These responses include the range of feelings experienced by the person or family preoccupied with an anticipated loss. The term *morbid grief reaction* described delayed and dysfunctional reactions to loss; a variety of debilitating health problems were seen in people who displayed excessive or delayed responses to loss.

Caplan: Stress and Loss

Caplan's (1990) theory of stress and its relationship to loss is useful in understanding the grief process. He expanded the focus of the grief process to include not only bereavement but also other episodes of stress that people experience, such as may result from surgery or childbirth. Caplan described these periods as "psychological crises precipitated by hazardous circumstances that lead to a temporary upset in the normal homeostatic balance of forces that characterizes transactions between an individual and his environment" (p. 28). He believed these "hazardous circumstances" lead to psychologic disequilibrium in some people because their coping skills are inadequate in helping them gain mastery over their predicament.

Caplan described three factors that influence the person's ability to deal with a loss. He believed these factors might cause distress for a year or more following the loss.

- The psychic pain of the broken bond and the agony of coming to terms with the loss.
- Living without the assets and guidance of the lost person or resource.
- The reduced cognitive and problem-solving effectiveness associated with the distressing emotional arousal.

Caplan described the process of building new attachments to replace those that have been lost. This process involves two elements: a feeling of hope and the assumption of regular activity as a form of participating in ordinary living.

Kübler-Ross: Stages of Coping with Loss

Kübler-Ross's (1969, 1978) research on death and dying provided a framework for gaining insight about the stages of coping with an impending or actual loss. According to Kübler-Ross, not all people dealing with a loss go through these stages, and those who do may not experience the stages in the sequence described. In identifying the stages of death and dying, Kübler-Ross (1978) repeatedly stressed the danger of prematurely labeling a "stage" and emphasized that her goal was to describe her observations of how people come to terms with situations of loss.

Some or all of the following reactions may occur during the grieving process and may reappear as the person experiences the loss:

- *Denial.* A person may react with shock and disbelief after receiving word of an actual or potential loss. After receiving a terminal diagnosis, notification of a death, or other serious loss, people may make such statements as "This can't be happening to me" or "This can't be true." This initial stage of denial serves as a buffer in helping the person or family mobilize defenses to cope with the situation.

- *Anger.* In the anger stage, the person resists the loss. The anger is often directed toward family and health care providers.

- *Bargaining.* The bargaining stage serves as an attempt to postpone the reality of the loss. The person makes a secret bargain with God, expressing a willingness to do anything to postpone the loss or change the prognosis. This is the individual's plea for an extension of life or the chance to "make everything right" with a dying family member or friend.

- *Depression.* The person enters a stage of depression as the full impact of the actual or perceived loss is realized. The person prepares for the impending loss by working through the struggle of separation. While grieving over "what cannot be," the person may either talk freely about the loss or withdraw from others.

- *Acceptance.* The person begins to come to terms with the loss and resumes activities with an air of hopefulness for the future. Some dying people reach a stage of acceptance in which they may appear to be almost devoid of emotion. The struggle is past, and the emotional pain is gone.

Carter: Themes of Bereavement

Carter (1989) focused on identifying themes of bereavement expressed by grieving persons. She identified themes disclosed by people who had experienced the death of a loved one as:

- Grief's changing character, including "waves" of intense pain that may be triggered years after the death by a photograph of the loved one, a favorite song, a fragrance, or anything that calls the loved one to mind.

- Holding, an individual process of preserving the fact and the meaning of the loved one's existence.

- Expectations, both social and personal, regarding how the bereaved should react to the experience.

- The critical importance of personal history in affecting the quality and meaning of individual bereavement.

Factors Affecting Responses to Loss

A variety of factors affect a person's responses to loss. These include age, social support, families, spirituality, and rituals of mourning.

Age

The understanding of and reaction to loss is influenced by the age of the person experiencing the loss. In general, as people experience life transitions, their ability to understand and accept the losses associated with the transitions increases. From the age of three years, the development of the concept of death as a loss proceeds rapidly.

Social Support

Grieving is painful and lonely. One's social support system is important because of its potentially positive influence on the successful resolution of grief. Some losses may lead to social isolation, placing clients at high risk for dysfunctional grief reactions. For example, survivors of people with AIDS often report feeling excluded by the deceased person's family and by health care providers. Characteristic factors that can interfere with successful grieving include the following:

- Perceived inability to share the loss.
- Lack of social recognition of the loss.
- Ambivalent relationships prior to the loss.
- Traumatic circumstances of the loss.

A move, a divorce, or even the death of a pet can cause a person to feel extremely isolated, yet the person experiencing these types of loss does not ordinarily receive the same social support offered to the person mourning the death of a loved one. A woman having an abortion or giving up a child for adoption seldom receives the same social support as the mother of a child who died at birth. It is therefore especially important that the nurse does not place a value on the client's loss when assessing the need for support.

The painful nature of grief can cause the client to withdraw from a previously established social support system, thereby increasing the feelings of loneliness caused by the loss. A recently widowed woman, for example, may refuse invitations involving married couples with whom she had socialized while her husband was alive. The client's needs for social interaction remain similar to those established before the loss.

Families

A well-functioning family usually rallies after the initial shock and disbelief and provides support for each other during all phases of the grieving process. After a loss, the functional family is able to shift roles, levels of responsibility, and ways of communicating.

The family may have negative as well as positive effects. For example, the dying client may request that someone the family perceives as an outsider be near, and the family may respond with anger to the perceived "intrusion." Similarly, certain family members may express hurt feelings or anger if the client is unresponsive to other family members. Well-meaning family members may also try to shield the client from the pain of grieving. It is rare for the family and the client to experience anger, denial, and acceptance in unison. While one member is in denial, another may be angry because "not enough is being done."

Spirituality

Spirituality is at the core of human existence, integrating and transcending the physical, emotional, intellectual, and social dimensions (Reed, 1996). The principles, values, personal philosophy, and meaning of life by which the client has pursued goals and self-actualization, however, may be called into question when the client responds to an actual or perceived loss. Because of a fear of intruding on the personal spiritual beliefs and practices of the client, the nurse often feels at a loss in implementing interventions that would be helpful to the client responding to a loss.

Rituals of Mourning

Through the participation in religious ceremonies, such as baptism, confirmation, and Bat or Bar Mitzvah, people joyously celebrate progression to a new stage of life and loss of a former way of being. The funeral ceremony serves many of the same purposes in meeting the needs of the bereaved as people gather to share loss. Through the ceremony, people symbolically express triumph over death and deny the fear of death. Culture is the primary factor that dictates the rituals of mourning.

Nurses' Self-Assessment

Nurses care for clients and families at various stages of the grief process and may feel that crisis situations are not the time for self-reflection. However, because the nurse's conscious or unconscious reactions to the client's responses to the loss will influence the outcome of any interventions, nurses need to take time to analyze their own feelings and values related to loss and the expression of grief. The nurse can promote self-awareness by reflecting on the following questions:

* What are my personal feelings about how grief should be expressed?
* Am I making judgments about the meaning of this loss to the client?
* Are unresolved losses in my own life preventing me from relating therapeutically to the client?

End-of-Life Considerations

Nurses care for the dying client in intensive care units, emergency rooms, hospital units, long-term care facilities, and the home. Regardless of the setting, the client's wishes about death should be respected. The Dying Person's Bill of Rights states that each person has "the right to be cared for by caring, sensitive, knowledgeable people who will attempt to understand my needs and will be able to gain some satisfaction in helping me face my death" (Barbus, 1975).

Legal and Ethical Issues

Issues such as those involved in advance directives and living wills, euthanasia, and quality of life are especially important to nurses in upholding the specific care requests of their clients.

Advance Directives and Living Wills

Advance directives are legal documents that allow a person to plan for health care and/or financial affairs in the event of incapacity. A **durable power of attorney for health care** (or health care proxy) is a legal document written by a competent (mentally healthy) adult that gives another competent adult the right to make health care decisions on his or her behalf if he or she cannot. The legal authority is limited to decisions about health care.

A **living will** is a legal document that formally expresses a person's wishes regarding life-sustaining treatment in the event of terminal illness or permanent unconsciousness. It is not a type of durable power of attorney and usually does not designate a substitute decision maker. It is the responsibility of the nurse as client advocate to request and record the client's preference for care and include it in the plan of care. The nurse's documentation helps communicate these preferences to the other members of the health care team.

All facilities that receive Medicare and Medicaid funds are required to provide all clients with written information and counseling about advance directives and the institution's policies governing them. The specific terms of this requirement are found in the Patient Self-Determination Act (PSDA). A copy of the signed advance directive must be kept in the client's medical record, but clients do not have to sign it in order to be treated. Nurses are the ones in close contact with clients, so they are often left with unresolved feelings about the moral, ethical, and legal aspects of their actions. Although advance directives do not ease the pain of seeing clients die, they do help nurses provide clients with the care that the clients have chosen.

Do-Not-Resuscitate Orders

A **do-not-resuscitate (DNR, or "no-code") order** is written by the physician for the client who is near death. This order is usually based on the wishes of the client and family that no cardiopulmonary resuscitation be performed for respiratory or cardiac arrest. A **comfort measures only order** indicates that no further life-sustaining interventions are necessary and that the goal of care is a comfortable, dignified death. Confusing or conflicting DNR orders create dilemmas, because nurses are involved in resuscitation and either begin CPR or ensure that unwanted attempts do not occur. The ANA has made specific recommendations related to a DNR order.

The ANA further recommends that guidelines and policies be developed to help resolve conflicts between clients and their families, between clients and health care professionals, and among health care professionals.

Euthanasia

Euthanasia (from the Greek for painless, easy, gentle, or good death) is now commonly used to signify a killing prompted by some humanitarian motive. There are many arguments for and against euthanasia, and nurses have often found themselves at the center of the debate. As a result, nurses have pushed for the development of appropriate guidelines and procedures for DNR orders. When no such orders exist, the nurse faces a dilemma. Certainly, there are situations in which the nurse's role is clear. For example, it is considered malpractice to participate in "slow codes" (in which the nurse does not hurry to alert the emergency team when a terminally ill client who does not have a DNR order stops breathing).

The natural death laws seek to preserve the notion of voluntary versus involuntary euthanasia. In *voluntary euthanasia,* the competent adult client and a physician, nurse, or adult friend or relative make the decision to terminate life. *Involuntary euthanasia* ("mercy killing") is performed without the client's consent. Because care settings offer many complex and technologic interventions, it is not likely that the ethical aspects of euthanasia will soon be resolved. However, advance directives do give clients a much more active role in decisions about their own care.

Hospice

Hospice is a model of care (rather than a place of care) for clients and their families when faced with a limited life expectancy. Hospice care is initiated for clients as they near the end of life, emphasizing quality rather than quantity of life. Emotional, spiritual, and practical support is provided based on the wishes of the client and the needs of the family. Hospice regards dying as a normal part of life and provides support for a dignified and peaceful death.

The American hospice movement was originally led by volunteers (many of whom were nurses) who wanted to make life better for those who were dying. These devoted volunteers promoted the dignity of patients during their death and decreased their institutionalization. In 1986, Congress passed the Medicare Hospice Benefit and also gave states the option of including hospice services in their Medicaid programs. Since then, patients dying of cancer or any other terminal illness may receive hospice care in the comfort of their homes with their families.

Hospice care usually begins when the patient has six months or less to live and ends with the family one year after the death. Nurses providing hospice care work with an interdisciplinary team of other health professionals, such as social workers, pastoral counselors, home health aides, and volunteers, to provide comprehensive palliative care. The hospice nurse must combine all of the skills of the home care nurse with the ability to provide daily emotional support to dying patients and their families. Hospice nurses are especially skilled in pain and symptom management. Their focus is on improving quality of life and preserving dignity for the patient in death.

End-of-Life Care

End-of-life nursing care that ensures a peaceful death was mandated by the International Council of Nurses' (1997) and further supported by the American Association of Colleges of Nursing (AACN; 1999). The principles of hospice care are basic to end-of-life care: that people live until the moment they die; that care until death may be offered by a variety of health care professionals; and that such care is coordinated, is sensitive to diversity, offered around the clock, and incorporates the physical, psychological, social, and spiritual concerns of the patient and the patient's family. Following are selected competencies necessary for nurses to provide high-quality end-of-life care as defined by the AACN (1999).

- Promote the provision of comfort care to the dying as an active, desirable, and important skill, and an integral component of nursing care.
- Communicate effectively and compassionately with the patient, family, and health care team members about end-of-life issues.
- Recognize one's own attitudes, feelings, values, and expectations about death and the individual, cultural, and spiritual diversity existing in those beliefs and customs.
- Demonstrate respect for the patient's views and wishes during end-of-life care.
- Use scientifically based standardized tools to assess symptoms (e.g., pain, dyspnea, constipation, anxiety, fatigue, nausea/vomiting, and altered cognition) experienced by patients at the end of life.
- Use data from symptom assessment to plan and intervene in symptom management using state-of-the-art traditional and complementary approaches.
- Assist the patient, family, colleagues, and one's self to cope with suffering, grief, loss, and bereavement in end-of-life care.

Physiological Changes in the Dying Client

Death may occur rapidly or slowly. Physiological changes are a part of the dying process.

- *Weakness and fatigue.* Weakness and fatigue cause discomfort, especially in joints, and contribute to an increased risk for pressure ulcers.
- *Anorexia and decreased food intake.* Although anorexia and a decrease in food intake are normal in the dying client, the family often views this as "giving up." Anorexia may be

a protective mechanism; the breakdown of body fats results in ketosis, which leads to a sense of well-being and helps decrease pain. Parenteral or enteral feedings do not improve symptoms or prolong life and may actually cause discomfort. As weakness and difficulty swallowing progress, the gag reflex is decreased and clients are at increased risk for aspiration if oral foods are given.

- *Fluid and electrolyte imbalances.* Decreased oral fluid intake is normal at the end of life and does not cause distress. Parenteral fluids are sometimes given to decrease delirium, but they may cause increased edema, breathlessness, cough, and respiratory secretions. If the client has edema or ascites (a collection of fluid in the abdominal cavity), excess body water is present so dehydration is not a problem.

- *Hypotension and renal failure.* As cardiac output decreases, so does intravascular blood volume. As a result, renal perfusion decreases and the kidneys cease to function. Urinary output is scanty. The client will have tachycardia, hypotension, cool extremities, and cyanosis with skin mottling.

- *Neurologic dysfunction.* Neurologic dysfunction results from any or all of the following: decreased cerebral perfusion, hypoxemia, metabolic acidosis, sepsis, an accumulation of toxins from liver and renal failure, the effects of medications, and disease-related factors. These changes may result in decreased level of consciousness or agitated delirium. Clients with terminal delirium may be confused, restless, or agitated. Moaning, groaning, and grimacing often accompany the agitation and are often misinterpreted as pain. Level of consciousness often decreases to the point where the client cannot be aroused. Although decreased consciousness and agitation are both normal states at the end of life, they are very distressing to the client's family. A client near death often has altered cerebral function, so the nurse must stand near the bedside and speak clearly. Hearing is thought to be the last sense a dying client loses; the nurse should never whisper or engage in conversation with the family as if the client were not there.

- *Respiratory changes.* Respiratory changes are normal at this time. The client may have dyspnea, apnea, or Cheyne-Stokes respirations, and may use accessory muscles to breathe. Fluids accumulated in the lungs and oropharynx may lead to what is sometimes called "the death rattle." Oxygen may not relieve these manifestations.

- *Bowel and/or bladder incontinence.* Loss of sphincter control may lead to incontinence of feces or urine.

- *Pain.* A common problem for clients at the end of life, pain is what people often say they fear the most. It is of utmost importance to keep the client comfortable through general comfort measures and by administering ordered medications for pain and anxiety.

Support for the Client and Family

As the client's condition deteriorates, the nurse's knowledge of the client and family guides the care provided. It may be necessary to provide opportunities for clients to express personal preferences about where they want to die and about funeral and burial arrangements. If the family feels that this is morbid, the nurse explains that it helps clients to keep a sense of control as they approach death.

The client needs the opportunity to say goodbye to others. The nurse encourages and supports the client and family as they terminate relationships as a necessary part of the grief process. The nurse acknowledges that termination is painful and, if the client or family desires, stays with them during this time. Family members are often afraid to be present at the moment of death, yet dying alone is the greatest fear expressed by clients.

Death

Pronouncement of death is legally required by a physician or other health care provider to confirm death. The time of death, with any related data, is documented in the client's chart.

The nurse may also fear being present at the moment of the client's death. In fact, Kübler-Ross (1969) noted that the nurse's fear of death frequently interferes with the ability to provide support for the dying client and family. Thoughts such as, "Please, God, don't let him die on my shift," are common, and they express the nurse's emotional turmoil in dealing with the task. Nurses who have worked through their own feelings about death and dying are more at ease in assisting the dying client toward a peaceful death.

After the death, the family is encouraged to acknowledge the pain of loss. The nurse's presence and support as the bereaved express their sorrow, anger, or guilt can help them resolve their grief. It is important for the bereaved not to suppress the pain of grieving with drugs. By accepting variations in the expression of grief, the nurse supports the family's grief reactions and helps prevent dysfunctional grieving. Dysfunctional grieving is an extended and unsuccessful resolution of grief.

Resolution of grief begins with acceptance of the loss. The nurse can encourage this acceptance by maintaining open, honest dialogue and by providing the family with the opportunity to view, touch, hold, and kiss the person's body (Carpenito, 2000). As family members realize the finality of the death, they are often comforted by the presence of the nurse who cared for the client during the final days.

Postmortem Care

The nurse documents the time of death (required for the death certificate and all official records), notifies the physician, and assists the family (if needed) in choice of a funeral home. If the client dies at home, death must be pronounced before the body is removed. In some states and in some situations, nurses can pronounce death; for specifics, consult state practice acts, laws, and agency policy. All jewelry is removed and given to the family unless they ask that it be left on. The body is kept in place until the family is ready and gives permission. If an autopsy is required or requested, the body must be left undisturbed (e.g., do not remove any tubes) for transportation to the medical examiner.

Documentation of the death is completed by sending a completed death certificate to the funeral home (for a death in the home), or by completing the required paperwork and sending the body to the morgue or funeral home (for a death in the hospital or long-term care setting).

Nurses' Grief

The nurse who has developed a close relationship with the client who has died may experience strong feelings of grief. Sharing grief with the family after the death of a loved one helps both the nurse and family to cope with their feelings about the loss. Taking time to grieve after the death of a client provides a release that can help prevent "blunting" of feelings, a problem often experienced by nurses who care for clients who are terminally ill.

Nurses working with critically or terminally ill clients should be aware that witnessing a client's death and the family's grief may reactivate feelings about some unresolved grief in their own lives. In these cases, nurses may need to reflect on their responses to their own losses. Also, nurses who work with dying clients need support from peers and other professionals to work through the often overwhelming feelings that result from dealing with death, grief, and loss.

Collaborative Care

Interventions for loss and grief may be planned and implemented by any or all members of the health care team. Nurses and social workers provide interventions to help clients or families adapt to a loss. They also make referrals to mental health professionals (grief counselors, social services), support groups, chaplains, or legal or financial assistance agencies. Grieving clients frequently enter the health care system with significant somatic symptoms. In some cases, the symptoms of grief and loss are overlooked until the client reaches a crisis state requiring psychiatric medical intervention. Collaborative care by the physician and the nurse early in the normal grieving process can help the client achieve an early and effective resolution of grief and avoid physical or psychiatric health problems.

Nursing Care

Nurses practicing in all types of settings care for clients who are in various stages of the grieving process. Grief is highly individual. The grief process may range from uncomfortable to debilitating, and it may last for a day or a lifetime, depending on what the loss means to the person experiencing it.

Health Promotion

In planning and implementing nursing care for the client experiencing a loss, the nurse considers the individual responses, which may vary greatly. In an era of short acute care stays for clients, nurses may feel that an elaborate grief assessment is impossible or, at the least, impractical. But research and clinical experience suggest that clients who delay the grieving process after a loss are prone to have health problems that may last a lifetime.

Assessment

Knowledge of the expected physical reactions to loss provides the nurse with a basis for identifying reactions requiring further assessment. To assess the extent of somatic distress, the nurse observes for changes in sensory processes and asks questions about the client's sleeping and eating patterns, activities of daily living, general health status, and pain.

Physical Assessment

Clients may experience one or more predictable somatic symptoms as they become aware of a loss. Gastrointestinal symptoms occur frequently. They may include indigestion, nausea or vomiting, anorexia, weight gain or loss, constipation, or diarrhea. The shock and disbelief that accompany a loss may cause shortness of breath, a choking sensation, hyperventilation, or loss of strength. Some clients also report insomnia, preoccupation with sleep, fatigue, and decreased or increased activity level.

Crying and sadness are observed during normal grief states. Crying may make the client feel exhausted and interfere with carrying out activities of daily living. However, a person who is unable to cry may have difficulty completing the mourning process. If the client does not express feelings of grief, somatic symptoms may increase.

It is imperative that the client's concerns about pain be assessed, especially if the client has cancer or another painful illness. Knowledge of pain theories and pain assessment can help the nurse assess the need for pain medication. During the last stages of dying, the client usually becomes very weak, and sensations and reflexes decrease; these changes call for careful assessment of the client's physical needs.

Reactions to loss are not always obvious. For example, in clients who experience an illness following a serious loss, assessment may reveal somatic complaints related to the grief state as well as the illness. When a person who has been healthy begins to develop patterns of increased illness, the nurse should be aware that this may signal dysfunctional grieving. This is especially common in the loss and grieving associated with a change in body image. In addition to making a physical assessment, assess the client's perception of the alteration in body image. The loss of a body part, weight gain or loss, and scars from surgery or trauma can be difficult for the client to accept. Some clients may grieve hair loss that accompanies chemotherapy used in cancer treatment.

Spiritual Assessment

Because spiritual beliefs and practices greatly influence people's reaction to loss, it is important to explore them with the client when assessing a loss. The spiritually healthy client has inner resources that help work through the grief process. Faith, prayer, trust in God or a superior being, perception of a purpose in life, or belief in immortality are examples of the inner resources that may sustain the client during an actual or perceived loss (Reed, 1996).

Assessing the client's spiritual life and its significance to the client and family helps identify spiritual support systems. Some nurses are uncomfortable with assessing the client's spiritual needs; the following questions may be helpful:

- What are the spiritual aspects of the client's philosophy about life? Death?
- Are the values and beliefs about life and death congruent with those of people who are important to the client?
- Which spiritual resources and rituals have significance for the client?

Belief systems that are incompatible with those of family members can be an additional source of stress for clients dealing with a loss. The anger and resentment often observed among families faced with decisions concerning dying members may be avoided if the nurse assesses the potential impact of differing beliefs.

Clients coping with a loss often perceive that it is a punishment from God for their wrongdoing or for their failure to remain faithful to their religious practices. Therefore, it is important to assess the level of guilt the client or family expresses. Assessing the client's comments regarding feelings of responsibility for the loss helps determine whether these feelings are an expected phase of grieving or indicate dysfunctional grieving.

Clients who had not considered themselves religious before the actual or perceived loss often turn to religion to seek comfort or to cope with feelings of despair, helplessness, hopelessness, or guilt. They may utter anguished statements such as "Why, God?" or "Please help me, God." The nurse continues to assess the client's verbalization of such feelings to determine the best interventions to help the client cope with the loss.

Psychosocial Assessment

When working through the grief process, clients can be overwhelmed by the fears associated with the loss and the changes it will produce. The client responding to an actual or perceived loss commonly expresses anxiety (fear of the unknown). An extreme level of anxiety can threaten the client's well-being. Assessment includes helping clients openly acknowledge their fears. Some clients may fear the feelings they experience while proceeding through the grief process more than the loss itself. The most common fear expressed by clients facing a loss is that of losing self-control.

Focusing on the meaning of the loss to the client is more important than attempting to place the client in a sequence or phase of grief. The degree of caring and sensitivity shown when asking questions about the meaning of the loss influences the amount of information the client will be willing to reveal. Asking such questions as, "Why do you feel this way?" or "What does this loss mean to you?" is less helpful than making a statement such as, "This must be difficult for you." The latter more effectively conveys a genuine interest in hearing how the client feels about the loss.

Awareness of the altered sensorium observed during the stage of shock and disbelief provides parameters for assessment. The nurse may note in the client feelings of numbness, unreality, emotional distance, intense preoccupation with the lost object, helplessness, loneliness, and disorganization. As awareness of the loss begins to develop, preoccupation with the lost person or object may increase, and self-accusation and ambivalence toward the lost person or object may follow.

Nursing Diagnoses and Interventions

A variety of nursing diagnoses may be appropriate for the client experiencing loss and grief, as well as for the client who is nearing death. Nurses practicing medical-surgical nursing will most often provide interventions for anticipatory grieving, chronic sorrow, and death anxiety

Anticipatory Grieving

Anticipatory grieving is a combination of intellectual and emotional responses and behaviors by which people adjust their self-concept in the face of a potential loss. Anticipatory grieving may be a response to one's own future death; to potential loss of body parts or functions; to potential loss of a significant person, animal, or possession; or to potential loss of a social role. Nursing interventions are designed to assist with grief resolution.

- Assess for factors causing or contributing to the grief. Ask about support systems, how many losses have occurred, relationship with the lost person, significance of the body part, and previous experiences with loss and grief. *Grief and mourning occur when a person experiences any type of loss.*

- Use open-ended questions to encourage the person to share concerns and the possible effect on the family. *Grief resolution cannot occur until the client acknowledges the loss.*

- Promote a trusting nurse-client relationship: Allow enough time for communications; speak clearly, simply, and concisely; listen; be honest in responses to questions; do not give unrealistic hope; offer support; and demonstrate respect for the person's age, culture, religion, race, and values. *An effective nurse-client relationship begins with acceptance of the client's feelings, attitudes, and values related to the loss. If the client is ready to talk, listening and being present are the most appropriate interventions.*

- Ask about strengths and weakness in coping with the anticipated loss. *Current responses are influenced by past experiences with loss, illness, and death. Socioeconomic and cultural background, as well as cultural and spiritual beliefs and values, affect a person's ability to adapt to loss.*

- Teach the client and family the stages of grief. *This helps them to be aware of their emotions in each stage and reassures them that their reactions are normal.*

- Provide time for decision making. *In periods of stress, people may need extra time to make informed decisions.*

- Provide information about appropriate resources, including support from family, friends, and support groups, community resources, and legal/financial aides. *Support from others decreases feelings of loneliness and isolation and facilitates grief work.*

Chronic Sorrow

Chronic sorrow is a cyclical, recurring, and potentially progressive pattern of pervasive sadness experienced in response to continual loss, throughout the trajectory of an illness or disability. It is triggered by situations that bring to mind the person's losses, disappointments, or fears. It may be experienced by a client, parent or caregiver, or person with chronic illness or disability.

- Explain the difference between chronic sorrow and chronic grieving. *Grieving is time-limited and ends in adaptation to the loss. Chronic sorrow may vary in intensity, but it persists as long as the person with the disability or chronic sorrow condition lives.*

- Encourage verbalization of feelings about the loss, and about the personal relevance of the changes to hopes for the future. *Expressing feelings is normal and necessary to decrease the emotional pain.*

- Help identify triggers that intensify the sorrow, such as birthdays, anniversaries, and holidays. *When triggers have been identified, role-playing may make the events less painful.*

- Refer to appropriate community support groups. *Participating in support groups with others experiencing grief is helpful in coping with loss.*

- Encourage use of personal, family, significant other, and spiritual support systems *to facilitate coping with loss.*

Death Anxiety

Death anxiety is worry or fear related to death or dying. It may be present in clients who have an acute life-threatening illness, who have a terminal illness, who have experienced the death of a family member or friend, or who have experienced multiple deaths in the same family.

- Explore the client's knowledge of the situation. For example, ask, "What has your doctor told you about your condition?" *This informs you of the client's knowledge base about the condition and about his or her ability to make informed decisions.*

- Ask the client to identify specific fears about death. *This provides data about any unrealistic expectations or misperceptions.*

- Determine the client's perceptions of strengths and weakness in coping with death. *Identifying past strengths can help the client cope with loss, illness, and death.*

- Ask the client to identify needed help. *This determines whether available resources are adequate.*

- Encourage independence and control in decisions about treatment and care. *This promotes self-esteem, decreases feelings of powerlessness, and allows the client to retain dignity in dying.*

- Facilitate access to culturally appropriate spiritual rituals and practices. *This provides spiritual comfort.*

- Explain advance directives and assist with them if necessary. *Advance directives help ensure that the client's wishes for end-of-life care are carried out.*

- Encourage life review and reminiscence. *Life review is self-affirming.*

- Encourage activities, such as listening to music, aromatherapy, massage, or relaxation exercises. *These activities decrease anxiety.*

- Suggest keeping a journal or leaving a written legacy. *A written document provides continuing support to others after death.*

Home Care

In addition to teaching clients and families to carry out the physical skills that are necessary to the client's care, nurses also provide information on identifying signs of deterioration and additional sources of support.

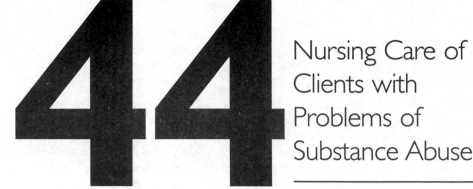

Nursing Care of Clients with Problems of Substance Abuse

Substance abuse refers to the use of any chemical in a fashion inconsistent with medical or culturally defined social norms despite physical, psychological, or social adverse effects. Anxiety and depressive disorders frequently occur with substance abuse and more than 90% of people who commit suicide have a depressive or substance abuse disorder (National Institute of Mental Health [NIMH], 2001).

In a recent report of the surgeon general, 6% of the adult U.S. population are estimated to have an addictive disorder and 3% have both mental and addictive disorders (U.S. Department of Health and Human Services [USDHHS], 1999). Consequently, 9% of the population (15.4 million) have a substance abuse disorder. The costs of addictive disorders are exceedingly high. Direct costs of all mental health services in the United States totaled $69 billion with nearly 20% ($12.6 billion) spent on substance abuse treatment (USDHHS, 1999).

Alcohol is the most commonly used and abused substance in the United States. One of every 10 persons in America is alleged to be alcoholic (American Psychiatric Association [APA], 2000a). Two thirds of the nation's adult population consume alcohol regularly. When used in moderation, alcohol can have positive physiological effects by decreasing coronary artery disease and protecting against stroke; however, when consumed in excess, alcohol can severely diminish one's ability to function and will ultimately lead to life-threatening conditions.

The *Diagnostic and Statistical Manual of Mental Disorders,* fourth edition, text revision (DSM-IV-TR) (APA, 2000b) includes a classification scheme for distinguishing between substance abuse and substance dependence. **Substance dependence** refers to a severe condition occurring when the use of the chemical substance is no longer under an individual's control for at least three months. Continued use of the substance usually persists despite adverse effects on the person's physical condition, psychological health, and interpersonal relationships. The DSM-IV-TR criteria deals with the behavioral aspects and the maladaptive patterns of substance use, emphasizing the physical symptoms of **tolerance** and **withdrawal.** Tolerance is a cumulative state in which a particular dose of the chemical elicits a smaller response than before. With increased tolerance, the individual needs higher and higher doses to obtain the desired effect. When a person is physically addicted to the drug and stops taking it, **withdrawal symptoms** can occur within hours. Withdrawal is an uncomfortable state lasting several days, manifested by tremors, diaphoresis, anxiety, high blood pressure, tachycardia, and possibly convulsions.

Risk Factors

Various risk factors help explain why one person becomes addicted while another does not. Biological, psychological, and sociocultural factors shed light on how a person may abuse or become dependent on a substance.

- *Biological factors* include an apparent hereditary factor, especially with alcohol. Studies have shown that children of alcoholic parents are more likely to develop alcoholism than children of nonalcoholic parents (Kutlenios, 1998). This is primarily true with male relatives. One type of alcoholism seen mostly in the sons of alcoholic fathers is thought to be connected with an early onset, inability to abstain, and an antisocial personality (Stuart & Laraia, 2001). Another type of alcoholism may be more environmentally influenced and is linked with onset after the age of 25, inability to stop after one drink, and a passive-dependent personality (Stuart & Laraia, 2001). More recent studies have demonstrated that alcohol and drug use has specific effects on selected biochemicals in the brain. Alcohol and other CNS depressants, such as benzodiazepines and barbiturates, act on gamma-aminobutyric acid (GABA). This may be why additive and cross-tolerance effects occur when alcohol and other CNS depressants are used in combination (Varcarolis, 2002).

- *Psychological factors* attempt to explain substance abuse through a combination of psychoanalytic, behavioral, and family system theories. Psychoanalytic theorists view substance abuse as a fixation at the oral stage of development, while behavioral theorists see addiction as a learned, maladaptive behavior. Family system theory focuses on the pattern of family relationships throughout several generations. No addictive personality type has been identified; however, several common factors seem to exist among alcoholics and drug users. Many substance abusers have experienced sexual or physical abuse in their childhood and, as a result, have low self-esteem and difficulty expressing emotions. A link also exists between substance abuse and psychiatric disorders, such as depression, anxiety, and antisocial and dependent personalities. The habit of using a substance becomes a form of self-medication to cope with day-to-day problems, and over time develops into an addiction.

- *Sociocultural factors* often influence individuals' decisions as to when, what, and how they use substances. Many Asian people do not drink alcohol because of an uncomfortable physiological response characterized by flushing and tachycardia. About half of the Asian population have a deficiency of aldehyde dehydrogenase, the chemical that breaks down alcohol acetaldehyde (APA, 2000b). A buildup of acetaldehyde causes toxic symptoms and therefore keeps the prevalence rate of alcoholism lower in Asians. Europeans, on the other hand, have higher alcoholism rates. Religious background may also correlate with the likelihood that a person will abuse alcohol. Among major religions, people of Jewish faith have the lowest rate of alcoholism, while Roman Catholics have the highest rate. Many people have a desire for social acceptance and initiate drug use to "fit in" with a peer group. Others may suffer from social anxiety and need drugs or alcohol to feel less inhibited while interacting with others.

Many factors place a person at risk for substance use, abuse, and dependence. No single cause can explain why one individual develops a pattern of drug use and another person does not. Thorough assessment of these factors is necessary to understand the whole person and plan appropriate interventions.

Characteristics of Abusers

As mentioned, no addictive personality type exists; however, many abusers have several characteristics in common. There is a tendency for drug users to indulge in impulsive, risk-taking behaviors. Abusers often have a low tolerance for frustration and pain. The human tendency to seek pleasure and avoid stress and pain is partially responsible for substance abuse. The reinforcing properties of drugs can create a pleasurable experience and reduce the intensity of unpleasant experiences. Often, drug users are rebellious against social norms and engage in antisocial behaviors, such as stealing, promiscuity, driving while intoxicated, and violence against others.

There is also a tendency toward anxiety, anger, and low self-esteem in substance abusers. Although there is no greater prevalence of psychiatric illness in substance abusers than in the general population, dual diagnosis is often present. **Dual diagnosis,** or **dual disorder,** refers to the coexistence of substance abuse or dependence and a psychiatric disorder in one individual. One disorder can be an indication of another, such as the relationship with alcoholism and depression. A depressed person may use self-medication in the form of alcohol to treat the depression, or the alcoholic person may become depressed. One recent study described the prevalence and characteristics of co-occurring serious mental illness (SMI) and substance abuse or dependence (Virgo, et al., 2001). Most dual diagnoses in adult mental health patients were (1) alcohol and/or cannabis abuse with psychoses and heroin and/or (2) alcohol abuse or dependence with depression. Compared with other SMI patients, those who were dually diagnosed were younger, more often male, in less stable accommodation, more likely to be unemployed, and more likely to have more than one psychiatric diagnosis and personality disorder. They also tended to have more crises and pose greater risk to themselves and others (Virgo, et al., 2001).

Addictive Substances and Their Effects

Nicotine

Nicotine enters the system via the lungs (cigarettes and cigars) and oral mucous membranes (smokeless tobacco as well as smoking). In low doses, nicotine stimulates nicotinic receptors in the brain to release norepinephrine and epinephrine, causing vasoconstriction. As a result, the heart rate accelerates and the force of ventricular contractions increases. Gastrointestinal (GI) effects include an increase in gastric acid secretion, tone and motility of GI smooth muscle, and promotion of vomiting. Nicotine acts on the central nervous system (CNS) as a stimulant, increasing respiration and arousal. Nicotine also activates the pleasure system in the mesolimbic system (Lehne, 2001). Moderate doses of nicotine can cause tremors. With high doses, such as acute poisoning from insecticides, convulsions and death can occur.

Tolerance can develop to nausea and dizziness, but not to the cardiovascular effects. Nicotine dependence results from chronic use with withdrawal seen as craving, nervousness, restlessness, irritability, impatience, increased hostility, insomnia, impaired concentration, increased appetite, and weight gain. Gradual reduction in nicotine use seems to prolong suffering. Chronic toxicity from smoking has been well established in the form of vascular diseases; chronic lung disease; and cancers of the larynx, esophagus, oral cavity, lung, bladder, and pancreas (Lehne, 2001). In addition, secondhand effects from smoking have been demonstrated, especially to fetuses during pregnancy. Smoking during pregnancy leads to increased risks for infants, such as low birth weight, spontaneous abortions, perinatal mortality, and sudden infant death.

Table 44-1. Terminology Associated with Substance Abuse

Term	Definition
Abstinence	Voluntarily going without drugs
Addiction	A disease process characterized by the continued use of a specific chemical substance despite physical, psychological, or social harm (used interchangeably with substance dependence)
Codependence	A cluster of maladaptive behaviors exhibited by significant others of a substance abusing individual that serves to enable and protect the abuse at the expense of living a full and satisfying life
Cross dependence	Ability of one drug to support physical dependence on another drug
Cross-tolerance	Tolerance to one drug confers tolerance to another
Delirium tremens	A medical emergency usually occurring three to five days following alcohol withdrawal and lasting two to three days. Characterized by paranoia, disorientation, delusions, visual hallucinations, elevated vital signs, vomiting, diarrhea, and diaphoresis.
Detoxification	The process of helping an addicted individual safely through withdrawal
Dual diagnosis	The coexistence of substance abuse/dependence and a psychiatric disorder in one individual (used interchangeably with dual disorder)
Dual disorder	Concurrent diagnosis of a substance use disorder and a psychiatric disorder. One disorder can precede and cause the other, such as the relationship between alcoholism and depression.
Korsakoff's psychosis	Secondary dementia caused by thiamine (B_1) deficiency that may be associated with chronic alcoholism; characterized by progressive cognitive deterioration, confabulation, peripheral neuropathy, and myopathy
Physical dependence	A state in which withdrawal syndrome will occur if drug use is discontinued
Polysubstance abuse	The simultaneous use of many substances
Psychologic dependence	An intensive subjective need for a particular psychoactive drug
Substance abuse	Continued use of a chemical substance in a fashion inconsistent with medical or social norms, for at least one month, despite related problems
Substance dependence	A severe condition occurring when the use of the chemical substance is no longer under control, for at least three months; continued use persists despite adverse effects (used interchangeably with addiction)
Tolerance	State in which a particular dose elicits a smaller response than it formerly did. With increased tolerance the individual needs higher and higher doses to obtain the desired response.
Wernicke's encephalopathy	Caused by thiamine (B_1) deficiency, characterized by nystagmus, ptosis, ataxia, confusion, coma, and possible death. Thiamine deficiency is common in chronic alcoholism.
Withdrawal syndrome	Constellation of signs and symptoms that occurs in physically dependent individuals when they discontinue drug use

Cannabis

Cannabis sativa is the source of marijuana. Use of cannabis is on the rise in the United States, with 10% of children age 12 to 17 using marijuana (Lehne, 2001). One recent study revealed that lifetime use of marijuana in a sample of 918 adolescents aged 12 to 21 years was 59%, while 18.4% reported frequent weekly use (Siqueira, Diab, Bodian, & Rolnitzky, 2001). Contributing factors to marijuana use in this population were negative life events, anger, and less parental support. The greatest psychoactive substances are in the flowering tops of the cannabis plant. Marijuana (also know as grass, weed, pot, dope, joint, and reefer) and hashish are the most common derivatives. The psychoactive component of marijuana is an oily chemical known as delta-9-tetrahydrocannabinol (THC). THC activates specific cannabinoid receptors in the brain. Recent evidence suggests that marijuana may act like opioids and cocaine in producing a pleasurable sensation, probably by causing release of endogenous opioids and then dopamine (Lehne, 2001).

Physiologic effects of cannabis are dose related and can cause an increase in heart rate and bronchodilation in short-term use, but airway constriction with chronic use leading to bronchitis, sinusitis, asthma, and possibly cancer. The reproductive system is also affected by marijuana; it causes decreased spermatogenesis and testosterone levels in males and decreased levels of follicle-stimulating, luteinizing, and prolactin hormones in females. Birth defects may also be associated with cannabis use. Subjective effects of marijuana include euphoria, sedation, and hallucinations. In addition, chronic use of marijuana can result in amotivational behaviors, such as apathy, dullness, poor grooming, reduced interest in achievement, and disinterest. At extremely high doses, tolerance and physical dependence result.

Alcohol

Alcohol acts as a CNS depressant and enhances the action of gamma aminobutyric acid (GABA). Chronic use of alcohol can cause severe neurologic and psychiatric disorders. Severe damage to the liver occurs with chronic alcohol abuse, and can progress from fatty liver to other liver diseases, such as hepatitis or cirrhosis. Chronic alcoholism is the major cause of fatal cirrhosis. Alcohol causes damaging effects to many other systems; its effects include myocardial disease, erosive gastritis, acute and chronic pancreatitis, sexual dysfunction, and an increased risk of breast cancer.

Malnutrition is another serious complication of chronic alcoholism, especially thiamine (B_1) deficiency that can result in neurological impairments. Thiamine depletion is thought to cause the Wernicke-Korsakoff syndrome observed in chronic alcoholics (Stuart & Laraia, 2001). Severe cognitive impairment is a principal feature of **Wernicke's encephalopathy** and **Korsakoff's psychosis.** Although alcohol is a CNS depressant, it actually disrupts sleep, thus altering the sleep cycle, decreasing the quality of sleep, intensifying obstructive sleep apnea, and reducing total sleeping time. Heavy drinkers have a higher mortality rate and many fatalities occur from alcohol-related accidents. Blood alcohol levels (BALs) are highly predictive of CNS effects. Euphoria, reduced inhibitions, impaired judgment, and increased confidence are seen at 0.05% (Vacarolis, 2002). The legal level of intoxication in most states is 0.10%. Toxic levels in excess of 0.5% can cause coma, respiratory depression, peripheral collapse, and death (Vacarolis, 2002). Chronic consumption of alcohol produces tolerance and creates cross-tolerance to general anesthetics, barbiturates, benzodiazepines, and other CNS depressants. If alcohol is withdrawn abruptly, withdrawal symptoms, such as tachycardia, hypertension, diaphoresis, nausea, vomiting, tremors, sleeplessness, irritability, **delirium tremens (DT),** seizures, and convulsions result.

CNS Depressants

Central nervous system depressants including barbiturates, benzodiazepines, paraldehyde, meprobamate, and chloral hydrate are also subject to abuse. Cross dependence exists among all CNS depressants and cross-tolerance can develop to alcohol and general anesthetics. Chronic users of barbiturates require progressively higher doses to achieve subjective effects as tolerance develops, but they develop little tolerance to respiratory depression. The depressant effects related to barbiturates are dose dependent and range from mild sedation to sleep to coma to death. With larger doses over time and a combination of alcohol and barbiturates, the risk of death increases greatly. Benzodiazepines alone are safer than barbiturates, because an overdose of oral benzodiazepines rarely results in death.

Psychostimulants

Psychostimulants, such as cocaine and amphetamines, have a high potential for abuse. Euphoria is the main subjective effect associated with cocaine and amphetamines, leading to addiction. Cocaine base (freebase, cocaine, or "crack") is heat stable and is usually smoked (freebasing). Cocaine hydrochloride (HCl) is diluted or cut before sale and the pure form ("rocks") is administered intranasally (snorted) or injected intravenously. "Skin popping" is a method many substance abusers are using to administer drugs, perhaps leading to the formation of abscesses under the skin. The use of crack cocaine reached epidemic proportions, especially in teens (who have a high risk of lethal overdose) in 1985, but has declined in use over the past few years (Lehne, 2001). Mild overdose of cocaine produces agitation, dizziness, tremor, and blurred vision. Severe overdose produces anxiety, hyperpyrexia, convulsions, ventricular dysrhythmias, severe hypertension, and hemorrhagic stroke with possible angina or myocardial infarction (MI). The use of cocaine during pregnancy is especially problematic, because the drug crosses the placenta and enters the fetal bloodstream. Spontaneous abortion, premature delivery, retardation of intrauterine growth, congenital abnormalities, and fetal addiction can result. Long-term intranasal use of cocaine can cause atrophy of the nasal mucosa, necrosis and perforation of the nasal septum, and lung damage.

Amphetamine use is on the rise in the United States and poses a severe health risk to society. Between 1993 and 1999, amphetamine treatment admission rates increased by 250% or more in 14 states and 100% to 249% in another 10 states (USDHHS, 2001). Dextroamphetamine, methamphetamine, and amphetamine can be taken orally or intravenously. Methamphetamine is the primary form of amphetamine seen in the United States, comprising 94% of all amphetamine treatment admissions in 1999 (USDHHS, 2001). A form of dextroamphetamine ("ice" or "crystal meth") can be smoked. Amphetamines cause arousal and an elevation of mood with a sense of increased strength, mental capacity, self-confidence, and a decreased need for food and sleep. A psychotic state with hallucinations and paranoia are common with long-term use, requiring treatment similar to other psychotic disorders. The cardiovascular effects of amphetamines are comparable to those of cocaine, including vasoconstriction, tachycardia, hypertension, angina, and dysrhythmias. Tolerance to mood elevation, appetite suppression, and cardiovascular effects develops with amphetamines; however, dependence is more psychological than physical. Withdrawal from amphetamines produces dysphoria and craving with fatigue, prolonged sleep, excessive eating, and depression.

Opiates

Opiates, such as morphine and heroin, have been abused for many centuries and are major drugs of abuse. The urban poor constitute the majority of abusers, although opiates are used and abused by people of all socioeconomic status. A small percentage of individuals are originally exposed to opiates in the context of pain management; however, most people use opiates under social or illicit circumstances. Heroin is usually the opiate of choice, except among health care workers, who usually select meperidine (Demerol). Health care professionals have a higher risk for opiate abuse than other professionals due to the high accessibility of opiates in their line of work. If colleagues are showing signs of a substance abuse problem, information about impaired nurse programs is available through state boards of nursing to help individual nurses.

Heroin is usually administered intravenously and induces a "rush" or "kick" that lasts less than a minute, followed by a sense of euphoria for an extended period. Tolerance develops to the euphoria, respiratory depression, and nausea, but not to constipation and miosis. Physical dependence occurs with long-term use of opiates. Initial withdrawal symptoms, such as drug craving, lacrimation, rhinorrhea, yawning, and diaphoresis usually take ten days to run their course, with the second phase of opiate withdrawal lasting for months with insomnia, irritability, fatigue, and potential GI hyperactivity and premature ejaculation as problems.

Hallucinogens

Hallucinogens are also called psychedelics or psychotomimetics and include d-lysergic acid diethylamide (LSD), mescaline, dimethyltryptamine (DMT), and psilocin. Psychedelics bring on the same types of thoughts, perceptions, and feelings that occur in dreams. LSD was first used to simulate psychosis. It affects serotonin receptors at multiple sites in the brain and spinal cord. LSD is usually taken orally, but can be injected or smoked. The individual's response to a "trip," the experience of being high on LSD, cannot be predicted and psychological effects and "flashbacks" are common. Ecstasy (3,4-methylenediosy-methamphetamine or MDMA) had extensive use in the 1980s as a popular recreational "rave" drug, and has reappeared in recent years as a date or rape drug. Current research has revealed that women might be more susceptible to the neurotoxic effects on serotonin neurons when using MDMA (Reneman, et al., 2001). Serotonin imbalance is thought to affect impulse control and may be responsible for uninhibited sexual responses in women who have been given the drug without their knowledge. Phencyclidine (PCP, also called angel dust and peace pill) was formerly an anesthetic similar to ketamine used for animals, but caused emergence delirium in humans. Other hallucinogens are similar to LSD, but with different potency and time course of action.

Inhalants

Inhalants are categorized into three types: anesthetics, volatile nitrites, and organic solvents. Nitrous oxide (laughing gas) and ether are the most abused anesthetics. Amyl nitrite, butyl nitrite, and isobutyl nitrite are volatile nitrites used especially by homosexual males to induce venodilation and anal sphincter relaxation. Amyl nitrite is manufactured for medical use, but butyl and isobutyl nitrites are sold for recreational use. Other names for butyl and isobutyl nitrites are climax, rush, and locker room. Street names for amyl nitrite are "poppers" or "snappers." Brain damage or sudden death can occur from the first, tenth, or hundredth time an individual uses an inhalant, resulting in "sudden sniffing death." This danger makes the use of inhalants more hazardous than some other substances.

Organic solvents are ingested in three different methods: bagging, huffing, or sniffing. *Bagging* involves pouring the solvent in a plastic bag and inhaling the vapor. *Huffing* refers to pouring the solvent on a rag and inhaling. *Sniffing* refers to inhaling the solvent directly from the container. Common organic solvents are toluene, gasoline, lighter fluid, paint thinner, nail polish remover, benzene, acetone, chloroform, and model airplane glue. The effects from inhaling organic solvents are similar to alcohol, with prolonged use leading to multiple toxicity. There are no antidotes for these inhalants; therefore, management of toxicity is supportive.

Collaborative Care

Effective treatment of substance abuse and dependence results from the collaborative efforts of an interdisciplinary team specializing in the treatment of psychiatric and substance abuse disorders. Therapies may include detoxification, aversion therapy to maintain abstinence, group and/or individual psychotherapy, psychotropic medications, cognitive-behavioral strategies, family counseling, and self-help groups. Clients suffering from substance abuse can be treated in either inpatient or outpatient settings. A substance overdose is a life-threatening condition that requires emergency hospitalization to stabilize the client medically before implementing any of the above interventions. Several diagnostic tests can provide valuable information about the patients physical condition and set the course for treatment.

Diagnostic Tests

The body fluids most often tested for drug content are blood and urine. A urine drug screen (UDS) and/or blood alcohol level (BAL) are useful biological measures for assessment purposes. The length of time that drugs can be found in blood and urine varies according to dosage and metabolic properties of the drug. All traces of the drug may disappear within 24 hours or may still be detectable 30 days later. Knowledge of the BAL is helpful in ascertaining the level of intoxication, the level of tolerance, and whether the person accurately reported recent drinking. At 0.10% (after 5 to 6 drinks in 1 to 2 hours), voluntary motor action becomes clumsy and reaction time is impaired. The degree of impairment varies with gender, weight, and food ingestion. Small women who drink alcohol on an empty stomach will experience intoxication more rapidly than large males who have eaten a full meal. At 0.20% (after 10 to 12 drinks in 2 to 4 hours), function of the motor area in the brain is depressed, causing staggering and ataxia (Vacarolis, 2002). A level above 0.10% without associated behavioral symptoms indicates the presence of tolerance. A BAL greater than 0.10% is considered legal intoxication in most states. High tolerance is a sign of physical dependence. Assessing for withdrawal symptoms is important when the BAL is high. Medications given for treatment of withdrawal from alcohol are usually not started until the BAL is below a set norm (usually below 0.10%) unless withdrawal symptoms become severe. BAL may be repeated several times, several hours apart, to determine the body's metabolism of alcohol and when it is safe to give the patient medication to minimize the withdrawal symptoms.

Emergency Care for Overdose

The care of a patient who has overdosed on any substance is a serious medical emergency. Respiratory depression may require mechanical ventilation. The patient may become severely sedated and difficult to arouse. Every effort must be made to keep the patient awake; however, stupor and coma may often result. A seizure is another serious complication that requires emergency treatment. If the overdose was intentional, the patient must be constantly monitored for further signs of suicidal ideation. Never leave an actively suicidal patient alone. Signs of overdose and withdrawal from major substances are summarized in Table 44-2 along with their recommended treatments.

Table 44-2. Signs and Treatment of Overdose and Withdrawal

Drug	Overdose Signs	Overdose Treatment	Withdrawal Signs	Withdrawal Treatment
CNS Depressants:	Cardiovascular or respiratory depression or arrest (mostly with barbiturates)	*If awake:* Keep awake	Nausea and vomiting	Carefully titrated detoxification with similar drug
Alcohol		Induce vomiting	Tachycardia	NOTE: Abrupt withdrawal can lead to death.
Barbiturates	Coma	Activated charcoal to absorb drug	Diaphoresis	
Benzodiazepines	Shock	VS q 15 minutes	Anxiety or agitation	
	Convulsions	*Coma:*	Tremors	
	Death	Clear airway, intubate IV fluids	Marked insomnia	
		Gastric lavage	Grand mal seizures	
		Seizure precautions	Delirium	
		Possible hemo or peritoneal dialysis	(after 5–15 years of heavy use)	
		Frequent VS		
		Assess for shock and cardiac arrest		
Stimulants:	Respiratory distress	Antipsychotics Management for:	Fatigue	Antidepressants (desipramine)
Cocaine-crack	Ataxia Hyperpyrexia	1. Hyperpyrexia	Depression	Dopamine agonist
Amphetamines	Convulsions	2. Convulsions	Agitation	Bromocriptine
	Coma	3. Respiratory distress	Apathy	
	Stroke	4. Cardiovascular shock	Anxiety	
	Myocardial infarction (MI)	5. Acidify urine (ammonium CI for amphetamine)	Sleepiness	
	Death		Disorientation	
			Lethargy	
			Craving	

Continued on the next page

Table 44-2. Continued

Drug	Signs	Treatment	Signs	Treatment
		Overdose	**Withdrawal**	
Opiates: Heroin Meperidine Morphine Methadone	Pupil dilation due to anoxia Respiratory depression-arrest Coma Shock Convulsions Death	Narcotic antagonist, (Narcan) quickly reverses CNS depression	Yawning, insomnia Irritability Rhinorrhea Panic Diaphoresis Cramps Nausea and vomiting Muscle aches Chills and fever Lacrimation Diarrhea	Methadone tapering Clonidine naltrexone detoxification Buprenorphine substitution
Hallucinogens: Lysergic acid diethylamide (LSD)	LSD: Psychosis Brain damage Death	Low stimuli with minimal light, sound, activity Have one person "talk down client," reassure Speak slowly and clearly Diazepam or chloral hydrate for anxiety	No pattern of withdrawal	
Phencyclidine piperidine (PCP)	Possible hypertensive crisis Respiratory arrest Hyperthermia Seizures	Acidify urine to help excrete drug (cranberry juice, ascorbic acid); in acute stage: ammonium chloride Minimal stimulis Do NOT attempt to talk down, speak slowly in low voice Diazepam or Haldol		

Table 44-2. Continued

Drug	Signs	Overdose	Withdrawal	
		Treatment	**Signs**	**Treatment**
Inhalants: Volatile Solvents, such as butane, paint thinner, airplane glue, or nail polish remover	Intoxication: 1. Excitation 2. Drowsiness 3. Disinhibition 4. Staggering 5. Lightheadedness 6. Agitation Side Effects: 1. Damage to nervous system 2. Death	Support affected systems	No pattern of withdrawal	
Nitrates	Enhance sexual pleasure	Neurological symptoms may respond to vitamin B_{12} and folate		
Anesthetics, such as nitrous oxide	Giggling, laughter Euphoria	Chronic users may experience polyneuropathy and myelopathy		

Table 44-3. Drugs Used in the Treatment of Substance Withdrawal/Abuse

Drug	*Dose*	*Purpose*
Benzodiazepines		
1. Clordiazepoxide (Librium)	15–100 mg	Diminishes anxiety and has anticonvulsant
2. Diazepam (Valium)	4–40 mg	qualities to provide safe withdrawal. May
3. Oxazepam (Serax)	30–120 mg	be ordered q4h or prn to manage adverse
4. Lorazepam (Ativan)	2–6 mg	effects from withdrawal, then dose is
		tapered to zero.
Vitamins		
1. Thiamine (Vitamin B$_1$)	100 mg/day	Prevents Wernicke's encephalopathy
2. Folic acid	1 mg/day	Corrects vitamin deficiency caused by
3. Multivitamins	I tab/cap daily	heavy long-term alcohol abuse
Anticonvulsants		
1. Phenobarbital	30–320 mg	For seizure control and sedation
2. Magnesium sulfate	1 g q6h	Reduces postwithdrawal seizures
Abstinence medications		
1. Disulfiram (Antabuse)	250 mg/day	Prevents breakdown of alcohol
2. Naltrexone (ReVia)	50 mg/day	Diminishes cravings for alcohol and opioids
3. Methadone	40 mg/day	Blocks craving for heroin
Antidepressants		
1. Fluoxetine (Prozac)	20–80 mg/day	Enhances and stabilizes mood and
2. Sertraline (Zoloft)	50–200 mg/day	diminishes anxiety

Treatment of Withdrawal

All CNS depressants, including alcohol, benzodiazepines, and barbiturates, have a potentially dangerous progression of withdrawal. Alcohol and the entire class of CNS depressants share the same withdrawal syndrome. Early signs of withdrawal appear within a few hours following cessation of the drug, peak after 24 to 48 hours, and then rapidly disappear unless the withdrawal progresses to delirium tremens. Severe withdrawal or delirium tremens is a medical emergency that usually occurs two to five days following alcohol withdrawal and persists two to three days. The symptoms of severe withdrawal include disorientation, paranoid delusions, visual hallucinations, and marked withdrawal symptoms. Seizures may also occur, requiring the use of emergency equipment. Treatment of severe withdrawal during detoxification is mostly symptomatic through acetaminophen, vitamins, and medications to minimize discomfort. Withdrawal symptoms from opiates and stimulants can be very unpleasant but are generally not life threatening. The patient experiencing an acute phase of cocaine withdrawal may become suicidal. Common drugs used in the treatment of substance abuse and withdrawal are presented in Table 44-3.

Nursing Care

Health Promotion

Nursing care of the client with substance abuse or dependence is challenging and requires a nonjudgmental atmosphere promoting trust and respect. Health promotion efforts are aimed at preventing drug use among children and adolescents and reducing the risks among adults. Adolescence is the most common phase for the first experience with drugs (Stuart & Laraia, 2001), therefore teenagers are a vulnerable population, often succumbing to peer pressure. Healthy lifestyles, parental support, stress management, good nutrition, and information about ways to steer clear of peer pressure are important topics for the nurse to provide in school programs.

Nurses should provide adults with information on healthy coping mechanisms, relaxation, and stress reduction techniques to decrease the risks of substance abuse. Nurses have a responsibility to educate their clients about the physiological effects of substances on the body as well as ways to manage stress and anxiety. Nurses must encourage and support periods of abstinence while assisting clients to make major changes in lifestyles, habits, relationships, and coping methods.

Assessment

A comprehensive approach to the assessment of substance use is essential to ensure adequate and appropriate intervention. Three important areas to be assessed are a history of the client's past substance use, medical and psychiatric history, and the presence of psychosocial concerns. Ask questions in a nonthreatening, matter-of-fact manner, phrased as to not imply wrongdoing (Henderson-Martin, 2000). For instance, a nonthreatening question such as, "How much alcohol do you drink?" is preferable to the judgmental question, "You don't drink too much alcohol, do you?" Open-ended questions that elicit more than a simple yes or no answer help to determine the direction of future counseling.

Use therapeutic communication techniques to establish trust prior to the assessment process.

History of Past Substance Use

A thorough history of the client's past substance use is important to ascertain the possibility of tolerance, physical dependence, or withdrawal syndrome. The following questions are helpful in eliciting a pattern of substance use behavior:

- How many substances has the client used simultaneously (**polysubstance abuse** or simultaneous use of many substances) in the past?
- How often, how much, and when did the client first use the substance(s)?
- Is there a history of blackouts, delirium, or seizures?
- Is there a history of withdrawal syndrome, overdoses, and complications from previous substance use?
- Has the client ever been treated in an alcohol or drug abuse clinic?
- Has the client ever been arrested for driving under the influence (DUI) or charged with any criminal offense while using drugs or alcohol?
- Is there a family history of drug or alcohol use?

Medical and Psychiatric History

The client's medical history is another important area for assessment and should include the existence of any concomitant physical or mental condition (e.g., HIV, hepatitis, cirrhosis, esophageal varices, pancreatitis, gastritis, Wernicke-Korsakoff syndrome, depression, schizophrenia, anxiety, or personality disorder). Ask about prescribed and over-the-counter medications as well as any allergies or sensitivity to drugs. A brief overview of the client's current mental status is also significant.

- Is there a history of abuse (physical or sexual) or family violence?
- Has the client ever tried to commit suicide?
- Is the client currently having suicidal or homicidal ideation?

Psychosocial Issues

Information about the client's level of stress and other psychosocial concerns can help in the assessment of substance use problems.

- Has the client's substance use affected his or her ability to hold a job?
- Has the client's substance use affected relationships with spouse, family, friends, or coworkers?
- How does the client usually cope with stress?
- Does the client have a support system that helps in time of need?
- How does the client spend his or her leisure time?

Assessment Tools Several screening tools such as the Michigan Alcohol Screening Test (MAST) (Pokorny, Miller, & Kaplan, 1972), Drug Abuse Screening Test (DAST) (Skinner, 1982), and the CAGE questionnaire (Ewing, 1984) may help the nurse determine the degree of severity of substance abuse or dependence. These screening tools provide a nonjudgmental, brief, and easy method to ascertain patterns of substance abuse behaviors.

- *Michigan Alcohol Screening Test (MAST) Brief Version* is a 10-question, dichotomous, self-administered questionnaire that takes 10 to 15 minutes to complete. An answer of yes to three or more questions indicates a potentially dangerous pattern of alcohol abuse.
- *CAGE questionnaire* is more useful when the client may not recognize he or she has an alcohol problem, or is uncomfortable acknowledging it. This questionnaire is designed to be a self-report of drinking behavior or may be administered by a professional. One affirmative response indicates the need for further discussion and follow-up. Two or more yes answers signify a problem with alcohol that may require treatment.

  Have you ever felt you should *cut* down on your drinking?

  Have people *annoyed* you by criticizing your drinking?

  Have you ever felt bad or *guilty* about your drinking?

  Have you ever had a drink first thing in the morning (an "*eye-opener*") to steady your nerves or to get rid of a hangover?

- *Drug Abuse Screening Test (DAST)* is a yes/no self-administered questionnaire that is useful in identifying people who are possibly addicted to drugs other than alcohol. A positive response to one or more questions suggests significant drug abuse problems and warrants further evaluation. Because the tools can be incorrect if the client is not answering truthfully, all clients who are screened positive for drug addiction should be evaluated according to diagnostic criteria.

Nursing Diagnoses and Interventions

The primary nursing diagnoses and interventions for clients with substance abuse problems are listed below. Implications for nursing care in acute and home care settings are combined in this discussion.

Risk for Injury

- Assess client's level of disorientation to determine specific risks to safety. *Knowledge of the client's level of cognitive functioning is essential to the development of an appropriate plan of care.*
- Obtain a drug history, as well as urine and blood samples for laboratory analysis of substance content. *Subjective history is often not accurate and knowledge regarding substance use is important for accurate assessment.*
- Place client in a quiet, private room to decrease excessive stimuli, but do not leave client alone if excessive hyperactivity or suicidal ideation is present. *Excessive stimuli increase client's agitation.*
- Frequently orient client to reality and the environment, ensuring that potentially harmful objects are stored outside the client's access. *Client may harm self or others if disoriented and confused.*
- Monitor vital signs every 15 minutes until stable and assess for signs of intoxication or withdrawal. *The most reliable information about withdrawal symptoms are vital signs; they provide information about the need for medication during detoxification.*

Ineffective Denial

- Be genuine, honest, and respectful of client. Keep all promises and convey an attitude of acceptance of the client. *The development of a nonjudgmental, therapeutic nurse-client relationship is essential to gain the client's trust.*
- Identify maladaptive behaviors or situations that have occurred in client's life and discuss how the use of substances may have been a contributing factor. *The first step in combating denial is for the client to recognize the relationship between substance use and personal problems.*
- Do not accept the use of defense mechanisms, such as rationalization or projection, as the client attempts to blame others or make excuses for his or her behavior. Use confrontation with caring to avoid placing client on the defensive. *Confrontation interferes with the client's ability to use denial.*
- Encourage client participation in therapeutic group activities, such as dual diagnosis or Alcoholics Anonymous (AA) meetings, with other people who are experiencing or have experienced similar problems. *Peer feedback is often more accepted than feedback from authority figures.*

Ineffective Individual Coping

- Establish trusting relationship. *Trust is essential to the nurse-client relationship.*
- Set limits on manipulative behavior and maintain consistency in responses. *Client is unable to set own limits and must begin to accept responsibility without being manipulative.*
- Encourage client to verbalize feelings, fears, or anxieties. Use attentive listening and validate client's feelings with observations or statements that acknowledge feelings. *Verbalization of feelings helps client to develop insight into behaviors and long-standing problems.*
- Explore methods of dealing with stressful situations other than resorting to substance use. Provide encouragement for changing to a healthier lifestyle. Teach healthy coping mechanisms (e.g., physical exercise, progressive muscle relaxation, deep breathing

exercises, meditation, and imagery). *Client needs knowledge about how to adapt to stress without resorting to drug use.*

Imbalanced Nutrition: Less Than Body Requirements

* Administer vitamins and dietary supplements as ordered by physician. *Vitamin B_1 is necessary to prevent complications from chronic alcoholism, such as Wernicke's syndrome.*

* Monitor lab work (e.g., total albumin, complete blood count, urinalysis, electrolytes, and liver enzymes) and report significant changes to physician. *Objective laboratory tests provide necessary information to determine the extent of malnourishment.*

* Collaborate with dietitian to determine number of calories needed to provide adequate nutrition and realistic weight gain. Document intake, output, and calorie count. Weigh daily if condition warrants. *Weight loss or gain is important assessment information so that an appropriate plan of care can be developed.*

* Teach the importance of adequate nutrition by explaining the food guide pyramid and relating the physical effects of malnutrition on body systems. *Client may have inadequate knowledge of proper nutritional habits.*

Low Self-Esteem

* Spend time with client and convey an attitude of acceptance. Encourage client to accept responsibility for own behaviors and feelings. *An attitude of acceptance enhances self-worth.*

* Encourage client to focus on strengths and accomplishments rather than weaknesses and failures. *Minimize attention to negative ruminations.*

* Encourage participation in therapeutic group activities. Offer recognition and positive feedback for actual achievements. *Success and recognition increase self-esteem.*

* Teach assertiveness techniques and effective communication techniques, such as the use of "I feel" rather than "You make me feel" statements. *Previous patterns of communication may have been aggressive and accusatory, causing barriers to interpersonal relationships.*

Deficient Knowledge

* Assess client's level of knowledge and readiness to learn the effects of drugs and alcohol on the body. *Baseline assessment is required to develop appropriate teaching material.*

* Develop teaching plan that includes measurable objectives. Include significant others, if possible. *Lifestyle changes often affect all family members.*

* Begin with simple concepts and progress to more complex issues. Use interactive teaching strategies and written materials appropriate to the client's educational level. Include information on physiological effects of substances, the propensity for physical and psychological dependence, and the risks to a fetus if the client is pregnant. *Active participation and handouts enhance retention of important concepts.*

Disturbed Sensory Perceptions

* Observe for withdrawal symptoms. Monitor vital signs. Provide adequate nutrition and hydration. Place on seizure precautions. *These actions provide supportive physical care during detoxification.*

* Assess level of orientation frequently. Orient and reassure client of safety in presence of hallucinations, delusions, or illusions. *Client may be frightened.*

- Explain all interventions before approaching client. Avoid loud noises and talk softly to client. Decrease external stimuli by dimming lights. *Excessive stimuli increase agitation.*
- Administer PRN medications according to detoxification schedule. *Benzodiazepines help to minimize the discomfort of withdrawal symptoms.*

Disturbed Thought Processes

- Give positive reinforcement when thinking and behavior are appropriate or when client recognizes that delusions are not based in reality. *Drugs and alcohol can interfere with client's perception of reality.*
- Use simple, step-by-step instructions and face-to-face interaction when communicating with client. *Client may be confused or disoriented.*
- Express reasonable doubt if client relays suspicious or paranoid beliefs. Reinforce accurate perception of people or situations. *It is important to communicate that you do not share that false belief as reality.*
- Do not argue with delusions or hallucinations. Convey acceptance that the client believes a situation to be true, but that the nurse does not see or hear what is not there. *Arguing with the client or denying the belief serves no useful purpose, because delusions are not eliminated.*
- Talk to client about real events and real people. Respond to feelings and reassure client that he or she is safe from harm. *Discussions that focus on the delusions may aggravate the condition. Verbalization of feelings in a nonthreatening environment may help the client develop insight.*

Home Care

Teaching the client and family includes:

- The negative effects of substance abuse including physical and psychological complications of substance abuse.
- The signs of relapse and the importance of after care programs and self-help groups to prevent relapse. An acronym that can assist the client in recognizing behaviors that lead to relapse is HALT: **h**ungry, **a**ngry, **l**onely, and **t**ired. Stress the importance of adequate sleep and nutrition, healthy recreation activities, and a caring support system in managing stressful situations.
- Information about specific medications that help to reduce the craving for alcohol (naltrexone [ReVia]) and maintain abstinence (disulfiram [Antabuse]), including the potential side effects, possible drug interactions, and any special precautions to be taken (e.g., avoiding over-the-counter medications such as cough syrup that may have alcohol content).
- Stress management techniques, such as progressive muscle relaxation, abdominal breathing techniques, imagery, meditation, and effective coping skills.

In addition, suggest the following resources:

1. Self-help groups
2. Employee assistance programs
3. Individual, group, and/or family counseling
4. Community rehabilitation programs
5. National Alliance for the Mentally Ill.

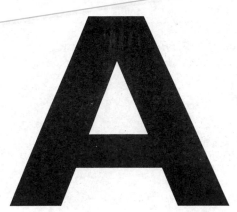

Appendix A
Bibliography

Chapter 1

American Hospital Association. (1990). *A patient's bill of rights*. Chicago: Author.

American Nurses Association. (2001). *Code of ethics for nurses with interpretive statements*. Washington, D.C.: American Nurses Publishing.

American Nurses Association. (2003). *Nursing: Scope and standards of practice*. Washington, D.C.: American Nurses Publishing.

American Nurses Association. (2003). *Nursing's social policy statement* (2nd ed.). Washington, D.C.: American Nurses Publishing.

Beauchamp, T. L., & Childress, J. F. (2001). *Principles of biomedical ethics* (5th ed.). New York: Oxford University Press.

Daly, B. J. (1996). Ethics in critical care. In J. M. Clochesey, C. Breu, S. Cardin, A. A. Whittaker, & E. B. Rudy (Eds.), *Critical care nursing* (2nd ed., pp. 1375–1383). Philadelphia: Saunders.

Trandel-Korenchuk, D. M., & Trandel-Korenchuk, K. M. (1997). *Nursing & the law* (5th ed.). Gaithersburg, MD: Aspen.

Chapter 2

Aguilera, D. C. (1998). *Crisis intervention: Theory and methodology* (8th ed.). St. Louis, MO: Mosby.

Bandura, A. (1986). *Social foundations of thought and action: A social cognitive theory*. Englewood Cliffs, NJ: Prentice-Hall.

Bowen, M. (1978). *Family therapy in clinical practice*. New York: Jason Aronson.

Bridges, W. (1991). *Managing transitions: Making the most of change*. Reading, MA: Addison-Wesley.

Burr, W. R., Leigh, G. K., Day, R. D., & Constantine, J. (1979). Symbolic interaction and the family. In W. R. Burr, R. Hill, F. I. Nye, & I. L. Reiss (Eds.), *Contemporary theories about the family* (pp. 42–111). New York: Free Press.

Chinn, P. L., & Jacobs, M. K. (1987). *Theory and nursing: A systematic approach* (2nd ed.). St. Louis, MO: Mosby.

Erikson, E. H. (1955). Growth and crises of the healthy personality. In C. Kluckhorn, H. A. Murray, & D. M. Scheider (Eds.), *Personality in nature, society and culture* (pp. 185–225). New York: Knopf.

Fawcett, J., & Downs, F. S. (1992). *The relationship of theory and research* (2nd ed.). Philadelphia: F.A. Davis.

Fishbein, M., & Azjen, I. (1975). *Belief, attitude, intention, and behavior: An introduction to theory and research.* Reading, MA: Addison-Wesley.

Huber, D. (1996). *Leadership and nursing care management.* Philadelphia: WB Saunders.

King, K. M., Humen, D. P., Smith, H. L., Phan, C. L., & Teo, K. K. (2001). Psychosocial components of cardiac recovery and rehabilitation attendance. *Heart, 85*(3), 290–294.

Lewin, K. (1951). *Field theory in social science.* New York: Harper & Row.

Pender, N. J. (1996). *Health promotion in nursing practice* (3rd ed.). Norwalk, CT: Appleton & Lange.

Prochaska, J. O., & DiClemente, C. C. (1984). *The transtheoretical approach: Crossing traditional boundaries of change.* Homewood, IL: Dow-Jones-Irwin.

Rosenstock, I. M. (1974). Historical origins of the health belief model. In M. H. Becker (Ed.), *The health belief model and personal health behavior* (pp. 1–8). Thorofare, NJ: Slack.

Roy, C., & Roberts, S. L. (1981). *Theory construction in nursing: An adaptation model.* Englewood Cliffs, NJ: Prentice-Hall.

Smith, J. (1983). *The idea of health: Implications for the nursing profession.* New York: Teachers College.

Sullivan, M. D., LaCroix, A. Z., Russo, J., & Katon, W. J. (1998). Self-efficacy and self-reported functional status in coronary heart disease: A six-month study. *Psychosomatic Medicine, 60*(4), 473–478.

Chapter 3

Bleich, M. R. (1999). Managing and leading. In P. Yoder-Wise (Ed.), *Leading and managing in nursing* (pp. 2–20). St. Louis: Mosby.

Burns, J. (1978). *Leadership.* New York: Harper & Row.

Case Management Society of America. (2001). *Definition of case management.* Retrieved from www.cmsa.org

Coile, R. C. (1999). Nursing case management in the new millennium: Two perspectives. *Nursing Case Management, 4*(6), 244–251.

Idvall, E., Rooke, L., & Hamrin, E. (1997). Quality indicators in clinical nursing: A review of the literature. *Journal of Advanced Nursing, 25*(1), 6–17.

McCallin, A. (2001). Interdisciplinary practice—A matter of teamwork: An integrated literature review. *Journal of Clinical Nursing, 10*(4), 419–428.

Millward, L. J., & Jeffries, N. (2001). The team survey: A tool for health care team development. *Journal of Advanced Nursing, 35*(2), 276–287.

Spradley, B., & Allender, J. (2001). The community health nurse as leader, change agent, and case manager. In J. Allender & B. Spradley (Eds.), *Community health nursing.* Philadelphia: Lippincott.

Swansburg, R. C., & Swansburg, R. J. (1999). *Introductory management and leadership for nurses* (2nd ed.). Sudbury, MA: Jones & Barlett.

Urden, L. D. (2001). Outcome evaluation: An essential component of CNS practice. *Clinical Nurse Specialist, 15*(6), 260–268.

Chapter 4

Abraham, I., Bottrell, M. M., Fulmer, T., & Mezey, M. D. (Eds.). (2003). *Geriatric nursing protocols for best practice* (2nd ed.). New York: Springer.

Burns, N., & Gove, S. K. (1997). *The practice of nursing research: Conduct, critique & utilization* (3rd ed.). Philadelphia: Saunders.

Mateo, M. A., & Kirchoff, K. T. (Eds.) (1999). *Using and conducting nursing research in the clinical setting* (2nd ed.). Philadelphia: Saunders.

Mateo, M. A., & Newton, C. (1999). Progressing from an idea to a research question. In M. A. Mateo & K. T. Kirchoff (Eds.), *Using and conducting nursing research in the clinical setting* (2nd ed.. Philadelphia: Saunders.

Norman, E. M. (1999). *We band of angels: The untold story of American nurses trapped on Bataan by the Japanese.* New York: Random House.

Chapter 5

Bandura, A. (1986). *Social foundations of thought & action: A social cognitive theory.* Englewood Cliffs NJ: Prentice-Hall.

Knowles, M. (1975). *The modern practice of adult education.* New York: Associated Press.

North American Nursing Diagnosis Association. (2001). *Nursing diagnoses: Definitions & classification 2001–2002.* Philadelphia: Author.

Pender, N. (1987). *Health promotion in nursing practice* (2nd ed.). Los Altos, CA: Appleton & Lange.

Rankin, S. H., & Stallings, K. D. (2001). *Patient education: Principles & practice* (4th ed.). Philadelphia: Lippincott..

Redman, B. K. (2001). *The practice of patient education* (9th ed.). St. Louis, MO: Mosby.

Report of the U.S. Preventive Services Task Force. (1996). *Guide to clinical preventive services* (2nd ed.). Baltimore: Williams & Wilkins

Rotter, J. B. (1966). Generalized expectancies for internal versus external control of reinforcement. *Psychological Monographs, 80,* 1.

Chapter 6

Administration on Aging. (2000). *Older Americans 2000.* Retrieved from www.aoa.gov

American Heart Association. (2001a) *My heart watch.* Retrieved from www.americanheart.org

American Heart Association. (2001b). *Take wellness to heart.* Retrieved from www.women.americanheart.org.

American Heart Association. (2001c). *Operation heartbeat.* Retrieved from www.americanheart.org

Maddox, P. J. (2001). Bioterrorism: A renewed public health threat. *Dermatology Nursing, 13*(6), 437–441.

The Mended Hearts. (2002). *The purpose of mended hearts.* Retrieved from www.mendedhearts.org

National Heart, Lung, and Blood Institute. (2001a). *Act in Time to Heart Attack Signs.* www.nhlbi.nih.gov

National Heart, Lung, and Blood Institute. (2001b). *National high blood pressure education program.* Retrieved fromwww.nhlbi.nih.gov

National Heart, Lung, and Blood Institute. (2001c). *Detection, evaluation, and treatment of high blood cholesterol in adults.* Retrieved from www.nhlbi.nih.gov

National Heart, Lung, and Blood Institute. (2001d). *Obesity education initiative.* Retrieved from www.nhlbi.nih.gov.

National Heart, Lung, and Blood Institute. (2001e). *Developing a woman's heart health education action plan.* Retrieved from www.nhlbi.nih.gov

Spardley, B., & Allender, J. (2001). Opportunities and challenges of community health nursing. In J. Allender & B. Spradley (Eds.), *Community health nursing.* Philadelphia: Lippincott.

U.S. Census Bureau. (2001). *Population Projections.* Retrieved from www.census.gov.states

U.S. Department of Health and Human Services. (2000). *Healthy People 2010: With understanding and improving health and objectives for improving health* (2nd ed.). Washington, D.C.: US Government Printing Office. Available online at www.health.gov/healthypeople

U. S. Department of Health and Human Services. (2001). *Healthy people in healthy communities.* Retrieved from www.health.gov/healthypeople

Chapter 7

Farla, S., & Flannery, J. (1999). Assessment of the patient in heart failure. *Home Care Provider,* *4*(5), 184–188.

Kirton, C. (1997a). Assessing bowel sounds. *Nursing97, 27*(3), 64.

_____. (1996a). Assessing breath sounds. *Nursing, 26*(6), 50–51.

_____. (1996b). Assessing for ascites. *Nursing 96, 26*(4), 53.

_____. (1996c). Assessing normal heart sounds. *Nursing96, 26*(2), 56–57.

_____. (1997b). Assessing a heart murmur. *Nursing97, 27*(9), 51.

_____. (1997c). Assessing S_3 and S_4 heart sounds. *Nursing97, 27*(7), 52–53.

Ludwig, L. (1998). Cardiovascular assessment for home healthcare nurses: Part 1. *Home Healthcare Nurse, 16*(7), 450–456.

McAvoy, J. (2000). Cardiac pain: Discover the unexpected. *Nursing, 30*(3), 34–40.

McGrath, A., & Cox, C. (1998). Cardiac and circulatory assessment in intensive care units. *Intensive & Critical Care Nursing, 14*(6), 283–287.

Norrie, P. (1999). The parameters that cardiothoracic intensive care nurses use to assess the progress or deterioration of their patients. *Nursing in Critical Care, 4*(3), 133–137.

O'Hanlon-Nichols, T. (1997). Basic assessment series: The adult cardiovascular system. *American Journal of Nursing, 97*(12), 34–40.

Scrima, D. (1997). Foundations of arrhythmia interpretation. *MEDSURG Nursing, 6*(4), 193–202.

Weber, J., & Kelley, J. (2002). *Health assessment in nursing* (2nd ed.). Philadelphia: Lippincott.

Wilson, S., & Giddens, J. (2001). *Health assessment for nursing practice.* St. Louis: Mosby.

Chapter 8

Ackley, B. J., & Ladwig, G. B. (2002). *Nursing diagnosis handbook: A guide to planning care* (5th ed.). St. Louis, MO: Mosby.

Artinian, N. T. (2001). Perceived benefits and barriers of eating heart healthy. *MEDSURG Nursing, 10*(3), 129–138

Ayers, D. M. M. (2002). EBCT: Beaming in on coronary artery disease. *Nursing, 32*(4), 81.

Beattie, S. (2000). A portrait of postop a-fib. *RN, 63*(3), 26–29.

Braunwald, E., Fauci, A. S., Kasper, D. L., Hauser, S. L., Longo, D. L., & Jameson, J. L. (2001). *Harrison's Principles of internal medicine* (15th ed.). New York: McGraw-Hill.

Bubien, R. S. (2000). A new beat on an old rhythm. *American Journal of Nursing, 100*(1), 42–50.

Bullock, B. A., & Henze, R. L. (2000). *Focus on pathophysiology.* Philadelphia: Lippincott.

Copstead, L. C., and Banasik, J. L. (2000). *Pathophysiology: Biological and behavioral perspectives* (2nd ed.). Philadelphia: Saunders.

Cowan, M. J., Pike, K. C., & Budzynski, H. K. (2001). Psychosocial nursing therapy following sudden cardiac arrest: Impact on two-year survival. *Nursing Research, 50*(2), 68–76.

Crumlish, C. M., Bracken, J., Hand, M. M., Keenan, K., Ruggiero, H., & Simmons, D. (2000). When time is muscle. *American Journal of Nursing, 100*(1), 26–33.

Deglin, J. H., & Vallerand, A. H. (2003). *Davis's drug guide for nurses* (8th ed.). Philadelphia: F.A. Davis.

Dracup, K., & Moser, D. K. (1997). Beyond sociodemographics: Factors influencing the decision to seek treatment for symptoms of acute myocardial infarction. *Heart & Lung, 26*(4), 253–262.

Fontaine, K. L. (2000). *Healing practices: Alternative therapies for nursing.* Upper Saddle River, NJ: Prentice Hall Health.

Gallo, J. J., Busby-Whitehead, J., Rabins, P. V., Silliman, R. A., & Murphy, J. B. (Eds.). (1999). *Reichel's care of the elderly: Clinical aspects of aging* (5th ed.). Philadelphia: Lippincott Williams & Wilkins.

Glessner, T. M., & Walker, M. K. (2001). Standardized measures: Documenting processes and outcomes of care for patients undergoing coronary artery bypass grafting. *MEDSURG Nursing, 10*(1), 23–29.

Goodman, D. (2001). Automatic external defibrillation. *MEDSURG Nursing, 10*(5), 251–253, 276, 278.

Granger, B. B., & Miller, C. M. (2001). Acute coronary syndrome. *Nursing, 31*(11), 36–43.

Humphreys, D. R. (2001). Enhanced external counter pulsation: Beating angina. *Nursing, 31*(10), 54–55.

Incredibly easy! Understanding chest pain. (2001). *Nursing, 31*(12), 28.

Johnson, M., Bulechek, G., Dochterman, J. M., Maas, M., & Moorhead, S. (2001). *Nursing diagnoses, outcomes, & interventions.* St. Louis: Mosby.

Johnson, M., Maas, M., & Moorhead, S. (Eds.). (2000). *Nursing outcomes classification (NOC)* (2nd ed.). St. Louis: Mosby.

Kuhn, M. A. (1999). *Complementary therapies for health care providers.* Philadelphia: Lippincott.

Lehne, R. A. (2001). *Pharmacology for nursing care* (4th ed.). Philadelphia: Saunders.

Malarkey, L. M., & McMorrow, M. E. (2000). *Nurse's manual of laboratory tests and diagnostic procedures* (2nd ed.). Philadelphia: Saunders.

Mancini, M. E., & Kaye, W. (1999). AEDs: Changing the way you respond to cardiac arrest. *American Journal of Nursing, 99*(5), 26–30.

McAvoy, J. A. (2000). Cardiac pain: Discover the unexpected. *Nursing, 30*(1), 34–39.

McCance, K. L., & Huether, S. E. (2002). *Pathophysiology: The biologic basis for disease in adults and children* (4th ed.). St. Louis: Mosby.

McCloskey, J. C., & Bulechek, G. M. (Eds.) (2000). *Nursing interventions classification (NIC)* (3rd ed.). St. Louis: Mosby.

Meeker, M. H., & Rothrock, J. C. (1999). *Alexander's care of the patient in surgery* (11th ed.). St. Louis: Mosby.

National Cholesterol Education Program. (2001). *Adult treatment panel III report.* National Cholesterol Education Program Expert Panel on Detection, Evaluation, and Treatment of High Blood Cholesterol in Adults. Bethesda, MD: National Heart, Lung, and Blood Institute.

National Heart, Lung, and Blood Institute. National Institutes of Health. (2002). *Morbidity & mortality: 2002 chart book of cardiovascular, lung, and blood diseases.* Bethesda, MD: Author.

Navuluri, R. (2001). Antiplatelet and fibrinolytic therapy. *American Journal of Nursing, 101*(10), Hospital Extra 24A, 24D.

North American Nursing Diagnosis Association. (2001). *NANDA nursing diagnoses: Definitions & classification 2001–2002.* Philadelphia: NANDA.

Palatnik, A. M. (2001). Critical care. Acute coronary syndrome: New advances and nursing strategies. *Nursing, 31*(5), 32cc1–32cc2, 32cc4, 32cc6.

Photo guide. How to perform 3- or 5-lead monitoring. (2002). *Nursing, 32*(4), 50–52.

Porth, C. M. (2002). *Pathophysiology: Concepts of altered health states* (6th ed.). Philadelphia: Lippincott.

Robinson, A. W. (1999). Getting to the heart of denial. *American Journal of Nursing, 99*(5), 38–42.

Shaffer, R. S. (2002). ICD therapy: The patient's perspective. *American Journal of Nursing, 102*(2), 46–49.

Siomko, A. J. (2000). Demystifying cardiac markers. *American Journal of Nursing, 100*(1), 36–40.

Snowberger, P. (2001). VT or SVT? You can tell at the bedside. *RN, 64*(2), 26–31.

Steinke, E. E. (2000). Sexual counseling after myocardial infarction. *American Journal of Nursing, 100*(12), 38–43.

Sullivan, C. (2000). Critical care. Easing severe angina with laser surgery. *Nursing, 30*(4), 32cc1–32cc2, 32cc4.

Tierney, L. M., McPhee, S. J., & Papadakis, M. A. (2001). *Current medical diagnosis & treatment* (40th ed.). New York: Lange Medical Books/McGraw-Hill.

Urden, L. D., Stacy, K. M., & Lough, M. E. (2002). *Thelan's critical care nursing: Diagnosis and management* (4th ed.). St. Louis: Mosby.

U. S. Preventive Services Task Force. (2002). Aspirin for the primary prevention of cardiovascular events: Recommendations and rationale. *American Journal of Nursing, 102*(3), 67, 69–70.

————. (2002). Screening for lipid disorders in adults: Recommendations and rationale. *American Journal of Nursing, 102*(6), 91, 93, 95.

Whitney, E. N., & Rolfes, S. R. (2002). Understanding nutrition (9th ed.). Belmont, CA: Wadsworth.

Wilkinson, J. M. (2000). *Nursing diagnosis handbook with NIC interventions and NOC outcomes* (7th ed.). Upper Saddle River, NJ: Prentice Hall Health.

Woods, S. L., Froelicher, E. S. S., & Motzer, S. U. (2000). *Cardiac nursing* (4th ed.). Philadelphia: Lippincott.

Writing Group for the Women's Health Initiative Investigators. (2002). Risks and benefits of estrogen plus progestin in healthy postmenopausal women. [On-line]. *JAMA, 288*(3). Available: http://jama.ama-assn.org/issues/v288n3/fffull/joc21036.html

Chapter 9

Ackley, B. J., & Ladwig, G. B. (2002). *Nursing diagnosis handbook: A guide to planning care* (5th ed.). St. Louis: Mosby.

American Heart Association. (2001). *2002 heart and stroke statistical update.* Dallas, TX: Author.

Ammon, S. (2001). Managing patients with heart failure. *American Journal of Nursing, 101*(12), 34–40.

Baptiste, M. M. (2001). Aortic valve replacement. *RN, 64*(1), 58–63.

Bither, C. J., & Apple, S. (2001). Home management of the failing heart. *American Journal of Nursing, 101*(12), 41–45.

Braunwald, E., Fauci, A. S., Kasper, D. L., Hauser, S. L., Longo, D. L., & Jameson, J. L. (2001). *Harrison's principles of internal medicine* (15th ed.). New York: McGraw-Hill.

Bullock, B. A., & Henze, R. L. (2000). *Focus on pathophysiology.* Philadelphia: Lippincott.

Capriotti, T. (2002). Current concepts and pharmacologic treatment of heart failure. *MEDSURG Nursing, 11*(2), 71–83.

Carelock, J., & Clark, A. P. (2001). Heart failure: Pathophysiologic mechanisms. *American Journal of Nursing, 101*(12), 26–33.

Copstead, L. C., and Bansik, J. L. (2000). *Pathophysiology: Biological and behavioral perspectives* (2nd ed.). Philadelphia: Saunders.

Deglin, J. H., & Vallerand, A. H. (2003). *Davis's drug guide for nurses* (8th ed.). Philadelphia: F.A. Davis.

Fontaine, K. L. (2000). *Healing practices: Alternative therapies for nursing.* Upper Saddle River, NJ: Prentice Hall Health.

Gallo, J. J., Busby-Whitehead, J., Rabins, P. V., Silliman, R. A., & Murphy, J. B. (Eds.). (1999). *Reichel's care of the elderly: Clinical aspects of aging* (5th ed.). Philadelphia: Lippincott Williams & Wilkins.

Hunt, S. A., Baker, D. W., Chin, M. H., Ciquegrani, M. P., Feldman, A. M., Francis, G. S., Ganiats, T. G., Goldstein, S., Gregoratos, G., Jessup, M. L., Noble, R. J., Packer, M., Silver, M. A., and Stevenson, L. W. (2001). ACC/AHA guidelines for the evaluation and management of chronic heart failure in the adult: Executive summary: A report of the American College of Cardiology / American Heart Association Task Force on Practice Guidelines (Committee to Revise the 1995 Guidelines for the Evaluation and Management of Heart Failure). *Circulation, 104,* 2996–3007.

Johnson, M., Bulechek, G., Dochterman, J. M., Maas, M., & Moorhead, S. (2001). *Nursing diagnoses, outcomes, & interventions.* St. Louis: Mosby.

Johnson, M., Maas, M., & Moorhead, S. (Eds.). (2000). *Nursing outcomes classification (NOC)* (2nd ed.). St. Louis: Mosby.

Kearney, K. (2000). Emergency. Digitalis toxicity. *American Journal of Nursing, 100*(6), 51–52.

Kuhn, M. A. (1999). *Complementary therapies for health care providers.* Philadelphia: Lippincott.

Lehne, R. A. (2001). *Pharmacology for nursing care* (4th ed.). Philadelphia: Saunders.

Malarkey, L. M., & McMorrow, M. E. (2000). *Nurse's manual of laboratory tests and diagnostic procedures* (2nd ed.). Philadelphia: Saunders.

McCance, K. L., & Huether, S. E. (2002). *Pathophysiology: The biologic basis for disease in adults and children* (4th ed.). St. Louis: Mosby.

McCloskey, J. C., & Bulechek, G. M. (Eds.) (2000). *Nursing interventions classification (NIC)* (3rd ed.). St. Louis: Mosby.

Meeker, M. H., & Rothrock, J. C. (1999). *Alexander's care of the patient in surgery* (11th ed.). St. Louis: Mosby.

Miracle, V. A. (2001). Put the brakes on pericarditis. *Nursing, 31*(4), 44–45.

Myers, T. A., Eichhorn, D. J., Guzzetta, C. E., Clark, A. P., Klein, J. D., Taliaferro, E., & Calvin, A. (2000). Family presence during invasive procedures and resuscitation: The experience of family members, nurses, and physicians. *American Journal of Nursing, 100*(2), 32–42.

National Heart, Lung, and Blood Institute. National Institutes of Health. (2002). *Morbidity & mortality: 2002 chart book of cardiovascular, lung, and blood diseases.* Bethesda, MD: Author.

North American Nursing Diagnosis Association. (2001). *NANDA nursing diagnoses: Definitions & classification 2001–2002.* Philadelphia: NANDA.

Porth, C. M. (2002). *Pathophysiology: Concepts of altered health states* (6th ed.). Philadelphia: Lippincott.

Pugh, L. C., Havens, D. S., Xie, S., Robinson, J. M., & Blaha, C. (2001). Case management for elderly persons with heart failure: The quality of life and cost outcomes. *MEDSURG Nursing, 10*(2), 71–75.

Springhouse. (1999). *Nurse's handbook of alternative & complementary therapies.* Springhouse, PA: Author.

Tierney, L. M., McPhee, S. J., & Papadakis, M. A. (2001). *Current medical diagnosis & treatment* (40th ed.). New York: Lange Medical Books/McGraw-Hill.

Urden, L. D., Stacy, K. M., & Lough, M. E. (2002). *Thelan's critical care nursing: Diagnosis and management* (4th ed.). St. Louis: Mosby

Way, L. W., & Dahoerty, G. M. (2003). *Current surgical diagnosis & treatment* (11th ed.). New York: Lange Medical/McGraw-Hill.

Wilkinson, J. M. (2000). *Nursing diagnosis handbook with NIC interventions and NOC outcomes* (7th ed.). Upper Saddle River, NJ: Prentice Hall Health.

Woods, S. L., Froelicher, E. S. S., & Motzer, S. U. (2000). *Cardiac nursing* (4th ed.). Philadelphia: Lippincott.

Chapter 10

Andresen, G. (1998). Assessing the older patient. *RN, 61*(3), 46–56.

Ayello, E. (2000). On the lookout for peripheral vascular disease. *Nursing, 30*(6 Home Health), 64hh1–2, 64hh4.

Ayello, E. (2001). Why is pressure ulcer risk assessment so important? *Nursing, 31*(11), 74–80.

Faria, S. (1999). Assessment of peripheral arterial pulses. *Home Care Provider, 4*(4), 140–141.

Hoskins, M. (1997). Using dopplers. *Community Nurse, 3*(3), 17–18.

MacLaren, J. (2001). Skin changes in lymphoedema: Pathophysiology and management options. *International Journal of Palliative Nursing, 7*(8), 381–382, 384–388.

McConnell, E. A. (1997). Performing Allen's test. *Nursing, 17*(11), 26.

Watson, R. (2000). Assessing cardiovascular functioning in older people. *Nursing Older People, 12*(6), 27–28.

Weber, J., & Kelley, J. (2002). *Health assessment in nursing* (2nd ed.). Philadelphia: Lippincott.

Willis, K. (2001). Gaining perspective on peripheral vascular disease. *Nursing, 31*(2 Hospital Nursing), 32hn1–4.

Wilson, S., & Giddens, J. (2001). *Health assessment for nursing practice.* St. Louis: Mosby.

Young, T. (2001). Leg ulcer assessment. *Practice Nurse, 21*(7), 50, 52.

Chapter 11

Ackley, B. J., & Ladwig, G. B. (2002). *Nursing diagnosis handbook: A guide to planning care* (5th ed.). St. Louis: Mosby.

Alcoser, P. W., & Burchett, S. (1999). Bone marrow transplantation: Immune system suppression and reconstitution. *American Journal of Nursing, 99*(6), 26–31.

American Cancer Society. (2002a). *Cancer facts and figures 2002.* Atlanta: Author.

_____ . (2002b). *Gleevec's new successes show growing promise of targeted therapies.* Available: www.cancer.org/eprise/main/docroot/NWS/content/NWS_1_1x_Gleevec

Braunwald, E., Fauci, A. S., Kasper, D. L., Hauser, S. L., Longo, D. L., & Jameson, J. L. (2001). *Harrison's principles of internal medicine* (15th ed.). New York: McGraw-Hill.

Bullock, B. A., & Henze, R. L. (2000). *Focus on pathophysiology.* Philadelphia: Lippincott.

Copstead, L. C., & Banasik, J. L. (2000). *Pathophysiology: Biological and behavioral perspectives* (2nd ed.). Philadephia: Saunders.

Day, S. W., & Wynn, L. W. (2000). Sickle cell pain & hydroxyurea. *American Journal of Nursing, 100*(11), 34–38.

Druker, B. J., Sawyers, C. L., Capdeville, R., Ford, J. M., Baccarani, M., & Goldman, J. M. (2001). Chronic myelogenous leukemia. *Hematology (American Society of Hematology Education Program),* 87–113. Abstract from National Cancer Institute. Available: www.nci.nih.gov/cancerinformation/doc_cit.aspx?args= 22; 11722980

Fontaine, K. L. (2000). *Healing practices: Alternative therapies for nursing.* Upper Saddle River, NJ: Prentice Hall Health.

Gorman, K. (1999). Sickle cell disease. *American Journal of Nursing, 99*(3), 38–43.

Gutaj, D. (2000). Oncology today: Lymphoma. *RN, 63*(8), 32–37.

Johnson, M., Bulechek, G., Dochterman, J. M., Maas, M., & Moorhead, S. (2001). *Nursing diagnoses, outcomes, & interventions.* St. Louis: Mosby.

Johnson, M., Maas, M., & Moorhead, S. (Eds.). (2000). *Nursing outcomes classification (NOC)* (2nd ed.). St. Louis: Mosby.

Kuhn, M. A. (1999). *Complementary therapies for health care providers.* Philadelphia: Lippincott.

Lea, D. H., & Williams, J. K. (2002). Genetic testing and screening. *American Journal of Nursing, 102*(7), 36–43.

Lehne, R. A. (2001). *Pharmacology for nursing care* (4th ed.). Philadelphia: Saunders.

Malarkey, L. M., & McMorrow, M. E. (2000). *Nurse's manual of laboratory tests and diagnostic procedures* (2nd ed.). Philadelphia: Saunders.

McCance, K. L., & Huether, S. E. (2002). Pathophysiology: *The biologic basis for disease in adults & children* (4th ed.). St. Louis: Mosby.

McCloskey, J. C., & Bulechek, G. M. (Eds.) (2000). *Nursing interventions classification (NIC)* (3rd ed.). St. Louis: Mosby.

Medoff, E. (2000). Oncology today: Leukemia. *RN, 63*(9), 42–49.

Mitchell, R. (1999). AJN Clinical Snapshot. Sickle cell anemia. *American Journal of Nursing, 99*(5), 36.

National Heart, Lung, and Blood Institute, National Institutes of Health. (2002). *Morbidity & mortality: 2002 chart book of cardiovascular, lung, and blood diseases.* Bethesda, MD: Author.

Navuluri, R. (2001). Understanding hemostasis. *American Journal of Nursing, 101*(9), Hospital extra: 24B, 24C.

North American Nursing Diagnosis Association. (2001). *NANDA nursing diagnoses: Definitions & classification 2001–2002.* Philadelphia: NANDA.

Persson, L., Hallberg, I. R., & Ohlsson, O. (1997). Survivors of acute leukemia and highly malignant lymphoma—retrospective views of daily life problems during treatment and when in remission. *Journal of Advanced Nursing, 25*(1), 68–78.

Porth, C. M. (2002). *Pathophysiology: Concepts of altered health states* (6th ed.). Philadelphia: Lippincott.

Spahis, J. (2002). Human genetics: Constructing a family pedigree. *American Journal of Nursing, 102*(7), 44–49.

Spatto, G. R., & Woods, A. L. (2003). *2003 edition PDR® nurse's drug handbook.* Clifton Park, NY: Delmar.

Springhouse. (1999). *Nurse's handbook of alternative & complementary therapies.* Springhouse, PA: Author.

Thompson, K. A. (1999). Adolescent health: Detecting Hodgkin's disease. *American Journal of Nursing, 99*(5), 61–64.

Tierney, L. M., McPhee, S. J., & Papadakis, M. A. (2001). *Current medical diagnosis & treatment* (40th ed.). New York: Lange Medical Books/McGraw-Hill.

U. S. Food and Drug Administration, Center for Drug Evaluation and Research. (2001). *Drug information. Gleevec (imatinib mesylate) questions and answers.* Available: www.fda.gov/cder/drug/infopage/gleevec/qa.htm

Wilkinson, J. M. (2000). *Nursing diagnosis handbook with NIC interventions and NOC outcomes* (7th ed.). Upper Saddle River, NJ: Prentice Hall Health.

Chapter 12

Ackley, B. J., & Ladwig, G. B. (2002). *Nursing diagnosis handbook: A guide to planning care* (5th ed.). St. Louis: Mosby.

Braunwald, E., Fauci, A. S., Kasper, D. L., Hauser, S. L., Longo, D. L., & Jameson, J. L. (2001). *Harrison's principles of internal medicine* (15th ed.). New York: McGraw-Hill.

Breen, P. (2000). DVT: What every nurse should know. *RN, 63*(4), 58–62.

Chase, S. L. (2000). Hypertensive crisis. *RN, 63*(6), 62–67.

Church, V. (2000). Staying on guard for DVT & PE. *Nursing, 30*(2), 34–42.

Deglin, J. H., & Vallerand, A. H. (2003). *Davis's drug guide for nurses* (8th ed.). Philadelphia: F.A. Davis.

Ferguson, M., Cook, A., Rimmasch, H., Bender, S., & Voss, A. (2000). Pressure ulcer management: The importance of nutrition. *MEDSURG Nursing, 9*(4), 163–175.

Fontaine, K. L. (2000). *Healing practices: Alternative therapies for nursing.* Upper Saddle River, NJ: Prentice Hall Health.

Gallo, J. J., Busby-Whitehead, J., Rabins, P. V., Silliman, R. A., & Murphy, J. B. (Eds.). (1999). *Reichel's care of the elderly: Clinical aspects of aging* (5th ed.). Philadelphia: Lippincott Williams & Wilkins.

Gibson, J. M., & Kenrick, M. (1998). Pain and powerlessness: The experience of living with peripheral vascular disease. *Journal of Advanced Nursing, 27*(4), 737–745.

Hess, C. T. (2001). Putting the squeeze on venous ulcers. *Nursing, 31*(9), 58–63.

Johnson, M., Bulechek, G., Dochterman, J. M., Maas, M., & Moorhead, S. (2001). *Nursing diagnoses, outcomes, & interventions.* St. Louis: Mosby.

Johnson, M., Maas, M., & Moorhead, S. (Eds.). (2000). *Nursing outcomes classification (NOC)* (2nd ed.). St. Louis: Mosby.

Kuhn, M. A. (1999). *Complementary therapies for health care providers.* Philadelphia: Lippincott.

Lehne, R. A. (2001). *Pharmacology for nursing care* (4th ed.). Philadelphia: Saunders.

Malarkey, L. M., & McMorrow, M. E. (2000). *Nurse's manual of laboratory tests and diagnostic procedures* (2nd ed.). Philadelphia: Saunders.

McCance, K. L., & Huether, S. E. (2002). *Pathophysiology: The biologic basis for disease in adults and children* (4th ed.). St. Louis: Mosby.

McCloskey, J. C., & Bulechek, G. M. (Eds.) (2000). *Nursing interventions classification (NIC)* (3rd ed.). St. Louis: Mosby.

McConnell, E. A. (2002). Clinical do's & don'ts. Applying antiembolism stockings. *Nursing, 32*(4), 17.

Meeker, M. H., & Rothrock, J. C. (1999). *Alexander's care of the patient in surgery* (11th ed.). St. Louis: Mosby.

Miracle, V. A. (2001). Act fast during a hypertensive crisis. *Nursing, 31*(9), 50–51.

National Heart, Lung, and Blood Institute: National High Blood Pressure Education Program. (1997). *The sixth report of the Joint National Committee on Prevention, Detection, Evaluation, and Treatment of High Blood Pressure.* Bethesda, MD: National Institutes of Health.

National Heart, Lung, and Blood Institute, National Institutes of Health. (2002). *Morbidity & mortality: 2002 chart book of cardiovascular, lung, and blood diseases.* Bethesda, MD: Author.

Navuluri, R. (2001a). Anticoagulant therapy. *American Journal of Nursing, 101*(11), 24A–24D.

Navuluri, R. (2001b). Nursing implications of anticoagulant therapy. *American Journal of Nursing, 101*(12), 24A–B.

North American Nursing Diagnosis Association. (2001). *NANDA nursing diagnoses: Definitions & classification 2001–2002.* Philadelphia: NANDA.

Patel, C. T. C., Kinsey, G. C., Koperski-Moen, K. J., & Bungum, L. D. (2000). Vacuum-assisted wound closure. *American Journal of Nursing, 100*(12), 45–48.

Porth, C. M. (2002). *Pathophysiology: Concepts of altered health states* (6th ed.). Philadelphia: Lippincott.

Spratto, G. R., & Woods, A. L. (2003). *2003 edition PDR® nurse's drug handbook™*. Clifton Park, NY: Delmar Learning.

Tierney, L. M., McPhee, S. J., & Papadakis, M. A. (2001). *Current medical diagnosis & treatment* (40th ed.). New York: Lange Medical Books/McGraw-Hill.

Wipke-Tevis, D. D., Stotts, N. A., Williams, D. A., Froelicher, E. S., & Hunt, T. K. (2001). Tissue oxygenation, perfusion, and position in patients with venous leg ulcers. *Nursing Research, 50*(1), 24–32.

Woods, S. L., Froelicher, E. S. S., & Motzer, S. U. (2000). *Cardiac nursing* (4th ed.). Philadelphia: Lippincott.

Woods, A. (2002). Patient education series. High blood pressure (hypertension). *Nursing, 32*(4), 54–55.

Chapter 13

Andresen, G. (1998). Assessing the older patient. *RN, 61*(3), 46–56.

Basfield-Holland, E. (1997). Assessing pulmonary status: It's more than listening to breath sounds. *Nursing, 27*(8), 1–2, 4–9.

Connolly, M. (2001). Chest x-rays: Completing the picture. *RN, 64*(6), 56–62, 64.

Jevon, P., & Ewens, B. (2001). Assessment of a breathless patient. *Nursing Standard, 15*(16), 48–53.

Lyneham, J. (2001). Physical examination (abdomen, thorax and lungs): A review. *Australian Journal of Advanced Nursing, 18*(3), 31.

O'Hanlon-Nichols, T. (1998). Basic assessment series: The adult pulmonary system. *American Journal of Nursing, 98*(2), 39–45.

Walton, J., & Miller, J. (1998). Evaluating physical and behavioral changes in older adults. *MEDSURG Nursing, 7*(2), 85–90.

Watson, R. (2000). Assessing pulmonary function in older people. *Nursing Older People, 12*(8), 27–28.

Weber, J., & Kelley, J. (2002). *Health assessment in nursing* (2nd ed). Philadelphia: Lippincott.

Wilson, S., & Giddens, J. (2001). *Health assessment for nursing practice*. St. Louis: Mosby.

Chapter 14

Ackley, B. J., & Ladwig, G. B. (2002). *Nursing diagnosis handbook: A guide to planning care* (5th ed.). St. Louis: Mosby.

American Cancer Society. (2002a). *Cancer facts and figures 2002*. Atlanta: Author.

_____.(2002b). *Laryngeal and hypopharyngeal cancer*. Available: www.cancer.org

Atkinson, W., Wolfe, C., Humiston, S., & Nelson, R. (Eds.). (2000). *Epidemiology and prevention of vaccine-preventable diseases* (6th ed.) Atlanta: Centers for Disease Control and Prevention.

Braunwald, E., Fauci, A. S., Kasper, D. L., Hauser, S. L., Longo, D. L., & Jameson, J. L. (2001). *Harrison's principles of internal medicine* (15th ed.). New York: McGraw-Hill.

Bullock, B. A., & Henze, R. L. (2000). *Focus on pathophysiology.* Philadelphia: Lippincott.

Conn, V. (1991). Self-care actions taken by older adults for influenza and colds. *Nursing Research, 40*(3), 176–181.

Deglin, J. H., & Vallerand, A. H. (2001). *Davis's drug guide for nurses* (7th ed.). Philadelphia: F.A. Davis.

Fontaine, K. L. (2000). *Healing practices: Alternative therapies for nursing.* Upper Saddle River, NJ: Prentice Hall Health.

Hakemi, A. (2001). Diagnosing and managing rhinosinusitis. *Physician Assistant, 25*(11), 16–25.

Hughes, D. L., & Tartasky, D. (1996). Implementation of a flu immunization program for homebound elders: A graduate student practicum. *Geriatric Nursing, 17*(5), 217–221.

Johnson, M., Bulechek, G., Dochterman, J. M., Maas, M., & Moorhead, S. (2001). *Nursing diagnoses, outcomes, & interventions.* St. Louis: Mosby.

Johnson, M., Maas, M., & Moorhead, S. (Eds.). (2000). *Nursing outcomes classification (NOC)* (2nd ed.). St. Louis: Mosby.

Kearney, K. (2001). Emergency. Epiglottitis. *American Journal of Nursing, 101*(8), 37–38.

Kirchner, J. T. (1999). Manifestations of pertussis in immunized children and adults. *American Family Physician, 60*(7), 2148–2149.

Klein, L. (2001). Sinusitis: When to treat and how. *RN, 64*(1), 42–44, 46, 48.

Kuhn, M. A. (1999). *Complementary therapies for health care providers.* Philadelphia: Lippincott.

Lehne, R. A. (2001). *Pharmacology for nursing care* (4th ed.). Philadelphia: Saunders.

Loud, B. (2001). A water pick to clear sinuses? *RN, 64*(1), 48–49.

Malarkey, L. M., & McMorrow, M. E. (2000). *Nurse's manual of laboratory tests and diagnostic procedures* (2nd ed.). Philadelphia: Saunders.

Marchiondo, K. (2000). Pickwickian syndrome: The challenge of severe sleep apnea. *MEDSURG Nursing, 9*(4), 183–188.

McCloskey, J. C., & Bulechek, G. M. (Eds.). (2000). *Nursing interventions classification (NIC)* (3rd ed.). St. Louis: Mosby.

Meeker, M. H., & Rothrock, J. C. (1999). *Alexander's care of the patient in surgery* (11th ed.). St. Louis: Mosby.

Merritt, S. L. (2000). Putting sleep disorders to rest. *RN, 63*(7), 26–30.

North American Nursing Diagnosis Association. (2001). *NANDA nursing diagnoses: Definitions & classification 2001–2002.* Philadelphia: NANDA.

Porth, C. M. (2002). *Pathophysiology: Concepts of altered health states* (6th ed.). Philadelphia: Lippincott.

Seay, S. J., Gay, S. L., & Strauss, M. (2002). Emergency. Tracheostomy emergencies. *American Journal of Nursing, 102*(3), 59, 61, 63.

Shellenbarger, T., & Wolfe, S. (2000). Nosebleeds: Not just kids' stuff. *RN, 63*(2), 50–55.

Springhouse. (1999). *Nurse's handbook of alternative & complementary therapies.* Springhouse, PA: Author.

Tierney, L. M., McPhee, S. J., & Papadakis, M. A. (2001). *Current medical diagnosis & treatment* (40th ed.). New York: Lange Medical Books/McGraw-Hill.

Urden, L. D., Stacy, K. M., & Lough, M. E. (2002). *Thelan's critical care nursing: Diagnosis and management* (4th ed.). St. Louis: Mosby.

The Voice Center. (2002). Speech after a total laryngectomy. Available: www.voice-center.com/alaryngeal_speech.htm

Way, L. W., & Doherty, G. M. (2003). *Current surgical diagnosis and treatment* (11th ed.). New York: McGraw-Hill.

Whitney, E. N., & Rolfes, S. R. (2002). *Understanding nutrition* (9th ed.). Belmont, CA: Wadsworth.

Wilkinson, J. M. (2000). *Nursing diagnosis handbook with NIC interventions and NOC outcomes* (7th ed.). Upper Saddle River, NJ: Prentice Hall Health.

Yantis, M. A. (2002). Pain control. Obstructive sleep apnea syndrome. *American Journal of Nursing, 102*(6), 83, 85.

Chapter 15

Ackley, B. J., & Ladwig, G. B. (2002). *Nursing diagnosis handbook: A guide to planning care* (5th ed.). St. Louis: Mosby.

Adatsi, G. (1999). Health going up in smoke: How can you prevent it? *American Journal of Nursing, 99*(3), 63–64, 66, 67–68.

Adiutori, D. M. (2000). Primary pulmonary hypertension: A review for advanced practice nurses. *MEDSURG Nursing, 9*(5), 255–264.

American Cancer Society. (2002). *Cancer facts and figures 2002.* Atlanta: Author.

Belza, B., Steele, B. G., Hunziker, J., Lakshminaryan, S., Holt, L., & Buchner, D. M. (2001). Correlates of physical activity in chronic obstructive pulmonary disease. *Nursing Research, 50*(4), 195–202.

Braunwald, E., Fauci, A. S., Kasper, D. L., Hauser, S. L., Longo, D. L., & Jameson, J. L. (2001). *Harrison's principles of internal medicine* (15th ed.). New York: McGraw-Hill.

Carroll, P. (2000). Exploring chest drain options. *RN, 63*(10), 50–54.

Centers for Disease Control and Prevention. (2003a). *Guidelines and recommendations. Interim domestic guidance for management of exposures to severe acute respiratory syndrome (SARS) for healthcare and other institutional settings.* Author: Department of Health and Human Services.

_____. (2003b). *Guidelines and recommendations. Interim guidance on infection control precautions for patients with suspected severe acute respiratory syndrome (SARS) and close contacts in households.* Author: Department of Health and Human Services.

_____. (2003c). *Fact sheet. Basic information about SARS.* Author: Department of Health and Human Services.

Chernecky, C. (2001). Pulmonary complications in patients with cancer. *American Journal of Nursing, 101*(5), 24A, 24E, 24G–24H.

Deglin, J. H., & Vallerand, A. H. (2003). *Davis's drug guide for nurses* (8th ed.). Philadelphia: F. A. Davis.

Dest, V. (2000). Ocology today: Lung cancer. *RN, 63*(5), 32–34, 36, 38.

Dunn, N. A. (2001). Keeping COPD patients out of the ED. *RN, 64*(2), 33–37.

Evans, T. (2000). Neuromuscular blockade: When and how. *RN, 63*(5), 56–60.

Fontaine, K. L. (2000). *Healing practices: Alternative therapies for nursing.* Upper Saddle River, NJ: Prentice Hall Health.

Goldsmith, C., & Haban, M. (2002). Lung cancer: A preventable tragedy. *NurseWeek, 3*(2), 17–18.

Goodfellow, L. T., & Jones, M. (2002). Bronchial hygiene therapy. *American Journal of Nursing, 102*(1), 37–43.

Hayes, D. D. (2001). Stemming the tide of pleural effusions. *Nursing2001, 31*(5), 49–52.

Higgins, P. A. (1998). Patient perception of fatigue while undergoing long-term mechanical ventilation: Incidence and associated factors. *Heart & Lung, 27*(3), 177–183.

Johnson, M., Bulechek, G., Dochterman, J. M., Maas, M., & Moorhead, S. (2001). *Nursing diagnoses, outcomes, & interventions.* St. Louis: Mosby.

Johnson, M., Maas, M., & Moorhead, S. (Eds.). (2000). *Nursing outcomes classification (NOC)* (2nd ed.). St. Louis: Mosby.

Kuhn, M. A. (1999). *Complementary therapies for health care providers.* Philadelphia: Lippincott.

LaDuke, S. (2001). Terminal dyspnca & palliative care. *American Journal of Nursing, 101*(11), 26–31.

Lehne, R. A. (2001). *Pharmacology for nursing care* (4th ed.). Philadelphia: Saunders.

Leifer, G. (2001). Hyperbaric oxygen therapy. *American Journal of Nursing, 101*(8), 26–34.

Lenaghan, N. A. (2000). The nurse's role in smoking cessation. *MEDSURG Nursing, 9*(6), 298–302.

Little, C. (2001). What you need to know about chronic bronchitis. *Nursing2001, 31*(9), 52–55.

Malarkey, L. M., & McMorrow, M. E. (2000). *Nurse's manual of laboratory tests and diagnostic procedures* (2nd ed.). Philadelphia: Saunders.

Marion, B. S. (2001). A turn for the better: 'Prone positioning' of patients with ARDS. *American Journal of Nursing, 101*(5), 26–34.

Martin, B., Llewellyn, J., Faut-Callahan, M., & Meyer, P. (2000). The use of telemetric oximetry in the clinical setting. *MEDSURG Nursing, 9*(2), 71–76.

McCance, K. L., & Huether, S. E. (2002). *Pathophysiology: The biologic basis for disease in adults and children* (4th ed.). St. Louis: Mosby.

McCloskey, J. C., & Bulechek, G. M. (Eds.) (2000). *Nursing interventions classification (NIC)* (3rd ed.). St. Louis: Mosby.

Miracle, V., & Winston, M. (2000). Take the wind out of asthma. *Nursing2000, 30*(8), 34–41.

Morrison, C., & Lew, E. (2001). Aspergillosis. *American Journal of Nursing, 101*(8), 40–48.

National Center for HIV, STD, and TB Prevention, Division of Tuberculosis Elimination. (2002). *Surveillance reports. Reported tuberculosis in the United States 2001.* Atlanta, GA: Centers for Disease Control and Prevention.

National Heart, Lung, and Blood Institute, National Institutes of Health. (2002). *Morbidity & mortality: 2002 chart book of cardiovascular, lung, and blood diseases.* Bethesda, MD: Author.

North American Nursing Diagnosis Association. (2001). *NANDA nursing diagnoses: Definitions & classification 2001–2002.* Philadelphia: NANDA.

Owen, C. L. (1999). New directions in asthma management. *American Journal of Nursing, 99*(3), 26–33.

Persell, D. J., Arangie, P., Young, C., Stokes, E. N., Payne, W. C., Skorga, P., & Gilbert-Palmer, D. (2002). Preparing for bioterrorism. *Nursing, 32*(2), 37–43.

Pope, B. B. (2002). Patient education series. Asthma. *Nursing2002, 32*(5), 44–45.

Porth, C. M. (2002). *Pathophysiology: Concepts of altered health states* (6th ed.). Philadelphia: Lippincott.

Ruppert, R. A. (1999). The last smoke. *American Journal of Nursing, 99*(11), 26–32.

Schultz, T. R. (2002). Straight talk about community-acquired pneumonia. *Nursing2002, 32*(1), 46–49.

Sellers, K. F., Hargrove, B., & Jenkins, P. (2000). Asthma disease management programs improve clinical and economic outcomes. *MEDSURG Nursing, 9*(4), 201–203, 207.

Tierney, L. M., McPhee, S. J., & Papadakis, M. A. (2001). *Current medical diagnosis & treatment* (40th ed.). New York: Lange Medical Books/McGraw-Hill.

Trogger, D. A., & Brenner, P. S. (2001). Metered dose inhalers. *American Journal of Nursing, 101*(10), 26–32.

Trudeau, M. E., & Solano-McGuire, S. M. (1999). Evaluating the quality of COPD care. *American Journal of Nursing, 99*(3), 47–50.

Truesdell, S. (2000). Helping patients with COPD manage episodes of acute shortness of breath. *MEDSURG Nursing, 9*(4), 178–182.

Urden, L. D., Stacy, K. M., & Lough, M. E. (2002). *Thelan's critical care nursing: Diagnosis and management* (4th ed.). St. Louis: Mosby.

Way, L. W., & Doherty, G. M. (2003). *Current surgical diagnosis & treatment* (11th ed.). New York: Lange Medical Books/McGraw-Hill.

Whitney, E. N., & Rolfes, S. R. (2002). Understanding nutrition (9th ed.). Belmont, CA: Wadsworth.

Wilkinson, J. M. (2000). *Nursing diagnosis handbook with NIC interventions and NOC outcomes* (7th ed.). Upper Saddle River, NJ: Prentice Hall Health.

Woods, S. L., Froelicher, E. S. S., & Motzer, S. U. (2000). *Cardiac nursing* (4th ed.). Philadelphia: Lippincott.

World Health Organization. (2003). Cumulative number of reported probable cases of severe acute respiratory syndrome (SARS). *Communicable disease surveillance & response (CSR)*. Author.

Chapter 16

Curl, P., & Warren, J. (1997). Nutritional screening for the elderly: A CNS role. *Clinical Nurse Specialist, 11*(4), 153–158.

Evans-Stoner, N. (1997). Nutrition assessment: A practical approach. *Nursing Clinics of North America, 32*(4), 637–650.

Langan, J. (1998). Abdominal assessment in the home: From A to Zzz. *Home Healthcare Nurse, 16*(1), 50–58.

O'Hanlon-Nichols, T. (1998). Basic assessment series: The gastrointestinal system. *American Journal of Nursing, 98*(4), 48–53.

Watson, J., Miller, J., & Tordecilla, L. (2001). Elder oral assessment and care. *MEDSURG Nursing, 10*(1), 37–44.

Watson, R. (2000a). Assessing the gastrointestinal tract in older people: The lower GI tract. *Nursing Older People, 13*(1), 27–28.

_____. (2000b). Assessing the gastrointestinal tract in older people: The upper GI tract. *Nursing Older People, 12*(10), 27–28.

Weber, J., & Kelley, J. (2002). *Health assessment in nursing* (2nd ed). Philadelphia: Lippincott-Raven.

Wood, S. (1998). Nutrition assessment. *Nursing Times, 94*(29), insert 2p.

Wright, J. (1997). Seven abdominal assessment signs every emergency nurse should know. *Journal of Emergency Nursing, 23*(5), 446–450.

Chapter 17

Ackley, B. J., & Ladwig, G. B. (2002). *Nursing diagnosis handbook: A guide to planning care* (5th ed.). St. Louis: Mosby.

Ainley, H. (2001). Analysis°managing obesity. *Practice Nurse, 22*(3), 14–15.

Bender, S., Pusateri, M., Cook, A., Ferguson, M., & Hall, J. C. (2000). Malnutrition: Role of the TwoCal® HN med pass program. *MEDSURG Nursing, 9*(6), 284–295.

Braunwald, E., Fauci, A. S., Kasper, D. L., Hauser, S. L., Longo, D. L., & Jameson, J. L. (2001). *Harrison's principles of internal medicine* (15th ed.). New York: McGraw-Hill.

Bullock, B. A., & Henze, R. L. (2000). *Focus on pathophysiology.* Philadelphia: Lippincott.

Cammons, A. R., & Hackshaw, H.S. (2000). Are we starving our patients? *American Journal of Nursing, 100*(5), 43–46.

Crogan, N. L., Shultz, J. A., & Massey, L. K. (2001). Nutrition knowledge of nurses in long-term care facilties. *Journal of Continuing Education in Nursing, 32*(4), 171–176.

Deglin, J. H., & Vallerand, A. H. (2001). *Davis's drug guide for nurses* (7th ed.). Philadelphia: F.A. Davis.

Devlin, M. (2000). The nutritional needs of the older person. *Professional Nurse, 16*(3), 951–955.

Dudek, S. G. (2000). Malnutrition in hospitals: Who's assessing what patients eat? *American Journal of Nursing, 100*(4), 36–42.

Ferguson, M., Cook, A, Bender, S., Rimmasch, H., & Voss, A. (2001). Diagnosing and treating involuntary weight loss. *MEDSURG Nursing, 10*(4), 165–175.

Gallo, J. J., Busby-Whitehead, J., Rabins, P. V., Silliman, R. A., & Murphy, J. B. (Eds.). (1999). *Reichel's care of the elderly: Clinical aspects of aging* (5th ed.). Philadelphia: Lippincott Williams & Wilkins.

Green, S., & O'Kane, M. (2001). Obesity. *Practice Nurse, 22*(3), 20, 22, 24.

Jeffrey, S. (2001). The role of the nurse in obesity management. *Journal of Community Nursing, 15*(3), 20, 22, 26.

Johnson, M., Bulechek, G., Dochterman, J. M., Maas, M., & Moorhead, S. (2001). *Nursing diagnoses, outcomes, & interventions.* St. Louis: Mosby.

Ledsham, J., & Gough, A. (2000). Screening and monitoring patients for malnutrition. *Professional Nurse, 15*(11), 695–698.

Lehne, R. A. (2001). *Pharmacology for nursing care* (4th ed.). Philadelphia: Saunders.

Malarkey, L.M., & McMorrow, M.E. (2000). *Nurse's manual of laboratory tests and diagnostic procedures* (2nd ed.). Philadelphia: Saunders.

Meeker, M. H., & Rothrock, J. C. (1999). *Alexander's care of the patient in surgery* (11th ed.). St. Louis: Mosby.

Metheny, N. A., & Titler, M. G. (2001). Assessing placement of feeding tubes. *American Journal of Nursing, 101*(5), 36–45.

Metheny, N., Wehrle, M., Wiersema, L., & Clark, J. (1998). pH, color, and feeding tubes. *RN, 61*(1), 25–27.

North American Nursing Diagnosis Association. (2001). *NANDA nursing diagnoses: Definitions & classification 2001–2002.* Philadelphia: NANDA.

Nutrition. Clinical guidelines to manage malnutrition in nursing homes. (2001). *Geriatric Nursing, 22*(1), 46.

Orbanic, S. (2001). Understanding bulimia. *American Journal of Nursing, 101*(3), 35–41.

Porth, C. M. (2002). *Pathophysiology: Concepts of altered health states* (5th ed.). Philadelphia: Lippincott.

Robinson, F. (2001). Analysis: Management of excess weight in primary care. *Practice Nurse, 21*(5), 16, 19.

Saunders, C. S. (2001). Diet and nutrition in your practice. Intervening in the obesity epidemic. *Patient Care for the Nurse Practitioner, 4*(3), 12–14, 16, 18+.

Tierney, L. M., McPhee, S. J., & Papadakis, M. A. (2001). *Current medical diagnosis & treatment* (40th ed.). New York: Lange Medical Books/McGraw-Hill.

Vender, S., Pusateri, M., Cook, A., Ferguson, M., & Hall, J.C. (2000). Malnutrition: Role of the TwoCal® med pass program. *MEDSURG Nursing, 9*(6), 284–295.

Chapter 18

Ackley, B.J., & Ladwig, G. B. (2002). *Nursing diagnosis handbook: A guide to planning care* (5th ed.). St. Louis: Mosby.

Ahya, S. N., Flood, K., & Paranjothi, S. (Eds.). (2001). *The Washington manual of medical therapeutics* (30th ed.). Philadelphia: Lippincott Williams & Wilkins.

Braunwald, E., Fauci, A. S., Kasper, D. L., Hauser, S. L., Longo, D. L., & Jameson, J. L. (2001). *Harrison's principles of internal medicine* (15th ed.). New York: McGraw-Hill.

Brooks-Brunn, J. A. (2000). Esophageal cancer: An overview. *MEDSURG Nursing, 9*(5), 248–254.

Bullock, B. A., & Henze, R. L. (2000). *Focus on pathophysiology.* Philadelphia: Lippincott.

Chait, M. M. (2000). The many complications of gastroesophageal reflux disease. *Home Health Care Consultant, 7*(1), 25–27.

Edwards, S. J., & Metheny, N. A. (2000). Measurement of gastric residual volume: State of the science. *MEDSURG Nursing, 9*(3), 125–128.

Gallo, J. J., Busby-Whitehead, J., Rabins, P. V., Silliman, R. A., & Murphy, J. B. (Eds.). (1999). *Reichel's care of the elderly: Clinical aspects of aging* (5th ed.). Philadelphia: Lippincott Williams & Wilkins.

Galvin, T. J. (2001). Dysphagia: Going down and staying down. *American Journal of Nursing, 101*(1), 37–42.

Johnson, M., Bulechek, G., Dochterman, J. M., Maas, M., & Moorhead, S. (2001). *Nursing diagnoses, outcomes, & interventions.* St. Louis: Mosby.

Malarkey, L. M., & McMorrow, M. E. (2000). *Nurse's manual of laboratory tests and diagnostic procedures* (2nd ed.). Philadelphia: Saunders.

Mattonen, M. C. (2001). Managing heartburn in adults. *MEDSURG Nursing, 10*(5), 269–276.

McManus, T. J. (2000). *Helicobacter pylori.* An emerging infectious disease. *Nurse Practitioner,* 25(8), 40, 43–44, 47–48+

Meeker, M. H., & Rothrock, J. C. (1999). *Alexander's care of the patient in surgery* (11th ed.). St. Louis: Mosby.

Metheny, N. A., & Titler, M. G. (2001). Assessing placement of feeding tubes. *American Journal of Nursing, 101*(5), 36–45.

North American Nursing Diagnosis Association. (2001). *NANDA Nursing diagnoses: Definitions & classification 2001–2002.* Philadelphia: NANDA.

Porth, C. M. (2002). *Pathophysiology: Concepts of altered health states* (6th ed.). Philadelphia: Lippincott.

Resto, M. A. (2000). Hospital extra. Gastroesophageal reflux disease. *American Journal of Nursing, 100*(9), 24D, 24F, 24H.

Terrado, M., Russell, C., & Bowman, J. B. (2001). Dysphagia: An overview. *MEDSURG Nursing, 10*(5), 233–248.

Tierney, L. M., McPhee, S. J., & Papadakis, M. A. (2001). *Current medical diagnosis & treatment* (40th ed.). New York: Lange Medical Books/McGraw-Hill.

Walton, J. C., Miller, J., & Tordecilla, L. (2001). Elder oral assessment and care. *MEDSURG Nursing, 10*(1), 37–44.

Wilkinson, J. M. (2000). *Nursing diagnosis handbook with NIC interventions and NOC outcomes* (7th ed.). Upper Saddle River, NJ: Prentice Hall Health.

Chapter 19

Ackley, B.J., & Ladwig, G. B. (2002). *Nursing diagnosis handbook: A guide to planning care* (5th ed.). St. Louis: Mosby.

American Cancer Society. (2002). *Cancer facts and figures 2002.* Atlanta: Author.

Atkinson, W., Wolfe, C., Humiston, S., & Nelson, R. (Eds.). (2000). *Epidemiology and prevention of vaccine-preventable diseases* (6th ed.). Atlanta: Centers for Disease Control.

Bockhold, K. M. (2000). Who's afraid of hepatitis C? *American Journal of Nursing, 100*(5), 26–31.

Braunwald, E., Fauci, A. S., Kasper, D. L., Hauser, S. L., Longo, D. L., & Jameson, J. L. (2001). *Harrison's principles of internal medicine* (15th ed.). New York: McGraw-Hill.

Bullock, B. A., & Henze, R. L. (2000). *Focus on pathophysiology.* Philadelphia: Lippincott.

Cole, L. (2001). Acute pancreatitis. *Nursing, 31*(12), 58–63.

Deglin, J. H., & Vallerand, A. H. (2001). *Davis's drug guide for nurses* (7th ed.). Philadelphia: F.A. Davis.

Dill, B., Dill, J. E., Berkhouse, L., & Palmer, S. T. (1999). Endoscopic ultrasound for chronic abdominal pain and gallbladder disease. *Gastroenterology Nursing, 22*(5), 209–212.

Dougherty, A. S., & Dreher, H. M. (2001). Hepatitis C: Current treatment strategies for an emerging epidemic. *MEDSURG Nursing, 10*(1), 9–13.

Farrar, J. A. (2001). Emergency! Acute cholecystitis. *American Journal of Nursing, 101*(1), 35–36.

Fontaine, K. L. (2000). *Healing practices: Alternative therapies for nursing.* Upper Saddle River, NJ: Prentice Hall Health.

Hession, M. C. (1998). Factors influencing successful discharge after outpatient laparoscopic sholecystectomy. *Journal of Perianesthesia Nursing, 13*(1), 11–15.

Johnson, M., Bulechek, G., Dochterman, J. M., Maas, M., & Moorhead, S. (2001). *Nursing diagnoses, outcomes, & interventions.* St. Louis: Mosby.

Johnson, M., Maas, M., & Moorhead, S. (Eds.). (2000). *Nursing outcomes classification (NOC)* (2nd ed.). St. Louis: Mosby.

Klainberg, M. (1999). Primary biliary cirrhosis. *American Journal of Nursing, 99*(12), 38–39.

Kuhn, M. A. (1999). *Complementary therapies for health care providers.* Philadelphia: Lippincott.

Lehne, R. A. (2001). *Pharmacology for nursing care* (4th ed.). Philadelphia: Saunders.

Malarkey, L. M., & McMorrow, M. E. (2000). *Nurse's manual of laboratory tests and diagnostic procedures* (2nd ed.). Philadelphia: Saunders.

Marx, J. F. (1998). Understanding the varieties of viral hepatitis. *Nursing, 28*(7), 43–49.

McCloskey, J. C., & Bulechek, G. M. (Eds.). (2000). *Nursing interventions classification (NIC)* (3rd ed.). St. Louis: Mosby.

Meeker, M. H., & Rothrock, J. C. (1999). *Alexander's care of the patient in surgery* (11th ed.). St. Louis: Mosby.

North American Nursing Diagnosis Association. (2001). *NANDA nursing diagnoses: Definitions & classification 2001–2002.* Philadelphia: NANDA.

Porth, C. M. (2002). *Pathophysiology: Concepts of altered health states* (6th ed.). Philadelphia: Lippincott.

Savage, R. B., Hussey, M. J., & Hurie, M. B. (2000). A successful approach to immunizing men who have sex with men against hepatitis B. *Public Health Nursing, 17*(3), 202–206.

Shovein, J. T., Damazo, R. J., & Hyams, I. (2000). Hepatitis A: How benign is it? *American Journal of Nursing, 100*(3), 43–47.

Springhouse. (1999). *Nurse's handbook of alternative & complementary therapies.* Springhouse, PA: Author.

Thorn, K. (1999). Hepatitis C: The lurking dragon. *Case Manager, 10*(4), 55–62.

Tierney, L. M., McPhee, S. J., & Papadakis, M. A. (2001). *Current medical diagnosis & treatment* (40th ed.). New York: Lange Medical Books/McGraw-Hill.

Urden, L. D., Stacy, K. M., & Lough, M. E. (2002). *Thelan's critical care nursing: Diagnosis and management* (4th ed.). St. Louis: Mosby

Wilkinson, J. M. (2000). *Nursing diagnosis handbook with NIC interventions and NOC outcomes* (7th ed.). Upper Saddle River, NJ: Prentice Hall Health.

Williamson, L. (1998). Self-destruction in the pancreas. *Nursing Times, 94*(29), 57–59.

Wrobleski, D. M., Barth, M. M., & Oyen, L. J. (1999). Necrotizing pancreatitis: Pathophysiology, diagnosis, and acute care management. *AACN Clinical Issues, 10*(4), 464–477.

Chapter 20

Dammel, T. (1997). Fecal occult-blood testing: Looking for hidden danger. *Nursing97, 27*(7), 44–45.

Goff, K. (1997). Assessment of the gastrointestinal tract. *Support Line, 19*(2), 3–7.

Hall, G., Karstens, M., Rakel, B., Swanson, E., & Davidson, A. (1995). Managing constipation using a research-based protocol. *MEDSURG Nursing, 4*(1), 11–18.

Langan, J. (1998). Abdominal assessment in the home: From A to Zzz. *Home Healthcare Nurse, 16*(1), 50–58.

Lyneham, J. (2001). Physical examination (abdomen, thorax and lungs): A review. *Australian Journal of Advanced Nursing, 18*(3), 31.

Watson, R. (2001). Assessing the gastrointestinal tract in older people. 2: The lower GI tract. *Nursing Older People, 13*(1), 27–28.

Weber, J., & Kelley, J. (2002). *Health assessment in nursing* (2nd ed.). Philadelphia: Lippincott.

Wilson, S., & Giddens, J. (2001). *Health assessment for nursing practice* (2nd ed.). St. Louis: Mosby.

Wright, J. (1997). Seven abdominal assessment signs every emergency nurse should know. *Journal of Emergency Nursing, 23*(5), 446–450.

Chapter 21

Ackley, B.J., & Ladwig, G. B. (2002). *Nursing diagnosis handbook: A guide to planning care* (5th ed.). St. Louis: Mosby.

American Cancer Society. (2002). *Cancer reference information: What are the key statistics for colon and rectum cancer?* Available http://www.cancer.org

Bailey, C. (2001). Focus. Older patients' experiences of pre-treatment discussions: An analysis of qualitative data from a study of colorectal cancer. *NT Research, 6*(4), 736–746.

Baker, D. (2001). Current surgical management of colorectal cancer. *Nursing Clinics of North America, 36*(3), 579–592.

Ball, E. M. (2000). Ostomy guide, part two. A teaching guide for continent ileostomy. *RN, 63*(12), 35–36, 38, 40.

Bliss, D. Z., Jung, H., Savik, K., Lowry, A., LeMoine, M., Jensen, L., Werner, C., & Schaffer, K. (2001). Supplementation with dietary fiber improves fecal incontinence. *Nursing Research, 50*(4), 203–213.

Braunwald, E., Fauci, A. S., Kasper, D. L., Hauser, S. L., Longo, D. L., & Jameson, J. L. (2001). *Harrison's principles of internal medicine* (15th ed.). New York: McGraw-Hill.

Breeze, J. (2001). Colorectal cancer. *Nursing Times, 97*(11), 39–41.

Bullock, B. A., & Henze, R. L. (2000). *Focus on pathophysiology.* Philadelphia: Lippincott.

Burger, E. T. (2001). Preparing adult patients for international travel. *Nurse Practitioner: American Journal of Primary Health Care, 26*(5), 13–15, 19–25.

Cox, J. A., Rogers, M. A., & Cox, S. D. (2001). Treating benign colon disorders using laparoscopic colectomy. *AORN Journal, 73*(2), 375, 377–380, 382+.

Deglin, J. H., & Vallerand, A. H. (2001). *Davis's drug guide for nurses* (7th ed.). Philadelphia: F.A. Davis.

Dest, V. M. (2000). Oncology today: New horizons. Colorectal cancer. *RN, 63*(3), 53–59.

Erwin-Toth, P. (2001). Caring for a stoma is more than skin deep. *Nursing, 31*(5), 36–40.

Fontaine, K. L. (2000). *Healing practices: Alternative therapies for nursing.* Upper Saddle River, NJ: Prentice Hall Health.

Gallo, J. J., Busby-Whitehead, J., Rabins, P. V., Silliman, R. A., & Murphy, J. B. (Eds.). (1999). *Reichel's care of the elderly: Clinical aspects of aging* (5th ed.). Philadelphia: Lippincott Williams & Wilkins.

Gauf, C. L. (2000). Diagnosing appendicitis across the life span. *Journal of the American Academy of Nurse Practitioners, 12*(4), 129–133.

Heuschkel, R., Afzal, N., Wuerth, A., Zurakowski, D., Leichtner, A., Kemper, K., & Tolia, V. (2002). Complementary medicine use in children and young adults with inflammatory bowel disease. *American Journal of Gastroenterology, 97*(2), 382–388.

Jenks, J. M., Morin, K. H., & Tomaselli, N. (1997). The influence of ostomy surgery on body image in patients with cancer. *Applied Nursing Research, 10*(4), 174–180.

Joachim, G. (2000). Responses of people with inflammatory bowel disease to foods consumed. *Gastroenterology Nursing, 23*(4), 160–167.

Johnson, M., Bulechek, G., Dochterman, J. M., Maas, M., & Moorhead, S. (2001). *Nursing diagnoses, outcomes, & interventions.* St. Louis: Mosby.

Johnson, M., Maas, M., & Moorhead, S. (Eds.). (2000). *Nursing outcomes classification (NOC)* (2nd ed.). St. Louis: Mosby.

Kinney, A. Y., Choi, Y., DeVellis, B., Millikan, R., Kobetz, E., & Sandler, R. S. (2000). Attitudes toward genetic testing in patients with colorectal cancer. *Cancer Practice: A Multidisciplinary Journal of Cancer Care, 8*(4), 178–186.

Kuhn, M. A. (1999). *Complementary therapies for health care providers.* Philadelphia: Lippincott.

Langmead, L., Dawson, C., Hawkins, C., Banna, N., Loo, S., & Rampton, D. S. (2002). Antioxidant effects of herbal therapies used by patients with inflammatory bowel disease: An in vitro study. *Alimentary Pharmacologic Therapy, 16*(2), 197–205.

Lehne, R. A. (2001). *Pharmacology for nursing care* (4th ed.). Philadelphia: Saunders.

Levine, C. D. (1999). Toxic megacolon: Diagnosis and treatment challenges. *AACN Clinical Issues: Advanced Practice in Acute and Critical Care, 10*(4), 492–499.

Lord, L. M., Schaffner, R., DeCross, A. J., & Sax, H. C. (2000). Management of the patient with short bowel syndrome. *AACN Clinical Issues: Advanced Practice in Acute and Critical Care, 11*(4), 604–618.

Malarkey, L.M., & McMorrow, M.E. (2000). *Nurse's manual of laboratory tests and diagnostic procedures* (2nd ed.). Philadelphia: Saunders.

Mason, I. (2001). Inflammatory bowel disease. *Nursing Times, 97*(9), 33–35.

McCloskey, J. C., & Bulechek, G. M. (Eds.) (2000). *Nursing interventions classification (NIC)* (3rd ed.). St. Louis: Mosby.

McConnell, E. A. (2001). Appendicitis: What a pain! *Nursing, 31*(8), 32hn1–3.

_____. (2001). What's behind intestinal obstruction? *Nursing, 31*(10), 58–63.

Meeker, M. H., & Rothrock, J. C. (1999). *Alexander's care of the patient in surgery* (11th ed.). St. Louis: Mosby.

North American Nursing Diagnosis Association. (2001). *NANDA nursing diagnoses: Definitions & classification 2001–2002.* Philadelphia: NANDA.

Olson, S. J., & Zawacki, K. (2000). Hereditary colorectal cancer. *Nursing Clinics of North America, 35*(3), 671–685.

Pontieri-Lewis, V. (2000). Colorectal cancer: Prevention and screening. *MEDSURG Nursing, 9*(1), 9–15, 20.

Porth, C. M. (2002). *Pathophysiology: Concepts of altered health states* (6th ed.). Philadelphia: Lippincott.

Rankin-Box, D. (2000). An alternative approach to bowel disorders. *Nursing Times, 96*(19), NT-plus 24, 26.

Rayhorn, N. (1999). Understanding inflammatory bowel disease. *Nursing, 29*(12), 57–61.

Sercombe, J. (2000). Inflammatory bowel disease and smoking. *Professional Nurse, 15*(7), 439–442.

_____. (2001). Surgical therapy for inflammatory bowel disease. *Nursing Times, 97*(10), 34–36.

Shepherd, M. (2000). Treating diarrhea and constipation. *Nursing Times, 96*(6), NTplus 15–16.

Tierney, L. M., McPhee, S. J., & Papadakis, M. A. (2001). *Current medical diagnosis & treatment* (40th ed.). New York: Lange Medical Books/McGraw-Hill.

Verhoef, M. J., Rapchuk, I., Liew, T., Weir, V., & Hilsden, R. J. (2002). Complementary practitioners' views of treatment for inflammatory bowel disease. *Canadian Journal of Gastroenterology, 16*(2), 95–100.

Whitney, E. N., & Rolfes, S. R. (2002). *Understanding nutrition* (9th ed.). Belmont, CA: Wadsworth.

Wilkinson, J. M. (2000). *Nursing diagnosis handbook with NIC interventions and NOC outcomes* (7th ed.). Upper Saddle River, NJ: Prentice Hall Health.

Wood, M. C., & Ryan, C. T. (2000). Patient resources. Resources on colorectal cancer for patients. *Cancer Practice: A Multidisciplinary Journal of Cancer Care, 8*(6), 308–310.

Young, M. (2000). Caring for patients with coloanal reservoirs for rectal cancer. *MEDSURG Nursing, 9*(4), 193–197.

Chapter 22

Bevan, M. (2001). Assessing renal function in older people. *Nursing Older People, 13*(2), 27–28.

Criner, J. (2001). Urinary incontinence in a vulnerable population: Older women. *Seminars in Perioperative Nursing, 10*(1), 33–37.

Edwards, S. (2000). Fluid overload and monitoring indices. *Professional Nurse, 15*(9), 568–572.

Godfrey, K. (1997). Continence: Incontinence in ethnic groups. *Community Nurse, 3*(5), 42.

Gray, M. (2000). Urinary retention. Management in the acute care setting. *American Journal of Nursing, 100*(7), 40–47.

Irwin, B. (2001). Incontinence. *Practice Nurse, 22*(4), 31–32, 43.

Johnson, S. (2000). From incontinence to confidence. *American Journal of Nursing, 100*(2), 69–76.

Kirton, C. (1997). Assessing for bladder distention. *Nursing97, 27*(4), 64.

Lyneham, J. (2001). Physical examination (abdomen, thorax, and lungs): A review. *Australian Journal of Advanced Nursing, 18*(3), 31.

Sheppard, M. (2001). Assessing fluid balance. *Nursing Times, 97* (6 Ntplus), XI–XII.

Weber, J., & Kelley, J. (2002). *Health assessment in nursing.* (2nd ed.). Philadelphia: Lippincott.

Wilson, S., & Giddens, J. (2001). *Health assessment for nursing practice.* St. Louis: Mosby.

Chapter 23

Ackley, B. J., & Ladwig, G. B. (2002). *Nursing diagnosis handbook: A guide to planning care* (5th ed.). St. Louis: Mosby.

Ahya, S. N., Flood, K., & Paranjothi, S. (Eds.). (2001). *The Washington manual of medical therapeutics* (30th ed.). Philadelphia: Lippincott Williams & Wilkins.

American Cancer Society. (2002). *Cancer facts and figures 2002.* Atlanta: Author.

Bardsley, A. (1999). Assessment of incontinence. *Elder Care, 11*(9), 36–39.

Baxter, A. (1999). Bladder cancer: Its diagnosis and treatment. *Nursing Times, 95*(41), 42–44.

Braunwald, E., Fauci, A. S., Kasper, D. L., Hauser, S. L., Longo, D. L., & Jameson, J. L. (2001). *Harrison's principles of internal medicine* (15th ed.). New York: McGraw-Hill.

Bullock, B. A., & Henze, R. L. (2000). *Focus on pathophysiology.* Philadelphia: Lippincott.

Fontaine, K. L. (2000). *Healing practices: Alternative therapies for nursing.* Upper Saddle River, NJ: Prentice Hall Health.

Gallo, J. J., Busby-Whitehead, J., Rabins, P. V., Silliman, R. A., & Murphy, J. B. (Eds.). (1999). *Reichel's care of the elderly: Clinical aspects of aging* (5th ed.). Philadelphia: Lippincott Williams & Wilkins.

Gray, M. (2000a). Urinary retention: Management in the acute care setting. Part 1. *American Journal of Nursing, 100*(7), 40–47.

_____. (2000b). Urinary retention: Management in the acute care setting. Part 2. *American Journal of Nursing, 100*(8), 36–43.

Gray, M., McClain, R., Peruggia, M., Patrie, J., & Steers, W. D. (2001). A model for predicting motor urge urinary incontinence. *Nursing Research, 50*(2), 116–122.

Hanchett, M. (2002). Techniques for stabilizing urinary catheters. *American Journal of Nursing, 102*(3), 44–48.

Johnson, M., Bulechek, G., Dochterman, J. M., Maas, M., & Moorhead, S. (2001). *Nursing diagnoses, outcomes, & interventions.* St. Louis: Mosby.

Johnson, M., Maas, M., & Moorhead, S. (Eds.). (2000). *Nursing outcomes classification (NOC)* (2nd ed.). St. Louis: Mosby.

Johnson, S. T. (2000). From incontinence to confidence. *American Journal of Nursing, 100*(2), 69–70, 72–75.

Lekan-Rutledge, D. (2000). Diffusion of innovation. A model for implementation of prompted voiding in long-term care settings. *Journal of Gerontology Nursing, 26*(4), 25–33.

Lyons, S. S., & Specht, J. K. (2000). Prompted voiding protocol for individuals with urinary incontinence. *Journal of Gerontology Nursing, 26*(6), 5–13.

Malarkey, L.M., & McMorrow, M.E. (2000). *Nurse's manual of laboratory tests and diagnostic procedures* (2nd ed.). Philadelphia: Saunders.

Maloney, C., & Cafiero, M. R. (1999). Urinary incontinence. Noninvasive treatment options. *Advance for Nurse Practitioners, 7*(6), 36–42.

McCloskey, J. C., & Bulechek, G. M. (Eds.) (2000). *Nursing interventions classification (NIC)* (3rd ed.). St. Louis: Mosby.

McConnell, E. A. (2001). Myths & facts ... about kidney stones. *Nursing, 31*(1), 73.

Meeker, M. H., & Rothrock, J. C. (1999). *Alexander's care of the patient in surgery* (11th ed.). St. Louis: Mosby.

National Kidney and Urologic Diseases Information Clearinghouse. (1998). *Urinary incontinence in women.* National Institute of Diabetes and Digestive and Kidney Diseases (NIDDK), National Institutes of Health. Available www.niddk.nih.gov/health/urolog/pubs/uiwomen/uiwomen.htm

Nicolle, L. E. (2001). Urinary tract infections in long-term care facilities. *Infections Control & Hospital Epidemiology, 22*(3), 167–175.

North American Nursing Diagnosis Association. (2001). *NANDA nursing diagnoses: Definitions & classification 2001–2002.* Philadelphia: NANDA.

Porth, C. M. (2002). *Pathophysiology: Concepts of altered health states* (6th ed.). Philadelphia: Lippincott.

Prieto-Fingerhut, T., Banovac, K., & Lynne, C. M. (1997). A study comparing sterile and nonsterile urethral catheterization in patients with spinal cord injury. *Rehabilitation Nursing, 22*(6), 299–302.

Ratliff, C. R., & Donovan, A. M. (2001). Frequency of peristomal complications. *Ostomy & Wound Management, 47*(8), 26–29.

Springhouse. (1999). *Nurse's handbook of alternative & complementary therapies.* Springhouse, PA: Author.

Suchinski, G. A., Piano, M. R., Rosenberg, N., & Zerwic, J. J. (1999). Treating urinary tract infections in the elderly. *Dimensions of Critical Care Nursing, 18*(1), 21–27.

Tierney, L. M., McPhee, S. J., & Papadakis, M. A. (2001). *Current medical diagnosis & treatment* (40th ed.). New York: Lange Medical Books/McGraw-Hill.

Vinsnes, A. G., Harkless, G. E., Haltbakk, J., Bohm, J., & Hunskaar, S. (2001). Healthcare personnel's attitudes towards patients with urinary incontinence. *Journal of Clinical Nursing, 10*(4), 455–462.

Young. J. (2000). Action stat. Kidney stone. *Nursing, 30*(7), 33.

Chapter 24

Ackley, B. J., & Ladwig, G. B. (2002). *Nursing diagnosis handbook: A guide to planning care* (5th ed.). St. Louis: Mosby.

American Cancer Society. (2002). *Cancer facts and figures 2002.* Atlanta: Author.

Bartucci, M. R. (1999). Kidney transplantation: State of the art. *AACN Clinical Issues: Advanced Practice in Acute and Critical Care, 10*(2), 153–163.

Braunwald, E., Fauci, A. S., Kasper, D. L., Hauser, S. L., Longo, D. L., & Jameson, J. L. (2001). *Harrison's principles of internal medicine* (15th ed.). New York: McGraw-Hill.

Bullock, B. A., & Henze, R. L. (2000). *Focus on pathophysiology.* Philadelphia: Lippincott.

Deglin, J. H., & Vallerand, A. H. (2001). *Davis's drug guide for nurses* (7th ed.). Philadelphia: F.A. Davis.

Fontaine, K. L. (2000). *Healing practices: Alternative therapies for nursing.* Upper Saddle River, NJ: Prentice Hall Health.

Fox, H. L., & Swann, D. (2001). Goodpasture syndrome: Pathophysiology, diagnosis, and management. *Nephrology Nursing Journal, 28*(3), 305–312.

Gallo, J. J., Busby-Whitehead, J., Rabins, P. V., Silliman, R. A., & Murphy, J. B. (Eds.). (1999). *Reichel's care of the elderly: Clinical aspects of aging* (5th ed.). Philadelphia: Lippincott Williams & Wilkins.

Hagren, B., Pettersen, I. M., Severinsson, E., Lutzen, K., & Clyne, N. (2001). The haemodialysis machine as a lifeline: Experiences of suffering from end-stage renal disease. *Journal of Advanced Nursing, 34*(2), 196–202.

Hayes, D. D. (2000). Caring for your patient with a permanent hemodialysis access. *Nursing, 30*(3), 41–46.

Johnson, M., Bulechek, G., Dochterman, J. M., Maas, M., & Moorhead, S. (2001). *Nursing diagnoses, outcomes, & interventions.* St. Louis: Mosby.

Johnson, M., Maas, M., & Moorhead, S. (Eds.). (2000). *Nursing outcomes classification (NOC)* (2nd ed.). St. Louis: Mosby.

King, B. (2000). Meds and the dialysis patient. *RN, 63*(7), 54–59.

Kostadaras, A. (2001). Erythropoietin for the anemia of chronic renal failure. *Home Health Care Consultant, 8*(7), 27–31.

Lang, M. M., & Towers, C. (2001). Identifying poststreptococcal glomerulonephritis. *Nurse Practitioner: American Journal of Primary Health Care, 26*(8), 34, 37–38, 40–42+.

Lehne, R. A. (2001). *Pharmacology for nursing care* (4th ed.). Philadelphia: Saunders.

Little, C. (2000). Renovascular hypertension. *American Journal of Nursing, 100*(2), 46–51.

Mackenzie, D. L. (1999). When *E. coli* turns deadly. *RN, 62*(7), 28–31.

Malarkey, L. M., & McMorrow, M. E. (2000). *Nurse's manual of laboratory tests and diagnostic procedures* (2nd ed.). Philadelphia: Saunders.

Mallick, N., & El Marasi, A. (1999). Chronic renal failure. *Care of the Critically Ill, 15*(3), 80, 82–84.

McCann, K., & Boore, J. R. (2000). Fatigue in persons with renal failure who require maintenance haemodialysis. *Journal of Advanced Nursing, 32*(5), 1132–1142.

McCloskey, J. C., & Bulechek, G. M. (Eds.) (2000). *Nursing interventions classification (NIC)* (3rd ed.). St. Louis: Mosby.

Meeker, M. H., & Rothrock, J. C. (1999). *Alexander's care of the patient in surgery* (11th ed.). St. Louis: Mosby.

Meister, J., & Reddy, K. (2002). Rhabdomyolysis: An overview. *American Journal of Nursing, 102*(2), 75, 77, 79.

Myhre, M. J. (2000). Herbal remedies, nephropathies, and renal disease. *Nephrology Nursing Journal, 27*(5), 473–480.

National Kidney and Urologic Diseases Information Clearinghouse. (2001). *Kidney and urologic disease statistics for the United States.* NIH Publication No. 02-3895. Available www.niddk.nih.gov/health/kidney/pubs/kustats

North American Nursing Diagnosis Association. (2001). *NANDA Nursing diagnoses: Definitions & classification 2001–2002.* Philadelphia: NANDA.

Porth, C. M. (2002). *Pathophysiology: Concepts of altered health states* (6th ed.). Philadelphia: Lippincott.

Ross, C. A. (2000). Emergency. Dialysis disequilibrium syndrome. *American Journal of Nursing, 100*(2), 53–54.

Schmelzer, M., & Stam, M. A. (2000). A hidden menace: Hemolytic uremic syndrome. *American Journal of Nursing, 100*(11), 26–32.

Seaton-Mills, D. (1999). Acute renal failure: Causes and considerations in the critically ill patient. *Nursing in Critical Care, 4*(6), 293–297.

Sprauve, D. (2000). Understanding chronic renal failure. *Nursing, 30*(4), Hosp Nurs 32hn12, 32hn14.

Tierney, L. M., McPhee, S. J., & Papadakis, M. A. (2001). *Current medical diagnosis & treatment* (40th ed.). New York: Lange Medical Books/McGraw-Hill.

United Network for Organ Sharing. (2002a). *All about UNOS.* Available www.unos.org/Newsroom/allabout_main.htm

———. (2002b). *Critical data. U. S. facts about transplantation.* Available www.unos.org/Newsroom/critdata_main.htm

———. (2002c). *Living donation outpaces cadaveric in 2001.* Available www.unos.org/Newsroom/archive_story_20020426_2001donornumbers.htm

Urden, L. D., Stacy, K. M., & Lough, M. E. (2002). *Thelan's critical care nursing: Diagnosis and management* (4th ed.). St. Louis: Mosby.

U. S. Renal Data System. (2001). *USRDS 2001 annual data report: Atlas of end-stage renal disease in the United States.* Bethesda, MD: National Institute of Diabetes and Digestive and Kidney Diseases (NIDDK).

Welch, J. L., & Davis, J. (2000). Self-care strategies to reduce fluid intake and control thirst in hemodialysis patients. *Nephrology Nursing Journal, 27*(4), 393–395.

Whitney, E. N., & Rolfes, S. R. (2002). *Understanding nutrition* (9th ed.). Belmont, CA: Wadsworth.

Wise, L. C., Mersch, J., Racioppi, J., Crosier, J., & Thompson, C. (2000). Evaluating the reliability and utility of cumulative intake and output. *Journal of Nursing Care Quality, 14*(3), 37–42.

Wallace, L. S. (2001). Rhabdomyolysis: A case study *Medsurg Nursing, 10*(3), 113–120.

Chapter 25

Andresen, G. (1998). Assessing the older patient. *RN, 61*(3), 46–56.

Loriaux, T. (1996). Endocrine assessment: Red flags for those on the front line. *Nursing Clinics of North America, 31*(4), 695–713.

Rusterholtz, A. (1996). Interpretation of diagnostic laboratory tests in selected endocrine disorders. *Nursing Clinics of North America, 31*(4), 715–724.

Watson, R. (2001). Assessing endocrine system function in older people. *Nursing Older People, 12*(9), 27–28.

Weber, J., & Kelley, J. (2002). *Health assessment in nursing* (2nd ed.). Philadelphia: Lippincott-Raven.

Wilson, S., & Giddens, J. (2001). *Health assessment for nursing practice.* St. Louis: Mosby.

Winger, J., & Hornick, T. (1996). Age-associated changes in the endocrine system. *Nursing Clinics of North America, 31*(4), 827–844.

Chapter 26

American Cancer Society. (2002). *Cancer facts & figures.* New York: American Cancer Society.

Burton, M. (1997). Emergency! Pheochromocytoma. *American Journal of Nursing, 97*(11), 57.

Clayton, L., & Dilley, K. (1998). Cushing's syndrome. *American Journal of Nursing, 98*(7), 40–41.

Cooper, D. S. (Ed.). (2001). *Medical management of thyroid disease.* New York: Marcel Dekker, Inc.

Gumowski, J., & Loughran, M. (1996). Disease of the adrenal gland. *Nursing Clinics of North America, 31*(4), 747–768.

Johnson, M., & Maas, M. (Eds.). (1997). *Nursing outcomes classification (NOC).* St. Louis: Mosby.

Kee, J. (2001). *Handbook of laboratory and diagnostic tests with nursing implications* (4th ed.). Upper Saddle River, NJ: Prentice Hall.

McCloskey, J., & Bulechek, G. (Eds.). (2000). *Iowa intervention project: Nursing interventions classification (NIC)* (3rd ed.). St. Louis: Mosby.

McKenry, L., & Salerno, E. (1998). *Pharmacology in nursing* (20th ed.). St. Louis: Mosby.

McPhee, S., Lingappa, V., Ganong, W., & Lange, J. (2000). *Pathophysiology of disease: An introduction to clinical medicine.* New York: Appleton & Lange.

Mead, M. (2000). Thyroid function tests. *Practice Nurse, 19*(6), 283.

New guidelines for detecting thyroid dysfunction. (2000). *Consultant, 40*(9), 1676.

North American Nursing Diagnosis Association. (2001). *Nursing diagnoses: Definitions & classification 2001–2002.* Philadelphia: NANDA.

O'Donnell, M. (1997). Emergency! Addisonian crisis. *American Journal of Nursing, 97*(3), 41.

Porth, C. (2002). *Pathophysiology: Concepts of altered health states* (6th ed.). Philadelphia: Lippincott.

Romeo, J. (1996). Hyperfunction and hypofunction of the anterior pituitary. *Nursing Clinics of North America, 31*(4), 769–778.

Sabol, V. (2001). Addisonian crisis: This life-threatening condition may be triggered by a variety of stressors. *American Journal of Nursing, 101*(7, Advanced Practice Extra), 24AAA, 24CCC–DDD.

Sache, D. (2001). Acromegaly. *American Journal of Nursing, 101*(11), 69, 71, 73–75, 77.

Schilling, J. (1997). Hyperthyroidism: Diagnosis and management of Graves' disease. *Nurse Practitioner, 22*(6), 72, 74–75, 78.

Shannon, M., Wilson, B., & Stang, C. (2002). *Health professional's drug guide 2002.* Upper Saddle River, NJ: Prentice Hall.

Sheppard, M. (2001). Assessing fluid balance. *Nursing Times, 97*(6 Ntplus), XI–XII.

Terpstra, T., & Terpstra, T. L. (2000). Syndrome of inappropriate antidiuretic hormone secretion: Recognition and management. *MEDSURG Nursing, 9*(2), 61–70.

Thyroid disorders and women's health. (2000). *National women's health report, 22*(5), 1–2, 4–6.

Tierney, L., McPhee, S., & Papadakis, M. (Eds.). (2001). *Current medical diagnosis & treatment* (40th ed.). Stamford, CT: Appleton & Lange.

Tiesinga, L., Dassen, T., & Halfens, R. (1996). Fatigue: A summary of the definitions, dimensions, and indicators. *Nursing Diagnosis, 7*(2), 51–62.

Trotto, N. (1999). Hypothyroidism, hyperthyroidism, hyperparathyroidism. *Patient Care, 33*(14), 186–188, 191, 195–200.

Wartofsky, L. (1998). Q & A...Thyroid tests and food. *New Choices: Living Even Better After 50, 38*(1), 79.

Yarbro, C., Frogge, M., Goodman, M., & Broenwald, S. (2001). *Cancer nursing: Principles and practice.* Sudbury, MA: Jones and Bartlett.

Chapter 27

American Diabetes Association. (2002). *Clinical practice recommendations 2002, 25* (Supplement 1).

Batts, M., Gary, T., Huss, K., Hill, M., Bone, L., & Brancatt, F. (2001). Patient priorities and needs for diabetes care among urban African American adults. *Diabetes Educator, 27*(3), 405–412.

Bohannon, N. (1998). Treatment of vulvovaginal candidiasis in patients with diabetes. *Diabetes Care, 21*(3), 451–456.

Bulpitt, C., Palmer, A., Battersby, C., & Fletcher, A. (1998). Association of symptoms of type 2 diabetic patients with severity of disease, obesity, and blood pressure. *Diabetes Care, 21*(1), 111–115.

Burke, D. (2001). Diabetes education for the Native American Population. *Diabetes Educator, 27*(2), 181–189.

Cameron, B. (2002). Making diabetes management routine. *American Journal of Nursing, 102*(2), 26–33.

Carter, J., Gilliland, S., Perez, G., Levin, S., Broussand, B., Valdez, L., Cunningham-Sabo, L., & Davis, S. (1997). Tool chest. Native American Diabetes Project: Designing culturally relevant education materials. *Diabetes Educator, 23*(2), 133–134.

Fishman, T., Freedline, A., & Town, L. (1997). Helping diabetic patients treat their feet right. *Nursing97, 27*(6), 10–12.

Goldberg, J. M. (2001). Nutrition and exercise. *RN, 64*(7), 34–39.

Guthrie, D., & Guthrie, R. (1997). *Nursing management of diabetes mellitus* (4th ed.). New York: Springer.

Haire-Joshu, D. (Ed.) (1996). *Management of diabetes mellitus: Perspectives of care across the life span* (2nd ed.). St. Louis: Mosby.

Hanna, K., & Guthrie, D. (2001). Healthcompromising behavior and diabetes mismanagement among adolescents and young adults. *Diabetes Educator, 27*(2), 223–230.

Hernandez, D. (1998). Microvascular complications of diabetes: Nursing assessment and intervention. *American Journal of Nursing, 98*(6), 26–31.

Johnson, M., & Maas, M. (Eds). (1997). *Nursing outcomes classification (NOC).* St. Louis: Mosby.

Kee, J. (1999). *Laboratory & diagnostic tests with nursing implications* (5th ed.). East Norwalk, CT: Appleton & Lange.

Lipton, R., Losy, L., Giachello, A., Mendez, J., & Girotti, M. (1998). Attitudes and issues in treating Latino patients with type 2 diabetes. *Diabetes Educator, 24*(1), 67–71.

Lupo, M. (1997). An overview of foot disease associated with diabetes mellitus. *MEDSURG Nursing, 6*(4), 225–229.

McCance, K., & Huether, S. (2002). *Pathophysiology: The biologic basis for disease in adults and children.* (4th ed.). St. Louis: Mosby.

McCloskey, J. C., & Bulechek, G. M. (Eds.). (2000). *Nursing interventions classification (NIC).* St. Louis: Mosby.

McKenry, L., & Salerno, E. (1998). *Pharmacology in nursing* (20th ed.). St. Louis: Mosby.

National Institutes of Health. (2002). *Diabetes statistics in the United States.* NIH Publication No. 99–3892. Washington, DC: NIH.

North American Nursing Diagnosis Association. (2001). *Nursing diagnoses: Definitions & Classification 2001–2002.* Philadelphia: NANDA.

Passanza, C. (2001). Diabetes update: Monitor options. *RN, 64*(6), 36–43.

Paterson, B., Thorne, S., & Dewis, M. (1998). Adapting to and managing diabetes. *Image: Journal of Nursing Scholarship, 30*(1), 57–62.

Porth, C. (2002). *Pathophysiology: Concepts of altered health states* (6th ed.). Philadelphia: Lippincott.

Robertson, C. (1998). When your patient is on an insulin pump. *RN, 61*(3), 30–33.

Shannon, M., Wilson, B., & Stang, C. (2002). *Health professional's drug guide 2002.* Upper Saddle River, NJ: Prentice Hall.

Stanley, K. (1998). Assessing the nutritional needs of the geriatric patient with diabetes. *Diabetes Educator, 24*(1), 29–30, 35–36, 38.

Strowig, S. (2001). Insulin therapy. *RN, 64*(9), 38–44.

Sullivan, E., & Joseph, D. (1998). Struggling with behavior changes: A special case for clients with diabetes. *Diabetes Educator, 24*(1), 72–77.

Tierney, L., McPhee, S., & Papadakis, M. (Eds.). (2001). *Current medical diagnosis & treatment* (40th ed.). Stamford, CT: Appleton & Lange.

Tkacs, N. (2002). Hypoglycemia unawarenesss. *American Journal of Nursing, 102*(2), 34–41.

Whittemore, R. (2000). Strategies to facilitate lifestyle change associated with diabetes mellitus. *Journal of Nursing Scholarship, 32*(3), 225–232.

Chapter 28

Andresen, G. (1998). Assessing the older patient. *RN, 61*(3), 46–56.

Bynum, D. (1997). Clinical snapshot: Gout. *American Journal of Nursing, 97*(7), 36–37.

Campbell-Giovaniello, K. (1997). Clinical snapshot: Plantar fasciitis. *American Journal of Nursing, 97*(9), 38–39.

Krug, B. (1997). Rheumatoid arthritis and osteoarthritis: A basic comparison. *Orthopedic Nursing, 16*(5), 73–75.

Ludwidk, R., Dieckman, B., & Snelson, C. (1999). Assessment of the geriatric orthopaedic trauma patient. *Orthopaedic Nursing, 18(6), 11–20.*

Mangini, M. (1998). Physical assessment of the musculoskeletal system. *Nursing Clinics of North America, 33*(4), 643–652.

McDougall, T. (1999). Orthopedic update: Assessment of limb injury. *Australian Emergency Nursing Journal, 2*(1), 26–28.

Neal, L. (1997). Basic musculoskeletal assessment: Tips for the home health nurse. *Home Healthcare Nurse, 15*(4), 227–235.

O'Hanlon-Nichols, T. (1998). A review of the adult musculoskeletal system: A guide to a key aspect of patient care. *American Journal of Nursing, 98*(6), 48–52.

Watson, R. (2001). Assessing the musculoskeletal system in older people. *Nursing Older People, 13*(5), 29–30.

Weber, J., & Kelley, J. (2002). *Health assessment in nursing* (2nd ed.) Philadelphia: Lippincott.

Wilson, S., & Giddens, J. (2001). *Health assessment for nursing practice.* St. Louis: Mosby.

Chapter 29

Amputation. (2001). Available www.hendrickhealth.org/healthy/0037150.html

A parents guide to first aid. Amputation. (2002). Available www.choa.org/first_aid/amputation.shtml

Black, C. (1997). Wound management in patients with traumatic injuries. *Journal of Wound Care, 6*(5), 209–211.

Davis, P., & Barr, L. (1999). Principles of traction. *Journal of Orthopaedic Nursing, 3*(4), 222–227.

Electrical stimulation and bone healing. (2001). *Foot & Ankle Quarterly—The Seminar Journal, 14*(1), 1–37.

Falls and hip fractures among older adults. (2000). National Center for Injury Prevention & Control, CDC. Available www.cdc.gov/ncipc/factsheets/falls.htm

Hager, C. A., & Brncick, N. (1998). Fat embolism syndrome: A complication of orthopaedic trauma. *Orthopaedic Nursing, 17*(2), 41–43, 46, 58.

Hess, D. (1997). Employee perceived stress. Relationship to the development of repetitive strain injury symptoms. *AAOHN Journal, 45*(3), 115–123.

Johnson, M., & Maas, M. (Eds.). (1997). *Nursing outcomes classification (NOC).* St. Louis: Mosby.

Junge, T. (2000). Fat embolism: A complication of long bone fracture. *Surgical Technologist, 32*(11), 34–41.

Love, C. (2001). Using assisted walking devices. *Journal of Orthopaedic Nursing, 5*(1), 45–53.

Maher, A., Salmond, S., & Pellino, T. (2002). *Orthopedic nursing* (3rd ed.). Philadelphia: Saunders.

McCloskey, J. C., & Bulechek, G. M. (Eds.). (2000). *Nursing interventions classification (NIC)* (3rd ed.). St. Louis: Mosby.

Milisen, K., Abraham, I. L., & Broos, P. L. (1998). Postoperative variation in neurocognitive and functional status in elderly hip fracture patients. *Journal of Advanced Nursing, 27*(1), 59–67.

Mooney, N. (2001). Pain management in the orthopaedic patient. *Pain Management Nursing, 2*(1), 4–5.

Moss Rehab Resource Net. (2002). *Amputation fact sheet.* Available www.mossresourcenet.org/amputa.htm

North American Nursing Diagnosis Association. (2001). *NANDA nursing diagnoses: Definitions and classification, 2001–2002.* Philadelphia: Author.

National Center for Injury Prevention and Control. (2000). *Preventing falls among seniors.* Atlanta: Author.

O'Neill, M. (2001). Developing a clinically effective DVT prophylaxis protocol. *Journal of Orthopaedic Nursing, 5*(4), 186–191.

Pachucki-Hyde, L. (2001). Assessment of risk factors for osteoporosis and fracture. *Nursing Clinics of North America, 36*(3), 401–408.

Parsons, L., Krau, S., & Ward, K. (2001). Orthopedic trauma: Managing secondary medical problems. *Nursing Clinics of North America, 13*(3), 433–442.

Porth, C. M. (2002). *Pathophysiology: Concepts of altered health states* (6th ed.). Philadelphia: Lippincott.

Santy, J., & Mackintosh, C. (2001). A phenomenological study of pain following fractured shaft of femur. *Journal of Clinical Nursing, 10*(4), 521–527.

Scott, J. (1998). Mending broken bones. *Nursing Times, 94*(12), 28–30.

Shannon, M., Wilson, B., & Stang, C. (2002). *Health professionals drug guide 2002.* Upper Saddle River, NJ: Prentice Hall.

Sydell, W. (1999). Care of patients in casts. *Nursing Standard, 14*(8), 55.

Thompson, J., McFarland, G., Hirsch, J., & Tucker, S. (2002). *Mosby's clinical nursing* (5th ed.). St. Louis: Mosby.

Walls, M. (2002). Orthopedic trauma. *RN, 65*(7), 53–56.

Walsh, C. R., & McBryde, A. M., Jr. (1997). A joint protocol for home skeletal traction. *Orthopaedic Nursing, 16*(3), 28–33.

Weiss, S. A., & Lindell, B. (1996). Phantom limb pain and etiology of amputation in unilateral lower extremity amputees. *Journal of Pain and Symptom Management, 11*(1), 3–17.

Williams, M. A., Hughes, S. H., Bjorklund, B. C., & Oberst, M. T. (1996). Family caregiving in cases of hip fracture. *Rehabilitation Nursing, 21*(3), 124–131, 138.

Yarnold, B. (1999). Hip fracture: Caring for a fragile population. *American Journal of Nursing, 99*(2), 36–41.

Yetzer, E. A. (1996). Helping the patient through the experience of an amputation. *Orthopaedic Nursing, 15*(6), 45–49.

Chapter 30

Adler, P., Good, M., Roberts, B., & Snyder, S. (2000). Abstract: The effects of Tai Chi on older adults with chronic arthritis pain. *Journal of Nursing Scholarship, 32*(4), 377.

American Cancer Society. (2001). *What is bone cancer?* Available www.cancer.org

Barbieri, R. L. (1998). A step-by-step approach to osteoporosis treatment. *Patient Care, 32*(8), 138–147.

Curry, L., & Hogstel, M. (2002). Osteoporosis. *American Journal of Nursing, 102*(1), 26–33.

Delmas, P. D., & Meunier, P. J. (1997). The management of Paget's disease of bone. *The New England Journal of Medicine, 336*(8), 558–567.

Drugay, M. (1997). Breaking the silence: A health promotion approach to osteoporosis. *Journal of Gerontological Nursing, 23*(6), 36–43.

Garfin, J., & Garfin, S. (2002). Low back pain: Exercises to prevent recurrence. *Consultant, 42*(3), 357–358.

Hill, N., & Davis, P. (2000). Nursing care of total joint replacement. *Journal of Orthopaedic Nursing, 4*(1), 41–45.

Holmes, S. (1998). Osteoporosis: The hidden illness. *Nursing Times, 94*(1), 20–23.

Johnson, M., & Maas, M. (Eds.). (1997). *Nursing outcomes classification (NOC).* St. Louis: Mosby.

Katz, W. A., & Sherman, C. (1998). Osteoporosis: The role of exercise in optimal management. *The Physician and Sportsmedicine, 26*(2), 33–41.

Kee, C. C., McCoy, S., Rouser, G., Booth, L. A., & Harris, S. (1998). Perspectives on the nursing management of osteoarthritis. *Geriatric Nursing, 19*(1), 19–26.

Kee, J. (2001). *Handbook of laboratory and diagnostic tests with nursing implications* (4th ed.). Upper Saddle River, NJ: Prentice Hall.

Krug, B. (1997). Rheumatoid arthritis and osteoarthritis: A basic comparison. *Orthopaedic Nursing, 16*(5), 73–75.

Mahat, G. (1997). Perceived stressors and coping strategies among individuals with rheumatoid arthritis. *Journal of Advanced Nursing, 25*(6), 1144–1150.

Maher, A., Salmond, S., & Pellino, T. (2002). *Orthopaedic nursing* (3rd ed.). Philadelphia: Saunders.

Mayo Clinic. (2002). *Osteoporosis.* Available www.mayoclinic.com/invoke.cfm?id5DS00128

Matula, P., & Shollenberger, D. (1999). Total joint project: Acute care to home care. *MEDSURG Nursing, 8*(2), 92–98.

McCance, K., & Huether, S. (2002). *Pathophysiology: The biologic basis for disease in adults & children* (4th ed.). St. Louis: Mosby.

McCloskey, J., & Bulechek, G. (Eds.). (2000). *Nursing interventions classification (NIC)* (3rd ed.). St. Louis: Mosby.

Mooney, N. (2001). Pain management in the orthopaedic patient. *Pain Management Nursing, 2*(1), 4–5.

Moss Rehab Resource Net. (2002). *Arthritis fact sheet.* Available www.mossresourcenet.org/arthritis.htm

National Center for Chronic Disease Prevention and Health Promotion. (2002a). *Arthritis.* Available www.cdc.gov/ncedphp/arthritis/index.htm

_____. (2002b). *Chronic diseases and conditions: Arthritis.* Available www.cdc.gov/needphp/major.htm

_____. (2002c). *Healthy aging: Preventing disease and improving quality of life among older Americans.* Available www.cdc.gov/nccdphp/aag-aging.htm

National Institute of Arthritis and Musculoskeletal and Skin Diseases. (2002). *Questions and answers about fibromyalgia.* Available www.niams.nih.gov/i/topics/fibromyalgia/fibrofs.htm

National Institute of Neurological Disorders and Stroke. (2001). *NINDS back pain information page.* Available www.ninds.nih.gov/health_ and_medical disorders/back pain_doc.htm

National Institutes of Health. (2002). *Osteoporosis overview.* Available www.osteo.org/osteo.html

Neuberger, G. B., Press, A. N., Lindsley, H. B., Hinton, R., Cagle, P. E., Carlson, K., Scott, S., Dahl, J., & Kramer, B. (1997). Effects of exercise on fatigue, aerobic fitness, and disease activity measures in persons with rheumatoid arthritis. *Research in Nursing and Health, 20*(3), 195–204.

North American Nursing Diagnosis Association. (2001). *Nursing diagnoses: Definitions and classification, 2001–2002.* Philadelphia: Author.

Overdorf, J., Pachuki-Hyde, L., Kressenich, C., McClung, B., & Lucasey, C. (2001). Osteoporosis: There's so much we can do. *RN, 64*(12), 30–35,

Pachucki-Hyde, L. (2001). Assessment of risk factors for osteoporosis and fracture. *Nursing Clinics of North America, 36*(3), 401–408.

Porth, C. M. (2002). *Pathophysiology: Concepts of altered health states* (6th ed.). Philadelphia: Lippincott.

Raak, R., & Wahren, L. (2002). Background pain in fribromyalgia patients affecting clinical examination of the skin. *Journal of Clinical Nursing, 11*(1), 58–64.

Ramsburg, K. (2000). Rheumatoid arthritis. *American Journal of Nursing, 100*(11), 40–43.

Reuters Health. (2002). *Arthroscopic surgery for knee arthritis doubted.* Available www.reutershealth.com

Rizzoli, R., Schaad, M., & Uebelhart, B. (2001). Osteoporosis in men. *Nursing Clinics of North America, 36*(3), 467–479.

Rossiter, R. (2000). Understanding the special needs of the patient with scleroderma. *Australian Nursing Journal, 8*(3), Insert 1–4 (27–30).

Ryan, S. (1996). The role of the nurse in the management of scleroderma. *Nursing Standard, 10*(48), 39–42.

Sedlak, C., & Dohehy, M. (2000). Fashion tips for women with osteoporosis. *Orthopedic Nursing, 19*(5), 31–35.

Shannon, M., Wilson, B., & Stang, C. (2002). *Health professional's drug guide 2002.* Upper Saddle River, NJ: Prentice Hall.

Solomon, J. (1998). Osteoporosis. When supports weaken. *RN, 61*(5), 37–40.

Springhouse. (1998). *Nurse's handbook of alternative & complementary therapies.* Springhouse, PA: Springhouse Corp.

Tierney, L. M., McPhee, S. J., & Papadakis, M. A. (Eds.). (2001). *Current medical diagnosis & treatment (40th ed.).* Stamford, CT: Appleton & Lange.

Weinstein, R. S. (1997). Advances in the treatment of Paget's bone disease. *Hospital Practice, 32*(3), 63–76.

Wright, A. (1998). Nursing interventions with advanced osteoporosis. *Home Healthcare Nurse, 16*(3), 144–151.

Chapter 31

Jagoda, A., & Riggio, S. (1999). The rapid neurologic examination, part 1. History, mental status, cranial nerves. An orderly search identifies problems requiring immediate care. *Journal of Critical Illness, 14*(6), 325–331.

Maher, L. (2000). A quick neurologic examination. *Patient Care, 34*(3), 161–162, 165–168, 171–172.

O'Hanlon-Nichols, T. (1999). Neurologic assessment. *American Journal of Nursing, 99*(6), 44–50.

Riggio, S., & Jagoda A. (1999). The rapid neurologic examination, part 2: Movement, reflexes, sensation, balance. Know the signs that lead to the site of the pathologic process. *Journal of Critical Illness, 14*(7), 368–372.

Weber, J., & Kelley, J. (2002). *Health assessment in nursing* (2nd ed.). Philadelphia: Lippincott.

Chapter 32

Breteton, L., & Nolan, M. (2000). "You do know he's had a stroke, don't you?" Preparation for family care-giving: The neglected dimension. *Journal of Clinical Nursing, 9*(4), 498–506.

Bucher, L. & Melander, S. (1999). *Critical care nursing.* Philadelphia: Saunders.

Buckley, D., & Guanci, M. (1999). Spinal cord trauma. *Nursing Clinics of North America, 34*(3), 661–687.

Chotikul, L. (2000). Spinal implants. *RN, 63*(5), 28–31.

Christensen, J., Cook, E., & Martin, B. (1997). Identifying denial in stroke patients. *Clinical Nursing Research, 6*(1), 105–118.

Davies, S. (1999). Dysphagia in acute strokes. *Nursing Standard, 13*(30), 49–55.

DeLisa, J., & Kirshblum, S. (1997). A review: Frustrations and needs in clinical care of spinal cord injury patients. *Journal of Spinal Cord Medicine, 20*(4), 384–390.

Duncan, P., & Lai, S. (1997). Stroke recovery. *Topics in Stroke Rehabilitation, 4*(3), 51–58.

Garner, C. (1999). Cancer-related spinal cord compression. *American Journal of Nursing, 99*(7), 34–35.

Gendreau-Webb, R. (2001). Action stat: Ischemic stroke. *Nursing, 31*(11), 120.

Gerhart, K., Charlifue, S., Weitzenkamp, D., Menter, R., & Whiteneck, G. (1997). Aging with spinal cord injury. *American Rehabilitation, 23*(1), 19–25.

Harding-Okimoto, M. (1997). Pressure ulcers, self-concept and body image in spinal cord injury patients. *SCI Nursing, 14*(4), 111–117.

Hayn, M., & Fisher, T. (1997). Stroke rehabilitation: Salvaging ability after the storm. *Nursing97, 27*(3), 40–46, 48.

Hickey, J. (2003). *The clinical practice of neurological and neurosurgical nursing* (4th ed.). Philadelphia: Lippincott.

Hock, N. (1999). Brain attack: The stroke continuum. *Nursing Clinics of North America, 34*(3), 689–723.

Huston, C. (1998). Cervical spine injury. *American Journal of Nursing, 98*(6), 33.

Identification and nursing management of dysphagia in adults with neurological impairment. *Best Practice, 4*(2), 1–6.

John, C. (1997). Time is of the essence: "Brain attack: Treating acute ischemic CVA." *Nursing97, 27*(6), 9–10.

Johnson, M., & Maas, M. (Eds). (1997). *Iowa outcome project: Nursing outcomes classification (NOC)*. St. Louis: Mosby.

Krause, J. (1998). Skin sores after spinal cord injury: Relationship to life adjustment. *Spinal Cord, 36*(1), 51–56.

LaFavor, K., & Ang, R. (1997). Managing autonomic dysreflexia through the use of clinical practice guidelines. *SCI Nursing, 14*(3), 83–86.

McAweeney, M., Tate, D., & McAweeney, W. (1997). Psychosocial interventions in the rehabilitation of people with spinal cord injury: A comprehensive methodologic inquiry. *SCI Psychosocial Process, 10*(2), 58–66.

McCloskey, J., & Bulechek, G. (Eds.). (2000). *Iowa intervention project: Nursing interventions classification (NIC)* (3rd ed.). St. Louis: Mosby.

McColl, M., Walker, J., Stirling, P., Wilkins, R., & Corey, P. (1997). Expectations of life and health among spinal cord injured adults. *Spinal Cord, 35*(12), 818–828.

McHale, J., Phipps, M., Horvath, K., & Schmelz, J. (1998). Expert nursing knowledge in the care of patients at risk of impaired swallowing. *Image: Journal of Nursing Scholarship, 30*(2), 137–141.

Mower, D. (1997). Brain attack: Treating acute ischemic CVA. *Nursing97, 27*(3), 34–39, 47–48.

National Spinal Cord Injury Association (1998). *Spinal cord injury statistics.* Available www. eskimo.com/~jlubin/disabled/nscia/fact02.html

Perry, L. (2001). Screening swallowing function of patients with acute stroke. Part 2. Detailed evaluation of the tool used by nurses. *Journal of Clinical Nursing, 10*(4), 474–481.

Petterson, M. (1997). Thrombolytic therapy in stroke management. *Critical Care Nurse, 17*(5), 88–93.

Porth, C. (2002). *Pathophysiology: Concepts of altered health states* (6th ed.). Philadelphia: Lippincott.

Routh, J. (1997). Consumer's perspective: Dressing and undressing following a stroke. *Topics in Stroke Rehabilitation, 4*(2), 94–98.

Sander, R. (1998). Stroke: The hidden problems. *Elderly Care, 10*(1), 27–32.

Shannon, M., Wilson, B., & Stang, C. (2002). *Health professionals drug guide 2002.* Upper Saddle River, NJ: Prentice Hall

Sipski, M. (1997). Sexuality and spinal cord injury: Where we are and where we are going. *American Rehabilitation, 23*(1), 26–28.

Thompson, J., McFarland, G., Hirsch, J., & Tucker, S. (2002). *Mosby's clinical nursing* (5th ed.). St. Louis: Mosby.

Tierney, L., McPhee, S., & Papadakis, M. (Eds.). (2001). *Current medical diagnosis & treatment.* Stamford, CT: Appleton & Lange.

Westergren, A., Ohlsson, O., & Halberg, I. (2001). Eating difficulties, complications, and nursing interventions during a period of three months after a stroke. *Journal of Advanced Nursing, 35*(3), 416–426.

Whipple, B., & Komisarck, B. (1997). Sexuality and women with complete spinal cord injury. *Spinal Cord, 35*(3), 136–138.

Chapter 33

American Cancer Society. (2001). *Cancer facts and figures–2001.* Atlanta: ACS.

Barker, E. (1998). The xenon CT: A new neuro tool. *RN, 61*(2), 22–25.

Brain Trauma Foundation and the Joint Section on Neurotrauma and Critical Care of the American Association of Neurological Surgeons and the Congress of Neurological Surgeons. (1995). *Guidelines for the management of severe head injury.* Park Ridge, IL: The Brain Trauma Foundation.

Bucher, L., & Melander, S. (1999). *Critical Care Nursing.* Philadelphia: Saunders

Chiocca, E. (1997). Action stat! Bacterial meningitis. *Nursing, 27*(9), 33.

Dodick, D. (1997). Headache as a symptom of ominous disease: What are the warning signals? *Postgraduate Medicine, 101*(5), 46–50, 55–56, 62.

Duff, D., & Wells, D. (1997). Postcomatose unawareness/vegetative state following severe brain injury: A content methodology. *Journal of Neuroscience Nursing, 29*(5), 305–307, 312–317.

Edmeads, J. (1997). Headaches in older people: How are they different in this age group? *Postgraduate Medicine, 101*(5), 91–94, 98, 100.

Fettes, I. (1997). Menstrual migraine: Methods of prevention and control. *Postgraduate Medicine, 101*(5), 67–70, 73–75, 77.

Hickey, J. (2003). *The clinical practice of neurological and neurosurgical nursing* (5th ed.). Philadelphia: Lippincott.

Hilton, G. (2001). Emergency: Acute head injury. *American Journal of Nursing, 101*(9), 51–52.

———.(1997). Seizure disorder in adults: Evaluation and management of new onset seizures. *Nurse Practitioner: American Journal of Primary Health Care, 22*(9), 42, 54, 49–50.

Horowitz, S., Passik, S., & Malkin, M. (1996). "In sickness and in health": A group intervention for spouses caring for patients with brain tumors. *Journal of Psychosocial Oncology, 14*(2), 43–56.

Johnson, M., & Maas, M. (Eds.). (1997). *Nursing outcomes classification (NOC).* St. Louis: Mosby.

Kee, J. (2001). *Handbook of laboratory and diagnostic tests* (4th ed.). Upper Saddle River, NJ: Prentice Hall.

Kidd, P., & Wagner, K. (2001). *High-acuity nursing* (3rd ed.). Upper Saddle River, NJ: Prentice Hall.

King, D. (1999). Central nervous system infections. Basic concepts. *Nursing Clinics of North America, 34*(3), 761–771.

Levitt, M., Lamb, S., & Voss, B. (1996). Brain tumor support group: Content themes and mechanisms of support. *Oncology Nursing Forum, 23*(8), 1247–1356.

Lin, Jong-mi. (2001). Overview of migraine. *Journal of Neuroscience Nursing, 33*(1), 6–13.

Liporace, J. (1997). Women's issues in epilepsy: Menses, childbearing and more. *Postgraduate Medicine, 102*(1), 123–124, 127–129, 133–135.

Long, L., & McAuley, J. (1996). Epilepsy: A review of seizure types, etiologies, diagnosis, treatment, and nursing implications. *Critical Care Nurse, 16*(4), 83–92.

Long, L., & Reeves, A. (1997). The practical aspects of epilepsy: Critical components of comprehensive patient care. *Journal of Neuroscience Nursing, 29*(4), 249–254.

McCance, K., & Huether, S. (2002). *Pathophysiology: The biologic basis for disease in adults and children* (4th ed.). St. Louis: Mosby.

McCloskey, J., & Bulechek, G. (Eds.). (2000). *Nursing interventions classification (NIC)* (3rd ed.). St. Louis: Mosby.

McKenry, L., & Salerno, E. (1998). *Pharmacology in nursing* (20th ed.). St. Louis: Mosby.

McNair, N. (1999). Traumatic brain injury. *Nursing Clinics of North America, 34*(3), 637–659.

McNew, C., Hunt, S., & Warner, L. (1997). How to help your patient with epilepsy. *Nursing, 27*(9), 56–63.

Miller, L, & Chol, C. (1997). Meningitis in older patients: How to diagnose and treat a deadly infection. *Geriatrics, 52*(8), 43–44, 47–50, 55.

Myers, F. (2000). Meningitis: The fears, the facts. *RN, 63*(11), 53–57.

North American Nursing Diagnosis Association. (2001). *Nursing diagnoses: Definitions & classification 2001–2002.* Philadelphia: NANDA.

Porth, C. (2002). *Pathophysiology: Concepts of altered health states* (6th ed.). Philadelphia: Lippincott.

Schultz, R. (1997). Eggs and brains—The basics of head trauma. *Emergency Medical Services, 26*(4), 29–34, 75.

Shafer, P. (1999). Epilepsy and seizures. *Nursing Clinics of North America, 34*(3), 743–759.

Shannon, M., Wilson, B., & Stang, C. (2002). *Drug guide 2002.* Upper Saddle River, NJ: Prentice Hall.

Sullivan, J. (2000). Positioning of patients with severe traumatic brain injury: Research-based practice. *Journal of Neuroscience Nursing, 32*(4), 204–209.

Tierney, L., McPhee, S., & Papadakis, M. (Eds.). (2001). *Current medical diagnosis & treatment* (40th ed). New York: McGraw-Hill.

Wall, B., Howard, J., & Perry-Phillips, J. (1995). Validation of two nursing diagnoses: Increased intracranial pressure and high risk for increased intracranial pressure. In M. Rantz & P. LeMone (Eds). *Classification of nursing diagnoses: Proceedings of the 11th conference* (pp. 166–170). Glendate, CA: CINAHL.

Wright, M. (1999). Resuscitation of the multitrauma patient with head injury. *AACN Clinical Issues, 10*(1), 32–45.

Yarbo, C., Frogge, M., Goodman, M., & Groenwald, S. (Eds.). (2001). *Cancer nursing: Principles and practice* (5th ed.). Sudbury, MA: Jones & Bartlett.

Chapter 34

Alzheimer's Disease and Related Disorders Association, Inc. (2000). Available www.Alzheimers.org

Andresen, G. (1998). Dx dementia. But what kind? *RN, 61*(6), 26–29.

Baker, L. (1998). Sense making in multiple sclerosis: The information needs of people during an acute exacerbation. *Qualitative Health Research, 8*(1), 106–120.

Bell, V., & Troxel, D. (2001). Spirituality and the person with dementia—A view from the field. *Alzheimer's Care Quarterly, 2*(2), 31–45.

Boyden, K. (2000). The pathophysiology of demyelination and the ionic basis of nerve conduction in multiple sclerosis: An overview. *Journal of Neuroscience Nursing, 32*(1), 49–53, 60.

Center for Disease Control. (2001). *Bovine spongiform encephalopathy and Creutzfeldt-Jakob disease.* Available www.cdc.gov/ncidod/diseases

Charles, T., & Swash, M. (2001). Amyotrophic lateral sclerosis: Current understanding. *Journal of Neuroscience Nursing, 33*(5), 245–253.

Costa, M. (1998). Trigeminal neuralgia. *American Journal of Nursing, 98*(6), 42–43.

Dewing, J. (2001). Care for older people with a dementia in acute hospital settings. *Nursing Older People, 13*(3), 18–20.

Epps, C. (2001). Recognizing pain in the institutionalized elder with dementia. *Geriatric Nursing, 22*(2), 71–79.

Fontaine, K. (2000). *Healing practices: Alternative therapies for nursing.* Upper Saddle River, NJ: Prentice Hall.

Fowler, S. (1997). Hope and a health-promoting lifestyle in persons with Parkinson's disease. *Journal of Neuroscience Nursing, 29*(2), 111–116.

Gerdner, L., & Hall. G. (2001). Chronic confusion. In M. Maas, K. Buckwalter, M. Hardy, T. Tripp-Reimer, M. Titler, & J. Specht (Eds.), *Nursing care of older adults: Diagnoses, outcomes, & interventions* (pp. 421–441). St. Louis: Mosby.

Gray, P., & Hildebrand, K. (2000). Fall risk factors in Parkinson's disease. *Journal of Neuroscience Nursing, 32*(4), 222–228.

Greenway, M., & Walker, A. (1998). Home health: Helping caregivers cope with Alzheimer's disease. *Nursing98, 28*(2), 32hh 1–2, 4–6.

Gulick, E. (1997). Correlates of quality of life among persons with multiple sclerosis. *Nursing Research, 46*(6), 305–311.

Herndon, C., Young, K., Herndon, A., & Dole, E. (2000). Parkinson's disease revisited. *Journal of Neuroscience Nursing, 32*(4), 216–221.

Hickey, J. (2002). *The clinical practice of neurological and neurosurgical nursing* (5th ed.). Philadelphia: Lippincott.

Johnson, M., & Maas, M. (Eds.). (1997). *Nursing outcomes classification (NOC).* St. Louis: Mosby.

Kee, J. (1998). *Handbook of laboratory and diagnostic tests with nursing implications* (4th ed.). Upper Saddle River, NJ: Prentice Hall.

Lisak, D. (2001). Overview of symptomatic management of multiple sclerosis. *Journal of Neuroscience Nursing, 33*(5), 224–230.

McCance, K., & Huether, S. (2002). *Pathophysiology: The biologic basis for disease in adults and children.* St. Louis: Mosby.

McCloskey, J., & Bulechek, G. (Eds.). (2000). *Nursing interventions classification (NIC)* (3rd ed.). St. Louis: Mosby.

McKenry, L., & Salerno, E. (1998). *Pharmacology in nursing* (20th ed.). St. Louis: Mosby.

McMahon-Parkes, K., & Cornock, M. (1997). Guillain-Barré syndrome: Biological basis, treatment and care. *Intensive & Critical Care Nursing, 13*(1), 42–48.

Mini-mental state exam. (1975). *The Journal of Psychiatric Research, 12*, 189–198.

National Parkinson Foundation. (2001). *New approaches for treating tremor.* Available www.Parkinson.org/treatment.htm

North American Nursing Diagnosis Association. (2001). *Nursing diagnoses: Definitions & classification 2001–2002.* Philadelphia: NANDA.

O'Donnell, L. (1997). Immune-mediated neurological diseases. Management of myasthenia gravis—An overview. *Journal of Care Management, 3*(6 Disease Management Digest), 4–5, 17–18.

Porth, C. (2002). *Pathophysiology: Concepts of altered health states* (6th ed.). Philadelphia: Lippincott.

Ross, A. (1999). Neurologic degenerative disorders. *Nursing Clinics of North America, 34*(3), 725–742.

Schutte, D., Williams, J., Schutte, B., & Maas, M. (1998). Alzheimer's disease genetics: Practice and education implications for special care unit nurses. *Journal of Gerontological Nursing, 24*(1), 40–48, 58–64.

Segatore, M. (1998). Managing the surgical orthopaedic patient with Parkinson's disease. *Orthopaedic Nursing, 17*(1), 13–22.

Shannon, M., Wilson, B., & Stang, C. (2002). *Health professional's drug guide 2002.* Upper Saddle River, NJ: Prentice Hall.

Spratto, G., & Woods, A. (1998). *Delmar's therapeutic class drug guide for nurses 1998.* Albany, NY: Delmar.

Tierney, L., McPhee, S., & Papadakis, M. (Eds.). (2001). *Current medical diagnosis & treatment* (40th ed.). Stamford, CT: Appleton & Lange.

Worsham, T. (2000). Easing the course of Guilllain-Barre syndrome. *RN, 63*(3), 46–50.

Zaveruha, A., Bishop, D., St. Clair, A., & Moreau, K. (1997). Rabies update for nurse practitioners. *Clinical Excellence for Nurse Practitioners, 1*(6), 367–375.

Chapter 35

Andresen, G. (1998). Assessing the older patient. *RN, 61*(3), 46–56.

Lawton, S. (2001). Assessing the patient with a skin condition. *Journal of Tissue Viability, 11*(3), 113–115.

McConnell, E. (1996). Assessing pruritus. *Nursing 96, 26*(12), 32.

Rupp, J., & Kaplan, D. (1999). Scratching the surface of pruritic disorders. *Consultant, 39*(11), 3161–3164, 3167.

Talbot, L., & Curtis, L. (1996). The challenge of assessing skin indicators in people of color. *Home Healthcare Nurse,14*(3), 167–173.

Weber, J., & Kelley, J. (2002). *Health assessment in nursing* (2nd ed). Philadelphia: Lippincott-Raven.

Wilson, S., & Giddens, J. (2001). *Health assessment for nursing practice* (2nd ed.). St. Louis: Mosby.

Young, T. (1997). Skin assessment and usual presentations. *Community Nurse, 3*(5), 33–36.

Chapter 36

Agency for Health Care Policy and Research. (1992). *Pressure ulcers in adults: Prediction and prevention.* Rockville, MD: USDHHS.

_____ . (1994). *Treatment of pressure ulcers.* Rockville, MD: USDHHS.

American Cancer Society. (2002). *Cancer facts and figures 2002.* Atlanta: American Cancer Society.

American Melanoma Foundation/National Cancer Institute. (2001). *Skin cancer treatment.* Available http://cancernet.nci.nih.gov

Appling, S. (1997). Promoting healthy skin. *MEDSURG Nursing, 6*(6), 377–378.

Bielan, B. (1997a). What's your assessment—Papular urticaria. *Dermatology Nursing, 9*(3), 191, 201.

_____ . (1997b). What's your assessment—Tinea pedis. *Dermatology Nursing, 9*(2), 105, 117.

Bjorgen, S. (1998). Clinical snapshot: Herpes zoster. *American Journal of Nursing, 98* (2 Continuing Care Extra), 46–47.

Blawat, D., & Banks, P. (1997). Comforting touch: Using topical skin preparations. *Nursing 97, 27*(5), 46–48.

Center for Disease Control. (2001). *Cancer prevention and control.* Available www.cdc.gov/cancer/nscpep/skin

Boston, M. (1997). Acne: Avoiding permanent damage. *Community Nurse, 3*(4), 15–16.

Davis, P. (1998). Pain from herpes zoster and postherapetic neuralgia. *American Journal of Nursing, 98*(2 Continuing Care Extra), 18, 20.

Hardy, M. (1996). What can you do about your patient's dry skin? *Journal of Gerontological Nursing, 22*(5), 10–18, 52–53.

Johnson, M., & Maas, M. (1997). *Iowa outcome project: Nursing outcomes classification (NOC).* St. Louis: Mosby.

Landow, K. (1998). Hand dermatitis: The perennial scourge. *Postgraduate Medicine, 103*(1), 141–142, 145–148, 151–152.

Lapka, D. (2000). Oncology today. New horizons: Skin cancer. *RN, 63*(7), 32–40.

Lebwohl, M. (1997). Understanding psoriasis. *Women's Health Digest, 3*(3), 159–164.

Leshaw, S. (1998). Itching in active patients: Causes and cures. *Physician & Sportsmedicine, 26*(1), 47–50.

Marghoob, A. (1997). Basal and squamous cell carcinomas. *Postgraduate Medicine, 102*(2), 139–142.

McCloskey, J., & Bulechek, G. (Eds.). (2000). *Iowa intervention project: Nursing interventions classification (NIC)* (3rd ed.). St. Louis: Mosby.

McKay, S. (2000). Why we need to worry about warts. *RN, 63*(9), 68–74.

Metules, T. (2000). Tips for nurses who wash too much. *RN, 63*(3), 34–37.

North American Nursing Diagnosis Association. (2001) *Nursing diagnoses: Definitions & classification 2001–2002.* Philadelphia: NANDA.

Penzer, R., & Finch, M. (2001). Promoting healthy skin in older people. *Nursing Standard, 15*(34), 46–52.

Pieper, B., & Weiland, M. (1997). Pressure ulcer prevention within 72 hours of admission in a rehabilitation setting. *Ostomy Wound Management, 43*(8), 14–16, 18, 20.

Pieper, B., Sugrue, M., Weiland, M., Sprague, K., & Heimann, C. (1997). Presence of ulcer prevention methods used among patients considered at-risk versus those considered not-at-risk. *Journal of WOCN, 24*(4), 191–199.

Porth, C. (2002). *Pathophysiology: Concepts of altered health states* (6th ed.). Philadelphia: Lippincott.

Reifsnider, E. (1997). Common adult infectious skin conditions. *Nursing Practitioner: American Journal of Primary Health Care, 22*(11), 17–18, 20, 23–24.

Rigel, D., & Carucci, J. (2000). Malignant melanoma: Prevention, early detection, and treatment in the 21st century. *CA: A Cancer Journal for Clinicians, 50*(4), 209–213.

Russell, J. (2000). Topical therapy for acne. *American Family Physician, 61*(2), 357–366.

Sarver-Steffensen, J. (1999). When MRSA reaches into long-term care. *RN, 62*(3), 39–41.

Tierney, L., McPhee, S., & Papadakis, M. (Eds.). (2001). *Current medical diagnosis & treatment* (40th ed.). Stamford, CT: Appleton & Lange.

Wilson, B., Shannon, M., & Stang, C. (2001). *Nursing drug guide 2001.* Upper Saddle River, NJ: Prentice Hall.

Yarbo, C., Frogge, M, Goodman, M., & Groenwald, S. (Eds.) (2001). *Cancer nursing: Principles and practice* (5th ed.). Sudbury, MA: Jones & Bartlett.

Chapter 37

Badger, J. (2001). Burns: The psychological aspects. *American Journal of Nursing, 101*(11), 38–44.

Barnes, A., & Budd, L. (1999). Family-centered burn care. *Canadian Nurse, 95*(6), 24–27.

Braunwald, E., & Fauci, A. (2001). *Harrison's principles of internal medicine* (15th ed.). New York: McGraw-Hill.

Bucher, L., & Melander, S. (1999). *Critical Care Nursing.* Philadelphia: Saunders.

Carrougher, G. (1998). *Burn care and therapy.* St. Louis: Mosby.

Davis, S., & Sheely-Adolphson, P. (1997). Psychosocial interventions: Pharmacologic and psychologic modalities. *Nursing Clinics of North America, 32*(2), 331–342.

DeBoer, S. (2001). Pain control for burn victims: Don't be afraid to administer more morphine than is usual. *American Journal of Nursing, 101*(3), 56.

deRios, M., Novac, A., & Achauer, B. (1997). Sexual dysfunction and the patient with burns. *Journal of Burn Care & Rehabilitation, 18*(1, Pt 1), 37–42.

Docking, P. (1999). Trauma. Electrical burn injuries. *Accident & Emergency Nursing, 7*(2), 70–76.

Eakes, G., Burke, M., & Hainsworth, M. (1998). Middle-range theory of chronic sorrow. *Image: Journal of Nursing Scholarship, 30*(2), 179–184.

Fowler, A. (1998). Nursing management of minor burn injuries. *Emergency Nurse, 6*(6), 31–39.

Greenfield, E., & McManus, A. (1997). Infectious complications—Prevention and strategies for their control. *Nursing Clinics of North America, 32*(2), 297–309.

Hilton, G. (2001). Emergency: Thermal burns. *American Journal of Nursing, 101*(11), 32–34.

Holm, C., Horbrand, F., von Donnersmarck, G., & Muhlbauer, W. (1999). Acute renal failure in severely burned patients. *Burns, 25*(2), 171–178.

Johnson, M., & Maas, M. (1997). *Nursing outcomes classification (NOC)*. St. Louis: Mosby.

Kagan, R., & Smith, S. (2000). Evaluation and treatment of thermal injuries. *Dermatology Nursing, 12*(5), 334–335, 338–344, 347–350.

Kee, J. (2001). *Handbook of laboratory and diagnostic tests* (4th ed.). Upper Saddle River, NJ: Prentice Hall.

Kidd, P., & Wagner, K. (2001). *High-acuity nursing* (3rd ed.). Upper Saddle River, NJ: Prentice Hall.

Lim, J., Rehma, S., & Elmore, P. (1998). Rapid response: Care of burn victims. *AAOHN Journal, 46*(4), 169–180.

Mayes, T., Gottschlich, M., & Warden, G. (1997). Clinical nutrition protocols for continuous quality improvements in the outcomes of patients with burns. *Journal of Burn Care & Rehabilitation, 18*(4), 365–368.

McKirdy, L. (2001). Burn wound cleansing. *Journal of Community Nursing, 15*(5), 24, 26–27, 29.

Menzies, V. (2000). Depression and burn wounds. *Archives of Psychiatric Nursing, 14*(4), 199–206.

McCloskey, J., & Bulechek, G. (Eds.). *Nursing interventions classification (NIC)* (3rd ed.). St. Louis: Mosby.

McKenry, L., & Salerno, E. (1998). *Pharmacology in nursing* (20th ed.). St. Louis: Mosby.

Mertens, D., Jenkins, M., & Warden, G. (1997). Outpatient burn management. *Nursing Clinics of North America, 32*(2), 343–374.

Milner, S., Mottar, R., & Smith, C. (2001). The burn wheel. *American Journal of Nursing, 101*(11), 35–37.

North American Nursing Diagnosis Association. (2001). *Nursing diagnoses: Definitions & classification 2001–2002*. Philadelphia: NANDA.

Porth, C. (2002). *Pathophysiology: Concepts of altered health states* (6th ed.). Philadelphia: Lippincott.

Richard, R. (1999). Assessment and diagnosis of burn wounds. *Advances in Wound Care, 12*(9), 468–471.

Richard, R. (1999). The physiology of burns. *Nursing Times, 95*(34), 25–31.

Rutan, R. (1998). Physiologic response to cutaneous burn injury. In G. Carrougher (Ed.), *Burn care and therapy* (pp. 1–33). St. Louis: Mosby.

Tierney, L., McPhee, S., & Papadakis, M. (Eds.). (2001). *Current medical diagnosis & treatment* (40th ed.). Stamford, CT: Appleton & Lange.

Wiebelhaus, P., & Hansen, S. (2001). Another choice for burn victims. *RN, 64*(9), 34–37.

Wiebelhaus, P., & Hansen, S. (2001). What you should know about managing burn emergencies. *Nursing, 31*(1), 36–42.

Wiebelhaus, P., Hansen, S., & Hill, H. (2001). Helping patients survive inhalation injuries. *RN, 64*(10), 28–32.

Chapter 38

Acello, B. (2000). Controlling pain. Facing fears about opioid addiction. *Nursing, 30*(5), 72.

Ackerman, C., & Turkoski, B. (2000). Using guided imagery to reduce pain and anxiety. *Home Healthcare Nurse, 18*(8), 524–530.

American Pain Society. 2001. *Pain: The fifth vital sign.* Available www.ampainsoc.org

American Pain Society Quality of Care Committee. (1995). Quality improvement guidelines for the treatment of acute pain and cancer pain. *Journal of the American Medical Association, 274*(23), 1874–1880.

Anonymous. (1997). The use of opioids for the treatment of chronic pain: A consensus statement from the American Academy of Pain Medicine and the American Pain Society. *Clinical Journal of Pain, 13*(1), 6–8.

Berkowitz, C. (1997). Epidural pain control—Your job, too. *RN, 60*(8), 22–27.

Carpenito, L. (2000). *Nursing diagnosis: Application to clinical practice* (8th ed.). Philadelphia: Lippincott.

Coyne, M., Smith, J., Stein, D., Hieser, M., & Hoover, L. (1998). Describing pain management documentation. *MEDSURG Nursing, 7*(1), 45–51.

Dellasega, C., & Keiser, C. (1997). Pharmacologic approaches to chronic pain in the older adult. *American Journal of Primary Health Care, 22*(5), 20, 22–24, 26.

Joint Commission on Accreditation of Healthcare Organizations. (2000). *Joint Commission on Accreditation of Healthcare Organizations pain standards for 2001.* Available www.jcaho.org

Kodiath, M. (1997). Chronic pain: Contrasting two cultures. *Clinical Excellence for Nurse Practitioners, 1*(1), 59–61.

Lipson, J., Dibble, S., & Minarik, P. (1996). *Culture & nursing care: A pocket guide.* San Francisco: UCSF Nursing Press.

McCaffery, M. (1979). *Nursing management of the patient with pain.* Philadelphia: Lippincott.

McCaffery, M., & Beebe, A. (1999). *Pain: Clinical manual.* St. Louis: Mosby.

McCance, K., & Huether, S. (2002). *Pathophysiology: The biologic basic for disease in adults and children* (4th ed.). St. Louis: Mosby.

McKenry, L., & Salerno, E. (1998). *Pharmacology in nursing* (20th ed.). St. Louis: Mosby.

Melzack, R. (1975). The McGill Pain Questionnaire: Major properties and scoring methods. *Pain, 1,* 277.

Melzack, R., & Wall, P. (1965). Pain mechanisms: A new theory. *Science, 150,* 971–979.

_____ . (1968). Gate control theory of pain. In A. Soulairac, J. Cahn, & J. Carpentier (Eds.), *Pain: Proceedings of the International Association on Pain.* Baltimore: Williams & Wilkins.

Merboth, M. K., & Barnason, S (2000). Managing pain: The fifth vital sign. *Nursing Clinics of North America, 35*(2), 375–383.

Pasero, C. (1999). Using agonist-antagonist opioids and antagonist drugs. *American Journal of Nursing, 99*(1), 20–21.

_____ . (2000). Oral patient-controlled analgesia. *American Journal of Nursing, 100*(3), 24.

Pasero, C., & McCaffrey, M. (1999). Opioids by the rectal route. *American Journal of Nursing, 99*(11), 20.

_____ . (2000). When patients can't report pain. *American Journal of Nursing, 100*(9), 22–23.

Porth, C. (2002). *Pathophysiology: Concepts of altered health states* (6th ed.). Philadelphia: Lippincott.

Seal, R. (1997). Choosing the right step on the analgesic ladder. *Community Nurse, 3*(2), 58–59.

U.S. Department of Health and Human Services. (1992). *Acute pain management: Operative or medical procedures and trauma* (AHCPR Publication No. 92-0032). Rockville, MD: Agency for Health Care Policy and Research, Public Health Service, USDHHS.

Victor, K. (2001). Properly assessing pain in the elderly. *RN, 64*(5), 45–49.

Waitman, J., & McCaffery, M. (2001). Meperidine—A liability. *American Journal of Nursing, 101*(1), 57–58.

Watt-Watson, J., Garfinkel, P., Gallop, R., Stevens, B., & Streiner, D. (2000). The impact of nurses' empathic responses on patients' pain management in acute care. *Nursing Research, 49*(4), 191–200.

Wilson, B. A., Shannon, M. T., & Stang, C. L. (2001). *Nursing drug guide 2001.* Upper Saddle River, NJ: Prentice Hall.

World Health Organization. (1986/1990). *Cancer pain relief.* Geneva: WHO.

Chapter 39

Ackley, B. J., & Ladwig, G. B. (2002). *Nursing diagnosis handbook: A guide to planning care* (5th ed.). St. Louis: Mosby.

Braunwald, E., Fauci, A. S., Kasper, D. L., Hauser, S. L., Longo, D. L., & Jameson, J. L. (2001). *Harrison's principles of internal medicine* (15th ed.). New York: McGraw-Hill.

Bullock, B. A., & Henze, R. L. (2000). *Focus on pathophysiology.* Philadelphia: Lippincott.

Call-Schmidt, T. (2001). Interpreting lab results: A primer. *MEDSURG Nursing, 10*(4), 179–184.

Castiglione, V. (2000). Emergency. Hyperkalemia. *American Journal of Nursing, 100*(1), 55–56.

Cook, L. (1999). The value of lab values. *American Journal of Nursing, 99*(5), 66–69, 71, 73, 75.

Danner, K. (2000). Acid/base balance: Making sense of pH. *CIN PLUS* (On-line serial), *3*(1), 3.

Deglin, J. H., & Vallerand, A. H. (2001). *Davis's drug guide for nurses* (7th ed.). Philadelphia: F. A. Davis.

Edwards, S. (2001). Regulation of water, sodium and potassium: Implications for practice. *Nursing Standard, 15*(22), 36–44.

Gallo, J. J., Busby-Whitehead, J., Rabins, P. V., Silliman, R. A., & Murphy, J. B. (Eds.). (1999). *Reichel's care of the elderly: Clinical aspects of aging* (5th ed.). Philadelphia: Lippincott Williams & Wilkins.

Heater, D. W. (1999). If ADH goes out of balance: Diabetes insipidus. *RN, 62*(7), 42–46.

_____. (1999). If ADH goes out of balance: SIADH. *RN, 62*(7), 47–49.

Horne, C., & Derrico, D. (1999). Mastering ABGs. *American Journal of Nursing, 99*(8), 26–32.

Iggulden, H. (1999). Dehydration and electrolyte balance. *Nursing Standard, 13*(19), 48–56.

Incredibly easy! Understanding imbalances caused by GI fluid loss. (1999). *Nursing, 29*(8), 72.

Johnson, M., Bulechek, G., Dochterman, J. M., Maas, M., & Moorhead, S. (2001). *Nursing diagnoses, outcomes, & interventions: NANDA, NOC, and NIC linkages.* St. Louis: Mosby.

Kuhn, M. A. (1999). *Complementary therapies for health care providers.* Philadelphia: Lippincott.

Lehne, R. A. (2001). *Pharmacology for nursing care* (4th ed.). Philadelphia: Saunders.

Malarkey, L. M., & McMorrow, M. E. (2000). *Nurse's manual of laboratory tests and diagnostic procedures* (2nd ed.). Philadelphia: Saunders.

Meeker, M. H., & Rothrock, J. C. (1999). *Alexander's care of the patient in surgery* (11th ed.). St. Louis: Mosby.

Metheny, N. M. (2000). *Fluid and electrolyte balance: Nursing considerations* (4th ed.). Philadelphia: Lippincott.

Morrison, C. (2000). Helping patients maintain a healthy fluid balance. *Nursing Times,* (NTplus), *96*(31), 3–4.

Naxarko, L. (2000). How age affects fluid intake. *Nursing Times* (NTplus), *96*(31), 11–12.

North American Nursing Diagnosis Association. (2001). *NANDA nursing diagnoses: Definitions & classification 2001–2002.* Philadelphia: NANDA.

Porth, C. M. (2002). *Pathophysiology: Concepts of altered health states* (6th ed.). Philadelphia: Lippincott.

Powers, F. (1999). The role of chloride in acid-base balance. *Journal of Intravenous Nursing, 22*(5), 286–291.

Roper, M. (1996). Assessing orthostatic vital signs. *American Journal of Nursing, 96*(8), 43–46.

Rosenberger, K. (1998). Pharmacology update. Management of electrolyte abnormalities: Hypocalcemia, hypomagnesemia, and hypokalemia. *Journal of the American Academy of Nurse Practitioners, 10*(5), 209–217.

Sheehy, C. M., Perry, P. A., & Cromwell, S. L. (1999). Dehydration: Biological considerations, age-related changes, and risk factors in older adults. *Biological Research for Nuring, 1*(1), 30–37.

Shepherd, E. (2000). Fluids: A balancing act. *Nursing Times* (NTplus), *96*(31), 1.

Sheppard, M. (2001). Assessing fluid balance. *Nursing Times* (NTplus), *97*(6), XI–XII.

Shoulders-Odom, B. (2000). Using an algorithm to interpret arterial blood gases. *Dimensions of Critical Care Nursing, 19*(1), 36–41.

Springhouse. (1999). *Nurse's handbook of alternative & complementary therapies.* Springhouse, PA: Author.

Tasota, F. J., & Wesmiller, S. W. (1998). Balancing act: Keeping blood pH in equilibrium. *Nursing, 28*(12), 34–41.

Terpstra, T. L., & Terpstra, T. L. (2000). Syndrome of inappropriate antidiuretic hormone secretion: Recognition and management. *MEDSURG Nursing, 9*(2), 61–68.

Tierney, L. M., McPhee, S. J., & Papadakis, M. A. (2001). *Current medical diagnosis & treatment* (40th ed.). New York: Lange Medical Books/McGraw-Hill.

Wallace, L. S. (2000). Using color to simplify ABG interpretation. *MEDSURG Nursing, 9*(4), 205–208.

Whitney, E. N., & Rolfes, S. R. (2002). *Understanding nutrition* (9th ed.). Belmont, CA: Wadsworth.

Wilkinson, J. M. (2000). *Nursing diagnosis handbook with NIC interventions and NOC outcomes* (7th ed.). Upper Saddle River, NJ: Prentice Hall Health.

Wise, L. C., Mersch, J., Racioppi, J., Crosier, J., & Thompson, C. (2000). Evaluating the reliability and utility of cumulative intake and output. *Journal of Nursing Care Quality, 14*(3), 37–42.

Wong, F. W. (1999). A new approach to ABG interpretation. *American Journal of Nursing, 99*(8), 34–36.

Chapter 40

A crash course in skin trauma. (1998). *Homecare Education Management, 3*(2), 24–25.

American College of Surgeons. Committee on Trauma. (1997). *Advanced trauma life support manual.* Chicago: ACS.

Asuncion, M., & Koushik, V. (2000). Shock states in the elderly. *Clinical Geriatriacs, 8*(8), 40–42, 45–48.

Bucher, L., & Melander, S. (1999). *Critical care nursing.* Philadelphia: Saunders.

Carpenito, L. (2000). *Nursing diagnoses: Application to clinical practice* (8th ed.). Philadelphia: Lippincott.

Champion, H., Copes, W., Gann, D., Gennarelli, T., & Flanagan, M. (1989). A revision of the trauma score. *Journal of Trauma, 29*(5), 624.

Craven, A. (1998). Trauma. In C. Hudak, B. Gall, & P. Morton (Eds.), *Critical care nursing: A holistic approach* (7th ed.) (pp. 973–990). Philadelphia: Lippincott-Raven.

DeJong, M. (1997). Emergency! Cardiogenic shock. *American Journal of Nursing, 97*(6), 40–41.

Emergency Nurses Association. (1992). *Trauma resource document.* Park Ridge, IL: ENA.

Fitzpatrick, L., & Fitzpatrick, T. (1997). Blood transfusions: Keeping your patient safe. *Nursing 97, 27*(8), 34–42.

Hupcey, J. (2000). Feeling safe: The psychosocial needs of ICU patients. *Journal of Nursing Scholarship, 32*(4), 361–367.

Huston, C. (1996). Emergency! Hemolytic transfusion reaction. *American Journal of Nursing, 96*(3), 47.

Johnson, M., & Maas, M. (Eds.). (1997). *Nursing outcomes classification (NOC).* St. Louis: Mosby.

Jordan, K. S. (2000). Fluid resuscitation in acutely injured patients. *Journal of Intravenous Nursing, 23*(2), 81–87.

Labovich, T. (1997). Transfusion therapy: Nursing implications. *Clinical Journal of Oncology Nursing, 1*(3), 61–72.

Liepert, D., & Rosenthal, M. (2000). Management of cardiogenic, hypovolemic, and hyperdynamic shock. *Current Reviews for Perianesthesia Nurses, 22*(9), 1–3, 113, back cover.

Lisanti, P. (1996). Emergency! Anaphylaxis. *American Journal of Nursing, 96*(11), 51.

McCloskey, J. C., & Bulechek, G. M. (Eds.). (2000). *Nursing interventions classification (NIC).* St. Louis: Mosby.

McConnell, E. (1997). Safely administering a blood transfusion. *Nursing 97, 27*(6), 30.

McCracken, L. (2001). The forensic ABC's of trauma care. *Canadian Nurse, 97*(3), 30–33.

McKenny, L., & Salerno, E. (1998). *Pharmacology in nursing* (20th ed.). St. Louis: Mosby.

Mower-Wade, D., Bartley, M., & Chiari-Allwein, J. (2001). How to respond to shock. *Dimensions of Critical Care Nursing, 20*(2), 22–27.

North American Nursing Diagnosis Association. (2001). *Nursing diagnoses: Definitions & classification 2001–2002.* Philadelphia: NANDA.

Porth, C. (2002). *Pathophysiology: Concepts of altered health states* (6th ed.). Philadelphia: Lippincott.

Sole, M., Lamborn, M., & Hartshorn, J. (2001). *Introduction to critical care nursing* (3rd ed.). Philadelphia: Saunders.

Speck, P., & Whalley, A. (1996). Domestic violence: Role of the RN. *Tennessee Nurse, 59*(3), 27, 31.

Stamatos, C., Sorensen, P., & Tefler, K. (1996). Meeting the challenge of the older trauma patient. *American Journal of Nursing, 96*(5), 40–47.

Stoll, E. (2001). Sepsis and septic shock. *Clinical Journal of Oncology Nursing, 5*(2), 71–72.

Tierney, L., McPhee, S., & Papadakis, M. (Eds.). (2001). *Current diagnosis & treatment* (40th ed.). Stamford, CT: Appleton & Lange.

Waldsburger, W. J. (1999). Massive transfusion in trauma. *AACN Clinical Issues: Advanced Practice in Acute & Critical Care, 10*(1), 69–84.

Watts, D., Abrahams, E., MacMillan, C., Sanat, J., Silver, R., VanGorder, S., Waller, M., & York, D. (1998). Insult after injury: Pressure ulcers in trauma patients. *Orthopaedic Nursing, 17*(4), 84–91.

Wilson, B., Shannon, M., & Stang, C. (2001). *Nursing drug guide 2001.* Upper Saddle River, NJ: Prentice Hall.

Chapter 41

Ackley, B. J., & Ladwig, G. B. (2002). *Nursing diagnosis handbook* (5th ed.). St. Louis: Mosby.

American Hospital Association. (2001). *ATS: Hospital-acquired pneumonia remains a serious problem.* Available http://www.ahanews.com

Andreoli, T., Bennett, J., Carpenter, C., & Plum, F. (Eds.). (1997). *Cecil essentials of medicine* (4th ed.). Philadelphia: Saunders.

Biggs, A. J., & Freed, P. E. (2000). Nutrition and older adults What do family caregivers know and do? *Journal of Gerontological Nursing, 26*(8), 6–14.

Bullock, B. L., & Henze, R. L. (2000). *Focus on pathophysiology.* Philadelphia: Lippincott.

Burggraf, V., & Weinstein, B. F. (2000). Don't miss this opportunity: Promote adult immunizations. *MEDSURG Nursing, 9*(6), 198–200.

Centers for Disease Control. (1996). Guidelines for isolation precautions in hospitals. *American Journal of Infection Control, 24* (1), 32–52.

_____. (2000a). *Preventing emerging infectious diseases. A strategy for the 21st century.* Atlanta: CDC.

_____. (2000b). *Vaccine-preventable adult diseases.* Atlanta: CDC.

_____. (2001, October). Update: Investigation of anthrax associated with intentional exposure and interim public health guidelines. *MMWR, 50*(41), 889–897.

_____. (2002). *Recommended adult immunization schedule, United States, 2002–2003.* Atlanta: CDC.

Coleman, E. A. (2001). Anthrax. *American Journal of Nursing, 101*(12), 48–52.

Copstead, L. C., & Banasik, J. L. (2000). *Pathophysiology, biological, and behavioral responses* (2nd ed.). Philadelphia: W.B. Saunders.

Eliopoulous, C. (2000). *Gerontological nursing* (5th ed.). Philadelphia: Lippincott.

Fauci, A., et al. (1998). *Harrison's principles of internal medicine* (14th ed.). New York: McGraw-Hill.

Fraser, D. (1997). Assessing the elderly for infections. *Journal of Gerontological Nursing, 23*(11), 5–10, 52–58.

Glover, T. L. (2000). How drug-resistant microorganisms affect nursing. *Orthopaedic Nursing, 19*(2), 19–27.

Gylys, K. H. (1999). Antimicrobial resistance. *Journal of Cardiovascular Nursing, 13*(2), 66–69.

Hazzard, W., Bierman, E., Blass, J., Ettinger, W., & Halter, J. (Eds.). (1994). *Principles of geriatric medicine and gerontology* (3rd ed.). New York: McGraw-Hill.

Inman, W. B. (2000). Pathogens invade 21st century. *Nursing 2000, 30*(8), 22–23.

Jackson, M. M., Rickman, L. S., & Pugliese, G. (1999). Pathogens, old and new: An update for cardiovascular nurses. *Journal of Cardiovascular Nursing, 13*(2), 1–22.

Johnson, M., Maas, M., & Moorhead, S. (2000). *Iowa outcomes project: Nursing outcomes classification (NOC)* (2nd ed.). St. Louis: Mosby.

Kee, J. (2001). *Handbook of laboratory & diagnostic tests with nursing implications* (4th ed.). Upper Saddle River, NJ: Prentice Hall.

Lueckenotte, A. G. (2000). *Gerontologic nursing* (2nd ed.). St. Louis: Mosby.

Lutz, C., & Przytulski, K. (2001). *Nutrition and diet therapy* (3rd ed.) Philadelphia: F.A. Davis.

Markis, A. T., Morgan, L., Gaber, D. J., Richter, A., & Rubino, J. R. (2000). Effect of comprehensive infection control program on the incidence of infections in long-term care facilities. *American Journal of Infection Control, 28*(1), 3–7.

McCance, K., & Huether, S. (1998). *Pathophysiology: The biologic basis for disease in adults and children.* St. Louis: Mosby.

McCloskey, J., & Bulechek, G. (2000). *Iowa intervention project: Nursing interventions classification (NIC)* (3rd ed.). St. Louis: Mosby.

Miller, J. M., Walton, J. C., & Tordicella, L. L. (1998). Recognizing and managing *Clostridium difficile*–associated diarrhea. *MEDSURG Nursing, 7*(6), 348–356.

Miller, N. C., & Rudoy, R. C. (2000). Vancomycin intermediate-resistant *Staphylococcus aureus* (VISA). *Orthopaedic Nursing, 19*(6), 45–50.

National Institute of Allergy and Infectious Diseases. (2000). *Antimicrobial resistance.* Bethesda, MD: National Institutes of Health.

Porth, C. (2002). *Pathophysiology: Concepts of altered health states* (6th ed.). Philadelphia: Lippincott.

Price, S., & Wilson, L. (2003). *Pathophysiology: Clinical concepts of disease processes* (6th ed.). St. Louis: Mosby.

Reece, S. M. (1999). The emerging threat of antimicrobial resistance: Strategies for change. *The Nurse Practitioner, 24*(11), 70, 73, 77–80, 85–86.

Roitt, I. (1994). *Essential immunology* (8th ed.). London: Blackwell.

Rowsey, P. J. (1997a). Pathophysiology of fever. Part 1: The role of cytokines. *Dimensions of Critical Care Nursing, 16*(4), 202–207.

_____ . (1997b). Pathophysiology of fever. Part 2: Relooking at cooling interventions. *Dimensions of Critical Care Nursing, 16*(5), 251–256.

Sandhu, S. K., & Mossad, S. B. (2001). Influenza in the older adult. *Geriatrics, 56*(1), 43–44, 47–48, 51.

Schlossberg, D. (2001). *Current therapy of infectious disease* (2nd ed.). St. Louis: Mosby.

Shannon, M., Wilson, B., & Stang, C. (2001). *Nursing drug guide 2001.* Upper Saddle River, NJ: Prentice Hall.

Sheff, B. (1998). VRE & MRSA: Putting bad bugs out of business. *Nursing 98, 28*(3), 40–45.

_____ . (1999). Minimizing the threat of *C. difficile. Nursing 99, 29*(2), 33–39.

Silverblatt, F. J., Tibert, C., Mikolich, D., Blazek-D'Arezzo, J., Alves, J., Tack, M., & Agatiello, P. (2000). Preventing the spread of vancomycin-resistant enterococci in a long-term care facility. *Journal of the American Geriatrics Society, 48*(10), 1211–1214.

Smith, S. F., Duell, D. J., & Martin, B. C. (2000). *Clinical nursing skills* (5th ed.). Upper Saddle River: Prentice Hall.

Tenover, F. C., & McGownan, J. E. (1997). Antimicrobial resistance. *Infectious Disease Clinics of North America, 11*(4), 813–928.

Tierney, L., McPhee, S., & Papadakis, M. (Eds). (2001). *Current medical diagnosis & treatment* (40th ed.). Stamford, CT: Appleton & Lange.

Wenzel, R. P., & Edmond, M. B. (2001). The impact of hospital-acquired bloodstream infections. *Emerging Infectious Diseases, 7*(2), 174–177.

Chapter 42

Abramowicz, M. (Ed.). (2000). *Drugs for HIV infection.* New Rochelle, NY: The Medical Letter, Inc.

Abrams, A. C. (2001). *Clinical drug therapy: Rationales for practice* (6th ed.). Philadelphia: Lippincott.

Ackley, B. J., & Ladwig, G. B. (2002). *Nursing diagnosis handbook* (5th ed.). St. Louis: Mosby.

American Nurses Association. (1997). *Position statement: Needle exchange and HIV.* Washington, DC: ANA.

Bihari, B., Levin, S., Malebranche, D., & Valdez, H. (2000). Caring for diverse populations: Identifying HIV infection. *Patient Care, 34*(9), 55–56, 58, 60–62, 65–66, 68, 73, 76–77.

Braunwald, E., Fauci, A. S., Kasper, D. L., Hauser, S. L., Longo, D. L., & Jameson, J. L. (2001). *Harrison's Principles of internal medicine* (15th ed.). New York: McGraw-Hill.

Bullock, B. A., & Henze, R. L. (2000). *Focus on pathophysiology.* Philadelphia: Lippincott.

Carrico, R.M. (2001). What to do if you're exposed to a bloodborne pathogen. *Home Healthcare Nurse, 19*(6), 362–368.

Centers for Disease Control. (1992). 1993 Revised classification system for HIV infection and expanded case definition for AIDS among adolescents and adults. *MMWR, CDC Recommendations and Reports, 41*(RR-17), 1–19.

_____ . (1996). Update: Provisional public health recommendations for chemoprophylaxis after occupational exposure to HIV. *MMWR, 45,* 468–472.

Cheng, C., & Umland, E.M. (2001). A practical update on antiretroviral therapy. *Patient Care, 35*(10), 99–106.

Chernecky, R., & Berger, B. (1997). *Laboratory tests and diagnostic procedures* (2nd ed.). Philadelphia: Saunders.

Cournoyer, S. (1997). How much do you know about the opportunistic diseases of AIDS? *Nursing97, 27*(6), 1–2, 4, 6.

Early HIV Infection Guideline Panel. (1994). *Evaluation and management of early HIV infection: Clinical practice guidelines* (AHCPR Publication No. 94-0572). Rockville, MD: AHCPR Public Health Service, USDHHS.

Esch, J. F., & Frank, S. V. (2001). HIV drug resistance and nursing practice. *American Journal of Nursing, 101*(6), 30–36.

Fryback, P., & Reinert, B. (1997). Alternative therapies and control for health in cancer and AIDS. *Clinical Nurse Specialist, 11*(2), 64–69.

Joint United Nations Programme on HIV/AIDS. (2000). Men make a difference. Press kit: world AIDS day. HIV/AIDS in Africa. Available http://www.unaids.org/wac/2000/wad00/files/FS_Africa.htm

Kee, J. (1999). *Laboratory & diagnostic tests with nursing implications* (5th ed.). Upper Saddle River, NJ: Prentice Hall.

Kirton, C.A., Ferri, R.S., & Eleftherakis, V. (1999). Primary care and case management of persons with HIV/AIDS. *Nursing Clinics of North America, 34*(1), 71–94.

Johnson, M., Maas, M., & Moorhead, S. (2000). *Iowa outcomes project: Nursing outcomes classification (NOC)* (2nd ed.). Upper Saddle River, NJ: Prentice Hall.

Lueckenotte, A.G. (2000). *Gerontologic nursing* (2nd ed.). St. Louis: Mosby.

Lutz, C., & Przytulski, K. (2001). *Nutrition and diet therapy* (3rd ed.). Philadelphia: F.A. Davis.

Lyon, D. E., & Munro, C. (2001). Disease severity and symptoms of depression in black Americans infected with HIV. *Applied Nursing Research, 14*(1), 3–10.

McCloskey, J. C., & Bulechek, G. M. (2000). *Iowa interventions project: Nursing interventions classifications (NIC)* (3rd ed.). Upper Saddle River, NJ: Prentice Hall.

Muehlbauer, P., & White, R. (1998). Are you prepared for interleukin-2? *RN, 61*(2), 34, 36–38.

National Institute of Allergy and Infectious Diseases. (2000). *HIV infection in women.* Bethesda, MD: National Institutes of Health.

_____ . (2001). *HIV/AIDS statistics (fact sheet)*. Available http://www.niaid.nih.gov/factsheets/aidstat.htm

National Institute of Occupational Safety and Health. (1997). *Preventing allergic reactions to natural rubber latex in the workplace*. Washington, DC: USDHHS.

Novello, A. (1993, June). *Surgeon General's report to the American public on HIV infection and AIDS—extracts*. Rockville, MD: CDC National AIDS Clearinghouse.

Panel on Clinical Practices for Treatment of HIV Infection. (2000). *Guidelines for the use of antiretroviral agents in HIV-infected adults and adolescents*. Available http://www.hivatis.org

Porche, D. J. (1999). State of the art: Antiretroviral and prophylactic treatments in HIV/AIDS. *Nursing Clinics of North America, 34*(1), 95–112.

Porth, C. (2002). *Pathophysiology: Concepts of altered health states* (6th ed.). Philadelphia: Lippincott.

Roitt, I. (1994). *Essential immunology* (8th ed.). London: Blackwell.

Shannon, M. T., Wilson, B. A., & Stang, C. L. (2001). *Nursing drug guide 2001*. Upper Saddle River, NJ: Prentice Hall.

Sherman, D. (1996). Nurses' willingness to care for AIDS patients and spirituality, social support, and death anxiety. *Image: Journal of Nursing Scholarship, 28*(3), 205–213.

Sowell, R. L., Moneyham, L., & Aranda-Naranjo, B. (1999). The care of women with AIDS. *Nursing Clinics of North America, 34*(1), 179–199.

Swenson, M. R. (2000). Autoimmunity and immunotherapy. *Journal of Intravenous Nursing, 23*(5S), S8–S13.

Szirony, T. A. (1999). Infection with HIV in the elderly population. *Journal of Gerontological Nursing, 25*(10), 25–31.

Thurlow, K. L. (2001). Latex allergies: Management and clinical responsibilities. *Home Healthcare Nurse, 19*(6), 369–376.

Tierney, L., McPhee, S., & Papadakis, M. (Eds). (2001). *Current medical diagnosis & treatment* (40th ed.). New York: Lange Medical Books/McGrawHill.

Trzcianowska, H., & Mortensen, E. (2001). HIV and AIDS: Separating fact from fiction. *American Journal of Nursing, 101*(6), 53, 55, 57, 59.

Ungvarski, P. (1996). Waging war on HIV wasting. *RN, 59*(2), 26–32.

_____ . (2001). The past 20 years of AIDS. *American Journal of Nursing, 101*(6), 26–29.

Valdez, M. R. (2001). A metaphor for HIV-positive Mexican and Puerto Rican women. *Western Journal of Nursing Research, 23*(5), 517–535.

Williams, A. B. (2001). Adherence to HIV regimens: 10 vital lessons. *American Journal of Nursing, 101*(6), 37–44.

Chapter 43

American Association of Colleges of Nursing. (1999). *Peaceful death: Recommended competencies and curricular guidelines for end-of-life nursing care*. Washington, DC: AACN.

American Nurses Association. (1992). *Position statement on nursing and the Patient Self Determination Act*. Kansas City: ANA.

_____. (1992). *Report from the task force on the nurse's role in end of life decisions*. Kansas City: ANA.

Barbus, A. J. (1975). The dying person's bill of rights. *The American Journal of Nursing, 75* (1), 99.

Bowlby, J. (1973). Attachment and loss. *In Separation, anxiety, and anger* (Vol. 2). New York: Basic Books.

_____. (1980). Attachment and loss. *In Loss, sadness, and depression* (Vol. 3). New York: Basic Books.

Caplan, G. (1990). Loss, stress, and mental health. *Community Mental Health Journal, 26*(1), 27–48.

Carpenito, L. (2000). *Nursing diagnoses: Application to clinical practice* (8th ed.). Philadelphia: Lippincott.

Carter, S. (1989). Themes of grief. *Nursing Research, 36*(6), 354–358.

Collins, D. (2001). Grief and loss experienced by patients with Alzheimer's disease and their caregivers. *Geriaction, 19*(1), 17–20.

Duffield, P. (1998). Advance directives in primary care. *American Journal of Nursing, 61*(4), 16CCC–16DDD.

Durham, E., & Weiss, L. (1997). How patients die. *American Journal of Nursing, 97*(12), 41–46.

Engel, G. (1964). Grief and grieving. *American Journal of Nursing, 64*, 93.

Freud, S. (1917/1957). Mourning and melancholia. In J. Strachey & A. Tyson (Eds.), *The complete psychological works of Sigmund Freud* (Vol. 14). London: Hogarth Press.

Goetschius, S. (1997). Families and end-of-life care: How do we meet their needs? *Journal of Gerontological Nursing, 23*(3), 43–49.

International Council of Nurses. (1997). *Basic principles of nursing care*. Washington, DC: American Nurses Publishing.

Johnson, M., & Maas, M. (Eds.). (1997). *Nursing outcomes classification (NOC)*. St. Louis: Mosby.

Kaunonen, M., Tarkka, M., Paunonen, M., & Laippala, P. (1999). Grief and social support after the death of a spouse. *Journal of Advanced Nursing, 30*(6), 1304–1311.

Kübler-Ross, E. (1969). *On death and dying*. New York: Macmillan.

_____. (1978). *To live until we say goodbye*. Englewood Cliffs, NJ: Prentice Hall.

Libson, J., Dibble, S., & Minarik, P. (1996). *Culture & nursing care: A pocket guide.* San Francisco: UCSF Nursing Press.

Lindemann, E. (1944). Symptomatology and management of acute grief . *American Journal of Psychiatry, 32,* 141.

Matzo, P. L., & Sherman, D. W. (Eds.). (2001). *Palliative care nursing: Quality care to the end of life.* New York: Springer.

McCloskey, J. C., & Bulechek, G. M. (Eds.). (2000). *Nursing interventions classification (NIC)* (3rd ed.). St. Louis: Mosby.

McCorkle, R., Robinson, L., Nuamah, I., Lev, E., & Benoliel, J. (1998). The effects of home nursing care for patients during terminal illness on the bereaved's psychological distress. *Nursing Research, 47*(1), 2–10.

Ott, B., & Hardie, T. (1997). Readability of advance directive documents. *Image: Journal of Nursing Scholarship, 29*(1), 53–57.

Perrin, K. (1997). Giving voice to the wishes of elders for end-of-life care. *Journal of Gerontological Nursing, 23*(3), 18–27.

Poor, B., & Poirrier, G. (2001). *End of life nursing care.* Boston: Jones & Bartlett.

Reed, P. G. (1996). Transcendence: Formulating nursing perspectives. *Nursing Science Quarterly, 9*(1), 2–4.

Rushton, C., & Scanlon, C. (1998). A road map for navigating end-of-life care. *MEDSURG Nursing, 7*(1), 57–59.

Tierney, L. M., McPhee, S. J., & Papadakis, M. A. (2001). *Current medical diagnosis & treatment* (40th ed.). New York: McGraw Hill.

Tipton, K. (1997). How to discuss death with patients and families. *Nursing97, 27*(32), 10–12.

Ufema, J. (2000). Terminal illness: Compassion and raspberry tea. *Nursing, 30*(12), 66–67.

Chapter 44

Adams, W. L., & Cox, N. S. (1995). Epidemiology of problem drinking among elderly people. *International Journal of the Addictions, 30,* 1693–1716.

Adams, W. L., & Kinney, J. (1995). *The clinical manual of substance abuse.* St. Louis: Mosby.

American Psychiatric Association. (2000a). *Practice guidelines for the treatment of psychiatric disorders compendium 2000.* Washington, DC: APA.

_____ (2000b). *Diagnostic and statistical manual of mental disorders* (4th ed., text revision) (DSM-IV-TR). Washington, DC: APA.

Beresford, T. P., Blow, F. C., & Brower, K. J. (1990). Alcoholism in the elderly. *Comprehensive Therapeutics, 16,* 38–43.

Blixen, C. E., McDougall, G. J., & Suen, L. J. (1997). Dual diagnosis in elders discharged from a psychiatric hospital. *International Journal of Geriatric Psychiatry, 12*(3), 307–313.

Ewing, J. A. (1984). Detecting alcoholism: The CAGE questionnaire. *Journal of the American Medical Association, 252*(14), 1905–1907.

Henderson-Martin, B. (2000). No more surprises: Screening patients for alcohol abuse. *American Journal of Nursing, 100*(9), 26–32.

Johnson, M., & Maas, M. (Eds.). (1997). *Nursing outcomes classification (NOC).* St. Louis: Mosby.

Kutlenios, R.M. (1998). Genetics and alcoholism—Implications for advance practice psychiatric/mental health nursing. *Archives of Psychiatric Nursing, 12*(3), 154.

Lehne, R. A. (2001). *Pharmacology for nursing care.* Philadelphia: W.B. Saunders.

McCloskey, J. C., & Bulechek, G. M. (Eds.). (2000). *Nursing interventions classification (NIC).* St. Louis: Mosby.

National Institute of Mental Health. (2001). *Mental disorders in America.* NIH Publication No. 01-4584. Bethesda, MD: NIMH. Available http://www.nimh.nih.gov/publicat/numbers.cfm.

North American Nursing Diagnosis Association. (2001). *Nursing diagnoses: Definitions & classification 2001–2002.* Philadelphia: NANDA.

Ondus, K. A., Hujer, M. E., Mann, A. E., & Mion, L. C. (1999). Substance abuse and the hospitalized elderly. *Orthopaedic Nursing, 18*(4), 27–36.

Pokorny, A. D., Miller, B. A., & Kaplan, H. B. (1972). The brief MAST: A shortened version of the Michigan Alcohol Screening Test. *American Journal of Psychiatry, 129*: 342–345.

Reneman, L., Booij, J., de Bruin, K., Reitsma, J. B., de Wolff, F. A., Gunning, W. B., den Heeten, G. J., & van den Brink, W. (2001). Effects of dose, sex, and long-term abstention from use on toxic effects of MDMA (ecstasy) on brain serotonin neurons. *Lancet, 358*(9296), 1864–1869.

Siqueira, L., Diab, M., Bodian, C., & Rolnitzky, L. (2001). The relationship of stress and coping methods to adolescent use. *Substance Abuse, 22*(3), 157–166.

Skinner, H. A. (1982). *Drug Abuse Screening Test (DAST)* (p. 363). Langford Lance, England: Elsevier Science Ltd.

Stuart, G. W., & Laraia, M. T. (2001). *Stuart & Sundeen's principles and practice of psychiatric nursing* (7th ed.). St. Louis: Mosby.

U.S. Department of Health and Human Services. (1999). *Mental health: A report of the surgeon general—Executive summary.* Rockville, MD: USDHHS, Substance Abuse and Mental Health Services Administration, Center for Mental Health Services, National Institutes of Health, National Institute of Mental Health. Available http://www.surgeongeneral.gov/Library/MentalHealth.

_____ (2001). *The DASIS Report: Amphetamine treatment admission increase: 1993–1999.* Rockville, MD: USDHHS, Substance Abuse and Mental Health Services Administration, Center for Mental Health Services, National Institutes of Health, National Institute of Mental Health. Available http://www.samhsa.gov/oas/facts/speed.cfm.

Varcarolis, E. (2002). *Foundations of psychiatric mental health nursing: A clinical approach* (4th ed). Philadelphia: W.B. Saunders.

Virgo, N., Bennett, G., Higgins, D., Bennett, L., & Thomas, P. (2001). The prevalence and characteristics of co-occurring serious mental illness (SMI) and substance abuse or dependence in the patients of Adult Mental Health and Addictions Services in eastern Dorset. *Journal of Mental Health, 10*(2), 175–188.

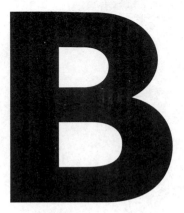

Appendix B
Practice Questions

1. Dopamine is produced in which location?
   a. Locus ceruleus
   b. Nucleus basalis
   c. Raphi nuclei
   d. Substantia nigra

2. Which best describes metabolic syndrome?
   a. An advanced disturbance of fluid and electrolytes in diabetics
   b. The constellation of lipid and non-lipid risk factors linked to insulin resistance
   c. Evidence of impaired renal function in patients with hypertension
   d. The occurrence of dyslipidemia in patients with obesity

3. Which statement best describes the practice of community health nurses?
   a. Community health nurses work as clinicians to care for patients in their home.
   b. The major responsibility of community health nurses is public education.
   c. Community health nursing practice includes the roles of clinician, leader, collaborator, researcher, and educator.
   d. The responsibilities of community health nurses include traditional nursing roles such as administrator and arbitrator.

4. A 74-year-old man with vascular dementia is admitted to the hospital from the nursing home with dehydration. He has difficulty swallowing liquids and has been restricted to thickened liquids. He does not have any advance directives and his wife believes a feeding tube is in his best interest. This situation poses an ethical dilemma based on which ethical principles?
   a. Justice versus autonomy
   b. Beneficence versus autonomy
   c. Beneficence versus nonmaleficence
   d. This situation does not represent an ethical dilemma

5. Which is an example of a middle-range theory?
   a. Roy's Adaptation Model
   b. Plastic model of the heart
   c. Health Belief Model
   d. Symbolic Interaction Theory

6. Adequate sample size for a study is defined by:
   a. a minimum of 10 subjects per variable.
   b. anticipated effect size, power of the statistical tests, and significance level.
   c. a minimum of 30 subjects for a descriptive study.
   d. maturity of the concepts being studied.

7. Coronary heart disease (CHD) in women can be characterized by:
   a. presenting equally as angina, myocardial infarction (MI), and sudden death.
   b. 25% of women dying within one year after having an initial recognized MI.
   c. presenting less frequently than breast cancer.
   d. events lagging behind those of men by 10 to 15 years.

8. Which is a nonmodifiable risk factor for CHD?
   a. Hypertension
   b. Diet
   c. Family History
   d. Weight

9. Which skin condition is noted in Addison's disease?
   a. Jaundice
   b. Hyperpigmentation
   c. Psoriasis
   d. Hypopigmentation

10. Which symptom is common among patients with Crohn's disease?
    a. Dry, hard stools
    b. Blood in stools
    c. Free of anorectal lesions
    d. Anemia

11. Trimethoprim is contraindicated for clients with which medical condition?
    a. Hypothyroidism
    b. Lung cancer
    c. Hyperaldosteronism
    d. Liver failure

12. Metolazone (Zaroxolyn) promotes diuresis by affecting which part of the kidneys?
    a. Ascending loop
    b. Distal tubule
    c. Descending loop
    d. Collecting tubule

13. Which is a symptom of urinary retention and overflow?
    a. Decrease in total amounts of urine voided
    b. Frequency secondary to inability to empty bladder
    c. Continual incontinence
    d. Oliguria and edema

14. When a patients states that everything appears "yellowish in color," the nurse suspects:
    a. glaucoma.
    b. digoxin toxicity.
    c. cataracts.
    d. dementia.

15. Which is a common complication of myocardial infarctions?
    a. Cardiac arrhythmias
    b. Anaphylactic shock
    c. Heart enlargement
    d. Hypokalemia

16. Which might a patient receiving propranolol (Inderal) experience?
    a. Dizziness with strenuous exercise
    b. A flushing sensation for a few minutes after taking the medication
    c. Palpatations for a few minutes after taking the medication
    d. Tremors after long-term use

17. Which medication is contraindicated for patients receiving anticoagulants?
    a. Isoxsuprine (Vasodilan)
    b. Chloral hydrate
    c. Chlorpromazine (Thorazine)
    d. Aspirin

18. Which is a cause of leg cramps during the night?
    a. Low bone density
    b. Gait problems
    c. Decreased extracellular potassium
    d. Thickening of synovial fluid

19. Making a choice between two equally desirable or undesirable alternatives is called:
    a. beneficence.
    b. utilitarianism.
    c. maleficience.
    d. ethical dilemma.

20. An irreversible loss of central vision occurs in:
    a. cataracts.
    b. macular degeneration.
    c. glaucoma.
    d. presbycusis.

21. Which class of medications can cause hyperkalemia and neutropenia?
    a. Beta blockers
    b. Angiotensin-converting enzyme (ACE) inhibitors
    c. Calcium channel blockers
    d. Diuretics

22. Encouraging school-age children to engage in non-competitive activities such as kayaking or swimming is an example of:
    a. primary prevention.
    b. secondary prevention.
    c. tertiary prevention
    d. lifetime prevention.

23. Which term best defines a community that is a group of people seeking to solve a problem?
    a. Geographic community
    b. Common interest community
    c. Community of solution
    d. Population

24. Which strategy is most likely to be effective when teaching a patient to fill his Mediset?
    a. Lecture with discussion
    b. Role playing with feedback
    c. Demonstration with return demonstration
    d. Instructional manual or booklet with illustrations

25. When assessing heart sounds, which disease process can be signaled by an accentuated S_1 is heard?
    a. Hypoparathyroidism
    b. Liver failure
    c. Hyperthyroidism
    d. Encephalitis

26. A 32-year-old male is admitted to the hospital with complaints of nausea, vomiting, and diarrhea for three days. His EKG reveals significant bradycardia with widening QRS complexes. The patient is taking spironolactone (Aldactone) for Conn's disease. Which electrolyte level does the nurse review first?
    a. Chloride
    b. Potassium
    c. Sodium
    d. Magnesium

27. A patient is admitted with the following ABG results: pH 7.25, $PaCO_2$ 50, PaO_2 90, HCO_3 28, and Base Excess 1. These results indicate:
    a. Metabolic alkalosis
    b. Metabolic acidosis
    c. Respiratory acidosis
    d. Respiratory alkalosis

28. Which term best defines an unintentional tort?
    a. Beneficence
    b. Autonomy
    c. Maleficence
    d. Negligence

29. The compulsive use of a substance in spite of its consequences is called:
    a. Addiction
    b. Tolerance
    c. Dependence
    d. Abuse

30. Patients with valvular disorders scheduled for dental procedures need to have:
    a. anti-inflammatories to prevent gingival infections.
    b. aspirin to prevent clot formation.
    c. antibiotics for endocarditis prophylaxis.
    d. analgesics for pain management.

31. When a 68-year-old patient returns to the post-operative unit after surgical repair of an abdominal aneurysm, which nursing intervention has the highest priority?
    a. Assessing the level of pain and providing appropriate analgesia
    b. Providing emotional support
    c. Encouraging the patient to cough and breathe deeply
    d. Monitoring urine output

32. Which hormone regulates potassium elimination through the kidneys?
    a. Progesterone
    b. Cortisol
    c. Aldosterone
    d. Testosterone

33. What is the recommended daily intake for iron?
    a. 15 mg
    b. 150 mg
    c. 30 mg
    d. 300 mg

34. A syndrome that results in the failure of the heart as a pump to meet the metabolic demands of the body is:
    a. myocardial infarction.
    b. cardiogenic shock.
    c. metabolic syndrome.
    d. pancreatitis.

35. While conducting a health assessment, the nurse discovers that a female patient has a waist circumference of 36 inches, a fasting glucose level of 124 mg/dL, and blood pressure of 140/90 mm Hg. From this information the nurse concluded that the patient has:
    a. obesity.
    b. hypertension.
    c. metabolic syndrome.
    d. hyperlipidemia.

36. Which type of angina is considered unpredictable and occurs primarily at night?
    a. Stable
    b. Unstable
    c. Prinzmetal
    d. Asymptomatic

37. The usual sequence of examination techniques is:
    a. Inspection, palpation, percussion, and auscultation
    b. Palpation, auscultation, inspection, and percussion
    c. Auscultation, inspection, percussion, and palpation
    d. Inspection, auscultation, palpation, and percussion

38. What is the ideal body weight for a female who is 5 ft 6 in tall?
    a. 110 lb
    b. 120 lb
    c. 130 lb
    d. 140 lb

39. When a client begins to explore ways to quit smoking he is at which stage of change?
    a. Contemplation
    b. Preparation
    c. Action
    d. Termination

40. Which case management model focuses on employee health and wellness and return to work?
    a. Long-term health care
    b. Occupational health
    c. Managed care
    d. Private

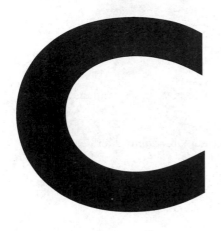

Appendix C
Practice Questions
Answers

1. **Correct Answer: D.** The locus ceruleus is an area of the brain stem with many norepinephrine-containing neurons; the nucleus basalis is the gray matter of the forebrain that consists of cholinergic neurons; and the raphe nuclei is an area of the brain stem that releases serotonin to the rest of the brain.

2. **Correct Answer: B.** The underlying pathology of insulin resistance is central to the metabolic syndrome. There are no associated fluid or electrolyte disturbances. Patients may have hypertension. Obese patients may or may not have dyslipidemia to meet one of three qualifying criteria.

3. **Correct Answer: C.** Community health nurses have multiple roles that are used to coordinate the services needed by individuals and families.

4. **Correct Answer: D.** An ethical dilemma requires a choice between courses of action that involve fundamental concepts of right and wrong.

5. **Correct Answer: C.** The Health Belief Model is an example of a middle-range theory. Middle-range theories have a narrower scope and contain few concepts. The HBM seeks to explain health-related behavior of individuals.

6. **Correct Answer: B.** Adequate sample size depends on how big an effect the researcher anticipates, the power of the statistical test to detect small but reliable differences, and the probability of making a type I error (p-value).

7. **Correct Answer: D.** The onset of CHD in women is about ten years later than onset in men because of the heart-protective effect of estrogen; women's risk is equal to that of men after menopause.

8. **Correct Answer: C.** Family history is the only nonmodifiable risk factor among these options.

9. **Correct Answer: B.** Hyperpigmentation is seen in Addison's disease. Jaundice and hypopigmentation are seen in thyroid disease.

10. **Correct Answer: D.** Bloody stools are not a common feature among clients with Crohn's disease.

11. **Correct Answer: D.** Trimethoprim is a urinary anti-infective, and is contraindicated for use in clients with hepatic impairment.

12. **Correct Answer: B.** Metolazone promotes the exrection of sodium, chloride, postassium, and water by decreasing absorption in the distal tubule.

13. **Correct Answer: B.** Overflow is characterized by an inability to empty the bladder, resulting in overdistention and frequent loss of small amounts of urine.

14. **Correct Answer: B.** A manifestation of digoxin toxicity is yellow halos around objects. People with glaucoma generally have no symptoms until vision loss; clients with cataracts may experience blurry vision or see faded colors.

15. **Correct Answer: A.** Stress on the heart may result in hypertension, arrhythmias, tachycardia, and congestive heart failure.

16. **Correct Answer: A.** Adverse effects of beta blockers include bradycardia, decreased cardiac output, heart failure, heart block, bronchoconstriction, or altered blood glucose levels.

17. **Correct Answer: D.** Aspirin, which thins the blood, should not be used while the patient is using anticoagulants unless advised to do so by a physician.

18. **Correct Answer: C.** In addition to weakness, lethargy, thirst, depression, and vomiting, muscle cramps are a manifestation of potassium deficiency.

19. **Correct Answer: D.** Beneficence is the doing of good; maleficience is the doing of harm; utilitarianism is the belief that action should be directed toward achieving the greatest happiness for the greatest number of people.

20. **Correct Answer: B.** Macular degeneration results in loss of vision in the central portion of the retina. Cataracts result in opacity of the lens of the eye or the membrane that covers it; glaucoma is characterized by fluid pressure in the eye. Presbycusis is a loss of hearing.

21. **Correct Answer: B.** Nurses should monitor serum potassium levels for hyperkalemia, and white blood cell count for neutropenia.

22. **Correct Answer: A.** Primary prevention is concerned with promoting health and delaying or preventing disease in the general population.

23. **Correct Answer: C.** A geographic community is defined by the boundaries of towns, cities, or neighborhoods while a common interest community is composed of people with similar interests.

24. **Correct Answer: C.** Demonstration with return demonstration is an effective strategy for teaching psychomotor skills. Information, discussion, cuing, and feedback may all be used with this strategy to enhance learning and build skill.

25. **Correct Answer: C.** Increased amplitude of the S_1 ("lub") may occur with hyperkinetic states, such as anxiety, hyperthyroidism, and anemia.

26. **Correct Answer: B.** All of the patient's symptoms indicate hyperkalemia. Spironolactone is a potassium-sparing diuretic.

27. **Correct Answer: B.** Metabolic acidosis results from impaired hydrogen ion elimination by the kidneys; metabolic alkalosis results from increased hydrogen ion elimination. Respiratory acidosis develops when carbon dioxide levels rise; respiratory alkalosis develops from falling carbon dioxide levels.

28. **Correct Answer: D.** A tort is a civil action for financial damages for injury to a person, property, or reputation. Negligence is the most common cause of cases involving nurses.

29. **Correct Answer: A.** The habit of using a substance becomes a form of self-medication to cope with day-to-day problems. Addiction is a disease process characterized by the continued use of a specific chemical substance despite physical, psychological, or social harm.

30. **Correct Answer: C.** Patients with valvular disorders are at risk for endocarditis and should receive antibiotic prophylaxis.

31. **Correct Answer: A.** Only about 10% to 20% of clients survive rupture of an abdominal aortic aneurysm. Severe pain may indicate impending rupture of the aneurysm, so assessing the level of pain is paramount.

32. **Correct Answer: C.** Aldosterone causes the kidneys to reabsorb water and sodium and to lose potassium. Progesterone and testosterone are female and male, respectively, sex hormones. Cortisol stimulates coversion of proteins to carbohydrates, raises blood sugar levels, and promotes glycogen storage in the liver.

33. **Correct Answer: A.** An adequate supply of minerals, including 15 mg of iron daily, is necessary to health.

34. **Correct Answer: B.** CHD is the cause for approximately two-thirds of the people with systolic dysfunction.

35. Correct Answer: C. Metabolic syndrome is defined clinically as the presence of at least 3 of the following factors abdominal obesity (waist circumference > 35 inches in women; > 40 inches in men), triglycerides > 150 mg/dL, low HDL cholesterol (< 50 mg/dL in women; < 40 mg/dL in men), elevated blood pressure (> 130/ 85 mm Hg) and a fasting blood glucose > 110 mg/dL. The other answers are incorrect because obesity is defined by body mass index (BMI > 30), hypertension can not be diagnosed from a single reading, and there is no information provided about lipid levels.

36. Correct Answer: C. Prinzmetal is unrelated to activity, and is caused by coronary artery spasm with or without an atherosclerotic lesion. Stable angina occurs with a predictable amount of activity of stress; unstable angina occurs with increasing frequency, severity, and duration, and may occur at rest; asymptomatic ischemia may occur with either activity or with mental stress.

Index

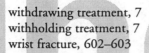

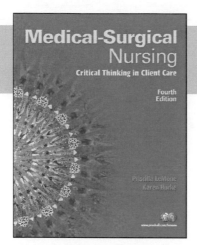

Medical-Surgical Nursing
Critical Thinking in Client Care
Fourth Edition

Priscilla LeMone
Karen Burke

Priscilla LeMone, Emeritus,
University of Missouri, Columbia

Karen Burke,
Oregon State Board of Nursing

0-13-171308-6
© 2008

For more information visit
www.prenhall.com /health

Need to contact your
local Prentice Hall Sales
Representative?
Please call **1.800.526.0485.**

Medical Surgical Nursing: Critical Thinking in Client Care, 4/e

Turning great students into excellent nurses takes dedication and exceptional resources. We know you are dedicated to making a difference in your students' lives and Prentice Hall Health is committed to providing the resources to make that happen.

EXCELLENCE IN THE CLASSROOM

5 new chapters including *Genetic Implications of Adult Health Nursing* and *Nursing Care of Clients Experiencing Disasters* bring the latest information to students.

Assessment Chapters present techniques, normal, and abnormal findings seamlessly so students can easily recognize findings.

EXCELLENCE IN CLINICAL

Building Clinical Competence reinforces content and helps students synthesize unit knowledge through clinical scenarios and case studies.

Concept Mapping software tool on the Student DVD helps students create and organize their concept maps.

EXCELLENCE ON THE NCLEX-RN®

Over 30 NCLEX® style review questions per chapter are available. These questions found in the text, the companion website (www.prenhall.com/berman), and the student DVD help students prepare for and become familiar with the NCLEX-RN® exam.

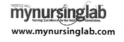

www.mynursinglab.com